Compendium for the Antenatal Care of High-Risk Pregnancies

Compendium for the Antenatal Care of High-Risk Pregnancies

Harini Narayan FRCOG

Consultant Obstetrician and Gynaecologist
Great Western Hospitals NHS Foundation Trust, Swindon, UK
and Honorary Consultant in Feto-Maternal Medicine
Oxford University Hospitals NHS Trust, Oxford, UK

OXFORD
UNIVERSITY PRESS

OXFORD
UNIVERSITY PRESS

Great Clarendon Street, Oxford, OX2 6DP,
United Kingdom

Oxford University Press is a department of the University of Oxford.
It furthers the University's objective of excellence in research, scholarship,
and education by publishing worldwide. Oxford is a registered trade mark of
Oxford University Press in the UK and in certain other countries

Impression: 1

Published in the United States of America by Oxford University Press
198 Madison Avenue, New York, NY 10016, United States of America

British Library Cataloguing in Publication Data

Data available

Library of Congress Control Number: 2014949677

ISBN 978–0–19–967364–3

Printed in Great Britain by
Clays Ltd, St Ives plc

FOREWORD

I would like to congratulate Dr Harini Narayan for this high-calibre book that is rich in evidence-based information and practical pathways of high-risk obstetric conditions.

Although there are a number of well-regarded conventional textbooks available on high-risk pregnancy, there are no other similar books that are set up like this *Compendium*, covering a vast range of conditions that can complicate pregnancies. Dr Narayan has written an impressive book that presents management of high-risk pregnancy in a comprehensive but accessible way. The remarkable manner in which the chapters are planned in this manual hand-book, makes it useful to dip into for an experienced obstetrician who wants to remind themselves of some area of care, and for trainees preparing for the MRCOG examination or doing Advanced Antenatal Care and Maternal Medicine advanced training specialist modules (ATSMs).

This book adopts a condition-based and patient-centred approach to allow an integration and seamless delivery of antenatal care provided in all settings. Midwives wanting to learn about complex obstetrics and inform their patients about possible plans will also recognize the value of such a *Compendium*. The strength of this book is its practical and easy use by health professionals who look after pregnant women in all clinical settings.

The chapters are well written and clearly explained. It successfully achieves the aim of presenting the latest knowledge based on current best evidence and good practice recommendations from the Royal College of Obstetricians and Gynaecologists (RCOG) and the National Institute for Health and Clinical Excellence (NICE) guidelines.

Modernizing maternity services is part of the new vision for NHS. Maternity units will be required to have clear care pathways for how different groups of women are managed. This will ensure the best care for patients, while also ensuring that visits, staff time, and resources are not wasted where they are not required; resulting in an evidence-based high quality service for information-empowered women. This book could not have become available at a better time. It is also seen as increasingly important that women are informed participants in their care; thus the concept of including a very wide range of good quality patient information leaflets that could be adapted for local use as required, is invaluable.

I do think that this book will be useful and very popular. It is certainly one that I would buy myself and for my unit in hard copy and on-line versions. It would be a beneficial source for helping units to design their antenatal services based on evidence based care pathways and produce good quality patient information which should also make the book very attractive to staff and units that may not have time to develop such information for themselves.

It is important to note the contents could also be easily transferrable from the UK to abroad, with the appropriate adaptation for local services. This will be a timely addition to trainees in the UK and abroad in particular as the RCOG is due to pilot some ATSM modules abroad. Focussing on the different high-risk obstetrics ATSM modules will set the standard for the level of detail in the book, whilst also attracting specialist allied health professionals and junior trainees alike.

On a final note, I would like to congratulate Dr Narayan and her team for the national awards and international recognition achieved for their radical restructuring of antenatal care for high-risk pregnancies provided in Swindon, for which this *Compendium* served as the keystone.

Mr Hassan Shehata FRCOG FRCPI

Consultant and Head of the Maternal Medicine Unit and Clinical Director for Women and Children Services, Deputy Director of Research & Development, Epsom & St Helier University Hospitals NHS Trust, Wrythe Lane, Carshalton, Surrey SM5 1AA, UK

Honorary Senior Lecturer, Obstetrics & Gynaecology Division, St George's Hospital Medical School, Blackshaw Road, Tooting, London SW17 0QT, UK

Royal College of Obstetricians & Gynaecologists Ambassador to the Gulf Region, RCOG, 27 Sussex Place, London NW1 4RG

CONTENTS

Contents

ABBREVIATIONS

AC	abdominal circumference
ACE	angiotensin converting enzyme
ACIP	Advisory Committee on Immunization Practices
aCL	anticardiolipin antibodies
ACOG	American College of Obstetricians and Gynaecologists
ACS	acute chest syndrome
ACT	assisted conception techniques
ADPKD	autosomal dominant polycystic kidney disease
AED	antiepileptic drug
AF	atrial flutter
AFI	amniotic fluid index
AFP	alp ha-fetoprotein
AIH	autoimmune hepatitis
AIP	acute intermittent porphyria
ALP	alkaline phosphatase
ALT	alanine aminotransferase
AMC	arthrogryposis multiplex congenita
AP	acute pancreatitis
APD	antero-posterior diameter
APH	antepartum haemorrhage
aPL	antiphospholipid antibodies
APS	antiphospholipid syndrome
APTT	activated partial thromboplastin time
ARB	angiotensin receptor blocker
ARPKD	autosomal recessive polycystic kidney disease
ART	assisted reproductive techniques
AST	aspartate aminotransferase or aspartate transaminase
AZT	azathioprine
BCSH	British Committee for Standards in Haematology
BMI	body mass index
BP	blood pressure
BPP	biophysical profile
BV	bacterial vaginosis
C&S	culture and sensitivity
CAH	congenital adrenal hyperplasia
CBT	cognitive behavioural therapy
CCAM	congenital cystic adenomatoid malformation
CDH	congenital diaphragmatic hernia
CEMACH	Confidential Enquiry into Maternal and Child Health
CESDI	Confidential Enquiry into Stillbirths and Deaths in Infancy
CF	cystic fibrosis
CFS	chronic fatigue syndrome
CH	cystic hygroma
CHB	complete heart block
CHD	congenital heart disease
CHF	congenital hepatic fibrosis
CIN	cervical intraepithelial neoplasia
CK	creatinine kinase
CKD	chronic kidney disease
CMD	congenital muscular dystrophy
CMV	cytomegalovirus
CNS	central nervous system
COCP	combined oral contraceptive pill
CP	cerebral palsy
CPC	choroid plexus cysts
CRP	C-reactive protein
CSF	cerebrospinal fluid
CT	computed tomography
CTG	cardiotocography
CVS	chorionic villus sampling
CVT	cerebral venous thrombosis
DAT	direct antiglobin test
DDAVP	desmopressin acetate (1-deamino-8-D-arginine vasopressin)
DGH	district general hospital
DH	Department of Health
DIC	disseminated intravascular coagulopathy
DMD	Duchenne muscular dystrophy
DV	ductus venosus
DVT	deep vein thrombosis
EB	epidermolysis bullosa
ECG	electrocardiography
ECHO	echocardiogram
ECS	endocervical swab
ECV	external cephalic version
EEG	electroencephalography
EFW	estimated fetal weight
ELISA	enzyme-linked immunosorbent assay
EMG	electromyography
ERCP	endoscopic retrograde cholangiopancreatography
ERCS	elective repeat Caesarean section
ET	essential thrombocythaemia
EU	endoscopic ultrasonography
EXIT	ex-intrapartum treatment
FAS	fetal alcohol syndrome
FBC	full blood count
FBS	fetal blood sampling
FFP	fresh frozen plasma
FGM	female genital mutilation
FGR	fetal growth restriction
FMU	fetal medicine unit
FSE	fetal scalp electrode
FVS	fetal varicella syndrome
G…P…	gravida…para…
GAS	group A streptococcus
GBS	group B streptococcus
GCS	Glasgow coma score
GDM	gestational diabetes mellitus
GGT	gamma-glutamyl transpeptidase or gamma-glutamyl transferase
GTT	glucose tolerance test
HAART	highly active antiretroviral therapy
Hb	haemoglobin
HBV	hepatitis B virus
HC	head circumference
HCV	hepatitis C virus
HDFN	haemolytic disease of the fetus and newborn
HDN	haemolytic disease of the newborn
HDU	high-dependency unit
HELLP	haemolysis, elevated liver enzymes, and low platelets (syndrome)
HFEA	Human Fertilization and Embryology Authority
HG	hyperemesis gravidarum

HH	hereditary haemochromatosis
HHT	hereditary haemorrhagic telangiectasia
HIV	human immunodeficiency virus
HPV	human papillomavirus
HRT	hormone replacement therapy
HS	hereditary spherocytosis
HSV	herpes simplex virus
HUS	haemolytic uremic syndrome
HVS	high vaginal swab
HZ	herpes zoster
IBD	inflammatory bowel disease
ICH	intracranial haemorrhage
ICS	inhaled corticosteroids
ICU	intensive care unit
Ig	immunoglobulin
IGE	idiopathic generalized epilepsy
IGF	insulin-like growth factor
IIH	idiopathic intracranial hypertension
IM	intramuscular
INR	international normalised ratio
IOL	induction of labour
ITP	idiopathic thrombocytopenia
IUCD	intrauterine contraceptive device
IUD	intrauterine death
IUGR	intrauterine growth restriction
IUT	in-utero transfusion
IV	intravenous
IVC	inferior vena cava
IVF	in-vitro fertilization
IVIG	intravenous immunoglobulin
IVU	intravenous urethrography
LAGB	laparoscopic adjustable gastric band
LFT	liver function test
Lg-IUS	levonorgestrel intrauterine system
LGMD	limb-girdle muscular dystrophy
LHR	lung-to-head ratio
LLETZ	large loop excision of transformation zone
LMP	last menstrual period
LMWH	low molecular weight heparin
LSCS	lower segment Caesarean section
LV	liquor volume
MAP	mean arterial pressure
MCA	middle cerebral artery
MCV	mean corpuscular volume
MEOWS	Modified Early Obstetric Warning Score
MFI	Multidimensional Fatigue Inventory
MG	myasthenia gravis
MI	myocardial infarction
MLC	midwifery led care
MMR	measles, mumps, and rubella (vaccination)
MoM	multiples of the median
MRI	magnetic resonance imaging
MROP	manual removal of placenta
MRSA	meticillin-resistant *Staphyloccus aureus*
MS	multiple sclerosis
MSU	midstream urine
MVPD	maximum vertical pool depth
M/W	midwife
NAS	neonatal abstinence syndrome
NHL	non-Hodgkin's lymphoma
NICE	National Institute for Health and Care Excellence
NICU	neonatal intensive care unit
NIHF	non-immune hydrops fetalis
NRT	nicotine replacement therapy
NSAID	non-steroidal anti-inflammatory drug
NT	nuchal thickness
NTD	neural tube defect
OASIS	obstetric anal sphincteric injuries
OC	obstetric cholestasis
OCP	oral contraceptive pill
OI	osteogenesis imperfecta
PAC	premature atrial contractions
PAH	phenylalanine hydroxylase
PAS	para-aminosalicylic acid
PCP	pneumocystis pneumonia
PCR	protein-creatinine ratio
PE	pulmonary embolism
PEEP	positive end expiratory pressure
PFO	patent foramen ovale
PG	prostaglandin
PGD	pre-implantation genetic diagnosis
PI	pulsatility index
PKD	polycystic kidney disease
PlGF	placental growth factor
PND	postnatal depression
PNMR	perinatal mortality rate
PO	per oral (by mouth)
POCT	point of care test
PPH	postpartum haemorrhage
PPROM	preterm prelabour rupture of membranes
PSV	peak systolic velocity
PUO	pelviureteric obstruction
PUPPP	pruritic urticarial papules and plaques of pregnancy
RA	rheumatoid arthritis
RAADP	routine antenatal anti-D prophylaxis
RAIU	radioactive iodine uptake
RBC	red blood cells
RCOG	Royal College of Obstetricians and Gynaecologists
RFM	reduced fetal movements
RFT	renal function tests
RI	resistance index
RPR	rapid plasma reagin
RVT	radical vaginal trachelectomy
RYGB	Roux-en-Y gastric bypass
SARS	severe acute respiratory syndrome
SC	subcutaneous
SCD	sickle cell disease
SFH	symphysio-fundal height
SGA	small for gestational age
SLE	systemic lupus erythematosus
SNRI	serotonin norepinephrine reuptake inhibitors
SPD	symphysis pubis dysfunction
SROM	spontaneous rupture of membranes
SSRI	selective serotonin reuptake inhibitor
STI	sexually transmitted infection
SVT	supraventricular tachycardia
TBII	TSH-binding inhibitory immunoglobulins
TED	thromboembolic disease
TFT	thyroid function test
TIBC	total iron binding capacity
TOP	termination of pregnancy
TP	*Treponema pallidum*
TPA	tissue plasminogen activator
TPN	total parenteral nutrition
TRH	thyrotropin receptor hormone
TS	tuberous sclerosis
TSH	thyroid stimulating hormone
TTP	thrombotic thrombocytopenic purpura
TTTS	twin-to-twin transfusion syndrome
TVS	transvaginal scan
UA	umbilical artery

UC	ulcerative colitis
U&E	urea and electrolytes
URSO	ursodeoxycholic acid
U/S	ultrasound
UTI	urinary tract infection
UV	umbilical vein
VBAC	vaginal birth after Caesarean
VEGF	vascular endothelial growth factor
VL	viral load
VT	ventricular tachycardia
VTE	venous thromboembolism
VUR	vesicoureteral (or vesicoureteric) reflux
vWD (vWF)	von Willebrand disease (factor)
VZIG	varicella zoster immune globulin
VZV	varicella zoster virus
WBC	white blood cells
WHO	World Health Organization
ZDV	zidovudine

CONTRIBUTORS

I am very grateful to my colleagues who have contributed to some of the chapters in this compendium. Their contributions highlight the essential multidisciplinary and multiprofessional management that is so vital in the care of high-risk pregnancies.

Mrs Susan Tucker, Antenatal Screening Co-ordinator and Senior Midwife, The Great Western Hospitals NHS Foundation Trust, for her contribution to 'Abnormal biochemistry markers from first/second-trimester screening' (Chapter 28.4)

ACKNOWLEDGEMENTS

I thank all the pregnant women and their babies who have been the reason that this book was created. I am also grateful to all the obstetricians, midwives, and colleagues from other specialities with whom I have enjoyed working in the last three decades in the UK.

On a personal note, this book is dedicated to ***my 3 As—Amma, Appa, and Arun***—for their infinite patience and unstinting support as well as to ***Bonnie*** for her long-distance enthusiastic motivation!

Harini Narayan
Swindon, October 2014

DISCLAIMER

The author and publishers are not responsible for the contents of the linked external websites or third party information and do not necessarily endorse any product, views, or processes expressed within them. Listing should not be taken as endorsement of any kind. Knowledge and best practice in this field are dynamic. Changes in practice, treatment and drug therapy come into effect with emerging research. It is the reader's responsibility to keep abreast.

INTRODUCTION

BACKGROUND

High-risk pregnancies form a significant and increasing proportion of any pregnant population. Women with serious medical disorders, who would previously have been unable to conceive or would have been advised not to, are now increasingly seen in antenatal clinics. The rising incidence of obesity, diabetes, hypertension, multiple pregnancies due to assisted reproduction techniques, pregnancies in older mothers, increasing social deprivation and a 25% Caesarean section rate (in the UK) have ensured that more than 50% of all pregnancies in any population would now merit the label of 'high risk' or 'complex' pregnancies.

In the current era, when there have been important advances in obstetrics, patient expectations are at an all-time high. All maternity units are working under serious financial and staffing constraints in an increasingly litigious environment.

Until recently the focus, quite rightly, of obstetricians, midwives, maternity care providers, and bodies such as the NHS Litigation Authority (NHSLA), has been on the development and implementation of intrapartum guidelines. Regular audit of adherence to such uniform guidelines, multidisciplinary and multiprofessional team training sessions in obstetric emergencies, 'skills and drills', etc. are the norm in any maternity unit in the UK that offers a safe service.

There has been comparatively less emphasis, however, on the structure and value **of antenatal care of high-risk pregnancies**; yet it is the quality of care of these pregnancies that is the keystone for eventual good maternal and fetal outcomes.[1] The recent MBRRACE-UK report unequivocally endorses the prime importance of high-standard antenatal care in those with pre-existing co-morbidities as have previous successive Reports of the Confidential Enquiry into Maternal and Infant Health.[2,3]

The vast majority of high-risk pregnancies come under one of three categories:

- Where there is a pre-existent medical or surgical condition or the therapy involved which could have a potentially serious impact on maternal/fetal outcome of any pregnancy and where specific management plans with multispeciality input are essential.
- Where the pregnancy itself could cause worsening of a pre-existent medical/mental disorder which had hitherto remained stable or in remission.
- Where complications experienced during a previous pregnancy, or those that develop in the course of the present pregnancy, are either likely to recur or adversely affect maternal and/or fetal outcome.

Evidence-based clinical guidelines published by the Royal College of Obstetricians and Gynaecologists (RCOG) in UK including the Green-top Guidelines, Good Practice guidelines, Working Party reports, Study Group Consensus Statements, Scientific Impact Papers as well as those from the National Institute for Health and Care Excellence (NICE) have, to date, addressed about 50 topics dealing solely with the antenatal care of high-risk pregnancies. These are mainly related to care delivered in the hospital setting (secondary or tertiary level).

The content and structure of antenatal care for individual high-risk pregnancies continues however, in many instances, to be opinion-based, according to the individual opinions of various consultants or non-consultant grade doctors and trainees, rather than on up-to-date evidence-based guidelines which are uniformly applicable in both primary and secondary care.

This invariably results in differing care plans as well as confusing and sometimes conflicting advice. Unnecessary follow-up appointments, investigations, and/or interventions and increased ward admissions are the norm in many maternity units. Such repetitive clinical activities, often duplicated in the community, are often of little proven clinical value and cause considerable inconvenience and anxiety for women and their families as well as placing great strain on already overstretched resources.

THE NEED FOR A COMPENDIUM

A unified and integrated framework covering all aspects of antenatal care for individual high-risk conditions of pregnancy provided both in primary care and in district general hospitals and/or tertiary centres is difficult to find.

Antenatal services are no different from any other specialist service where every penny spent needs to be worthwhile and accountable for. Especially with the enhanced focus on the new tariff of Payment By Results (PbR),[4] maternity care providers need to work from a template that provides best-practice care models that are up to date and evidence based for every high-risk pregnancy.

Obstetrics/maternity care provision for high-risk pregnancies is invariably multidisciplinary and multiprofessional. It must represent cohesive and seamless continuum from pre-pregnancy to post-delivery. Antenatal care has to bridge traditional boundaries of primary/secondary/tertiary centre settings to be truly patient centred.

In the UK, the majority of high-risk pregnancies are managed in district general hospitals (DGH). In practice, only a small proportion of these pregnancies are referred from the DGH maternity unit to a tertiary centre for antenatal management and/or delivery. Such cases are mainly, but not exclusively, for serious maternal cardiovascular or haematological conditions or where there is an anticipated need for specialist neonatal services that are not generally available at the DGH level.

There is often much misunderstanding about the label '***high-risk pregnancy***' by both hospital and community healthcare professionals. Considerable anxiety can be created for the pregnant woman and her family. Not infrequently, the mere label of 'high-risk pregnancy' can result in unwarranted, unnecessary, and sometimes potentially risky interventions such as early induction of labour or Caesarean section being undertaken without any valid obstetric indication.

The 'high-risk' label often leads to community midwives almost entirely disengaging from the ongoing routine antenatal care, with the mistaken impression that their own input is unnecessary. This denies the normality that exists even in the most complex of pregnancies.

The converse is equally true. Just because a pregnancy is deemed 'high risk', there is often unnecessary duplication of appointments, sometimes within the same week or even on the same day, between the hospital antenatal clinic and the community midwife in primary care. This not only creates significant disruption and inconvenience for patients, but highlights how a lack of coordination and of shared-care pathways in a fragmented service can waste valuable resources.

This Compendium is the first of its kind, designed to integrate antenatal care for women with high-risk pregnancies. The aim is to provide an individualized framework of up-to-date knowledge for professionals, offer model care pathways, and incorporate condition-specific information for patients for nearly 150 high-risk conditions of pregnancy. These include a wide range of conditions, both common problems which any obstetrician may meet in everyday practice, as well as some rare conditions and eponymous syndromes that are bound to perplex most clinicians.

WHO IS THE COMPENDIUM IS DESIGNED FOR?

This compendium is meant to be multipurpose and user-friendly. It offers up-to-date information about each condition for the busy clinician, whether a generalist obstetric consultant or a trainee in a clinic setting, while also providing easy-to-assimilate knowledge for those preparing for higher examinations such as the MRCOG or undertaking the Royal College of Obstetricians and Gynaecologists (RCOG) Advanced Training Skills Modules (ATSM) in Obstetrics.[5]

The compendium will serve obstetricians of all grades from trainees to consultants, midwives working in hospitals and community, and specialists from other disciplines (e.g. neurology, haematology, anaesthetics, gastroenterology) who have an integral role in the care of such complex pregnancies. GPs, service commissioners, and even interested patients, will find it provides a practical and systematic guide to the antenatal care of high-risk pregnancies.

Service structures and processes can be built or remodelled on the basis of this compendium, as has been possible and successful in our DGH maternity unit at the Great Western Hospital in Swindon.

Healthcare professionals can obtain as much information as they wish to derive from this compendium in order to inform their own field of practice. The underlying, unifying theme is that it provides a structured format for multidisciplinary antenatal service based on evidence or good practice for an extensive range of high-risk pregnancies, working within available resources. Contributions from midwifery, GP, anaesthetic, and paediatric colleagues exemplify the multidisciplinary, multiprofessional antenatal care that high-risk pregnancies deserve.

It is anticipated that obstetric trainees, especially those intending to be or are already registered for the RCOG ATSM in maternal medicine, Advanced Antenatal Practice, or Fetomaternal medicine, will find this compendium particularly valuable. The extensive range of topics covered as well as the practical risk management and clinical governance principles that each chapter refers to will be valuable for their future roles as specialists in fetomaternal medicine or consultants with a special interest in high-risk obstetrics.

Although it is set against the backdrop of the UK National Health Service, this compendium is equally applicable to and adaptable by other healthcare systems internationally as well as to the individual clinical practice of high-risk obstetrics worldwide.

HOW THIS COMPENDIUM CAN BE USED TO HELP CLINICAL PRACTICE AND PATIENT CARE

Uniquely, almost all high-risk conditions of pregnancy in this compendium are dealt with as a triad of a fact file, a care pathway and information for the patient.

Fact files

The **fact file** for each condition deals with basic facts as well as more advanced information that the busy clinician needs to know. Each fact file is generously referenced so that further reading is facilitated and the basis for the Care pathway that follows is well-evidenced.

For the nearly 150 high-risk conditions of pregnancy covered in this compendium, there are extensive references to up-to-date published literature, international guidelines, Cochrane reviews, and good practice publications, in addition to UK national guidelines. Evidence-based guidelines and good practice recommendations from the RCOG,[6] NICE,[7] BCSH,[8]

BASHH,[9] BTS,[10] etc., are incorporated and fully referenced in the relevant fact files, ensuring concordance with current national guidelines.

Although the readership is mainly expected to be in the UK and countries with similar obstetric training schemes and systems of care delivery, the comprehensive referencing of each chapter offers a transatlantic flavour as well.

Care pathways

The clinical algorithm or **care pathway** for each high-risk condition covers the entire journey from essential pre-pregnancy assessment and counselling, antenatal preparation for labour and delivery to specific contraceptive advice before discharge.

For each condition, the care pathway addresses the why, where, what, and when of every antenatal appointment, specifying the purpose of each visit, the assessments, the tests, and any referrals required.

Each of the care pathways demonstrates how the antenatal service can be shaped to be truly patient-oriented, integrated and coordinated between primary and secondary/tertiary care. The care pathways make explicit reference to the content, purpose, and structure of every appointment in the specialist hospital-based antenatal clinic, as well as care provided in the community with avoidance of unnecessary follow-up visits or unwarranted interventions.

The suggested frequency of follow-up visits specific to the individual condition is presented as a working model in each care pathway.

The care pathways presented here are model algorithms that can be easily adapted by individual maternity units to suit local population profiles, resources, and staffing levels. Thye are not meant to be prescriptive or proscriptive. They are meant to serve as a workable model for each high-risk pregnancy condition, easily adaptable to individual units in the UK or for individual practice internationally.

The care pathways designed for each condition offer clear and coordinated flowcharts, representing true integration of hospital care (in the DGH or tertiary referral centre) with community-based antenatal care.

Each antenatal visit is designed to be more meaningful and productive for the patient and her family.

Each care pathway is entirely constructed on the basis of the evidence and references presented in the preceding fact file for the relevant high-risk pregnancy condition.

Information for Patients

Information for patients is essential in order to engage and invite participation from the very start of the pregnancy. Engagement and active involvement of the woman (and her family) with complex medical needs should be encouraged from even before conception. Specific pre-pregnancy assessment and counselling are referred to under different high-risk conditions in this compendium. The patient information also refers to reliable websites and/or support groups.

As there are certain sources of good-quality information for patients accessible on the internet, these have been cited, as I see no point in reinventing the wheel. Others have been developed with the collaboration of patients themselves. Each patient information leaflet that I have developed was reviewed by two patients, one with and the other without that particular high-risk pregnancy condition. Their comments helped shape the final version, and I am hugely indebted to them.

WHAT THIS COMPENDIUM DOES NOT OFFER

This compendium does not profess to be a substitute for specialist textbooks or reference works on medical disorders of pregnancy or fetal medicine, neither is it intended to deflect referrals away from tertiary centres in those instances where the patient's care should ideally be managed in such large specialist units. Essential referral to tertiary units or regional centres is cited as and when this is necessary for various high-risk conditions.

As this is a Compendium for Antenatal rather than intrapartum management, only those aspects of care during labour that require detailed discussion and pre-planning are elaborated in each topic. The reader will notice that I have not unnecessarily replicated topics such as antenatal management of certain common conditions such as aneuploidy screening or breech presentation at term, as every unit will no doubt have their own version of the RCOG guidelines that have been active for several years. Likewise, I have not included mental health as a separate chapter, given that comprehensive and specialized NICE perinatal mental health guidelines already exist.[7]

WHAT THIS COMPENDIUM DOES OFFER

The compendium provides an easily accessible, integrated and practical step-by-step model of management. Along with the relevant information section for patients, for most conditions, this will enable the clinician in any maternity unit to provide high quality, coordinated antenatal care for complex pregnancies while working within existing resources.

The topics dealt with here are not limited to maternal medical disorders but encompass a wide variety of conditions that make a pregnancy 'high risk', whether due to previous uterocervical surgery, fetal conditions, or previous adverse pregnancy outcomes.

The unique theme of this compendium is that it provides a structure for a seamless continuum of antenatal care but also highlights the normality that is present in even the most complex pregnancies. This is why each Care pathway carries reference to continued community midwfery antenatal visits, without overlap, according to the' standard' NICE protocol.[14]

This compendium also addresses key recommendations of CEMACH (2007, 2011), MBRRACE (2014) ref 3)[2] and the RCOG *Standards for Maternity Care: Report of a Joint Working Party*,[11] for example:

- To provide multidisciplinary, multiprofessional, consistent and coordinated care pathways with good communication and interface between primary and secondary health care providers (CEMACH 2007, Chapter 1, RCOG 2008, Standards 5 and 6).
- To offer individualized and clear management plans for all women with medically complex pregnancies (CEMACH 2007, Chapter 1, RCOG 2008, Standards 5 and 6).
- To improve clinical knowledge amongst healthcare providers (CEMACH 2007, Chapter 1).
- To offer continuity of care with patient involvement, thereby leading to increased patient trust and satisfaction (CEMACH 2007, Chapter 1).
- To provide pre-conception counselling and support, both opportunistic and planned, for women of childbearing age with pre-existing serious medical or mental health conditions which may be aggravated by pregnancy. This includes obesity. (CEMACH 2007, The 'top ten' key recommendations).

The compendium also incorporates key recommendations and guidelines of *NSF: Maternity*,[12] *Maternity Matters* (Department of Health 2007),[13] *Standards for Maternity Care: Report of a Working Party* (RCOG 2008),[11] and relevant NICE[7] and RCOG Green-top guidelines.[6]

Each chapter illustrates how robust **risk management and clinical governance principles** should be woven into the pattern of day-to-day obstetric practice. Essential pointers such as clear and comprehensive documentation to avoid **medico-legal** pitfalls are highlighted in both the fact files and the accompanying care pathways.

A few conditions are so diverse (e.g. muscular and myotonic dystrophies) that it is impossible to construct a single care pathway to include all the variables. In such cases, where the antenatal care must be individualized according to the specific manifestation of the condition in a particular pregnant woman, the general principles of management are highlighted within the fact file itself.

Clinicians will find the 'ready reckoner' style of the fact files and care pathways reassuringly simple in a busy clinical setting. Nothing is more likely to undermine the patient's trust or confidence than hearing the doctor caring for her pregnancy confessing that he/she is unfamiliar with the rare condition, perhaps even unable to pronounce its name! Designed with the busy clinic in mind, the fact files and care pathways provide enough information to help the clinician face such situations.

In those rare conditions where little literature exists to inform practice, care pathways have been designed based on personal or collective experience, adopting a pragmatic, commonsense and best practice approach. The rarer the condition, the more comprehensive the fact file and references, in order to encourage the reader to learn more about these diseases.

Every one of the high-risk conditions in this compendium has been encountered and personally managed by the author in over three decades of obstetric practice. This might explain the rather idiosyncratic inclusion of certain rare conditions that are infrequently met with in clinical practice!

REFERENCES

1. Rosene-Montella K, et al. The growing importance of medical problems in pregnancy (editorial). Obstet Med 2010; 3: 1.
2. The Confidential Enquiry into Maternal and Child Health (CEMACH): Saving Mothers Lives: reviewing maternal deaths to make motherhood safer (2003–2005), Seventh Report and 2006–2008, Eighth Report. London: CEMACH, 2007 and 2011.
3. MBRRACE - UK Report: Saving Lives, Improving Mothers' Care - Dec 2014 https://www.npeu.ox.ac.uk/.../mbrrace-uk/reports/
4. Department of Health. Maternity services pathway payment system—a simple guide 2012–2013 <https://www.gov.uk/government/publications/maternity-care-services-pathway-payment-system-a-simple-guide-2012-2013>
5. Royal College of Obstetricians and Gynaecologists. Advanced Training Skills Modules (ATSMs) <https://www.rcog.org.uk/en/careers-training/specialty-training-curriculum/atsms/>
6. Royal College of Obstetricians and Gynaecologists. Green-top guidelines <https://www.rcog.org.uk/en/guidelines-research-services/guidelines/>
7. National Institute for Health and Clinical Excellence. Clinical guidelines <http://www.guidance.nice.org.uk/CG>
8. British Committee for Standards in Haematology (BCSH). <http://www.bcshguidelines.com/guidelines>
9. British Association for Sexual Health and HIV (BASHH). <http://www.bashh.org.guidelines>
10. British Thoracic Society. Guidelines <http://www.brit-thoracic.org.uk>
11. Royal College of Obstetricians and Gynaecologists. Standards for maternity care: report of a joint working Party. London: RCOG Press, 2008.
12. National service framework for children, young people and maternity services: core standards. London: Department of Health, 2004.
13. Maternity matters: choice, access and continuity of care in a safe service. London: Department of Health, 2007.
14. National Institute for Health and Clinical Excellence. Antenatal care:routine care for the healthy pregnant woman. CG 62. London: NICE, 2008, last modified 2014.

1 Maternal Haematological and Vascular Conditions

1.1 Refractory Anaemia

FACT FILE

Definitions and epidemiology

- **WHO definition** of **anaemia during pregnancy** is a haemoglobin (Hb) level of less than 110 g/litre (in pre-March 2013 terminology, 11 g/dl)[1] and postpartum anaemia as Hb less than 100 g/litre.[2]
- Iron deficiency, particularly during pregnancy, is the most common nutrient deficiency in the world, especially in developing and resource-poor countries. Even in developed countries, it is estimated that about 30–40% of pregnant women have iron deficiency anaemia.[3]
- **British Committee for Standards in Haematology guidelines:** Hb of less than 110 g/litre in the first and third trimesters, less than 105 g/litre in the second trimester, and less than 100 g/litre in the postpartum period.[4,5]

Physiological changes

- Low Hb concentrations are part of the normal physiological response to pregnancy due to a dilution effect.
- Hb concentrations fall from early pregnancy to the lowest point at about 36 weeks gestation, when compared with a non-pregnant state. Maternal haematocrit follows a similar pattern.
- Mean Hb and the haematocrit usually return to normal within 3 months in healthy women after a normal delivery.
- Each normal pregnancy and delivery requires about 1 g of iron.

Refractory iron deficiency anaemia (microcytic hypochromic)

Surveillance

- One-third to one-half of all pregnant women who are not on iron supplements will have a haemoglobin of less than 110 g/litre. Those on a healthy diet do not suffer serious clinical problems or develop symptoms. Women with multiple gestations or grand multiparas as well as those who smoke and/or have poor nutrition can develop symptomatic iron deficiency anaemia.
- Other indications for checking serum ferritin levels in pregnant women not previously known to be anaemic include those with a high risk of iron depletion or poor stores,[3] such as
  - previous anaemia
  - multiple pregnancies
  - multiparity >P3
  - short interpregnancy interval of <1 year
  - recent history of bleeding
  - teenage pregnancies
  - Jehovah's witnesses.
- Effective management is needed to prevent adverse outcomes during pregnancy, delivery, and the postnatal period, including increased susceptibility to infections and altered immune responses.[4]
- Maternal iron depletion also increases the risk of neonatal iron deficiency in the first 3 months of life,[6] although the fetus is largely protected due to the up-regulation of placental transport proteins.[7]
- Some[8] have suggested the use of routine iron supplementation for all pregnant women irrespective of their status. However, additional iron supplementation for women who have normal levels of iron may even be associated with increased blood viscosity, impaired placental circulation, and therefore restricted fetal growth.
- Where there are facilities for regular Hb monitoring in pregnancy, as in the UK, iron supplements are offered only to those who have demonstrable iron deficiency anaemia. **Routine iron supplementation for all pregnant women is not currently recommended in the UK except in those areas with a particularly large population of 'at risk' women with haemoglobinopathies.**

Clinical symptoms

- Clinical symptoms and signs of severe iron deficiency anaemia in pregnancy include fatigue as the most common symptom as well as dyspnoea, palpitations, headaches, weakness, irritability, and pallor.

Diagnosis and management

- A trial of oral iron should be the first-line diagnostic test, as an increment seen at 2 weeks is a positive result for iron deficiency anaemia. The Hb concentration should rise by approximately 20 g/litre over 3–4 weeks.[9]
- Serum ferritin is the best indicator of iron deficiency. Serum iron, transferrin saturation and total iron binding capacity (TIBC) are less reliable indicators due to the wide fluctuation in levels from recent ingestion of iron, diurnal variation, infections, etc.[10]
- Measurement of red cell zinc protoporphyrin (ZPP) levels, a rarely performed test, is more sensitive than serum ferritin levels, bearing an inverse relationship with the degree of iron availability.[11]
- Serum ferritin levels in women with adequate iron stores at conception initially rises, followed by a progressive fall by 32 weeks to about 50% pre-pregnancy levels due to haemodilution and utilization of iron. There is a small increase again in the third trimester.[12]
- Women with known haemoglobinopathies should have their serum ferritin checked and offered oral supplements if the ferritin level is less than 30 micrograms/litre.[4,13]
- Women with established iron deficiency anaemia must be prescribed 100–200 mg of **elemental** iron/day (200 mg of either ferrous sulfate or fumarate contains 65 mg of elemental iron; 300 mg of ferrous gluconate has 35 mg of elemental iron) with advice regarding the correct administration to optimize absorption.[4]
- In those who are not anaemic as yet, but are found to be iron deficient, a daily dose of 65 mg elemental iron may be offered. Hb and serum ferritin test must be repeated after 8 weeks, as these women have little iron stores to utilize should additional iron be required.
- Referral to secondary care is advisable if there are significant symptoms and/or severe anaemia (Hb <70–80 g/litre) or if found in late gestation (>34 weeks) or if there is failure to respond to a trial of oral iron (refractory anaemia).[4]
- After restoration of the Hb level to the normal range, it is important to advise that iron supplementation be continued for 3 months during pregnancy and at least until 6 weeks postpartum to replenish iron stores.[4]
- In those with severe anaemia, additional intrapartum precautions are needed and must be documented, including need for delivery in a hospital setting, blood group-and-save on admission, prompt establishment of IV access, active management of the third stage of labour, and pre-planning in the event of postpartum haemorrhage **(see also Chapter 24.3 for women refusing blood and blood products)**.

- Suggested Hb cut-offs are around 100 g/litre for delivery in hospital (including midwifery-led co-located birthing units) and less than 95 g/litre for delivery in an obstetrician-led unit.[4]

Role of IV parenteral iron in iron deficiency anaemia

- Parenteral iron should be considered from the latter part of the second trimester onwards and during the postpartum period for women with refractory iron deficiency who are either totally non-compliant with or intolerant of oral iron therapy or have proven malabsorption.[14]
- Contraindications for parenteral iron include a history of anaphylaxis, adverse reactions to a test dose of parenteral iron, the first trimester of pregnancy, active acute or chronic infection, chronic liver disease.[15]
- Facilities and staff trained in management of anaphylaxis should be available.
- Women should be informed of potential side effects and written information should be provided.[4]
- IV parenteral iron has little added advantage over oral iron therapy except the certainty of administration. Some studies[16,17,18] have, however, shown a more rapid rise of Hb and better replenishment of iron stores compared with oral therapy.

Blood transfusion

- This should be reserved for only those women who have developed severe anaemia (<70 g/litre at ≥36 weeks gestation), especially if associated with repeated APHs.
- Though transfusion will 'improve' the Hb level, transfused red blood cells have a shorter lifespan and a reduced oxygen-carrying capacity.
- Transfusion of blood has often been found to trigger onset of uterine contractions, a factor to be borne in mind before a decision regarding transfusion is taken.
- Blood transfusion should be reserved for those with continued bleeding or have a risk of further bleeding, imminent cardiac compromise or symptoms requiring immediate action.[14]

Planning intrapartum management

- If anaemia persists with Hb levels 95 g/litre or less after 36–37 weeks gestation, even average blood loss in the third stage may not be adequately tolerated.
- It is essential that an intrapartum care plan is discussed and documented.[19] The following documentation should be clear in the notes regarding PPH prophylaxis: 'Active management of third stage with high-dose oxytocin infusion for a minimum of 2–4 h in addition to the routine bolus of IM oxytocin.'

Megaloblastic anaemia: folate deficiency, vitamin B_{12} deficiency

- Folate is a generic term for a naturally occurring family of B-group vitamins found in a variety of foods including green leafy vegetables, fruit, liver, yeast, etc. Folic acid is the synthetic form of folate which is widely used in supplements and for fortification.
- Folate is vital for the growth of the fetus, placenta, and maternal tissues. The fetus actively accumulates folate reserves.[20]
- ***The incidence of megaloblastic anaemia in pregnancy in the UK is estimated to be at least 0.2–5%, with most cases caused by folate deficiency rather than that of vitamin B_{12}.***[21]
- This quoted prevalence rate is based on serum folate levels and is likely to be a significant underestimate due to megaloblastic changes already present in the bone marrow, detectable only by bone marrow aspiration.
- The prevalence of megaloblastic anaemia during pregnancy is influenced by nutritional and socio-economic status[21] and therefore varies between different population groups.
- The normal dietary folate intake in some countries is inadequate to supply the recommended amount required during pregnancy to prevent megaloblastic anaemia in one-quarter of all pregnant women.
- In Europe, the recommended daily intake ranges from 200 to 400 micrograms of folate for adults. For a normal singleton pregnancy, it ranges from 300 to 600 micrograms/day and from 260 to 600 micrograms/day during lactation.[22]
- The average daily intake in unsupplemented women in a UK study is 237 micrograms/day.[23]
- **Metabolism during pregnancy** is associated with a negative folate balance[24] due to fetal requirements and increased folate breakdown. Megaloblastic anaemia occurs following 17–19 weeks of a negative folate balance, so is usually encountered in late gestation.
- Due to a combination of physiological haemodilution and a negative folate balance, there is normally a progressive fall in serum folate levels as pregnancy advances.
- In a normal pregnancy, the serum folate concentration at term may be only 50% of non-pregnancy values.

Diagnostic tests

- Serum folate levels in pregnancy are, however, not particularly useful in the diagnosis of megaloblastic anaemia associated with folate deficiency as postprandial and day-to-day variations are common.[24]
- There is also considerable overlap in the range of serum folate concentrations in pregnant women with normal haematopoiesis and those with megaloblastic anaemia.
- **Red cell folate** is a more reliable indicator of the folate status in pregnancy as it displays less short-term variation and is a better indicator of folate stores.

Management

- Without folate supplementation during pregnancy, one-third of women will have low folate levels in the puerperium and around 10% will develop macrocytic anaemia. There are currently no DH recommendations in the UK for all women to take folate supplements throughout pregnancy.
- It must be noted that pregnant women with severe iron deficiency may also have coexisting folate deficiency, and simultaneous folate supplementation with that of iron must be borne in mind. If only iron supplementation is given, the resultant increase in red cell production may further deplete folate stores, resulting in severe megaloblastic anaemia.
- Apart from the well- established link between maternal folate deficiency and fetal neural tube and cleft defects, an association has also been found with other adverse pregnancy outcomes such as abruption, recurrent miscarriage, fetal growth restriction, preterm delivery, and low birth weight.[25]
- A higher dose of folate supplementation (5 mg/day) is advisable for women with a previous pregnancy with neural tube/cleft abnormality, a strong family history of neural tube defect (NTD), those on folate-antagonist drugs such as antiepileptics, and those with diabetes.
- A similar high dose must also be considered for women at greater risk of deficiency, such as those with malabsorption disorders, as well as in cases of excessive folate utilization such as multiple pregnancies.[26]
- Certain drugs, such as several antiepileptics, sulfasalazine, and azathioprine, have antifolate effects and a higher dose of folic acid (5 mg/day) is recommended throughout pregnancy.
- Similarly, those with coeliac disease, inflammatory bowel disorders such as Crohn's or ulcerative colitis, malabsorption syndromes, those with multiple gestations or severe prolonged hyperemesis gravidarum may need higher doses of folic acid supplementation throughout pregnancy.
- Previous concerns that widespread use of folate supplementation in pregnancy may lead to neurological sequelae because of an unmasking of vitamin B_{12} deficiency appear largely unfounded.[21,24]
- Because active transport of folate across the placenta continues despite severe maternal folate deficiency, term neonates usually have a normal full blood count,[20] although preterm babies of these mothers may display megaloblastic anaemia.[21]
- **Vitamin B_{12} deficiency** may be a rare cause of megaloblastic anaemia.
- Clinical vitamin B_{12} deficiency may be a cause of infertility or recurrent spontaneous abortion.
- Inadequate vitamin B_{12} status periconceptually may increase the risk of birth defects such as NTD, and may contribute to preterm delivery, although further research is required.[26]

- Inadequate vitamin B_{12} status in the mother may lead to frank deficiency in the infant if sufficient fetal stores are not accumulated during pregnancy or are not available in breast milk.
- In those known to have pernicious anaemia, the 3-monthly intramuscular hydroxocobalamin injections can be safely continued during pregnancy and lactation.

Refractory anaemia—in general

Investigations

- In those with refractory anaemia, further investigations are required to establish aetiology and to guide management.
- In such cases the following conditions need to be considered:
  - Any underlying **renal disease**—chronic UTIs, nephrotic syndrome, repeated pyelonephritis, etc. **Investigations:** MSU, microscopic haematuria, renal function tests and maternal renal scan as indicated.
  - Any underlying **bowel disease** (e.g. coeliac disease, inflammatory bowel disease, malabsorption syndromes, etc.). **Investigations** may include stool samples (× 3) for evidence of parasites or melena, markers for coeliac disease such as IgA and IgG, serum gliadin antibody assay, and tissue transglutaminase antibody assays.
  - Hypothyroidism—thyroid function tests (**TFTs)** to be checked.
  - Haemoglobinopathies—check **electrophoresis.**
  - Aplastic anaemia, hereditary spherocytosis, myeloproliferative disorders, etc. to be excluded.
  - Autoimmune haemolytic anaemia—these women are usually diagnosed before pregnancy or have associated conditions such as systemic lupus erythematosus (SLE).
  - Malaria—the patient may have arrived from a country where falciparum malaria is endemic. Peripheral blood films may be required.

Suggested laboratory investigations

- Recheck serum ferritin, red cell folate and vitamin B12 levels along with haematocrit and blood film.
- Renal function tests, urine examination, MSU.
- Liver function tests.
- Peripheral blood smear for malarial parasites, RBC fragmentation, spherocytosis.
- TFTs.
- Antiphospholipid antibodies and lupus anticoagulant.
- Coeliac disease markers: serological diagnosis by IgA and IgG, gliadin antibody assay.
- Stool samples (× 3) to exclude parasites, chronic melena, malabsorption syndrome.
- ***Early discussion with haematologists is highly recommended when dealing with refractory anaemia.***

Information for patients

Please see Information for patients: Anaemia and pregnancy (p. 493)

References

1. <http://www.pathologyharmony.co.uk>.
2. WHO Iron deficiency anaemia: assessment, prevention and control. WHO/NHD/01.3, Geneva: World Health Organization, 2001.
3. de Benoist B, et al. WHO global database on anaemia. Worldwide prevalence of anaemia 1993–2005. Geneva: World Health Organization, 2008.
4. BCSH UK guidelines on the management of iron deficiency in pregnancy. London: British Committee for Standards in Haematology, 2011.
5. Ramsey M, et al. Normal values in pregnancy, 2nd ed. London: WB Saunders, 2000.
6. Colomer J, et al. Anaemia during pregnancy as a risk factor for infant iron deficiency: report from the Valencia Infant Anaemia Cohort (VIAC) study. Paediatr Perinatal Epidemiol 1990;4: 196–204
7. Gambling L, et al. Effect of iron deficiency on placental transfer of iron and expression of iron transport proteins in vivo and in vitro. Biochem J 2001;356: 883–889.
8. Hemminki E, Rimpela U. A Randomised comparison of routine versus selective iron supplementation during pregnancy. J Am Coll Nutr 1991;10: 3–10.
9. British National Formulary 64; Sept 2012:599.
10. Adams PC, et al. Biological variability of transferrin saturation and unsaturated iron binding capacity. Am J Med 2007;120: 999.
11. Schifman RB, et al. Role of ferritin supported in diagnosis of anemias of pregnancy. Am J Obstet Gynecol 1989;161: 258–259.
12. Asif N, et al. Comparison of serum ferritin levels in three trimesters of pregnancy and their correlation with increasing gravidity. Int J Pathol 2007;5: 26–30.
13. Van den Broek NR, et al. Iron status in pregnant women: which measurements are valid? Br J Haematol 1998;103: 817–824.
14. RCOG Green-top guideline No. 47. Blood transfusions in obstetrics. London: Royal College of Obstetricians and Gynaecologists, 2008.
15. Perewusnyk G, et al. Parenteral iron therapy in obstetrics: 8 years experience with iron-sucrose complex. Br J Nutr 2002;88: 3–10.
16. Al, RA, et al. Intravenous versus oral iron for treatment of anemia in pregnancy: a randomized trial. Obstet Gynecol 2005;106: 1335–1340.
17. Bayoumeu F, et al. Iron therapy in iron deficiency anaemia in pregnancy: Intravenous route versus oral route. Eur J Obstet Gynecol Reprod Biol 2005;123: S15–S19.
18. Van Wyk DB, Martens MG Intravenous ferric carboxymaltose compared with oral iron in the treatment of postpartum anaemia: a randomized controlled trial. Obstet Gynecol 2007;110: 267–278.
19. RCOG Green-top guideline No. 52. Postpartum haemorrhage, prevention and management. London: Royal College of Obstetricians and Gynaecologists, 2009, updated 2011.
20. Burton R, et al. Severe folate deficiency in pregnancy with normal red cell folate level. Clin Lab Haematol 2006;28: 66–68
21. Letsky EA Blood volume, haematinics, anaemia. In:de Swiet M, ed.., Medical disorders in obstetric practice 4th ed. Oxford: Blackwell Science, 2002, pp. 20–60.
22. EFSA ESCO report prepared by the EFSA Scientific Cooperation Working Group on Analysis of Risks and Benefits of Fortification of Food with Folic Acid. Parma: European Food Safety Authority, 2009.
23. Langley-Evans SC, Langley-Evans AJ Use of folic acid supplements in the first trimester of pregnancy. J Roy Soc Health 2002;122: 181–186.
24. Chanarin I Megaloblastic anaemia associated with pregnancy. In: The megaloblastic anaemias, 2nd ed. Oxford: Blackwell, 1979.
25. Scholl TO, Johnson WG Folic acid: influence on the outcome of pregnancy. Am J Clin Nutr 2000;71: 1295s–1303s.
26. Molloy AM, et al. Effects of folate and vitamin B12 deficiencies during pregnancy on fetal, infant, and child development. Food Nutr Bull 2008;29: 101–111.

CARE PATHWAY

Persistent anaemia in pregnancy* not responding to oral iron ± folic acid supplementation
*Hb persists at less than 85 g/litre

↓

Community midwife/GP refers patient to hospital specialist antenatal clinic

↓

First visit to hospital antenatal clinic

- Detailed history of any haemoglobinopathies, chronic or acute infections, malabsorption disorders, medication history, etc.
- Confirm compliance with medication, assess whether high-dose folic acid (5 mg/day) is required (e.g. in those on antifolate antiepilepsy medication)
- If a smoker, smoking cessation advice and support to be offered
- **Blood tests:**
  - repeat FBC, peripheral blood film for reticulocytes, fragmented RBCs, spherocytosis, and for malarial parasites, if indicated by history and symptomatology
  - serum ferritin, red cell folate levels, serum vitamin B_{12} levels
  - check electrophoresis for haemoglobinopathy
  - thyroid function tests
  - liver function tests
  - anticardiolipin antibodies and lupus anticoagulant
  - total blood picture for any evidence of myeloproliferative disorders, aplastic anaemia
  - coeliac disease markers: serum IgA, IgG, gliadin antibody assay
- MSU—chronic infections, microscopic haematuria
- Stool samples, if indicated by history—for detection of parasites, melena
- Growth scans at about 28–30 and 34–36 weeks gestation with same-day review in specialist antenatal clinic
- Routine antenatal care continues in the community according to NICE guidelines for normal pregnancy
- Treat aetiology if detected and treatment is feasible (e.g. hypothyroidism, UTI, antiparasitic medication, pernicious anaemia)
- While investigations are in progress, further management in severe cases to be discussed with haematologist
- If Hb level is restored to normal during pregnancy, advise continuation of oral iron ± folic acid for at least 3 months during pregnancy and 6 weeks postpartum
- Parenteral iron or blood transfusion in selected cases after discussions with haematologist. Contraindications to be noted. All facilities and trained personnel to manage anaphylaxis to be readily available. Inform patient of potential risks, give printed information
- Antenatal blood transfusion only if Hb is <70 g/litre and $\geq$ 36 weeks pregnancy
- Caution: Antenatal blood transfusion may trigger uterine contractions, resulting in iatrogenic preterm birth
- ***No indication for early IOL or for LSCS based solely on refractory anaemia***
- Clear discussion and documentation in notes regarding need for hospital delivery and plans for intrapartum care
- Document precautions for PPH prophylaxis including: establishing IV access early in labour, group and save, active management of third stage with high-dose oxytocin infusion for a minimum of 2–4 h in addition to bolus dose of oxytocin/oxytocin with ergometrine
- If any unusual blood group or antibodies interfering with routine cross-matching are present, prearrange availability of compatible blood
- Advise continuation postpartum and during lactation of supplemental iron ± folic acid and of **Vit B_{12}** injections in those with pernicious anaemia
- Advise effective contraception to avoid short interpregnancy interval

1.2 Inherited Thrombophilias

FACT FILE

- **Thrombophilias** are **inherited** or **acquired** conditions that predispose the affected individual to venous thromboembolism (VTE) such as deep vein thrombosis (DVT) and pulmonary embolism (PE).
- For **acquired thrombophilias such as lupus (SLE) and antiphospholipid syndrome (APS)** refer to specific fact files and care pathways in Chapter 13.1.
- **Inherited (heritable) thrombophilias (e.g. factor V Leiden mutation, protein C and protein S deficiencies, antithrombin deficiency, prothrombin gene mutation)** are not uncommon and when taken together affect around 15% of the Western population.[1,2]
- ***Normal pregnancy itself induces a state of hypercoagulability with a 10-fold increase in thrombotic risk throughout pregnancy and the puerperium.***
- VTE or TED (thromboembolic disease) remains one of the main direct causes of maternal death in the UK.[3]
- VTE complicates 1 in 1000 pregnancies.
- Thrombophilias cause more than one-third to one-half of all maternal VTE. Inherited thrombophilia is found in 20–50% of pregnancy-related VTE.[1,4]
- The risk of VTE is greater postpartum than antepartum.
- At present there is no good evidence to suggest that heritable thrombophilias increase the risk of arterial diseases such as myocardial infarction or strokes.
- Thrombophilias are also implicated in other adverse obstetric outcomes such as:
  - early-onset and severe pre-eclampsia requiring delivery before 34 weeks gestation[5,6,7,8].
  - severe IUGR, especially early-onset, requiring delivery before 34 weeks gestation[9]
  - stillbirth[10,11,12]
  - recurrent miscarriages[10,11,12,13,14,15]
  - placental abruption.[16]

Heritable thrombophilias

Antithrombin deficiency

- Previously called **antithrombin III deficiency**.
- Antithrombin is synthesized by the liver. Its action inhibits not only thrombin but also the activated clotting factors IXa, Xa, XIa, and XIIa.[17]
- Antithrombin levels are significantly reduced if the patient is on heparin therapy and in those who have a current thrombosis. Profound decrease in antithrombin levels is also seen in those with disseminated intravascular coagulopathy (DIC), liver disease, and nephrotic syndrome.
- There are two major types of antithrombin deficiency:
  - In **type I** there is a quantitative reduction of functionally normal antithrombin protein.
  - **Type II** is due to production of a qualitatively abnormal protein.
- Incidence of thrombosis is higher in those with type I antithrombin deficiency. The prevalence of type I antithrombin deficiency is about 0.02% in the general population and about 1% in patients with thrombosis (Table 1.1).
- The relative risk of VTE in an individual with antithrombin deficiency is increased by 25–50-fold.

Protein C deficiency

- Protein C is a vitamin K-dependent glycoprotein, synthesized in the liver.
- In normal pregnancy, there is a naturally occurring reduction of protein C levels.
- Reduced protein C levels are also seen in DIC and liver disease, and in those on warfarin.

Table 1.1 Relative risk of VTE in various thrombophilias in the general population (men and women)

Type of thrombophilia	*Relative risk increase for VTE*
Type I antithrombin deficiency	25–50-fold (35% chance of VTE in a pregnancy)
Protein C deficiency	10–15-fold
Protein S deficiency	2-fold
Factor V Leiden heterozygous carrier	3–8-fold
Factor V Leiden homozygotes	10–40-fold

Data from Walker DW et al., 'Investigation and Management of Heritable Thrombophilia', British Journal of Haematology, 2001, 114, pp. 512–528; and RCOG Green-top Guideline No. 37a, 'Reducing the risk of thrombosis and embolism during pregnancy and the puerperium', 2009, London: RCOG press

- Prevalence of heritable protein C deficiency in the general population is approximately 0.2–0.3% and about 3% in patients with VTE.
- The relative risk of VTE in an individual with protein C deficiency is increased by 10–15-fold.

Protein S deficiency

- Protein S is a vitamin K-dependent protein and is also a cofactor of protein C.
- Protein S levels fall progressively during pregnancy.[16,18]
- Reduced levels are seen in DIC, liver disease, APS, or those on warfarin.
- Prevalence of protein S deficiency in the general population is unknown. Deficiency of protein S has a mild effect on the risk of venous thrombosis, increasing the risk by around twofold.

Factor V Leiden mutation

- Factor V Leiden mutation is the most common heritable thrombophilia in white people, especially those of northern European extraction.
- Prevalence in the general population is 2–15%.
- Factor V Leiden mutation is found in 20–50% of those presenting with a first episode of VTE. Heterozygous carriers have a 3–8-fold increased risk of venous thrombosis; homozygous carriers have an 80-fold increased risk.

Prothrombin G20210A mutation

- The prevalence of prothrombin *G20210A* mutation in northern European general population is about 2%, and 6% in those with a first thrombosis.
- Prevalence is greater in southern European populations, in whom this is the most common form of hereditable thrombophilia
- The risk of VTE in heterozygous carriers of the prothrombin *G20210A* mutation is estimated to be around three times that of non-carriers.

Combined thrombophilias

- Due to the high prevalence of factor V Leiden and prothrombin *G20210A* mutations in many populations, it is not uncommon to have more than one heritable thrombophilic factor in an individual or in family members. The risk of VTE is also increased in families with combinations of thrombophilic conditions.[19,20]

Screening for inherited thrombophilias

- Levels of protein C and protein S are reduced during a normal pregnancy without indicating a thrombophilic state. There is little use, therefore, in screening for these conditions during pregnancy. Such patients must be screened at least 8–12 weeks postpartum to get accurate levels of proteins C and S.[17]

- Similarly, protein C, protein S, and antithrombin are reduced in the acute post-thrombotic state and assay results are affected by the use of anticoagulants.
- There is little point, therefore, in seeking to test for most heritable thrombophilia factors when the patient presents with an acute VTE or is already on anticoagulants.
- Testing is best delayed until at least 4 weeks after completion of the course of anticoagulation.
- PCR-based tests for factor V Leiden and the prothrombin *G20210A* allele are, however, unaffected by factors such as pregnancy, acute VTE, or the presence of anticoagulants.
- ***Who should be screened for thrombophilia?***
  - Those with a previous personal history of VTE.
  - Those with a family history of VTE in a first-degree relative under 50 years of age.

Pregnancy-associated VTE risk stratification in those with known inherited thrombophilia

High risk of clinical VTE (>1:40)

- Women who are on long-term anticoagulation thromboprophylaxis [17,21]
- Those with a known **antithrombin deficiency**, whether or not they have had a previous VTE. This is because the relative risk of VTE is increased 25–50-fold if the patient has type I antithrombin deficiency.
- In all such high-risk women, anticoagulant prophylaxis must be continued throughout pregnancy and puerperium along with the use of below knee compression stockings. They should be a advised to immediately switch from warfarin to low molecular weight heparin (LMWH) (or to start LMWH if not previously on warfarin) when a pregnancy is confirmed with a positive pregnancy test.
- The dose of LMWH prescribed in such cases is **usually closer to that used for treatment of VTE rather than for prophylaxis only**. The dose of the SC LMWH is based on the early pregnancy weight as well.
- Platelet counts should be checked before and 1 week after starting LMWH.

Moderately high risk of clinical VTE (1:40–1:200)

- Women with a previous VTE, who have an underlying thrombophilia but do not belong to the previous high-risk category.
- Women with no personal history of VTE but who, before pregnancy, have been found to be protein C deficient (usually discovered on screening initiated due to a family history), or those with a combination of thrombophilic defects, or those who are homozygous for a thrombophilia disorder.
- LMWH prophylaxis should be commenced as soon as pregnancy is confirmed and continued throughout pregnancy and puerperium along with the use of below knee compression stockings in all such women.

Slightly increased risk of clinical VTE (1:200–1:400)

- Women with no personal history of venous thrombosis but who have had a thrombophilic defect identified pre-pregnancy (usually because of a family history) and who do not belong to the previous high or moderately high risk categories (**e.g. those who are heterozygous for protein S or factor V Leiden deficiency or for prothrombin *G20210A* mutations). These women do not usually require routine antenatal anticoagulant prophylaxis but must be given anticoagulant prophylaxis for at least 6 weeks following delivery.** Below knee compression stockings are advisable throughout pregnancy and for at least 6 weeks postnatally.
- Women with a history of previous venous thrombosis occurring in association with a temporary risk factor which is no longer present and who have no identifiable thrombophilic defect also belong to this low-risk group.
- ***Documentation in the notes after antenatal discussions about special points for labour, delivery, and puerperium is essential. This should include:***
  - Advice regarding LMWH dosage, duration of postnatal thromboprophylaxis, etc. Referral for haematology review is recommended.
  - Anaesthetic review regarding when to stop pharmacological thromboprophylaxis before labour. An epidural or spinal should not be sited less than 12 h after last dose of LMWH. Also, LMWH should not be given within 2–3 h of siting an epidural or spinal anaesthesia or of catheter removal.
  - Providing there is no excessive bleeding, LMWH can be introduced or reintroduced within 12 h after delivery in fixed prophylactic doses.
  - Advice regarding postnatal thromboprophylaxis: If the woman does not wish to continue injections throughout her puerperium, she may change to oral warfarin. Generally, oral warfarin is introduced on the first or second postpartum day and the LMWH is withdrawn when the INR is within the recommended therapeutic range (usually 2.0–3.0) for two consecutive days. Warfarin will need to be continued for at least 6 weeks after delivery along with the below-knee compression stockings.
  - The woman may opt to continue LMWH in the puerperium and she needs to be advised to do so for at least 6 weeks, along with wearing the below-knee compression stockings.
  - No contraindication for breastfeeding either with LMWH or warfarin.
  - Contraception advice: The combined oral contraceptive must be avoided. Levonorgestrel intrauterine system (Mirena®) is probably the contraception of choice.
- ***Treatment of VTE during pregnancy and the puerperium in a woman with an inherited thrombophilic disorder is no different from the management of VTE due to any cause in pregnancy (see Chapter 1.10).***

Information for patients

Please see Information for patients: Inherited thrombophilia (p. 494)

References

1. Greer IA Inherited thrombophilia and venous thromboembolism. Best Pract Res Clin Obstet Gynaecol 2003;17: 413–425.
2. Lockwood CJ, Silver R Thrombophilias in pregnancy. In:Creasy RK et al., ed., Maternal-fetal medicine 5th ed. Philadelphia, PA: WB Saunders, 2004, pp. 1005–1021.
3. Centre for Maternal and Child Enquiry Saving Mothers' Lives: Reviewing maternal deaths to make motherhood safer—2006-2008, The Eighth Report of the Confidential Enquiries into Maternal Deaths in the United Kingdom. London: RCOG Press, 2011.
4. McColl MD, et al. The role of inherited thrombophilia in venous thromboembolism associated with pregnancy. BJOG 1999;75: 387–388.
5. Sibai BM. Thrombophilia and severe preeclampsia: time to screen and treat in future pregnancies? Hypertension 2005;46: 1252–1253.
6. Lin J, August P Genetic thrombophilias and preeclampsia. a meta-analysis. Obstet Gynecol 2005;105: 182–192.
7. Kupferminc MJ Thrombophilia and preeclampsia: the evidence so far. Clin Obstet Gynecol 2005;48: 406–415.
8. Mello G, et al. Thrombophilia is significantly associated with severe preeclampsia. Results of a large scale, care-controlled study. Hypertension 2005;46: 1270–1274.
9. Dizon-Townson D The relationship of the factor V Leiden mutation and pregnancy outcomes for mother and fetus. Obstet Gynecol 2005;106: 517–524.
10. Preston FE, et al. Increased fetal loss in women with heritable thrombophilia. Lancet 1996;348: 913–916.
11. Brenner B Inherited thrombophilia and pregnancy loss. Best Pract Res Clin Haematol 2003;16: 311–320.
12. Sarig G, et al. Thrombophilia is common in women with pregnancy loss and is associated with late pregnancy wastage. Fertil Steril 2002;77: 342–347.
13. Paidas MJ, et al. Screening and management of inherited thrombophilias in the setting of adverse pregnancy outcome. Clin Perinatol 2004;31: 783–805.
14. Blumenfeld Z, Brenner B Thrombophilia-associated pregnancy wastage. Fert Steril 1999;72: 765–774.
15. Middeldorp S. Thrombophilia and pregnancy complications: cause or association? J Thromb Haemost 2007;5: 276–282.
16. Walker MC, et al. Heparin for pregnant women with acquired or inherited thrombophilias. Cochrane Database Syst Rev 2003;2: CD003580.

17. Walker DW, et al. Investigation and management of heritable thrombophilia. Br J Haematol 2001;114: 512–528.
18. Clarke P, et al. Activated protein C sensitivity, protein C, protein and coagulation in normal pregnancy. Thromb Haemost 1998;79: 1166–1170.
19. Folkeringa N, et al High-risk of pregnancy-related venous thromboembolism in women with multiple thrombophilic defects. Br J Haematol 2007;138: 110–116.
20. Vossen CY, et al. Risk of a first venous thrombotic event in carriers of a familial thrombophilic defect. The European Prospective Cohort on Thrombophilia (EPCOT). J Thromb Haemost 2005;3: 459–464.
21. RCOG Green-top Guideline No. 37a. Reducing the risk of thrombosis and embolism during pregnancy and the puerperium. London: Royal College of Obstetircians and Haematologists, 2009.

CARE PATHWAY

As soon as pregnancy is confirmed, any woman with the following should be referred by community midwife/GP to maternal medicine/specialist antenatal clinic:

- A personal history of venous thromboembolism (VTE)
- A family history of VTE in a 1st-degree relative <50 years of age
- Any known history of a thrombophilic disorder, e.g.
  - Antithrombin deficiency, especially type 1
  - Protein C or protein S deficiency
  - Factor V Leiden mutation (homozygote or heterozygote)
- A known history of lupus/antiphospholipid syndrome
- Those on long-term anticoagulation
- ***Women on long-term anticoagulation with warfarin should have had it switched to low molecular weight heparin (LMWH) as soon as a pregnancy is confirmed and even before a hospital appointment***

↓

First visit to maternal medicine antenatal clinic

Detailed history to include:

- Detailed family history: DVT? thrombophilia?
- personal history of previous DVT: provoked? idiopathic?
- length of time previous anticoagulation therapy had been prescribed for
- any pre-pregnancy screening for thrombophilias—attempt to get results if in an another unit
- previous adverse obstetric problems (e.g. IUGR, severe pre-eclampsia, IUD, abruption, recurrent miscarriage, etc.)
- *Screening tests (if not yet preformed)*
  - anticardiolipin antibodies
  - lupus anticoagulant
  - factor V Leiden mutation
  - If pre-pregnancy screening has not been performed based on a family history of VTE/thrombophilia then screening for heritable thrombophilia during early pregnancy is confined only to factor V Leiden mutation, as there is a normal drop of antithrombin, protein C, and protein S during pregnancy
- If patient is still on warfarin—change immediately to SC LMWH, urgent referral to anticoagulation team and consultant haematologist
- For those women who do not have a thrombophilic disorder but who have had a previous history of confirmed VTE (either idiopathic or during COCP use or during a previous pregnancy), antenatal thromboprophylaxis with LMWH should be commenced from as early in pregnancy as possible and continued throughout pregnancy along with use of below knee compression stockings and for at least 6 weeks postnatal
- For women who have had a previous isolated VTE episode not associated with COC or pregnancy but post trauma or surgery, with no identifiable thrombophilia and no additional risk factors in this pregnancy* such as obesity, smoking, hyperemesis, dehydration, or relative immobility, **antenatal** anticoagulant thromboprophylaxis may be omitted but is required **postnatally** for at least 6 weeks. below knee compression stockings and low-dose aspirin during pregnancy should be advised instead
- *If any additional risks are identified in this category either at the start of pregnancy (e.g. obesity, smoking) or develop during pregnancy (e.g. immobility, dehydration, pre-eclampsia), antenatal thromboprophylaxis with LMWH is essential
- Discuss and document an individualized management plan for care during rest of pregnancy and for labour and delivery, as well as for the puerperium
- Refer all such women on LMWH to the anaesthetic high-risk clinic as soon as possible for advice regarding omitting anticoagulation injection once labour starts, timing of epidural/spinal, and restarting anticoagulation thromboprophylaxis a few hours after delivery, etc.
- Discuss small (though reversible) risk of osteoporosis with long-term LMWH, thrombocytopenia induced by heparin etc., along with benefits. Heparin/LMWH does not cross the placenta and is therefore safe for the baby
- Arrange serial growth scans at about 26, 30, 34, and 37 weeks if screen positive for thrombophilia, lupus/APS *(frequency of serial growth scans depending on unit's protocol)*
- Antenatal clinic appointment for subsequent visits to tally with date for scan
- Advise patient to continue routine appointments with community midwife in between hospital visits, avoiding overlap

↓

Antenatal checks by community midwife to continue as usual

↓

Subsequent visits to specialist antenatal clinic (or joint obstetric/haematology antenatal clinic)

Suggested intervals: 26, 30, 34, and 37 weeks gestation with serial growth scans (frequency depends on the individual unit's protocol for serial scans)

- Check patient is continuing thromboprophylaxis with prescribed LMWH, below knee compression stockings
- Assessment of fetal growth and liquor ± Dopplers
- Check for pre-eclampsia signs/symptoms
- Continue close liaison with haematologists and anticoagulation clinic
- If patient is on anticoagulant thromboprophylaxis with a history/screen positive for thrombophilia, consider delivery at 38–40 weeks. Plan date for IOL if appropriate and advise stopping anticoagulation prophylaxis at least 12 h before IOL or to miss the due dose if spontaneous labour commences meanwhile
- ***LSCS only for obstetric indications***
- Reassure patient regarding safety of breastfeeding—no contraindication with either heparin or warfarin
- Advise continuation of thromboprophylaxis for at least 6 weeks after birth, either SC LMWH or after conversion to oral warfarin. below knee compression stockings for at least 6 weeks
- Advise regarding contraception —**not for combined OCP**. LNG-IUS, progesterone implant, or barrier method are alternatives

Risk stratification for VTE in those with thrombophilic disorder at first visit to maternal medicine/specialist antenatal clinic

High Risk
>1:40

- Women on long-term anticoagulation prophylaxis after previous VTE
- Women with known **type 1 antithrombin deficiency** whether or not they have had previous VTE

↓

- Antenatal LMWH from as early as possible in pregnancy at doses closer to treatment doses than of prophylaxis doses. Switch from warfarin to LMWH once pregnancy confirmed
- Advise below knee compression stockings in pregnancy and puerperium
- Thromboprophylaxis to continue with either LMWH or warfarin for at least 6 weeks postpartum
- Below knee compression stockings for at least 6 weeks postnatally
- Platelet count before LMWH and 1 week later.
- ***Close liaison with anticoagulation clinic team and consultant haematologist***

Moderate Risk
1:40 to 1:200

- Those who have had a previous VTE and have an underlying thrombophilic disorder which is not of the very high risk type
- Those who have **not** had a personal history of VTE but are screen positive in pre-pregnancy testing for **protein C deficiency, combination disorders, or are homozygous for protein S or for Factor V Leiden mutation**

↓

- Antenatal LMWH from as early as possible in pregnancy at prophylactic doses, continued throughout pregnancy and for at least 6 weeks postpartum, with below knee compression stockings in pregnancy and postpartum
- Platelet count before LMWH and 1 week later
- ***Close liaison with anticoagulation team and consultant haematologist***

Low Risk
1:200 to 1:400

- Those with no personal history of VTE but who are screen positive for a thrombophilic disorder not belonging to very high or moderately high risk categories. For example, **no personal history of VTE but are protein C (or S) deficient or heterozygotic for Factor V Leiden mutation**

↓

- Antenatal LMWH thromboprophylaxis **not** needed
- Below knee compression stockings during pregnancy
- ***LMWH thromboprophylaxis with below knee compression stockings for 6 weeks postnatal***

1.3 Thrombocythaemia or Thrombocytosis.

FACT FILE

Definition and incidence in pregnancy

- **Thrombocytosis (thrombocythaemia)** or a platelet count in excess of 450 × 10^9/litre is a common finding. The normal platelet count in pregnancy is between 150 and 400 × 10^9/litre.
- There is a normal physiological rise in platelets postpartum, called **reactive thrombocythaemia**, an essential part of maternal haemostasis.
- Wide variations can occur; involvement of the haematologist is recommended if the platelet count is 600 × 10^9/litre or higher.
- Thrombocytosis can be either *primary or secondary (reactive)*
- See Table 1.2 for the causes of thrombocytosis.[1]
- If platelet counts range between 450 and 600 × 10^9/litre, low-dose aspirin and graded elastic compression stockings are advisable during pregnancy and for at least 6 weeks postpartum.

Essential thrombocythaemia

- Essential thrombocythaemia **(ET)** is one of a group of disorders known as ***myeloproliferative diseases***. In ET, there is an overproduction of blood cells, especially of platelets in the bone marrow, although any combination of the three cell lines producing red and white blood cells as well as platelets may be affected to some degree.
- ET is rare in women of childbearing age.[2]
- Diagnosis made when is there is **sustained** thrombocytosis in excess of 450 × 10^9/litre and reactive causes of thrombocythaemia have been excluded. The blood film will show thrombocytosis with varying degrees of platelet anisocytosis.[1]
- When platelets occur in very high numbers they may not function normally, leading to thrombus production or to a failure of the normal clotting process causing bleeding problems. Thrombosis is a more common complication of ET than is bleeding.
- The major risk related to ET which may impact on long-term survival of patients is the occurrence of thrombosis, and rarely transformation to leukaemia or myelofibrosis.
- Careful thrombotic risk stratification is therefore essential to prevent thrombosis.
- Patients with ET should be screened for hypertension, hyperlipidaemia, diabetes, and a history of smoking and of any cardiovascular risk factors.
- ET should be excluded in women with unexplained miscarriages, stillbirths, severe pre-eclampsia, fetal growth restriction, etc. even if the woman has never had a thromboembolic episode. FBC must be performed to establish pre-pregnancy platelet counts in such wome

Table 1.2 Causes of thrombocytosis

Primary	*Secondary or reactive*
Essential thrombocythaemia	Infection[a]
Polycythaemia vera	Inflammation[a]
Myeloproliferative neoplasms	Tissue damage[a]
Myelodysplastic syndromes	Haemorrhage[a]
	Iron deficiency[a]
	Postoperative[a]
	Haemolysis[a]
	Drug therapy (corticosteroids, etc.)*
	Malignancy
	Splenectomy

[a] All these could be relevant in pregnancy or intra- or postpartum causing reactive thrombocytosis.

Data from Harrison CN, et al., for British Committee for Standards in Haematology, Guideline for investigation and management of adults and children presenting with a thrombocytosis, *British Journal of Haematology*, 2010, 149, pp. 352–375.

Pregnancy in women with ET

- ***The diagnosis of ET has usually been established before pregnancy.***
- Pre-pregnancy counselling is very important given that there is only about a 60–65% live birth rate, even with various treatment modalities.[1,2,3] The increased maternal risks of arterial and venous thrombosis as well as haemorrhage must also be discussed. All patients known to have ET should be advised to continue low-dose aspirin throughout pregnancy.[2]
- **Hydroxycarbamide**, which is often used for cytoreduction in ET, is teratogenic and effective contraception should be advised if it is prescribed. If either partner is using hydroxycarbamide, it should be discontinued 3–6 months before cessation of contraception.[1,4].
- The presence of the ***JAK2 V617F*** mutation in patients with ET is associated with an increased risk of thrombosis and may also increase the risk of pregnancy loss.[6]
- Other risk factors (e.g. obesity, diabetes, smoking, hypertension, prolonged immobility) increase the risks of thrombosis in pregnancy in women with ET.
- In women with ET, stratification of risk factors for complications in pregnancy and to plan appropriate management strategies for ET in pregnancy should be based on the patients' disease status and previous obstetric history.

Risk factors for pregnancy complications in women with ET

- Previous venous or arterial thrombosis (during a previous pregnancy or in the non-pregnant state)
- Previous haemorrhage attributed to ET(whether pregnant or not)
- Previous pregnancy complication that may have been caused by ET, e.g.:
  - unexplained recurrent first-trimester pregnancy losses
  - IUGR
  - intrauterine death (IUD) and stillbirth (with no other obvious cause)
  - severe pre-eclampsia, especially if of early onset
  - placental abruption
  - significant antepartum or postpartum haemorrhage (requiring RBC transfusion)
- Marked and sustained rise in platelet count rising to above 1500 × 10^9/litre.
- Development of severe pre-eclampsia, especially before 34 weeks gestation, in this index pregnancy
- *When one or more of the above risk factors are present in a pregnant woman known to have ET*, there is a high risk of maternal and/or fetal complications (Table 1.3).[1,2,3,4,5,6]
- ***Untreated ET can result in severe pregnancy complications such that only 50–60% have a successful pregnancy outcome.***[3,7–9]
- *Placental infarction due to thrombosis is the most consistent pathological event.*[13]

Diagnosis of ET during pregnancy

- ET may be identified in symptom-free patients when a routine blood count shows platelet counts in excess of 600 × 10^9/litre and the count remains high over a period of observation, with no underlying reason detected.
- ET may come to light when haematological investigations are performed for a patient who develops a blood clot (arterial or venous) or has unexpected bleeding or a mildly enlarged spleen or has symptoms of transient ischaemic attacks (headaches, dizziness, weakness/numbness of one side of the body, slurred speech, etc.).

Table 1.3 Increased rates of pregnancy complications in untreated ET

Adverse event	*Risk*	*References*
Miscarriage	26–36% (in the first trimester)	
Recurrent miscarriages (≥3 losses)	1–2%	10,11
Late pregnancy loss, IUD, stillbirth	5–9.6%	11–12
Preterm delivery	8%	13
Pre-eclampsia	5%	
IUGR	5%	13,14
Abruption of placenta	3%	
Maternal haemorrhage (PPH)	4–6%	8
Maternal thrombosis: cerebral, cardiac, abdominal, arterial thrombi, also DVT	5%	8

Management of ET during pregnancy

- ***Prevention of maternal thrombosis is key. In ET, neither a previous history of a thrombotic event nor the pre-conception platelet count nor aspirin prophylaxis during pregnancy seem to significantly influence pregnancy outcomes. Management modalities are mainly to reduce risks of maternal thrombosis (arterial or venous) during and after pregnancy.***
- Immediate referral to consultant haematologist.
- Advice and support regarding smoking cessation.
- Low-dose aspirin (75 mg od) to inhibit platelet aggregation and thrombosis, to be continued throughout pregnancy. Pregnancy outcomes, however, do not appear to be changed even with use of aspirin.[2,3]
- Low-dose aspirin and graded elastic compression stockings are recommended throughout pregnancy and at least 6 weeks postpartum.
- The use of low-dose aspirin and LMWH in regimes as for APS has been advocated for ET by some, but clear data is as yet unavailable.[1,15]
- Continued risk assessment for venous thrombotic risk should be maintained throughout pregnancy.[16]
- ***If the patient has had previous venous thromboembolism, prophylactic LMWH should be advised throughout pregnancy and for at least 6 weeks postpartum.***
- Cytoreductive therapy with hydroxycarbamide is not recommended due to the risk of teratogenicity. All myelosuppressive drugs, such as hydroxyurea or anagrelide, are contraindicated during pregnancy.
- If treatment is deemed necessary, interferon alfa (**IFN-α**) is the drug of choice, and this may be either continued or instituted during pregnancy.[1,3]
- Referral for anaesthetic assessment is recommended, particularly if the patient is on LMWH.[1]
- **Reduction of the risk of PPH must be documented in the records, e.g:** 'Active management of the third stage with IV oxytocin infusion continued for 3–4 h, in addition to the initial bolus dose of oxytocin.' Carboprost and misoprostol are both safe to use, but **tranexemic acid is contraindicated**[4] due to the risk of thrombosis in these patients who are already prothrombotic.
- If the patient needs to have cytotoxic agents for myelosuppression (e.g. hydroxycarbamide or anagrelide) **postpartum**, breastfeeding is relatively contraindicated. Given the benefits of breastfeeding, however, any decision should be made on an individual basis after full explanation of the benefits and the risks.[1]
- ***The patient must be advised that the combined oral contraceptive pill is contraindicated in her case.***

Information for patients

Please see Information for patients: High platelet counts also called thrombocytosis or thrombocythaemia (p. 495)

References

1. Harrison CN, et al for British Committee for Standards in Haematology. Guideline for investigation and management of adults and children presenting with a thrombocytosis. Br J Haematol 2010;149: 352–375.
2. Ruggeri Z, et al. Pregnancy in essential thrombocythaemia during aspirin treatment. Acta Gynecol Obstet 2003;268: 209–210.
3. Vantroyen B, Vanstraelen D Management of essential thrombocythemia during pregnancy with aspirin, interferon alpha-2a and no treatment: a comparative analysis of the literature. Acta Haematol 2002;107: 158–169.
4. Walker ID Myeloproliferative disorders. In:Greer I A et al., ed., Medical problems in pregnancy. Edinburgh: Churchill Livingstone Elsevier 2007, pp. 142–145
5. Passamonti F, et al. Increased risk of pregnancy complications in patients with essential thrombocythemia carrying the JAK2 (617VF) mutation. Blood 2007;110: 485–489.
6. Niittyvuopio RC et al. Pregnancy in essential thrombocythemia: experience with 40 pregnancies. Obstet Gynecol Surv 2005;60: 344–346.
7. Griesshammer M, et al. Fertility, pregnancy and the management of myeloproliferative disorders. Baillieres Clin Haematol 1998;11: 859–874.
8. Griesshammer M, et al. Acquired thrombophilia in pregnancy: essential thrombocythemia. Semin Thromb Hemost 2003;29: 205–212.
9. Griesshammer M, et al. Essential thrombocythemia and pregnancy. Leuk Lymphoma 1996;22: 57–63.
10. Hatasaka HH Recurrent miscarriage: epidemiologic factors, definitions, and incidence. Clin Obstet Gynecol 1994;37: 625–634.
11. Cook CL, Pridham DD Recurrent pregnancy loss. Curr Opin Obstet Gynecol 1995;7: 357–366.
12. Martinelli I, et al. Mutations in coagulation factors in women with unexplained late fetal loss. N Engl J Med 2000;343: 1015–1018.
13. Pagliaro P, et al. Primary thrombocythemia and pregnancy: treatment and outcome in fifteen cases. Am J Hematol 1996;53: 6–10.
14. Falconer J, et al. Essential thrombocythemia associated with recurrent abortions and fetal growth retardation. Am J Hematol 1987;25: 345–347.
15. Robinson S, et al. The management and outcome of 18 pregnancies in women with polycythaemia vera. Haematologica 2005;90: 1477–1483.
16. RCOG Green-top Guideline No. 37. Reducing the risk of thrombosis and embolism during pregnancy and the puerperium. London: Royal College of Obstetricians and Gynaecologists, 2009 London. <http://www.rcog.org.uk/womens-health/clinicalguidance/reducing-risk-of-thrombosis-greentop37>.

CARE PATHWAY

Secondary thrombocythaemia excluded

↓

Primary or essential thrombocythaemia (ET)

ET diagnosed for the first time during pregnancy: platelet count consistently >600 × 10^9/litre

↓

Referral from community midwife, GP, or any source to maternal medicine clinic or joint obstetric–haematology clinic

Known ET

↓

- Pre-pregnancy counselling vital:
  - advise to stop smoking, weight loss if high BMI
  - if on hydroxycarbamide, advise discontinuation at least 3–6 months before stopping contraception
  - discuss increased risks of pregnancy loss, thrombosis
  - low-dose aspirin 75 mg if not already on it
  - discuss plan of care during future pregnancy

↓

First visit to specialist antenatal clinic

Urgent referral to haematologist

- Obtain detailed history of any previous obstetric complications, e.g. recurrent miscarriages, severe early pre-eclampsia, previous IUGR, IUD, APH, PPH, any previous VTE in or outside of pregnancy
- Check for splenomegaly
- Explain risks of pregnancy, also of thromboembolism
- Start low-dose aspirin 75 mg od to continue till end of pregnancy, advise graduated elasticated compression stockings throughout pregnancy and at least 6 weeks postpartum
- Advise to stop smoking
- Baseline blood tests including routine booking bloods if not already done
- Vigilance for pre-eclampsia, abruption—inform patient of warning symptoms
- Arrange serial growth scans ± Doppler at 24, 28, 32, 36 weeks with clinic visits in the same session (Note: the frequency of scans may depend on the protocols of the individual unit)

Refer to anaesthetic high-risk clinic

- Documentation: High risk of intrapartum blood loss and PPH. Active management of third stage with additional o infusion for at least 2–4 h. Avoid dehydration during labour
- Document: thromboprophylaxis (LMWH and below knee compression stockings) for 6–8 weeks postpartum
- Close liaison with haematologist
- May need treatment with interferon alfa as advised by haematologists
- Suggested frequency of subsequent specialist antenatal clinic appointments : 24, 28, 32, 36, and 38 weeks
- **Routine community antenatal care to continue** with vigilance for pre-eclampsia, preterm labour, DVT, bleeding, fetal movement enquiry, etc
- Continued community midwife checks suggested at 20, 26, 30, 34, 35, and 37 weeks gestation

↓

Subsequent visits to specialist antenatal clinic (24, 28, 32, 36, and 38 weeks)

- Pregnancy assessment: vigilance for complications such as pre-eclampsia, IUGR, thrombosis
- Assessment of serial growth and Dopplers
- Ensure continued use of low-dose aspirin and below knee compression stockings
- Note anaesthetic and haematology advice and recommendations
- If alpha-interferon commenced, inform paediatricians and anaesthetist
- LMWH may be required in addition to aspirin during pregnancy and puerperium as directed by haematologist—ensure anaesthetist aware
- IOL at 39–40 weeks if no pregnancy complications thus far. *Aim for vaginal delivery.* Remind patient about thromboprophylaxis for at least 6 weeks postpartum
- If cytotoxic drugs required postnatally, relative contraindication for breastfeeding, but decision to be individualized, based on haematologist's advice, explaining benefits and risks
- ***Discuss and document contraception advice—no COCP***

Routine community antenatal care to continue with vigilance for pre-eclampsia, preterm labour, DVT, bleeding, fetal movement enquiry, etc.

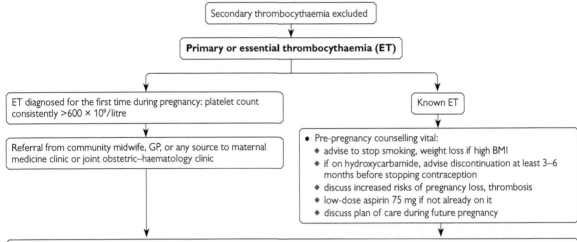

Management of high platelet counts in pregnancy in women not previously known to have ET

If counts consistently 400–600 × 10^9/litre and rest of blood parameters normal:

- Low dose aspirin-throughout pregnancy
- Advise below knee compression stockings throughout pregnancy and for 6 weeks after delivery
- Monitor trend of platelet counts monthly till 28 weeks, then fortnightly till delivery
- Re-check for any underlying causes to exclude secondary or reactive thrombocythaemia, e.g. iron deficiency anaemia, infection
- Check for splenic enlargement
- Arrange serial fetal growth scans
- Advise regarding smoking cessation
- Document active management of third stage with high-dose oxytocinon infusion for 2–4 h in addition to initial bolus dose. Carboprost or misoprostol can be used. **Tranexemic acid must be avoided**
- Thromboprophylaxis postpartum with below knee compression stockings. LMWH to be considered based on haematologist's advice
- **No change in obstetric management in labour/delivery**
- **COCP contraindicated for contraception**

If platelet counts are consistently ≥600 × 10^9 on two occasions, 4 weeks apart:

- *Immediate referral to haematologists* in **addition to all above actions**
- Check rest of haematological parameters; exclude causes of secondary or reactive thrombocythaemia
- Low-dose aspirin throughout pregnancy
- Below knee compression stockings throughout pregnancy and for at least 6 weeks postpartum
- Vigilance for pre-eclampsia, preterm labour, abruption, thromboembolism
- Serial scans, Dopplers for IUGR detection
- Refer to high-risk anaesthetic clinic
- May require LMWH/interferon alfa as advised by haematologist; if so, inform neonatologists and anaesthetist
- ***May need delivery timed according to alpha-interferon course; consult with haematologist. Avoid prolongation of pregnancy past 39–40 weeks due to higher risk of IUD***
- Avoid dehydration during labour
- **Vigilance for PPH:** Active management of third stage with additional high-dose oxytocin infusion; Carboprost, misoprostol can be used. **Avoid tranexemic acid**
- Puerperal thromboprophylaxis with below knee compression stockings as well as LMWH for at least 6 weeks depending on haematologist's advice.
- If after delivery, cytotoxic drugs are commenced, decision regarding breastfeeding needs to be individualized after full discussion of benefits and risks of
- ***COCP is contraindicated***

1.4 Thrombocytopenia (Including ITP)

FACT FILE

Definition and classification

- **Thrombocytopenia** is defined as a platelet count **of less than 150 × 10⁹/litre** caused by either accelerated platelet destruction or reduced production.
- In both the pregnant and non-pregnant state, mature platelets circulate for 8–9 days.
- Thrombocytopenia is classified as:[1,2]
  - **mild** when platelet counts are 100–150 × 10^9/litre
  - **moderate** when counts are 50–100 × 10^9/litre
  - **severe** when counts are below 50 × 10^9/litre.
- Thrombocytopenia is the second most common haematological abnormality, next to anaemia, to be found in pregnancy. Maternal thrombocytopenia is found in 5–10% of all pregnancies.[3,4,5]
- The most common cause for thrombocytopenia in pregnancy is the benign condition of **gestational thrombocytopenia (GTP)**, which accounts for 75% of cases.[6]
- **Hypertensive disorders, such as severe pre-eclampsia and eclampsia with HELLP,** account for about 21% of pregnancy-related thrombocytopenia.[4,7]
- Till recently, the acronym ITP was used for idiopathic thrombocytopenic purpura which is immune mediated. An International Consensus Group in 2007,[8] however, recommended that the acronym **ITP** should stand for **immune thrombocytopenia**, omitting the term 'purpura' as bleeding disorders are absent in the majority of cases.
- The Consensus Group also recommended a platelet count of less than 100 × 10^9/litre to support a diagnosis of ITP, thus avoiding the inclusion of most women with GTP.[8,9]
- ITP and neonatal alloimmune thrombocytopenia (NAITP), though responsible for only 3–5% of all cases of thrombocytopenia in pregnancy,[5,6,10,11] can cause significant maternal and neonatal morbidity and sometimes mortality.

Platelet count in normal pregnancy

- **Most cases of thrombocytopenia in pregnancy come to light as incidental findings in routine full blood counts.**
- Platelet counts tend to fall by about 10% during a normal, healthy pregnancy compared with pre-pregnancy levels,[12] although usually remaining within the normal range for the non-pregnant. Incidence of low platelets at booking is about 0.4% and at term it is about 7.6%.
- Mild thrombocytopenia in the range of 120–150 × 10^9/litre is not uncommon,[13,14] especially in the third trimester in about 10% of normal, healthy pregnant women.[15]
- **Any sudden and significant fall of platelets causing moderate to severe thrombocytopenia (≤100 × 10^9/litre)** requires thorough clinical and laboratory assessment and consultation with the haematologist.

Causes of maternal thrombocytopenia in pregnancy

Spurious

- Lab error/clotted sample, or sample taken in the wrong bottle, such as one with EDTA anticoagulant.

'Benign'/GTP

- Accounts for 75% of all thrombocytopenia cases and is found in 5% of all pregnancies.[6,16,17]
- GTP is mainly a diagnosis of exclusion where the patient is asymptomatic and has no history of bleeding problems.
- Review of maternal platelet counts, if available, from a previous pregnancy as well as pre-pregnancy and first-trimester counts are useful in narrowing the diagnosis in GTP.
- There is no pre-pregnancy thrombocytopenia in GTP. At booking, the platelet count in early gestation is invariably normal.
- If the platelet count is known to have been low before pregnancy or during the first trimester, GTP is unlikely to be the cause.
- GTP has a tendency to recur in each pregnancy, usually in the second and third trimesters. The degree of thrombocytopenia is usually mild to moderate, rarely falling below 70 × 10^9/litre. Thrombocytopenia of a similar degree may have been identified in a previous pregnancy.
- No other causes are detected to explain low platelets (e.g. HIV, medications, HELLP/severe pre-eclampsia, SLE/APS, etc.).
- GTP has no clinical consequences for mother or baby,[14] therefore no change in pregnancy management is required, other than periodic monitoring either once in each trimester or monthly.[2,18] Any unnecessary medical or obstetric interventions should be avoided.
- Provided the platelet counts are higher than 80 × 10^9/litre, most anaesthetists will offer epidural or spinal.
- Refer patient to the anaesthetic high-risk clinic during the third trimester if the platelet count is around 80 × 10^9/litre.
- In GTP, the outcomes are very good and the platelet counts return to normal between 4 and 12 weeks postpartum.
- Occasionally, it may be difficult in the more severe cases, to differentiate GTP from ITP. The opinion of a haematologist should be sought.
- Cord blood for fetal platelet level is essential at delivery, and instructions to this effect needs to be documented in the notes. The fetal platelet count is expected to be normal in GTP.
- Discharge information should be sent to the GP to request a repeat FBC 6–8 weeks after delivery to ensure resolution. Women with persistent thrombocytopenia should be referred to haematology clinic.

Pre-eclampsia, eclampsia, HELLP syndrome, DIC

- Thrombocytopenia occurs in 15–18% of those with moderate–severe pre-eclampsia and in about 30% of cases of eclampsia.[4] About 4–12% of those with severe pre-eclampsia will also have characteristics of HELLP syndrome.
- Thrombocytopenia could be an indication of worsening pre-eclampsia and can sometimes precede development of clinical manifestations.
- If thrombocytopenia is also associated with haemolysis and elevated liver enzymes, HELLP syndrome is diagnosed.
- Maternal platelet counts return to normal usually within 5 days after delivery.[19]
- Preterm, though not term, babies of mothers with thrombocytopenia due to severe pre-eclampsia, eclampsia, or HELLP syndrome are at risk of neonatal thrombocytopenia with bleeding complications.[2]
- If DIC results, catastrophic bleeding can occur due to rapid consumption of platelets and coagulation factors.

Immune thrombocytopenia (previously known as Immune Thrombocytopenic Purpura)

- ITP constitutes about 3–5% of all cases of thrombocytopenia in pregnancy.[3,10,17]
- It may be secondary to lupus or APS.

Other causes of maternal thrombocytopenia in pregnancy

- Folate deficiency
- DIC
- Haemolytic–uraemic syndrome (HUS)/thrombotic thrombocytopenic purpura
- Secondary to HIV
- Rarer causes include congenital platelet disorders or hypersplenism.
- Medication-induced by certain drugs, including: [6]
  - **antibiotics**—ampicillin, penicillin
  - **analgesics**—aspirin, paracetamol, indometacin
  - **anticonvulsants**—valproic acid, phenytoin, carbamazepine

- **others**—methyldopa, heparin, ranitidine, cimetidine, ciclosporin, procainamide, furosemide.

Immune thrombocytopenia (ITP)

- In ITP, IgG antiplatelet antibodies are produced against the patient's own platelet membrane glycoproteins, resulting in increased platelet destruction which outstrips production.

Incidence in pregnancy

- ITP is about 100 times less common than GTP.
- Incidence is about 0.1–1 case per 1000 pregnancies.[5,11]
- A history of thrombocytopenia when not pregnant or in early pregnancy is very useful in differentiating between ITP and GTP.
- ITP is most common in women of childbearing age.

Diagnosis

- Exclusion of SLE, APS, pre-eclampsia, etc. is necessary.
- Diagnosis is one of exclusion of other systemic diseases or medications that might induce thrombocytopenia.
- Most patients have had ITP diagnosed before pregnancy.

Pre-pregnancy assessment and counselling

- Ideally, women known to have ITP should be referred for pre-pregnancy counselling[9] to clarify the diagnosis, obtain a history of bleeding, whether a splenectomy has been performed, previous obstetric history and details of a previous neonate's platelet count at birth, etc.
- Discussions should include plans for platelet monitoring; management of pregnancy, labour, and delivery; the fact that antenatal treatment is required in about one-third of women; indications and options available for such treatment; and the small risk of maternal/neonatal complications.
- The patient should be reassured about the generally favourable outcomes in the majority of pregnancies.
- Although pregnancy does not appear to worsen the course of pre-existent ITP, significant morbidity and on rare occasions even maternal/neonatal mortality could result.

Presentation during pregnancy

- In practice, in the absence of a recorded platelet count prior to pregnancy or information from any previous pregnancy, moderate to severe thrombocytopenia in the first trimester with a falling count with advancing gestation suggests a diagnosis of ITP.[7]
- Autoimmune thrombocytopenia may present with bruising seen in 1 in 10 000 cases, but the most common presentation is an asymptomatic low platelet count of 50–100 × 10^9/litre from early pregnancy or even preceding pregnancy.
- Moderate or severe levels of platelet counts (50–100 × 10^9/litre or <50 × 10^9/litre) are seen in ITP.
- Patients must be examined for hepatosplenomegaly or lymphadenopathy. Splenomegaly is usually absent in ITP.[20,21]
- ***IgG antibody can cross the placenta, especially in late gestation, thereby causing fetal/neonatal thrombocytopenia in about 15% of these infants. This can present as neonatal purpura, ecchymosis, and even intracranial haemorrhage.***[2,22]
- Despite this, fetal or neonatal intracranial haemorrhage is rare (1–2% of neonates in mothers with ITP). Overall, the risk of maternal ITP being the cause of neonatal intracranial haemorrhage is about 2 in 100 000 births.
- Patients occasionally present for the first time with severe thrombocytopenia in pregnancy, not having been diagnosed to have ITP prior to pregnancy.
- Some with previously diagnosed ITP may experience an exacerbation, especially in the third trimester.
- Bone marrow examination is unnecessary unless there is suspicion of leukaemia or lymphoma.

Workup in maternal thrombocytopenia

Detailed history

- This should include family or personal history of bleeding abnormalities, medication history, any history of maternal thrombocytopaenia in a previous pregnancy or of neonatal thrombocytopenia, previous pregnancy complicated by pre-eclampsia, any autoimmune conditions (eg SLE/APS), or viral disease (HIV).

Clinical examination

- Look for signs of any mucocutaneous bleeding, tenderness in the right upper quadrant of the abdomen, other features of pre-eclampsia, hepatosplenomegaly, etc.

Investigations

- FBC and peripheral blood film.
- SLE and APS screening, if not previously done.
- If a severe degree of thrombocytopenia is diagnosed in later gestation or postpartum, a complete pre-eclampsia screen including coagulation profile and LFTs is required to exclude pre-eclampsia, thrombotic thrombocytopenic purpura, and DIC.
  - ***Recent recommendations include screening for hepatitis C if primary ITP has been identified.***[23]
  - HIV and hepatitis B screening may be re-offered if not previously done at booking.
  - Further tests, as directed by the history and clinical examination, may include kidney and TFTs, folate levels, etc.
- Platelet-associated IgG levels are of little diagnostic value as they are elevated in both GTP and ITP.
- Antiplatelet antibody tests are not useful in distinguishing ITP from GTP, therefore not recommended for routine use.[24]

Management

- Optimum management requires multidisciplinary collaboration between the obstetrician, haematologist, anaesthetist, midwives, and neonatologist.

Principles of management

- The aim is to reduce bleeding complications associated with severe thrombocytopenia.
- It is generally recommended that the platelet counts are checked monthly till 28 weeks, then fortnightly till 36 weeks and weekly thereafter. The frequency of monitoring will, however, vary according to the degree ITP and if the patient develops symptoms.[9]
- Antenatal assessments need to continue at regular intervals. At 34–36 weeks, assessment needs to be targeted to review any indication for treatment including the degree and trend of ITP, any obstetric complication which might increase the risk of peripartum haemorrhage, or development of symptoms related to low platelet counts.
- Referral to the high-risk anaesthetic assessment clinic is vital.
- There is no strong evidence that maternal treatment with steroids or IVIG improves fetal/neonatal platelet counts.[25,26]

The critical limit

- The current international consensus[23,27] is that in asymptomatic patients or when no intervention is planned in the first or second trimester (which would then warrant treatment), as long as the platelet counts remain higher than 20–30 × 10^9/litre, treatment is not indicated unless miscarriage/preterm delivery is imminent. Careful clinical and haematological monitoring is essential.
- Platelet counts of 50 × 10^9/litre or more are generally safe for both vaginal delivery and operative delivery, including Caesarean section,[18,20,23,27,28] although regional blocks such as spinal/epidural analgesia are generally considered safe if platelet counts are greater than 80 × 10^9/litre at the time of labour with a normal coagulation profile.[27]
- Haemorrhage due to thrombocytopenia is very unlikely if the platelet count is greater than 50 × 10^9/litre at time of delivery. The earlier in pregnancy that the fall in platelets becomes apparent, the greater the risks of bleeding.
- Risk of spontaneous fetal haemorrhage in utero and during normal vaginal delivery is low.
- Maternal clinical characteristics or degree of thrombocytopenia do not predict neonatal thrombocytopenia.[7]

Timing and indications for treatment in ITP

- The decision to treat the mother depends on the platelet count, the development of obstetric problems which might pose an increased risk of haemorrhage, the gestational age, and whether she develops any **symptoms like bruising or petechiae, when treatment is always indicated.**
- ***In general, treatment is considered necessary if platelet counts are less than 50 × 10^9/litre close to the time of delivery, or an elective Caesarean is planned for other obstetric indications.***

Mode of delivery

- There is no evidence that Caesarean section is safer for the neonate than an uncomplicated vaginal delivery. Vaginal delivery is the preferred option unless there are obstetric reasons requiring Caesarean section..
- The incidence of fetal thrombocytopenia with maternal ITP is low; **the nadir of platelet counts in any affected fetus is reached 2–5 days after delivery, therefore no additional advantage is conferred by Caesarean section.**

Maternal treatment

- ***Oral corticosteroids and IV immunoglobulin (IVIG) form the first-line treatment for maternal ITP.***[24]
- The choice between corticosteroids and IVIG should be case-based and depends on consideration of potential side effects, how quickly an increase of platelet count is deemed necessary, and for how long this increased level needs to be maintained to reduce the risk of haemorrhage.
- Steroids are appropriate if the duration of treatment is likely to be short, particularly if a low maintenance dose of steroids proves adequate to maintain steady levels of platelet count.
- If the duration of treatment is likely to be prolonged or if the maintenance dose of steroids is unacceptably high, IV IgG may need to be considered.
- Initial therapy usually starts with oral prednisolone at doses of 10–20 mg once a day,[4,9] with tapering of the dose to maintain effective haemostatic platelet levels.
- The initial response to oral steroids could take 3–7 days and a maximal response is not usually achieved until 2–3 weeks. 80% of patients will respond to steroids within 3–6 weeks.
- If this time lag is unacceptable, especially if the pregnancy is approaching term, IV IgG may be the option especially in preparation for delivery.[7]
- The treatment dose of IVIG is 2 g/kg divided over 2–5 days.[9]
- The response to IVIG is more rapid than with oral steroids. With IV IgG, 70% of cases will show a platelet response within 3–6 days but the initial administration needs to be given over 2–5 days.
- This treatment very expensive; the increase in platelet count lasts only for 1–4 weeks and repeat doses may be required.
- Side effects of steroids and IVIG must be considered and discussed by the haematologist and obstetrician. Side effects of IVIG, which is a pooled plasma product, may include infusion reactions, aseptic meningitis, and headache.
- In some refractory cases, a combination of high-dose methylprednisolone and Ivlg may be required as advised by the haematologist.
- Second-line therapy with drugs such as azathioprine is indicated only as advised by the haematologist.
- Splenectomy for ITP performed during pregnancy is rarely necessary with modern management modalities.
- ***Rationale for any decision must be clearly recorded in the notes, as should instructions for labour and delivery.***
- If the woman has been on maintenance doses of steroids for more than 2 weeks, bolus doses of IV hydrocortisone 100 mg are required 6–8 hourly for labour and delivery, irrespective of the mode of delivery.
- Fetal blood sampling (FBS), fetal scalp electrodes (FSE), ventouse, and rotational forceps are to be avoided.
- Active management of the third stage is recommended.
- In the case of unexpected delivery and major haemorrhage in the face of platelet counts less than 20–30 × 10^9/litre, early involvement of the haematologist and provision of platelets must be sought without delay.
- In the case of major PPH, in addition to all standard medical and surgical haemostatic measures, IVIG ± IV methylprednisolone may be required as advised by the haematologist.
- Neonatal staff to be alerted.
- Pain relief, as indicated by prior anaesthetic consultation notes, or as assessed in the course of labour, depending on the platelet counts.
- Routine antibiotics are not required.
- Avoid NSAIDs throughout pregnancy, especially diclofenac for postpartum analgesia/anti-inflammatory use.
- Routine postpartum risk assessment for thromboprophylaxis is required. If the platelet count is more than 50 × 10^9/litre with expected average postpartum blood loss, well-contracted uterus, and no signs of bleeding from other sites, routine thromboprophylaxis can be considered.
- If the platelet counts is less than 50 × 10^9/litre, or there is evidence of bleeding from other sites, even though the uterus remains well contracted with no signs of PPH, immediate consultation with the haematologist is advisable before routine thromboprophylaxis is administered.[9]
- **Cord bloods are necessary for neonatal platelet counts.** Infants with subnormal counts, irrespective of the mode of delivery, should be closely observed clinically and haematologically as platelet count tends to fall further to a nadir between 2–5 days after birth.
- Oral rather than IM vitamin K should be given until neonatal thrombocytopenia is excluded.
- ***Severe neonatal thrombocytopenia (< 50 × 10^9/litre) with intracranial haemorrhage in neonates is very unusual, occurring in less than 5%[29] of neonates of mothers with ITP. When they occur, NAITP should be excluded by laboratory testing.***
- ***This is essential not only for the management of the neonate but also in relation to antenatal management of subsequent pregnancies. In neonatal alloimmune thrombocytopenia, the maternal platelet count is normal and the mother therefore does not have idiopathic thrombocytopenia.***

Information for patients

Please see Information for patients: Low platelet counts or thrombocytopenia (p. 495)

References

1. Parnas M, et al. Moderate to severe thrombocytopenia during pregnancy. Eur J Obstet Gynecol Reprod Biol 2006;128: 163–168.
2. Levy JA, Murphy LD Thrombocytopenia in pregnancy. J Am Board Fam Prac 2002;15: 290–297.
3. McCrae KR, et al Pregnancy-associated thrombocytopenia: pathogenesis and management. Blood 1992;80: 2697–2714.
4. Sullivan CA, Martin JN Management of the obstetric patient with thrombocytopenia. J Clin Obstet Gynecol 1995;38: 521–534.
5. Sainio S, et al. Maternal thrombocytopenia: a population based study. Acta Obstet Gynecol Scand 2000;79: 744–749.
6. Shehata N, et al. Gestational thrombocytopenia. Clin Obstet Gynecol 1999;42: 327–334.
7. McCrae KR Thrombocytopenia in pregnancy: differential diagnosis, pathogenesis and management. Blood Rev 2003;17: 7–14.
8. Rodeghiero F, et al. Standardization of terminology, definitions and outcome criteria in immune thrombocytopenic purpura of adults and children: report from an international working group. Blood 2009;113: 2386–2393.
9. Sankaran S, Robinson S E. Immune thrombocytopenia and pregnancy. Obstet Med 2011;4: 140–146.
10. Gill KK, Kelton JG Management of idiopathic thrombocytopenic purpura in pregnancy. Semin Hematol 2000;37: 275–289.
11. Segal JB, Powe NR Prevalence of immune thrombocytopenia: analyses of administrative data. J Thromb Haemost 2006;4: 2377–2383

12. Verdy E, et al. Longitudinal analysis of platelet count and platelet volume in normal pregnancy. Thromb Haemost 1997;77: 806–807.
13. Sill PR, et al. Platelet values during normal pregnancy. Br J Obstet Gynaecol 1985;92: 480–483.
14. Burrows RF, Kelton JG Incidentally detected thrombocytopenia in healthy mothers and their infants. N Engl J Med 1998;319: 142–145.
15. Boehlen F, et al. Platelet count at term pregnancy: a reappraisal of the threshold. Obstet Gynecol 2000;95: 29–33.
16. Kam PC, et al. Review article, thrombocytopenia in the parturient. Anaesthesia 2004;59: 255–264.
17. Crowther MA, et al. Thrombocytopenia in pregnancy: diagnosis, pathogenesis and management. Blood 1996;10: 8–16.
18. Silver R, et al. Thrombocytopenia in pregnancy. ACOG Practice Bulletin, No 6 Chicago, IL: American College of Obstetrics and Gynecology, 1999.
19. Cunningham FG, et al. Hematological disorders. In: Williams Obstetrics, 21st ed. New York, McGraw-Hill, 2001, pp. 1307–1338.
20. Johnson JR, Samuels P Review of autoimmune thrombocytopenia: pathogenesis, diagnosis, and management in pregnancy. Clin Obstet Gynecol 1999;42: 317–326.
21. Silver RM, et al. Maternal thrombocytopenia in pregnancy: time for a reassessment. Am J Obstet Gynecol 1995;173: 479–482.
22. Payne SD, et al. Maternal characteristics and risk of severe neonatal thrombocytopenia and intracranial hemorrhage in pregnancies complicated by autoimmune thrombocytopenia. Am J Obstet Gynecol 1997;177: 149–155.
23. Provan D, et al. International consensus report on the investigation and management of primary immune thrombocytopenia. Blood 2010;115: 168–186.
24. Skupski DW, Bussel JB Alloimmune thrombocytopenia. Clin Obstet Gynecol 1999;42: 335–348.
25. Christiaens GC, et al. Idiopathic thrombocytopenic purpura in pregnancy: a randomized trial on the effect of antenatal low dose corticosteroids on neonatal platelet count. Br J Obstet Gynaecol 1990;97: 893–898.
26. Nicolini U, et al. Continuing controversy in alloimmune thrombocytopenia: fetal hyperimmunoglobinemia fails to prevent thrombocytopenia. Am J Obstet Gynecol. 1990;163: 1144–1146.
27. Provan D, et al. Guidelines for the investigation and management of idiopathic thrombocytopenic purpura in adults, children and pregnancy. Br J Haematol 2003;120: 574–596.
28. George JN, et al. Idiopathic thrombocytopenic purpura: a practice developed by explicit methods for the American Society of Hematology. Blood 1996;88: 3–40.
29. Samuels P, et al. Estimation of the risk of thrombocytopenia in the offspring of pregnant women with presumed immune thrombocytopenic purpura. New Engl J Med 1990;323: 229–235.

Thrombocytopenia in pregnancy

Low platelet count (<150 × 10^9/litre)

- Found at any stage during pregnancy
- Referral from community or any other antenatal clinic to **maternal medicine clinic/specialist antenatal clinic**

Patient known to have ITP

- ***Ideally, pre-pregnancy assessment and counselling***
- Referral by GP or community midwife to maternal medicine antenatal clinic or joint obstetric–haematology clinic

➡ ***Refer to next pathway for patients known to have ITP***

Maternal medicine clinic/specialist antenatal clinic

- Exclude 'spurious' result
- Obtain detailed personal and family history of any bleeding abnormalities
- Elicit any relevant h/o medications, medical disorders, autoimmune conditions (e.g. lupus, APS), whether she has had a splenectomy
- Obtain previous obstetric history of low maternal or neonatal platelet count, or of pre-eclampsia/HELLP
- Compare with platelet counts from any previous pregnancy or in a non-pregnant state, if available
- In low platelet count identified in 2nd/3rd trimesters, compare with early pregnancy platelet count at booking.
- Grade level of thrombocytopenia
- Further monitoring and investigations directed by history and clinical examination (mucocutaneous bleeding, hepatosplenomegaly, signs of pre-eclampsia, etc.)
- SLE and APS: Check if not already done. If HIV test has not been performed at booking, consider re-offering
- Repeat FBC and peripheral blood film
- If platelet count <100 × 10^9/litre—check clotting and full pre-eclampsia lab investigations

Gestational thrombocytopenia (GTP)

Most likely if:

- No SLE/APS/pre-eclampsia, HELLP
- Earlier counts were normal, or similar trend during last pregnancy
- Other FBC parameters normal

SLE/APS

➡ Refer SLE/APS care pathway (pp. 272–273)

Idiopathic thrombocytopenia (ITP)

➡ See next care pathway for ITP

(GTP:)

- Follow-up in maternal medicine antenatal clinic 4 weeks after initial visit and then at 36 weeks
- Reassure mother that GTP is limited to pregnancy and has no clinical consequences for her or the baby, and good outcomes can be expected
- No change in pregnancy management necessary other than periodic platelet count monitoring at monthly intervals
- Routine community midwife antenatal checks meanwhile if counts continue ≥100 × 10^9/litre
- Repeat FBC monthly, either in hospital or at surgery
- Refer for anaesthetic review if counts ≤100 × 10^9/litre
- Refer to haematologist if counts ≤ 50 × 10^9/litre, although in GTP levels usually remain above 70–80 × 10^9/litre
- Alert paediatricians if maternal platelet counts ≤ 50 × 10^9/litre, rarely do levels fall <50 × 10^9/litre in GTP
- Discuss and document mode of delivery. No indication for early IOL or for LSCS unless for other obstetric reasons
- Cord bloods at delivery for fetal platelet count
- Postnatal platelet count recommended at 6–8 weeks to ensure return to normal values. Arrange with primary care team and inform patient

Immune thrombocytopenia (ITP)

ITP confirmed by

- Previously diagnosed ITP
- Exclusion of SLE/APS/pre-eclampsia/HELLP and other causes for thrombocytopenia
- Low count from before or in early pregnancy. Moderate to severe thrombocytopaenia as pregnancy advances suggests ITP
- ***Community midwife/GP or other antenatal clinic to refer patient asap to maternal medicine or joint obstetric–haematology clinic***

Platelet count $>80 \times 10^9$/litre

Subsequent antenatal visits at 28, 32, 36, and 40 weeks

- Routine antenatal review by community midwife meanwhile
- Platelet counts checked every month till 28 weeks, then every fortnight till 36 weeks, then weekly till delivery
- ***Referral to anaesthetist, haematologist, neonatologist if counts drop <80 × 10⁹ litre***

- Frequency of subsequent visits to maternal medicine clinic to be individualized for each case
- Routine community midwife antenatal checks meanwhile

Subsequent counts

Remain $>80 \times 10^9$/litre

- No change in obstetric management
- Discuss and document mode of delivery. ***LSCS or early IOL only for obstetric reasons. Vaginal delivery preferable***
- Avoid FSE/FBS/ventouse/rotational forceps
- Cord bloods
- Paediatric check of baby to exclude signs of bruising, purpura, etc.
- NSAIDs (e.g. diclofenac) contraindicated

Platelet count $<80 \times 10^9$/litre

Refer to:

- Anaesthetist
- Haematologist
- Neonatologist

- FBC every 2 weeks

Drop to $\leq 50 \times 10^9$/litre

- ***If in 3rd trimester, urgent referral to haematologist***
- Anaesthetic assessment, if not done already
- Steroids or intravenous IgG as advised by haematologist
- Alert paediatricians
- *Document*: Hydrocortisone bolus IV 100 mg 6–8 hourly during labour and for any mode of delivery if patient is on or has been on steroids
- *Document*: No FBS, FSE, ventouse, or rotational forceps; also to institute **active management of 3rd stage**
- If treatment required, **timing of delivery** can be crucial.
- Elective IOL at term timed to ensure adequate haemostatic platelet count are reached and maintained. Caesarean section only for other obstetric reasons
- NSAIDs (e.g. diclofenac) contraindicated
- **Postpartum thromboprophylaxis risk assessment:** If counts $<50 \times 10^9$/litre, but evidence of bleeding from other sites though uterus well contracted and no PPH—**immediate advice to be sought from haematologist** before routine thromboprophylaxis offered
- Cord bloods for fetal platelet levels
- Paediatric check of baby for bruising, purpura
- Daily neonatal platelet counts in those babies with subnormal cord blood levels until after lowest level is reached (usually 2–5 days after birth).

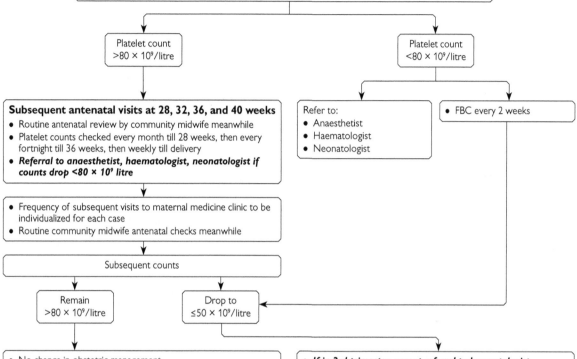

1.5 Inherited Bleeding Disorders: Haemophilia

FACT FILE

Incidence and inheritance

- The four most common conditions, accounting for almost 90% of all inherited bleeding disorders in women,[1] are:
  - von Willebrand disease (vWD)
  - Haemophilia A (deficiency of factor VIII)
  - Haemophilia B (deficiency of factor IX)
  - Factor XI deficiency (deficiency of serine protease), encoded on chromosome 4, found most often in Ashkenazi Jews.
- vWD is the most common inherited bleeding disorder affecting women, with a prevalence rate of 1–1.3%. vWD is due to deficiency of the carrier glycoprotein for factor VIII, resulting in deficiency of factor VIII. Both men and women are affected, with autosomal inheritance.
- Patients with vWD have a combined platelet and coagulation defect, characterized by a prolonged bleeding time and mucosal bleeding.
- Haemophilia A and B are less common than vWD but the most common severe inherited bleeding disorders.
- **Haemophilia A** is a congenital disorder of coagulation characterized by a deficiency of factor VIII.
- **Haemophilia B** (also known as *Christmas disease*) is an identical condition caused by a deficiency of factor IX.
- Both haemophilias are X-linked recessive disorders; men inherit the condition and women are carriers.
- Prevalence in the UK is 1–2 in 10 000 of the population. Haemophilia A affects about 1 in 5000 live male births. Haemophilia B occurs in 1 in 50 000 live male births.
- Haemophilia occurs in all ethnic groups.
- The prevalence rate of female carriers is unknown. Female carriers have only one affected chromosome, therefore the clotting factor level is usually about 20–50% of normal.[1,2]
- Some female carriers can have very low factor levels due to extreme lyonization of the normal chromosome.[1]
- The daughters of males with haemophilia A or B are obligate carriers who have a 50:50 chance of passing the disease state to a son and a 50:50 chance of passing the carrier state to a daughter.
- One-third of cases arise as fresh mutations without any family history.[3]

Clinical presentation

- Clinical presentation depends on the degree of deficiency of the coagulation factor in the blood. Severe haemophilia is associated with a level of less than 1% of normal levels of the coagulation factors. The severity of haemophilia remains constant within families.
- Severe haemophilia is characterized by repeated spontaneous bleeding into joints, especially the knees, elbows, and ankles, leading to disabling arthritis at a young age as well as bleeding into deep muscles and soft tissues.
- Advances in the management of haemophilia have meant an improvement in life expectancy.
- Female carriers with low levels of factors VIII or IX are at risk of excessive bleeding when undergoing dental procedures or surgery, even minor procedures.
- Desmopressin (DDAVP®) or recombinant coagulation factor concentrates are the products of choice for haemostatic support.

Pre-pregnancy counselling

- Pre-pregnancy counselling is best done by a multidisciplinary team of genetics, haematology, and obstetrics sited in the regional tertiary haemophilia centre.
- Such pre-pregnancy counselling is essential for female members of families with inherited bleeding disorders especially for carriers of haemophilia or type 3 vWD in order to identify either the disease or the carrier state.
- During this pre-pregnancy counselling:
  - The woman must be helped to understand the genetic implications of the disorder.
  - Implications of inheritance should ideally be discussed well in advance of pregnancy.
  - Options of prenatal diagnosis must be discussed.
  - Plans for the multidisciplinary management of future pregnancy must be discussed.
  - If appropriate, a trial of desmopressin (DDAVP®) may be organized by haematologists.
  - Pre-implantation genetic diagnosis and in-vitro fertilization (IVF) to identify unaffected embryos for transfer into the uterus may need to be considered, if appropriate.[4,5]
- Women who are likely to require blood products must be immunized against hepatitis A and B. General advice regarding peri-pregnancy folic acid must be offered.

Prenatal diagnosis

- Genetic testing with informed consent after sharing written information.
- CVS (chorionic villus sampling) at 11–14 weeks carries a miscarriage rate of about 1% and is the principle method currently used for prenatal diagnosis of haemophilia—preferable to amniocentesis.
- Analysis of full fetal DNA in the maternal circulation for the presence or absence of *SRY* loci is a non-invasive method to determine fetal sex.[6,7]
- If the mother declines invasive testing, fetal sex determination by ultrasound by about 14 weeks gestation is feasible and needs to be offered.
- Determination of the fetal sex is vital information for planning management of labour and delivery. The parents may choose not to be made aware of the baby's sex during pregnancy though agreeing to have antenatal sex determination performed to help healthcare professionals plan for labour and delivery.
- If the fetus is male, parents may or may not want to determine whether the baby is affected.
- If the male infant is affected, termination of pregnancy may be an acceptable option for some couples. In vWD the option of prenatal diagnosis is usually offered only to pregnant women of families affected by the severe forms of the disease, mainly type 3.
- Before any invasive test for prenatal diagnosis, the mother's clotting factors should be checked and prophylactic haemostatic support instituted to avoid the risk of haemorrhage.

Antenatal management

- ***Multidisciplinary management with close liaison between obstetricians, midwives, haematologists, neonatologist, and anaesthetist is essential.***[1]
- Pregnancy and labour to be managed closely with the regional haemophilia centre. Advice from the haemophilia team is essential for the necessary blood tests and arrangement of prophylactic or replacement treatment, especially when there is a bleeding complication.
- Women with mild or moderate bleeding disorders can be managed in the local hospital with close links maintained with the tertiary centre. Those with severe or rare disorders or those carrying an affected/ potentially affected infant need to be managed in a tertiary haemophilia centre.[8]
- Levels of factor VIII and type 1 von Willebrand factor (vWF) **increase** in normal pregnancy, especially during the third trimester.[9] Baseline levels need to be checked early in pregnancy and repeated at 28 and 34 weeks gestation.

- Measurement is especially important during the third trimester so that postpartum haemorrhage (PPH) prophylaxis can be planned. This is even more important in those who have had previous rapid labours and deliveries.
- The levels of factors IX and XI do not, however, increase significantly during pregnancy. Carriers of haemophilia B are therefore likely to require haemostatic support to prevent excess bleeding in situations such as invasive prenatal testing, miscarriages and delivery, especially by Caesarean section.[2,8,10,11]

Analgesia requirements

- Antenatal referral for anaesthetic consultation is mandatory.
- Regional analgesia is generally provided if the relevant factor level at 34–36 weeks gestation is at least 50 IU/dl.[12]
- Provided the coagulation status is normal, there is usually no contraindication for regional analgesia.
- It is very important to check the factor levels have been more than 50 IU/dl before removal of the epidural catheter.

Preparation for labour

- ***Individualized management plans must be prepared in advance and be readily available and shared with all involved in the care. A copy must be given to the woman and preferably enclosed with the patient's hand-held notes. Instructions for labour, delivery, and postnatal care must be clearly documented.***
- The safest mode of delivery for the affected infant is still controversial.[8,13,14]
- Caesarean section is not routinely indicated for suspected fetal haemophilia and is performed for obstetric indications only.
- At the beginning of labour: FBC and coagulation screen as well as saving serum for crossmatch purposes. Factor levels are not usually measurable in the acute setting and planning for delivery is usually based on the levels found at 34–36 weeks gestation.
- IV access must be established.
- If the factor level is less than 50 IU/dl (factors VIII, IX, vWF) or less than 70 IU/dl (factor XI), prophylactic treatment with coagulation factor concentrates for labour and postpartum is indicated, Levels above these cut-offs must be maintained for at least 3 days after a vaginal delivery and at least 5 days after Caesarean section.
- If treatment is indicated in carriers of haemophilia A or B, recombinant coagulation factor, clotting factor concentrate, tranexemic acid, or desmopressin (DDAVP®) may be required depending on the bleeding condition.[15]
- Desmopressin (DDAVP®), a synthetic analogue of the antidiuretic hormone vasopressin, is useful to boost levels of factor VIII and vWF in the blood, but not that of factor IX. It is therefore of no value in haemophilia B carriers. It can be used as a nasal spray or be given parenterally by the IV or SC route.[16]
- Avoid FBS and FSE during labour in case the fetus is affected.
- Prolonged labour, especially prolonged second stage should be avoided. Ventouse delivery and difficult or rotational forceps must be avoided. Early recourse to Caesarean section is recommended instead.
- Delivery must be conducted by an experienced obstetrician and/ or senior midwife.
- Ventouse delivery is contraindicated because it carries the maximum risk of intracranial haemorrhage.[8]
- Low forceps delivery is less traumatic than a Caesarean section performed at full dilatation.

Third stage and puerperium

- High incidence of primary PPH in inherited bleeding disorders (22% in vWD and 19% in carriers of haemophilia vs 5% of general population).[17]
- Active management of third stage with IV syntocinon infusion in addition to initial bolus. Carboprost/misoprostol as required.
- Risk of secondary PPH even higher due to the rapid physiological fall of maternal clotting factor activity after delivery[9] (20–30% in vWD and 11% in haemophilia carriers vs 0–7% in general population).
- The risk is lessened by minimizing maternal genital and perineal trauma at delivery and prophylactic treatment with the specific clotting factor concentrate or with desmopressin (DDAVP®).
- Desmopressin (DDAVP®) can boost levels of factor VIII and vWF in the blood, but not that of factor IX. It can be used as a nasal spray or given parenterally by IV or SC route. Care must be taken to prevent fluid overload, curtailing fluid input to 1.5 litres in 24 h. Repeated doses of desmopressin (DDAVP®) must be avoided.[1]
- VTE risk[18] assessment must be individualized with advice from the haematologists. Below-knee compression stockings, and avoiding dehydration and prolonged immobility, are general measures.

Neonate

- Three to four per cent of infants with haemophilia can suffer intracranial bleeding during labour and delivery.[19,20]
- Cord bloods for coagulation factor assay should be taken in an anticoagulated bottle and should be sent to the regional haemophilia centre.
- Till the result of the coagulation assay is known, IM injections such as IM vitamin K should be withheld and oral vitamin K given instead.
- A cranial ultrasound must be performed without delay in cases of a traumatic delivery or if neonatal intracranial haemorrhage is suspected.
- In such cases, the neonate may require prophylactic haemostatic support.
- Coagulation factors VIII and IX do not cross the placenta, therefore any recombinant coagulation factor concentrate given to the mother does not offer protection to the infant. If there is any increased risk of intracranial haemorrhage, an infusion of recombinant coagulation factor concentrate may be given to the neonate.

Information for patients

Please see Information for patients: Haemophilia and pregnancy (p. 495)

References

1. Chi C, Kadir RA Management of women with inherited bleeding disorders in pregnancy. Obstetrician and Gynaecologist 2007;9: 27–33.
2. Gringeri A Congenital bleeding disorders and pregnancy. Haematol Rep 2005;1: 43–46.
3. Giannelli F, Green PM The molecular basis of haemophilia A and B. Bailieres Haematol 1996;9: 211–228.
4. Michaelides K, et al. Live birth following the first mutation specific pre-implantation genetic diagnosis for haemophilia A. Thromb Haemost 2006;95: 373–379.
5. Lavery S Preimplantation genetic diagnosis of haemophilia. Br J Haematol 2009;144: 303–307.
6. Chi C, et al. Non-invasive first trimester determination of fetal gender: a new approach for prenatal diagnosis of haemophilia. BJOG 2006;113: 239–242.
7. Honda H, et al. Fetal gender determination in early pregnancy through qualitative and quantitative analysis of fetal DNA in maternal serum Hum Genet 2002;110: 75–79.
8. Huq FY, Kadir RA Management of pregnancy, labour and delivery in women with inherited bleeding disorders. Haemophilia 2011;17: 20–30.
9. Kadir RA, et al. The obstetric experience of carriers of haemophilia. Br J Obstet Gynaecol 1997;104: 803–810.
10. Ljung R The optimal mode of delivery for the haemophilia carrier expecting an affected infant is vaginal delivery. Haemophilia 2010;16: 415–419.
11. Yang MY, Ragni MV Clinical manifestations and management of labour and delivery in women with factor IX deficiency. Haemophilia 2004;10: 483–490.
12. Letsky EA. Haemostasis and epidural anaesthesia Int J Obstet Anesth 1991;1: 51–54.
13. Kulkarni R, Lusher. Intracranial and extracranial hemorrhages in newborns with hemophilia. J Pediatr Hematol Oncol 1999;21: 289–295.
14. Dunkley SM, et al, on behalf of the Australian Haemophilia Centre Directors Organisation. A consensus statement on the management

of pregnancy and delivery in women who are carriers of or have bleeding disorders. Med J Aust 2009;191: 460–463.
15. United Kingdom Haemophilia Centre Doctors' Organisation (UKHCDO). Guidelines on the selection and use of therapeutic products to treat haemophilia and other hereditary bleeding disorders Haemophilia 2003;9: 1–23.
16. Lethagen S, et al, Intranasal and intravenous administration of desmopressin: effect on F VIII/vWF, pharmacokinetics and reproducibility. Thromb Haemost 1987;58: 1033–1036.
17. Plug I, et al. Bleeding in carriers of hemophilia. Blood 2006;108: 52–56.
18. Dargaud Y, et al. Haemophilia and thrombophilia: an unexpected association! Haemophilia 2004;10: 319–326.
19. Chalmers E, et al for the Paediatric Working Party of the United Kingdom Haemophilia Doctors' Organization. Guideline on the management of haemophilia in the fetus and neonate. Br J Haematol 2011;154: 208–215.
20. Lee CA, et al. The obstetric and gynaecological management of women with inherited bleeding disorders—review with guidelines produced by a task force of UK Haemophilia Centre Doctors' Organisation. Haemophilia 2006;12: 301–336.

CARE PATHWAY

Haemophilia

Pre-pregnancy counselling

- Joint consultation (genetics, haematology, obstetrics) to discuss:
  - genetic implications of condition, and inheritance pattern
  - options for prenatal diagnosis
  - multidisciplinary management in future pregnancy
- pre-implantation genetic diagnosis and IVF if appropriate
- In those likely to require blood products, advise Hep A and B immunization
- Routine peripregnancy folic acid

↓

Multidisciplinary joint management, close liaison with regional haemophilia centre

- Early referral, dating scan; offer genetic testing with written information—informed consent for CVS at 11–14 weeks
- Test maternal coagulation factors pre-CVS as mother may need haemostatic support if levels <50 iu/dl, anti-D if Rh negative
- Non-invasive fetal DNA analysis from cells in maternal circulation may be possible, if CVS declined
- Offer early 2nd-trimester ultrasound scan. Parents might not wish to be told sex

↓

Continuation of pregnancy

- Antenatal care and delivery in DGH working closely with regional centre in cases of mild–moderate haemophilia where the fetus is not known to be affected
- If severe maternal disease or fetus known/suspected to be affected, antenatal care and delivery in tertiary centre with haemophilia unit

If affected male fetus identified, discuss implications and options about continuation of pregnancy or TOP

↓

First trimester

- Check level of coagulation factor at booking, routine bloods
- If miscarriage or any invasive procedure during pregnancy, mother may need haemostatic support with coagulation factors to control excess bleeding if has <50 iu/dl of VIII, IX, or vWF—joint care with haematologists
- Antenatal care in community continues as per normal pattern

↓

28 weeks: antenatal assessment and joint consultation with haematologist in DGH or tertiary centre

- Assess factor levels
- Refer to anaesthetic high risk clinic
- Refer to neonatologists
- Routine antenatal assessment, bloods at 28 weeks
- Routine care continues with community midwife, avoiding overlap.

↓

34 and 36 weeks: antenatal assessment and joint consultation with haematologist in DGH or tertiary centre

- Assess factor levels,
- Formulate joint management plan for place of delivery, plans for labour, delivery and neonatal care, the latter involving neonatologists in local DGH/tertiary centre
- Management plan to be shared with all involved in patient care and copy to her, include in hand-held notes
- **Clear documentation of all discussions and instructions is vital**
- Vaginal delivery safe, Caesarean section only for other obstetric indications
- Safest mode of delivery for **affected** fetus remains controversial

→

Labour and delivery

- FBC, coagulation screen, factor level assay if available round the clock.
- Establish IV access
- Inform senior anaesthetist, neonatologist, obstetrician, and haematologist
- Avoid FSE, FBS, ventouse, difficult forceps or prolonged labour. Early recourse to LSCS to avoid prolonged labour
- If factor levels very low at 34–36 weeks, may need prophylactic haemostatic support with recombinant coagulation factor concentrate—liaise with haematologist
- Delivery to be conducted by experienced obstetrician or midwife
- Outlet forceps may be less traumatic than LSCS at full dilatation
- Aim to minimize genital tract trauma
- **Active management of 3rd stage**, IV bolus oxytocin, high-dose oxytocin infusion to continue for 2–4 h. Vigilance for atonic PPH
- Desmopressin (DDAVP®) may be used to boost factor VIII or vWF levels (as intradermal route for immunization of neonate nasal spray or IV/SC route) but does not boost factor IX levels
- **Cord bloods** in citrate bottle for urgent fetal coagulation factor assay
- VTE risk assessment and general measures. Discuss LMWH thromboprophylaxis with haematologist
- Vigilance for secondary PPH

↓

Neonate

- Until results of coagulation assay, avoid IM injections, employ intradermal route for immunizations
- Oral vitamin K
- If traumatic delivery or intracranial haemorrhage suspected, immediate cranial ultrasound. Infusion of recombinant factor to be considered in such cases

1.6 Inherited Bleeding Disorders: Von Willebrand Disease

FACT FILE

- **vWD** is the most common inherited bleeding disorder and is caused by quantitative (types 1 and 3) or qualitative (type 2) defects of vWF.
- vWF is essential for platelet adhesion to endothelial cells as well as to protect factor VIII from degradation. In vWD there is a combination of both platelet and coagulation defects, characterized by mucosal bleeding, easy bruising, and prolonged bleeding time. Epistaxis and menorrhagia are common.
- There are several different types of vWD, all resulting in a defect in primary haemostasis. Type I is the most prevalent subtype, accounting for about 80% of all cases of vWD. Type 2 is divided into subtypes: 2A, 2B, 2M, and 2N each caused by different gene mutations.
- The expression of vWF is also affected by the blood group. Those with group O have the lowest levels and those with group AB the highest. This can lead to variable degrees of severity within the same family, in contrast to haemophilia where the severity remains constant within the same family.
- There is a virtual absence of vWF in the most severe form of vWD (type 3).[1]
- Incidence is 1–2% of the population, affecting both men and women.
- Inheritance is as autosomal dominant in types 1 and 2 but recessive in type 3. In type 3, affected individuals are either homozygotes or compound heterozygotes.[1]
- Prenatal diagnosis in vWD is offered when the fetus is at risk of inheriting the severe form of the disease, mainly type 3.
- In Type 1 vWD the bleeding time is prolonged. APPT may be prolonged and vWF and factor VIII may be reduced.
- **Type 2B vWD** may be associated with **thrombocytopenia**, which can develop or worsen during pregnancy. In this subtype, additional monitoring for thrombocytopenia is indicated.
- Factor VIII levels are often used as a surrogate marker for vWF levels.
- During pregnancy, the level of vWF usually increases 3–4-fold to within the normal range by the third trimester and haemostatic support is rarely required.
- There might not be a significant rise in the levels during the first or second trimester, therefore miscarriages, ectopic pregnancy, interventions (e.g. CVS), or early preterm delivery may be associated with excessive bleeding.
- Baseline factor VIII and vWF should be checked at booking and repeated at 28 and 34 weeks gestation.
- The vWF levels fall rapidly after delivery, thereby increasing the risk of both primary and secondary PPH.
- ***Clinical presentation in relation to pregnancy could include postpartum haemorrhage and postoperative bleeding as well as excessive bruising.***
- vWD per se does not increase the risk of APH or miscarriage.

Management of pregnancy

- Management of pregnancy in vWD should be in close collaboration with haematologists, in both local and tertiary/regional haemophilia unit.
- Referral to the anaesthetic high-risk clinic must be made in a timely manner and the anaesthetic assessment completed before the third trimester.
- Determination of the subtype of vWD is essential either pre-pregnancy or as early as possible in the first trimester, as is ascertaining whether the disease responds to desmopressin (DDAVP®) or not.
- If the subtype of vWF responds to desmopressin (DDAVP®), this may need to be given as an IV infusion to boost levels of vWF and factor VIII in certain specific circumstances:[2,3,4,5] for example, before delivery or Caesarean section.
- Caution is advised in the use of desmopressin (DDAVP®) **antenatally** as there are a few reports of it causing preterm labour and hyponatraemia.[3]
- Desmopressin (DDAVP®) is not effective in boosting levels of VWF in other types of vWD such as 2A, 2B, and 3 (the most severe form), which together account for 20% of vWD.
- In type 3, vWF levels do not increase at any stage of the pregnancy.
- If haemostatic support is needed in those subtypes of vWD that are not responsive to desmopressin (DDAVP®), then FFP or plasma-derived factor concentrates containing vWF and factor VIII are required to prevent or control severe bleeding.
- No recombinant vWF concentration is available as yet.

Preparations for labour, delivery, and postnatal care

- During labour, FSE, FBS, ventouse, and rotational forceps must be avoided because of the risk of severe fetal or neonatal bleeding in the event of the fetus being affected with this autosomal dominant condition.
- Active management of the third stage (as detailed in section 1.5. 'Inherited bleeding disorders: haemophilia') should be instituted.
- Clear documentation regarding intrapartum management is required and the management plan shared with those involved with the care of the mother and the neonate. A copy is given to the patient and also enclosed with the hand-held notes.
- In the absence of other obstetric complications, vaginal delivery is safest in most cases of vWD, especially in type 1.[3,4,5,6,7]
- In certain circumstances however, an elective Caesarean section to avoid the risks of either an emergency Caesarean or an instrumental delivery may need to be considered.
- In general, in women with heritable bleeding disorders like vWD or in haemophilia carriers, a clotting factor activity level greater than 50 IU/ml is usually safe for either a vaginal delivery or Caesarean section as well as for regional analgesia.
- ***The risk of both primary PPH (found to occur in 16–29%) and secondary PPH (in 20–29%) is significant in those with vWD, especially in types 2 and 3, more so than in carriers of haemophilia.***[4,7,8]
- Perineal or vulvar haematomas can also manifest in vWD.[9]
- Daily postnatal monitoring of factor VIII levels (surrogate for vWF) should therefore continue in order to ensure the levels remain above 50 IU/ml for 3–4 days following an uncomplicated vaginal delivery or 4–5 days following a Caesarean section.[3,7,9]
- If the levels fall significantly soon after delivery, an infusion of desmopressin (DDAVP®) may be indicated. As desmopressin (DDAVP®) is present only in insignificant amounts in breast milk, it is safe for breastfeeding mothers.

Neonatal care

- The neonatologists need to be alerted to pregnant women with vWD and an antenatal referral made.
- **Cord bloods** must be sent urgently for clotting factor assay.
- **IM injections must be avoided in the neonate till an inherited bleeding disorder is excluded.** While awaiting the clotting factor assay of the neonate, oral vitamin K must be given and immunizations given intradermally.
- In the severe form (type 3), the diagnosis is readily made from cord blood. In the more common varieties of vWD, neonatal diagnosis cannot be entirely excluded by testing cord blood as the levels of vWF rise significantly during labour and remain elevated for several months.[10] It is therefore necessary to test the infant for varieties of vWD other than type 3 at about 6 months of age.

Information for patients

Please see Information for patients: von Willebrand disease and other bleeding disorders (p. 495)

References

1. Chi C, Kadir RA. Management of women with inherited bleeding disorders in pregnancy. Obstetrician and Gynaecologist 2007;9: 27–33.
2. Giangrande PLF Carriers of haemophilia. In: Pregnancy in women with inherited bleeding disorders. Treatment of haemophilia, No. 29 Montreal: World Federation of Haemophilia, 2003, pp. 1–5. <http://www.haemophilia.ie/PDF/Pregnancy.pdf>.
3. Chediak JR, et al. von Willebrand's disease and pregnancy: Management during delivery and outcome of offspring. Am J Obstet Gynecol 1986;155: 618–624.
4. Ramsahoye RH, et al. Obstetric management of von Willebrand's disease: a report of 24 cases and a review of the literature. Haemophilia 1995;1: 140–144.
5. Ragni MV, et al. von Willebrand disease and bleeding in women. Haemophilia 1999;5: 313–317.
6. Ljung R. The optimal mode of delivery for the haemophilia carrier expecting an affected infant is vaginal delivery. Haemophilia 2010;16: 415–419.
7. Kadir RA, Aledort LM. Obstetrical and gynaecological bleeding: a common presenting symptom. Clin Lab Haematol 2004;22: 12–16.
8. Kadir RA, et al. Pregnancy in women with von Willebrand's disease or factor XI deficiency. Br J Obstet Gynaecol 1998;105: 314–321.
9. James AH. More than menorrhagia: a review of the obstetric and gynaecological manifestations of bleeding disorders. Haemophilia 2005;11: 295–307.
10. Gringeri A. Congenital bleeding disorders and pregnancy. Haematol Rep 2005; 1(10): 43–46.

CARE PATHWAY

Pre-pregnancy counselling for vWD

- This should ideally include
  - autosomal dominant inheritance in types 1 and 2, therefore 50% chance of baby with vWD
  - determining subtype of vWD; in type 3 (the most severe), prenatal diagnosis to be offered
  - ascertaining whether responsive to desmopressin (DDAVP®) or not
  - discussion of increased risk of 1st/2nd trimester bleeding if ectopic, miscarriage or CVS, etc.
- vWD itself does not increase risk of miscarriages or abruption—reassure patient
- Discuss pregnancy management, prophylaxis and management options for risk of PPH, neonatal issues etc.
- Multidisciplinary care during pregnancy with haematologists at both the local hospital and tertiary centre/regional haemophilia centre

↓

- Any pregnancy in a vWD patient is to be referred by community as soon as possible in the 1st trimester to **maternal medicine** antenatal clinic or **joint obstetric–haematology** antenatal clinic

↓

First visit to joint obstetric–haematology or maternal medicine antenatal clinic in early 1st trimester

- Steps mentioned under pre-pregnancy counselling (above) should be instituted without delay, if not done already
- Routine viability and anomaly scan, clotting factor assay as directed by regional haemophilia unit, local haematologists
- If vWD type 2B identified, continued monitoring for thrombocytopenia
- Subsequent visits to specialist antenatal clinics—to be individualized
- Routine NICE-based 'low-risk' care to continue with community midwife

↓

Subsequent antenatal clinic visits at individualized frequency

- Coagulation factor levels rechecked at 28 and 34 weeks
- Assay particularly important before labour starts to ensure levels >50 iu/dl
- Consider desmopressin (DDAVP®) or plasma-derived factor concentrates of vWF and factor VIII before delivery/LSCS in selected cases
- Referral to anaesthetic high-risk clinic: day assessment unit
- Antenatal referral made to paediatricians about patient with vWF
- Management plan for labour, delivery, postpartum to be finalized after coagulation factor level assays at about 34 weeks and made easily available to all involved in care; a copy of this is given to the patient and included in hand-held notes
- Discuss mode of delivery—vaginal delivery, Caesarean section, regional analgesia are safe if vWF levels >50 iu/dl
- Vaginal delivery in the absence of other obstetric complications. Caesarean section for other obstetric indications in most cases
- In desmopressin (DDAVP®)-responsive cases, prophylactic infusion of desmopressin (DDAVP®) before delivery (vaginal or by Caesarean) if levels <50 iu/dl

Document the following:

- Avoid FSE, FBS in labour
- Avoid ventouse, rotational forceps delivery, prolonged labour
- Outlet forceps preferable to a difficult 2nd-stage Caesarean section
- Active management of 3rd stage with additional high-dose oxytocin infusion for 2–4 h after delivery
- Vigilance for primary and secondary PPH, for vulvar or perineal haematomas
- Cord bloods to be sent urgently for neonate's clotting factor assay
- Type 3 vWD, the most severe form, is easily diagnosed from cord blood assay; milder forms cannot be excluded till infant is about 6 months of age
- Avoid IM injections for neonate till clotting assay is known. Oral vitamin K, not IM till result obtained, intradermal route for immunizations
- Daily maternal clotting factor activity level to be checked for 3–4 days after normal vaginal delivery and for 4–5 days after either assisted vaginal delivery or LSCS to ensure daily levels are >50iu/dl
- Baby to be screened by paediatricians at age of 6 months for vWD

1.7 Haemoglobinopathies: Sickle Cell Disease

FACT FILE

Epidemiology

- **Sickle cell disease (SCD)** is the most common inherited condition worldwide,[1] seen most commonly in those of African descent including African Caribbeans, and also those of Mediterranean, Middle Eastern, northern Indian, and Central and South American descent.
- It is estimated that there are over 300 infants born with SCD per year in the UK with a prevalence rate of 1 in 2000 live births.[2]
- SCD refers to a group of inherited single-gene autosomal recessive disorders caused by the 'sickle' gene affecting the structure of Hb. The presence of HbS causes red cells to deform into the characteristic sickle shape.
- Hb S combined with normal HbA results in sickle trait (AS), which is usually asymptomatic except for an increased risk of UTIs and microscopic haematuria.
- Included in SCD are homozygous sickle cell anaemia (HbSS) and the heterozygous conditions as a result of a combination of HbS with other clinical abnormal haemoglobins such as HbC (HbSC), with beta-thalassaemia (HbSB thalassaemia), and others such as HbD Punjab, E, O Arab, Lepore, etc., all with clinically similar presentations but with varying degrees of severity.[3]
- ***In homozygous (SS) sickle cell anaemia:***
  - Hb concentration of 60–80 g/litre is often well tolerated.
  - Patients may suffer episodes of localized or generalized pain due to microscopic tissue infarctions resulting from vaso-occlusion in the small blood vessels. The sickle-shaped red cells are more readily broken down, resulting in haemolytic anaemia.
- Clinical manifestation in SCD can include acute chest symptoms, pulmonary hypertension, renal disease, leg ulcers, retinal disease, pyrexia, leucocytosis, mild elevation of liver enzymes, pleuritic pain, tachypnoea, and stroke.
- Sickle crisis is brought on by dehydration, exertion, or infection.
- Treatment involves hydration and analgesia.

Sickle cell disease and pregnancy outcomes

- Pregnancy increases risks for women with SCD.[3,4,5,6,7,8,9,10,11] A recent study showed complications of SCD occurred in 25% of pregnancies.[3]
- Maternal mortality rates are increased to about 2.5% in SCD.[10]
- Perinatal mortality is increased 4–6-fold.[10]
- Increased fetal risks are due to placental hypoperfusion and poor oxygen delivery to the fetus.
- **Sickle cell crisis** complicates about 35% of pregnancies in women with SSD.
- Pregnancy-induced hypertension and pre-eclampsia are more common and of earlier onset and have an accelerated course.[4,10,12]
- Spontaneous miscarriage rate in SCD is 9–24%.
- Placental abruption, IUGR, and preterm labour and delivery are more common.[10]
- Increased incidence of pulmonary thrombosis and thromboembolism, also acute stroke, especially intrapartum, are seen in SCD.
- SCD pregnant or postnatal patients are more prone to infections such as UTI, pneumonia, and puerperal sepsis.
- Routine prophylactic transfusion is not recommended during pregnancy in those with SCD unless there is an acute sickle complication.

Pre-conception counselling

- Women with SCD should be referred pre-conceptually to a specialist sickle cell unit where genetic counselling and availability of prenatal testing can be discussed.
- The aim of pre-pregnancy assessment and counselling also includes optimization of management of the SCD and screening for any complications of chronic disease seen as end-organ damage.[1]
- Advisability of early booking in pregnancy should be emphasized.
- Every effort must be made to ascertain the partner's Hb type before a pregnancy so that pre-pregnancy counselling and advice about reproductive options, including pre-implantation genetic diagnosis, can be offered. This will also facilitate an offer of early screening with CVS in a future pregnancy.
- ***If the partner's sickle status is unknown, the fetus and neonate need to be treated as high risk for SCD.***
- Discussions should include the chances of the baby being affected by SCD, how pregnancy could precipitate sickle cell crisis, acute chest syndrome (ACS), worsening anaemia, infections, etc.
- Penicillin (or erythromycin in case of allergy to penicillin) prophylaxis must be prescribed because of the presence of hyposplenia and therefore increased risk of infections.[13]
- Pregnancy vaccinations (hepatitis B, conjugated meningococcal C, and *Haemophilus influenzae*) as well as yearly combined influenza and swine flu vaccine and 5-yearly pneumococcal vaccine) should be advised as SCD patients are more prone to infections as a result of hyposplenism.
- Factors that could activate a SCD crisis include dehydration (especially if hyperemesis develops), cold stress, or exertion.
- Fetal risks such as growth restriction or preterm birth must also be discussed.
- SCD patients require high-dose folic acid in view of the haemolytic anaemia. High-dose folic acid (5 mg/day) should be prescribed pre-conceptually with advice to continue throughout a future pregnancy.
- Pre-pregnancy end-organ damage screening includes tests for pulmonary hypertension, BP and urine analysis, liver and renal function tests, retinal screening, and tests for any iron overload and red cell antibodies.[13,14,15,16]
- If **hydroxycarbamide** is being used by either partner to reduce the incidence of acute painful crisis, and the couple wish to conceive, advise that it should be stopped preferably 3 months before unprotected intercourse due to its **potential teratogenicity**. Termination of pregnancy, however, is not necessary on the basis of exposure to hydroxycarbamide alone as there have been a few more recent reassuring reports.[17,18] Detailed (level 3) anomaly scanning is mandatory.[1]
- If the SCD woman's hypertension is being treated with ACE inhibitors or angiotensin receptor blockers (ARB), these should be stopped before conception, replaced with labetalol and/or methyldopa, and need to be continued throughout pregnancy.

Antenatal management

- Multidisciplinary team working in close liaison with the regional haemoglobinopathy referral unit.
- Specialist obstetrician, midwives, haematologist, anaesthetist, and neonatologist must be involved in the antenatal care as well as during labour, delivery, and puerperium.
- ***Referral to a regional centre with a multidisciplinary Sickle Cell team is essential in those with SCD. Shared care, if offered in local units, should involve close liaison and common management protocols with the Regional Unit.***[1]
- Although care must be individualized for each patient, general antenatal management principles[1] include:
  - Daily folic acid 5 mg and prophylactic antibiotics (if no contraindications) to be continued throughout pregnancy.
  - Ensure ACE inhibitors or ARBs have been replaced by labetalol or methyldopa.
  - Partner testing encouraged if not done pre-conceptually.

- Renal, retinal, or cardiac screening (ECHO to exclude pulmonary hypertension), must be offered if not done in the previous year.
- Low-dose aspirin from the 13th week of gestation and continued throughout pregnancy is advisable to reduce risk of pre-eclampsia.[19]
- Serum ferritin levels are required. Iron supplementation only if there is clear evidence of deficiency
- Baseline renal function tests including PCR, liver function tests, and oxygen saturation in the first trimester.
- Graduated compression stockings to reduce risk of DVT. Prophylactic LMWH if admitted to hospital or any period of relative immobility.
- Routine BP and urine checks at each antenatal visit, as well as midstream urine (MSU) for culture and sensitivity (C&S) once a month.
- Ultrasound scans are recommended at 7–9 weeks for viability and dates especially if CVS is being considered for fetal SCD screening; routine first-trimester scan and anomaly scan at 20 weeks followed by fetal biometric scans from 24–26 weeks at monthly intervals.
- If there has been exposure to hydroxycarbamide, additional scan for the spine at 16 weeks and a detailed cardiac scan ± fetal ECHO may be considered.
- Referral for senior anaesthetist review is mandatory.
- Referral to the neonatologists to discuss neonatal care is mandatory.
- Management of acute sickle crisis and ACS.
- Delivery recommended at 38–40 weeks. SCD itself is not a contraindication for either vaginal delivery or for a VBAC.
- Crossmatch blood for delivery if atypical antibodies are present, otherwise group-and-save is sufficient.[1]
- Caesarean section only for obstetric reasons such as severe IUGR or pre-eclampsia. GA to be avoided if possible.

• ***Documentation in the patient records for multidisciplinary labour management should include:***
  - Vigilance for SC crisis, acute anaemia, or ACS as these are more frequent intrapartum and may require transfer for urgent intensive care.
  - **Avoidance of pethidine** as this can trigger seizures in SCD, though other opiate analgesia can be used.
  - Regional analgesia for Caesarean section.
  - Avoidance of cold and dehydration in labour and postnatally.
  - Avoidance of protracted labour; in the event of slow progress earlier recourse to Caesarean section must be considered.
  - Continuous CTG recommended as increased rate of fetal distress may warrant operative delivery.[1,10]
  - Pulse oximetry and oxygen therapy, if oxygen saturation is below 94%.
  - Any signs of pyrexia should be actively investigated and broad-spectrum antibiotics administered.
  - Capillary sample from the neonate must be sent to the regional sickle cell centre if the baby is at high risk of SCD (if the father is a carrier or affected or his status is unknown).
  - LMWH for thromboprophylaxis postnatally and for 7 days post-discharge after a vaginal delivery and for 6 weeks following a Caesarean section. Antiembolic stockings to be continued to be worn in the puerperium.
  - NSAIDs for analgesia after delivery, safe during breastfeeding.
  - Breastfeeding to be encouraged
  - In SCD, the combined oral contraceptive pill and intrauterine contraceptive devices (inert or copper IUCDs) come under UKMEC[20] Category 2 (where the advantages of using the method generally outweigh the theoretical or proven risk). Such risks in this context are of thromboembolism with the combined OCP and menorrhagia or pelvic infection with IUCDs.
  - Progesteroneonly-contraceptive methods including the levonorgestrel- intrauterine system (Mirena®) and barrier methods are UKMEC Category 1, where there is no contraindication for use in SCD.

Information for patients

Please see **Information for patients: Sickle cell and thalassaemia** (p. 496)

References

1. RCOG Green-top Guideline No. 61. Management of sickle cell disease in pregnancy. London: Royal College of Obstetricians and Gynaecologists, 2011.
2. Streetley A, et al. Implementation of universal newborn bloodspot screening for sickle cell disease and other clinically significant haemoglobinopathies in England: screening results for 2005-7. J Clin Pathol 2009;62: 26–30.
3. Chase AR, et al. Pregnancy outcomes in sickle cell disease: a retrospective cohort study from two tertiary centres in the UK. Obstet Med 2010;3: 110–112.
4. Smith JA, et al. Pregnancy in sickle cell disease: experience of the Cooperative Study of Sickle Cell Disease. Obstet Gynecol 1996;87: 199–204.
5. Rajab KE, et al. Sickle cell disease and pregnancy in Bahrain. Int J Gynaecol Obstet 2006;93: 171–175.
6. Afolabi BB, et al. Morbidity and mortality in sickle cell pregnancies in Lagos, Nigeria: a case control study. J Obstet Gynaecol 2009;29: 104–106.
7. Sun PM, et al. Sickle cell disease in pregnancy: twenty years of experience at Grady Memorial Hospital, Atlanta, Georgia. Am J Obstet Gynecol 2001;184: 1127–1130.
8. Hassell K. Pregnancy and sickle cell disease. Haematol Oncol Clin North Am 2005;19: 903–916
9. Howard RJ, et al. Pregnancy in sickle cell disease in the UK: results of a multicentre survey of the effect of prophylactic blood transfusion on maternal and fetal outcome. Br J Obstet Gynaecol 1995; 102; 947–951.
10. Villers MS, et al. Morbidity associated with sickle cell disease in pregnancy. Am J Obstet Gynecol 2008;199:125. e 1–5
11. Serjeant GR, et al. Outcome of pregnancy in homozygous sickle cell disease. Obstet Gynecol 2004;103: 1278–1285.
12. Al Jama FE, et al. Pregnancy outcome in patients with homozygous sickle cell disease in a university hospital, Eastern Saudi Arabia. Arch Gynecol Obstet 2009;280: 793–797.
13. Sickle Cell Society Standards for the clinical care of adults with sickle cell disease in the UK. London: Sickle Cell Society; 2008.
14. Ataga KI, et al. Pulmonary hypertension in patients with sickle cell disease: a longitudinal study. Br J Haematol 2006;134: 109–15.
15. Gladwin MT, et al. Pulmonary hypertension as a risk factor for death in patients with sickle cell disease. N Engl J Med 2004;350: 886–895.
16. Clarkson JG The ocular manifestations of sickle-cell disease: a prevalence and natural history study. Trans Am Ophthalmol Soc 1992;90: 481–504.
17. Diav-Citrin O, et al. Hydroxyurea use during pregnancy: a case report in sickle cell disease and review of the literature. Am J Hematol 1999;60: 148–150.
18. Byrd DC, et al. Hydroxyurea in two pregnant women with sickle cell anemia. Pharmacotherapy 1999;19: 1459–1462.
19. NICE Clinical Guideline. Hypertension in pregnancy. The management of hypertensive disorders during pregnancy. CG107. London: NICE, 2010 <http://guidance.nice.org.uk/CG107>.
20. FSRH The UK medical eligibility criteria for contraceptive use. London: Faculty of Sexual and Reproductive Healthcare, 2009.

CARE PATHWAY

Women with sickle cell disease (SCD) must be referred to a Regional Haemoglobinopathy Unit which has a multidisciplinary specialist team. Antenatal care can be managed between the local hospital and the tertiary referral centre with shared protocols and close communication. Pre-pregnancy assessment and counselling must be arranged in the referral centre

Pre-pregnancy

- Clinical tests and laboratory investigations for assessment of BP, renal, cardiovascular system, LFTs, oxygen saturation, serum ferritin for iron overload are needed for any evidence of end-organ damage and to allow pre-pregnancy optimization of management
- Discussion of genetic counselling, partner testing, discussions about chances of an affected baby, pre-implantation genetic diagnosis, available prenatal screening for fetal SC status, etc.
- Discussion of increased risk of acute crisis, acute chest syndrome, acute anaemia during pregnancy, labour, delivery and the puerperium, fetal risks of IUGR, preterm birth, etc.
- Prophylactic penicillin (or erythromycin if penicillin allergy) advised throughout pregnancy
- High-dose folic acid (5 mg/day) to be started before pregnancy and continued throughout.
- Advise to stop hydroxycarbamide for at least 3 months before a pregnancy
- Replace ACE inhibitors or ARBs with labetalol/methyldopa pre-pregnancy and to continue throughout pregnancy
- Discussions about importance of early booking in pregnancy, avoidance of SC crisis precipitating factors (e.g. cold, dehydration, exertion, stress)
- Ensure up to-date with vaccinations, immunizations (meningococcal, Hib, H1N1, pneumococcal, Hep B)

Antenatal management

- Either entirely in Regional Centre or shared with DGH and community midwife; must be individualized
- General principles include:

First visit

- Discuss how SCD can affect pregnancy and vice versa. Advise to avoid dehydration, keep warm, etc.
- In hyperemesis, prompt antiemetics and oral or IV fluids to correct dehydration
- Early booking at about 7–9 weeks gestation, ensure on high-dose folic acid (5 mg/day) and advise continuation throughout pregnancy. Ensure has stopped hydroxycarbamide, ACE inhibitors, ARBs, obtain detailed history of any recent attacks, etc.
- Encourage partner testing, if not already done
- Arrange early scan asap to confirm viability, discuss and arrange CVS if indicated, and if patient opts for prenatal diagnosis
- ECHO, renal and retinal assessment if not performed within previous year
- Baseline BP, renal function (including PCR), MSU, LFTs, oxygen saturation, serum ferritin with routine pregnancy booking blood tests
- Consider low-dose aspirin for pre-eclampsia prophylaxis. If hypertensive, preferred drugs in pregnancy in addition to low-dose aspirin are M-dopa or labetalol

Subsequent visits

- At 16, 20, 24, 28, 32, 36, and 38 weeks gestation seen by multidisciplinary team, with scans at 20, 24, 28, 32, and 36 weeks. Community midwife routine visits, MSU sent each time at 26, 30, 34, and 39 weeks gestation
- Referral to anaesthetic high-risk clinic
- If fetus likely to have SCD, antenatal referral to neonatologist
- MSU at each visit
- FBC—repeat at 20 weeks
- Full antibody screen at booking, repeated at 28 weeks. If any rising titres in those likely to cause HDN, close monitoring of titres and scans—see separate HDN pathway (p. 39)
- **At 36 weeks**—Biometry scan, MSU, FBC. Discuss timing, mode of delivery and management of birth and puerperium. Discussions with neonatologist to include care and investigations of neonate
- **At 38 weeks**—Recommend IOL at 38–40 weeks gestation. If patient declines, discuss and document risks. Arrange for continue fetal monitoring at close intervals till IOL is accepted or spontaneous labour starts

1.8 Haemoglobinopathies: Thalassaemia

FACT FILE

- Haemoglobinopathies are autosomal recessive inherited disorders of Hb synthesis (thalassaemias) or of structure (sickle cell disorders).
- Haemoglobinopathies are one of the most common inherited disorders.
- Increasing global migration has led to increased prevalence of haemoglobinopathies in countries where they were not previously endemic.[1]

Thalassaemias

- Worldwide, more than 70 000 babies with thalassaemia are born each year and about 100 million people live as asymptomatic carriers.[2]
- There are normally two active alpha-globin genes on both copies of chromosome 16, thus four genes control the production of alpha chain; two inherited from the father and two from the mother.
- Production of normal beta chain is under the control of two genes located on chromosome 11; one inherited from the father and the other from the mother.
- Thalassaemias are single-gene disorders characterized by a quantitative defect in globin chain production. There is a decrease or absence of synthesis of one of the two polypeptide chains (alpha or beta) that form the normal adult haemoglobin molecule (haemoglobin A, $alpha_2/beta_2$). This results in reduced haemoglobin content in red cells and therefore anaemia.[1]
- In thalassaemia syndromes due to significantly defective erythropoiesis, there is a release of damaged red cells and red cell precursors into the peripheral circulation. The resulting extravascular haemolysis characterizes thalassaemias.[2]
- Beta-globin gene defects may cause beta-thalassaemia while those of the alpha-globin gene may cause alpha-thalassaemia.
- Beta-thalassaemia is prevalent in areas around the Mediterranean, in the Middle East, parts of China and South-east Asia. Alpha-thalassaemia is found in South-east Asia, India, and Africa.
- There is a high prevalence of alpha- and beta-thalassaemia in regions where *Plasmodium falciparum* malaria is endemic.
- Thalassaemias pose increased risks to both the mother and the baby including maternal cardiomyopathy due to iron overload and fetal growth restriction.
- As iron chelation has to be restricted during pregnancy, those with thalassaemia major may even develop de-novo endocrine problems such as diabetes mellitus, hypothyroidism, or hypoparathyroidism.[2]

Defects of alpha-globin

- One defective gene = alpha-thal$^+$ trait: Usually asymptomatic, there is mild hypochromic, microcytic anaemia with target cells in peripheral blood films. Mean cell volume (MCV) is often less than 80 fl.
- Two defective genes = **either alpha-thal^0 trait** (both defective genes from one parent) **or homozygous alpha-thal$^+$ trait** (one defective gene from each parent).
- The patient is asymptomatic alpha-thal$^+$ trait, alpha-thal^0 trait, and homozygous alpha-thal$^+$ trait).
- If three defective genes are inherited, two from one parent and one from the other) the result is mild to moderate haemolytic anaemia **(HbH disease).** The newborn with HbH may have moderate haemolytic anaemia but not needing blood transfusion as severe anaemia and infections are not usually seen.[1,2]
- **Homozygous alpha-thalassaemia**, where all four alpha-globin genes are completely absent or defective from both alleles, hence no globin production is possible, the result is fetal anaemia, heart failure, and fetal hydrops, also called **Hb Barts hydrops**. This is almost always incompatible with life; the fetus shows severe hydrops and dies in utero during the second or third trimester or shortly after birth.
- **Hb Barts hydrops is incompatible with survival** unless intrauterine transfusion is performed. Those babies born alive remain transfusion dependent for life. The pregnant mother is at risk of developing severe polyhydramnios/severe pre-eclampsia as well as intrapartum problems including PPH. Women who have had previous affected fetuses/infants are at risk of further affected infants.

Defects of beta-globin

- If one beta-globin gene is defective the outcome is **beta-thalassaemia trait (beta-thal minor or heterozygous beta-thalassaemia)**, which results in mild, microcytic anaemia. The woman is usually symptom-free but may become anaemic during pregnancy with Hb values 90–110 g/litre.
- **Homozygous beta-thalassaemia (beta-thalassaemia major):** If both beta-globin genes are defective, no beta-globin can be produced, resulting in beta-thalassaemia major.
- If both parents are heterozygotic for beta-thalassaemia, the chances are 1 in 2 of producing a child with heterozygous beta-thalassaemia, 1 in 4 of a child with homozygous beta-thalassaemia major, and 1 in 4 of a normal child.
- Such couples must be referred to a tertiary referral centre for prenatal counselling and subsequent prenatal diagnosis during pregnancy.
- Homozygous affected infants with beta-thalassaemia major show markedly severe haemolysis and anaemia. If not treated, the children will have complications of severe haemolytic anaemia with growth failure, hepatosplenomegaly, and iron overload in almost all organs due to increased gastrointestinal absorption. Life expectancy without treatment is about 5–10 years.[1] The affected individuals are transfusion dependent for life but transfusion therapy itself can lead to iron overload with end-organ damage (e.g. liver and cardiac haemosiderosis). Iron chelation therapy is required.[4,5]
- There is a third form, a milder variety of homozygous beta-thalassaemia called **beta-thalassaemia intermedia**, where the disease severity varies.
  - In the more severe form of beta-thalassaemia intermedia, diagnosis is often made between the ages of 2–6 years and although these children survive without blood transfusion, their growth and development are affected.[2]
  - In the milder variety of beta-thalassaemia intermedia, affected individuals are entirely asymptomatic till adulthood when they may present with mild anaemia or chance finding of splenomegaly. A haemoglobin concentration above 70 g/litre is usually maintained without blood transfusions.[1,2,6,7]
- Previously, splenectomy was the mainstay of treatment for those with thalassaemia major or severe forms of thalassaemia intermedia. This has now been replaced by blood transfusions and iron chelation therapy.

Screening and pre-pregnancy counselling: prenatal diagnosis

- *A universal antenatal and neonatal screening programme for haemoglobinopathies is operational in UK, allowing early identification of couples at risk and prompt diagnosis of newborns* (<http://www.sct.screening.nhs.uk>).
- Ideally screening and counselling will have taken place before pregnancy, although this occurs only rarely.
- In women with beta-thalassaemia major or intermedia, pre-pregnancy assessment of iron levels is advisable to ensure lowest possible levels before the chelating agents are stopped before conception. Screening for end-organ damage and limiting complications while optimizing thalassaemia management are vital before a pregnancy is commenced. This might involve aggressive chelation therapy before conception.

- Due to repeated transfusions, alloimmunity occurs in nearly 17%[2,8] of those with thalassaemia, thereby increasing the risks of fetal anaemia and haemorrhagic disease of the newborn. Prenatal determination of maternal ABO and full blood genotyping and antibody titres is essential.

Screening for end-organ damage and interventions before pregnancy

- Expert cardiological assessment to exclude cardiomyopathy secondary to myocardial iron deposition. Investigations should include ECHO and ECG as well as T2* cardiac MRI.[2,9]
- Diabetes is common in people with thalassaemia due to factors including iron-induced impairment of pancreatic islet-cell function and insulin resistance. The ideal pre-pregnancy target should be a serum fructosamine level of less than 300 nmol/litre for at least 3 months prior to conception (equivalent to an HbA_{1c} of less than 43 mmol/mol). **In thalassaemic women who have had blood transfusions, HbA_{1c} is not a reliable marker due to dilution: instead, serum fructosamine levels are chosen for monitoring glycaemia control.**[10]
- Hypothyroidism is similarly not uncommon in those with thalassaemia and prenatal thyroid function screening is essential, with treatment aimed at achieving an euthyroid state before pregnancy.[11]
- Liver iron concentrations must be assessed pre-pregnancy with a FerriScan or liver T2* with target levels below 7 mg/g (dry weight or dw).[2] An intensive course of pre-conceptual iron chelation may be required if the levels exceed this. Ultrasound detection of gallstones or a cirrhotic appearance of the liver is also recommended.
- Pre-conceptual bone density scan and vitamin D supplements, if necessary, to improve serum vitamin D levels are recommended,[2] as osteoporosis is common in thalassaemias. vitamin D supplementation should be continued during pregnancy.
- If the woman is on **deferasirox** and **deferiprone** these should be discontinued some 3 months before conception, substituted by desferrioxamine iron chelation. All biphosphonates should be stopped at least 3 months before conception and are contraindicated in pregnancy.[2]
- Viral hepatitis, especially active hepatitis C, related to repeated blood transfusions must be screened for before conception: if positive, expert hepatology review is indicated.[2]
- Those who have had a previous splenectomy should be vaccinated for pneumococcus (every 5 years) as well as receive the *Haemophilus influenzae* type b (Hib) and the conjugated meningococcal C vaccine, if not previously done.
- Daily penicillin (or erythromycin, if allergic to penicillin) prophylaxis should be continued indefinitely in those who have had a previous splenectomy.
- Time is of the essence to enable partner testing, counselling, prenatal diagnosis if opted for by the parents, and the offer of the option of termination.
- Referral to the regional centre for prenatal diagnosis is indicated if both parents are found to have alpha- or beta-thalassaemia trait.
- Prenatal diagnosis by DNA analysis is optimally from a CVS sample in the first trimester rather than from amniotic fluid sampling.[7] Uptake of prenatal diagnosis is not universal, only 80% in those at risk of the baby having thalassaemia major and less (30–50%) for sickle cell disease.[5,12]
- Pre-implantation genetic diagnosis (PGD) in high-risk couples offers an alternative to invasive testing and termination of pregnancy in affected cases.[13]
- Pre-pregnancy high-dose folic acid (5 mg/day) should be prescribed. This should be commenced 3 months before conception and continued till the end of the first trimester due to the higher demand for folic acid in thalassaemic women.[2]

Pregnancy management in those with alpha- or beta-thalassaemia

- ***Multidisciplinary management involving the Regional Haemoglobinopathy centre is essential. In general, monthly reviews till 28 weeks gestation, then fortnightly, are to be provided by the multidisciplinary team offering both routine antenatal care and specialist haemoglobinopathy advice.***[2]
- ***Care should be individualized; more frequent reviews are required for those who have significant cardiac or hepatic damage.***

Beta-thalassaemia major

- Pregnancy is rare in women with **beta-thalassaemia major**, though with intensive pre-pregnancy transfusion and chelation therapy or bone marrow transplant, favourable perinatal outcomes have been reported. If the woman is on desferrioxamine, this should be avoided in the first trimester although it can be used in low doses after 20 weeks gestation.[14]
- The antenatal care in women with beta-thalassaemia major is best managed jointly with a regional referral centre with a multidisciplinary team with expertise in haemoglobinopathy management.
- Urgent partner screening for haemoglobinopathy carrier status, as well as establishing maternal iron levels and cardiological assessment, are required if pregnancy has occurred before pre-conceptual assessment and counselling.
- Chelating agents are contraindicated in the first trimester due to potential teratogenicity. Of the available chelating agents, there is evidence regarding safety of use in the second and third trimesters only for desferrioxamine.[14]
- Folic acid 5 mg daily supplementation is required throughout pregnancy. Anaemia during pregnancy in women with beta-thalassaemia major should be treated with transfusion if necessary, **but not with oral iron**.
- Women with **beta-thalassaemia major** should have regular blood transfusions to maintain their pre-transfusion Hb of 100 g/litre with Hb monitoring continued every 2–3 weeks.[2]
- Women with **beta-thalassaemia intermedia**, who have worsening anaemia, or develop fetal growth problems, should receive regular transfusions with Hb targets similar to beta-thalassaemia major.
- Women with beta-thalassaemia intermedia who have low Hb but are asymptomatic with normal fetal growth should have a documented formalized plan regarding blood transfusion in late pregnancy.[2] If the Hb is over 80 g/litre at 36 weeks gestation, there is no need for transfusion before delivery although postnatal transfusion may be required. If the Hb is less than 80 g/litre at 36 weeks of gestation, two units of blood can be given at 37–38 weeks.
- In those who have had previous splenectomy, high platelet counts are not uncommon. This thrombocythaemia along with the fragmented red cells in thalassaemia can provoke thromboembolism; thromboprophylaxis must be considered
- If a woman has had a splenectomy **and** has a platelet count in excess of 600 × 10^9/litre, thromboprophylaxis in the form of LMWH as well as low-dose aspirin is recommended along with below-knee elasticated compression stockings.
- If a woman has had a previous splenectomy **or** has a platelet count in excess of 600 × 10^9/litre, thromboprophylaxis in the form of low-dose aspirin must be advised along with below-knee elasticated compression stockings.
- Should a woman with beta-thalassaemia major or severe forms of thalassaemia intermedia and not on LMWH require hospital admission and be relatively immobile, LMWH thromboprophylaxis should be initiated for the duration.[2]
- ***Due to multiple previous transfusions, several maternal red cell alloantibodies are likely to be present, increasing the risk of haemolytic disease of the newborn. Regular measurement of antibody titres is essential and vigilance maintained for ultrasound and Doppler evidence of fetal hydrops, IUGR, and anaemia (middle cerebral artery peak systolic velocity).***[7]
- In the presence of diabetes, hypothyroidism, liver or cardiac end-organ damage associated with thalassaemia, multispeciality and multidisciplinary management individualized to each case is essential with close involvement of the regional haemoglobinopathy referral centre.

- In the presence of myocardial iron overload or severe liver iron load, chelation therapy in a regional referral centre is essential.[2]
- Clear plans for intrapartum and postnatal management should be documented.[2]
  - Senior obstetric, midwifery, anaesthetic, haematology, and neonatology staff must be informed as soon as admission takes place and remain involved.
  - Continuous intrapartum fetal monitoring.
  - In beta-thalassaemia major, IV desferrioxamine 2 g over 24 h should be instituted for the duration of labour.
  - Active management of the third stage to minimize blood loss.
  - Thalassaemia is itself **not** an indication for Caesarean section in the absence of obstetric indications.
  - Postnatal thromboprophylaxis with thromboembolic stockings and LMWH is required during the period of hospital stay, irrespective of the mode of delivery.
  - Women who have had a vaginal delivery should have LMWH thromboprophylaxis with thromboembolic stockings continued for 7 days after hospital discharge.
  - Those who had had a Caesarean section should continue LMWH thromboprophylaxis with thromboembolic stockings for 6 weeks after hospital discharge.
  - In those with beta-thalassaemia major, desferrioxamine should be restarted as soon as the initial 24-h infusion is completed after delivery.
  - Mothers with thalassaemia major who choose to breastfeed must be reassured that desferrioxamine is not orally absorbed by the neonate and is therefore safe.
  - There is no contraindication for any form of hormonal methods of contraception in women with thalassaemia including the combined pill, progesterone-only pill, implant, or Mirena®.[15]

The fetus and the neonate

- If the parents choose to continue a pregnancy even if the fetus is known to be affected by alpha- or beta-thalassaemia major, or when couples decline prenatal diagnosis though both parents have alpha- or beta-thalassaemia trait, the antenatal care needs to be managed with close links with the regional referral centre and care individualized for each case. Delivery must be arranged in a tertiary unit in such cases.
- Apart from the routine first-trimester and mid-pregnancy anomaly scans, additional scans in early pregnancy (7–9 weeks) and serial growth and liquor scans at 4-week intervals from about 24 weeks gestation should be offered.
- The paediatricians at the local hospital must be informed early about such a pregnancy and be given an opportunity to meet the couple for further discussions as well.

Alpha- or beta-thalassaemia trait

- In women with **alpha- or beta-thalassaemia trait**, anaemia may develop during pregnancy. If iron deficiency is proven, iron and folic acid (5 mg/day) oral supplementation is indicated, but **not** parenteral iron. Antenatal transfusion is hardly ever required to correct the anaemia.
- Women with HbH thalassaemia have chronic haemolytic anaemia and need high-dose (5 mg/day) folic acid supplementation in pregnancy.
- If the fetus has Hb Barts hydrops, vigilance is essential for maternal complications including early-onset severe pre-eclampsia.
- Serial growth and liquor scans to exclude IUGR.
- ***In the absence of complications, pregnancy, labour, and delivery need not be managed any differently from routine.***

Information for patients

Please see Information for patients: Sickle cell and thalassaemia (p. 496)

References

1. Peters M, et al. Diagnosis and management of thalassaemia. BMJ 2012;344: 40–44.
2. RCOG Green-top Guideline No.66. Management of beta-thalassaemia in pregnancy. London: Royal College of Obstetricians and Gynaecologists, 2014.
3. Lal A, et al. Heterogeneity of haemoglobin H disease in childhood. N Engl J Med 2011;364: 710–718
4. Borgna-Pignatti C, et al. Survival and complications in thalassaemia. Ann N Y Acad Sci 2005;1054: 40–47.
5. Modell B, et al. Survival in beta-thalassaemia major in the UK: data from the UK Thalassaemia Register. Lancet 2000;355: 2051–2052.
6. Taher AT, et al. Overview on practices in thalassaemia intermedia management aiming for lowering complication rates across a region of endemicity: the OPTIMAL CARE study. Blood 2010;115: 1886–1892.
7. Johnston TA Haemoglobinopathies in pregnancy. Obstetrician and Gynaecologist 2005;7: 149–157.
8. Thompson AA, et al; for the Thalassemia Clinical Research Network Investigators. Red cell alloimmunization in a diverse population of transfused patients with thalassaemia. Br J Haematol 2011;153: 121–128.
9. Kirk P, et al. Cardiac T2* magnetic resonance for prediction of cardiac complications in thalassemia major. Circulation 2009;120: 1961–1968.
10. Spencer DH, et al. Red cell transfusion decreases hemoglobin A1c in patients with diabetes [letter]. Clin Chem 2011;57: 344–346.
11. Abalovich M, et al. Management of thyroid dysfunction during pregnancy and postpartum: an Endocrine Society Clinical Practice Guideline. J Clin Endocrinol Metab 2007: 92Suppl: S 1–47.
12. Petrou M, et al. Factors affecting the uptake of prenatal diagnosis for sickle cell disease. J Med Genet 1992;29: 820–823
13. Xu K, et al. First unaffected pregnancy using pre-implantation genetic diagnosis for sickle cell anemia. JAMA 1999;281: 1701–1706.
14. Singer ST, Vichinsky EP Deferoxamine treatment during pregnancy: is it harmful? Am J Hematol 1999;60: 24–26.
15. FRSH UK medical eligibility criteria for contraceptive use. London: Faculty of Reproductive and Sexual Healthcare, 2009.

CARE PATHWAY

Thalassaemia Prenatal screening, counselling, and optimizing management

- Ideally includes screening of both partners.
- If woman has beta-thalassaemia major or intermedia, prenatal assessment of maternal iron levels.
- Screening and optimal management of diabetes, hypothyroidism, hypoparathyroidism, end-organ damage including cardiological, hepatological assessments, maternal ABO and full red cell genotype and antibody titres, bone density scan, vitamin D supplements, screening for Hep C; vaccination updates if previous splenectomy
- Stop biphosphonates, deferasirox/deferiprone at least 3 months before conception, start desferrioxamine iron chelation pre-pregnancy and withdraw in first trimester
- Discuss prenatal diagnosis or pre-implantation diagnosis in high-risk couples.
- Discuss TOP option if fetus is affected

↓

Ongoing pregnancy management of women with beta-thalassaemia major or severe form of thalassaemia intermedia

- Multidisciplinary management jointly with regional referral centre

↓

Referral in 1st trimester from primary care to DGH or directly to regional referral centre

First visit

- Discuss effect of thalassaemia on pregnancy, offer information and advice, outline management plans
- Urgent partner testing if not done previously, review results if available
- Prenatal diagnosis—CVS, amniocentesis, or cell-free fetal DNA if appropriate
- Clinical history and relevant investigations to assess extent of thalassaemia sequelae
- Review and advice on medications—ensure:
  - high-dose folic acid (5 mg/day), advise to continue throughout pregnancy
  - chelators should have been stopped 3 months pre-pregnancy
  - antibiotic prophylaxis if previous splenectomy
  - thromboprophylaxis with below knee compression stockings, low-dose aspirin ± LMWH if previous splenectomy and/or thrombocythaemia of > 600 × 10^9/litre respectively
- If diabetic, refer for joint care with diabetologist, optimize treatment, monitor control with serum fructosamine
- If previous splenectomy, ensure has had relevant vaccinations (pneumococci, Hib, meningococci, Hep B, etc.) before conception
- Offer MRI heart and liver (T2* and FerriScan) in women with thalassaemia major if not done in previous year
- Determine presence of any red cell antibody, genotype and titre
- Routine antenatal checks—BP, urine, viability scan. Reiterate primary care advice regarding healthy eating, smoking cessation, healthy lifestyle, etc.; offer requisite support
- Refer for senior anaesthetic review during pregnancy

↓

Subsequent multidisciplinary hospital and community midwife antenatal assessments

- Monthly till 28 weeks, then fortnightly reviews—more frequent if heart or liver iron overload found
- If diabetic, joint care with diabetes team; maximize control; monitored with serum fructosamine
- Routine 1st-trimester screenings tests and scan; detailed anomaly scan at around 20 weeks gestation
- Monthly fetal biometry scans from 24 weeks if alloimmune red cell antibodies
- Specialist cardiology reviews at 20–24 weeks and at 28 weeks—if increased risk of cardiac decompensation, desferrioxamine SC or infusion according to T2* levels and as directed by haematology expert in iron chelation. Delivery plans formulated based on cardiac function
- Continued routine antenatal assessments with regular review of medications
- Regular blood transfusion regime for all women with beta-thalassaemia major, aiming for pre-transfusion Hb of 100 g/litre
- In women with beta-thalassaemia intermedia, transfusions based on presence or absence of maternal anaemia and evidence of fetal growth restriction
- *If rising maternal red-cell antibody titres*, scans and Doppler studies for assessment of signs of fetal anaemia, hydrops—timing and mode of delivery to be individualized
- Continue thromboprophylaxis as appropriate in cases of splenectomy and/or thrombocytosis >600 × 10^9/litre
- **At 36 weeks**—Fetal biometry scan, routine maternal assessments. Intrapartum care plan formulated after discussions with patient by multidisciplinary team including anaesthetist and neonatologist, and documented in notes
- **At 38 weeks**—Delivery if woman has diabetes.
- **At 38–41 weeks**—Weekly routine pregnancy assessments to continue in non-diabetics
- If normal fetal growth and no complications, IOL as per unit policy for postdated pregnancy
- Discuss contraception before hospital discharge
- Postnatal LMWH thromboprophylaxis for 7 days if vaginal delivery and 6 weeks if Caesarean section

1.9 Red Cell Antibodies (ABO and Other Blood Group Incompatibilities)

FACT FILE

- ***All patients found to have red cell antibodies need to be referred to a high-risk specialist antenatal clinic.***
- Pre-pregnancy counselling with a specialist must be offered to all women known to have red cell antibodies where there is a potential risk of fetal anaemia resulting in fetal hydrops as well as haemolytic disease of the fetus and newborn (HDFN).
- Management of such sensitized pregnancies needs close liaison with regional haematology and blood transfusion services, with local haematology consultants as well as with neonatologists in cases where HDFN is likely.
- The risk of HDFN is greatest with anti-D, anti-c, anti-K antibodies as well as coexisting presence of anti-c and anti-E antibodies. Others that pose a significant risk of HDFN include anti-E, -Fy^a, -Jk^a, -C, and -Ce.
- In addition to the risk of HDFN, maternal red cell antibodies may pose a problem for crossmatching and therefore the timely provision of blood and blood components.
- Identification of any of the antibodies that has a potential to cause HDFN marks the pregnancy as being at increased risk. Regular, frequent scans may be required for early detection of haemolytic problems, if maternal antibody titres are rising.
- Referral to a fetal medicine specialist should be arranged whenever there are rising antibody titres or if the titre is above a specific cut-off or if there are ultrasound features suggestive of fetal anaemia.
- Timing of delivery needs to be individualized with advice from the regional blood transfusion services. In those cases where severe HDFN is likely, referral to the tertiary referral centre for the latter part of antenatal care and for delivery is recommended.

Haemolytic disease of the fetus and newborn

- ***Pregnancies potentially affected by HDFN should be cared for by specialist teams with facilities for early diagnosis, intrauterine transfusion, and support for high-dependency neonates.***
- It is estimated that in England and Wales about 500 fetuses per year develop HDFN,[1] and unfortunately 25–30 babies die each year.
- HDFN occurs when the mother has anti-red cell IgG antibodies in her plasma that cross the placenta and bind to fetal red cells which carry the corresponding antigen.
- ***The three most common red cell alloantibodies which cause significant HDFN are anti-D, anti-c and anti-Kell (anti-K).***
- Approximately 1% of all pregnant women are found to have clinically significant red cell antibodies.[2] Of these, the commonest is anti-D. With the universal introduction of routine antenatal anti-D prophylaxis (RAADP) offered to all RhD-negative women in the UK without any detectable immune anti-D, the rate of sensitization has decreased significantly.
- When fetal red cells are bound to maternal IgG antibodies, they are destroyed in the fetal reticuloendothelial system, producing haemolysis and varying degrees of fetal anaemia.
- In severe cases the fetus may die in utero of high-output heart failure (**hydrops fetalis**). If the fetus survives birth, the neonate rapidly develops jaundice and is at increased risk of neurological damage due to the high bilirubin level.
- Development of red cell antibodies in the mother may occur either as a result of previous pregnancy/ies with a fetus that is **RhD, c, or K positive** or as a result of a previous blood transfusion. The latter is an important cause of alloimmunization with resultant HDFN in those mothers with non-anti-D antibodies.
- In general, the timing, mode, and place of delivery in pregnancies with red cell antibodies that can cause fetal anaemia depends on antibody titres, rate of their rise, whether in-utero transfusion was required, and whether neonatal exchange transfusion is anticipated.

HDFN due to anti-D antibodies

- Only IgG antibodies are capable of entering the fetal circulation.
- The most important cause of HDFN is the development of maternal antibodies to fetal RhD antigen. This occurs in RhD-negative women who either have had a previous pregnancy of a RhD-positive fetus or who have developed antibodies to RhD in this pregnancy directed at fetal cells normally found in maternal circulation.
- While HDFN only rarely occurs in a first pregnancy, the mother could be sensitized so that subsequent pregnancies with RhD-positive babies boost antibody production progressively, putting later pregnancies at increasing risk. Smaller family sizes and the introduction of prophylaxis with RhD immunoglobulin have reduced the incidence and severity of this condition.
- The fetus is only at risk if its red blood cells bear the antigen against which the mother's antibody is directed (e.g. if a RhD-negative woman with anti-D is carrying a RhD-positive fetus there is a risk that the fetus will be affected, but if the fetus is RhD negative there is no risk of HDFN).
- ***All women who have previously had a fetus or an infant affected by HDFN should be referred before 20 weeks to a specialist unit for advice and for assessment of fetal haemolysis, irrespective of antibody level.***[4]
- *Routine direct antiglobin test (DAT) on the cord samples of D-positive infants born to D-negative women who have had RAADP is not recommended.*
- ***All infants born to women who have clinically significant antibodies should, however, be closely observed for evidence of HDFN. A DAT should be performed and if positive, haemoglobin and bilirubin levels should be measured.***[4]
- Some infants may remain anaemic for a few weeks after birth or develop late anaemia due to hyporegeneration.

Antenatal routine testing protocols

- All pregnant women should have samples taken early in pregnancy, ideally at 10–12 weeks gestation, for ABO and RhD typing and screening for the presence of other red cell alloantibodies. When an antibody screen is positive, further tests should be carried out to determine the antibody specificity and significance.[4]
- *All pregnant women, whether D positive or D negative, should have a further blood sample taken at 28 weeks gestation for rechecking the ABO and D group and further screening for other red cell alloantibodies. RhD-positive women are just as likely as RhD-negative women to form antibodies to other red cell antigens such as c, K, etc.*
- No further routine blood grouping or antibody screening is necessary after 28 weeks in women who are RhD negative if the booking and 28-week screening has not shown anti-D antibodies. It is not possible at present to differentiate between prophylactic and immune anti-D.[6] While prophylactic anti-D levels will fall with time, immune anti-D levels will usually remain stable or rise if there is restimulation of the antibody. The level of anti-D in maternal samples post-prophylaxis rarely exceeds 1 IU/ml unless a dose (or doses) of more than1250 IU has been administered. **Also, antibodies detected only in the third trimester do not appear to cause HDN.**[7,8]
- Potentially sensitizing episodes during pregnancy which require anti-D prophylaxis in RhD-negative women:
  - amniocentesis
  - cordocentesis
  - other in-utero therapeutic intervention/surgery (e.g. intrauterine transfusion, shunting)
  - antepartum haemorrhage (APH)

Figure 1.1

Anti-D administration checklist

Always confirm:
- ***the woman's identity***
- ***that the woman is RhD negative using the latest laboratory report***
- ***that the woman does not have immune anti-D using the latest laboratory report***
- ***that informed consent for administration of anti-D Ig is recorded in notes***

Potentially sensitizing events during pregnancy

Gestation <12 weeks	
Vaginal bleeding associated with severe pain ERPC/instrumentation of the uterus Termination of pregnancy (surgical or medical) Ectopic/molar pregnancy CVS	Administer at least 250 IU anti-D Ig within 72 h of event *Confirm product, dose, expiry, and patient ID before administration*

Gestation 12–20 weeks	
For any potentially sensitizing event	Administer at least 250 IU anti-D Ig within 72 h of event *Confirm product, dose, expiry, and patient ID before administration*

Gestation 20 weeks to term	
For any potentially sensitizing event (irrespective of whether RAADP has been given)	Request a Kleihauer test (FMH test) and administer at least 500 IU anti-D Ig within 72 h of event *Confirm product, dose, expiry, and patient ID before administration*
Does the Kleihauer/FMH test indicate that further anti-D Ig is required?	Administer more anti-D Ig following discussion with laboratory
For continuous vaginal bleeding at least 500 IU anti-D Ig should be administered at a minimum of 6-weekly intervals, irrespective of the presence of detectable anti-D, and a Kleihauer/FMH test requested every 2 weeks in case more anti-D is needed	

Routine antenatal anti-D prophylaxis (RAADP)

For RAADP (irrespective of whether anti-D Ig already given for a potentially sensitizing event)	Take a blood sample to confirm group and check antibody screen. Do not wait for results before administering anti-D Ig Administer 1500 IU anti-D Ig at 28–30 weeks **or** Administer at least 500 IU anti-D Ig at 28 weeks and then administer at least 500 IU anti-D at 34 weeks *Confirm product, dose, expiry, and patient ID before administration*

At delivery (or at both diagnosis and delivery of intrauterine death >20 weeks)

Is the baby's group confirmed as RhD positive? **or** Are cord samples not available?	Request a Kleihauer test (FMH test) Administer at least 500 IU anti-D Ig within 72 h of delivery *Confirm product, dose, expiry, and patient ID before administration*
Does the Kleihauer/FMH test indicate that further anti-D Ig is required?	Administer more anti-D Ig following discussion with laboratory

Adapted with kind permission from Serious Hazards of Transfusion (SHOT), <http://www.shotuk.org/wp-content/uploads/2010/03/SHOT-Anti-D-Administration-Checklist-v12-Oct-2012.pdf>

    - CVS
    - ectopic pregnancy
    - external cephalic version
    - fall or abdominal trauma
    - intrauterine death
    - miscarriage
    - termination of pregnancy.
- See Figure 1.1 for a SHOT flowchart to guide the appropriate administration of anti-D Ig9 (<http://www.shotuk.org>).
- The following anti-D levels[4] serve as a guide to management:
    - ***Anti-D less than 4 IU/ml: HDFN unlikely***
    - ***Anti-D 4–15 IU/ml: Moderate risk of HDFN***
    - ***Anti-D more than 15 IU/ml: High risk of hydrops fetalis***
    - A significant anti-D level (>4 IU/ml) should trigger referral to a specialist fetomaternal unit.
- In cases of allo-immunization, non-invasive techniques of assessing fetal anaemia such as weekly ultrasound specifically measuring the middle cerebral artery peak systolic volume (MCA-PSV) are applicable, not only in anti-D alloimmunization, but in other atypical antibodies such as Kell alloimmunization.[10,11] When the MCA -PSV is more than 1.5 multiples of the median, the fetus is likely to have moderate–severe anaemia. In such circumstances, or if there are other signs of fetal anaemia such as hydrops, urgent referral to a tertiary unit is required as cordocentesis and in-utero transfusion may be required.
- MCA-PSV Doppler assessment is the primary test of choice for detection of fetal anaemia in alloimmunization.[12]
- A woman whose anti-D level is 4 IU/ml or greater and/or who has a rising anti-D level and/or has a history of previous HDFN-affected offspring must be referred to a specialist fetal medicine unit.[4]

HDN due to other antibodies: anti-c, anti-K

- The incidence of **non-anti D** antibodies in Western countries has been estimated to be about 1–2% of all pregnancies.[13,14] The prevalence of a positive antibody screen was found to be 1 in 80 of all pregnancies, with a 1 in 300 prevalence of clinically relevant alloantibodies other than anti-D.[15]
- The other common causes of severe HDFN are the **anti-c** or **anti-K antibodies**. In HDFN due to **anti-K**, the maternal

antibodies not only cause haemolysis of fetal red cells but can significantly suppress fetal red cell production; in such cases the anaemia is often very severe while jaundice may be minimal.[16]

- The incidence of **anti-K alloimmunization** is low in the obstetric population, 0.1–0.2%.[16]
- The majority of cases of **anti-K** in pregnant women are the consequence of previous K-positive transfusions. The incidence of anti-K could be reduced by using K-negative units for transfusion to women of childbearing age.
- Once anti-K is detected, referral to fetal medicine should occur as severe anaemia can occur even with low titres.[17] The development of or severity of HDFN due to anti-K does not always correlate with titres of anti-K antibody or with a previous obstetric history of an affected infant. Affected pregnancies, however, appear to be associated with anti-K titres of at least 1 in 32.[18]
- The transfusion history of women with anti-K should be established and a sample from the father of the fetus should be K-typed. If there is no history of blood transfusion, and the father is K positive, levels should continue to be checked at monthly intervals up to 28 weeks and at fortnightly intervals thereafter.
- **Anti-c** belongs to the rhesus group of antibodies. About 14–21% of babies born to mothers with anti-c antibodies require exchange transfusion.[3,19]
- Anti-c may cause delayed anaemia in the neonate and it is imperative that the neonatal team is informed before delivery
- Women with identified anti-c and anti-K antibodies should be retested at the same frequency as women with anti-D, i.e. at least monthly up to 28 weeks gestation and every 2 weeks thereafter until delivery, or as requested by the blood bank service.
- The following levels of anti-c are a guide to management.[19] Cases where the antibody reaches the critical level and/or the level is rising significantly must be promptly referred to a specialist fetal medicine unit.[4]
- ***Anti-c levels:***
  - ***Less than 7.5 IU/ml: Continue to monitor.***
  - ***7.5–20 IU/ml: Risk of moderate HDFN; refer to specialist unit.***
  - ***More than 20 IU/ml: Risk of severe HDFN; refer to specialist unit.***
- **In addition to anti-D, anti-K, and anti-c, the following IgG antibodies could also be implicated in causing HDFN**: anti-C [Ce], -E [-cE], -Fy^a, and -Jk^a.[20,21,22] In these cases, the frequency of antibody testing, apart from at booking and 28 weeks, should be individualized.[12] Women who have had a previous pregnancy affected by HDFN should be referred early to a fetal medicine specialist.[17]
- The presence of anti-E can enhance the severity of the fetal anaemia caused by anti-c antibodies, therefore referral to specialist fetal medicine must be made at lower levels (titres) unless the fetus has only one of these antigens.[17]
- **Anti-E** antibodies with a titre greater than 1 in 32 should prompt further evaluation for fetal anaemia with Doppler assessments of MCA-PSV.[23]
- As in the case of anti-D alloimmunization, MCA-PSV Doppler assessment is the primary test of choice for detection of fetal anaemia due to anti-c, anti-Kell, or anti -E.

In-utero transfusion for fetal anaemia

- In-utero transfusion (IUT) must be performed only in specialist fetal medicine units with requisite perinatal haematological expertise.[17] Blood used for in-utero transfusion is always irradiated and should have plasma removed by the blood centre to increase the haematocrit to 0.70–0.85. Red cell preparations for IUT should be group O or ABO identical with the fetus (if known) and negative for the antigen(s) corresponding to maternal cell antibodies.[17]
- In red cell alloimmunization, IUT can be performed up to 35 weeks gestation and delivery planned for 37–38 weeks.[24] Vaginal delivery can be attempted despite the prior IUTs.
- Immediate delivery, once viability is reached, is required if complications arise during the process of IUT. Antenatal steroids are therefore recommended once viability is attained.

HDFN due to ABO incompatibility

- ***Although not usually severe, the most common form of HDFN is that caused by ABO incompatibility.***
- In women of blood group O, there are naturally occurring anti-A and anti-B IgG antibodies which can cross the placenta.
- HDFN due to ABO incompatibility occurs when a group O mother with IgG anti-A or IgG anti-B antibodies is carrying a fetus of blood group A or blood group B respectively.
- The most common presentations of ABO-incompatibility HDFN include mild to moderate anaemia and jaundice (unconjugated hyperbilirubinaemia). The DAT is usually (but not always) positive.
- Severe fetal/neonatal anaemia can rarely result from transplacental transfer of maternal anti-A or anti-B of the IgG subclass in a group O mother, thus causing haemolysis of fetal erythrocytes. This is uncommon in white women in the UK, but is more common in some other ethnic groups, especially among women of African Caribbean origin.
- ***Unlike in anti-D alloimmunization, no prophylaxis is available for atypical antibodies, so alloimmunization will continue to occur.***[4]

Maternal antibodies that can potentially cause problems with crossmatching

- These antibodies are not usually implicated in causing significant HDFN but may cause problems with crossmatching and issues with availability of appropriate blood.
- These antibodies include Fy^3, Jk^b, Duffy, H(Bombay), Kidd, MNS, and P systems.
- Discussion with the transfusion laboratory and/or consultant haematologist is advisable regarding frequency of antenatal testing and arrangements for availability of blood at short notice.[17] This is particularly important in those at high risk of requiring transfusion such as placenta praevia, sickle cell disease, etc.
- Women with such antibodies are at increased risk of requiring significant amounts of transfused blood either antenatally, intrapartum, or postnatally. Transferring their care to a regional centre should therefore be considered. Rapid processing of crossmatched samples and rapid provision of compatible blood is possible in these centres.[17]

Information for patients

Please see Information for patients: Red cell antibodies and pregnancy (p. 496)

References

1. Poole J, Daniels G Blood group antibodies and their significance in transfusion medicine. Transfus Med Rev 2007;21: 58–71.
2. Howard H, et al. Consequences for fetus and neonate of maternal red cell allo-immunisation. Arch Dis Child Fetal Neonatal Ed 1998;78:
3. Daniels G Blood group antibodies in haemolytic disease of the fetus and newborn. In:Hadley A, Soothill P, ed., Alloimmune disorders of pregnancy. Cambridge: Cambridge University Press, 2002, pp. 21–40.
4. Gooch J, et al. British Committee for Standards in Haematology Blood Transfusion Task Force. Guideline for blood grouping and antibody testing in pregnancy. Transfus Med 2007;17: 252–262.
5. Thompson S, et al. Late developing red cell antibodies in pregnancy. Transfus Med 2003; 13suppl: 8–9.
6. New HV, et al. Antenatal antibody screening [letter]. Lancet 2001;357: 1295.
7. Rothenberg JM, et al. Is a third-trimester antibody screen for Rh+ women necessary? Am J Managed Care 1999;5: 1145–1150.
8. Heddle NM, et al. A retrospective study to determine the risk of red cell alloimmunization and transfusion during pregnancy. Transfusion 1993;33: 217–220.
9. Qureshi H, et al. BCSH guideline for the use of anti-D immunoglobulin for the prevention of haemolytic disease of the newborn. Transfus Med 2014;24: 8–20.
10. Van Dongen H, et al. Non-invasive tests to predict fetal anemia in Kell-alloimmunized pregnancies. Ultrasound Obstet Gynecol 2005;25: 341–345.
11. Scheier M, et al. Prediction of fetal anemia in rhesus disease by measurement of fetal middle cerebral artery peak systolic velocity. Ultrasound Obstet Gynecol 2004;23: 432–436.

12. Gajjar K, Spencer C. Diagnosis and management of non-anti-D red cell antibodies in pregnancy. Obstetrician and Gynaecologist 2009;11: 89–95.
13. Weinstein L Irregular antibodies causing hemolytic disease of the newborn: a continuing problem. Clin Obstet Gynecol 1982;25: 321–332.
14. Weinstein L Irregular antibodies causing haemolytic disease of the newborn. Obstet Gynecol Surv 1976;31: 581–591.
15. Koelewijn JM, et al. Effect of screening for red cell antibodies, other than anti-D, to detect hemolytic disease of the fetus and newborn: a population study in the Netherlands. Transfusion 2008;48: 941–952.
16. Vaughan JI, et al. Inhibition of erythroid progenitor cells by anti-Kell antibodies in fetal alloimmune anemia. N Engl J Med 1998;338: 798–803.
17. RCOG Green-top Guideline, no.65. The management of women with red cell antibodies during pregnancy. London: Royal College of Obstetricians and Gynaecologists, 2014
18. Ahaded A, et al. Quantitative determination of anti-K (KEL1) IgG and IgG subclasses in the serum of severely alloimmunized pregnant women by ELISA. Transfusion 2000;40: 1239–1245.
19. Kozlowski CL, et al. Quantification of anti-c in haemolytic disease of the newborn. Transfus Med 1995;5: 37–42.
20. Moise KJ Non-anti-D antibodies in red cell alloimmunisation. Eur J Obstet Gynecol Reprod Biol 2000;92: 75–81.
21. Moran, P, et al. Anti-E in pregnancy. BJOG 2000;107: 1436–1438.
22. Goodrick, M. J, et al. Haemolytic disease of the fetus and newborn due to anti-Fya and the potential clinical value of Duffy genotyping in pregnancies at risk. Transfus Med 1997;7: 301–304.
23. Joy SD, et al. Management of pregnancies complicated by anti-E alloimmunisation. Obstet Gynecol 2005;105: 24–28.
24. Klumper FJ, et al. Benefits and risks of fetal red cell transfusion after 32 weeks gestation. Eur J Obstet Gynecol Reprod Biol 2000;92: 91–96.

CARE PATHWAY

ABO/Blood Group Antibody Screening

All pregnancies—booking bloods
- ABO group and Rh (D) typing
- Antibody screening

Positive clinically significant (of maternal or fetal significance) **antibody screen** (e.g. anti-D, anti-c, anti-K, also anti-E, -Fy^a, -Jk^a, -C and -Ce)

Anti-D, anti-c, or anti-K antibodies (highest risk of HFDN):
- test monthly till 28 weeks; then fortnightly till delivery
- if antibody titres suggestive of moderate or high risk of HDFN—early assessment and referral to fetal medicine specialist unit

Other antibodies including anti-E, anti-Fy^a, -Jk^a, -C, -Ce found at booking:
- paternal/fetal genotyping for specific antigen to be considered

Repeat antibody screen at 28 weeks

Cord bloods for direct antiglobin test (DAT), fetal Hb, and bilirubin levels

No clinically significant antibodies (of either maternal or fetal significance) found:

Repeat antibody testing at 28 weeks

Clinically significant antibodies (of maternal or fetal significance) found

No antibodies found—no further action required

Reproduced from: Royal College of Obstetricians and Gynaecologists. Red cell antibodies during pregnancy. Green-top Guideline No. 65. London: RCOG; 2014, with the permission of the Royal College of Obstetricians and Gynaecologists.

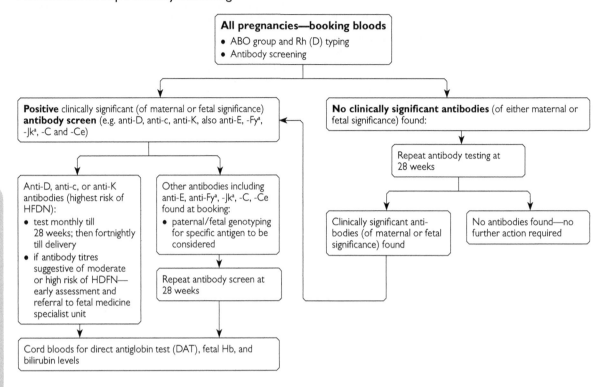

Management of Anti-D, Anti-K, or Anti-c Alloimmunization

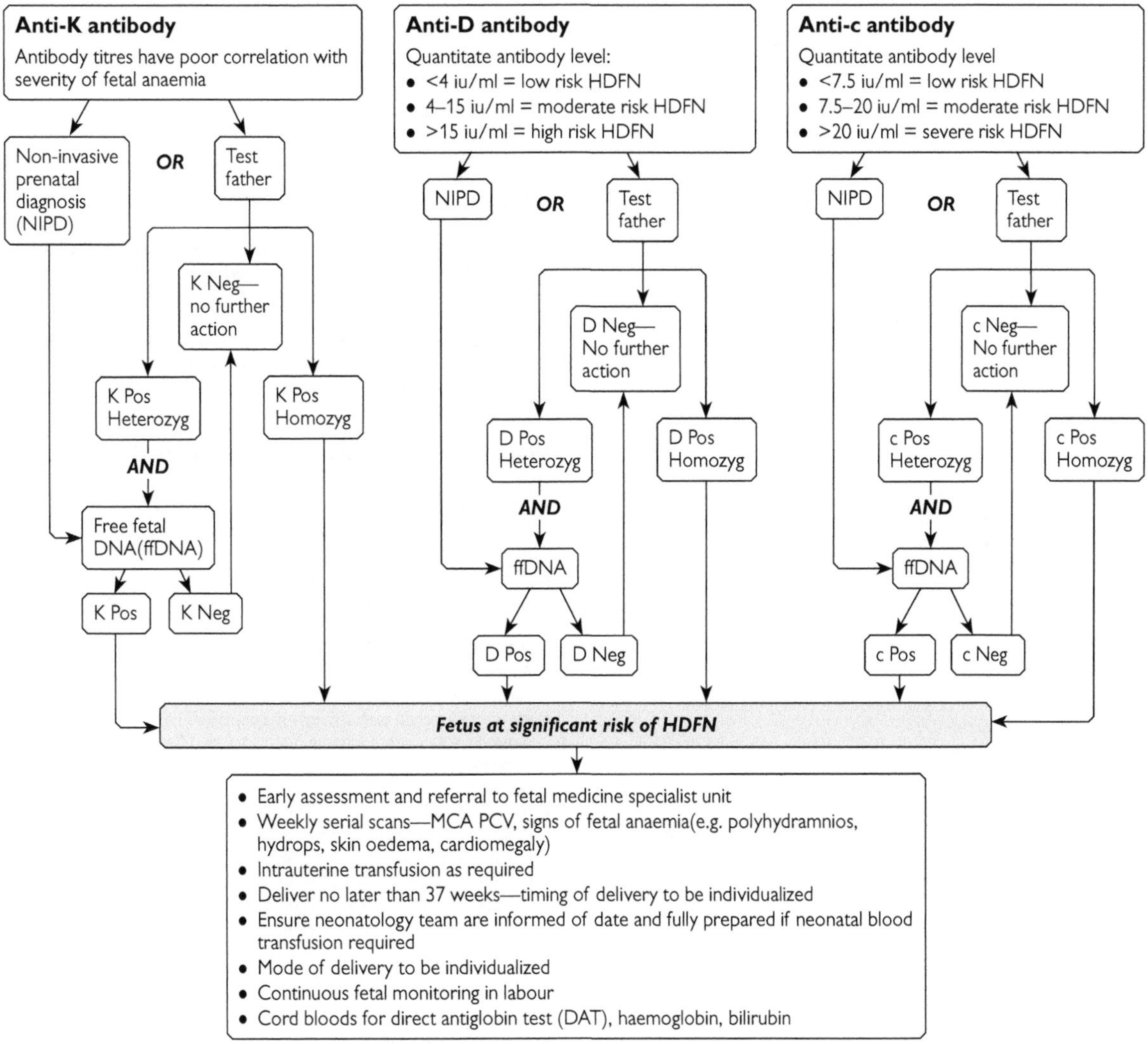

Reproduced from: Royal College of Obstetricians and Gynaecologists. Red cell antibodies during pregnancy. Green-top Guideline No. 65. London: RCOG; 2014, with the permission of the Royal College of Obstetricians and Gynaecologists.

1.10 Venous Thromboembolism

FACT FILE

Epidemiology

- The overall incidence of **venous thromboembolism (VTE)** in pregnancy and in the puerperium is about 1–2 in 1000.[1,2,3,4]
- In the UK, the incidence of PE (pulmonary embolism) during pregnancy is 1.3 in 10 000 maternities with a case fatality rate of 3.5%.[5]
- PE has consistently remained one of the top five direct causes of maternal mortality. In the 2007 CEMACH report, 11% of maternal deaths were due to PE.[6]
- Identifiable risk factors have been found in 70–79% of pregnancy-related PE.[5,6]
- It is estimated that the risk of TED could be reduced by up to 75% with LMWH prophylaxis.[1,2,3,4]
- If risk factors for TED are identified, LMWH prophylaxis needs to be started early in pregnancy as many fatal events of TED can occur in the first trimester.[7]
- 55% of fatal PEs occur in women who have had vaginal deliveries.[6]
- The greatest risk period for TED, especially PE, is postpartum. A 60% increase in the risk of VTE has been found in the first 12 weeks after delivery[8] compared with non-pregnant controls.

Risk factors for VTE in pregnancy and puerperium

- *All women should have a documented risk assessment for VTE performed in early pregnancy, repeated if admission to hospital is required for any indication or if any intercurrent problems should develop. Risk assessment should be repeated intrapartum or immediately postpartum.*[1]
- **Pre-existing risk factors:**
  - smoking
  - age >35 years
  - obesity (BMI >30 kg/m^2) pre-pregnancy or in early pregnancy
  - multiparity (≥P3)
  - previous VTE: 10–11% increased risk of recurrence during subsequent pregnancy and puerperium.
  - *Heritable thrombophilias* (account for 20–50% of pregnancy-related VTE):[9,10]
    - antithrombin deficiency
    - protein C deficiency
    - protein S deficiency
    - factor V Leiden
    - prothrombin gene *G20210A*.
  - *Acquired thrombophilias:*
    - persistent lupus anticoagulant
    - persistent anticardiolipin antibodies or beta$_2$ glycoprotein-1 antibodies
  - *Medical comorbidities*: Including heart or lung disease, SLE, cancer, inflammatory conditions (inflammatory bowel disease or inflammatory polyarthropathy), nephrotic syndrome (proteinuria >3 g/day), sickle cell disease, IV drug use, paraplegia, gross varicosities.
- **Current obstetric risk factors:**
  - multiple pregnancy, assisted reproductive therapy
  - pre-eclampsia
  - Caesarean section
  - prolonged labour, mid-cavity rotational operative delivery
  - PPH (>1 litre) requiring transfusion.
- **New-onset/transient risks—potentially reversible:**
  - surgical procedure in pregnancy or puerperium (e.g. ERPC, appendicectomy, postpartum sterilization)
  - hyperemesis, dehydration
  - ovarian hyperstimulation syndrome
  - admission or immobility (≥3 days bed rest), e.g. symphysis pubis dysfunction restricting mobility
  - systemic infection (requiring antibiotics or admission to hospital), e.g. pneumonia, pyelonephritis, postpartum wound infection
  - long-distance travel (>4 h).
- ***If a woman has three or more of current or persisting risk factors mentioned above (other than previous VTE or thrombophilia), prophylactic LMWH should be considered antenatally and will invariably need to be continued for 6 weeks postnatally, but a postnatal risk assessment must be performed.***
- ***If there are two or more of current or persisting risk factors mentioned above (other than previous VTE or thrombophilia), prophylactic LMWH should be considered for at least 7 days postpartum.***[1]

Women with a history of previous VTE: thrombosis risk assessment and management

- *All women should have a documented assessment of risk factors for VTE before pregnancy or in early pregnancy as well as repeated at each hospital admission.*[1]
- Women with a previous non-oestrogen-related VTE provoked by a minor risk factor should undergo testing for thrombophilia before pregnancy to enable appropriate antenatal management plans regarding thromboprophylaxis.
- At the first booking visit by the midwife, women should be specifically asked about any personal or family history of VTE.
- Ideally all women with a family history of VTE in first- or second-degree relatives should have been screened for thrombophilias (inherited or acquired) *before conception, and received pre-conceptual counselling.*
- If a personal history of VTE is obtained, enquire whether the diagnosis was confirmed by scans or radiographs. If this information is not available, ask how long any anticoagulant treatment was prescribed and continued for. When prolonged anticoagulant therapy (>6 weeks) has been prescribed, in keeping with the management of VTE, it is safe to assume this has been a definite VTE episode.
- If there is a personal history of previous VTE, stratification of the risk is important for thromboprophylaxis management during the current pregnancy and puerperium.
- **Stratification of risk** in those with a history of previous VTE into three categories (**very high risk**, **high risk**, and **intermediate risk**) is based on international and national guidelines.[1,11,12,13]
- Thrombophilia testing must be offered to women who have had a previous VTE that was not related to oestrogen (combined OCP or pregnancy-related), especially if the precipitating cause was a 'minor risk' such as long-distance travel (>4 h) or a period of restricted mobility (>3 days).
- Women who have had a previous unprovoked or oestrogen-related VTE already qualify for thromboprophylaxis during this pregnancy and puerperium. It can therefore be argued that thrombophilia screening is not required in such patients as this would not alter management.[1] *The increasing evidence of the role played by thrombophilias in placental deficiency, growth restriction, and intrauterine fetal death must, however, be considered. Identification of thrombophilia (acquired or inherited) may alter plans for fetal surveillance and management during the present pregnancy.*
- Thrombophilia testing in women with previous history of VTE is best offered pre-pregnancy. *Due to the normal fall in the naturally occurring anticoagulants protein C, protein S, and antithrombin factor in any pregnancy, thrombophilia screening is limited during pregnancy to factor V Leiden, prothrombin gene mutation, APS, and SLE.*

- *Also, screening results for certain thrombophilias, such as factor V Leiden deficiency or lupus anticoagulant, are not interpretable if patients are already on anticoagulants including both LMWHs and warfarin.*
- If there is a previous personal history of VTE but no identified thrombophilia and if the previous VTE event was oestrogen linked (e.g. combined OCP or during a pregnancy or puerperium), LMWH should be started as early as possible during pregnancy and continued throughout pregnancy and for at least 6 weeks postnatally. A gradual switch to oral warfarin may be made after delivery.
- Women with a previous single provoked (excluding oestrogen-related) VTE and no other risk factors require close surveillance during pregnancy and the puerperium. Antenatal LMWH is **not** routinely recommended but this is best decided by early referral to the haematology consultant.
- Each case should be judged on an individual basis, taking into account additional risk factors such as obesity, smoking, hyperemesis, relative dehydration, immobility, etc. The patient needs to be counselled about the potential risks and benefits of antenatal thromboprophylaxis and management options discussed.
- All women with VTE events during a previous pregnancy/ puerperium or when on the combined OCP, must have antenatal LMWH thromboprophylaxis (and antiembolic stockings) commenced as early as possible, even if no identifiable thrombophilia was found on previous testing. Thromboprophylaxis must be continued throughout pregnancy and for at least 6 weeks postnatally.
- All women with previous idiopathic (unprovoked) VTE should have antenatal thromboprophylaxis started as early as possible in pregnancy (even if previous thrombophilia screening was negative) and continued throughout pregnancy and for at least 6 weeks postnatally.
- In women with a history of previous VTE which was associated with a temporary risk factor which is no longer present (e.g. trauma or post-surgery) and who have no identifiable thrombophilia nor any current risk factors other than pregnancy, routine antenatal thromboprophylaxis is not required but they should be advised to wear graduated elasticated below-knee stockings during pregnancy and the puerperium. Thromboprophylaxis is, however, recommended in the puerperium for at least 6 weeks with LMWH.
- For those with a history of previous isolated VTE secondary to a temporary risk factor which is no longer present (e.g. trauma or post-surgery) in this pregnancy **but** who have additional risk factors in this pregnancy such as obesity, smoking, hyperemesis, ovarian hyperstimulation, relative dehydration, immobility, etc., antenatal thromboprophylaxis must be considered which is then continued for at least 6 weeks postnatally.
- Early referral to the anaesthetic high-risk clinic is required for any pregnant woman on anticoagulation either as prophylaxis or in therapeutic doses. Advice about the timing of interruption of LMWH for labour, delivery, or an elective Caesarean section should be discussed and documented.
- Women receiving antenatal LMWH should be advised that if they have any vaginal bleeding, or if spontaneous labour begins, they should not inject any further LMWH to allow for the use of regional analgesia or anaesthesia if requested or required. They should be reassessed on admission to hospital.[1]

Preparation for labour and delivery

- For women receiving high prophylactic or therapeutic doses of LMWH, the dose of heparin should be reduced to a prophylactic dose on the day before induction of labour and, if appropriate, continued in this dose during labour.[1]
- Regional techniques should not be used until at least 12 h after the previous prophylactic dose of LMWH.
- When a woman presents while on a therapeutic regimen of LMWH, regional techniques should not be used for at least 24 h after the last dose of LMWH.[14]
- LMWH should not be given for 4 h after use of spinal anaesthesia or after the epidural catheter has been removed. The cannula should not be removed within 10–12 h of the most recent injection.[14]
- For elective Caesarean section, a thromboprophylactic dose of LMWH can be administered on the day before the surgery, but the morning dose omitted on the day of the surgery. For such women every effort must be made to schedule the operation for the morning session. This allows the next thromboprophylactic dose of LMWH to be given 4 h postoperatively or 4 h after removal of the spinal/epidural catheter.
- Even with the above adjustments of the timing of LMWH, there is a 2% risk of wound haematoma in those on LMWH as well as unfractionated heparin. The patient should be warned of this when obtaining consent for the surgery.[15]
- In some women on treatment doses of LMWH, a planned induction of labour may need to be considered to help plan peripartum thromboprophylaxis.
- If regional analgesia cannot be provided for spontaneous labour due to the timing of the last LMWH, IV patient-controlled analgesia with opiates may be offered.
- In women at high risk of major APH or PPH, with advice obtained from haematologists, unfractionated heparin around the time of delivery and for the first postnatal day may need to be considered instead of LMWH. Unfractionated heparin has a shorter half-life and is more completely reversed by protamine sulfate than LMWH. Once the danger of haemorrhage has passed, LMWH can be resumed.

Postnatal thromboprophylaxis management

- Women with VTE before the current pregnancy should be offered LMWH for 6 weeks after delivery.[1]
- All women with class 3 obesity (i.e. BMI >40 kg/m^2), should be considered for thromboprophylaxis with LMWH for 7 days after delivery.
- All women who have had an emergency Caesarean section (category 1, 2, or 3) should be considered for thromboprophylaxis with LMWH for 7 days after delivery. Those who have had an elective (category 4) Caesarean section **and** have one or more additional risk factors (such as BMI >30, or smokers, or age >35) should also be considered for thromboprophylaxis with LMWH for 7 days after delivery.
- All women with asymptomatic heritable or acquired thrombophilia should be considered for LMWH for at least 7 days following delivery, even if they were not receiving antenatal thromboprophylaxis. This could be extended to 6 weeks if there is a family history or any other risk factors present.
- In women who have additional persistent (lasting >7 days postpartum) risk factors, such as prolonged admission or wound infection, thromboprophylaxis should be extended for up to 6 weeks or until additional risk factors are no longer present.
- Conversion from LMWH to warfarin should be gradual and the overlap time should be over 5–7 days after delivery, as warfarin is associated with a greater risk of PPH or perineal/wound haematomas.
- In those who develop skin allergy to heparin (both LMWH and unfractionated heparin), the haematologists may advice fondaparinux, a synthetic pentasaccharide which acts similarly to LMWH. Till further evidence is obtained, fondaparinux is not recommended for breastfeeding mothers.
- The woman should be reassured that both LMWH and warfarin are safe when breastfeeding.
- Where there are contraindications for LMWH,[1] expert advice from the haematologists must be sought without delay, regarding avoidance, postponement or discontinuation of LMWH. The likelihood of thromboembolism and the risk of bleeding must be weighed on a case-to-case basis, involving senior obstetricians and haematologists.
- *Risk factors that are contraindications for LMWH include:*[1]
  - active antenatal or postpartum bleeding
  - increased risk of major haemorrhage (such as placenta praevia)
  - known bleeding diathesis, such as vWD, haemophilia, or acquired coagulopathy

- Severe thrombocytopenia (platelet count <75 × 10^9/litre)
- acute stroke in the last 4 weeks (ischaemic or haemorrhagic)
- severe renal disease (glomerular filtration rate <30 ml/min/1.73 m^2)
- severe liver disease (prothrombin time above normal range)
- uncontrolled hypertension (blood pressure >200 mmHg systolic or >120 mmHg diastolic).

Women with a family history but no personal history of VTE

- Women who have no personal history or risk factors for VTE, but have a family history of VTE in a first-degree relative when aged under 50, that has been unprovoked or oestrogen-related, should be considered for thrombophilia testing.
- If the particular thrombophilia in the relative is known, this is particularly important information, but unfortunately in actual clinical practice this is not often the case.
- Under these circumstances, thrombophilia testing is best performed before pregnancy to include protein C, protein S, and antithrombin III levels as well as factor V Leiden and prothrombin gene variant. If such testing for inherited thrombophilias has not been performed before pregnancy, as is often the case, limited thrombophilia testing for factor V Leiden and prothrombin gene mutation should be considered in early pregnancy.
- There is a higher risk of pregnancy-related VTE in those who have deficient protein C, protein S, or antithrombin III, as well as those who are homozygous for factor V Leiden or for prothrombin gene mutation, compared with women who are heterozygous carriers for factor V Leiden and the prothrombin gene mutation. The risk is also higher in women who are compound heterozygotes for factor V Leiden and the prothrombin gene mutation.[16,17]
- Antenatal thromboprophylaxis is not routinely required in women with no previous personal history of VTE having a low-risk thrombophilic tendency such as heterozygous carriers for factor V Leiden and the prothrombin gene mutation, unless there are additional risk factors including a strong family history especially of pregnancy-related VTE.
- The decision to use LMWH thromboprophylaxis during pregnancy is best made jointly with advice from the haematologist and risk stratification.
- Women with a family history of VTE and an identified thrombophilia should be considered for 6 weeks postnatal thromboprophylaxis.
- ***For further information regarding prophylaxis of VTE and acute management of VTE in pregnancy and the puerperium, including care algorithms, the reader is referred to the RCOG Green-top Guidelines.***[1,2]

Information for patients

Please see Information for patients: Thrombosis or embolism and pregnancy (p. 496)

References

1. RCOG Green-top Guideline No. 37a. Reducing the risk of thrombosis and embolism during pregnancy and the puerperium. London: Royal College of Obstetricians and Gynaecologists, 2009.
2. RCOG Green-top Guideline No. 37b. The acute management of thrombosis and embolism during pregnancy and the puerperium. London: Royal College of Obstetricians and Gynaecologists, 2007, reviewed 2010.
3. Jacobsen AF, et al. Ante- and postnatal risk factors of venous thrombosis: a hospital-based case-control study. J Thromb Haemost 2008;6: 905–912.
4. James AH. Prevention and management of venous thromboembolism in pregnancy. Am J Med 2007;120: S26–34.
5. Knight M, on behalf of UKOSS. Antenatal pulmonary embolism: risk factors, management and outcomes. BJOG 2008;115: 453–461.
6. Confidential Enquiry into Maternal and Child Health. Saving mothers' lives: reviewing maternal deaths to make motherhood safer, 2003-2005. The Seventh Report of the Confidential Enquiries into Maternal Deaths in the United Kingdom. London: CEMACH, 2007.
7. James AH, et al. Thrombosis during pregnancy and the postpartum period. Am J Obstet Gynecol 2005;193: 216–219.
8. Pomp ER, et al. Pregnancy, the postpartum period and prothrombotic defects: risk of venous thrombosis in the MEGA study. J Thromb Haemost 2008;6: 632–637.
9. McColl MD, et al. The role of inherited thrombophilia in venous thromboembolism associated with pregnancy. Br J Obstet Gynaecol 1999;75: 387–388.
10. Gerhardt A, et al. Effect of hemostatic risk factors on the individual probability of thrombosis during pregnancy and the puerperium. Thromb Haemost 2003;90: 77–85.
11. Bates SM, et al. Venous thromboembolism, thrombophilia, antithrombotic therapy, and pregnancy: American College of Chest Physicians Evidence-Based Clinical Practice Guidelines (8th edition). Chest 2008; 6Suppl: 844S–846S.
12. Bauersachs RM, et al. Risk stratification and heparin prophylaxis to prevent venous thromboembolism in pregnant women. Thromb Haemost 2007;98: 1237–1245.
13. Duhl AJ, et al. Pregnancy and Thrombosis Working Group. Antithrombotic therapy and pregnancy: consensus report and recommendations for prevention and treatment of venous thromboembolism and adverse pregnancy outcomes. Am J Obstet Gynecol 2007;197: 457. e 1–21.
14. Horlocker TT, et al. Regional anesthesia in the anticoagulated patient: defining the risks (the second ASRA Consensus Conference on Neuraxial Anesthesia and Anticoagulation). Reg Anesth Pain Med 2003;28: 172–197.
15. Greer IA, Nelson-Piercy C Low-molecular-weight heparins for thromboprophylaxis and treatment of venous thromboembolism in pregnancy: a systematic review of safety and efficacy. Blood 2005;106: 401–407.
16. Rogenhofer N, et al. Prevention, management and extent of adverse pregnancy outcomes in women with hereditary antithrombin deficiency. Ann Hematol 2014;93: 385–392.
17. Jacobsen AF, et al. Risk of venous thrombosis in pregnancy among carriers of the factor V Leiden and the prothrombin gene G20210A polymorphisms. J Thromb Haemost 2010;8: 2443–2449.

CARE PATHWAY

Antenatal thromboprophylaxis risk assessment and management
At booking, and repeated later if admitted

- Single previous VTE +
  - thrombophilia or family history
  - unprovoked/oestrogen-related
- Previous recurrent VTE (>1)

→ ***High risk***
- Requires antenatal prophylaxis with LMWH
- Refer to trust-nominated thrombosis in pregnancy expert/team

- Single previous VTE with no family history or thrombophilia
- Thrombophilia + no VTE
- **Medical comorbities**, e.g. heart or lung disease, SLE, cancer, inflammatory conditions, nephrotic syndrome, sickle cell disease, IV drug use
- Surgical procedure, e.g. appendicectomy

→ ***Intermediate risk***
- Consider antenatal prophylaxis with LMWH
- Seek trust-nominated thrombosis in pregnancy expert/team advice

- Age >35 years
- Obesity (BMI >30 kg/m^2)
- Parity ≥3
- Smoker
- Gross varicose veins
- Current systemic infection
- Immobility, e.g. paraplegia, SPD, long-distance travel
- Pre-eclampsia
- Dehydration /hyperemesis/ovarian hyperstimulation syndrome
- Multiple pregnancy or assisted reproductive therapy

→ 3 or more risk factors
2 or more if admitted
→ (Intermediate risk)

→ <3 risk factors
→ ***Lower risk***
- Mobilization and avoidance of dehydration

Antenatal and postnatal prophylactic dose of LMWH
- Weight <50 kg = 20 mg enoxaparin/2500 units dalteparin/3500 units tinzaparin daily
- Weight 50–90 kg = 40 mg enoxaparin/5000 units dalteparin/4500 units tinzaparin daily
- Weight 91–130 kg = 60 mg enoxaparin/7500 units dalteparin/7000 units tinzaparin daily
- Weight 131–170 kg = 80 mg enoxaparin/10000 units dalteparin/9000 units tinzaparin daily
- Weight >170 kg = 0.6 mg/kg/day enoxaparin; 75 units/kg/day dalteparin/75 units/kg/day tinzaparin

Reproduced from: Royal College of Obstetricians and Gynaecologists. Reducing risk of thrombosis and embolism during pregnancy. Green-top Guideline No. 37a. London: RCOG; 2009, with the permission of the Royal College of Obstetricians and Gynaecologists

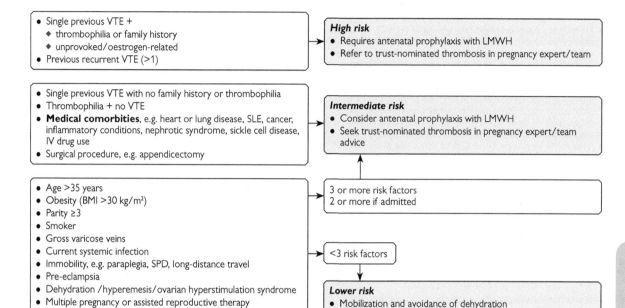

1.11 Hereditary Haemorrhagic Telangiectasia (Osler–Weber–Rendu Syndrome)

FACT FILE

Epidemiology and characteristics

- **Hereditary haemorrhagic telangiectasia (HHT), otherwise known as Osler–Weber–Rendu (OWR) syndrome** is an autosomal dominant syndrome characterized by an abnormal vasculature resulting in telangiectasia; arteriovenous malformations (AVM) are present in a variety of organs and tissues.
- HHT is characterized by the presence of multiple AVMs that lack intervening capillaries and result in direct connections between arteries and veins.[1] They appear as sharply demarcated reddish-purple spots on the skin, 1–2 mm in size, which disappear with slight pressure. They consist of a mat of tortuous vessels.
- Small AVMs (or telangiectases) close to the surface of the skin and mucous membranes often rupture and bleed after slight trauma.
- HHT is an autosomal dominant genetic condition that affects between 1 in 5000 and 1 in 8000 individuals and occurs in all ethnic groups and in both sexes.[2]
- Most patients are unaware that they have this condition, considering their nosebleeds or skin lesions to be 'common' occurrences,[3,4]

Clinical manifestations

- The main clinical manifestations are recurrent nosebleeds; characteristic mucocutaneous telangiectasia especially on the lips, tongue, oral mucosa, and fingertips; and anaemia.
- Most affected individuals will have an affected parent. Any child or sibling of an affected individual has a 50% chance of inheriting HHT. HHT can occur as de-novo mutations in individuals with no family history, but their offspring will have a 50% chance of inheriting HHT.
- Although HHT is a developmental disorder and infants are occasionally severely affected, in most people the features are age-dependent and the diagnosis is not suspected until adolescence or later.
- The manifestations of HHT do not usually appear at birth but symptoms develop with increasing age. Epistaxis appears earliest in childhood, pulmonary AVMs become apparent in puberty, mucocutaneous lesions in the 20s, and gastrointestinal telangiectasia develop with increasing age, usually after the age of 50 years.
- Mucocutaneous lesions mainly affect the hands and the wrists in about 40% and the face in about 33%.[5]
- HHT is a genetically heterogeneous condition, with considerable intrafamilial variability in its manifestations.
- Over 70% of those with HHT will have developed symptoms and signs of HHT by the age of 16 years. By the age of 40, nearly 90% of individuals display the manifestations of HHT.[3,5,6]
- Any offspring of a parent with HHT is at risk of having the disease since manifestations may not be seen until later in life. HHT can be excluded only by definitive molecular diagnosis.
- The gene locus for HHT type 1 is on 9q34, that for HHT type 2 is mapped to chromosome 12 and a third type, HHT3, is mapped to chromosome 5. Pulmonary hypertension is associated with HHT2.
- Genetic testing for patients and their families is based on identification of mutations within implicated genes, most commonly **endoglin** for HHT1 and **ALK1** for HHT2.
- Prenatal testing is possible for pregnancies at increased risk only if the gene mutation in the family has been identified.
- Gastrointestinal tract AVMs usually account for anaemia because of either chronic slow bleeding or acute haemorrhage. The anaemia may be profound enough to warrant repeated blood transfusions. GI bleeding is treated with iron replacement therapy and (if needed) endoscopic ablation, surgical resection of bleeding sites, and/or hormonal or antifibrinolytic therapy
- **Silent AVMs** are also common in HHT-affected individuals, and are found in pulmonary, hepatic, and cerebral circulations. AVMs are the second most common vascular abnormalities found in HHT.[3,7] They are considerably larger than telangiectasis and the morbidity/mortality associated with HHT is mainly due to AVMs in viscera such as the lungs, brain, GI tract, liver, and spine. Large AVMs often cause symptoms when they occur in the brain, liver, or lungs; complications from bleeding or shunting may be sudden and catastrophic.
- Pulmonary AVMs occur in at least 48% of women with HHT,[8,9] cerebral AVMs[10,11] in up to 10%, hepatic AVMs in about 30%,[12] GI tract AVMs in 11–40% (with or without bleeding), and spinal AVMs in about 0.3–1%.[4]

Curacao criteria for HHT diagnosis

- **Criteria:**
  - Epistaxis: spontaneous and recurrent
  - Telangiectasia: Multiple, at characteristic sites such as lips, tongue, oral cavity, nose, fingers
  - Visceral AVMs: Pulmonary, cerebral, gastrointestinal, hepatic, spine, bladder, bronchi, and even in the vagina.
  - Family history of a first-degree relative with HHT according to the criteria.
- The HHT **diagnosis** is:[13,14]
  - **Definite:** If three of the criteria are present
  - **Possible or suspected:** If two criteria are present
  - **Unlikely:** If fewer than two criteria are present.

Reproduced from CL Shovlin, 'Diagnostic criteria for hereditary hemorrhagic telangiectasia (Rendu-Osler syndrome)', *American Journal of Medical Genetics Part A, 91, 1, pp. 66–67, copyright 2000, with permission from Wiley-Liss, Inc*

HHT in the non-pregnant state

- **Epistaxis:** Due to telangiectasia of the nasal mucosa, usually requiring only iron supplements; occasionally nasal packing, even blood transfusion, may be required. Cauterization best avoided due to potential damage to the mucosa and vascular regrowth.[15] Individuals with significant epistaxis are advised to avoid vigorous nose blowing, lifting of heavy objects, straining during bowel movements, and finger manipulation in the nose.[1]
- **GI haemorrhage:** Seen in about 33% of patients with HHT. Iron supplementation is usually indicated but blood transfusions may be required. Antihaemorrhagic medical management and surgery have been tried with varying success in non-pregnant individuals, as has repeated laser therapy as a short-term measure of controlling bleeding.
- **Pulmonary AVMs:**Thin-walled bulbous vascular malformations that connect pulmonary arterial and venous circulations, replacing capillaries. Neurological sequelae due to paradoxical emboli or the risk of haemorrhage exist even in silent pulmonaryAVMs. A third of patients with pulmonary AVMs may show signs of right–left shunts**.** Treatment is by transcatheter embolization of the AVM. Prophylactic antibiotics are needed for any surgery or dental procedure to reduce the risk of brain abscess.
- **Cerebral AVMs:** Found in 10% of those with HHT; may lead to haemorrhage with catastrophic consequences. Neurological interventions may be required if cerebral AVM is detected by MRI.
- ***Patients with confirmed or suspected HHT should be screened for brain and lung AVMs using MRI of the brain and contrast echocardiography.***

HHT and pregnancy

- Women with treated pulmonary AVMs appear to be at no higher risk during pregnancy than those without pulmonary AVMs.
- While the majority of pregnancies in women with HHT proceed uneventfully, life-threatening events such as pulmonary AVM haemorrhage, myocardial infarction, and strokes can occur.[3]

- Prior awareness of the condition, especially of the presence of a pulmonary AVM, and appropriate advice could improve survival if such catastrophes occur in pregnancy.[3]
- Prenatal diagnosis for pregnancies at increased risk is possible by analysis of DNA extracted from fetal cells obtained by CVS or amniocentesis. However, prenatal testing can be offered only if the disease-causing allele of the affected family member has been identified.
- Pulmonary AVMs tend to enlarge during pregnancy and fatal haemorrhages have been described.
- Ideally, in HHT-affected women, screening and treatment of pulmonary AVMs should have taken place before pregnancy so as to reduce the risks of later problems such as haemorrhage or neurological sequelae due to paradoxical embolism.
- A pregnant woman who has not had a recent pulmonary evaluation should be evaluated as soon as pregnancy is recognized.[3,9] Chest CT, with abdominal shielding, should be delayed until the second trimester.
- Women not discovered to have pulmonary AVMs until they are already pregnant may be recommended to undergo occlusion during the second trimester.
- Complications are found to occur mainly in the second and third trimesters of pregnancy, probably linked to a decrease in the peripheral resistance and increased cardiac output.
- Pre-planning of management of any emergency complication is essential.
- Emergency interventions in the event of complications such as haemorrhage from a pulmonary AVM or cerebral AVM must be treated on a case-to-case basis with the immediate involvement of a multidisciplinary team.
- Any pregnancy in a woman with HHT must be considered as high risk. It is important that the patient, while being reassured that most pregnancies proceed uneventfully with good maternal and neonatal outcomes, is made aware that in a few cases complications might develop.
- She should be advised to be vigilant for any **haemoptysis or sudden severe dyspnoea**, when immediate hospital admission and care are indicated. These may be signposts of underlying AVMs.
- Due to the rarity of the condition, it is not unusual for general healthcare providers involved in the care of the pregnancy not to be fully aware of the HHT-specific pregnancy risks. It is essential, therefore, that all healthcare professionals involved in the care of the pregnancy are kept informed of the need for immediate referral in the event of haemoptysis or sudden severe dyspnoea.[3]
- Women must be referred antenatally for senior anaesthetic assessment to enable plans to be drawn up for analgesia/anaesthesia requirements for labour and delivery.[15]
- Caution is required before prescribing anticoagulant and anti-inflammatory agents (including aspirin) in individuals with significant epistaxis or GI bleeding from an underlying AVM in pregnancy and the puerperium.
- MRI scan during pregnancy is indicated to exclude spinal AVMs (found in 1–2%) of those with HHT, if regional analgesia is to be considered.
- If contrast echocardiography is positive for pulmonary shunting, even if no pulmonary AVM is demonstrated by chest CT, a lifetime recommendation for prophylactic antibiotics protocol for any dental, surgical, or obstetric procedure (including labour and delivery) is required because of the risk of brain abscess, associated with right-to-left shunting.
- Antibiotics such as those used for cardioprophylaxis are essential during labour and delivery to reduce the risk of brain abscess in these patients.[14,15]
- For the same reason, an air filter, or extreme caution not to introduce air bubbles, is recommended with IV lines.
- A prolonged second stage is preferably avoided to minimize the Valsalva manoeuvre.[3]

Long-term follow up—GP/respiratory physician

- Annual evaluation including interval history for epistaxis or other bleeding, shortness of breath or decreased exercise tolerance, and headache or other neurologic symptoms.
- Periodic haematocrit/haemoglobin determination with appropriate treatment for anaemia.
- Re-evaluation for pulmonary AVM at approximately 5-year intervals.

Information for patients

Please see Information for patients: Hereditary haemorrhagic telangiectasia (p. 496)

References

1. McDonald J, Pyeritz RE Hereditary hemorrhagic telangiectasia. 2000 Jun 26 [Updated 2012 Jan 5]. In: Pagon RA, et al., ed., GeneReviews [Internet]. Seattle,WA: University of Washington, Seattle, 1993-2013 <http://www.ncbi.nlm.nih.gov/books/NBK1351/>
2. Guttmacher AE, et al. Hereditary hemorrhagic telangiectasia. In:Rimoin DL, et al., ed. Principles and practice of medical genetics. Philadelphia, PA: Churchill Livingstone Elsevier, 2012.
3. Shovlin CL, et al. Estimates of maternal risks of pregnancy for women with hereditary haemorrhagic telangiectasia (Osler-Weber-Rendu syndrome): suggested approach for obstetric services. BJOG 2008;115: 1108–1115.
4. Shovlin CL Hereditary haemorrhagic telangiectasia: pathophysiology, diagnosis and treatment. Blood Rev 2010;24: 203–219.
5. Porteous ME, et al. Hereditary haemorrhagic telangiectasia: a clinical analysis. J Med Genet 1992;29: 527–530.
6. Shovlin CL, et al. Diagnostic criteria for hereditary haemorrhagic telangiectasia (Rendu-Osler-Weber syndrome). Am J Med Genet 2000;91: 66–67.
7. Sharathkumar AA, Shapiro A Hereditary haemorrhagic telangiectasia. Haemophilia 2008;14: 1269–1280.
8. Cottin V, et al. Pulmonary vascular manifestations of hereditary haemorrhagic telangiectasia (Rendu-Osler disease). Respiration 2007;74: 361–378.
9. Shovlin CL, et al. Medical complications of pregnancy in hereditary haemorrhagic telangiectasia. Q J Med 1995;88: 879–887.
10. Willemse RB Bleeding risk of cerebrovascular malformations in hereditary hemorrhagic telangiectasia. J Neurosurg 2000;92: 779–784.
11. Fulbright RK et al. MR of hereditary hemorrhagic telangiectasia: prevalence and spectrum of cerebrovascular malformations. Am J Neuroradiol 1998;19: 477–484.
12. Plauchu H, et al. Age-related clinical profile of hereditary hemorrhagic telangiectasia in an epidemiologically recruited population. Am J Med Genet 1989;32: 291–297.
13. Begbie ME, et al. Hereditary hemorrhagic telangiectasia (Osler-Weber-Rendu syndrome): a view from the 21st century. Postgrad Med J 2003;79: 18–24.
14. Faughnan ME, et al. International guidelines for the diagnosis and management of hereditary hemorrhagic telangiectasia. J Med Genet 2011;48: 73–87.
15. Waring PH, et al. Anesthetic management of a parturient with Osler-Weber-Rendu syndrome and rheumatic heart disease. Anesth Analg 1990;71: 96–99.

CARE PATHWAY

Pre-pregnancy assessment and advice in those previously diagnosed with HHT

- Screening for pulmonary, cerebral, or spinal arteriovenous malformations (AVMs) is ideally done before pregnancy and treated if found
- Discussion regarding prenatal diagnosis in familial HHT—possible only if gene mutation of family has been identified
- Treatment of anaemia, if present
- Reassure that most pregnancies proceed uneventfully with good fetal and maternal outcomes
- Multidisciplinary input is vital in management during pregnancy, involving consultants in obstetrics, radiology, thoracic medicine, anaesthetics, neurologist, gastroenterology, etc., depending on the site of any visceral AVM

HHT presenting for the first time in pregnancy

- Presenting features: Epistaxis, mucocutaneous telangiectasic spots, anaemia
- Enquiry regarding any suggestive family history
- Multidisciplinary involvement for assessment and appropriate investigations
- May require MRI scans to exclude cerebral, pulmonary, gastrointestinal, or spinal AVMs

↓

- In those who have not had pulmonary evaluation, CT of the chest(with shielding) may be required once in the 2nd trimester when organogenesis complete in 1st trimester
- Pulmonary AVMs may be treated in the 2nd trimester
- Iron supplementation if anaemic. Iron replacement is preferred for anaemia, but transfusion of packed red blood cells may be necessary for symptomatic anaemia
- Blood transfusion may be required, administered with an air filter in the giving set
- Urgent referral to senior anaesthetist
- If regional anaesthetic considered for labour/delivery, MRI scan of spine to exclude spinal AVMs
- Caution if prescribing aspirin or anticoagulants in those with GI bleeding or nose bleeds

↓

- **All healthcare staff need to be made aware of significance of symptoms: haemoptysis, sudden dyspnoea, sudden severe headache or visual disturbances, altered consciousness** may indicate bleeding from underlying GI, pulmonary, or cerebral AVMs, where immediate hospital admission is required
- Multidisciplinary pre-planning for any emergency such as haemorrhage from pulmonary or cerebral AVMs is essential
- Immediate transfer to a tertiary centre after initial stabilization is required
- Clear documentation of such plans and wide dissemination to all key personnel is essential
- Ensure there is a filter on all IV lines to prevent air bubbles from being inadvertently infused
- Antibiotic prophylaxis (as in cardioprophylaxis) required for labour and delivery
- Prolonged second stage to be avoided
- Combined oral contraception can be used
- Long-term follow up by annual evaluation of symptomatology, regular haematocrit measurements, and 5-yearly re-evaluation for pulmonary AVMs
- Reassure patient that most pregnancies proceed uneventfully with good fetal and maternal outcomes
- Advise patient to be vigilant for and to immediately report any **haemoptysis or sudden dyspnoea** (may signify bleeding from gastrointestinal or pulmonary AVM)

1.12 Henoch–Schönlein Purpura

FACT FILE

Epidemiology

- **Henoch–Schönlein purpura (HSP)** is an IgA-mediated systemic vasculitis of small-calibre blood vessels.
- Although HSP can occur at any age, it predominantly affects children below the age of 10 years.
- HSP is the most common systemic vasculitis in children, with a male to female ratio of 2:1 and a peak incidence between 2 and 5 years of age.
- It is predominantly found in white populations.[1]
- HSP is often triggered by upper respiratory tract infections, certain medications, or exposure to certain chemicals; sometimes aggravated by cold weather.
- An inappropriate immune response to environmental triggers is postulated as basis for the production of immune complexes by B-lymphocytes with IgA deposition within the walls of small vessels and the renal mesangium.[2]

Clinical manifestations

- The spectrum of HSP can range from minor petechial rash to severe gastrointestinal, renal, neurological, and joint disease.[3]
- The **classic presentation** and therefore the diagnostic criteria of HSP[4,5] include:
  - Palpable, slightly raised vascular cutaneous purpuric rash or papules, which usually affect the extensor aspects of the lower limbs but may extend to the trunk.[6] The lesions start as erythematous macules which develop into purple, non-pruritic, non-blanching purpuric papules which may become confluent in severe cases.[3] Localized oedema of the subcutaneous tissues may occur.
  - Polyarthralgia, especially of the knees, ankles, elbows, and wrists, seen in 75% of cases. The arthralgia of HSP is of a non-migratory, transient and non-destructive variety and may precede the purpuric rash in 25% of cases.
  - Abdominal symptoms including periumbilical colicky pain, nausea, vomiting, diarrhoea, and GI bleeding, may occur in 75% of HSP.[7] In about 5% of cases, severe abdominal complications such as intussusception, bowel ischaemia, and necrosis may occur. It is not uncommon for patients with HSP presenting with an acute abdomen to undergo an unnecessary laparotomy.
  - Haematuria (microscopic or overt) and proteinuria due to glomerulonephritis occur in 25–50%. Renal involvement occurs in one-third of children and in 63% of adults with HSP.[8]
  - Histology of the arterioles or venules shows marked IgA deposition.
- In children, HSP is usually self-limiting, with symptom relapses occurring over to 4–6 weeks, before spontaneous resolution.

Prognosis

- Prognosis is excellent in children, unless there is nephritis. In cases where there is severe nephritis, 10–20% will develop chronic renal impairment and of these, 1% will progress to end-stage renal damage[9] which can occur even after a long latent period of up to 20 years after HSP is first diagnosed.[10]
- HSP is uncommon in adults, and rare in pregnancy.[2] In adults, the purpuric lesions are more prominent and resolution takes longer.[11] Renal involvement is more common as well as more severe in adults,[12] and in such cases 28% may progress to chronic renal failure.
- Infrequently, atypical presentations may involve the lungs and CNS, haemorrhagic pancreatitis, or intracerebral haemorrhage, especially in adults.

Course of HSP in pregnancy

- HSP may be exacerbated during pregnancy or may undergo remission.[13]
- The occurrence of HSP for the first time during pregnancy is extremely rare.
- If there has been a past history of HSP in young women, vigilance must be maintained during pregnancy for signs of any relapse or complications.
- **Diagnosis in pregnancy** tends to be more difficult as the symptoms could initially be non-specific with headaches, pyrexia, joint pains, and abdominal cramps especially if renal, GI, or joint manifestations occur before the cutaneous purpuric lesions become evident.

Diagnosis

- Laboratory investigations are mainly useful to exclude other diagnostic possibilities of purpura, vasculitis, nephritis, etc. Skin biopsy can be performed during pregnancy. Raised serum IgA is found. Since the severity and persistence of proteinuria are predictors of long-term disease, urine testing is mandatory.[14]
- Diagnosis is however, based on clinical grounds.

Differential diagnosis

- HSP may then be mistaken for pre-eclampsia, pregnancy-related hypertension, nephrotic syndrome, or other causes for abdominal pain such as abruption or appendicitis which might even lead to unnecessary laparotomy.

Prognosis in pregnancy

- If there is no renal impairment of HSP in adult women, the obstetric prognosis is good.
- Complications such as hypertension, pre-eclampsia, and sequelae are associated with those with renal involvement of HSP; the degree of renal impairment may worsen during pregnancy.[15]

Management of HSP in pregnancy

- The aims of management of HSP are primarily to alleviate acute symptoms, reduce short-term morbidity such as acute abdominal complications that might otherwise lead to unnecessary surgery, and prevent chronic renal impairment.[16]
- Care during pregnancy must ideally be multidisciplinary, with involvement of the renal physician, rheumatologist, gastroenterologist, obstetrician, and midwife.
- The patient must be reassured that there is very little risk of IgA vasculitis in the fetus and newborn, as these immunoglobulins cannot pass through the placenta.[17]
- In those with no renal impairment, HSP can be managed symptomatically. NSAIDs which are effective in pain control in children and in the non-pregnant state are to be **avoided** during pregnancy and the woman must be specifically advised about this.
- Low-dose aspirin from the 12th week of gestation may be used to reduce risk of pre-eclampsia in this targeted high-risk group of patients.
- ACE inhibitors which might have been used to reduce proteinuria in adults with HSP nephritis are contraindicated in pregnancy and must, ideally, have been withdrawn prior to pregnancy.
- Corticosteroids (e.g. a 4-week tapering course of prednisolone) have been widely used in treating HSP, although their role is controversial. They have been shown, if used early in the disease process, to rapidly reduce the urticarial purpura,[17,18] abdominal symptoms,[19] and arthralgia, and hasten resolution of mild nephritis.[20]
- Available evidence does not indicate that steroids shorten the duration of HSP or prevent recurrence or nephritis from developing.[20,21]
- Other immunosuppressive medications (e.g. azathioprine or cyclophosphamide), as well as plasmapheresis have been used in

the treatment of HSP. The monoclonal antibody rituximab is not currently recommended for use during pregnancy or lactation.[2]

- While the disease is active, weekly urinalysis for proteinuria and haematuria must be performed, reducing to monthly urinalysis for 3 months after disease resolution.[9]
- Serial growth and liquor volume scans are advisable especially with evidence of any degree of renal impairment and if steroids are used during pregnancy.
- ***If steroids have been used within a few weeks of labour, bolus doses of 100 mg IM of hydrocortisone must be offered every 6–8 h during labour and for delivery.***

Information for patients

Please see Information for patients: Henoch–Schönlein purpura (p. 497)

References

1. Galla JHC et al. Racial differences in the prevalence of IgA-associated nephropathies. Lancet 1984; ii: 522
2. Tayabali SC et al. Diagnosis and management of Henoch-Schönlein purpura in pregnancy: a review of the literature. Arch Gynecol Obstet 2012;286: 825–829.
3. Rai A, et al. Henoch-Schönlein purpura nephritis. J Am Soc Nephrol 1999;10: 2637–2644.
4. Mills JAC et al. The American College of Rheumatology 1990 criteria for the classification of Henoch-Schönlein purpura. Arthritis Rheum. 1990;33: 1114–1121.
5. Ozen SC et al. EULR/PReS endorsed consensus criteria for the classification of childhood vasculitides. Ann Rheum Dis 2006;65: 936–941.
6. Tancrede-Bohin EC et al. Henoch-Schönlein purpura in adult patients. Arch Dermatol 1997;133: 438–442.
7. Choong CK, Beasley SW Intra-abdominal manifestations of Henoch-Schönlein purpura. J Paediatr Child Health 1998;34: 405–409.
8. Rieu P, Noel LH Henoch-Schönlein nephritis in children and adults: morphologic features and clinicopathological correlations. Ann Med Interne 1999;150: 151–159.
9. Saulsbury FT Clinical update: Henoch-Schönlein purpura. Lancet 2007;369: 976–978.
10. Goldstein ARC et al. Long-term follow-up of childhood. Henoch-Schönlein nephritis. Lancet 1992;339: 280–282.
11. Michel BA, et al. Hypersensitivity vasculitis and Henoch-Schönlein purpura: a comparison between the 2 disorders. J Rheumatol 1992;19: 721–728.
12. Blanco R, et al. Henoch-Schönlein purpura in adulthood and Childhood. Arthritis Rheum 1997;40: 859–864.
13. Merrill J, Lahita R. Henoch- Schönlein purpura remitting in pregnancy and during sex steroid therapy. Br J Rheumatol 1994;33: 586–588.
14. Rychlik I, et al. Clinical features and natural history of IgA nephropathy. Ann Med Interne 1999;150: 117–126.
15. Yasukawa K, et al. Henoch-Schönlein nephritis and nephrotic syndrome during pregnancy. Nihon Rinsho Meneki Gakkai Kaishi 1996;19: 505–511.
16. Weiss PF, et al. Effects of corticosteroid on Henoch-Schönlein purpura: a systematic review. Pediatrics 2007;120: 1079–1087.
17. Feldmann R, et al. Henoch-Schönlein purpura during pregnancy with successful outcome for mother and newborn. BMC Dermatol 2002;2: 1.
18. Kalmantis K, et al. Henoch-Schönlein purpura in pregnancy. J Obstet Gynaecol Res 2008;28: 403–405.
19. Itoh K, et al. A case of pregnancy with Henoch-Schönlein purpura. Nihon Sanka Fujinka Gakkai Zasshi 1994;46: 461–464.
20. Ronkainen J, et al. Early prednisolone therapy in Henoch-Schönlein purpura: a randomized, double- blind, placebo-controlled trial. J Pediatr 2006;149: 241–247.
21. Chartapisak W, et al. Prevention and treatment of renal disease in Henoch-Schönlein purpura: a systematic review. Arch Dis Child 2009;94: 132–137.

CARE PATHWAY

Patient known to have had HSP in the past

- Refer to maternal medicine/specialist antenatal clinic in pregnancy within 1st trimester

Pregnant patient without a known past history of HSP

- Presents with typical purpuric rash, arthralgia, abdominal symptoms, haematuria (macro- or microscopic) ± proteinuria. Consider HPS, though rare in pregnancy
- Lab tests to exclude other causes for symptoms
- Skin biopsy may be required—IgA deposition in walls of small blood vessels
- Refer to maternal medicine/specialist antenatal clinic

Multidisciplinary care with obstetrician, midwife, nephrologist, GI physician, rheumatologist as directed by disease presentation and severity

- If on ACE inhibitors, advise to stop them immediately
- Assess renal involvement in HPS. If present, assess severity based on weekly proteinuria measurement while disease is active, then monthly for 3 months
- Consider prophylactic low-dose aspirin as these patients are more prone to develop PIH and pre-eclampsia
- Vigilance for development of complications—pre-eclampsia, PIH, IUGR, worsening of renal impairment, etc.
- Reassure mother that there is very little chance of fetal/neonatal vasculitis as IgA does not cross placenta

Active disease relapse during pregnancy with renal involvement

- Weekly urine collection for total protein, after acute episode resolves, monthly checks for up to 3 months
- Most will require only symptomatic treatment with analgesia, but NSAIDs are not to be used during pregnancy
- Consider steroids—4 weeks of prednisolone in tapering doses if severe purpuric/abdominal manifestations
- Other immunosuppressants (e.g. azathioprine, cyclophosphamide) may be added as directed by multidisciplinary team
- Serial scans for growth and liquor volume
- In absence of obstetric complications such as PIH, pre-eclampsia, IUGR etc., **no change in management of pregnancy, labour, or delivery**
- Long-term follow-up by nephrologist of HSP nephritis patients is highly advisable

- Assessment of severity of HPS
- Assessment for renal involvement, degree of impairment to be assessed by amount of proteinuria
- Weekly proteinuria measurement while disease is active, then monthly for 3 months after resolution

- Most cases are mild and require only symptomatic treatment with analgesia, but NSAIDs are not to be used in pregnancy
- If severe purpuric rash, GI bleeding, or dense proteinuria, consider early commencement of steroids (prednisolone in tapering doses over 4 weeks)
- Vigilance for complications particularly in 3rd trimester (e.g. PIH, pre-eclampsia, IUGR, progressive renal impairment)
- If hypertensive, treat with methyldopa/labetalol
- Serial scans for growth and liquor volume
- Other immunosuppressants (e.g. azathioprine, cyclophosphamide) may be added as directed by multidisciplinary team
- In the absence of obstetric complications such as PIH, pre-eclampsia, IUGR, etc., **no change in management of pregnancy, labour or delivery**
- Reassure mother that very little chance of fetal/neonatal vasculitis as IgA does not cross the placenta
- Long-term follow-up of HSP nephritis by nephrologist is highly advisable. Ensure follow-up nephrology appointment is arranged before postnatal discharge

1.13 Hermansky–Pudlak Syndrome

FACT FILE

Epidemiology, genotypes, and clinical manifestations

- **Hermansky–Pudlak syndrome (HPS)** is an autosomal recessive multisystem disorder characterized by ocular and cutaneous albinism, bleeding diathesis, and visual impairment.[1,2,3,4,5,6]
- Those affected by HPS have tyrosinase-positive oculocutaneous albinism.
- Bleeding complications occur as a result of platelet dysfunction, the effects of which can range mild mucocutaneous bleeding to life-threatening haemorrhage, the latter encountered in about 15% of those with HPS.
- Tissue accumulation of ceroid pigment (a waxy lipoprotein complex), especially in the lysosomes, can lead to progressive restrictive pulmonary fibrosis (seen in up to 50% of HPS), inflammatory bowel disease resembling Crohn's disease (seen in 15% of HPS patients), and renal failure.[1,2,3,4,5,6]
- Premature mortality, around the fifth decade, can occur in about 50% of those with severe pulmonary fibrosis.[3]
- The worldwide prevalence is 1 in 500 000 to 1 in 1 000 000, with a preponderance in Puerto Rican communities where the reported prevalence is 1 in 1800.[5] Patients with various types of HPS have also been reported in other countries and populations.
- A variety of genotypes are found, HPS 1 located on chromosome 10 being the most common.
- Due to the variety of the various genotypes involved, skin colour in those with HPS can range from olive to white, transillumination of the iris with colours including blue, green or brown, and hair colour from white to brown.[6] In those with HPS3 there is only minimal cutaneous albinism but ocular signs predominate.
- Other skin conditions in HPS include excessive freckles, lentigines, and solar keratosis.
- Patients usually have congenital nystagmus, strabismus and decreased visual acuity.[8]
- In HPS, the platelet defect is a storage pool deficiency associated with decreased number or absence of **'dense'** bodies, although the platelets appear morphologically normal. 'Dense' bodies in the platelets store ATP, ADP, calcium, and serotonin, which when released activate the second wave of platelet aggregation required to maintain the normal bleeding time.[9]
- Coexistence of vWD must be excluded.
- Women with HPS often have prolonged heavy periods (seen in over 60%),[5] epistaxis, gingival bleeding, and easy bruising. Any woman with HPS needs early referral to the haematologist.
- A diagnosis of HPS must be considered in any pregnant woman presenting with albinism, particularly of the oculocutaneous variety.
- Referral to clinical genetics is recommended for evaluation of the patient with the syndrome and her family and for identification of the type of HPS gene mutation.

HPS in pregnancy

- **Antenatal diagnosis** of the underlying HPS facilitates multidisciplinary planning and limitation of risk.
- A **properly organized birth plan** has to be devised by a multidisciplinary team consisting of the haematologist, specialist obstetrician, anaesthetist, and senior midwife in charge of the delivery suite.
- All NSAIDs including aspirin and diclofenac are strictly contraindicated in any patient with HPS because of their antiplatelet effects.
- Since osteoporosis has been reported in patients with oculocutaneous albinism, pregnant patients with HPS may benefit from vitamin D and calcium supplementation.
- Two main issues arise in pregnancies complicated by HPS, The first is that **any form of regional analgesia is contraindicated, including an epidural to provide pain relief in labour and a spinal anaesthetic for Caesarean section, if one is required for any obstetric reason.** The patient must be made aware that if a Caesarean section is required for any obstetric indication, this would need to take place under general anaesthetic.
- Discussions about alternatives for labour analgesia need to be arranged during pregnancy by referral to the anaesthetic high-risk clinic. These alternatives may include Entonox®, opiates such as diamorphine or pethidine or patient-controlled analgesia using fentanyl.[7]
- The other serious risk lies in the increased **chance of postpartum haemorrhage** and prophylactic measures should be planned well ahead of time. These measures include:
  - Early engagement of the specialist obstetrician with the haematologist, senior midwife of delivery suite, and consultant anaesthetist.
  - Desmopressin (DDAVP®) (the synthetic analogue of the pituitary-secreted antidiuretic hormone, arginine vasopressin) at the standard dose of 0.3 micrograms/kg body weight in 50 ml normal saline IV over 20 min can be administered **immediately after delivery. The response to desmopressin (DDAVP®) is, however, not guaranteed and the patient may still require platelet transfusion.**[7,10]
  - A combination of desmopressin (DDAVP®) and tranexemic acid has also been suggested as being more effective in achieving haemostasis.[9]
  - During the antenatal period, HLA typing of the platelets is recommended to facilitate storage of the HLA-matched platelets for that particular patient if required at delivery and peripartum.
  - HLA-matched platelets must be kept ready and transfused promptly if there are any signs of excess bleeding after delivery.
  - Active management of the third stage with IV oxytocin as bolus as well as oxytocin high-dose infusion is continued for 4–6 h post-delivery, avoiding water intoxication.
  - Under the cover of desmopressin (DDAVP®) ± HLA-matched platelets, any perineal tear or episiotomy needs to be repaired without delay with attention to achieving good closure and surgical haemostasis as soon as possible. Similarly, manual removal of a retained or partially separated placenta must not be delayed because of the potential for severe PPH.

Information for patients

Please see Information for patients: Hermansky–Pudlak syndrome (p. 497)

References

1. Gahl WA, et al. Genetic defects and clinical characteristics of patients with a form of oculocutaneous albinism (Hermansky-Pudlak syndrome). N Engl J Med 1998;338: 1258–1264.
2. Tong IL, Bourjeily G Hermanksy-Pudlak syndrome in the peripartum period. Obstet Med 2008;1: 95–96.
3. Gahl WA, et al. Effect of pirfenidone on the pulmonary fibrosis of Hermansky-Pudlak syndrome. Mol Genet Metab 2002;76: 234–242.
4. Kouklakis G, et al. Complicated Crohn's-like colitis, associated with Hermansky-Pudlak syndrome, treated with Infliximab: a case report and brief review of the literature. J Med Case Rep 2007;1: 176.
5. Witkop CJ, et al. Albinism and Hermansky-Pudlak syndrome in Puerto Rico. Bol Asoc Med P R 1990;82: 333–339.
6. Reynolds SP, et al. Diffuse pulmonary fibrosis and the Hermansky-Pudlak syndrome: clinical course and postmortem findings. Thorax 1994;49: 617–618.
7. Poddar RK, et al. Hermansky-Pudlak syndrome in a pregnant patient. Br J Anaesth 2004;93: 740–742.
8. Gradstein L, et al. Eye movement abnormalities in Hermansky-Pudlak syndrome. () J AAPOS 2005;9: 369–378.
9. Saif MW, Hamilton JM. A 25 year old woman presenting with bleeding disorder and nystagmus. Postgrad Med J 2001;77: e6.
10. Trigg DE, et al. A systematic review: the use of desmopressin for treatment and prophylaxis of bleeding disorders in pregnancy. Haemophilia 2012;18: 25–33.

CARE PATHWAY

- Most cases already known to have **Hermansky–Pudlak syndrome (HPS)** before pregnancy
- Community midwife refers woman to a specialist antenatal clinic in the 1st trimester

No known renal involvement

- Routine antenatal assessment and booking blood tests; in addition, baseline renal function tests
- Reassure woman that pregnancy is likely to be relatively uncomplicated, with very little impact on fetus and neonate as these immunoglobulins do not cross the placenta
- Symptoms of HSP may be exacerbated or undergo remission in pregnancy
- Any acute symptoms(e.g. abdominal cramps, headaches, joint pains, pyrexia) should be treated symptomatically
- Consider low-dose aspirin 75 mg from 12 weeks gestation due to higher risk of pre-eclampsia
- All other NSAIDs (including adult-strength aspirin) must be avoided
- Continued vigilance maintained for pregnancy-induced hypertension (PIH) and pre-eclampsia
- ***In absence of pre-eclampsia or PIH, no need to change management during pregnancy, labour, or delivery***

Prior renal impairment

- Routine antenatal assessment and booking blood tests; in addition, baseline renal function tests
- Multidisciplinary care with renal physician as renal impairment may worsen during pregnancy
- If ACE inhibitors were used to reduce proteinuria in those with HSP nephritis, they should be stopped as soon as pregnancy confirmed, if not earlier. **Ensure that ACE inhibitors have been stopped**
- Prescribe low-dose aspirin 75 mg from 12 weeks gestation to end of pregnancy
- Repeat renal function tests in each trimester, more frequently as directed by renal physician
- If azathioprine is used as a disease-modifying agent in HSP nephritis, this can be continued in pregnancy
- Steroids may be needed during phase of active disease as advised by renal physicians—usually as a tapered-down course of 4 weeks
- If dense proteinuria present, prophylactic LMWH must be considered.

Subsequent antenatal clinic visits

- Frequency to be individualized
- During the active phase, frequent surveillance for worsening nephritis, repeat renal function tests including total protein loss/24 h
- Serial growth and liquor volume scans at frequencies according to individual unit's policy
- If long-term steroid use, GTT at 28 weeks to exclude steroid-induced gestational diabetes
- If steroids have been used during pregnancy, hydrocortisone cover required for labour and delivery—IM hydrocortisone 6–8 hourly during labour and for delivery
- Continued close vigilance maintained for pregnancy induced hypertension (PIH) and pre-eclampsia

- If PIH or pre-eclampsia develops, for further management see Chapter 5.1
- If IUGR, for further management see Chapter 26
- Timing of delivery depends on development and severity of PIH or pre-eclampsia or IUGR

1.14 Hereditary Spherocytosis

FACT FILE

Epidemiology

- **Hereditary spherocytosis (HS)** is the most common cause of haemolysis in northern Europe and the US. The incidence is about 1 in 2000 to 1 in 5000,[1,2,3]
- HS has been reported in all ethnic groups.
- Most cases (75%) will have a family history of HS.
- HS is inherited mainly as an autosomal dominant condition in about 75% and as a recessive condition in about a quarter of all HS cases. In a few, it can occur as a de-novo mutation, which, however, will be passed on to the offspring in an autosomal dominant pattern.[4,5]
- Mild cases may remain undetected till adulthood.
- The defect in HS lies in a destabilized red cell membrane. This leads to an abnormal morphology and a reduction in the red cell lifespan from the normal 120 days to a few days. The abnormal spherical red cells are less resistant to stress and tend to rupture, resulting in chronic haemolytic anaemia.
- The shorter the red cell lifespan, the worse the clinical effects.

Clinical features

- Clinical features of HS vary in severity from being mild and symptom-free to severe haemolysis, continued anaemia, and jaundice.[2,3]
- HS can present at any age from the neonatal period onwards, depending on the severity.
- The classic clinical features of haemolysis seen in HS include the triad of **anaemia, jaundice, and splenomegaly**.
- **Splenomegaly** in HS is a common feature, usually mild. There is no increased tendency for splenic rupture in those with the splenomegaly of HS compared with unaffected individuals.

Classification

- HS is classified as mild, moderate or severe.[3,6]

Mild HS (20–30%)

- No anaemia usually, modest reticulocytosis, jaundice and splenomegaly may be absent or mild. The disorder may not be diagnosed till adulthood and may come to light only when booking blood tests are performed in a first pregnancy or the incidental finding of splenomegaly.
- Anaemia is mild as the bone marrow compensates by increasing red cell production by some 6–8-fold. In these cases, the finding of raised reticulocytes (reflecting increased marrow output of red blood cells) may be the only clue.
- Jaundice may or may not be present in such compensated mild cases of HS. If, however, any intercurrent infection challenges the bone marrow, jaundice may come to light.[2]

Moderate HS (60–75%)

- Individuals have anaemia, high reticulocyte counts, and raised serum bilirubin and may require frequent blood transfusions. Usually detected in infancy or childhood.

Severe HS (5%)

- Characterized by marked haemolysis, persistent anaemia, jaundice (hyperbilirubinaemia), splenomegaly, and a regular requirement for red cell transfusions. Children with severe HS may be transfusion dependent, especially in the first few years of life.
- Haemolysis results in increased red cell turnover and increased hepatic pigment load. This can result in the early development of gall stones in the first or second decade.[2] The higher the reticulocyte count, greater the chances of early development of gallstones and this may be a pointer to consider splenectomy.

Laboratory diagnosis

- Finding spherocytes on the blood film and a raised reticulocyte count, with or without anaemia.
- Reduced MCV and increased red cell haemoglobin concentration (MCHC).
- Other haematological disorders such as beta-thalassaemia or sickle cell disease may sometimes confuse the diagnosis. Iron, folic acid or vitamin B_{12} deficiency can also mask the laboratory features.
- ***With these simple tests and a positive family history, no further investigations are required to make the diagnosis of HS. Confirmatory tests, if required in atypical cases, are by cryohaemolysis test and eosin-5-maleimide (EMA) binding.***[2,3]

Clinical management

- *Parvovirus B19 can result in a brief period of red cell aplasia, which in the individual (child or adult) can result in feeling unwell and a profound fall in haemoglobin levels, sometimes to 20–30 g/litre.*
- Once recovered, the individual carries lifelong immunity for parvovirus B19. No other infection produces such a profound fall in haemoglobin in those with HS as parvovirus B19.
- Women with HS who are not immune to parvovirus B19 who are planning a pregnancy or are pregnant must be warned about symptoms and severe anaemia which might warrant blood transfusion, should she contract parvovirus B19.
- Usually HS patients are on supplemental folic acid therapy of 5 mg/day, which should be continued throughout pregnancy.
- If the patient has had a previous splenectomy, lifelong prophylactic penicillin prophylaxis is necessary[3,8] as there is a continued susceptibility to overwhelming infection, particularly with the pneumococcal species. This risk is not completely eliminated by the presplenectomy vaccination.[3] Patients (and parents) must be informed of this and **splenectomy cards must be issued to patients.**
- Post-splenectomy, platelet counts rise sometimes to as high as 1000×10^9/litre; this does not in itself pose a threat for thrombosis in those with HS,[2,3] unless there are other risk factors.
- As pregnancy is a hypercoagulable state, use of below knee compression stockings as well as low-dose aspirin is usually recommended in pregnancy for women with HS who have postsplenectomy thrombocytosis.
- Perioperative and postpartum SC LMWH thromboprophylaxis with thromboembolic deterrent for at least 6 weeks postpartum may need to be considered.
- All women must be prescribed 5 mg folic acid preferably started pre-pregnancy and continued throughout pregnancy.
- During pregnancy, some non-splenectomized women may develop sufficiently severe anaemia to need blood transfusion.[3,9]
- There are some reports regarding laparoscopic splenectomy during the first half of pregnancy.[10,11,12,13]
- Maternal and fetal outcomes are better in women after a splenectomy than before.[9]

Information for patients

Please see Information for patients: Hereditary spherocytosis (p. 497)

References

1. Eber SW, et al. Prevalence of increased osmotic fragility of erythrocytes in German blood donors: screening using a modified glycerol lysis test. Ann Hematol 1992;64: 88–92.
2. Bolton-Maggs P Hereditary spherocytosis: new guidelines. Arch Dis Child 2004;89: 809–812.
3. Bolton-Maggs PHB, et al. Guidelines for the diagnosis and management of hereditary spherocytosis. London: British Committee for Standards in Haematology, 2011 <http://www.bcshguidelines.com>.
4. Gallagher PG, Lux SE Disorders of the erythrocyte membrane. In:Nathan DG, et al, ed., Nathan and Oski's hematology of infancy and childhood 6th ed. Philadelphia, PA: Saunders Elsevier, 2003, pp. 561–684.

5. Alloisio N, et al. Modulation of clinical expression and band 3 deficiency in hereditary spherocytosis. Blood 1997;90: 414–420.
6. Eber SW, et al. Variable clinical severity of hereditary spherocytosis: relation to erythrocytic spectrin concentration, osmotic fragility and autohemolysis. J Pediatr 1990;177: 409–411.
7. Tchernia G, et al. Recombinant erythropoietin therapy as an alternative to blood transfusions in infants with hereditary spherocytosis. Hematol J 2000;1: 146–152.
8. Davies KA, et al. Long-term management after splenectomy. Consider prophylaxis in systematic lupus erythematosus. BMJ 1994;308: 133.
9. Pajor A, et al. Pregnancy and hereditary spherocytosis; report of 8 patients and a review. Arch Gynecol Obstet 1993;253: 37–41.
10. Moore A, et al. Hereditary spherocytosis with hemolytic crisis during pregnancy. Treatment by splenectomy. Obstet Gynecol 1976;47: 19–21.
11. Maberry MC, et al. Pregnancy complicated by hereditary spherocytosis. Obstet Gynecol 1992;79: 735–738.
12. Allran C F Jr. Urgent laparoscopic splenectomy in a morbidly obese pregnant woman: case report and literature review. J Laparoendosc Adv Surg Tech A 2002;12: 445–447.
13. Khanna SB, Kiranbala D Hereditary spherocytosis with pregnancy—a case report. J Obst Gynecol 2011;61: 205–207.

CARE PATHWAY

Pregnant patient not previously known to have hereditary spherocytosis (HS)

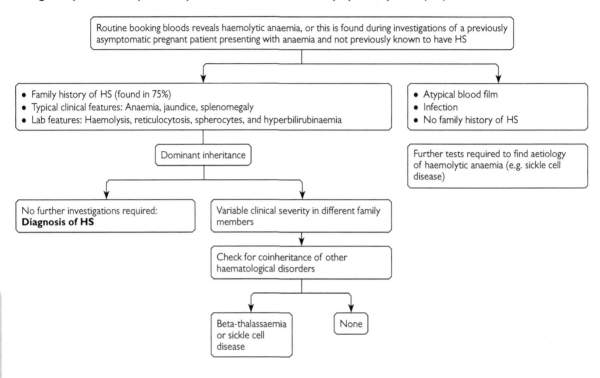

Routine booking bloods reveals haemolytic anaemia, or this is found during investigations of a previously asymptomatic pregnant patient presenting with anaemia and not previously known to have HS

- Family history of HS (found in 75%)
- Typical clinical features: Anaemia, jaundice, splenomegaly
- Lab features: Haemolysis, reticulocytosis, spherocytes, and hyperbilirubinaemia

Dominant inheritance

No further investigations required: **Diagnosis of HS**

Variable clinical severity in different family members

Check for coinheritance of other haematological disorders

Beta-thalassaemia or sickle cell disease

None

- Atypical blood film
- Infection
- No family history of HS

Further tests required to find aetiology of haemolytic anaemia (e.g. sickle cell disease)

Pregnant patient already known to have HS

Check has had genetic counselling

Previous splenectomy

- Long-term antibiotics to continue
- Folate 5 mg throughout pregnancy
- Check parvovirus B19 status: If susceptible, warn regarding chance of moderate temporary worsening of anaemia, usually spontaneous recovery if contracts infection during pregnancy. If immune, reassure
- Ensure patient carries splenectomy card
- Remind patient and family: Despite pre-splenectomy vaccinations as well as lifelong antibiotics, a small risk of increased susceptibility to severe sepsis persists
- Post-splenectomy thrombocytosis: Prescribe low-dose aspirin 75 mg daily throughout pregnancy, Thromboembolic deterrent stockings. Discuss post-delivery thromboprophylaxis with haematology consultant, document this in notes
- Anaesthetic referral, Haematology follow-up
- Rest of pregnancy care as normal
- No indication for early IOL or LSCS except for obstetric reasons

Spleen present

- Ensure early multidisciplinary involvement of haematologist, maternal medicine obstetrician, and midwife
- Degree of severity of HS to be established by obtaining careful history, clinical and haematological findings
- Folate 5 mg throughout pregnancy
- Check parvovirus B19 status: If susceptible, warn regarding chances of severe temporary worsening of haemolytic anaemia, may need blood transfusion, usually spontaneous recovery. If immune to parvovirus B19, reassure
- May develop episodes of abdominal pain if gallstones are present, confirmed by ultrasound scans; advise to report symptoms
- Advise patient that she may need blood transfusion if severe haemolysis due to intercurrent infection or persistent severe anaemia
- Fetal serial growth scans, Dopplers
- Anaesthetic referral, haematology follow-up
- Frequency of antenatal clinic visits to be individualized
- Interventions such as early IOL or LSCS for obstetric reasons only.

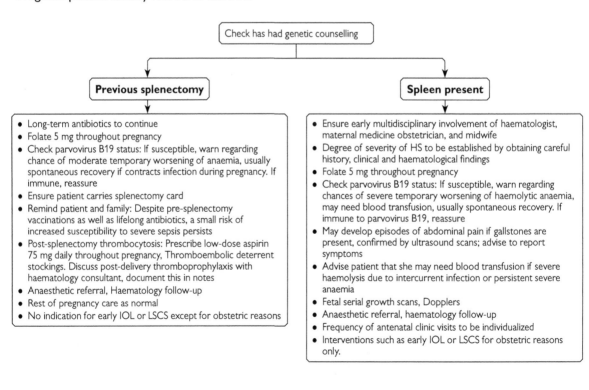

1.15 Thrombotic Thrombocytopenic Purpura—Haemolytic–Uraemic Syndrome

FACT FILE

Epidemiology

- **Thrombotic thrombocytopenic purpura (TTS) and haemolytic–uraemic syndrome (HUS)** are believed to be different clinical manifestations of the same underlying disease, and will be referred to as one entity, **TTP-HUS**, in this chapter.
- TTP is rare, with a reported incidence of 6 cases per million per year in the general population in the UK.[1]
- **TTP-HUS is a severe condition with high maternal morbidity and mortality rates.**
- Untreated mortality is 90%, which can be reduced with prompt **plasma exchange (PEX).** Tertiary referral centres and some larger district general hospitals have the capacity to institute the PEX programme and **prompt transfer to such a centre, as recommended by the haematologist from the local hospital, is mandatory.**
- Despite this, early death still occurs with about one-half of the deaths in the UK registry occurring within 24 h of presentation, primarily in women.[1]
- TTP-HUS is found more often in women. This is probably due to the greater incidence of autoimmune conditions among women, suggesting a potential autoimmune basis for TTP-HUS.[2]
- There is also an increased association of TTP-HUS and pregnancy, suggesting a causal association.[2,3,4,5] About 12–31% of TTP-HUS in women occurs during pregnancy and postpartum.[2,4,6,7,8,9]

Pathogenesis of TTP-HUS

- Microvascular platelet aggregation, causing blockages in the arterioles and capillaries, is the common pathology involved. With consumption of aggregated platelets at sites of endothelial inflammation or injury, both thrombocytopenia and microangiopathic haemolytic anaemia can ensue.
- In TTP-HUS, there is a diffuse endothelial insult and the blockage caused by aggregation of platelets at these sites, which can produce tissue ischaemia and infarction.
- In TTP, the platelet thrombi are found to contain increased amounts of an abnormal ultra-large form of vWF secreted by the endothelial cells, which in turn act as potent platelet aggregators. There is also a deficiency of the vWF-cleaving protease **(ADAMTS13)** and, in some patients, decreased levels of prostacyclin (PGI2) which is an antiplatelet aggregator normally produced in the endothelial cells, are also found.
- It is now recognized that congenital and acute acquired TTP are due to a deficiency of ADAMTS13.[10,11]
- Women who are heterozygous for ADAMTS13 deficiency may become severely deficient during pregnancy. Women, with additional risk factors for thrombosis in TTP-HUS factors, such as obesity and the factor V Leiden mutation, may be at additional risk for TTP-HUS, when there is moderate ADAMTS13 deficiency.
- If this process is extensive and the CNS bears the brunt, the condition is referred to as TTP and can occur at any stage of pregnancy and puerperium.
- Congenital TTP is due to an inherited deficiency of ADAMTS13, but acquired immune TTP is due to the reduction of ADAMTS13 by autoantibodies directed against ADAMTS13.[12]
- In some familial TTP-HUS cases there is congenital deficiency of ADAMTS13.[12,13] Though the affected individuals could suffer recurrent acute episodes of TTP-HUS during infancy, other events, such as infection, pregnancy, or surgery, appear to be the main precipitating factors.
- If platelet aggregation is less extensive and the renal manifestations are predominant, especially in the postnatal period, it is termed HUS. While 'typical' HUS is more common in children and usually preceded by a diarrhoeal illness caused by Shiga toxin-producing *E. coli*, in adults HUS is mainly of an 'atypical' variety.[14]
- Atypical HUS[14,15,16] is similar to TTP but with more severe renal involvement. There are a variety of causes of atypical HUS in adults, including autoimmune conditions such as SLE, APS, scleroderma, genetic abnormalities, infections such as HIV, and certain drugs such as tacrolimus, ciclosporin, etc.
- ***Atypical adult HUS can occur outside of pregnancy, and recur during and after pregnancy, as well as recurring in subsequent pregnancies.***

Clinical features in acute TTP–HUS

- **Classic features include the pentad of:**[17]
  - **Microangiopathic haemolytic anaemia (MAHA)**, resulting in jaundice and anaemia (median Hb levels at admission typically at 80–100 g/litre) with raised reticulocyte count and elevated lactate dehydrogenase (LDH) levels,
  - **Thrombocytopenia:** The median platelet count in acute TTP-HUS is typically 10–30 × 10^9/litre.[1,19, 20, 21] Epistaxis, petechiae, haematuria, gingival and gastrointestinal bleeding, and haemoptysis are often seen.
  - **Renal impairment/acute renal failure:** proteinuria, microhaematuria.
  - **Neurological manifestations:** These may be intermittent and variable, e.g. confusion, irritability, headaches, paresis, reduced cognition, visual problems, aphasia, dysarthria, irritability, drowsiness, seizures, encephalopathy, and coma
  - **Pyrexia** (>37.5 °C).
- In addition, **non-specific symptoms such as pallor, fatigue, chest pain, arthralgia, abdominal pain** may be present.
- All the above presenting symptoms and signs represent widespread multiorgan thrombosis.

Diagnosis

- ***Diagnosis can be difficult, as the clinical features of TTP-HUS may mimic and overlap with autoimmune disease and a spectrum of pregnancy-related problems including pre-eclampsia and particularly HELLP syndrome. In many cases the post-delivery course of the illness may be the only differentiating feature.***[5]
- While there is a gradual improvement following delivery with pre-eclampsia and HELLP, TTP-HUS usually worsens after delivery. Delivery is therefore no guarantee of TTP-HUS undergoing remission.
- However, TTP can present without the full pentad; up to 35% of patients do not have neurological signs at presentation and renal abnormalities and fever may not prominent features. **The revised diagnostic criteria therefore is that TTP must be considered in the presence of thrombocytopenia and microangiopathic haemolytic anaemia alone**, when there is no alternative clinically apparent aetiology.[21]

Investigations and diagnosis

- The initial diagnosis should be made on clinical history and examination as well as routine lab tests including a peripheral blood film.
- Blood film: Shows microangiopathic haemolytic anaemia with fragmented red cells.
- FBC: Thrombocytopenia may be severe. Also anaemia and reticulocytosis.
- Biochemistry: Increased Lactate dehydrogenase LDH and increased unconjugated bilirubin.
- Impaired renal function tests.

- Coagulation studies are usually normal including both clotting time and fibrinogen levels.
- Immunochemistry: Blood must be taken pre-treatment for baseline ADAMTS13 activity assay. **Severely reduced levels (<5%) ± the presence of an inhibitor or IgG antibodies confirms the diagnosis of TTP-HUS.**[17]

Treatment

- Multidisciplinary and immediate involvement of senior haematologists, obstetrician, anaesthetist, and intensive care specialists are mandatory in such a medical emergency.
- **PEX** is the essential therapy for adults with TTP-HUS, improving survival from less than 10%[22] to approximately 80%.[2,4]
- Due to the high risk of preventable early death,[23] early and aggressive treatment with PEX is required to reduce maternal morbidity and mortality. Large-volume FFP infusions are indicated if there is any delay in instituting PEX. Immediate transfer to a tertiary unit might need to be arranged for the PEX programme if such a facility does not exist in the local hospital.
- PEX is not always readily available in all hospitals and while awaiting transfer of the patient to a tertiary unit with facilities for PEX, high-dose plasma infusions serve as emergency initial treatment.[14] Care must be taken to avoid fluid overload when high volume and doses of plasma infusions are given (25–30 ml/kg/day).
- Daily PEX is the mainstay of initial treatment.
- ***Platelet transfusions are contraindicated in TTP-HUS.***
- Women with congenital TTP should have their care at a regional specialist centre where ADAMTS13 supplementation is carried out on a regular basis throughout pregnancy.[17]
- In acquired TTP, ADAMTS13 activity must be monitored throughout pregnancy to predict the need for adjuvant therapy.
- In acquired TTP, a reduced level of ADAMTS13 (<10%) at the start of pregnancy may indicate elective treatment to prevent microvascular thrombosis during pregnancy.
- Diagnosis of pregnancy-associated TTP is especially difficult if it develops postnatally. In any mother with a thrombotic microangiopathy (TMA) and an uncertain diagnosis (as both pre-eclampsia and HELLP can present for the first time during the postnatal period), PEX should be considered.[17]
- In pregnancy, thrombosis in placental vessels can lead to fetal growth restriction, intrauterine fetal death, and pre-eclampsia. Serial fetal monitoring with ultrasound and Doppler studies is therefore essential, as is vigilance for the development of pre-eclampsia.
- If TTP-HUS develops in the first trimester, it excludes a diagnosis of pre-eclampsia/HELLP syndrome. PEX is urgently indicated and may allow the continuation of the pregnancy even to term with delivery of a live baby.[1,24,25,26]
- In severe cases, if a woman presents with severe thrombocytopenia, microangiopathic haemolytic anaemia, oliguric acute renal failure, and mental state abnormalities this must be diagnosed as TTP-HUS.
- After delivery, if there is persistence or progression beyond day 3 of haematological, neurological, and renal abnormalities, this is characteristic of TTP-HUS and therefore there is need for immediate treatment with PEX.[27,28,29]
- Corticosteroids may be of benefit.
- Supportive measures to limit renal damage and cerebral symptoms
- Delivery does not guarantee remission of TTP-HUS.
- There is a continued risk of relapse in subsequent pregnancies, although women with normal levels of ADAMTS13 pre-pregnancy have a lower risk of recurrence.[30,31]
- Women with TTP should **not** be prescribed the combined OCP with oestrogen.[17]

Information for patients

Please see Information for patients: Thrombotic thrombocytopenic purpura and haemolytic uraemic syndrome (p. 498)

References

1. Scully M, et al. Regional UK TTP registry: correlation with laboratory ADAMTS13 analysis and clinical features. Br J Haematol 2008;142: 819–826.
2. George JN, et al Thrombotic thrombocytopenic purpura-hemolytic uremic syndrome following allogeneic HPC transplantation: a diagnostic dilemma. Transfusion 2004;44: 294–304.
3. Alqadah F Thrombotic thrombocytopenic purpura in pregnancy. Postgrad Med J 1996;72: 768.
4. George JN. How I treat patients with thrombotic thrombocytopenic purpura-hemolytic uremic syndrome. Blood 2000;96: 1223–1229.
5. McMinn JR, George JN Evaluation of women with clinically suspected thrombotic thrombocytopenic purpura-hemolytic uremic syndrome during pregnancy. J Clin Apheresis 2001;16: 202–209.
6. Ridolfi RL, Bell WR Thrombotic thrombocytopenic purpura. Report of 25 cases and review of the literature. Medicine (Baltimore) 1981;60: 413–428.
7. Bell WR, et al. Improved survival in thrombotic thrombocytopenic purpura-hemolytic uremic syndrome. N Engl J Med 1991;325: 398–403.
8. Thompson CE, et al. Thrombotic microangiopathies in the 1980s:Clinical features, response to treatment, and the impact of the human immunodeficiency virus epidemic. Blood 1992;80: 1890–1895.
9. Hayward CPM, et al. Treatment outcomes in patients with adult thrombotic thrombocytopenic purpura-hemolytic uremic syndrome. Arch Intern Med 1994;154: 982–987.
10. Fujikawa K, et al. Purification of human von Willebrand factor-cleaving protease and its identification asa new member of the metalloproteinase family. Blood 2001;98: 1662–1666.
11. Levy GG, et al. Mutations in a member of the ADAMTS gene family cause thrombotic thrombocytopenic purpura. Nature 2001;413: 488–494.
12. Furlan M, et al. Acquired deficiency of von Willebrand factor-cleaving protease in a patient with thrombotic thrombocytopenic purpura. Blood 1998;91: 2839–2846.
13. Uslu M, et al. Familial thrombotic thrombocytopenic purpura imitating HELLP syndrome (hemolysis, elevated liver enzymes, and low platelets) in two sisters during pregnancy. Am J Obstet Gynecol 1994;170: 699–700.
14. Egbor M, et al. Pregnancy- associated atypical haemolytic uraemic syndrome in the post-partum period: a case report and review of the literature. Obstet Med 2011;4: 83–85.
15. Fakhouri F, et al. Pregnancy associated hemolytic uremic syndrome revisited in the era of complement gene mutations. J Am Soc Nephrol 2010;21: 859–867.
16. Noris M, Remuzzi G Genetic abnormalities of the complement regulators in hemolytic uremic syndrome: how do they affect patient management? Nat Clin Prac Nephrol 2005;1: 2–3.
17. Scully M, et al. on behalf of British Committee for Standards in Haematology. Guidelines on the diagnosis and management of thrombotic thrombocytopenic purpura and other thrombotic microangiopathies. Br J Haematol 2012;158: 323–335.
18. Vesely SK, et al. ADAMTS13 activity in thrombotic thrombocytopenic purpura-hemolytic uremic syndrome: relation to presenting features and clinical outcomes in a prospective cohort of 142 patients. Blood 2003;102: 60–68.
19. Coppo P, et al. Prognostic value of inhibitory anti-ADAMTS13 antibodies in adult acquired thrombotic thrombocytopenic purpura. Br J Haematol 2006;132: 66–74.
20. Tuncer HH, et al. Predictors of response and relapse in a cohort of adults with thrombotic thrombocytopenic purpura-hemolytic uremic syndrome: a single-institution experience. Transfusion 2007;47: 107–114.
21. Galbusera M, et al. Thrombotic thrombocytopenic purpura—then and now. Semin Thromb Hemost 2006;32: 81–89.
22. Amoroso EL, Ultmann JE Thrombotic thrombocytopenic purpura: report of 16 cases and review of the literature. Medicine 1966: 45: 139–159.
23. Pereira A, et al. Thrombotic thrombocytopenic purpura/hemolytic uremic syndrome: a multivariate analysis of factors predicting the response to plasma exchange. Ann Hematol 1995;70: 319–323.
24. Rozdzinski E, et al. Thrombotic thrombocytopenic purpura in early pregnancy with maternal and fetal survival. Ann Hematol 1992;64: 245–248.
25. Ambrose A, et al. Thrombotic thrombocytopenic purpura in early pregnancy. Obstet Gynecol 1985;66: 267–272.

26. Mokrzycki MH, et al. Thrombotic thrombocytopenic purpura in pregnancy: successful treatment with plasma exchange. Case report and review of the literature. Blood Purification 1995;13: 271–282.
27. Katz VL, et al. The natural history of thrombocytopenia associated with preeclampsia. Am J Obstet Gynecol 1990;163: 1142–1143.
28. Chandran R, et al. Spontaneous resolution of pre-eclampsia-related thrombocytopenia. Br J Obstet Gynaecol 1992;99: 887–890.
29. Martin MG, et al. Thrombotic thrombocytopenic purpura induced by trimethoprim sulfamethoxazole in a Jehovah's Witness. Am J Hematol 2007;82: 679–681.
30. Ducloy-Bouthors AS, et al. Thrombotic thrombocytopenic purpura: medical and biological monitoring of six pregnancies. Eur J Obstet Gynecol Reprod Biol 2003;111: 146–152.
31. Scully M, et al. Successful management of pregnancy in women with a history of thrombotic thrombocytopaenic purpura. Blood Coag Fibrinolysis 2006;17: 459–463.

CARE PATHWAY

- Diagnosis suspected based on clinical signs and symptoms, and finding microangiopathic haemolytic anaemia and thrombocytopenia without any other identifiable cause such as pre-eclampsia, HELLP syndrome
- Differentiation may be difficult, especially if condition occurs postnatally

- In **TTP-HUS:** Urgent involvement of haematologist and intensive care physician
- Consider **immediate treatment with large volume FFP before transfer to tertiary centre for PEX**. If large volumes/ doses of FFP used, watch for fluid overload
- Care must be multidisciplinary, involving renal physician, neurologist, and cardiologist as indicated
- **Take bloods before PEX**—FBC, blood film (fragmented RBCs), reticulocytes, fibrinogen, U&Es, LFTs, amylase, troponin, calcium, blood group, antibody profile, ADAMTS13, autoimmune screen and, with patient's consent, HIV, Hep B/C screening
- ***Platelet transfusion contraindicated***
- Transfuse packed red cells, if indicated by significant anaemia

- Once PEX is commenced, give steroids either IV or oral, with oral proton pump inhibitor
- High-dose folic acid to meet increased demand due to haemolysis
- Daily PEX till at least 2 days after complete remission and platelet counts return >150 × 10^9/litre
- When PEX has increased platelet counts > 50 × 10^9/litre, consider prophylactic LMWH and low-dose oral aspirin
- Advise below-knee compression stockings

Continue close monitoring of maternal renal, cardiac function, coagulopathy, vigilance for neurological symptoms, early relapse of TTP-HUS within a few weeks. If cardiac/neurological symptoms, multidisciplinary consultation for further investigations and to consider rituximab

Close fetal surveillance—serial scans scans for fetal growth, liquor ± Doppler studies

Vigilance for development of pre-eclampsia, HELLP

Postnatal advice

- ***COCP contraindicated***
- Low risk of TTP recurrence in future pregnancy; atypical HUS can recur in subsequent pregnancies or out of pregnancy

Inform neonatologists

- Morbidity involving neonatal jaundice, red cell anisocytosis, tetany, thrombocythaemia, jaundice, even neonatal mortality

Data from Scully M, et al. on behalf of British Committee for Standards in Haematology, Guidelines on the diagnosis and management of thrombotic thrombocytopenic purpura and other thrombotic microangiopathies, *British Journal of Haematology*, 2012, 158, 3, pp. 323–335, doi:10.1111/j.1365-2141.2012.09167.x

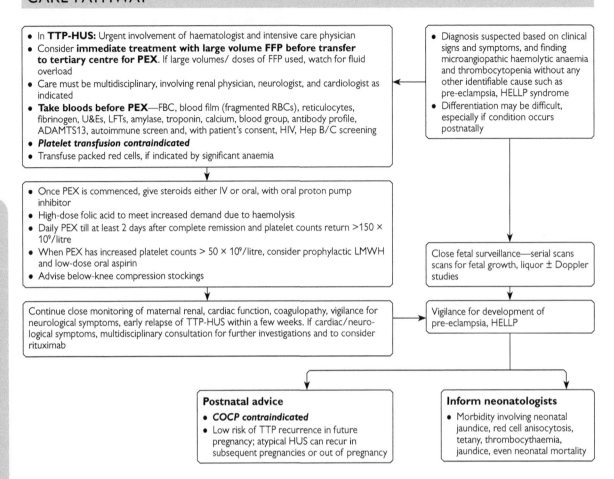

2 Maternal Infections

2.1 Bacterial Vaginosis

FACT FILE

Epidemiology

- **Bacterial vaginosis (BV)** is the most common lower genital tract disorder in women of reproductive age, with a prevalence rate of 4–60%, as well as the most common cause of vaginal discharge.
- BV has been reported in 6–35%[1,2,3] of **asymptomatic pregnant women** in the UK.
- ***BV is not an infectious condition caused by a single organism but represents an alteration of normal bacterial flora where the normal physiological lactobacilli-predominant flora are overcome by excessive growth of polymicrobials with anaerobic bacteria dominating.***
- Lactobacilli form 95% of the normal vaginal flora and the aerobic:anaerobic ratio is usually kept between 1:2 to 1:5.
- In BV, lactobacilli decrease, the vaginal pH increases from a normal value of less than 4.5 to as high as 7, and the aerobic:anaerobic ratio becomes 1:100 to 1:1000.[2]
- BV is caused by an overgrowth of predominantly **anaerobic** organisms such as *Mycoplasma hominis*, *Ureaplasma urealyticum*, *Gardnerella vaginalis*, *Bacteroides*, *Prevotella*, and *Moviluncus* species.
- The same organisms are also part of the normal vaginal flora except that when they become overabundant in numbers, BV results.
- BV is not believed to be sexually transmitted, so partner testing or treatment is not required.

Diagnosis

- Microbiological culture of vaginal secretions is **not** a reliable indicator of BV because BV is not caused by any single pathogen and represents an imbalance in the relative proportions of vaginal flora.
- Diagnosis of BV is instead made using the Gram stain method.[2]

Associated complications

- In pregnancy, BV is associated with a significant increase (5 to 7.5-fold) of various complications such as:[4,5,6,7]
  - late miscarriage (five fold increase)
  - preterm prelabour rupture of membranes (PPROM)
  - preterm delivery (BV doubles the risk of delivery <37 weeks gestation)[6,7]
  - low birth weight
  - postpartum endometritis.

Antibiotic prophylaxis and treatment

- Antibiotic prophylaxis for high-risk pregnant women, i.e. those with a previous history of any of the conditions listed above, as well as antibiotic treatment of pregnant women found to have BV in early pregnancy, has been shown in several studies[8,9,10,11] to significantly reduce the incidence of preterm birth and late miscarriages and to prolong gestation. Such a reduction has, however, not been seen in some other studies.[12,13]
- To be effective in reducing adverse pregnancy outcomes, **antibiotic prophylaxis/treatment must be used early in pregnancy (<17 weeks gestation)** before inflammation and tissue damage have occurred in cervical tissue.[10]
- If used only after 20 weeks gestation, antibiotic treatment or prophylaxis does not show a significant benefit in reducing either preterm birth or PPROM.[14]
- ***Vaginal clindamycin cream (2%) or oral clindamycin is the antibiotic of choice for BV in pregnancy.***
- Metronidazole, though used for treatment of BV out of pregnancy, is not the antibiotic of choice during pregnancy. In some studies, in fact, if oral metronidazole was the only antibiotic used in mid-trimester for BV, a higher incidence of preterm delivery was recorded.[15,16] Metronidazole is therefore best avoided during the second trimester of pregnancy. Metronidazole vaginal cream can, however, be used as an second choice.
- BV can recur within 3–4 months of treatment, therefore repeat doses may be recommended.
- In a **high-risk pregnancy**, the suggested schedule[3] for BV prophylaxis is clindamycin cream (2%) pv, one applicatorful daily for 5–7 days at 16 weeks gestation followed by a repeat course for 7 days at 22–24 weeks gestation.
- In a **low-risk asymptomatic pregnant woman,** if BV is found **at any stage of pregnancy**, immediate treatment with clindamycin pv as above for 7 days **or** oral clindamycin 300 mg bd for 5 days is required.
- Postpartum endometritis can occur after 2–5% of vaginal births and up to 10–15% of Caesarean deliveries. BV appears to be a significant risk factor in postpartum endometritis.[17] It might be prudent, even if BV has been detected only after 36 weeks gestation, to treat it in order to reduce the risk of postpartum endometritis.
- Repeat high vaginal swab (HVS) after 4–6 weeks to ensure eradication of BV is essential in this situation as repeat treatment would be indicated.

Mycoplasmas, ureaplasma

- *Mycoplasma hominis* and *Ureaplasma* spp. organisms (ureaplasma) are referred to as the **genital mycoplasmas**.
- Genital mycoplasmas are also implicated in causing adverse outcomes of pregnancy, acting as pathogens in their own right or in coexistence with BV. These complications include late miscarriages, chorioamnionitis,[18,19] preterm birth,[20,21,22,23,24] low birth weight, puerperal fever, neonatal conjunctivitis, and neonatal respiratory disease.[25]
- Infection with genital mycoplasmas is more common after rupture of membranes than with intact membranes.

Information for patients

Please see Information for patients: Bacterial vaginosis and pregnancy (p. 498)

References

1. Nelson DB, Macones G. Bacterial vaginosis in pregnancy: current findings and future directions. Epidemiol Rev 2002;24: 102–108.
2. Guaschino S, et al. Aetiology of preterm labour: bacterial vaginosis. BJOG 2006;113 Suppl 3: 46–51.
3. Lamont RF. Bacterial vaginosis. In: Critchley H, et al., ed., Preterm birth. London: RCOG Press, 2004.
4. Hillier SL, et al. Association between bacterial vaginosis and preterm delivery of a low-birth-weight infant. The Vaginal Infections and Prematurity Study Group. N Engl J Med 1995;333: 1737–1742.
5. Holst E, et al. Bacterial vaginosis and vaginal microorganisms in idiopathic premature labor and association with pregnancy outcome. J Clin Microbiol 1994;32: 176–186.
6. Leitich H, et al. Bacterial vaginosis as a risk factor for preterm delivery: a meta-analysis. Am J Obstet Gynecol 2003;189: 139–147.
7. Klebanoff MA, et al. Is bacterial vaginosis a stronger risk factor for preterm birth when it is diagnosed earlier in gestation? Am J Obstet Gynecol 2005;192: 470–477.

8. Kurkinen-Raty M, et al. A randomised controlled trial of vaginal clindamycin for early pregnancy bacterial vaginosis. BJOG 2000;107: 1427–1432.
9. Lamont RF, et al. Intravaginal clindamycin to reduce preterm birth in women with abnormal genital tract. Obstet Gynecol 2003;101: 516–522.
10. Ugwumadu A, et al. Effect of early oral Clindamycin on late miscarriage and preterm delivery in asymptomatic women with abnormal vaginal flora and bacterial vaginosis: a randomised controlled trial. Lancet 2003;361(9362): 983–988.
11. Kiss H, et al. Prospective randomised controlled trial of an infection screening programme to reduce the rate of preterm delivery. BMJ 2004;329: 371.
12. Guaschino S, et al. Treatment of asymptomatic bacterial vaginosis to prevent pre-term delivery: a randomised trial. Eur J Obstet Gynecol Reprod Biol 2003;110: 149–152.
13. Kekki M, et al. Vaginal clindamycin in preventing preterm birth and peripartal infections in asymptomatic women with bacterial vaginosis: a randomized, controlled trial. Obstet Gynecol 2001;97: 643–648.
14. Carey JC, et al. Metronidazole to prevent preterm delivery in pregnant women with asymptomatic bacterial vaginosis. National Institute of Child Health and Human Development Network of Maternal-Fetal Medicine Units. N Engl J Med 2000;342: 534–540.
15. Morency AM, Bujold E. The effect of second trimester antibiotic therapy on the rate of preterm birth. J Obstet Gynaecol Can 2007;29: 35–44.
16. Thinkhamrop J. Antibiotics for treating bacterial vaginosis in pregnancy: RHL commentary (last revised: 4 July 2007).The WHO Reproductive Health Library; Geneva: World Health Organization.
17. Watts DH, et al. Bacterial vaginosis as a risk factor for post Caesarean endometritis. Obstet Gynecol 1990;75: 52–58.
18. Namba F, et al. Placental features of chorioamnionitis colonized with Ureaplasma species in preterm delivery. Pediatr Res 2010;67: 166–172.
19. Yoon BH, et al. Isolation of Ureaplasma urealyticum from the amniotic cavity and adverse outcome in preterm labor. Obstet Gynecol 1998;92: 77–82.
20. Goldenberg RL, et al. The Alabama Preterm Birth Study: umbilical cord blood Ureaplasma urealyticum and Mycoplasma hominis cultures in very preterm newborn infants. Am J Obstet Gynecol 2008;198: 43–45.
21. Mitsunari M, et al. Cervical Ureaplasma urealyticum colonization might be associated with increased incidence of preterm delivery in pregnant women without prophlogistic microorganisms on routine examination. J Obstet Gynaecol Res 2005;31: 16–21.
22. Harada K, et al. Vaginal infection with Ureaplasma urealyticum accounts for preterm delivery via induction of inflammatory responses. Microbiol Immunol 2008;52: 297–304.
23. Pararas MV, et al. Preterm birth due to maternal infection: causative pathogens and modes of prevention. Eur J Clin Microbiol Infect Dis 2006;25: 562–569.
24. Kirchner L, et al. Amnionitis with Ureaplasma urealyticum or other microbes leads to increased morbidity and prolonged hospitalization in very low birth weight infants. Eur J Obstet Gynecol Reprod Biol 2007;134: 44–50.
25. Taylor-Robinson D, Lamont RF. Mycoplasmas in pregnancy. BJOG 2011;118: 164–174.

CARE PATHWAY

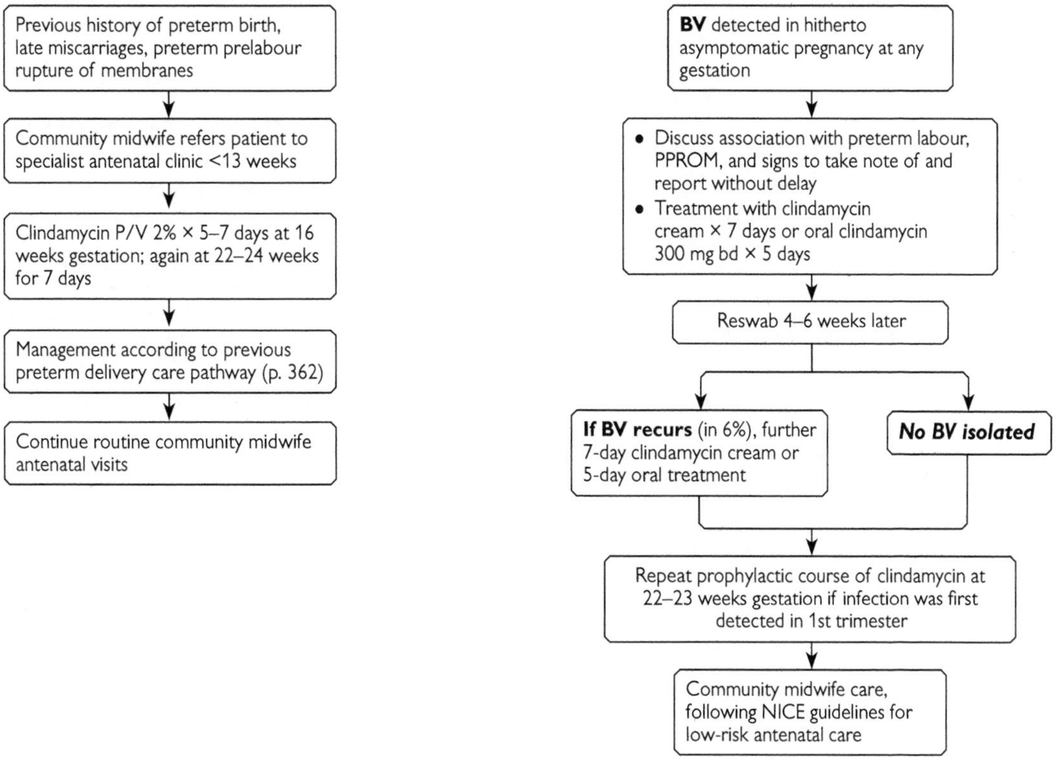
Previous history of preterm birth, late miscarriages, preterm prelabour rupture of membranes
Community midwife refers patient to specialist antenatal clinic <13 weeks
Clindamycin P/V 2% × 5–7 days at 16 weeks gestation; again at 22–24 weeks for 7 days
Management according to previous preterm delivery care pathway (p. 362)
Continue routine community midwife antenatal visits
BV detected in hitherto asymptomatic pregnancy at any gestation
• Discuss association with preterm labour, PPROM, and signs to take note of and report without delay
• Treatment with clindamycin cream × 7 days or oral clindamycin 300 mg bd × 5 days
Reswab 4–6 weeks later
If BV recurs (in 6%), further 7-day clindamycin cream or 5-day oral treatment
No BV isolated
Repeat prophylactic course of clindamycin at 22–23 weeks gestation if infection was first detected in 1st trimester
Community midwife care, following NICE guidelines for low-risk antenatal care

2.2 Chickenpox (Varicella Zoster)

FACT FILE

- **Chickenpox or varicella** is a highly contagious infection caused by herpes varicella zoster virus (VZV), a DNA virus of the herpes family.
- Primary VZV infection in pregnancy may lead to maternal morbidity, even mortality. Varicella infection in adults is associated with excess morbidity associated with pneumonia, hepatitis, and encephalitis and occasionally even mortality. Mortality rate is five times higher in pregnancy than in the non-pregnant state.[1]
- Up to 1 in 10 pregnant women with chickenpox develops pneumonia; the severity increases with later gestation, with a case fatality rate of 1% in the UK.[1,2]
- It may also cause the **fetal varicella syndrome (FVS)** as well as varicella infection in the neonate including congenital varicella and neonatal varicella.
- About 3 in 1000 pregnant women develop chickenpox.
- Incubation period is 1–3 weeks and the disease is infectious 48 hours before a rash appears and continues to be infectious until the vesicles crust over, which usually occurs within 5 days.[1]
- Transmission is through respiratory droplets or by personal contact with vesicular fluid or skin cells, clothing, bedding, etc.
- Primary VZV infection is common in children, which results in more than 90% of the adult population in the UK and Ireland being VZV IgG antibody seropositive, i.e. immune.[1,3,4] This immunity is lifelong.
- After a primary infection, the virus remains dormant but can be reactivated, resulting in herpes zoster (HZ) or shingles.
- At booking, enquiry should be made about previous VZV or shingles exposure. Those who have not had chickenpox or unsure of having had it, especially those from tropical and subtropical countries,[5] as well as women who are seronegative for VZV IgG, must be advised to avoid contact with chickenpox and shingles during pregnancy and to immediately inform their GP or midwife of any potential exposure.
- If there is a clear history of significant exposure to chickenpox or shingles in any of these groups of susceptible women, a blood test for VZV serological status must be sent. The lab turnaround time is usually 24–48 h.
- Pregnant women from tropical and subtropical countries are more likely to be seronegative for VZV IgG, thus more susceptible to chickenpox.[5]
- Universal antenatal testing for VZV IgG status is not recommended in the UK.[1]

Exposure during pregnancy

- Although contact with chickenpox is not uncommon in pregnancy, only a small number so exposed actually contract infection.[1,2]
- Seronegative pregnant women who have had significant exposure to confirmed infection in any trimester should be given varicella zoster immune globulin (VZIG) without delay.
- If the immune status is unknown, VZIG may be delayed till urgent serotesting results are available and the woman is found to be seronegative for VZV IgG.[1] VZIG is effective when given up to 10 days after contact.
- VZIG is derived from human donor plasma. It is beneficial in preventing or attenuating chickenpox and its sequelae in pregnant women, although some may still develop serious illness. At present, further evidence that this can actually prevent fetal infection is awaited.
- If VZIG is given, the pregnant woman should be managed as potentially infectious from 8 to 28 days after VZIG (8–21 days if no VZIG given).[1]
- Contact during pregnancy with a non-immunocompromised individual with shingles in an unexposed area of the body is highly unlikely to lead to infection. Exceptions to this are when there is exposure to an individual with shingles in an exposed site (e.g. ophthalmic) or in disseminated HZ infection in an immunocompromised person where more viral shedding may occur.[1,6,7]
- ***For management of VZV infection during pregnancy, see the care pathway.***

Fetal risks of maternal VZV infection

- If chickenpox occurs in the first trimester, the risk of spontaneous miscarriage does not seem to be increased.[6,7]
- There is a small risk of FVS if maternal VZV infection or seroconversion occurs in the first 28 weeks of gestation.
- FVS can occur in 0.55 % of cases of maternal varicella infection if contracted in the first trimester and less than 1% if contracted between 13–20 weeks. FVS is very rare following maternal infection between 20 and 28 weeks gestation and not reported when primary maternal infection has occurred after 28 weeks gestation.
- FVS is characterized by one or more of the following:[1,3]
  - skin scarring
  - eye defects (e.g. microphthalmia, chorioretinitis, cataracts)
  - limb hypoplasia
  - neurological abnormalities (microcephaly, cortical atrophy, dysfunction of bowel and bladder sphincters, learning difficulties, etc.).
- These sequelae develop in only a minority of infected fetuses and are due to subsequent HZ reactivation in utero.[1]
- For **prenatal diagnosis of FVS**, referral to a fetal medicine specialist is recommended at 16–20 weeks or 5 weeks after infection for further discussion and detailed ultrasound examination.[1]
- Detailed ultrasound imaging or MRI after at least 5 weeks after the primary infection can detect certain abnormalities of FVS such as limb deformity, microcephaly, hydrocephalus, soft tissue calcification, and intrauterine growth restriction (IUGR).[8] VZV DNA can be detected by polymerase chain reaction (PCR) in amniotic fluid, which has a high sensitivity but a low specificity for the development of FVS.[1]
- Severe maternal illness with varicella can cause fetal death or premature labour as a result of the severity of systemic infection of the mother rather than due to direct fetal infection.[7]
- Maternal infection in pregnancy may display no effect on the fetus or neonate at birth but can present as shingles in the first year of the child's life due to reactivation of the primary in-utero infection.[1]
- **Maternal infection in late pregnancy, especially the last 4 weeks before birth,** is associated with a high risk of perinatal infection in 20–60% of cases,[6,7] with a rash present either at birth or developing within the first few days of birth.

Neonatal varicella infection (previously called congenital varicella)

- Varicella infection of the newborn is VZV infection in the early neonatal period contracted from maternal infection close to the time of delivery or immediately postpartum or from neonatal contact with a person other than the mother with chickenpox or shingles.[1,10]
- Severe neonatal chickenpox is most likely to occur if the infant is born within 7 days of onset of the mother's rash or if the mother develops the rash up to 7 days after delivery when cord blood VZV IgG is low.[10,11] Under these circumstances, neonatal infection has a shorter incubation period and the onset of signs occurs at 5–10 days of age.
- ***IVIG is recommended for these infants to try to reduce the severity of neonatal infection.***[11]
- Severe maternal or neonatal infection should be treated with IV aciclovir which is safe and effective in improving the outcome.

Varicella vaccination in susceptible women

- Varicella vaccine containing live attenuated virus may be considered in women proven to be seronegative who are either planning a pregnancy or undergoing fertility investigations.
- Postpartum vaccination can be offered to women found to be seronegative for VZV IgG during pregnancy; breastfeeding is safe after vaccination.[12] After VZV vaccination, care must be taken to avoid pregnancy for a minimum of 3 months.[1]
- Vaccinated women who develop a post-vaccine rash should avoid contact with other susceptible pregnant women and should inform their GP. Transmission in the absence of a rash is very rare.

Information for patients

Please see Information for patients: Chickenpox and pregnancy (p. 499)

References

1. RCOG Green-top Guideline No. 13. Chickenpox in pregnancy. London: Royal College of Obstetricians and Gynaecologists, 2007.
2. Tan MP, Koren G. Chickenpox in pregnancy: revisited. Reprod Toxicol 2006;21: 410–420.
3. O'Riordan M, et al. Sera prevalence of varicella zoster virus in pregnant women in Dublin. Ir J Med Sci 2000;169: 288.
4. Manikkavasagan G, et al. Antenatal screening for susceptibility to varicella zoster virus (VZV) in the United Kingdom. A review commissioned by the National Screening Committee. London: MRC Centre of Epidemiology for Child Health, 2009.
5. Lee BW. Review of varicella zoster seroepidemiology in India and South-east Asia. Trop Med Int Health 1998;3: 886–890.
6. Lamont RF, et al. Varicella-zoster virus (chickenpox) infection in pregnancy. BJOG 2011;118: 1155–1162.
7. Enders G, Miller E.Varicella and herpes zoster in pregnancy and the newborn. In: Arvin AM, Gershon AA, ed. Varicella zoster virus: virology and clinical management. Cambridge: Cambridge University Press, 2000, pp. 317–347.
8. Verstralen H, et al. Prenatal ultrasound and magnetic resonance imaging in fetal varicella syndrome: correlation with pathology findings. Prenat Diagn 2003;23: 705–709.
9. Public Health England. Chickenpox: public health management and guidance, 2014 <https://www.gov.uk/government/collections/chickenpox-public-health-management-and-guidance>
10. Nathwani D, et al. Varicella infections in pregnancy and the newborn. J Infect 1998;36: 59–71.
11. Miller E, et al. Outcome in newborn babies given anti-varicella zoster immunoglobulin after perinatal maternal infection with varicella zoster virus. Lancet 1989; ii: 371–373.
12. Bohlke K, et al. Postpartum varicella vaccination: is the vaccine virus excreted in breast milk? Obstet Gynecol 2003;102: 970–977

CARE PATHWAY

- Check whether the patient had **chickenpox** in childhood
- Take a careful history to confirm significance of contact
- If any doubt about childhood chickenpox, arrange immediate blood test for VZV immunity. More than 85% will be IgG seropositive. Reassure regarding lifelong immunity. IgM in maternal serum indicates primary VZ infection
- If she is not immune to VZV and has had a significant exposure before 20 weeks gestation, give VZIG as soon as possible after contact (effective when given up to 10 days after contact)
- If VZIG given, the pregnant woman is potentially infectious from 8–28 days after VZIG (8–21 days if no VZIG is given)
- Whether given VZIG or not, women should be informed to notify their GP/midwife early if rash develops
- A second dose of VZIG may be required if further exposure is reported and 3 weeks have elapsed since last dose

Management of a pregnant woman who reports contact with chickenpox or shingles

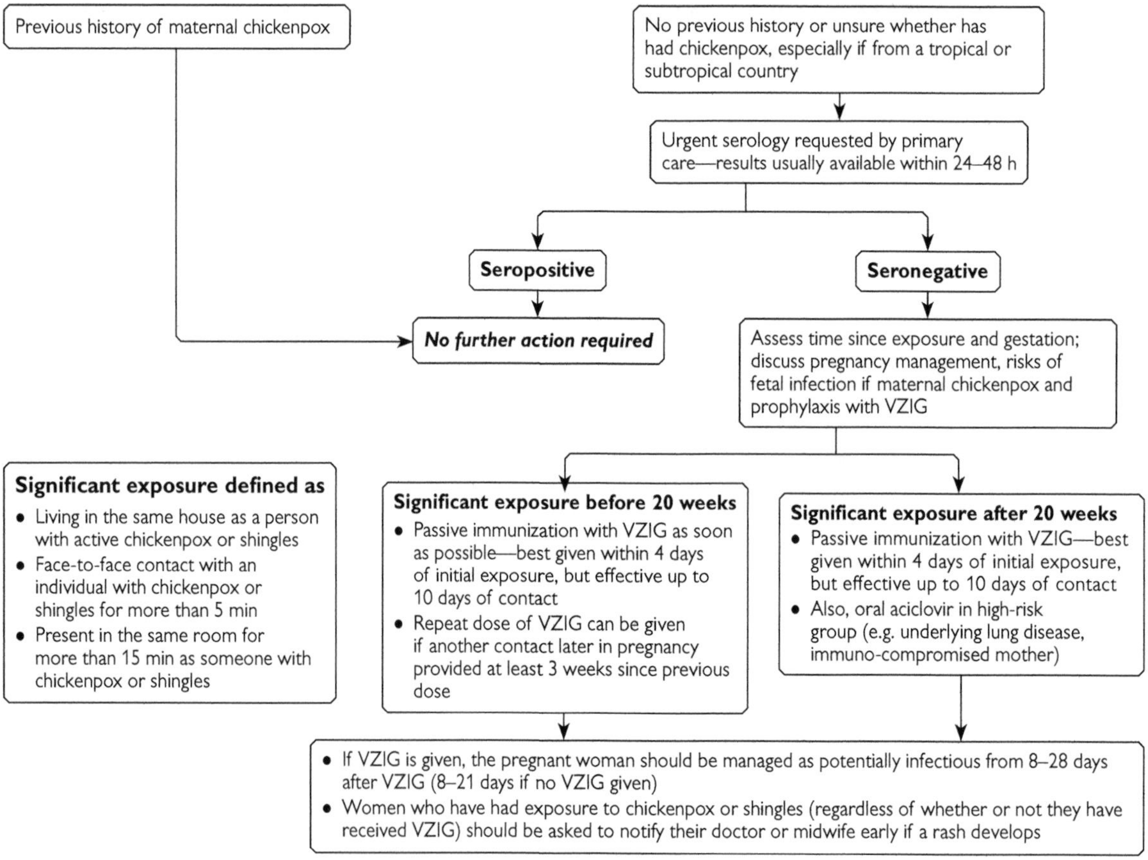

If a pregnant woman develops chickenpox during pregnancy

Urgent medical review needed in primary or secondary care, with advice to patient to stay away from other pregnant women and newborns until all the spots have crusted over (about 5–6 days after onset of rash). Discuss fetal risks of maternal infection dependent on gestation, serial scans, fetal varicella syndrome, and sequelae

Uncomplicated
Previously healthy pregnant woman, non-smoker, no respiratory disease, not immunocompromised by medications such as steroids

- Prescribe oral aciclovir if treatment within 24 h of rash appearing (after this time aciclovir is of little benefit)
- Can remain at home
- Advise to report any complication without delay to GP or midwife
- Describe symptoms of complications (e.g. breathing problems, bleeding from rashes, fever for > 5 days)
- Advise local hygiene to prevent secondary bacterial infection of lesions

If complications develop, i.e. respiratory symptoms, haemorrhagic rash, persistent pyrexia for >5 days, new eruptions developing after 6 days

Complications with chickenpox infection and/or high-risk group
Smokers, previous respiratory disease, immunocompromised individuals such as those on high dose steroids or other immunosuppressive medication

- Admission to hospital
- IV aciclovir
- Supportive therapy continues

Maternal chickenpox >7 days prior to delivery

- VZIG not required
- IV aciclovir for mother within 24 h of rash first appearing to reduce severity in both mother and baby
- Symptomatic therapy sufficient, care to avoid secondary bacterial infection of skin lesions
- If infection remote from delivery, serial ultrasound scans to detect abnormalities suggestive of fetal varicella syndrome
- Can breastfeed, no isolation required from baby
- No serious risk to baby unless very pre-term
- If very pre-term, neonate to receive IV aciclovir
- Paediatricians must be informed when mother admitted in labour

Maternal chickenpox ≤7 days prior to delivery

- IV aciclovir required immediately to curtail symptoms if severe maternal infection
- All other symptomatic therapy to continue
- Neonate will require IV VZIG ideally within 24 h of birth, but may be given up to 72 h
- In severe neonatal infection, IV aciclovir required for baby
- No isolation of mother from baby required
- Breastfeeding encouraged
- Isolate mother and neonate from pregnant or parturient women (including pregnant staff who have not had chickenpox previously or are unsure of having had it) and other neonates, with discharge of mother and baby as soon as possible and when safe to do so

Maternal chickenpox 0–28 days after delivery

- Neonate will require IV VZIG ideally within 24 h of development of maternal rash, but may be given up to 72 h
- In severe neonatal infection, IV aciclovir required for baby
- In severe maternal infection, IV aciclovir required
- No isolation of mother from baby required
- Breastfeeding encouraged
- Isolate mother and neonate from pregnant or parturient women (including pregnant staff who have not had chickenpox previously or are unsure of having had it) and other neonates. Discharge mother and baby as soon as possible and when safe to do so

Primary VZ infection confirmed before 20 weeks gestation

- Reassure that no increased risk of miscarriage if VZ infection in first trimester
- Explain that baby has 2% risk of congenital varicella syndrome and its implications
- Not an indication for TOP because risk is small and unpredictable
- Detailed scan at 16–20 weeks gestation or 5 weeks after Infection, whichever sooner
- Serial growth scans at 28, 32, and 36 weeks with clinic reviews on same day
- Continue routine care with community midwife in between hospital visits
- No indication to change obstetric management of labour or delivery
- Inform neonatologists about possibility of congenital VZ infection of newborn therefore neonatal ophthalmologic examination and further follow-up as indicated

Patient with chicken pox presenting within 24 h of onset of rash, after 20 weeks gestation

- Isolate from all pregnant women
- Reassure that no risk of fetal varicella syndrome
- Oral aciclovir (800 mg five times a day for 7 days) to reduce severity and duration of illness
- Referral to hospital mandatory for women who develop chest or neurological symptoms, haemorrhagic rash or bleeding, a dense rash ± mucosal lesion or those who have significant immunosuppression, smokers, those with chronic lung disease, those on steroids, etc.
- If respiratory symptoms suspicious of varicella pneumonia, IV aciclovir required, even ventilation in severe cases
- In seronegative pregnant women VZ IgG to mother asap after exposure (but before actual infection) needs to be considered. VZIG has no therapeutic benefit once VZ has developed
- If maternal infection occurs 5 days before or 2 days after delivery, 20–30% risk of varicella of new-born. Therefore, if feasible, delivery to be delayed until 5–7 days after onset of maternal illness to allow passive antibody transfer
- If delivery unavoidable within 5 days of maternal illness or if mother develops primary VZ within 2 days postpartum, treat neonate with VZ Ig as soon as possible after birth. Neonatal blood to be sent for passively acquired VZV IgM antibody
- Neonatal infection to be treated with IV aciclovir
- Follow-up sample of infant after 7 months of age for VZV IgG antibody

2.3 Cytomegalovirus

FACT FILE

Epidemiology

- **Cytomegalovirus (CMV),** a herpesvirus, is the most common cause of congenital viral infection in Western countries.[1]
- 40–80% of adults have been affected by CMV at some time in life, usually in childhood.
- In non-pregnant adults, CMV only becomes a problem if there is an immunosuppressed state: for example, coexistent HIV, those on immunosuppressant medication after organ transplant, those receiving chemotherapy, or on long-term oral steroids for more than 3 months.
- Once infected, CMV remains dormant in the body for life but may cause infection due to reactivation in pregnancy. About 2–2.5% of women seroconvert during the course of pregnancy.[2,3]
- In case of primary maternal infection, parents should be informed about a 30–40% risk for intrauterine transmission and fetal infection, and a 20–25% risk for development of sequelae postnatally if the fetus is infected.
- Transplacental infection[3] of the fetus occurs in 40% of mothers with primary CMV infection during pregnancy.
- While most primary CMV infections in adults are asymptomatic, some may present with flu-like illness or glandular fever with temperatures of 38 °C or above, fatigue, sore throat, swollen glands, muscle or joint pains, loss of appetite, shortness of breath, diarrhoea, large painful mouth ulcers, etc. Symptoms last for a couple of weeks.
- CMV is excreted in saliva, semen, blood, breast milk, cervicovaginal secretions, urine, tears, etc.

Congenital CMV

- Incidence of congenital CMV is 0.3–0.6% with the risk of transmission distributed across all trimesters.
- Most cases of congenital CMV resulting in serious neurological injury develop when a pregnant woman is infected by CMV for the first time during the first or early second trimester or just before conception.
- Infection in the first half of pregnancy is often characterized by a baby that is small for gestational age, with microcephaly and intracranial calcifications.
- Infection in late pregnancy is more likely to cause visceral damage such as hepatitis, purpura, pneumonia, or severe thrombocytopenia.
- If the mother is infected just before conception, the rate of transmission to the baby is at least 0.2–2%.
- Routes of transmission to the baby are transplacental during pregnancy, intrapartum due to swallowing of maternal cervicovaginal secretions, or postnatally through breast milk.
- In the majority of cases where CMV is transmitted from mother to the fetus, no damage is caused to the baby. In 10% of cases, however, the baby is born with symptoms at birth. These symptoms can have serious long-term neurological sequelae such as learning difficulties.
- A further 10% of babies who are born with congenital CMV will have no symptoms at birth but go on to develop sensorineural deafness by 5 years of age. The level of hearing loss can range from mild to total.
- A fetus affected by congenital CMV may be born with symptoms such as jaundice, pneumonia, hepatosplenomegaly, rash (red spots under the skin), chorioretinitis, low birth weight, microcephaly, seizures, and late developmental delay. It is estimated that 180 children are born every year in England and Wales will develop a severe handicap due to CMV infection.
- Such babies will also often show biochemical and haematological abnormalities suggestive of hepatitis, haemolytic anaemia, low platelet counts, and raised bilirubin levels.
- CMV infection can also cause **stillbirth** if the infection is contracted during the early stages of pregnancy. CMV has identified in 15% of fetal tissues or placentas, suggesting a strong association between CMV infection in pregnancy and stillbirth.[4]
- Long-term sequelae of congenital CMV seen in children can include microcephaly, impaired vision, blindness, hearing loss, seizures, lack of physical coordination, autism, epilepsy, or learning difficulties.
- As there are different strains of CMV, **previous infection does not exclude the possibility of infection with a new strain** followed by intrauterine infection.

Investigations and diagnosis

- Diagnosis of **primary CMV infection** made only on clinical grounds is not reliable as 90% are asymptomatic. Diagnosis is made by demonstration of **seroconversion of CMV-specific IgG antibodies from negative to positive.**[5] A rise of IgG titre is not useful as this can also occur with recurrent infection.
- Diagnosis of primary maternal CMV infection in pregnancy should therefore be based on de-novo appearance of virus-specific IgG in the serum of a pregnant woman who was previously seronegative, or on detection of specific IgM antibody associated with low IgG avidity.[5]
- IgM specific to CMV is not a reliable marker for diagnosis of primary infection because the CMV IgM, though suggestive of recent infection, can remain positive for many months. IgM can also indicate reactivation of a past infection.[6]
- The diagnosis of **secondary infection** should be based on a significant rise of IgG antibody titre with or without the presence of IgM and high IgG avidity.
- Certain ultrasonographic findings such as cerebral ventriculomegaly or periventricular calcification are suggestive but not specific for fetal CMV.
- Fetal CMV infection can be confirmed by positive amniotic fluid cultures after 21 weeks gestation. Greater viral loads are associated with a higher risk of an affected fetus.[7] **However, since no therapy is currently available for in-utero treatment of CMV, such an invasive process may not be entirely justified.**
- In cases of known primary CMV infection during pregnancy, it is essential that the **placenta** is sent for histology as the presence of **CMV inclusion bodies** found in some 10% of cases denotes a poor prognosis for the infant.
- At present there is no therapy for the in-utero treatment of primary infection. Antenatal management options include counselling followed by either expectant management or termination of pregnancy (TOP).

Neonatal management

- The neonatologists must be informed, before delivery, of the risk of congenital CMV infection of the neonate.
- Treatment strategies involve limiting sequelae after birth in infected babies. Ganciclovir, valaciclovir, etc. have been tried but have limitations due to toxicity.[7] CMV IgG-VF is currently undergoing trial.[9]
- All infants considered at risk for congenital CMV must be examined by the paediatricians.[7] Urine or saliva must be sent within the first 3 weeks of age for CMV culture or PCR, or by detecting CMV IgM in the neonate's blood (not cord blood).
- In addition, further newborn investigations are required, including hearing test, ocular examination, CT of the brain, full blood count (FBC), and liver function tests (LFT)s.

CMV and breastfeeding

- Though CMV can be passed through breast milk, the benefits of breastfeeding outweigh any risk posed by CMV. The only exception is if the baby is very premature, when the immune system may not be strong enough to control the infection.

Information for patients

Please see **Information for patients: Cytomegalovirus infection and pregnancy** (p. 499)

References

1. Gaytant MA, et al. Congenital cytomegalovirus infection: review of epidemiology and outcome. Obstet Gynecol Surv 2002;57: 245–256.
2. Raynor BD. Cytomegalovirus infection in pregnancy. Semin Perinatol 1993;17: 394–402.
3. Kenneson A, Cannon MJ.Review and meta-analysis of the epidemiology of congenital cytomegalovirus (CMV) infection. Rev Med Virol 2007;17: 253–276.
4. Iwasenko JM, et al. Human cytomegalovirus infection is detected frequently in stillbirths and is associated with fetal thrombotic vasculopathy. J Infect Dis 2011;203: 1526–1533.
5. SOGC Clinical Practice Guideline No. 240. Cytomegalovirus infection in pregnancy. Ottawa: Society of Obstetricians and Gynaecologists of Canada, 2010.
6. Adler SP. Screening for cytomegalovirus during pregnancy. Infect Dis Obstet Gynecol 2011;2011: 942937.
7. McCarthy FP, et al. Primary and secondary cytomegalovirus in pregnancy. Obstetrician and Gynaecologist 2009;11: 96–100.
8. Nigro G, et al. Congenital Cytomegalovirus Collaborating Group. Passive immunization during pregnancy for congenital cytomegalovirus infection. N Engl J Med 2005;353: 1350–1362.
9. Steininger C. Cytomegalovirus vaccine: light on the horizon. Lancet Infect Dis 2012;12: 257–259.

CARE PATHWAY

- Flu-like symptoms
- IgG (EIA, avidity) and IgM (EIA) seroconversion during or just before pregnancy (paired samples very useful)
- Direct detection of virus by PCR of CMV DNA or by CMV direct fluorescent antibody from blood, saliva , urine, or nasopharyngeal secretion
- Community midwife/GP refers patient to a specialist antenatal clinic

- **Primary CMV** confirmed during pregnancy—50% risk of transmission;
- Asymptomatic congenital CMV in 90% with risk of sequelae in 10% of these; symptomatic congenital CMV in 10% with risk of sequelae in 90% of these

- Non-primary reactivation of **past CMV** during pregnancy; risk of transmission is ≤1% for symptomatic congenital CMV ≤1% and ≥99% for asymptomatic congenital CMV

Specialist antenatal clinic, as soon as possible

- Discuss risks of fetal infection, short–medium–long-term effects and sequelae. Overall risk of fetal morbidity is 20–25%
- Discuss options including diagnostic test (amniocentesis and procedure-related risk) to diagnose whether fetus infected
- Quantitative PCR ± culture may identify infected fetuses at risk of symptomatic disease
- Give information leaflets to patient
- Amniocentesis (for PCR ± immunofluorescence test, culture) if opted for, after explanation of procedure-related risks
- Arrange detailed scan for signs of any periventricular calcification, ventriculomegaly, microcephaly, ascites, hydrops, pleural or pericardial effusion, intracranial or abdominal calcification, oligo- or polyhydramnios, etc.

Specialist antenatal clinic

- In only 1% does transplacental transfer take place
- Reassure patient
- Rest of care as indicated

Patient might choose TOP as an informed option

- Discuss post-mortem
- Placenta to be sent for histology

Patient chooses to continue pregnancy

- Arrange serial growth scans 28, 32, 36 weeks for evidence of IUGR or of oligo/polyhydramnios followed by ANC review on same day
- Inform paediatricians; arrange appointment if parents wish to see neonatologist during pregnancy
- Rest of antenatal care shared as usual with community
- No indication for early IOL or Caesarean section due to CMV
- Placenta to be sent for histology: request CMV inclusion bodies
- Neonatal tests and investigations by paediatricians; long-term follow-up

- Risk of congenital CMV infection after primary maternal CMV infection (overall risk = 12.7%) remains for up to 4 years post seroconversion , highest risk in first 2 years
- After 4 years of seroconversion, risk reduces to baseline 1%
- Counsel woman accordingly when planning a subsequent pregnancy

2.4 Genital Herpes

FACT FILE

- **Genital herpes** is a common sexually transmitted disease.
- The agent involved is the herpes simplex virus (HSV). Two strains of HSV can cause genital herpes, HSV-1 and HSV-2.
- Most HSV-2 seropositive individuals intermittently shed HSV from the genital mucosa, and may only have mild–moderate, recurrent symptoms.[1] Up to 90% of affected individuals with genital herpes are not aware of being infected as the manifestations are often subclinical.
- Although the initial clinical presentation of genital herpes is the same for HSV-1 and HSV-2, their later infectious course differs.
- **HSV-1 infection rarely recurs either symptomatically or asymptomatically after the first year of infection.**[2,3] HSV-1 reactivation may, however, occur after **mid-pregnancy**, when there is a physiological state of relative immunosuppression.
- Genital HSV-2 in contrast, may recur indefinitely and frequent reactivations are not uncommon.
- About 2% of women contract primary HSV infection during pregnancy; most of these infections are asymptomatic, therefore unrecognized.[3,4] The risk rises to about 20% if the woman's partner is HSV-positive.

Clinical presentation

- Symptoms of primary genital herpes infection (i.e. the first episode) can vary from mild discomfort and minimal lesions to widespread genital lesions associated with severe local pain described as 'burning', dysuria, even retention of urine, tender enlarged regional lymph nodes, and fever.
- Reactivations of HSV infection can similarly present a spectrum of symptoms, from very mild to severe, and lesions clinically indistinguishable from those of a primary infection.[5,6]
- In the first episode, lesions and lymphadenitis are usually bilateral.
- In recurrent disease, lesions tend to recur in previously affected sites. They may alternate between sides but are usually unilateral for each episode. Lymphadenitis occurs in around 30%.[7]
- Disseminated herpes is rare in adults but can occur in pregnant women due to relative immunosuppression. It carries a very high maternal mortality rate.
- Rarely, either a new or reactivated HSV infection in pregnancy can cause disseminated disease with hepatitis, encephalitis, or pneumonitis carrying a high mortality rate.[8] The diagnosis is confirmed by PCR testing of blood, cerebrospinal fluid, or positive serology.

Diagnosis

- **HSV culture** from genital ulcers or other mucocutaneous lesions is commonly done but actually has a relatively low sensitivity especially in recurrent lesions, with positive cultures declining rapidly after a day or two as lesions begin to heal.
- **PCR assays** for HSV DNA are more sensitive and can be used instead of viral culture.
- **Serology:** A negative result on culture or PCR does not rule out HSV infection, as viral shedding is intermittent. **Type-specific HSV serologic testing is an important diagnostic tool for women whose culture or PCR results are negative or who do not have active lesions at the time of presentation.**

Neonatal herpes

- Neonatal herpes is associated with high morbidity and mortality rates.
- Both HSV-1 and HSV-2 can cause neonatal infection.
- ***Infection is most commonly acquired at or near the time of delivery, although it can be acquired postnatally.***
- ***Incidence of neonatal herpes varies between 1 in 15 000 and 1 in 60 000.***[9]
- Factors influencing transmission include the type of maternal infection (primary or recurrent), the duration of ruptured membranes before delivery, use of fetal scalp electrodes, and mode of delivery.
- Risk of neonatal infection is greatest if the woman acquires primary (new) infection in the third trimester, especially within 6 weeks of delivery, as viral shedding will persist and the baby is likely to be born before the development of protective maternal antibodies.[10]
- Transplacental passage of maternal HSV antibodies, however, does **not** prevent viral spread to the neonate's brain.
- Neonatal infection can present as:
  - **Localized infection of the baby's skin, eyes, and/or mouth:** Morbidity is about 2%. With antiviral treatment, neonatal death is unusual.
  - **Encephalitis alone:** Presentation can be delayed by 10–30 days, with neurological sequelae in nearly 70% and neonatal mortality of about 6%.
  - **Disseminated herpes:** This has the worst prognosis with multiorgan involvement and mortality rates of more than 30% and long-term neurological damage in nearly 1 in 5 of survivors. It is more common in preterm babies and occurs almost exclusively due to primary infection.
- Rarely, neonatal infection could be acquired by the **transplacental route** rather than by direct contact with maternal secretions at the time of or leading up to delivery. This can result in all the three types of infections described above. Transplacental spread can also cause fetal growth restriction and intrauterine death.

Primary episode of genital herpes during pregnancy

- Immediate referral to genitourinary medicine. Advice about management and for screening for other sexually transmitted diseases will be given by the genitourinary physician.
- Saline baths, analgesia and topical anaesthetic agents (e.g. 5% lidocaine ointment) may be useful for local application, especially prior to micturition.
- **Antiviral drugs**: Oral antiviral drugs are indicated within 5 days of the start of the episode and while new lesions continue to be formed. Aciclovir, valaciclovir, and famciclovir can all reduce the severity and duration of episodes.[7]
- Although aciclovir is not licensed for use in pregnancy, there is substantial clinical experience supporting its safety.[9]
- The risks and benefits of antivirals should be explained to the patient.
- Topical agents are less effective than oral agents.
- Combined oral and topical treatment is of no benefit.
- IV therapy is indicated only when the patient cannot swallow or tolerate oral medication because of vomiting or lesions in the oral cavity, or in disseminated HSV infection.
- There is no evidence for benefit of courses longer than 5 days. However, it may be prudent to review the patient after 5 days and continue therapy if new lesions are still appearing at this time.
- If **primary infection occurs before 20 weeks of pregnancy** and the symptoms are severe, oral or IV aciclovir is recommended in standard doses. Thus far, there have been no reports of teratogenicity with use in the first trimester, though study numbers are limited.[9]
- Treatment with aciclovir is associated with a reduction in the duration and severity of symptoms and a decrease in the duration of viral shedding. Aciclovir is well tolerated in pregnancy.
- Treatment with oral aciclovir (400 mg three times a day for 5 days) should be considered in women with severe symptoms.
- It may be difficult at times to distinguish between recurrent and primary HSV infection, especially if a 'first episode' genital herpes infection occurs in the third trimester and within 6 weeks of delivery.
- In such cases, **immediate referral to the genitourinary physician for type-specific antibody testing** is recommended

since **this will influence the advice given regarding the mode of delivery and the risk of neonatal herpes**. If there are antibodies present of the same type as the HSV isolated from genital swabs, this would confirm that the present episode is a reactivation rather than a primary infection and there is no need for an elective Caesarean section to prevent neonatal transmission in such cases.

- ***Vaginal delivery can be anticipated if completion of treatment has been achieved well ahead of the time of delivery (a minimum of 6–8 weeks before the anticipated due date)***.
- Although there is insufficient evidence,[9] daily suppressive doses of aciclovir may be considered from 36 weeks gestation for women who have experienced a first episode of genital herpes earlier in pregnancy in order to reduce the likelihood of HSV lesions at term, and the necessity of performing a Caesarean section.[7]
- For primary genital herpes at the time of delivery or within 6 weeks of the expected due date, an elective Caesarean section is recommended in order to reduce the exposure of the fetus to HSV in genital secretions.
- Caesarean section may **not** be protective against neonatal herpes when membranes have been ruptured for more than 4 h. Therefore warn the women to present immediately after spontaneous rupture of membranes (SROM) to enable a prompt Caesarean section.
- For women who develop primary genital herpes lesions within 6 weeks of delivery but who opt for a vaginal birth, the membranes, if unruptured, must be left intact for as long as possible. Fetal scalp electrodes (FSE) or fetal blood sampling (FBS) need to be avoided.
- In such cases, IV aciclovir should be considered for the woman and subsequently for the neonate.
- The paediatrician should be informed well in time for prompt clinical evaluation of the neonate and to consider treatment with IV aciclovir.

Recurrent episodes of genital herpes

- Antiviral treatment is rarely indicated for treatment of recurrent episodes of genital herpes during pregnancy.
- Recurrence of genital herpes during the antenatal period is **not** an indication for delivery by Caesarean section.
- Cultures during late gestation to predict viral shedding at term are not indicated.
- **Daily suppressive aciclovir oral 200 mg qid from 36 weeks of gestation until delivery** in women with a history of recurrent genital herpes should be considered in order to further reduce the likelihood of HSV lesions at term.
- Aciclovir suppression was found in a meta-analysis [7,11,12] to reduce the risk of clinical HSV recurrence and thereby the need for delivery by Caesarean section in the majority of asymptomatic HSV-positive women.
- Although neutropenia is a recognized transient complication of aciclovir treatment of neonatal HSV infection, it has not been reported following maternal suppressive therapy. The aciclovir concentrations at which neutropenia occurred were approximately 5–30 times higher than were observed in umbilical vein plasma in a pharmacokinetic study of valaciclovir in pregnancy.[7]

Management of a pregnant woman with recurrent (active lesions) genital herpes at the onset of labour

- Advise a woman presenting with recurrent genital herpes lesions at the onset of labour that the risk to the baby of neonatal herpes is very small (about 1–3%).
- Caesarean section is not routinely recommended for women with recurrent genital herpes lesions at the onset of labour. The mode of delivery should be individualized according to the clinical circumstances and the patient's preferences.
- For a woman with a history of recurrent genital herpes, who would opt for Caesarean delivery if HSV lesions were to be detected at the onset of labour, daily suppressive aciclovir given from 36 weeks gestation until delivery may be given to reduce the likelihood of HSV lesions at term,[7,11,12,13]
- Women with recurrent genital herpes lesions and confirmed SROM at term should be advised to have delivery expedited by the appropriate means (augmentation). Avoid prolonged rupture of membranes.
- Avoid invasive procedures in labour for women with recurrent genital herpes lesions.
- Inform the neonatologist about babies born to mothers with recurrent genital herpes lesions at the time of labour.
- Even when recurrent genital herpes complicates PPROM, the risk of neonatal transmission is very small.

Prevention of postnatal HSV transmission to the neonate

- Mothers, family members and healthcare workers should be aware of the risk of neonatal transmission from active HSV lesions (e.g. orolabial herpes, herpetic whitlow).
- Breastfeeding is contraindicated only if there are herpetic lesions on the breast.

Summary of management of genital herpes in pregnancy

Primary episode of genital herpes during pregnancy

- Immediate referral to genitourinary physician for confirmation of diagnosis, advice on management, type-specific antibody testing, and screening for other STDs.
- Oral or IV aciclovir in standard doses after informing the woman of the potential risks and benefits of treatment.
- Local application of aciclovir cream on the active lesions maybe useful as an adjunct but insufficient treatment on its own. Local anaesthetic gel/cream application may be more useful.

Primary infection (active lesions) at the time of delivery

- Caesarean section recommended for any woman presenting with active lesions of a primary infection at the time of delivery or within 6 weeks of the expected date of delivery.
- The Caesarean section must be preferably performed within 4 hours of ruptured membranes.
- Therefore, advise women with primary infection in pregnancy to present as soon as possible, if SROM occurs before date set for elective Caesarean section.
- Alert paediatricians in good time; document clearly both in the hand-held notes and on the baby page of the main maternity notes.
- If women who have primary genital herpes lesions within 6 weeks of delivery, but opt for a vaginal delivery, document in the notes that artificial rupture or membranes (ARM), FSE, FBS should be avoided and that IV aciclovir for the mother and subsequently to the neonate should be considered. Clear documentation in baby's notes is required.

Recurrent episodes (secondary flare-ups) of genital herpes in pregnancy

- Antiviral treatment is rarely indicated.
- Most recurrent episodes are usually short lasting (7–10 days).
- Not an indication for Caesarean section.
- Viral cultures during late gestation are **not** indicated
- Consider suppressive aciclovir at oral doses of 200 mg qid from 36 weeks until delivery in these women. This has been shown to reduce the risk of clinical HSV lesions as well as asymptomatic viral shedding in the majority of cases.

Episode of recurrence (active lesions of a secondary flare-up) at onset of labour

- Inform the woman that the risk to baby of neonatal herpes is very small.
- Caesarean section is **not** routinely indicated.
- Document discussions about mode of delivery with mother, with notes of her clinical condition and individual preferences.
- Document in hand-held notes and in baby page of main notes about mother's recurrent episodes. Alert neonatologists well in time.

Information for patients

Please see Information for patients: Genital herpes and pregnancy (p. 499)

References

1. Wald A, et al. Reactivation of genital herpes simplex virus type 2 infection in asymptomatic HSV-2 seropositive persons. N Engl J Med 2000;342: 844–850.
2. Wald A, et al. Oral shedding of herpes simplex virus type 2. Sex Transm Infect 2004;80: 272–276.
3. Engelberg R, et al. Natural history of genital herpes simplex virus type 1 infection. Sex Transm Dis 2003;30: 174–177.
4. Wald A, et al. Frequent genital HSV-2 shedding in immunocompetent women. J Clin Invest 1997;99: 1092–1097.
5. Gardella C, Brown ZA. Managing genital herpes infections in pregnancy. Cleveland Clin J Med 2007; 74: 217–224.
6. Hensleigh P, et al. Genital herpes during pregnancy: inability to distinguish primary and recurrent infections clinically. Obstet Gynecol 1997;89: 891–895.
7. BASHH. National guideline for the management of genital herpes. London: British Association for Sexual Health and HIV, 2007.
8. Dupuis O, et al. Herpes simplex virus encephalitis in pregnancy. Obstet Gynecol 1999;94: 810–812.
9. RCOG Green-top Guideline No. 30. Management of genital herpes in pregnancy. London: Royal College of Obstetricians and Gynaecologists, 2007.
10. Brown ZA, et al. Effect of serologic status and abdominal deliveries on transmission rates of herpes simplex from mother to infant JAMA 2003;289: 203–209.
11. Hollier LM, Wendel GD; Third trimester antiviral prophylaxis for preventing maternal genital herpes simplex virus (HSV) recurrences and neonatal infection. Cochrane Database Syst Rev. 2008;1: CD004946.
12. Sheffield JS, et al. Acyclovir prophylaxis to prevent herpes simplex virus recurrence at delivery: a systematic review. Obstet Gynecol 2003;102: 1396–1403.
13. Prober CG, et al. Low risk of herpes simplex virus infections in neonates exposed to the virus at the time of delivery to mothers with recurrent genital herpes simplex virus infections. N Engl J Med 1987;316: 240–244.

CARE PATHWAYS

Management of genital herpes in pregnancy

Patient referred to general high-risk obstetric clinic

↓

Community midwife/GP refers patient with **previous history** of genital herpes to specialist antenatal clinic

↓

Reactivation during pregnancy, but remote from expected delivery date (EDD)

↓

First visit to specialist antenatal clinic

- Inform patient she could remain asymptomatic during pregnancy or could have short lasting episodes of recurrence (reactivation requiring treatment)
- Recurrent attacks do not usually require antiviral treatment. Analgesics and supportive management, local anaesthetic aciclovir cream may help
- Viral cultures **not** indicated
- Discuss and prescribe suppressive oral aciclovir 200 mg qid from about 36 weeks till delivery—recommended to prevent fresh reactivation at time of delivery
- Not an indication for routinely offering Caesarean section
- For further routine antenatal checks, can be transferred back to midwifery-led care

Recurrence of reactivated lesions close to EDD

↓

- Advise patient that risk of neonatal infection is very small (1–3%)
- **Caesarean section not routinely indicated. Discuss patient's preference and consider individual circumstances** to advise mode of delivery
- Clear documentation in notes—both hand-held and main notes to include:
  - If patient chooses vaginal delivery:
    - Expedite labour if SROM to avoid prolonged ROM
    - Avoid FSE, FBS
    - Inform neonatologists ahead of time for neonatal assessment and aciclovir if required
    - Breastfeeding contraindicated **only if** herpetic lesion on breast
  - If patients elects for planned LSCS:
    - Advise to come in immediately if SROM, to reduce exposure time
    - Inform neonatologist promptly
    - Breastfeeding contraindicated **only if** herpetic lesion on breast

Primary genital herpes infection during pregnancy

Urgent referral from primary care of patient with **primary** herpes infection during pregnancy to hospital specialist antenatal clinic or directly to genitourinary medicine (GUM) if diagnosis strongly suspected

If seen during 'office hours' in any specialist antenatal clinic:

- assess pregnancy
- visualize lesions
- if suspicious of HSV, refer patient immediately to GUM clinic

If seen out of hours in delivery suite and lesions are suspicious of HSV:

- take viral swabs from lesion
- send bloods for urgent HSV serology
- start aciclovir oral 400 mg tid for 5 days
- refer to first available GUM clinic

GUM clinic

Swabs taken, screening for other STI, type-specific antibody testing, treatment initiated if not already done; contact tracing

Severe infection—a life-threatening emergency

Admit. IV aciclovir and immediate multidisciplinary intensive treatment for disseminated maternal HSV infection

Subsequent visits to specialist antenatal clinic

- ***If primary HSV within 6 weeks of EDD, ensure is on or has completed treatment with aciclovir***
- ***IV aciclovir for mother may be required; seek advice from GUM consultant***
- ***Advise elective LSCS at 38–39 weeks***
- Advise patient to report urgently to delivery suite if SROM before operation date to enable prompt LSCS to curtail time of exposure. SROM to delivery interval should be <4 h to have any benefit of delivery by LSCS
- Alert paediatricians well in time
- IV aciclovir for neonate may be required
- Breastfeeding not contraindicated, unless herpetic lesions on breast

Subsequent visits to specialist antenatal clinic

- **If primary infection before 28–30 weeks gestation** and full treatment course completed, no further lesions present and if HSV antibodies have been found to be present on maternal serology, discuss option of vaginal delivery
- If vaginal delivery opted for, consider suppressive therapy with 200 mg qid of aciclovir daily from 36 weeks till delivery
- If vaginal delivery opted for:
  - Advise prompt admission after SROM and augmentation of labour to follow without delay
  - If membranes unruptured, keep intact as long as possible
  - Avoid FSE, FBS
  - IV aciclovir for mother and subsequently for the neonate
  - Inform paediatricans well ahead of time for neonatal assessment and IV aciclovir as indicated
  - Breastfeeding not contraindicated, unless herpetic lesions on breast

2.5 Group B Streptococcal Infection

FACT FILE

This fact file refers primarily to antenatally identified risk factors. For other risks that are identified during labour or delivery, refer to the labour ward guidelines of your unit and the RCOG guideline.[1]

Aetiology and incidence

- Colonization of the genital tract with **group B streptococci (GBS)** occurs in approximately 20% of all women.
- The incidence of neonatal early-onset GBS disease (within the first 7 days of birth) is about 0.5 per 1000 live births in the UK.[1,2,3]
- GBS is the most common cause of severe early-onset (<7 days of age) neonatal infection.
- There is no international consensus regarding screening and management of GBS and practice differs in different countries.
- In the UK, there is no universal screening programme for all pregnant women.
- UK practice generally follows the RCOG guidelines.[1,2,3]
- Current UK practice involves offering intrapartum antibiotic prophylaxis to those with high-risk factors, to help prevent early-onset GBS neonatal disease.
- Intrapartum antibiotics significantly reduce the risk of early-onset GBS neonatal infection, but do not protect against late-onset disease (>7 days after birth).

Risk factors

- ***If any one or more of the following risk factors is present, intrapartum antibiotic prophylaxis for early-onset GBS neonatal disease is essential:***
  - ***a previous baby affected by GBS***
  - ***preterm labour (<37 weeks)***
  - ***prolonged rupture of membranes (>18 h)***
  - ***intrapartum pyrexia (>38 °C).***
  - GBS bacteriuria or vaginal colonization (any colony count) detected in this pregnancy.
- Approximately 15% of all UK pregnancies have one or more of the risk factors emphasized above, and the same risk factors are operational in approximately 60% of early-onset GBS neonatal disease.

Screening, prophylaxis, and treatment

- If antenatal screening for GBS is performed **before** 35 weeks gestation, it does not reliably predict carrier state at term. The later in gestation that the swabs are tested, **preferably within 5 weeks of delivery,** the better the correlation with culture results at delivery.[4,5]
- GBS colonization is detected by swabs taken ideally from both lower vagina and rectum at between 35–37 weeks gestation. Detection rate with only a low vaginal swab is about 22%, which increases to 27% with dual swabs.
- ***Current evidence does not support either screening for GBS or the administration of intrapartum antibiotics to women in whom GBS carriage was detected in a previous pregnancy.***[2]
- Intrapartum antibiotics are to be offered if there has been an incidental detection antenatally of GBS,
- Intrapartum antibiotics are 80% effective in protecting against early-onset GBS neonatal disease.
- Antenatally detected GBS bacteriuria must be promptly treated with antibiotics at the time of diagnosis. **In addition**, prophylactic IV intrapartum antibiotics must be offered, because GBS bacteriuria carries a higher risk of neonatal disease.
- There is no need to routinely refer these patients to a specialist clinic in the absence of any previous history of neonatal morbidity or mortality caused by GBS. Pregnancy can remain under midwifery-led care in most of those cases where there were no adverse neonatal sequelae associated with GBS infection.
- ***If, however, there is a history of a previous baby affected with neonatal GBS disease, it is essential that intrapartum IV antibiotic prophylaxis is offered this time.***
- For women who are undergoing a planned Caesarean section, there is no need for GBS antibiotic prophylaxis, provided labour has not commenced and the membranes are intact.
- For those with preterm rupture of membranes, GBS antibiotic prophylaxis is not required till active labour commences. Once active labour commences, IV antibiotics must be given as soon as possible and continued until delivery according to the standard protocol.
- Once any high-risk factor for GBS early-onset neonatal disease has been detected antenatally, it is mandatory that there is clear documentation and identification with **Alert** stickers in the notes (both paper and electronic versions).
- When such a patient is in active labour, the paediatricians must be informed, so that appropriate neonatal checks and management can be undertaken.
- ***All information regarding GBS swabs or urine tests, prophylaxis, neonatal checks, and investigations must be shared with the patient and relevant information leaflets given.***
- The rest of antenatal care should continue as per the NICE guidelines for low-risk women, provided no other risk factors are identified in the course of the pregnancy.
- ***Note: Maternal carriage of GBS does not predict premature rupture of membranes or of preterm labour.***[6]

Information for patients

Please see Information for patients: Group B streptococcus infection and pregnancy (p. 499)

References

1. RCOG. The prevention of early-onset neonatal group B streptococcal disease in UK obstetric units. London: RCOG Press, 2007.
2. RCOG Green-top Guideline No. 36. Prevention of early onset neonatal group B streptococcal disease, 2nd ed. London: Royal College of Obstetricians and Gynaecologists, 2012.
3. Heath PT, et al. PHLS Group B Streptococcus Working Group. Group B streptococcal disease in UK and Irish infants younger than 90 days. Lancet 2004;363: 292–294.
4. Centers for Disease Control and Prevention. Prevention of perinatal group B streptococcal disease: a public health perspective. MMWR 1996;45: 1–24.
5. Yancey MK, et al. The accuracy of late antenatal screening cultures in predicting genital group B streptococcal colonization at delivery. Obstet Gynecol 1996;88: 811–815.
6. Garland SM, et al. Is antenatal group B streptococcal carriage a predictor of adverse obstetric outcome? Infect Dis Obstet Gynecol 2000;8: 138–142.

Group B streptococcal (GBS) infection found at any stage in present pregnancy

If found in **urine**

- Immediate treatment, and post-treatment check MSU
- Clear documentation and sticker in hand-held and main notes: 'For intrapartum GBS IV antibiotic prophylaxis in active labour.'
- If pregnancy otherwise uncomplicated, continue midwifery-led care
- Inform paediatricians when in labour
- After complete treatment of GBS bacteriuria during pregnancy, if an elective Caesarean section is planned for any other obstetric indication at term, there is no need for pre-op GBS antibiotics provided the membranes have been intact

If found only in a **vaginal swab (HVS)**

- No need for antenatal antibiotic treatment for the pregnant woman
- Clear documentation and alert/sticker in hand-held and main notes 'For intrapartum GBS IV antibiotic prophylaxis in active labour.'
- If pregnancy otherwise uncomplicated, continue midwifery-led care
- Inform paediatricians when in labour
- If elective Caesarean for any other obstetric indication, no need for pre-op GBS prophylaxis, if term and membranes intact

Note: The categories listed in the above care pathways are **in addition** to any other risk factors that would warrant standard IV antibiotic prophylaxis to prevent early-onset GBS neonatal infection, including:

- Previous baby affected with GBS infection
- Prematurity (<37 weeks)
- Prolonged ROM (>18 h)
- Pyrexia in labour (>38 °C)
- Diabetic mothers, etc.

Data from RCOG Green-top Guidelines No. 36, *The Prevention of Early-onset Neonatal Group B Streptococcal Disease*, 2012, Royal College of Obstetricians and Gynaecologists.

GBS identified either in a previous pregnancy or in a non-pregnant state

This care pathway refers only to the antenatal management and the necessary documentation in the labour and baby pages of the notes when GBS infection has been identified at any stage in:

- a previous pregnancy
- a non-pregnant HVS (Gyn swab) at any time prior to present pregnancy — No requirement for either screening or for intrapartum antibiotic prophylaxis

Was neonate infected with GBS?

Yes

- Clear documentation and 'ACTION REQUIRED' alert/sticker to be placed in maternity hand-held notes and main notes in labour and baby pages for IV antibiotic prophylaxis in labour
- Inform patient, give information leaflet
- If pregnancy otherwise uncomplicated, continue as midwifery-led care
- If elective Caesarean planned, no need for pre-op GBS prophylaxis if membranes intact
- Intrapartum prophylactic IV antibiotics required
- Inform paediatricians

No

No requirement for screening in this pregnancy or for intrapartum antibiotic prophylaxis

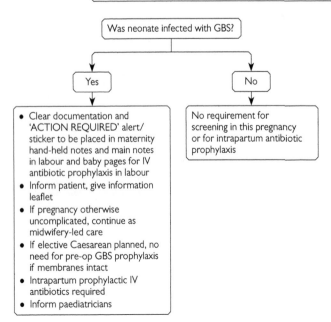

2.6 Hepatitis B

FACT FILE

This fact file deals mainly with the interpretation of the **hepatitis B (HBV, Hep B)** serology results of the pregnant woman and the requisite actions that need to be put in place to decrease the risk of vertical transmission of infection to the neonate.

Epidemiology

- A significant increase in the prevalence of hepatitis B infection has been experienced in most UK centres, particularly in the immigrant population.[1]
- HBV is a double-stranded DNA virus which, in infected individuals, is found in highest concentrations in the blood and in lower concentrations in saliva, vaginal secretions, semen, and wound exudates.
- HBV can remain viable on environmental surfaces at room temperature for up to 7 days.

Clinical presentation and transmission routes

- Average incubation period is 90 days from point of infection to onset of symptoms, though this may vary from 6 weeks to 6 months.
- Perinatal transmission is the most common form of HBV transmission worldwide.
- Sexual transmission accounts for the majority of cases of HBV infection in adults through percutaneous or mucous membrane exposure to infectious blood or body fluids.
- Acute infection produces clinical symptoms in 50% of cases in adults.
- In approximately 1% of reported cases acute liver failure and death can occur.
- Among those with chronic HBV infection, premature death from hepatocellular carcinoma or cirrhosis can occur in about 20%. **It is imperative that as soon as a pregnant woman is identified to be HBV positive, a referral is made to the hepatologist to initiate prompt review and long term follow up.**
- Symptoms in adults include loss of appetite, nausea, vomiting, fever, abdominal pain, and overt jaundice. Dark-coloured urine and grey stools may be noted.
- Approximately 10–20% of women who are seropositive for HBsAg (HBV surface antigen), in the absence of immunoprophylaxis, will transmit the virus to the neonates.[2]
- In pregnant women who are seropositive for both HBsAg and HBeAg, the vertical transmission rate, without immunoprophylaxis, is as high as 90%.[2,3]
- If a woman contracts acute hepatitis in the first trimester, the vertical transmission rate is about 10%, but up to 90% if the infection is acquired in the third trimester.
- Without immunoprophylaxis, most (>90%) of the infected infants would become chronic carriers by the age of 6 months if the mother is seropositive for both HBsAg and HBeAg.

Serological testing

- Clear understanding of the various serological tests and accurate interpretation of the results of maternal HBV serology results are crucial for further management planning to reduce the risk of vertical transmission (see Tables 2.1 and 2.2).
- Apart from the specific tests listed in Table 2.1, other liver tests (e.g. AST, ALT, GGT) may also be used to monitor the course of acute infection.
- Not all tests are performed in every pregnant woman. The result of an individual test has to be evaluated in the context of other Hep B specific tests.

Table 2.1 Specific hepatitis B tests and their clinical application

Test	*Relevance*	*Clinical application*
HBV surface antigen (HBsAg)	A protein present on surface of the virus-will be positive in both acute and chronic HBV infections	• Used to screen for and detect HBV infection • Earliest indicator of acute HBV infection, even before symptomatic • Becomes temporarily undetectable in blood during recovery phase • Primary method of detecting those with chronic infection • The presence of HBsAg indicates that the person is infectious
HBV surface antibody (Anti-HBs)	Antibody produced in response to HBV surface antigen; blood levels rise in recovery phase of acute infection Once positive after recovery from infection or after successful vaccination, remains so for life, indicating lifelong immunity of individual	• Used to detect previous exposure to HBV • Also positive after successful vaccination • Used to determine whether vaccination is required in susceptible individuals (if HBsAg is absent) • Used to determine whether infected individual has recovered and is now immune for life
Anti-HBV core antibody IgM (Anti-HBc IgM)	IgM antibody to HBV core antigen (HBV core antigen itself is present only in liver, cannot be detected in blood)	• Used to detect acute infection as it is the first antibody produced after infection • Positivity indicates recent infection (<6 months) and confirms acute infection
Anti-HBV total core antibody – both IgG and IgM (Anti-HBc IgG + IgM)	Both IgG and IgM to HBV core antigens	• Appear at the onset of symptoms in acute HBV • Presence of total HBV core antibody (both IgG and IgM) indicates either previous or current infection within an undefined time frame • Used to detect both acute and chronic HBV infections, persists for life
HBV e antigen (HBeAg)	Protein produced and detected in the blood in response to actively replicating HBV; is a marker of active infectivity	• Found in blood only during active replication of HBV in the blood (unlike HBsAg) • Used as a marker for infectivity and to monitor effectiveness of treatment • Certain strains of HBV (mostly found in Middle East and South-east Asia) do not produce e antigen, therefore absence of HBeAg in these strains does not indicate absence of HBV or lack of active infectivity
Anti-HBV e antibody	Detects antibody produced in response to Hep B 'e' antigen.	• Used to monitor recovery from acute infection;anti-HBe will be present along with anti-HBc and anti-HBs
Hep B viral DNA	Detects hepatitis B viral genetic material in blood	• A positive test indicates actively multiplying virus and that the person is highly contagious. Used to monitor effectiveness of antiviral therapy in those with chronic HBV infection.

Adapted from Lab Tests Online, http://labtestsonline.org.uk/understanding/analytes/hepatitis-b/tab/test/. © 2013 American Association for Clinical Chemistry, with permission http/labtestsonline.org/understanding/analytes/hepatitis-b/tab/test

Table 2.2 Interpretation of HBV serology results

HBV surface antigen (HBsAg)	*HBV surface antibody (Anti-HBs)*	*HBV core antibody (Anti-HBc IgM)*	*HBV core antibody total (Anti-HBc IgG+IgM)*	*HBV e antigen (HBeAg)*[a]	*HBV e antibody (Anti-HBe)*	*Stage of infection/interpretation*
Neg	Neg		Neg			No active or prior infection Is susceptible: vaccination to be considered
Pos	Neg	Neg	Neg	Pos	Neg	Early acute infection
Pos	Neg	Pos or Neg	Pos or Neg	Pos	Neg	Acute infection, usually symptomatic Contagious
Pos	Neg	Pos	Pos	Neg[a]	Pos	Late in acute stage of infection
Neg	Neg	Pos	Pos	Neg[a]	Pos	Resolving acute infection (convalescence)
Pos	Neg	Neg	Pos	Pos	Neg	May indicate active chronic infection (liver damage cannot be excluded)
Pos	Neg	Neg	Pos	Neg[a]	Pos	Chronic infection: carrier state Low risk of liver damage
Neg	Pos	Neg	Pos	Neg[a]	Pos	Infection resolved (recovery complete) Immunity acquired due to natural infection
Neg	Pos		Neg			Immunity acquired due to vaccination

[a] Some strains of HBV do not produce e antigen (usually those in the Middle East and South-east Asia). In such cases the individual may be infected with such a strain of HBV and may be infectious, yet the HBeAg will be negative. In such strains, therefore, testing for HBV e antigen is not useful.

Adapted from Lab Tests Online, http://labtestsonline.org.uk/understanding/analytes/hepatitis-b/tab/test/. © 2013 American Association for Clinical Chemistry, with permission http/labtestsonline.org/understanding/analytes/hepatitis-b/tab/test

HBV viral DNA

- A high count indicates active viral replication. The infection is contagious and there is a high risk of liver damage.
- A low HBV DNA result indicates such low viral count that it may not be detectable and, in general, that the infection is not contagious. If HBV DNA is being used to monitor treatment, a low count usually indicates that the therapy has been effective

Interventions to decrease vertical transmission to the neonate

- The risk of fetal hepatitis B infection through amniocentesis is low. However, if amniocentesis is required, every attempt must be made to avoid insertion of the needle through the placenta.[4]
- Mode of delivery does not appear to have a significant effect on HBV vertical transmission and Caesarean section is **not** recommended for the purpose of reducing mother–baby transmission.[2,3]
- ***Interventions such as internal monitoring with FSE or FBS should be avoided in labour. Documentation to this effect must appear clearly in the notes.***
- Babies born to infectious mothers are vaccinated at birth, usually in combination with HBV specific immunoglobulin 200 IU IM injection. This reduces vertical transmission rate by 90%.[1,5] The baby will need additional doses of HBV vaccine at 1 and 6 months of age to provide complete protection.
- Despite successful screening and the use of effective active and passive immunoprophylaxis, high maternal HBV DNA can lead to perinatal transmission. If the pregnant woman is found to be highly infectious with a high viral DNA count (>0.2×10^9 geq/ml), treatment with lamivudine may further reduce transmission rate,[6,7,8] although this needs further substantiation.[6] Lamivudine has also been shown to reduce the complications of HBV-infected women.[9,10]
- Indications for neonatal administration of HBV immunoglobulin with HBV vaccine within 24 h of birth must be evaluated during the antenatal period of pregnancy and clearly documented. These indications[6,11] include instances where the pregnant woman is:
    - HBsAg and HBe Ag positive
    - HBsAg positive and HBeAg negative; anti-HBe negative
    - HBsAg positive and e markers not available
    - HBsAg positive and HBV DNA level = 1×10^6 IU/ml, or
    - acute maternal hepatitis acquired during pregnancy.
- Good communication between hospital-based midwifery, obstetric, and neonatal staff and primary care (GPs, midwives, and health visitors) is important.
- Arrangements for HBV immunoglobulin for the neonate must be made available through the blood bank and must be actioned well ahead of time.
- Breastfeeding does not pose any additional risk of transmission.[6,12]

Information for patients

Please see Information for patients: Hepatitis B and pregnancy (p. 499)

References

1. Tehami N, et al. Outcome of the management of hepatitis B infection in pregnancy. Gut 2011;60: s248–s249.
2. ACOG Practice Bulletin No. 86. Viral hepatitis in pregnancy. Washington, DC: American College of Obstetriciansand Gynaecologists,D 2007.
3. Workowski KA, Berman SM. Sexually transmitted diseases treatment guidelines. Centers for Disease Control and Prevention. MMWR Recomm Rep 2006; 55(RR-11): 1–94.
4. Davies G, et al. Amniocentesis and women with hepatitis B, hepatitis C, or human immunodeficiency virus. Society of Obstetricians and Gynaecologists of Canada. J Obstet Gynaecol Can 2003;25: 145–148.
5. RCOG Query Bank. Hepatitis B in pregnancy. Royal College of Obstetricians and Gynaecologists, 2012. <http://www.rcog.org.uk/en/guidelines-research-services/guidelines/hepatitis-b-in-pregnancy-query-bank/>
6. Su GG, et al. Efficacy and safety of lamivudine treatment for chronic hepatitis. World J Gastroenterol 2004;10: 910–912.
7. Shi Z, et al. Lamivudine in late pregnancy to interrupt in utero transmission of hepatitis B virus: a systematic review and meta-analysis. Obstet Gynecol 2010; 116: 147–159.
8. Tran TT. Management of hepatitis B in pregnancy: Weighing the options. Cleveland Clin J Med 2009;76: s25–s29.
9. van Zonneveld M. Lamivudine treatment during pregnancy to prevent perinatal transmission of hepatitis B virus infection. J Viral Hepat 2003;10: 294–297.
10. Hung JH, et al. Lamivudine therapy in the treatment of chronic hepatitis B with acute exacerbation during pregnancy. J Chin Med Assoc 2008;71: 155–158.
11. BVHG Consensus Statement. UK Guidelines for management of babies born to women who are HBsAg positive. London: British Viral Hepatitis Group, 2008.
12. Wang JS, et al. Breastfeeding does not pose any additional risk of immunoprophylaxis failure on infants of HBV carrier mothers. Int J Clin Pract 2003;57: 100–102.

CARE PATHWAY

Maternal Hep B—management plans for infant

In the absence of immunoprophylaxis, if maternal serology shows:

- **HBsAg positive**—risk of vertical transmission to neonate is 10–20%
- **HBsAg and HBeAg positive**—risk of vertical transmission to neonate is nearly 90%
- 90% of infected infants become chronic carriers

↓

- Discuss risk of vertical transmission according to serology results with parents
- If amniocentesis performed, avoid needle insertion through placenta
- Antenatal evaluation for neonatal Hep B immunoglobulin (HBIg) and/or Hep B vaccine within 24 h of birth with clear documentation and communication with paediatricians and blood bank (for supply of HBIg and Hep B vaccine)
- No evidence that Caesarean section reduces risk of vertical transmission, therefore obstetric indications only for Caesarean section or early IOL
- Avoid FSE, FBS, ventouse for labour and delivery—clear documentation in notes
- No contraindication for breastfeeding—no increased neonatal transmission risk

↓

Low risk of neonatal infection

If the mother is anti-HBe positive and HBeAg negative, the baby requires Hep B vaccination after birth but not HBIg

↓

- ***Newborns at high risk of Hep B infection should receive both HBIg and the vaccine, ideally within 12–24 h of birth***
- High-risk neonates are those where:
  - the mother is HBsAg seropositive and HBeAg positive
  - the mother is HBsAg seropositive and HBeAg/anti-HBe negative
  - the mother is HBsAg seropositive and e markers are not available
  - the mother has acute hepatitis B in pregnancy
  - the mother is HBsAg seropositive and infant is born weighing ≤1500 g
- Usual dose of neonatal HBIg is 200 iu given as IM injection

↓

The infant is given further Hep B vaccines at 1 month, 2 months, and 12 months of age to complete the multidose schedule

↓

Follow-up serology at 12 months of age including HBsAg is mandatory

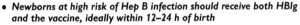

2.7 Hepatitis C

FACT FILE

Epidemiology

- **Hepatitis C virus (HCV, Hep C)** infection is a major global health problem. Worldwide prevalence in the general population is about 1%, but can be as high as 70–90% among high-risk groups such as IV drug users.[1]
- The main route of transmission of the single-stranded HCV is through infected blood (e.g. sharing of needles among injecting drug users, body piercing, tattooing) as well as inadvertent blood transfusion-acquired infection (pre-1992 in the UK).
- Sexual transmission is rare (<0.002%).[2]
- The average time frame from exposure to HCV to seroconversion is about 8–9 weeks.
- Patients with acute infection may present with mild jaundice, loss of appetite, nausea, vomiting, or abdominal pain, but 60–70% are asymptomatic.
- The diagnosis of HCV infection is made by the detection of anti-HCV antibodies by enzyme immunoassay (EIA) or enzyme-linked radioimmunosorbent assay (ELISA) The presence of HCV RNA detected by PCR is the gold standard test.
- HCV RNA is detectable in blood within 1–3 weeks after exposure.
- Anti-HCV antibodies can be detected in most patients (>97%) within 6 months of being infected.
- ***Once infected in adulthood, though HCV may remain quiescent for several years, approximately 85% of individuals will go on to develop chronic infection, 20% will suffer cirrhosis, and 1–4% will develop hepatocellular carcinoma.***[3,4]
- Most infected individual are unaware of their infection as they remain well for years, but they continue to be a source of infection, including perinatal infection.
- ***Mother-to-child vertical transmission is the most common route of acquisition of childhood infection.***[5,6]
- The prevalence of HCV infection **is low (<1%) in the general antenatal population in the UK.**[7]
- HCV infection is more prevalent among injecting drug users, especially in inner-city[1,8] pregnant populations within areas of deprivation.
- About one-third of HCV-infected pregnant women have usually been diagnosed prior to pregnancy but a substantial proportion of infected women do not report any risk factor.[7]
- In the UK, about 2% of HCV-positive women are coinfected with HIV.
- **The risk of vertical transmission of HCV is about 5%, but it is higher (up to 15%) for HCV/HIV coinfected women.**[9] More recently, the widespread use of highly active antiretroviral therapy (HAART) for HIV treatment, which results in improvement of the immune status of the affected woman, has also resulted in a significant decrease in the total viral load of HCV coinfection.[10]
- Risk factors for perinatal transmission include viral load and detectable viraemia during pregnancy, coinfection with HIV, and female gender of infant.[11]
- The virus does not usually appear to be transmitted when the mother's viral load is less than 10^6 copies/ml or the count is undetectable. However, there are several reports of vertical transmission despite the mother being non-viraemic.[11]
- In-utero acquisition of infection occurs in at least one-third to one-half of infected children, with the rest becoming infected intrapartum.[12]
- Amniocentesis in women infected with HCV does not appear to significantly increase the risk of vertical transmission, but the woman should be warned that very few studies have addressed this issue. If genetic amniocentesis is opted for, every attempt must be made to avoid insertion of the needle through the placenta.[13]
- During labour, procedures such as FSE, FBS or difficult instrumental delivery are best avoided.
- **Elective Caesarean section or withholding breastfeeding do not make any significant difference to HCV vertical transmission rate in women who are not HIV coinfected.**[4,6,14,15,16,17,18] Elective Caesarean section should be reserved for those women with dual infection of both HIV and HCV, where the HIV viral load is significant.

Screening/treatment for chronic HCV

- ***At present there is no vaccine, prophylactic measure, or treatment available during pregnancy. Interferon and ribavirin are contraindicated during pregnancy.***
- Also, as the prevalence rate among the pregnant population in the UK is low and the natural history of vertically acquired infection is largely unknown, routine antenatal HCV screening is not justified.
- ***Women with specific risk factors for HCV, such as IV drug users and HIV-positive women, must, however, be counselled and offered screening.***
- ***Referral to the gastroenterologist or hepatologist for long-term hepatological follow-up and treatment of the infected mother needs to made during pregnancy by the obstetrician and/or screening coordinator midwife.***

Treatment of infected children

- The natural history of vertically acquired infection in children born to HCV-infected mothers is, at present, incompletely defined.
- Spontaneous viral clearance has been noted in 7–27% within the first 3 years of life.[19,20]
- Most infected children remain HCV RNA positive though with little HCV-related morbidity. Only a small number (<2%) progress to severe morbidity.[19,20]
- Long-term follow-up of a minimum of 18 months after birth is needed for children suspected of having acquired perinatal HCV.
- Recent trials of combination of peg-interferon and ribavirin have been promising and sustained response rates of 50–60% have been reported.[21] Protease inhibitors such as telaprevir as an adjunct to standard combination therapy are under trial.

Information for patients

Please see Information for patients: Hepatitis C and pregnancy (p. 500)

References

1. Goldberg D, et al. Hepatitis C virus antibody prevalence among injecting drug users in Glasgow has fallen but remains high. Commun Dis Public Health 1998;1: 95–97.
2. Wejstal R. Sexual transmission of hepatitis C virus. J Hepatol 1999;31: 92–95.
3. Di Bisceglie AM. Hepatitis C. Lancet 1998;351: 351–355.
4. Centers for Disease Control and Prevention. Recommendations for prevention and control of hepatitis C virus (HCV) infection and HCV-related chronic disease. MMWR Recomm Rep 1998;47: 1–39.
5. Ohto H, et al. Transmission of hepatitis C virus from mothers to infants. The Vertical Transmission of Hepatitis C Virus Collaborative Study Group. N Engl J Med 1994; 330: 744–750.
6. Conte D, et al. Prevalence and clinical course of chronic hepatitis C virus (HCV) infection and rate of HCV vertical transmission in a cohort of 15, 250 pregnant women. Hepatology 2000; 31: 751–755.
7. UK Screening Portal. The UK National Screening Committee. Recommendation on hepatitis C screening in pregnancy, 2011.
8. Hutchinson SJ, et al. Hepatitis C virus among childbearing women in Scotland: prevalence, deprivation, and diagnosis. Gut 2004; 53: 593–598.
9. Pembrey L, et al. Antenatal hepatitis C virus screening and management of infected women and their children: policies in Europe. European Paediatric HCV Network. Eur J Pediatr 1999;158: 842–846.
10. Pappalardo BL. Influence of maternal human immunodeficiency virus (HIV) co-infection on vertical transmission of hepatitis C virus (HCV): a meta-analysis. Int J Epidemiol 2003;32: 293–299.

11. European Paediatric Hepatitis C Virus Network. A significant sex—but not elective cesarean section—effect on mother-to-child transmission of hepatitis C virus infection. J Infect Dis 2005; 192; 1872–1879.
12. Mok J, et al. When does mother to child transmission of hepatitis C virus occur? Arch Dis Child Fetal Neonatal Ed 2005;90: F156–F160.
13. Davies G, et al. Amniocentesis and women with hepatitis B, hepatitis C, or human immunodeficiency virus. J Obstet Gynaecol Can 2003; 25: 145–148.
14. McIntyre PG, et al. Caesarean section versus vaginal delivery for preventing mother to infant hepatitis C virus transmission. Cochrane Database Syst Rev 2006;4: CD 005546.
15. Tajiri H, et al. Prospective study of mother-to-infant transmission of hepatitis C virus. Pediatr Infect Dis J 2001;20: 10–14.
16. ACOG Committee Opinion. Breastfeeding and the risk of hepatitis C virus transmission. Int J Gynaecol Obstet 1999;66: 307–308.
17. American Academy of Pediatrics Committee on Infectious Diseases. Hepatitis C virus infection. Pediatrics 1998;101: 481–485.
18. Hunt CM, et al. Hepatitis C in pregnancy. Obstet Gynecol 1997;89: 883–890.
19. Resti M, et al. Guidelines for the screening and follow-up of infants born to anti-HCV positive mothers. Dig Liver Dis 2003;35: 453–457.
20. Bortolotti F. Long-term course of chronic hepatitis C in children: from viral clearance to end-stage liver disease. Gastroenterology 2008;134: 1900–1907.
21. Wirth S, et al. Recombinant alfa-interferon plus ribavirin therapy in children and adolescents with chronic hepatitis C. Hepatology 2002;36: 1280–1284.

Primary care healthcare professionals identify the following women for offer of **HCV** pre-test counselling. Test sent with booking bloods in 1st trimester of pregnancy from:
- Women already known to be Hep C positive
- Women who are at high risk for Hep C but whose status is unknown (e.g. current or past IV drug user, known abnormal LFTs, blood products received pre-1992, previous organ transplant/haemodialysis, partner Hep C + ve)
- All HIV-positive pregnant women (2% risk of HCV patients coinfected by HIV)

Known Hep C Ab positive (30%)

Confirmation that Hep C Ab +ve

If not already done, with patient's permission, counsel about testing for HIV and Hep B

- Referral to specialist antenatal clinic and to hepatologist.
- Implications for vertical transmission and maternal long-term hepatic impairment and treatment modalities discussed
- Baseline LFTs, also request Hep C RNA PCR

Hep C RNA PCR −ve

Hep C RNA PCR +ve

Reassure that low risk carrier, with no or very low risk of vertical transmission

Increased risk of vertical transmission of approx. 6% depending on viral load

- No evidence that Caesarean section reduces risk of vertical transmission.
- No indication for elective LSCS or for early IOL except for any other obstetric indication.
- Usual BBV precautions applicable for labour, delivery, postnatally
- **Breastfeeding not contraindicated** as no increased risk of transmission seen

---

Those in high-risk group whose HCV status is unknown

Pre-test counselling for Hep C, Hep B, and HIV testing

Hep C Ab +ve

Hep C Ab −ve

All HIV +ve pregnant women

Counselling for Hep C testing by Hep C RNA PCR irrespective of Ab serology which may be false −ve

Referral to specialist antenatal clinic, multidisciplinary input from GUM and hepatology

Hep C RNA PCR +ve

Hep C RNA PCR −ve

Increased risk of vertical transmission of Hep C when HIV +ve as well—15–45% risk of Hep C transmission

- Reassure that low risk carrier for Hep C with low risk of vertical transmission of Hep C to fetus
- Rest of care as in HIV care pathway (p. 89)

- Rest of antenatal care according to HIV guidelines, but hepatology long-term follow-up required in addition
- Referral to GI medicine/hepatology specialist mandatory in any Hep C +ve pregnancy

---

In all cases of Hep C positive mother, paediatricians must be informed for follow-up of the neonate and infant

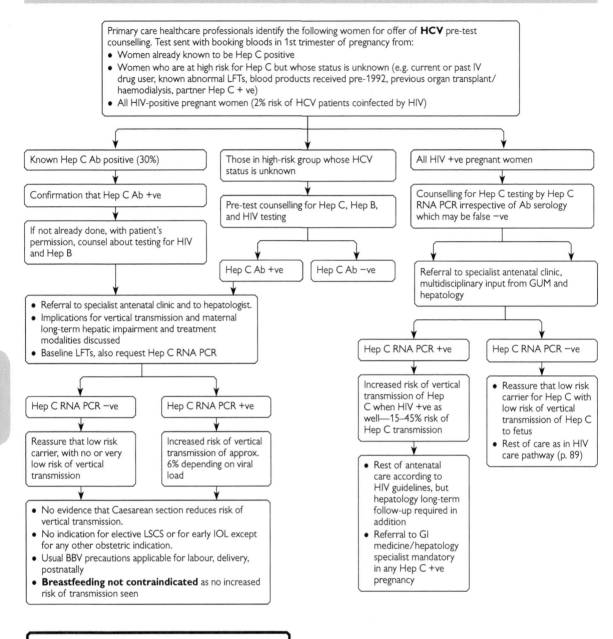

2.8 H1N1 Influenza (Swine Flu)

FACT FILE

Epidemiology

- Pregnant women are not known to be at increased risk of contracting **H1N1 influenza (swine flu)**.Once it is contracted, however, pregnancy, especially in the second and third trimesters as well as the early postpartum period, present high-risk factors for developing severe illness and respiratory complications.[1,2,3,4]
- Poor pregnancy outcomes with increased risk of preterm and very preterm delivery and high perinatal mortality rates are also recognized.[1]
- Pregnant women appear to be more susceptible to intracellular pathogens such as viruses,[2] due to the relative suppression of the immune system during pregnancy. The severity of the disease of the 2009 pandemic influenza A (H1N1) was recognized to be greater during pregnancy than in the non-pregnant population, a pattern similar to seasonal influenza and previous pandemics.[2,3,4,5]
- Pregnant women who contract H1N1 are four times more likely to require hospitalization than the general population,[4] with a significant proportion needing admission to level 2 (high dependency care) or level 3 (critical/intensive care).
- In a large study from California,[6] one-third of pregnant women who contracted H1N1 had other **underlying medical conditions** that were risk factors for the development of complications.
- In the CDC pan-US study[7] nearly 50% of pregnant or recently delivered women who contracted H1N1 had underlying medical conditions. Those who died were significantly more likely to have underlying conditions (about 62%) than those who survived H1N1 infection (47%).
- Such medical conditions include asthma, pre-gestational and gestational diabetes, obesity, haemoglobinopathy, hypertension, and chronic lung, cardiovascular, renal, autoimmune, and thyroid diseases. No differences were seen between intensive care unit (ICU) survivors or those who died in terms of ethnicity, age, or trimester of contracting H1N1 infection.[6]

Clinical presentation

- Symptoms could at first be mild or moderate in pregnancy and postpartum, but rapid deterioration is not uncommon.
- A substantial proportion of those who had severe illness needing ICU admission and, where a high rate of mortality was reported, had developed symptoms **within 2 weeks post-partum**.[6]

Prognosis

- **Pregnancy and perinatal outcomes** are poor in infected women.[1,6,7] Perinatal mortality is found to be more than five times greater, stillbirths four times greater, very preterm births (<32 weeks) increased by nearly five times, and neonatal deaths nearly six times more than in pregnancies without maternal H1N1 infection.[1]
- Similar outcomes have been noted in CDC US data[7] where, of liveborn babies of infected mothers, nearly 64% were either preterm or very preterm, 44% were of low birth weight, and 70% needed neonatal intensive care.
- ***Although the overall maternal mortality rate with H1N1 has not been determined, the mortality rate in all hospitalized adults is about 6%.***

Treatment

- ***Prompt antiviral treatment is essential and can be lifesaving for pregnant women or those within 2 weeks after delivery with either suspected or confirmed H1N1 influenza, ideally within 48 h of symptom onset.***[8,9]
- Pregnant women who received recommended antiviral treatment only after 48 h of symptom onset were four times more likely to need ICU admission and/or die compared with those treated within 48 h.[6,10,11]
- **Awaiting results of the PCR influenza diagnostic test (PCRIDT) introduces delayed initiation of treatment in suspected cases. Although rapid influenza antigen tests are widely available and can be done in about 15 min, they have a high false negative rate (nearly 40%),[6] making them unreliable in treatment initiation.**
- **Clinical decisions about the treatment of H1N1 influenza should therefore not be guided by or delayed because of negative results on rapid testing.**[12,13]
- **A high degree of suspicion based on clinical symptomatology in pregnant or recently delivered women should warrant prompt initiation of treatment with the neuraminidase inhibitors oseltamivir or zanamivir in uncomplicated cases.**[8]
- **Those with severe systemic disease or complications should be admitted and treated with oseltamivir.**
- Antibiotics should be considered in selected cases when there are signs of bacterial or respiratory tract infection, failure to respond to antiviral therapy, underlying disease, and in complicated, severe H1N1 infection.[8]
- Delay in treatment could arise due to various reasons including women attributing symptoms of myalgia or shortness of breath to pregnancy or to the recent delivery rather than influenza, or because of a delay in treatment initiation by healthcare professionals.
- **It is imperative to recognize that the onset of severe symptoms, rapid deterioration, and mortality can present postpartum.** The treatment guidelines above are therefore equally relevant in recently delivered women (within 2 weeks postpartum).
- **Severely ill women may require transfer to tertiary centres** depending on individual circumstances and facilities available, if the local hospitals cannot provide higher levels of ICU care.[14] **This decision must be made with top-level multidisciplinary input and according to previously agreed protocols of care.**
- The decision to deliver a critically ill pregnant woman where the baby is preterm in order to improve the outcome of ventilation should include the obstetric, critical care, and neonatal teams with involvement of the patient, or her partner and/or family if she is too ill to participate in decisions.[8]
- Delivery, in these circumstances usually by Caesarean section, needs to be performed only after the mother's clinical condition has been stabilized.
- A single course of antenatal steroids to accelerate fetal lung maturity has not been shown to cause maternal exacerbation of infection and is therefore recommended at least 24 h before the preterm delivery.[8]
- **Potential complications of severe H1N1 infection** include disseminated intravascular coagulation, viral and postviral encephalitis, thromboembolism, and cognitive and psychological effects after the recovery phase.[8]
- Breastfeeding is not contraindicated while the mother is on antiviral medications.
- ***The most important measure to reduce mortality and morbidity of H1N1 influenza in pregnant and recently delivered women is the promotion of vaccination, regardless of trimester. The monovalent vaccine has a well-recognized safety profile and all healthcare professionals in both primary and hospital-based care settings need to encourage this key public health priority.***[6,7,8]

Information for patients

See Information for patients: Swine flu (H1N1) and pregnancy (p. 500).

References

1. Pierce M, et al. On behalf of UKOSS. Perinatal outcomes after maternal 2009/H1N1 infection: national cohort study. BMJ 2011;342: 1351.
2. Rasmussen SA, et al. Pandemic influenza and pregnant women. Emerg Infect Dis 2008;14: 95–100.
3. Siston AM, et al. Pandemic 2009 influenza A (H1N1) virus illness among pregnant women in the United States. JAMA 2010;303: 1517–1525.
4. Jamieson DJ, et al. H1N1 2009 influenza virus infection during pregnancy in the USA. Lancet 2009;374: 451–458.
5. Saleeby E, et al. H1N1 influenza in pregnancy: cause for concern. Obstet Gynecol 2009;114: 885–891.
6. Louie JK, et al. for the California Pandemic (H1N1) Working Group. Severe 2009 H1N1 influenza in pregnant and postpartum women in California. N Engl J Med 2010;362: 27–35.
7. Centers for Disease Control and Prevention. Influenza vaccination coverage among pregnant women— United States,; 1; 2010–11 influenza season. MMWR 2011;60: 1078–1082.
8. DH/RCOG.Pandemic H1N1 2009 influenza: Clinical management guidelines for pregnancy. London: Department of Health and the Royal College of Obstetricians and Gynaecologists, 2009 <http://www.nhs.uk/news/Documents/Swine%20Flu-%20Pregnancy%20Clinical%20Guidelines.pdf>
9. Centers for Disease Control and Prevention. Updated interim recommendations for obstetric health care providers related to use of antiviral medications in the treatment and prevention of influenza for the 2009–2010 season. <http://www.cdc.gov/h1n1flu/pregnancy/antiviral_messages.htm>.
10. Rasmussen SA, et al. Preparing for influenza after 2009 H1 N1:special considerations for pregnant women and newborns. Am J Obstet Gynecol 2011;204: S13–20.
11. Centers for Disease Control and Prevention. Antiviral agents for the treatment and chemoprophylaxis of influenza: recommendations of the Advisory Committee on Immunization Practices (ACIP). MMWR 2011;60(No. RR-1). 11.
12. Centers for Disease Control and Prevention Health Alert Network (HAN) info service message: recommendations for early empiric antiviral treatment in persons with suspected influenza who are at increased risk of developing severe disease <http://www.cdc.gov/H1N1flu/HAN/101909.htm.>.
13. Vasoo S, et al. Rapid antigen tests for diagnosis of pandemic (swine) influenza A/H1 N1. Clin Infect Dis 2009;49: 1090–1093.
14. McNamee K, Dawood F. Severe H1N1 virus in pregnancy requiring extracorporeal membrane oxygenation and lobectomy. Obstet Med 2010;3: 156–157.

CARE PATHWAY

See guidelines for pregnancy prepared by the Department of Health and the Royal College of Obstetricians and Gynaecologists:

Pandemic H1N1 2009 influenza: clinical management guidelines for pregnancy v2, 2009 <http://www.nhs.uk/news/Documents/Swine%20Flu-%20Pregnancy%20Clinical%20Guidelines.pdf>

2.9 Human Immunodeficiency Virus (HIV)

FACT FILE

For more details see the British HIV Association 2012 guidelines,[1] current guidelines on the BHIVA website (<http://www.bhiva.org/Guidelines.aspx>), and the RCOG Green-top Guideline.[2]

Prevalence

- With the widespread implementation of routine antenatal screening for **Human Immunodeficiency Virus-HIV-1,** transmission of HIV-1 from mother to child is now a rare occurrence in the UK.
- Nationally, estimated prevalence increased gradually during the 1990s, more rapidly between 2000 and 2005, and has since stabilized.[1]
- At present, the majority of pregnant HIV-infected women in the UK come from sub-Saharan Africa where the prevalence of genital infections is high.
- Although prevalence among UK-born women giving birth remained low at about 0.46 per 1000 women (1 in 2200) in 2009, this represents a gradual increase since 2000 when it was 0.16 per 1000.
- In the UK, in 1993 when interventions were virtually non-existent, the rate of mother-to-child transmission in diagnosed women was 25.6%, vs about 2% at present, including both diagnosed and undiagnosed cases.[1]
- Between 2000 and 2004 the majority of HIV-infected women diagnosed before delivery were identified through antenatal screening. Since 2005, however, about 75% of women have already been aware of their infection before they conceived, many of them diagnosed in a previous pregnancy.
- Two-thirds of affected infants born in England between 2002 and 2005 were to women had not been diagnosed prior to delivery. About one-half of those undiagnosed women had declined antenatal testing.

Antenatal HIV screening

- All pregnant women should be advised screening for HIV infection,[2] syphilis, hepatitis B, and rubella in every pregnancy at their booking antenatal visit.
- If a woman declines an HIV test, this should be documented in the maternity notes, her reasons should be sensitively explored, and screening offered again at around 28 weeks
- If a woman tests HIV negative at booking but is judged by her clinician as being at continued high risk of acquiring HIV, offering a repeat HIV test should be considered.
- Midwives and doctors reviewing women during antenatal care should ensure that the HIV result is clearly documented.
- Fourth-generation laboratory assays are recommended as the first-line HIV test for antenatal screening. Where a woman books for antenatal care at 26 weeks of gestation or later, the test should be requested urgently and the result issued within 24 h.
- Rapid HIV tests use rapid-test devices to deliver results within 20 min of the sample being taken. These tests are recommended for all women with unknown HIV status in labour and a reactive result should be acted on immediately.

Management

- Management should be by a multidisciplinary team, including an HIV physician, obstetrician, specialist midwife, health advisor, and paediatrician.
- All women who are newly diagnosed HIV positive should have an early assessment of their social circumstances.
- Women should be reassured that their confidentiality will be maintained.
- Women should be encouraged to disclose their HIV status to their partner and given appropriate support.
- Care should be taken to avoid inadvertent disclosure to a woman's partner or family members, as they may be unaware of her HIV diagnosis, even though they may attend antenatal visits and be present at the delivery.
- Advice should be given about safer-sex practices and the use of condoms, to prevent transmission of HIV and other sexually transmitted infections to an uninfected partner.
- It is recommended that women with existing children of unknown HIV status should have them tested for HIV.
- In rare cases where women refuse interventions to reduce the risk of mother-to-child transmission, despite supportive guidance from the multidisciplinary team, a pre-birth planning meeting should be held with social services to discuss safeguarding issues.
- Each maternity unit in the UK and Ireland should have a named respondent who is responsible for notifying all HIV-positive pregnancies to the National Study of HIV in Pregnancy and Childhood (details at <www.nshpc.ucl.ac.uk>).
- The pregnancies of all women taking antiretroviral therapy should also be reported to the Antiretroviral Pregnancy Registry.
- Newly diagnosed HIV-positive pregnant women do not require any additional baseline investigations compared with non-pregnant HIV-positive women other than those routinely performed in the general antenatal clinic.

Interventions to prevent disease progression in the mother

- Women who require HIV treatment for their own health should take HAART, with treatment started as soon as possible according to the adult treatment guidelines.
- Treatment must continue postpartum.
- These women may also require prophylaxis against pneumocystis pneumonia (PCP), depending on their CD4 lymphocyte count.
- Women already taking HAART and/or PCP prophylaxis before pregnancy should not discontinue their medication.
- In women who either conceive on HAART or who do not require HAART for their own health, there should be a minimum of one CD4 count as baseline and one at delivery
- In women who commence HAART in pregnancy, a viral load should be performed 2–4 weeks after commencing HAART, at least once every trimester, at 36 weeks, and at delivery.
- In women commencing HAART in pregnancy, LFTs should be performed as for routine initiation of HAART and then at each antenatal visit.
- A three/four drug combination including **zidovudine plus lamivudine** (or tenofovir plus emtricitabine) **with nevirapine** are the most commonly used agents in HAART.

Interventions to prevent mother to child transmission of HIV

- **For women who require HIV treatment for their own health**, their prescribed HAART regimen should be continued throughout pregnancy and postpartum.[1,2]
- Women who do not require treatment for themselves should commence temporary HAART at 14/40 if the baseline viral load (VL) is more than 30 000 copies/ml and even earlier if VL is more than 100 000. All women should have commenced HAART by 24 weeks gestation.
- All women should be advised to take antiretroviral therapy.
- A woman who is not on treatment and presents late (i.e. after 28 weeks) should commence HAART without delay. If the VL is unknown or greater than 100 000, a three/four drug regimen that includes raltegravir is suggested.[1]
- An untreated woman presenting in labour at term should be given a stat dose of nevirapine and commence fixed-dose zidovudine with lamivudine and raltegravir. IV zidovudine should be considered for infusion for the duration of labour and delivery.
- **In women who do not require HIV treatment for their own health** and have a baseline VL less than 10 000 and a CD4

greater than 350, zidovudine (ZDV) monotherapy can be used if planning a Caesarean section. ZDV monotherapy should be initiated between 20 and 28 weeks, given orally, 250 mg twice daily, and IV at delivery.

- Delivery by elective Caesarean section at 38 weeks to prevent labour and/or ruptured membranes is recommended for
  - women taking HAART who have a plasma VL greater than 50 copies/ml
  - women taking ZDV monotherapy as an alternative to HAART
  - women with HIV and HCV coinfection.
- Avoidance of breastfeeding, use of antiretroviral therapy, and appropriate management of delivery has reduced mother-to-child transmission rates from 25–30% to less than 1%. All women in resource-rich countries should be advised not to breastfeed.

Antenatal care of pregnant women who are HIV positive

- Dating and anomaly scans should be offered to all women in accordance with national guidelines for the general population.[1,2]
- Pregnant women who are HIV positive are recommended to have screening for syphilis, hepatitis B, and rubella at their booking antenatal visit, in line with the general population. Women should be screened for genital infections at booking and again at 28 weeks. Any infection detected should be treated according to national guidelines, even if asymptomatic.
- Pregnant women who are HIV positive may be offered additional blood tests for hepatitis C, varicella zoster, measles, and toxoplasma.
- Screening for aneuploidy should be offered to all women in accordance with national guidelines for the general population. The combined screening test for trisomy 21 is recommended as this has the best sensitivity and specificity and will minimize the number of women who may need invasive testing.
- For women who present too late for the combined test, the most clinically and cost-effective serum screening test (triple or quadruple test) should be offered between 15^{+0} and 20^{+0} weeks.
- However, significantly increased levels of beta-hCG, and lower levels of oestriol (the elements of the 'triple test') have been observed in the HIV-positive population. This may increase the false-positive rate in women and thus increase the number of invasive tests offered compared with the uninfected population. Pregnancy-associated plasma protein A (PAPP-A) and nuchal translucency are unaltered by HIV infection or antiretroviral therapy (ART) and are thus the preferred screening modality.[1]
- Women who are HIV positive who are considering invasive diagnostic testing should be counselled and the advice of the HIV physicians sought about reducing the risk of HIV transmission.
- Invasive prenatal diagnostic testing should ideally not be done until after the HIV status of the mother is known and deferred until HIV VL has been adequately suppressed.
- If not on treatment and the invasive prenatal procedure cannot be delayed until viral suppression is achieved it is recommended that women should commence HAART to include raltegravir and are given a single dose of nevirapine 2–4 h before the procedure.
- *Women taking HAART at the time of booking should be screened for gestational diabetes.*
- Hepatitis B and pneumococcal vaccination is recommended for all individuals who are HIV positive and can be safely administered in pregnancy. Influenza vaccination can also be safely administered in pregnancy and the decision to immunize depends on the time of year.
- Varicella zoster and measles, mumps, and rubella (MMR) vaccines are contraindicated in pregnancy.
- Monitoring of plasma VL and drug toxicities will be undertaken by the HIV physicians.
- There is no contraindication for external cephalic version (ECV).
- ***A plan of care for antiretroviral therapy and mode of delivery should be made at 36 weeks following detailed discussion with the mother. This should be clearly documented.***
- Only women with plasma VLs of less than 50 copies/ml should be offered a planned vaginal delivery.
- ***In the absence of a documented mode of delivery plan, or in the event of uncertainty about VL results, urgent advice should be sought from the HIV physicians.***

Management of antenatal complications

- For any woman who is HIV positive who becomes acutely unwell in pregnancy, close liaison between the obstetricians and HIV physicians is mandatory to avoid diagnostic error.
- HIV-related complications should also be considered as a cause of acute illness in pregnant women whose HIV status is unknown, particularly those who are not booked for antenatal care. In these circumstances, a rapid HIV test should be considered.
- Women should be counselled about the small increased risk of preterm delivery associated with HAART

Management of preterm delivery and preterm prelabour rupture of membranes

- For women in preterm labour or threatened preterm labour, urgent multidisciplinary team (HIV physicians and paediatricians) advice should be sought about the choice of antiretroviral therapy. Infants born below 32 weeks of gestation may be unable to tolerate oral medication, so administering antiretroviral therapy to the mother just before and during delivery will provide prophylaxis for the neonate.
- Evidence of chorioamnionitis and fetal distress are indications for prompt delivery.
- If **PPROM occurs at <34 weeks**:
  - Prophylactic steroids to accelerate fetal lung maturity steroids.
  - Virological control should be optimized.
  - There should be multidisciplinary discussion about the timing and mode of delivery.
  - Oral erythromycin should be started in accordance with national guidelines for the general population.
  - IV antibiotics for GBS prophylaxis must be given according to national guidelines.
- Where **PPROM or SROM occurs any time after 34 weeks**, delivery should be expedited and IV antibiotics given according to national guidelines for GBS prophylaxis if less than 37 weeks gestation.

Management of delivery

- A plan of care for antiretroviral therapy and mode of delivery should be made at 36 weeks, following detailed discussion with the mother.
- Vaginal delivery is recommended for women on HAART with a VL less than 50 HIV RNA copies/ml plasma at 36 weeks gestation.[1,2]
- For women with a last measured plasma VL of 50–999 HIV RNA copies/ml, immediate Caesarean section should be considered.
- If maternal HIV VL is 1000 RNA copies/ml plasma or greater, immediate Caesarean section is recommended.
- Delivery by Caesarean section is recommended for women taking zidovudine monotherapy irrespective of plasma VL at the time of delivery and for women with VL greater than 400 RNA copies/ml regardless of antiretroviral therapy.
- **Use of intrapartum IV infusion of zidovudine** is recommended in the following circumstances:
  - For women with a VL greater than 10 000 who present in labour, or with ruptured membranes, or who are admitted for planned Caesarean section
  - For untreated women presenting in labour or with ruptured membranes in whom the current VL is not known.
- A maternal sample for plasma VL and CD4 count should be taken at delivery.
- Women taking HAART should have their medications prescribed and administered before delivery and, if indicated, after delivery.

Elective Caesarean section

- Where the indication for Caesarean section is the prevention of vertical transmission, it is best done at between 38 and 39 weeks gestation.

- Where Caesarean section is undertaken only for obstetric indications and plasma VL is less than 50 copies/mL, the usual obstetric considerations apply and timing will usually be at 39–40 weeks.
- If IV ZDV is indicated, the infusion should be started 4 h before beginning the Caesarean section and should continue until the umbilical cord has been clamped.
- The surgical field should be kept as haemostatic as possible and care should be taken if possible, to avoid rupturing the membranes until the head is delivered through the surgical incision.
- Peripartum antibiotics should be administered in accordance with national guidelines for the general population.

Planned vaginal delivery

- Planned vaginal delivery should only be offered to women taking HAART who have a VL of less than 50 copies/ml at 36 weeks gestation.
- In women in whom a vaginal delivery has been recommended and labour has commenced, obstetric management should follow the same guidelines as for the uninfected population observing universal blood borne virus (BBV) precautions.
- HAART should be prescribed and administered throughout labour.
- Invasive procedures such as FBS and FSE are contraindicated.
- If labour progress is normal, amniotomy should be avoided unless delivery is imminent.
- Amniotomy and use of oxytocin may be considered for augmentation of slow progress in labour.
- If instrumental delivery is indicated, low-cavity forceps are preferable to ventouse.
- If maternal HIV VL is less than 50 RNA copies/ml plasma, immediate augmentation of labour is recommended if there are no obstetric contraindications, with a low threshold for treatment of intrapartum pyrexia.
- If maternal HIV VL is 1000 RNA copies/ml plasma or more, immediate Caesarean section is recommended.
- Broad-spectrum IV antibiotics should be administered if there is evidence of genital infection or chorioamnionitis.

Prolonged pregnancy

- For women on HAART with plasma VL of less than 50 copies/ml, the decision regarding induction of labour for prolonged pregnancy should be individualized. There is no contraindication to membrane sweep or to use of prostaglandins.

Vaginal birth after Caesarean section

- Vaginal birth after Caesarean section (VBAC) can be offered to women with a VL of less than 50 copies/ml.

HIV diagnosed in labour

- Women presenting in labour/ROM/requiring delivery without a documented HIV result must be recommended to have a HIV diagnostic point of care test (POCT).
- **A reactive POCT result must be acted upon immediately** with initiation of the interventions for prevention of mother-to-child transmission without waiting for formal serological confirmation.[1]
- For women diagnosed HIV positive during labour, the paediatricians should be informed and urgent advice should be sought from the HIV physicians regarding optimum HAART.
- Delivery should be by Caesarean section and, where possible, this should be timed with respect to antiretroviral administration.

Postpartum management of women who are HIV positive

- Women should be given supportive advice about formula feeding.
- An immediate dose of oral cabergoline should be given to suppress lactation.
- Women taking HAART should have their medication prescribed and administered.
- Guidance about contraception should be given in the immediate postpartum period.
- MMR and varicella zoster immunization may be indicated, according to the CD4 lymphocyte count.
- Continuation of HAART is recommended after delivery in women with a baseline CD4 count of more than 350 cells/microlitre.

Management of the neonate

- ***Refer to the BHIVA guidelines.***[1]
- Neonates born to women who are HIV infected are reported to the National Study of HIV in Pregnancy and Childhood <http://www.nshpc.ucl.ac.uk/>.

Pre-pregnancy management

- Couples who are serodiscordant choosing to have intercourse should be advised to use condoms.
- Couples who are serodiscordant where the female partner is HIV negative should be advised that assisted conception with either donor insemination or sperm washing is significantly safer than timed unprotected intercourse.
- Couples should be advised to delay conception until plasma viraemia is suppressed, prophylaxis against PCP is no longer required, and any opportunistic infections have been treated.
- All women who are HIV positive are recommended to have annual cervical cytology.

Information for patients

Please see Information for patients: HIV and pregnancy (p. 501)

(Data from: RCOG Green-Top Guideline No. 39, *Management of HIV in pregnancy*, 2010, Royal College Obstetricians and Gynaecologists; and British HIV Association, British HIV Association Guidelines for the Management of HIV Infection in Pregnant Women, 2012, *HIV Medicine*, 2012, 13, Suppl. 2, pp. 87–157, DOI: 10.1111/j.1468-1293.2012.01030.x)

References

1. Taylor GP, et al. British HIV Association guidelines for the management of HIV infection in pregnant women, 2012. HIV Med 2012;13 Suppl 2: 87–157.
2. RCOG Green-top Guideline No. 39. Management of HIV in pregnancy. London: Royal College of Obstetricians and Gynaecologists, 2010.

CARE PATHWAY

- Modified from BHIVA and RCOG guidelines—refers only to antenatal management
- See the latest BHIVA and RCOG Guidelines for intrapartum and neonatal management of HIV mothers

Known HIV +ve woman

- Referred by GP/community midwife or HIV (GUM) clinic
- Screening for other genital infections, treated as per BASHH guidelines by GUM clinic
- Seen in designated antenatal clinic with members of the HIV team, obstetric consultant, HIV coordinating midwife
- Routine pregnancy booking blood tests
- Initial blood tests for known HIV +ve women: CD4, viral load, Hep C, varicella zoster, measles, toxoplasmosis screening, LFTs, U&E
- Initial retrovirus infection care plan formulated and commenced

HIV newly diagnosed in pregnancy (usually found after screening as part of booking bloods or later in pregnancy, with patient's consent)

- Referral to HIV team by virology and/or HIV midwife or nurse coordinator after alert from virology department
- Second confirmatory HIV test
- HIV baseline serology
- HIV resistance test
- CD4 count
- LFT, FBC, U&E
- Screening for Hep C, varicella zoster, measles, toxoplasmosis
- Hep B, influenza, pneumococcal vaccination recommended
- Screening for genital infections, treated according to BASHH guidelines

Those already on HAART treatment

- Dating and routine anomaly scans
- Routine screening for aneuploidy as per national guidelines for general population
- If invasive testing is opted for/indicated, counselling regarding theoretical risk of transmission to fetus, seek advice from GUM/ HIV consultants
- Neonatologist/paediatrician informed and introduced to pregnant woman, involved in developing plan of care with full discussion with woman

Further antenatal care

- Continue current treatment
- Close communication between all members of the HIV team
- Arrange GTT screening at 28 weeks
- Continued CD4 and viral load monitoring as per latest BHIVA guidelines and directed by HIV physicians
- Continue routine antenatal care with community midwife
- Fetal growth scans, suggested at 28 and 34 weeks gestation
- A joint multidisciplinary 'plan of care' for continued retroviral therapy, CD4 and viral load monitoring, LFTs, fetal growth scans, and the mode of delivery drawn up after discussion with the pregnant woman
- Clear documentation and joint plan circulated to those professionals directly involved with the care of the mother and the baby
- Only women with plasma viral loads <50 copies/ml should be offered a planned vaginal delivery
- See the BHIVA guidelines for management of labour and delivery in HIV +ve patients

Those not yet on HAART

- Selected HAART commenced as advised by HIV Physicians based on CD4 and viral loads
- Viral load measured 2–4 weeks after HAART commenced
- Close communication between all members of the HIV team
- Continued monitoring of CD4, viral loads
- LFTs at start of treatment and then at each antenatal visit as per BHIVA guidelines
- Fetal growth scans
- A joint multidisciplinary 'plan of care' for continued retroviral therapy, CD4 and viral load monitoring, LFTs and renal function tests, fetal growth scans, and the mode of delivery drawn up after discussion with the pregnant woman
- Clear documentation and joint plan circulated to those professionals directly involved with the care of the mother and baby
- Only women with plasma viral loads <50 copies/ ml at 36 weeks gestation should be offered a planned vaginal delivery

At 36 weeks

If viral load still detected or not < 50 HIV RNA copies/ml:

- Review patient's compliance with medication regime
- HIV team physicians may advise repeat resistance test as well as consider therapeutic drug monitoring (TDM)
- Optimize to best regimen
- Consider intensification
- If viral loads are still elevated, planned Caesarean section at 38 weeks advisable and inform neonatologist, anaesthetist
- Refer to BHIVA guidelines for management of labour and delivery in HIV +ve patients

Data from British HIV Association, British HIV Association Guidelines for the Management of HIV Infection in Pregnant Women, 2012, *HIV Medicine*, 2012, 13, Suppl. 2, pp. 87–157, DOI: 10.1111/j.1468-1293.2012.01030.x

2.10 Listeriosis

FACT FILE

Epidemiology

- **Listeriosis** is a rare disease that causes mild maternal illness, but can be fatal for the fetus, with a perinatal death rate of 20–30%.[1,2]
- Listeriosis is a rare aerobic infection, and is about 20 times more common in pregnant women than in the general population.[1] The incidence of listeriosis in pregnancy is 12 per 100 000, compared with a rate of 0.7 per 100 000 in the general population.[3]
- In 2010, there were an estimated 156 cases of listeriosis in England and Wales, 17 of which were in pregnant women.[2]
- Listeriosis is most often a food-borne illness.
- *Listeria monocytogenes* is a common organism in nature, easily isolated from soil, dust, water, processed foods, raw meat, and faeces of animals and humans.
- *Listeria monocytogenes* **can survive even at temperatures as low as 4 °C**, therefore contaminated refrigerated foods are potential sources of infection.
- Pregnant women may be able to reduce risk of listeria infection by observing hygienic food preparation, storage, and consumption guidelines
- Maternal listerial illness can be mild or even asymptomatic. Any condition that reduces cell-mediated immunity, such as pregnancy, can predispose to listerial infection.
- Although pregnant women with comorbidities are at increased risk of listeriosis, most cases occur in otherwise healthy pregnant women.[1]
- Comorbidities such as HIV infection, diabetes, or use of immunosuppressive medications including steroids, increase the risk for listerial infection due to a decrease in cell-mediated immunity. In such patients listerial infection can cause severe maternal illness, usually by spreading to the central nervous system (CNS)[1] with a fatality rate of 20–50%.
- *Listeria monocytogenes* has an intracellular life cycle and can therefore cross the placental barrier and the blood–brain barrier. It is an intracellular organism that hides within host cells.[1,2]
- The incubation period from 24 h to 70 days.[1]

Maternal symptoms

- Maternal symptoms include fever, flu-like malaise, headache, sore throat, conjunctivitis, abdominal or back pain, vomiting/diarrhoea.

Diagnosis

- ***Diagnosis is made only by culturing the Gram-positive bacilli from blood, CSF, amniotic fluid, or the placenta.***
- **Maternal vaginal secretions or stool cultures are not diagnostic** as they can occur in carriers of listeria, not necessarily indicating active infection.
- **Listeriosis must be suspected in any pregnant patient presenting with fever accompanied by gastrointestinal symptoms.** Blood culture is recommended.

Fetal/neonatal effects

- The incidence of listeriosis in the newborn is estimated as 8.6 per 100 000 live births.[1]
- Maternal listeriosis in the second or third trimester results in 40–50% fetal mortality.[4]
- Listeriosis characteristically causes meconium-stained liquor, even in preterm pregnancies less than 34 weeks.
- In later pregnancy fetal septicaemia may result in damage to multiple organs and stillbirth or neonatal death.[5]
- The mortality rate varies from 3% to 50% in liveborn neonates infected with listeria.[6]
- Perinatal listeria within 7 days of birth is often associated with prematurity and fulminant disease. Late-onset disease (7 days to 6 weeks) often presents with meningitis.[1,2,3,4]
- ***Transplacental passage can produce congenital listeriosis.***
- Neonatal infection can present with respiratory distress, rash, fever, or jaundice and can cause pneumonia, meningitis, or septicaemia.
- Early-onset listeriosis develops 1–2 days after birth, and the baby often has signs of a serious bacterial infection. Late-onset listeriosis occurs 1–2 weeks after birth and usually includes symptoms of meningitis.

Treatment

- If listeria chorioamnionitis is diagnosed preterm, treatment with high-dose IV antibiotics administered to the mother is possible, and preterm delivery may be avoided.[1,4,6,7]
- Penicillin, ampicillin, and amoxicillin and gentamicin have been used most extensively for treatment.[4] Erythromycin alone does not reach therapeutic levels in amniotic fluid and fetal serum.
- Whichever antibiotic is chosen, dosage is critical. A prolonged course of high doses of IV antibiotics (ampicillin and gentamicin) for at least 1 week after fever subsides is often recommended but continued treatment may be required in some cases for longer periods. A combination of amoxicillin and erythromycin can also be used. **Early consultation with the microbiologist is essential.**
- Optimal duration of therapy in pregnancy has not been established. In case reports, duration of therapy has varied from 2 weeks to continuous treatment until delivery.[7] Others have suggested at least 3–4 weeks of treatment in pregnancy.[4]

Prevention

- Epidemiological investigations have demonstrated that nearly all types of food can transmit listeria.[1,2]
- Most sporadic cases and all large outbreaks have been associated with manufactured foods such as paté.
- Dairy products, especially soft cheeses, have also been implicated in outbreaks. Pasteurization eliminates listeria from dairy products, and most dairy-associated outbreaks are from items that are inadequately pasteurized or contaminated after pasteurization.[1]
- Most cases of listeriosis are sporadic and not associated with an outbreak.
- Avoidance of cross-contamination is important for disease prevention, with all utensils and food preparation surfaces washed well after preparing meat dishes or cutting prepared foods.

Information for patients

Please see Information for patients: Listeriosis and pregnancy (p. 501)

References

1. Janakiraman V. Listeriosis in pregnancy: diagnosis, treatment and prevention. Rev Obstet Gynecol 2008;1: 179–185.
2. Gilbert GL. Infections in pregnant women. Med J Aust 2002;176: 229–236.
3. Hof H. History and epidemiology of listeriosis. FEMS Immunol Med Microbiol 2003;35: 199–202.
4. Palasanthiran P, et al. Management of perinatal infections. In: Palasanthiran P, et al., ed. Sydney: Australasian Society for Infectious Diseases (ASID) 2002.
5. Langford KS. Infectious disease and pregnancy. Curr Obstet Gynaecol 2002;12: 125–130.
6. Bortolussi R, Schlech WF. Listeriosis. In:Remington JS, Klein JO, ed., Infectious diseases of the fetus and newborn infant 5th ed. Philadelphia, PA: WB Saunders, 2001.
7. Temple ME, Nahata MC. Treatment of listeriosis. Ann Pharmacother 2000;34: 656–661.

CARE PATHWAY

In primary care

- A high degree of suspicion is required as Listeriosis infection is often asymptomatic or causes only mild flu-like illness with gastrointestinal symptoms in healthy pregnant women
- In pregnant women with comorbidities, awareness that the disease can take a severe form is essential
- Information regarding prevention of listeriosis is shared with all pregnant women at the booking visit by the community midwife as part of general healthy eating advice
- If the pregnant woman reports flu-like symptoms to GP or community midwife, a more detailed history needs to be obtained concerning whether she has had any contact in the last few days or weeks with animals, especially at calving or lambing time, whether there has been any consumption of meat-based paté, soft cheeses, etc.
- Remember: incubation period varies from 1 to 70 days
- If clinical suspicion, immediate blood tests should include urgent blood culture sent from primary care
- If blood cultures are reported positive, the patient is immediately sent to a specialist antenatal clinic for further management or treatment commenced in primary care after discussion with the microbiologist

↓

Hospital antenatal care with positive blood culture

- Patient and pregnancy assessment
- **HVS/ECS or stool culture are not specific** for acute infection due to carrier state found in 1–10% of individuals
- Depending on severity of maternal illness and after discussion with microbiologist, immediate treatment with antibiotics. If IV antibiotics required, admit away from other pregnant mothers
- Duration of treatment to be based on presence or absence of comorbidities, clinical severity, and as advised by microbiologist
- Further schedule of antenatal care must be individualized on a case-to-case basis
- The parents must be informed that though the maternal symptoms may subside, antibiotics may need to continue for longer (as advised by microbiologist)
- Discuss high pregnancy loss rate with 2nd-trimester miscarriages, IUD, preterm delivery, or early neonatal death. Almost 50% of all infected infants at or near term will die. Infants that do survive could suffer long-term neurological damage
- Parents must be warned that despite maternal treatment, the neonate could be severely ill with pneumonia, septicaemia, meningoencephalitis, meconium aspiration, etc.
- The neonatologists must be informed if delivery of the potentially infected but live baby is being considered as a viable option
- Samples must be sent for culture of *Listeria monocytogenes* from neonatal blood, urine and/or CSF. CT/MRI of the brain to demonstrate any CNS lesions as well as ECHO for vegetations may be required
- Placenta and amniotic fluid samples for culture must be sent
- Long-term neurology follow-up of those infected babies who survive is essential

Pregnant woman with flu-like illness or gastrointestinal symptoms

Detailed history of contact with animals, consumption of soft cheeses, paté, etc., infection with listeriosis to be anticipated

↓

Diagnosis

- Blood cultures and Gram stain for Gram-positive bacilli, **or**
- Amniotic fluid or CSF—culture and Gram stain

↓

Negative for *Listeria monocytogenes*
Investigate for other infections causing similar symptoms

Positive for Listeria monocytogenes

↓

Severe infection, chorioamnionitis

- Urgent consultation with microbiologist
- IV antibiotics as advised by microbiologist for about 14 days
- Dosage and duration of antibiotics as advised by microbiologist
- Discuss high perimortality rate of infected fetus/neonate with pregnant woman and partner/family, although early treatment of maternal infection can improve perinatal outcome

↓

- Delivery depending on severity of infection and gestational age
- Meconium staining of liquor, meconium aspiration, preterm delivery to be anticipated
- Inform neonatologist about potentially infected neonate
- Document need for placenta to be sent for microbiology culture and Gram staining

Mild infection

- Oral antibiotics after consultation with microbiologist—recommended antibiotics, dosage, and duration as recommended by microbiologist
- Antibiotics may need to be continued for 2 weeks or longer

↓

- Risk of **early** (within 7 days of birth) neonatal infection associated with preterm delivery or fulminant infection or **late-onset** (7 days–6 weeks of birth) neonatal infection to be anticipated by paediatricians

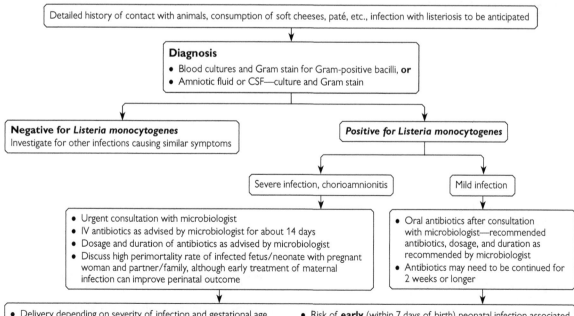

2.11 Malaria

FACT FILE

The following fact file and care pathway pertain only to general information and the ongoing obstetric antenatal management of those high-risk women who have already been diagnosed and have received/ or are receiving treatment for **malaria** during the pregnancy. For detailed information regarding the prevention, diagnosis, and treatment of malaria in pregnancy, see the RCOG Green-top Guidelines.[1]

Epidemiology

- Malaria is life threatening, but preventable and treatable.
- The highest prevalence of malaria is in tropical Africa, South-East Asia, and South America.
- The majority of imported infections in the UK are due to *Plasmodium falciparum* (79%), *P. vivax* (13%), *P. ovale* (5.5%), *P. malariae* (2%); the rest are mixed infections.[1]
- Most cases of *P. falciparum* imported into the UK are from West Africa, especially Ghana and Nigeria.
- Other malarial areas are the Indian subcontinent (*P. vivax*), South and Central America, Hispaniola, Papua New Guinea, South-East Asia, and the Middle East.
- *P. falciparum* is the most dangerous species of malaria, responsible for the most severe disease and nearly all mortality due to malaria.
- Worldwide, malaria is one of the causes of severe maternal and perinatal morbidity and mortality; for example, malaria accounts for up to 23% of maternal deaths and 18% of neonatal deaths in sub-Saharan Africa.[1,2,3,4,5,6] It affects about 32 million pregnancies per year in sub-Saharan Africa.[7]
- Most cases in the UK (1370 cases reported in 2008) are found in those who have travelled to or emigrated from malarial areas.
- Pregnant women are at higher risk of both acquiring malaria and of suffering from the more severe form of the disease, such as cerebral malaria, compared with non-pregnant women.
- ***Adverse effects of malaria in pregnancy are maternal and fetal mortality, severe anaemia, pregnancy loss due to miscarriages, stillbirth and premature labour, and low birth weight.***

Clinical features

- Pyrexia
- Rigors
- Nausea, abdominal pain
- Headache.

Maternal morbidity

Maternal morbidity caused by malaria includes:

- Severe refractory anaemia
- Hypoglycaemia
- Pulmonary oedema
- Hyperpyrexia
- Cerebral malaria

Fetal/neonatal morbidity

- Effects of malaria on the fetus include:
  - increased risk of second-trimester miscarriages
  - preterm labour
  - IUGR
  - stillbirth.
- **Congenital malaria** due to transplacental passage can lead to severe neonatal infection.
- Congenital malaria varies from 8% to 33%. Clinical features include fever, irritability, poor feeding, anaemia, jaundice and hepatosplenomegaly. Recommended treatment is quinine plus clindamycin for infants under 1 year of age.
- In pregnancy, the malarial parasites sequester in the placenta, where infection may be very heavy. Clearance of the parasite should therefore be the aim before delivery.
- Sickle cell trait has been associated with resistance to the severe forms of *P. falciparum* infection due to the increased sickling of parasitized red cells, promoting removal of these cells from circulation.[7]

Diagnosis

- The gold standard test is visualization of the parasite in a peripheral blood film by microscopy. The parasite count and type must be determined.
- Peripheral parasitaemia greater than 2% should be regarded as severe disease.
- A single negative film does not exclude the disease and repeat blood films should be taken and tested at intervals of 4–6 h. In a febrile patient, if there are three negative peripheral blood films 12–24 h apart, a diagnosis of malaria can be excluded.
- In women who are from endemic countries, the placenta may be heavily infected even though the peripheral film is negative.

Management

- **Admission** for treatment is often required due to increased risks of severe malaria.
  - Women who have arrived in the UK from endemic areas are usually immune and in the absence of severe disease may be managed as outpatients.
  - However, immigrants from sub-Saharan Africa who have lived in the UK for any length of time and visit Africa intermittently are likely to become non-immune and require admission for a possible severe form of the infection.
- Upon admission, **expert advice should be sought from microbiology**.
  - Regular check of haemoglobin and platelet counts.
  - Blood glucose check initially and 2-hourly once quinine is commenced.
  - Prompt treatment of fever with antipyretics is essential to prevent pyrexia-induced complications such as premature labour and fetal distress.
  - In women with severe anaemia, **slow** blood transfusion, preferably with packed cell and furosemide 20 mg.
- **Antimalarials:** Expert advice is required regarding choice of drug depending on the type of malarial parasite.[8, 9, 10]
- **WHO treatment protocol**[8] for *P. falciparum* malaria:
  - Admit to hospital.
  - *First trimester:* Quinine plus clindamycin for 7 days; if this fails, artesunate plus clindamycin for 7 days.
  - *Second and third trimesters:* Artemisinin-based combination therapy (ACT) known to be effective in the endemic country or region, or artesunate plus clindamycin for 7 days, or quinine plus clindamycin for 7 days.
  - *Breastfeeding:* Standard antimalarials (including ACTs) except dapsone, primaquine, and tetracyclines.
- **Chloroquine** is the drug of choice for *P. vivax*, *P. malariae*, and *P. ovale*.

(Reproduced from 'Guidelines for the Treatment of malaria, Second edition', World Health Organization, Box 7.5, 2010, © World Heath Organization, with permission Geneva: WHO. www.who.int/malaria/publications/atoz/0789241547925/en/index.html.)

- ***Severe malaria is a medical emergency requiring intensive care admission***, which is outside the remit of this antenatal fact file.

Antenatal care after an episode of malaria

- After recovery from an episode of malaria during pregnancy, **continued antenatal care should include:**
  - Regular antenatal care with assessment of haemoglobin, platelet count, glucose
  - Serial growth scans at 3–4-week intervals. If IUGR suspected, management as per IUGR guidelines.

Table 2.3 Antimalarial drug therapy in pregnancy

Severity	*Type of malaria*	*Drug regime*	*Dosage and route*	*Alternatives*	*Precautions*
Severe or complicated	All species	Artesunate with clindamycin or quinine with clindamycin	• IV loading dose at 2.4 mg/kg at 0, 12, and 24 h. Then daily thereafter. • When well enough to take oral medication, switch to daily oral artesunate 2 mg/kg (or IM artesunate 2.4 mg/kg) once daily, plus clindamycin	• Quinine IV 20 mg/kg loading dose (no loading dose if patient already taking quinine or mefloquine) in 5% glucose over 4 h and then 10 mg/kg IV over 4 h every 8 h plus clindamycin IV 450 mg every 8 h (max. dose quinine 1.4 g) • When well enough to take oral medication, switch to oral quinine 600 mg 3 times a day for 5–7 days and oral clindamycin 450 mg 3 times a day for 7 days (An alternative rapid quinine-loading regimen is 7 mg/kg quinine dihydrochloride IV over 30 min with infusion pump followed by 10 mg/kg over 4 h)	• Quinine dosing should be reduced to 12-hourly if IV therapy extends more than 48 h or if the patient has renal or hepatic dysfunction • Quinine is associated with severe and recurrent hypoglycaemia in late pregnancy
Uncomplicated malaria	*P. falciparum*	• Quinine with clindamycin **or** atovaquone-proguanil	• Oral quinine 600 mg 8-hourly and oral clindamycin 450 mg 8 hourly for 7 days (can be given together) **or** atovaquone-proguanil 4 standard tablets daily for 3 days	• If vomiting, but not severe or uncomplicated malaria, quinine 10 mg/kg dose IV in 5% glucose over 4 h every 8 h plus IV clindamycin 450 mg every 8 h • When the patient is well enough to take oral medication she can be switched to oral quinine 600 mg 3 times a day to complete 5–7 days and oral clindamycin can if needed be switched to 450 mg 3 times a day for 7 days	
Non-falciparum malaria	*P. vivax, P. ovale, P. malariae*		Oral chloroquine (base) 600 mg followed by 300 mg 68 h later. Then 300 mg on day 2 and again on day 3		
	Resistant *P. vivax*	As for uncomplicated *P. falciparum* malaria			
	Preventing relapse **during** pregnancy	Chloroquine	Chloroquine oral 300 mg weekly until delivery		
	Preventing relapse **after** delivery	Chloroquine	Postpone until 3 months after delivery and G6PD testing		
	P. ovale	Primaquine	Oral primaquine 15 mg single daily dose for 14 days		
	P. vivax	Primaquine	Oral primaquine 30 mg single daily dose for 14 days		
	G6PD (mild) for *P. vivax* or *P. ovale*	Primaquine	Primaquine oral 45–60 mg once a week for 8 weeks		

Data from: RCOG Green-top Guidelines No. 54a and No. 54b, 'The prevention of malaria in pregnancy' and 'The diagnosis and treatment of malaria in pregnancy', 2010, Royal College Obstetricians and Gynaecologists; World Health Organization, 'Assessment of the Safety of Artemisinin Compounds in Pregnancy', Report of two joint informal consultations convened in 2006 by the Special Programme for Research and Training in Tropical Diseases (TDR) sponsored by UNICEF/UNDP/World bank/WHO and The global Malaria Programme of the World Health Organization, Geneva, WHO, 2007; and Lalloo DG, et al., 'UK malaria treatment guidelines', *Journal of Infection*, 2007, 54, pp. 111–121.

- CTG and Doppler abnormalities may be observed due to maternal pyrexia and/or hypoglycaemia. Immediate treatment with antimalarials, antipyretics, and correction of hypoglycaemia, can reverse these signs.
- The patient must be informed of the risk of relapse, and a clear plan developed and documented in case of such relapse
- Uncomplicated malaria is not an indication for induction of labour (IOL). Preterm delivery may be required only in a few cases. Malaria by itself is not an indication for Caesarean section.
- ***Document the following in maternity hand-held and main notes for intrapartum management:***
- The paediatricians must be alerted well in time.
- Great care is required during labour, delivery, and postpartum to avoid pulmonary oedema, which carries a mortality rate of 50% in cases when an affected woman goes into labour with severe anaemia.
- Prompt treatment of secondary bacterial infections with signs of septicaemia.
- Assisted instrumental vaginal delivery is indicated if signs of maternal or fetal distress develop in the second stage.[1] The role of early elective Caesarean section in severe malaria with a viable fetus is unproven.[1]
- **The placenta must be sent for histology and microbiological studies.** If the placenta is positive for parasites, arrange weekly screening of the newborn for 28 days to allow early detection and treatment.
- Cord and baby blood films are essential for prompt detection of congenital malaria.
- If there is thrombocytopenia ($<10^9$/litre), routine pharmacological thromboprophylaxis must be withheld. Thrombocytopenia usually recovers with treatment.

Prophylaxis for travel and advice to pregnant women

- Pregnant women should be discouraged from travelling to malaria endemic areas.
- Immigrant women resident in the UK who wish to visit a malaria endemic area should be counselled likewise as their immunity will have declined, and the benefits of chemoprophylaxis outweigh the risk of malaria.
- The pregnant woman should be reminded that no malaria prophylaxis is 100% protective.
- The choice of drug and advice about chemoprophylaxis in pregnant women depends on the level of chloroquine-resistant

P. falciparum and *P. vivax* as well as the trimester of pregnancy. Specific guidelines can be accessed directly from the UK government website (<http://www.gov.uk/government/publications/malaria-prevention-guidelines-for-travellers-from-the-uk>). Drug dosages, adverse effects, contraindications, and interactions are listed in the British National Formulary (<http://www.bnf.org>). See Table 2.3.

- Warn pregnant women intending to travel that drugs for malaria prophylaxis may be cheaper over the internet or in endemic countries, **but may be counterfeit**.
- Proguanil and chloroquine: are not efficacious in chloroquine-resistant areas and most areas are now chloroquine resistant. **Doxycycline and primaquine are contraindicated in pregnancy**.
- **Mefloquine** is the recommended drug of choice for prophylaxis in the second and third trimester and it does not appear to increase the risk of teratogenicity at prophylactic doses. However, this has strict contraindications for those with a history of epilepsy, neuropsychiatric disorders, or depressive illness.
- **Advice for breastfeeding mothers wishing to travel to endemic areas** is the same as in pregnancy.

Information for patients

Please see Information for patients: Malaria and pregnancy (p. 501)

References

1. RCOG Green-top Guidelines No. 54A and No. 54B. The prevention of malaria in pregnancy; The diagnosis and treatment of malaria in pregnancy. London:Royal College of Obstetricians and Gynaecologists, 2010.
2. Dorman E, Shulman C. Malaria in pregnancy. Curr Obstet Gynaecol 2001;10: 181–189.
3. Nelson-Piercy C. Malaria in pregnancy. In: Handbook of obstetric medicine, 4th ed. London: Informa Healthcare, 2010, pp. 305–307.
4. Desai M, et al. Epidemiology and burden of malaria in pregnancy. Lancet Infect Dis 2007;7: 93–104.
5. Whitty CJ, et al. Malaria in pregnancy. BJOG 2005;112: 1189–1195.
6. Health Protection Agency Malaria Reference Laboratory. Malaria Epidemiological Data, 2006. <http://www.malaria-reference.co.uk>.
7. Soma-Pillay P, Macdonald AP. Malaria in pregnancy. Obstet Med 2012;5: 2–5.
8. WHO. Guidelines for the treatment of malaria, 2nd ed. Geneva: World Health Organization, 2010 <http://whqlibdoc.who.int/publications/2010/9789241547925_eng.pdf>
9. World Health Organization, 'Assessment of the Safety of Artemisinin Compounds in Pregnancy', Report of two joint informal consultations convened in 2006 by the Special Programme for Research and Training in Tropical Diseases (TDR) sponsored by UNICEF/UNDP/World bank/WHO and The global Malaria Programme of the World Health Organization, Geneva, WHO, 2007
10. Lalloo DG, et al., 'UK malaria treatment guidelines', Journal of Infection, 2007, 54, pp. 111–121.

After acute treatment of the malaria episode is complete, refer to the maternal medicine antenatal clinic

↓

The antenatal care pathway needs to be individualized according to severity and type of malaria, trimester of pregnancy, drug therapy, and risk of relapse in each case

↓

Maternal medicine antenatal clinic follow-up

- Regular antenatal checks and maternal assessment, including haemoglobin, platelet counts, glucose levels
- If severe anaemia, admit for slow blood transfusion with packed cells, taking precautions to avoid pulmonary oedema
- Serial growth scans at 3–4 week intervals
- If IUGR suspected, follow IUGR care pathway (see p. 421)
- If on proguanil or pyrimethamine—high-dose folic acid (5 mg/day)
- Further reviews in clinic to be individualized
- Inform patient of chances of relapse
- Multidisciplinary input for management plans in case of relapse to be clearly documented and shared with patient
- Inform paediatricians ahead of time for possibility of transplacental transmission and congenital malaria
- Early delivery may be indicated in a few cases but malaria per se is not an indication for routine LSCS or early IOL

Document the following instructions for intrapartum management in hand-held and main notes:

- Alert paediatrics well in time
- On admission, check haemoglobin, glucose, and platelet levels
- Care to avoid pulmonary oedema during labour, delivery, and postpartum
- Vigilance for fluid overload
- If signs of septicaemia, suspect secondary infection; active treatment with antibiotics, antipyretics
- If signs of maternal fatigue or fetal distress in 2nd stage, cut short 2nd stage with assisted instrumental delivery, if no contraindications
- PPH prophylaxis essential
- **Placenta must be sent** for urgent histological and microbiological examination
- Cord and neonatal blood films for prompt detection and treatment of congenital malaria
- If platelet count <100 x 10^9 withhold routine pharmacological thromboprophylaxis

2.12 Sexually Transmitted Infections (Excluding Syphilis)

FACT FILE

Gonorrhoea and pregnancy

- *Neisseria gonorrhoeae* is the second most common sexually transmitted infection (STI) in the UK, though still relatively uncommon and usually urban based.
- Gonorrhoea can affect the genitourinary tract, eye, rectum, and pharynx.
- It can be asymptomatic in women or be associated with dysuria and a mucopurulent vaginal discharge.
- Less frequently, in untreated cases a disseminated form of the disease can occur with septicaemia.
- *N. gonorrhoeae* can cause perinatal complications such as preterm premature rupture of membranes, preterm labour, chorioamnionitis, low birth weight, and ophthalmia neonatorum caused by neonatal transmission in 50% of exposed babies.
- ***As in any case of STI identified during pregnancy, immediate referral to genitourinary medicine is essential. Advice can also be sought from the microbiologist on call regarding swabs, treatment regimes, etc.***
- About 40–50% of women with gonorrhoea are coinfected with chlamydia, therefore concurrent treatment must be considered.
- Treatment is not different in pregnancy and the efficacy of treatment is the same as in non-pregnant patients.
- Treatment regimes should include chlamydia and syphilis as they can often coexist in gonococcal infection in pregnancy. Various antibiotic treatments (amoxicillin plus probenecid, spectinomycin, ceftriaxone, cefixime) are effective for curing gonorrhoea in pregnant women.[1] There are no reports of serious adverse effects.
- Recommended treatment of isolated gonorrhoea in pregnancy[1,2,3,4] is either cefixime 400 mg single oral dose[3] or ceftriaxone 250 mg IM or 3 g amoxicillin plus 1 g probenecid orally or cefotaxime 500 mg IM or spectinomycin 2 g IM.
- Tetracyclines and fluoroquinolones should be avoided in pregnancy

Chlamydia and pregnancy

- Most cases of chlamydia in women are found in those under 25 years of age, but in the last decade a doubling of cases has been seen in women in the 25–34 years age bracket.[5] Higher number of sexual partners and younger age are risk factors.
- The earlier in pregnancy the infection is acquired, the greater the perinatal risks may be.[4]
- Primary chlamydial infection contracted during pregnancy may cause PPROM and low birth weight.[4,6]
- Complications also include puerperal sepsis in one-third of untreated women and ophthalmia neonatorum in 50% of neonates, or neonatal chlamydial pneumonitis (15%).[4]
- There is no universal screening programme for chlamydia in the UK.
- Screening is recommended in high-risk groups such as when other STIs are detected, those with puerperal fever or women whose babies have developed ophthalmia neonatorum.
- Screening is usually performed by taking an endocervical swab (ECS). Care is essential to avoid inadvertent rupture of membranes or when there is known placenta praevia. Vulvovaginal swabs have been found to be as useful as ECS.
- Erythromycin and amoxicillin have all been found to be equally effective, but azithromycin has been found to have fewer side effects, hence better compliance.
- Erythromycin, 500 mg four times daily for 7 days, is the treatment of choice during pregnancy and lactation or azithromycin 1 g stat to treat *C. trachomatis* in pregnancy.[7]
- A test of cure needs to be performed 5–6 weeks after treatment completion.
- If chlamydia has been detected and treated early in pregnancy, repeat screening is advised in the third trimester.[4]

Anogenital warts (condyloma acuminata) and pregnancy

- Anogenital warts are the most common STI in the UK.
- Genital warts are very contagious and are spread during oral, genital, or anal sex with an infected partner. About 75% who have had sexual contact with a partner with genital warts will also develop warts, usually within 3 months of contact.
- Most often seen in young women aged 16–19 years.[4]
- Caused by human papillomavirus (HPV): 90% are caused by HPV 6 or 11 subtypes.
- In addition to warts in genital areas, HPV types 6 and 11 have been associated with conjunctival, nasal, oral, and laryngeal warts.
- Genital warts are usually asymptomatic, but depending on the size and anatomical location, they can be painful or pruritic. Genital warts are usually flat, papular, or pedunculated lesions on the genital mucosa.
- The primary reason for treating genital warts is the amelioration of symptoms. If left untreated in non-pregnant women, visible genital warts can resolve on their own, remain unchanged, or increase in size or number.
- Available therapies for genital warts can reduce, but not eradicate, HPV infectivity.
- No evidence indicates that the presence of genital warts or their treatment is associated with the development of cervical cancer.
- ***In pregnancy, due to decreased maternal immunity, infection can be symptomatic and spread rapidly.***
- The main concern is that the unborn baby of a mother infected with genital warts may contract laryngeal papillomatosis,[8] which is a life-threatening condition. Symptoms of this disease can lie dormant for as long as 3 years following birth. If a baby does become infected with laryngeal papillomatosis, laser therapy is required at regular intervals to eliminate it so that it does not obstruct breathing. Interferon therapy may also be used alongside with laser surgery.
- Although vertical transmission can cause neonatal laryngeal warts in about 1 in 80 cases, **routine elective Caesarean section is not recommended in anogenital warts.**
- Caesarean delivery is not indicated solely to prevent transmission of HPV infection to the newborn. Pregnant women with genital warts should be counselled concerning the small risk on warts on the larynx (recurrent respiratory papillomatosis) in their infants or children.
- Treatment of anogenital warts during pregnancy does **not**, in fact, reduce the risk of vertical transmission, but can improve symptoms.
- Podophyllin, podofilox, and fluorouracil are antimitotic, therefore contraindicated in pregnancy due to teratogenic and toxicity risks.
- Imiquimod is a topically active immune enhancer that stimulates production of interferon and other cytokines but has not been recommended due to lack of safety data. Sinecatechins similarly do not have enough safety data to be used in pregnancy.
- ***Treatment in pregnancy is limited to cryocautery, electrocautery, or application of liquid nitrogen to the warts.***[9]
- Pain followed by necrosis and sometimes blistering after application of liquid nitrogen is common. Local anaesthetic (topical or injected) might help therapy if warts are present in many areas or if the area of warts is large.
- Genital warts commonly recur after treatment, especially in the first 3 months.
- In rare cases when the warts are so extensive that they can cause actual obstruction to the delivery due to blockage of the vaginal outlet, or have a greater risk of local bleeding, a Caesarean section may have to be considered.

- Spontaneous and rapid resolution of even extensive warts occurs within 2–4 weeks of delivery as the relative suppression of the maternal immune system during pregnancy is restored to normal levels.

Trichomoniasis and pregnancy

- Caused by *Trichomonas vaginalis*.
- Most common non-viral STI in pregnancy.
- Can cause vulvovaginitis, but 10–15% are asymptomatic.
- Has been associated with preterm delivery and IUGR,[10] but very little neonatal morbidity.
- Metronidazole is the drug of choice outside of pregnancy though the British National Formulary (BNF) advises against its use in high doses during pregnancy.
- A Cochrane review[11] supports metronidazole in treating *Trichomonas vaginalis* during pregnancy.

Information for patients

Please see **Information for patients: Sexually transmitted infections and pregnancy (gonorrhoea, chlamydia, anogenital warts, and trichomonas)** (p. 501)

References

1. Brocklehurst P. Antibiotics for gonorrhoea in pregnancy. Cochrane Database Syst Rev 2002;2: CD000098
2. Prescriber 2005; 16 (6): 14–24.
3. BASHH. National guideline on the diagnosis and treatment of gonorrhoea in adults. London: British Association for Sexual Health and HIV, 2000.
4. Allstaff S, Wilson J. The management of sexually transmitted infections in pregnancy. Obstetrician and Gynaecologist 2012;14: 25–32.
5. Public Health England. National Chlamydia Screening Programme, 2013 <http://www.chlamydiascreening.nhs.uk/ps/data.asp>.
6. Harrison HR, et al. Cervical Chlamydia trachomatis and mycoplasmal infections in pregnancy. JAMA 1983;250: 1721–1727.
7. Lumbiganon P. Management of gonorrhoea and Chlamydia trachomatis infections in pregnancy: RHL commentary. (last revised: 15 September 2004). The WHO Reproductive Health Library; Geneva: World Health Organization.
8. Centers for Disease Control and Prevention. Sexually transmitted diseases treatment guidelines, 2010: Genital warts <http://www.cdc.gov/std/treatment/2010/genital-warts.htm>.
9. Scheinfeld N, Lehman DS. An evidence-based review of medical and surgical treatments of. An evidence-based review of medical and surgical treatments of genital warts. Dermatol Online J 2006;12:5 <http://dermatology.cdlib.org/123/reviews/warts/scheinfeld.html.>.
10. Cotch MF, et al. Trichomonas vaginalis associated with low birth weight and preterm delivery. Sex Trans Dis 1997;24: 353–360.
11. Gulmezoglu AM, Azhar M. Interventions for trichomoniasis in pregnancy. Cochrane Database Syst Rev 2011;5: CD 000220.

CARE PATHWAYS

Individual care pathways have to be constructed for sexually transmitted infections (gonorrhoea, chlamydia, anogenital warts, trichomoniasis) based on the following general principles:

- The stage of pregnancy at time of presentation and diagnosis
- Severity of presenting signs and symptoms
- Thorough counselling of pregnant patient, with discussions regarding organism involved, rates of reinfection, possible coexistence of other STIs, risk of transmission of infection to fetus and prevention of such transmission, treatment options with any side effects, importance of contact tracing
- Choice of drugs that are safe for use in pregnancy
- Notification required, as indicated, for genitourinary registers
- Multidisciplinary care with GUM and microbiology referral
- Confidentiality to be observed at all times; contact tracing by GUM with patient's permission
- Paediatricians to be made aware of mother's STI and any treatment received, so that specific neonatal examinations, investigations and follow-up can be instituted as appropriate
- Continuation of standard community antenatal checks with midwife
- Any impact of disease or treatment on pregnancy, labour, mode of delivery, and any puerperal problems that need to be anticipated
- Arrangements for post-treatment test of cure, if so indicated
- Advise patient about general sexual health, safety precautions, contraceptive and cervical cytology screening advice

Gonorrhoea

- Screening and, if detected, concomitant treatment for chlamydia, syphilis
- Inform patient about risk of premature labour, signs to note
- Neonatal ophthalmologic check by paediatricians
- Gonorrhoea in itself is **not an indication for early IOL or Caesarean section**

Chlamydia

- Care while taking ECS in pregnancy. A HVS may be as useful
- Test of cure in 5–6 weeks after end of treatment
- If detected and treated early in pregnancy, repeat screening at about 36 weeks
- Inform patient about risk of premature labour, signs to note
- Chlamydia itself is **not an indication for early IOL or Caesarean section**

Anogenital warts

- Treatment modalities during pregnancy limited to cautery, application of liquid nitrogen, or laser. Explain teratogenic risks or toxicity of podophyllin and some over-the-counter products during pregnancy
- Explain how dampened immunosuppression of pregnancy may cause warts to increase rapidly, but will settle after end of pregnancy
- Inform patient that rarely, neonatal laryngeal infection due to vertical transmission during delivery may occur
- Pain and blistering are common symptoms after local treatment with liquid nitrogen; local anaesthetic before procedure and analgesics are recommended
- Warn patient that despite treatment, recurrence possible within 3 months
- In rare cases due to very extensive spread, vaginal outlet may be virtually blocked or increased risk of bleeding at delivery. Caesarean section may need to be considered for such cases
- Anogenital warts per se, unless in extreme cases, are **not an indication for routine early IOL or Caesarean section** unless there are other obstetric indications

Trichomoniasis

- Inform patient about risk of premature labour, PPROM, and symptoms to be aware of

2.13 Parvovirus

FACT FILE

Epidemiology

- **Parvovirus infection,** caused by parvovirus B_{19}, is also known as **'slapped cheek syndrome' or 'Fifth disease'**. Outbreaks usually occur in nurseries or schools with seasonal peaks.
- In children it presents with mild fever and the typical 'slapped cheek' rash.
- Outbreaks occur in the late winter or early spring with cyclical peaks of incidence occurring every 4–7 years.
- Approximately 60% of women are immune to it by the age of 20 years, following infection sometime in the past.
- ***One attack confers immunity for life.***
- Parvovirus infections are transmitted by infected respiratory droplets and from mother to baby via the placenta. There is a 50% risk of transmission from an infected mother to her fetus in utero.[1,2,3,4,5,6,7,8]
- Transmission of parvovirus B_{19} is only through humans; cats and dogs cannot infect humans.
- Risk of infection in a susceptible pregnant woman after exposure at home is not preventable in practice and is up to 50%. The risk of infection of a susceptible pregnant woman who works as a teacher or with child care is up to 30%

Clinical presentation

- In adults, parvovirus infection can present as a flu-like illness with transient fever, malaise, and arthralgia, but 25% of parvovirus infections are asymptomatic.
- In adults, parvovirus infection can occasionally acute painful and swollen joints that could last for months.
- Congenital parvovirus B_{19} can cause severe fetal haemolytic anaemia, hydrops, cardiac failure, and intrauterine death.[1]
- About 15–30 % of patients develop erythema infectiosum giving rise to the appearance of 'slapped cheek'. The rash may spread to the arms and legs, and can fade quickly but may recur a few weeks later with exposure to sunlight.
- Incubation period for appearance of a clinical rash is 13–20 days. The illness is infective from 10 days pre-rash until the onset of the rash. **Once the rash appears, patients are no longer infectious.**
- Any pregnant woman who has come in contact with known or suspected parvovirus infection should have blood tests to check whether she is immune or susceptible. This will help determine whether or not any further intervention or investigations are required.

Serological diagnosis

- The finding of IgM antibodies to parvovirus B_{19} confirms that infection has occurred in the 4 weeks before sampling.[2,3,4]. This means that parvovirus infection cannot be excluded if investigation starts only after 4 weeks of the appearance of the rash. Test for parvovirus IgM or IgG should therefore be done as soon as possible after contact with or symptoms of rash.
- If IgM is detected in the first sample, a further sample should be taken immediately. Confirmation by an alternative method (DNA detection by PCR) is also required and this will be done at the central (regional) virology lab.
- The presence of parvovirus IgG antibodies alone, **without IgM**, indicates past infection which has conferred lifelong immunity to the patient.
- The absence of both parvovirus B_{19} IgG and IgM antibodies indicates there has been **no recent or previous infection** and that the patient is susceptible to the virus.
- In women with pre-existing chronic blood conditions like sickle cell anaemia or congenital spherocytosis, parvovirus can cause a temporary bone marrow disorder.[5]
- Those with previous immunosuppressive conditions could suffer chronic anaemia and remain infectious for weeks.

Fetal and neonatal prognosis

- If infection occurs within the first 4 weeks of gestation, there is no intrauterine transmission
- If infection occurs **before 20 weeks gestation,**[1,2,3,6,7,8,9] the adverse outcomes include:
  - miscarriage or fetal loss in 10–15%
  - fetal hydrops in 3–10%.
  - fetal anaemia and progressive cardiac failure.
- Mortality from untreated fetal hydrops is 50%, reduced to 18% by transfusion. Most deaths occur within 4–6 weeks of the maternal infection, but have been known to occur up to 3 months later.[1] **Once hydrops has resolved, there are no ongoing long-term sequelae and mothers should be reassured about this.**[1]
- The dead fetus usually displays signs of maceration.
- ***If infection occurs after 20 weeks gestation, fetal loss rate is 2% but hydrops is not a feature.***
- Parvovirus B_{19} infection is not associated with teratogenicity. **TOP is not recommended under these circumstances.**[2,3]
- If primary infection is confirmed by the finding of positive IgM antibodies or by DNA detected by PCR, serial scans should start from 2–4 weeks after the infection or seroconversion in order to detect any hydrops. Scanning needs to be repeated at 1–2 week intervals until 30–34 weeks gestation.
- ***Fetal hydrops can spontaneously resolve in one-third of cases but otherwise carries a poor prognosis due to fetal congestive cardiac failure resulting from severe anaemia.***

Management

- If there is any development of hydrops, the patient should be promptly referred to a tertiary fetal medicine centre for consideration of intrauterine transfusion.
- Tertiary care may provide:[1,2,4]
  - further assessment, using techniques such as Doppler assessment of the middle cerebral artery and parvovirus B_{19} genome detection in amniotic fluid
  - FBS and intrauterine transfusion by cordocentesis of erythrocytes, ideally after 22 weeks, though can be carried out from 18 weeks gestation[1]
  - early delivery of the baby if it is near term.
- Hydrops can resolve in 94% of cases within approximately 6 weeks of intrauterine transfusion.[1]
- At present there is no vaccination for parvovirus B_{19}, though clinical trials are in progress.
- Similarly, no antiviral prophylaxis is available at present. **Routine screening for parvovirus of all unselected pregnant women is therefore not recommended at present.**
- Only symptomatic treatment such as analgesia for painful joints can be offered at present.

Information for patients

Please see Information for patients: Parvovirus ('slapped cheek') infection in pregnancy (p. 502)

References

1. To M, et al. Prenatal diagnosis and management of fetal infections. Obstetrician and Gynaecologist 2009;11: 108–116.
2. RCOG Safety and Quality Committee. Safety Alert No. 3. Parvovirus in pregnancy. London: Royal College of Obstericians and Gynaecologists, 2012.

2.13 Parvovirus

3. Public Health England. Viral rash in pregnancy, 2011. <https://www.gov.uk/government/publications/viral-rash-in-pregnancy>
4. AAP. Parvovirus B^{19} (erythema infectiosum, fifth disease). In: Red Book 2006: Report of the Committee on Infectious Diseases, 27th ed. Elk Grove Village, IL: American Academy of Pediatrics, 2006, pp. 484–487.
5. Tolfvenstam T, Broliden K. Parvovirus B^{19} infection. Semin Fetal Neonatal Med 2009;14: 218–221.
6. Smith-Whitley K, et al. Epidemiology of human parvovirus B19 in children with sickle cell disease. Blood 2004;103: 422–427.
7. Young NS, Brown KE. Parvovirus B^{19}. N Engl J Med 2004;350: 586–597.
8. Katta R. Parvovirus B_{19}: a review. Dermatol Clin 2002;20: 333–342.
9. Palasanthiran P, et al. Management of perinatal infections. Sydney: Australasian Society for Infectious Diseases (ASID), 2014, pp. 51–55 <http://www.asid.net.au/documents/item/368.>

CARE PATHWAY

Rash or flu-like illness or exposure to an infected individual reported by patient to midwife/GP

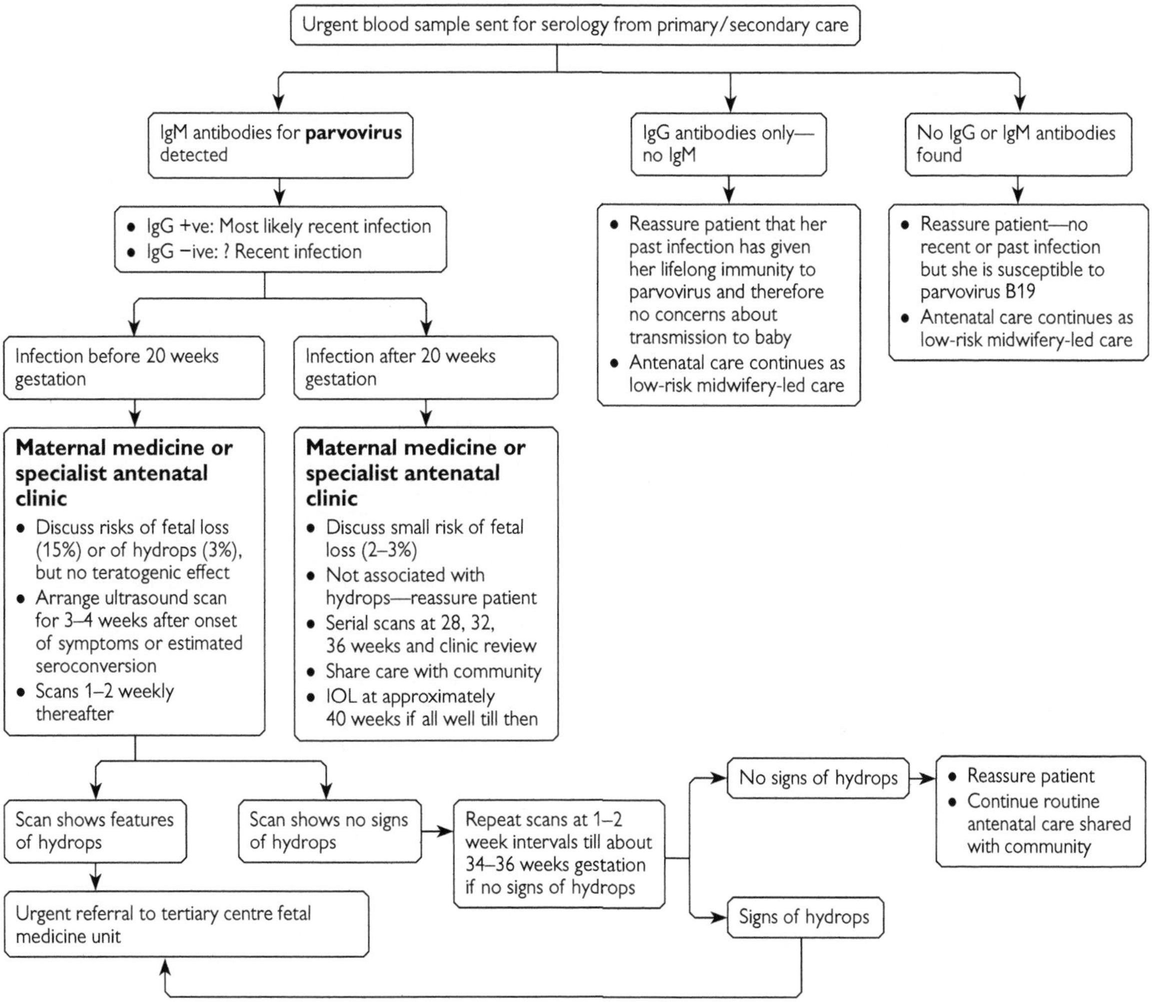
Urgent blood sample sent for serology from primary/secondary care
IgM antibodies for **parvovirus** detected
IgG antibodies only—no IgM
No IgG or IgM antibodies found
• IgG +ve: Most likely recent infection
• IgG −ive: ? Recent infection
• Reassure patient that her past infection has given her lifelong immunity to parvovirus and therefore no concerns about transmission to baby
• Antenatal care continues as low-risk midwifery-led care
• Reassure patient—no recent or past infection but she is susceptible to parvovirus B19
• Antenatal care continues as low-risk midwifery-led care
Infection before 20 weeks gestation
Infection after 20 weeks gestation
Maternal medicine or specialist antenatal clinic
• Discuss risks of fetal loss (15%) or of hydrops (3%), but no teratogenic effect
• Arrange ultrasound scan for 3–4 weeks after onset of symptoms or estimated seroconversion
• Scans 1–2 weekly thereafter
Maternal medicine or specialist antenatal clinic
• Discuss small risk of fetal loss (2–3%)
• Not associated with hydrops—reassure patient
• Serial scans at 28, 32, 36 weeks and clinic review
• Share care with community
• IOL at approximately 40 weeks if all well till then
Scan shows features of hydrops
Scan shows no signs of hydrops
Repeat scans at 1–2 week intervals till about 34–36 weeks gestation if no signs of hydrops
No signs of hydrops
• Reassure patient
• Continue routine antenatal care shared with community
Signs of hydrops
Urgent referral to tertiary centre fetal medicine unit

2.14 Syphilis

FACT FILE

- **Syphilis** is a sexually acquired disease caused by a bacteria-like organism, a spirochete called *Treponema pallidum* (TP).[1]
- Syphilis infection can cause miscarriages, stillbirths, hydrops, polyhydramnios, or fetal abnormalities.
- Approximately 30% of cases of infectious syphilis in pregnancy will end as miscarriages or stillbirths.
- A rapid increase of infectious syphilis has occurred in the UK between 1999 and 2008,[2] although this has been mainly in men who have sex with men.
- There was a reported fall in numbers of infectious syphilis in women between 2009 and 2010.[2]
- Maternal coinfection with HIV increases the transmission risk of syphilis.
- In 2009, there was a 96% uptake of antenatal screening for syphilis in the UK[3] (false-positive rate of 0.16%). The rate of congenital syphilis therefore remains low due to effective antenatal screening.

Stages of syphilis and transmission

- **Primary infection:** Painless but highly infectious sores disappear spontaneously in 2–6 weeks. Any sexual partner(s) within the past 3 months should be contacted, with the patient's consent, as the incubation period is up to 90 days.
- **Secondary infection:** Develops 6 weeks to 6 months after primary infection, may present with a rash on palms or soles, though very variable. Sexual partner contact, with the patient's permission, may need to be extended to up to 2 years.
- **Late syphilis:** Appears 4 years or more after an untreated primary. Multiorgan and system complications seen.
- TP can be transmitted to the fetus through the placenta at any stage of pregnancy (especially after 16 weeks) or during vaginal delivery.
- Transmission is most likely in primary, secondary, and early latent stages of syphilis.
- Risk of transmission depends on stage of maternal disease and duration of fetal exposure.[4] In early stage syphilis, there is up to a 100% transmission risk and a 50% rate of preterm birth, perinatal death, or long-term disability.
- In maternal late stage syphilis, only 10% of infants are born infected.
- Infection is detectable and can be treated, hence all pregnant women are screened for syphilis.

Diagnosis

- Diagnosis is by serology, either during antenatal screening or from a genital ulcer found during pregnancy. In the UK a very sensitive and specific enzyme immunoassay has been used for screening. Confirmation is obtained by a TP haemagglutination or TP particle agglutination study.
- The Venereal Disease Research Laboratory test (VDRL) is traditionally used to monitor disease and treatment response.[4] More recently, **VDRL has been replaced by the Rapid Plasma Reagin (RPR) test**.
- ***Other treponemal infections such as yaws or pinta can also give identical results but in these cases a RPR/VDRL is usually of low titre (<1:8) compared with active syphilis (>1:16).***[1]
- ***Biological false positives can occur with both VDRL and RPR testing with intercurrent viral or other infections, autoimmune diseases and, in a few, the state of pregnancy itself.***

Management in pregnancy

- Management in pregnancy must be multidisciplinary with the midwife, GP, specialist obstetrician, genitourinary physician, neonatologist, and microbiologist.
- Clinical assessment of the disease stage and prompt commencement of treatment is mandatory to reduce in-utero fetal exposure time.
- Benzathine benzylpenicillin is the first-line drug of choice. A second dose of benzathine benzylpenicillin is required if the pregnancy is in the third trimester. In those who are penicillin allergic, desensitization may need to be implemented as alternative drugs such as erythromycin and azithromycin have a high failure rate in syphilis.[5]
- Treatment of the baby at birth is recommended if maternal treatment was with macrolides.
- If delivery should take place within 30 days of treatment completion, the neonate needs empirical treatment.[1]
- The **Jarisch–Herxheimer reaction**can complicate about 40% of cases being treated for syphilis during pregnancy, a similar rate as in the non-pregnant state.[6,7] The reaction starts between 1 and 12 h after the first injection of antibiotics and lasts for a few hours or up to a day. Malaise, slight-to-moderate pyrexia, a flush due to vasodilation, tachycardia, and leucocytosis can occur. Any existing skin lesions become more prominent. Usually, the reaction resolves over a period of 6–12 hours.
- In pregnant women this can be accompanied by uterine contractions, preterm labour, and fetal heart rate decelerations. Therefore, timing of treatment to after 26–28 weeks and fetal heart monitoring should be considered. Supportive measures including antipyretics are required.
- Monthly maternal serology is required to monitor treatment response.
- The neonatologists must be informed about maternal syphilis so they can assess the neonate and treat if any evidence of congenital infection. Serological tests must be performed **on the infant's blood, not cord blood**. However, IgG antibodies may be positive due to passive transfer of maternal antibodies whether or not the baby is infected.
- If the neonate's serum is negative on screening and there are no signs of congenital syphilis, no further testing is necessary and the mother should be reassured.
- About 75% of infected babies may not show any symptoms at birth with signs of congenital syphilis surfacing only weeks, months, or even years after birth. These can then present as skin lesions, snuffles, hepatosplenomegaly, and lymphadenopathy, inflammation of bones and cartilages, and failure to thrive.

Information for patients

Please see Information for patients: Syphilis and pregnancy (p. 502)

References

1. BASHH.UK national guidelines on the management of syphilis. London: British Association for Sexual Health and HIV, 2008.
2. Public Health England. Sexually transmitted infections and chlamydia screening in England, 2013. Health Protection Report 2014; 8 (24), 20 June.
3. Public Health England Sexually transmitted infections (STIs): annual data tables. (2010; updated 2014) <https://www.gov.uk/government/statistics/sexually-transmitted-infections-stis-annual-data-tables>.
4. Allstaff S, Wilson J. The management of sexually transmitted infections in pregnancy. Obstetrician and Gynaecologist 2012;14: 25–32.
5. Centers for Disease Control and Prevention. Sexually transmitted diseases treatment guidelines. MMWR 2010; 59 <http://www.cdc.gov/std/treatment/2010/default.htm.>.
6. Kingston M, McAuliffe F. Update on management of syphilis in pregnancy. London: BASHH, 2011 <http://www.bashh.org/documents/3693.>.
7. De Santis M, et al. Syphilis infection during pregnancy: fetal risks and clinical management. Infect Dis Obstet Gynecol 2012; 2012: 430585.

CARE PATHWAY

Presumptive positive result, send sample to referral lab for **treponemal** specific tests—enzyme immunoassay (EIA)

Confirmed positive result
- Lab urgently informs designated midwife/consultant obstetrician according to locally agreed pathway
- Lab follows up with written report

Negative result

Patient informed at next visit to GP/midwife or hospital antenatal clinic

Specialist antenatal clinic
- Results discussed with GUM immediately
- Urgent appointment arranged for patient to see consultant obstetrician and specialist midwife
- Patient informed and urgent review arranged to be seen in GUM
- Dose of benzathine benzylpenicillin awareness of Jarisch–Herxheimer reaction
- Second dose of benzathine penicillin G if in 3rd trimester

Genitourinary medicine
- Stage of infection determined
- Treatment and risks explained
- Other STI screening
- Treatment organized in maternity ward according to prescribed schedule of drugs
- Follow-up monthly, serology
- Meanwhile, contact tracing and informing GP, both with the patient's permission
- Refer patient's other children for paediatric infectious diseases review
- Follow-up of all post-treatment bloods

Further visits to antenatal clinic
- Inform consultant paediatrician
- Refer patient to see paediatrician
- Follow-up: ensure that patient has had post-treatment bloods taken at appropriate times
- Follow up all missed appointments
- After 26 weeks, serial growth scans
- **document the following instructions** for labour, delivery, postnatal period:
  - Woman's syphilis titre should be re-checked at time of delivery
  - Paediatricians to be informed at time of delivery
  - Breastfeeding not contraindicated
  - Before discharge, ensure patient has 6-month post-treatment GUM appointment
  - If delivery within 30 days of end of treatment, neonate will require empirical treatment
- Attach paediatric care protocol to maternity notes

2.15 Tuberculosis

FACT FILE

Epidemiology

- **Tuberculosis (TB)** remains a global problem. TB is caused by the *Mycobacterium tuberculosis complex*, the most common being *M. tuberculosis* (99%), rarely *M. africanum* (0.5%) and *M. bovis* (0.4%).[1]
- Although the rate of TB in UK-born population has remained stable,[1] the incidence is increasing in the UK partly due to immigration patterns as well as the susceptibility of HIV-infected patients to TB.
- The risk of TB in pregnancy was estimated to be 1 per 24 000 maternities or 4.2 per 100 000 maternities in in 2005–2006.[2]
- TB is particularly common in non-UK-born immigrants from the Indian subcontinent and Africa as well as those from ethnic minorities who, though born in the UK, have close contact with families from endemic countries.[3]
- Previously treated TB is not a contraindication for pregnancy.
- **About 50–75% of immigrant pregnant women with TB are asymptomatic as the infection is in the latent phase** when clinical diagnosis is not possible.[2]

Clinical presentation

- The development, clinical presentation, and progress of TB are unaltered by pregnancy. Pregnancy is not associated with an increased risk of TB nor is the course of TB changed by pregnancy. The clinical signs and symptoms are the same in pregnant women as in the non-pregnant state.
- In pregnancy, TB can mimic certain features of normal pregnancy such as malaise, fatigue, weight loss in early pregnancy, loss of appetite. Fever and night sweats develop over a few weeks or months.
- Among pregnant women with TB, there is a **high prevalence (50%) of extrapulmonary TB** in sites such as lymph nodes (most common), liver, spleen, bone, caecum, CNS, or eye.[1,2,4]
- Pregnancy is no more likely to cause reactivation of the disease than any other time.[2]
- Symptomatology of TB in the pregnant woman usually includes cough, haemoptysis, weight loss, night sweats, and generalized and severe tiredness.
- Signs of any chest condition, lymphadenopathy, or erythema nodosum can suggest TB.

Effects of TB on pregnancy

- Higher rates of pre-eclampsia, preterm labour, or acute respiratory failure as well as perinatal mortality have been reported with pulmonary TB, especially when diagnosis has been delayed.[5,6]
- While maternal pulmonary TB or TB lymphadenitis in general pose little risk to the fetus, extrapulmonary TB especially in the spine, abdomen, and CNS may be associated with IUGR.[2,7]
- CNS infection carries significant maternal and fetal mortality and morbidity.[8]
- **Congenital TB** is exceptionally rare, seen mainly with widespread maternal miliary TB. Infants may present in the second or third week of life with respiratory distress, fever, poor feeding, weight loss, and irritability. Hepatosplenomegaly may be present.[5]
- Far greater risk lies in acquisition of neonatal infection due to exposure to an infected mother or any other family member.

Diagnosis

- Typical appearance on **chest radiograph** defines extent of pulmonary involvement, diagnoses active disease, and can be repeated to identify improvement post-treatment. Chest radiography should be performed with appropriate abdominal shielding.
- **Sputum examination** for acid-fast bacilli (Ziehl–Nielsen stain) is diagnostic.
- **Mycobacterium culture** from any tissue specimen or sputum can take up to 6 weeks.
- ***The Mantoux test, if positive, is representative of latent infection. This test result is not affected by pregnancy.***
- MRI/CT of non-pulmonary sites (e.g. spine/abdomen, brain) after due counselling, can identify extrapulmonary infection.

Principles of management

- Principles of management are similar in pregnancy to those in the non-pregnant state.
- Multidisciplinary team management with the microbiologist, respiratory physician, specialist TB nurse, anaesthetist, midwife, obstetrician, and neonatologist is essential.
- Untreated TB poses a far greater risk to the mother and baby than any risks associated with the treatment itself.
- Active identification and rigorous treatment of TB during pregnancy are essential.
- Active disease should receive treatment without delay with close surveillance by respiratory physicians and specialist TB nurse.
- Brief periods of hospitalization with due infection control precautions may be required in those ill with highly infectious multidrug-resistant disease.
- Women with suspected or confirmed multidrug-resistant TB should be admitted to a room with negative pressure ventilation.[9,10]
- Some drugs used in the treatment for TB have questionable teratogenic risks, though present data suggests that the most commonly used agents are safe in pregnancy.[1,2]
- A triple/quadruple model of supervised, prolonged therapy with **rifampicin**, **isoniazid**, **pyrazinamide**, and/or **ethambutol** is the standard recommendation for those with active TB.
- Isoniazid is used as both prophylaxis and treatment for those with latent TB. It is safe in pregnancy.
- Pyridoxine (doses of 25–50 mg/day) should be given with isoniazid to all pregnant and breastfeeding mothers as well as to the breastfed infants (5–10 mg/day).

Special issues of treatment in pregnancy

- Screening of all family members is essential to prevent neonatal infection.
- Antenatal referral to the anaesthetic high-risk clinic and communication with paediatricians is essential.
- Streptomycin is **not** to be used at any stage during pregnancy due to its high (>10%) risk of toxicity
- Duration of treatment with each drug may vary according to the resistance patterns and the form of the TB (e.g. longer for TB meningitis).
- **Isoniazid** and **ethambutol** may cause neuropathies and therefore patients should receive concurrent daily **pyridoxine** (25–50 mg/day). Most of the usual antenatal vitamins do not provide this dose, *so pyridoxine must be prescribed as a special supplement.*
- **Isoniazid** and **rifampicin** can interfere with vitamin K metabolism, so patients on these agents should also receive oral vitamin K 10 mg daily starting from 36 weeks until delivery to decrease the risk of postpartum haemorrhage (PPH) and haemorrhagic disease of the newborn.
- With **isoniazid** there is a small risk of maternal hepatotoxicity. Hepatic transaminase levels must therefore be tested at initiation of treatment and continued at monthly intervals thereafter. If these levels rise above three times normal values, isoniazid may need to be discontinued by the respiratory physician/microbiologist.
- **Ethambutol** may cause retrobulbar neuritis in 1% of patients, therefore at each monthly antenatal visit, the patient should be questioned regarding possible visual disturbances (e.g. blurred

vision, scotomata) and a monthly eye test for visual acuity and colour discrimination arranged.

- **Pyrazinamide**: Use in pregnancy supported by international recommendations in all pregnant patients with active TB **after** the first trimester, especially for multidrug-resistant TB and in HIV-positive patients
- ***Note: The BCG vaccine contains live attenuated strain of M. bovis and must not be offered to women during pregnancy. BCG vaccination should whenever possible be delayed until after childbirth.***[12]
- Serial growth and liquor volume scans at 28, 32, and 36 weeks.
- Routine community midwife antenatal checks should continue.
- TB itself is **not** an indication for either early induction of labour or Caesarean section unless there is severe respiratory compromise.
- Principles of infection control must be adhered to in all interactions with any pregnant women with active infection.

Postnatal care

- Neonatal infection can occur if the neonate is exposed to the mother or other family member with active TB.
- If the mother has had 3 months of treatment with negative sputum before delivery, the neonate should receive Bacille–Calmette–Guérin (BCG) vaccine and be examined monthly with tuberculin skin testing at 6, 12, and 24 months of life. BCG contains live attenuated strain of *M. bovis*.
- If the mother has sterile sputum, but has not completed 3 months of treatment before delivery, the neonate should be considered for isoniazid prophylaxis (with pyridoxine) in addition to the BCG.
- If the patient has untreated or incompletely treated sputum-positive TB by the time of delivery, the baby must be separated from her until she is no longer overtly infective. This is usually for a short time of about 10–14 days, by which time she usually becomes sputum negative with continued treatment with rifampicin and isoniazid.[9,10]
- In such situations, the neonate should be given isoniazid prophylaxis along with pyridoxine and have a tuberculin test at 6–12 weeks. If this is negative the baby can receive BCG vaccine and chemoprophylaxis can be stopped.[11]
- BCG should not be given to the babies of mothers who are HIV positive till the baby has been shown to be HIV negative.
- In general, the amount of anti-TB drugs excreted in breast milk is so small that **breastfeeding should be encouraged**. Mothers taking isoniazid should also receive pyridoxine supplements (25 mg/day).[13]
- **All anti-TB antimicrobial drugs can decrease the efficacy of oral contraception**. The use of **an alternative method of contraception** during the postpartum period should be recommended for women receiving the drugs before their discharge from the hospital (Table 2.4).

Antituberculosis drugs in pregnancy

First-line anti-TB drugs

See Table 2.4.

Second-line anti-TB drugs

To be used only on expert advice or **not to be used** in pregnancy:

- **Fluoroquinolines: Caution in pregnancy**. Use only when benefits outweigh risks and only after discussion with experts in anti-TB therapy; can cause fetal articular damage and long-term joint damage with prolonged course.

Table 2.4 First-line anti-TB drugs

Drug	*Dosage*	*Adverse effects*	*Maternofetal monitoring required*	*Fetal/neonatal effects*	*Comments*
Isoniazid	3–5 mg/kg up to 300 mg/day	Hepatotoxicity, skin rashes, fever, neurotoxicity in high doses	LFT monitoring at start of therapy, some recommend fortnightly for first 2 months, then monthly.[14] If LFTs are >3 times normal, cessation of drug may be considered by TB specialists	No increase in fetal malformation rate or IUGR	Safest, particularly for chemoprophylaxis in those at higher risk of developing disease, e.g. HIV coinfection
Pyridoxine	25–50 mg/day				Must be prescribed in conjunction with isoniazid either used on its own or combined with rifampicin, etc. Amount of pyridoxine contained in pregnancy multivitamins insufficient; must be prescribed individually
Ethambutol	15 mg/kg per day	Arthralgia, dose-related retro bulbar neuritis in 1%	Monthly eye tests recommended At each check, question whether any visual problems of acuity, colour discrimination, scotomata. Detailed anomaly scan and serial growth scans	Overall low-risk of teratogenicity, but crosses placenta. Theoretical risk of ocular toxicity Neonatal and paediatric ophthalmologic assessments	Safety record in pregnancy second only to isoniazid
Rifampicin	10–20 mg/kg per day up to 600 mg orally, four times a day	Liver enzyme inducer, cutaneous hypersensitivity, GI symptoms and thrombocytopenic purpura	LFTs, regular platelet counts Vit K 10 mg oral from 36–37 weeks of pregnancy Detailed anomaly and serial growth scans	Overall risk of teratogenicity low, Vit K to be given to protect against neonatal hypo-prothrombinaemia. Regular platelet counts Paeds to watch for problems of excessive or prolonged bleeding	
Pyrazinamide	20–30 mg/kg per day	Hepatotoxicity, GI symptoms, photosensitivity	LFTs Detailed anomaly and serial growth scans	Insufficient evidence for causing malformations but little overall data available	Used with caution in pregnancy, preferably after the first trimester; Especially useful in those with drug-resistant TB or HIV coinfection

GI, gastrointestinal; IUGR, intrauterine growth restriction; LFTs, liver function tests.

Data from Bothamley G, 'Drug treatment for tuberculosis during pregnancy: safety considerations', Drug Safety, 2001, 24, pp. 553–565

Second-line anti-TB drugs (Contd)

- **Para-aminosalicylic acid (PAS):** Not to be used in pregnancy unless benefits outweigh risks and only after discussion with experts in anti-TB therapy. Increased limb and ear abnormalities reported.
- **Aminoglycosides: Not recommended in pregnancy except as a last resort** and only after discussion with experts in anti-TB therapy: nephrotoxic and ototoxic effects.
- **Streptomycin: Avoid at any stage of pregnancy.** Can cause severe ototoxicity and vestibular abnormalities in baby.

Information for patients

Please see Information for patients: Tuberculosis (TB) and pregnancy (p. 502)

References

1. HPA. Tuberculosis in the UK: annual report on tuberculosis surveillance in the UK. London: Health Protection Agency Centre for Infections, 2009.
2. Knight M, et al. on behalf of UKOSS. Tuberculosis in pregnancy in the UK. BJOG 2009;116: 584–588.
3. Llewelyn M, et al. Tuberculosis diagnosed during pregnancy: a prospective study from London. Thorax 2000;55: 129–132.
4. Wilson EA, et al. Tuberculosis complicated by pregnancy. Am J Obstet Gynecol 1973; 115: 526–529.
5. Mahendru A, et al. Diagnosis and management of tuberculosis in pregnancy 6. Obstetrician and Gynaecologist 2010;12: 163–170.
6. Figueroa-Damian R, Arredondo-Garcia J. Pregnancy and tuberculosis: influence of treatment on perinatal outcome. Am J Perinatol 1998;15: 303–306.
7. Jana N, et al. Obstetrical outcomes among women with extra-pulmonary tuberculosis. N Engl J Med 1999;341: 645–649.
8. CEMACH. Saving mothers' lives: reviewing maternal deaths to make motherhood safer— 2003–2005. Lewis G, ed. The Seventh Report on Confidential Enquiries into Maternal Deaths in the United Kingdom. London: Confidential Enquiry into Maternal and Child Health 2007.
9. Joint Tuberculosis Committee of the British Thoracic Society. Control and prevention of tuberculosis in the United Kingdom: Code of Practice2000. Thorax 2000;55: 887–901.
10. Ormerod P. Tuberculosis in pregnancy and the puerperium. Thorax 2001;56: 494–499.
11. HPA. Pregnancy and tuberculosis: NHS Guidance for clinicians. London: Health Protection Agency, 2006.
12. Salisbury D, et al. Tuberculosis. In: Immunization against infectious disease. London: Department of Health, 2006, pp. 391–408.
13. Chung M, et al. Interventions in primary care to promote breastfeeding: an evidence review for the U. S. Preventive Services Task Force. Ann Intern Med 2008;149: 565–582.
14. Bothamley G. Drug treatment for tuberculosis during pregnancy: safety considerations. Drug Safety 2001;24: 553–565.

CARE PATHWAY

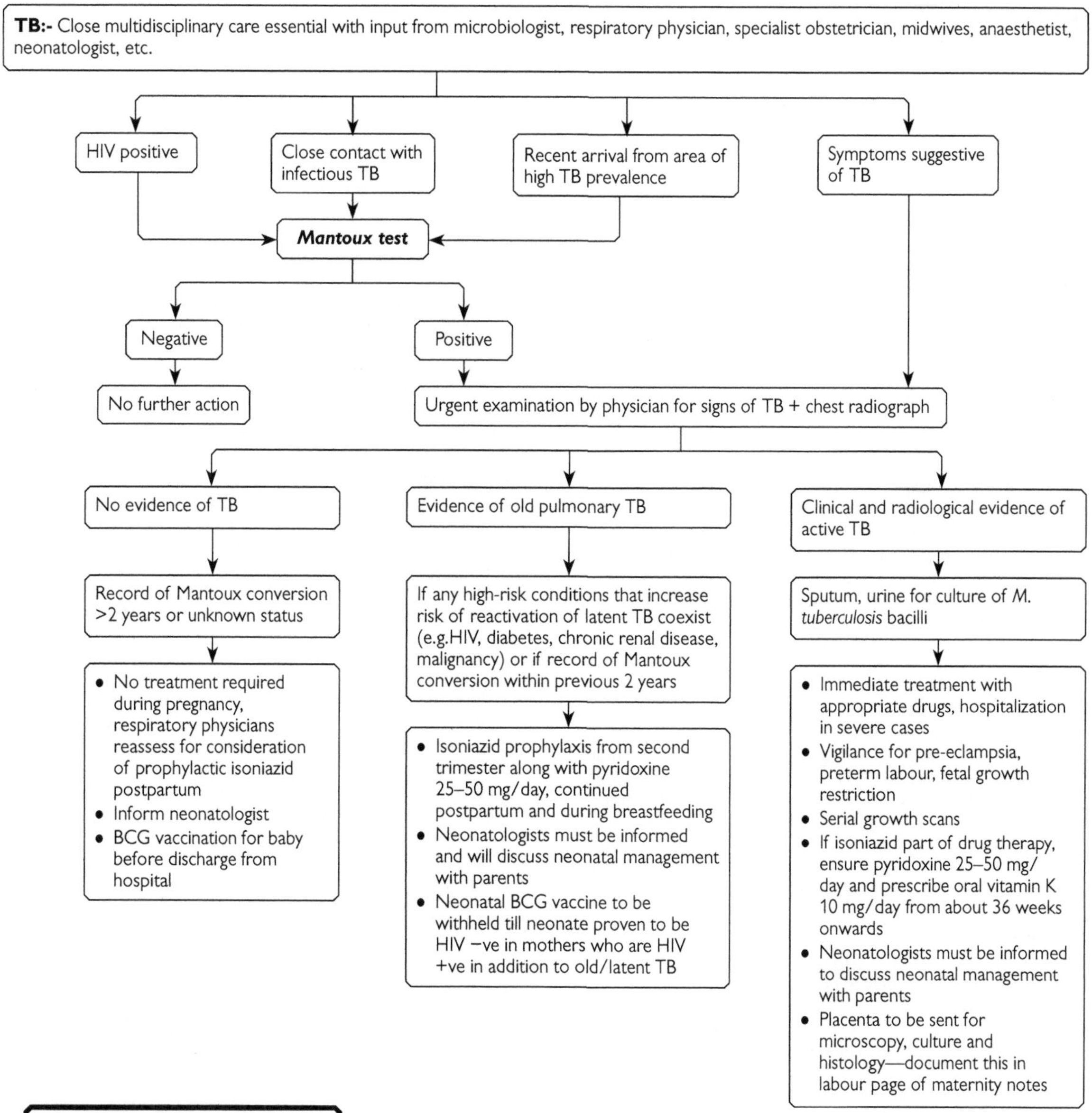
TB:- Close multidisciplinary care essential with input from microbiologist, respiratory physician, specialist obstetrician, midwives, anaesthetist, neonatologist, etc.
HIV positive
Close contact with infectious TB
Recent arrival from area of high TB prevalence
Symptoms suggestive of TB
Mantoux test
Negative
Positive
No further action
Urgent examination by physician for signs of TB + chest radiograph
No evidence of TB
Evidence of old pulmonary TB
Clinical and radiological evidence of active TB
Record of Mantoux conversion >2 years or unknown status
If any high-risk conditions that increase risk of reactivation of latent TB coexist (e.g.HIV, diabetes, chronic renal disease, malignancy) or if record of Mantoux conversion within previous 2 years
Sputum, urine for culture of *M. tuberculosis* bacilli
• No treatment required during pregnancy, respiratory physicians reassess for consideration of prophylactic isoniazid postpartum
• Inform neonatologist
• BCG vaccination for baby before discharge from hospital
• Isoniazid prophylaxis from second trimester along with pyridoxine 25–50 mg/day, continued postpartum and during breastfeeding
• Neonatologists must be informed and will discuss neonatal management with parents
• Neonatal BCG vaccine to be withheld till neonate proven to be HIV −ve in mothers who are HIV +ve in addition to old/latent TB
• Immediate treatment with appropriate drugs, hospitalization in severe cases
• Vigilance for pre-eclampsia, preterm labour, fetal growth restriction
• Serial growth scans
• If isoniazid part of drug therapy, ensure pyridoxine 25–50 mg/day and prescribe oral vitamin K 10 mg/day from about 36 weeks onwards
• Neonatologists must be informed to discuss neonatal management with parents
• Placenta to be sent for microscopy, culture and histology—document this in labour page of maternity notes

- ***All antimicrobials for TB decrease efficacy of oral contraceptives***
- ***Advice regarding alternative contraception till TB treatment is complete must be offered before hospital discharge***

Data from Palasanthiran P et al., 'Management of perinatal infections', In: Palasanthiran P, Starr M, and Jones (eds), 2002, Sydney: Australasian Society for Infectious Diseases

2.16 Toxoplasmosis

FACT FILE

Epidemiology

- Caused by protozoan ***Toxoplasma gondii***.
- Prevalence in the UK in pregnant population is 1–2 per 1000. Approximately 1–2 cases of congenital toxoplasma occur per 10 000 children born.[1]
- Often unrecognized in the pregnant woman, toxoplasmosis can produce a severe congenital infection with ocular and neurological damage.
- Maternal toxoplasmosis infection is usually asymptomatic, but 5–10% may experience flu-like symptoms with fever, fatigue and headache, and lymphadenopathy.[2,3]
- 85% of women of childbearing age are susceptible to infection at booking in the UK.
- The definitive host for the infection is the cat. Consumption of food (either inadequately cooked or in salads), contaminated with cat litter, or inadequate hand-washing after gardening or contact with cats are the main sources of infection.[2,4]
- Toxoplasmosis cannot be transmitted from person to person except transplacentally from mother to fetus.
- There is a 40–50% risk of vertical transmission.
- Risk of vertical transmission to the fetus is greatest if the mother is infected either immediately before conception or early in pregnancy. **The earlier in pregnancy that the fetus is infected, the more severe is the clinical disease in the infant**.
- If infection takes place later in the first trimester the risk of transmission to the fetus is 10–15%, causing either fetal loss or severe disease in the neonate.
- Risk of transmission in the second trimester, though up to 25–40%, usually has non-fatal sequelae. Similarly, infection in the third trimester can cause over 60% fetal infection with only mild or asymptomatic sequelae. Thus, although the frequency of vertical transmission is higher later in pregnancy, third-trimester congenital infections appear to be mild and very rarely result in a severely affected infant.[6]
- Risk of congenital fetal toxoplasmosis is very low in infants whose mothers have had toxoplasmosis of long-standing duration before pregnancy, except if the mother is immunocompromised.

Diagnosis

- Acute maternal infection is diagnosed by serological testing, although careful interpretation of the serology is required in reaching a definitive diagnosis of toxoplasmosis.
- In the UK, with a lower prevalence rate and where routine screening is not in practice, a single positive serologic test cannot differentiate between chronic infection and seroconversion after a recently contracted infection. In countries such as France and Austria, with a higher prevalence rate, women are screened as frequently as 1–3 monthly, whereby seroconversion is easily differentiated from chronic infection.
- Definitive diagnosis can be made only after rising IgG titres in serial samples are confirmed, apart from direct techniques using PCR amplification.
- IgG antibodies to toxoplasmosis appear 1–2 weeks after infection and they then persist at low levels for life.[3]
- **Rising IgG antibody titres (^{3}fourfold)**, 3 weeks apart tested in the same laboratory, indicates acute infection. This must be documented to diagnose a woman suspected of having contracted toxoplasmosis infection during pregnancy.[5]
- Stable IgG antibody titres indicate chronic infection, which poses no risk to the fetus.[5]
- IgG can be detected within the first 2 weeks of infection and can remain elevated for a year or even longer, hence is **not** diagnostic of recent infection. A single positive IgM titre can indicate infection acquired either during pregnancy or before conception.
- ***Absence of IgM excludes recent infection***.
- Absence of IgG antibodies in the first trimester identifies susceptible women.
- Women who are positive for IgG and negative for IgM are immune and no further follow-up is required, because the fetus is not at risk of congenital toxoplasmosis.[1]
- The gold standard test to determine whether the fetus has actually acquired *T. gondii* is the PCR identification of the protozoan in amniotic fluid. However, the procedure-related risk of miscarriage needs to be considered.
- **Toxoplasmosis can cause pregnancy complications such as miscarriages, prematurity, growth restriction, or stillbirth.**
- Serial ultrasound scans throughout the pregnancy at 2–4-week intervals can help identify hydrocephaly, ventriculomegaly and intracranial calcifications, symmetrical growth restriction, and non-immune hydrops.
- **The classic triad of signs associated with congenital toxoplasmosis is chorioretinitis, cerebral calcifications, and hydrocephalus.**
- Only 10–15% of congenitally infected infants display signs of toxoplasmosis at birth. The majority (90%) show no observable sequelae at birth but remain at high risk of developing symptoms months or even years after birth.
- **Neonatal toxoplasmosis** may present with hydrocephalus, intracranial calcifications, microcephaly, chorioretinitis, blindness, deafness, strabismus, epilepsy, psychomotor or mental retardation, petechiae, anaemia, or jaundice.[1,2,7]

Management during pregnancy

- TOP is an option that parents might choose if definitive diagnosis of the fetus having acquired toxoplasma infection in utero is made.
- **Spiramycin** is recommended as first-line treatment when the mother is diagnosed by serology as having contracted toxoplasma infection during pregnancy.
- Spiramycin is a macrolide antimicrobial that is safe to use in pregnancy and is concentrated in the placenta.
- Spiramycin is recommended at doses of 1–1.5 g oral bd from diagnosis until delivery. This reduces the risk of vertical transmission by almost 60%, but is not effective in treating an infected fetus or infant.[8]
- If fetal infection is confirmed (by amniocentesis or ultrasound findings) a combination of **pyrimethamine** (50 mg od) and **sulfadiazine** (1 g oral tid) is more effective. This treatment is generally continued till delivery. **Folic acid 5 mg/day** supplementation is required when the antifolate pyrimethamine is used. Pyrimethamine is contraindicated in the first trimester due to teratogenicity. While reducing the severity of congenital toxoplasmosis, these drugs will not be able to undo any damage that has already been done.[9]
- ***Treatment of the neonate with congenital toxoplasmosis with a regime of pyrimethamine and sulfadiazine alternating monthly with spiramycin, is usually continued for 12 months after birth***.[9]

Information for patients

Please see Information for patients: Toxoplasmosis and pregnancy (p. 502)

References

1. Foulon W, et al. Prevention of congenital toxoplasmosis. J Perinat Med 2000;28: 337–345.
2. Montoya JG, Liesenfield O. Toxoplasmosis. Lancet 2004;363: 1965–1976.
3. Wong SY, Remington JS. Toxoplasmosis in pregnancy. Clin Infect Dis 1994;18: 853–862.

4. Kapperud G, et al. Risk factors for Toxoplasma gondii infection in pregnancy: Results of a prospective case-control study in Norway. Am J Epidemiol 1996;144: 405.
5. Liesenfeld O, et al. Confirmatory serologic testing for acute toxoplasmosis and rate of induced abortions among women reported to have positive toxoplasma immunoglobulin M antibody titers. Am J Obstet Gynecol 2001;184: 140–145.
6. Dunn D, et al. Mother-to-child transmission of toxoplasmosis: risk estimates for clinical counseling. Lancet 1999;353: 1829–1836.
7. Sever JL. Toxoplasmosis: maternal and pediatric findings in 23, 000 pregnancies. Pediatrics 1988;82: 181–192.
8. Mombro M, et al. Congenital toxoplasmosis: 10-year follow-up. Eur J Paediatr 1995; 154: 635–639.
9. Montoya JG, Remington JS. Management of Toxoplasma gondii infection during pregnancy. Clin Infect Dis 2008;47: 554–566.

Toxoplasmosis screening

Blood sample sent for toxoplasma serology from pregnant woman with suspected infection/exposure in pregnancy

- IgG negative
- IgM negative
  - No past infection
  - Repeat if symptomatic or routine screening
  - IgG antibodies remains negative 1–2 weeks after presumed exposure or flu-like illness
  - Patient susceptible to toxoplasmosis
    - Advise eating only well-cooked food, proper hand-washing, avoiding contact with cat litter, etc.
      - Continue routine midwifery-led care

- Positive IgG
- Absent IgM
  - Indicates past infection,
  - Patient immune, fetus not at risk
    - Reassure patient
    - No further intervention required
    - Continue routine midwifery-led care

- Positive IgG
- Positive IgM
  - May indicate recent or chronic infection, but not definitive
    - Refer to hospital specialist antenatal clinic
      - **Repeat IgG titres 3 weeks later.** Same lab retests sera of both previous and second test for paired sample comparison on the same day
        - IgG titres show ≥ 4-fold increase between first and second samples and elevated IgM levels
          - Confirms **acute maternal toxoplasmosis infection**
            - **See next flowchart for further management**
        - Stable levels of IgG and IgM
          - Evidence of chronic infection
          - Fetus not at risk
          - Reassure patient
          - No further intervention required
          - Continue routine midwifery-led care

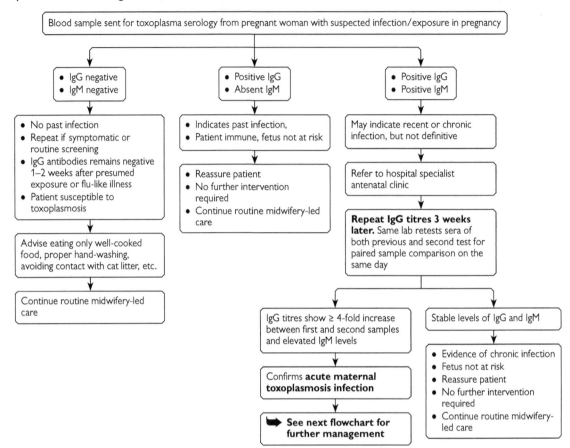

Maternal toxoplasmosis infection in pregnancy

Maternal acute toxoplasmosis infection confirmed by serology with paired sample testing 3 weeks apart showing a ≥ 4-fold increase in IgG titres

↓

- Discuss results with parents
- Risk of vertical transmission and congenital toxoplasmosis greater when maternal infection later in pregnancy **(20–25% in 2nd trimester rising to 60% in 3rd trimester)**, but generally milder sequelae in neonate
- The earlier the maternal infection in pregnancy, the lower the transmission rate but more severe clinical disease in neonate

↓

First visit to specialist antenatal clinic following definitive diagnosis of toxoplasmosis in mother

- Counsel patient about risks of miscarriage, stillbirth, congenital abnormalities; offer information leaflets
- Discuss amniocentesis for a definitive diagnosis of whether fetus has actually acquired in-utero infection by PCR identification of *T. gondii*. Explain procedure-related risk of miscarriage
- Arrange for detailed ultrasound scan to look for CNS abnormalities

→ Amniocentesis declined, but CNS abnormalities on scan, parents may opt for TOP

→ Amniocentesis accepted, confirms fetal infection, scan shows CNS abnormalities: parents counselled—may opt for TOP

→ Amniocentesis and scan findings indicate fetal infection abnormalities, but parents opt to continue pregnancy

↓

Subsequent visits to specialist antenatal clinic at 2–3 week intervals

- To try to limit damage, consider treatment with spiramycin or combination of pyrimethamine and sulfadiazine after discussions with microbiologist. Daily 5 mg folic acid supplementation, if pyrimethamine used
- Arrange serial scans at 2–3 week intervals for any signs of symmetrical IUGR, CNS abnormalities, hydrocephaly, etc. Review after each scan in specialist antenatal clinic
- Shared care with community midwife continues meanwhile
- Refer to paediatricians to discuss neonatal and infancy issues
- If non-immune hydrops on scan, refer to regional fetal medicine unit

→

- IOL at term, if no associated problems warranting earlier delivery (e.g. non-immune hydrops, IUGR, etc.)
- Inform paediatricians for neonatal assessment, serology, treatment if indicated and long-term follow-up
- Remind patient that she now has lifelong immunity to toxoplasmosis although her IgG and IgM could persist and be detectable for years. This does not signify fresh infection

2.17 Urinary Tract Infections

FACT FILE

- **Urinary tract infection (UTI)** is common, can be both symptomatic and asymptomatic, and can lead to adverse pregnancy outcomes, both maternal and perinatal.
- UTI can cause further impairment of any underlying renal disease during pregnancy, particularly if not promptly detected and treated.
- UTI is found in about 8% of all pregnancies.[1]
- Most individuals with UTI are found to have bacterial counts of more than 10^4–10^5/ml of urine and a count of 10^5/ml is used as the diagnostic criterion. Lower counts suggest contamination and a repeat sample of a clean-catch midstream specimen is required.
- When more than one strain of bacterial pathogen is found, this is more likely due to a contamination rather than true UTI where there is predominance of a single strain of pathogen. Similarly, if the same strain of bacterial species is isolated in a repeat specimen, this suggests significant bacteriuria.
- UTI can manifest as:[2]
  - asymptomatic bacteriuria (in 2–5% of pregnancies)
  - acute cystitis (about 1% of pregnancies)
  - acute pyelonephritis (in 2% of pregnancies, with a recurrence rate of up to 23% in the same pregnancy).
- Well-recognized physiological changes as well as the modified immune status of pregnancy aid the development of UTI.
- Most UTIs are caused by Gram-negative aerobes from the gastrointestinal tract. *Escherichia coli* accounts for 80–90% of UTI, followed by *Staphylococcus saprophyticus*, *Staph. aureus*, and the Gram-positive GBS.
- Organisms such as *Proteus mirabilis*, *Klebsiella*, and most enterococci have urease activity and can form calculi, which in turn increase the chances of further UTIs.
- UTI is more common when there are comorbidities such as diabetes, bladder or ureteric diverticulae, or sickle cell disease.

Asymptomatic bacteriuria

- This is associated with increased rates of subsequent pyelonephritis (in nearly one-third), anaemia, preterm labour (in about 13%), low birth weight, chorioamnionitis, increased perinatal mortality, developmental problems, etc.
- Screening with active treatment is shown to significantly reduce these risks.
- Routine midstream urine (MSU) screening for asymptomatic bacteriuria at the first booking visit is part of routine antenatal practice in the UK, applicable to all pregnancies.
- One-third of women with asymptomatic bacteriuria will go on to develop acute cystitis during pregnancy.
- Treatment is therefore recommended[3] with appropriate antibiotics for a minimum of 7 days.
- ***Post-treatment completion follow-up cultures are recommended to ensure clearance of asymptomatic bacteriuria. Repeat follow-up cultures may need to be performed once in each trimester in women identified to have asymptomatic bacteriuria in the first-trimester screening sample.***[4]

Acute cystitis

- Usual symptoms include dysuria, frequency, urgency, suprapubic discomfort or pain, and 'smelly' urine, but without pyrexia or other signs of systemic illness.
- Presence of nitrites in the dipstick test in symptomatic women is a good indicator of significant bacteriuria[2] and empirical antibiotic treatment should be initiated while awaiting culture and sensitivity results. Re-evaluation of the antibiotic treatment should be performed once the results are available, but treatment continued for a complete course of 7–10 days. Shorter courses have not only been found to be inadequate but could also lead to persistent infection, progressing to pyelonephritis.
- Follow-up cultures after treatment completion are essential and persistent infection or relapses must be treated with a second course of a different antimicrobial, depending on the sensitivity results.
- If there is urethral discharge in addition to other symptoms of acute cystitis but without bacteriuria, this should raise suspicion of gonococcal or non-gonococcal urethritis and further investigations are then required.
- Herpetic lesions involving the vulva, vagina, or cervix can mimic symptoms of acute cystitis.

Pyelonephritis

- This is the most severe form of UTI in pregnancy, responsible for most perinatal problems linked to bacteriuria and most frequent in the second and third trimesters of pregnancy.
- **Pyelonephritis** refers to infection of the renal papillae which can spread to the renal cortex if untreated. **Pyelonephrosis is infection of all of the kidney tissue**. Gram-negative septicaemia can result if the kidney capsule ruptures causing a sub-phrenic abscess. Overwhelming sepsis and multiorgan failure can result in maternal mortality.
- Symptoms include those of acute cystitis with systemic illness with pyrexia, tachycardia, rigors, nausea, vomiting and severe renal angle tenderness. Fetal tachycardia, secondary to maternal pyrexia and tachycardia, is also often found.
- Admission is required in most cases.
- A detailed history must be obtained followed by a thorough clinical examination. FBC, elevated C-reactive protein, blood, urine, and HVS must be sent before commencing treatment with parenteral broad-spectrum antibiotics. Treatment may need to be changed if so indicated by results of the culture and sensitivity tests.
- Parenteral treatment needs to continue till pyrexia has been absent for 24 h as a minimum. Meanwhile, following admission, analgesics and IV fluid hydration must be maintained. Simple analgesics, avoiding all NSAIDs, may sometimes need to be augmented with opioids, especially in the presence of renal colic.
- Antimicrobial treatment is required for a minimum of 10 days; some advocate even longer courses up to 14–21 days.
- After treatment completion, it is mandatory that further urine culture is checked to ensure it is sterile. Such follow-up cultures must be repeated at perhaps monthly intervals during the rest of the pregnancy.
- If there is dehydration and prolonged periods of reduced mobility, thromboprophylaxis must be considered.
- If preterm contractions develop secondary to the pyelonephritis, tocolysis and steroids may be required.
- In cases that do not respond to initial treatment, urgent consultation with the microbiologist is required for advice regarding change of antimicrobials. If treatment failure is noted despite appropriate antimicrobial being used, renal tract anomalies (e.g. calculi) must be suspected and the best imaging modality suitable for the stage of gestation must be discussed with radiology.
- Immediate investigations and resuscitation must be undertaken if severe sepsis or septic shock are suspected and multispecialty support then urgently obtained from microbiologist, intensive care consultant, nephrologist, urologist, etc.

Recurrent UTIs

- Occur in 3–4% of pregnancies.
- Renal tract calculi need to be excluded.
- Low-dose, long-term antibiotic therapy is advisable for the remainder of pregnancy if multiple attacks of UTI have occurred.
- A postpartum (>10–12 weeks after delivery) IV urethrogram may be required to delineate any renal tract anomalies.

Information for patients

Please see Information for patients: Urinary tract infection and pregnancy (p. 503)

References

1. Mikhail MS, Anyaegbunam A. Lower urinary tract dysfunction in pregnancy: a review. Obstet Gynecol Surv 1995;50: 675–683.
2. McCormick T, et al. Urinary tract infection in pregnancy. Obstetrician and Gynaecologist 2008;10: 156–162.
3. Smaill F, Vazquez JC. Antibiotics for asymptomatic bacteriuria in pregnancy. Cochrane Database Syst Rev, 2007;2: CD000490.
4. ACOG educational bulletin. Antimicrobial therapy for obstetric patients. No. 245. Int J Gynaecol Obstet 1998;61: 299–308.

CARE PATHWAY

Asymptomatic bacteriuria

↓

Appropriate oral antimicrobial therapy as indicated by culture, sensitivity result—continued for 7 days

↓

- Post- treatment check MSU
- Repeat follow-up cultures once in each trimester

Acute cystitis

↓

- Examine to exclude other causes for symptoms
- Dipstick shows nitrites
- Urine sent for C&S, start empirical oral antibiotics
- Re-evaluation after results of C&S; change antibiotics, if indicated
- Oral antibiotics to continue for 7–10 days
- Check MSU after treatment completion
- Persistent infection or relapse—treat with a further 7-day course of a different oral antibiotic according to sensitivity results
- Repeat follow-up urine cultures at suggested monthly intervals

Pyelonephritis

↓

- Admission in most cases; history and examination
- Investigations: FBC, CRP, blood cultures if pyrexial, MSU for C&S, vaginal swab
- IV fluids, parenteral empirical broad-spectrum antibiotics, simple analgesics (avoid any NSAID), opioids may be required especially with renal colic
- Continue IV antibiotics till results of blood and urine cultures available, change antibiotics if results so indicate
- Continue parenteral therapy till apyrexial for at least 24 h, then switch to oral route
- Continue antimicrobial therapy for minimum of 10 days—some advocate longer course of 14–21 days
- Consider thromboprophylaxis if dehydration and reduced mobility
- If preterm contractions due to UTI, tocolysis and steroids if appropriate
- Check MSU after treatment completion
- Repeat monthly follow-up urine cultures
- If not responding to initial treatment, consult microbiologist to discuss alternative antimicrobial therapy
- Imaging for calculi if not responding to usual initial treatment, seek radiology opinion for best imaging modality for that gestation
- If signs of severe sepsis/ septic shock, immediate management including urgent resuscitation and investigations
- Urgent multispecialty involvement required- microbiologist, nephrologist, urologist, intensive care specialist, etc.
- If repeated attacks of pyelonephritis in pregnancy, low-dose, long-term antibiotic for rest of pregnancy
- IVU 3 months post-delivery and follow-up by urologists if urinary calculi, diverticulum, etc.

2.18 Pneumonia

FACT FILE

- Respiratory complications are not uncommon in pregnancy and can be life-threatening. Prompt multidisciplinary input involving community and hospital-based care is essential.
- **Pneumonia has been found to be the most frequent cause of non-obstetric infection in the pregnant patient.**

Incidence

- Incidence ranges from 0.2 to 8.5 per 1000 deliveries,[1,2] reflecting a higher incidence of pneumonia in pregnancy from the pre-antibiotic era.
- The incidence of pneumonia in the pregnant patient is currently rising to about 1 in 660 deliveries,[2,3] attributable to a rising trend of women with serious underlying illnesses such as pre-existent diabetes or heart disease becoming pregnant, as well as the increased incidence of newer immune deficiencies, including HIV.[1,4]

Impact of pneumonia on pregnancy outcomes

- Depending on aetiology, particular types of pneumonia can have very different implications for the pregnant woman—especially pneumonia of viral origin.
- **Maternal death:** In the pre-antibiotic era, the maternal death rate was observed to be as high as 32% in all such cases. However, with the advent of antibiotics, there has been a reduction in maternal deaths although viral lung infection and opportunistic lung infection still carry a substantially high maternal mortality and morbidity.
- Pneumonia has been found to be the third most frequent cause of indirect obstetric death in North America.[5] In the UK, however, pneumonia is a rare cause of maternal death, even including women with cystic fibrosis. Mortality rates of 0–4% have been found in pregnant women who contract pneumonia in the UK,[1,6,7,8] which is similar to rates in the non-pregnant population.
- The relatively low mortality in this severely ill population probably reflects current therapeutic modalities and the overall good health of women of childbearing age.
- Pregnant women do not get pneumonia more frequently than non-pregnant women in general.
- However, there is increased morbidity compared with non-pregnant women due to normal anatomical, physiological, hormonal, and immunological changes that take place in pregnancy.[4] Increased level of surveillance and prompt interventions are therefore mandatory in this cohort of previously healthy women.[3]
- Pneumonia in the pregnant patient increases the **risk of preterm delivery** compared with pregnancies in which infection is absent. The incidence of preterm delivery in those who have developed pneumonia in pregnancy has been quoted as up to 1–43%.[8] The incidence of **small for gestational age** babies is also more frequent in this group,[2] as is **fetal distress** secondary to poor oxygenation.
- Poor fetal outcomes are more frequent in mothers with underlying comorbidities, such as chronic respiratory disease, diabetes, or HIV.
- Neonatal morbidity associated with maternal antepartum pneumonia ranges from 2% to 12%, mainly due to the impact of preterm delivery.[9]

Risk factors

- No significant differences with age or parity.
- Risk of pneumonia appears lowest in the first trimester.[1]
- Mean gestational age at admission for pneumonia is 24–31 weeks.[10,11]
- Both anaemia (a haematocrit of 30% or lower on admission) and asthma have been found to increase the risk of pneumonia during pregnancy by fivefold on multivariate analysis.[8]
- Smoking: Nearly one-third of pregnant women who are admitted with pneumonia have been found to be smokers.[11,12]
- Substance abuse.

Changes in pregnancy that predispose to pneumonia

- ***Anatomical changes:***
  - An outward flaring of the lower ribs, increase in the subcostal angle, and an increase of a maximum of about 2 cm in the transverse diameter of the chest.
  - The diaphragm rises by 4 cm in later pregnancy.[13]
- These changes decrease the ability of the pregnant woman to clear respiratory secretions. The elevation of the diaphragm leads to a decreased functional residual capacity.
- ***Physiological changes:***
  - A decrease in expiratory reserve volume.
  - A decrease in functional residual capacity from about 20 weeks gestation to a 10–20% reduction by term
  - Large airway function is not impaired by pregnancy. Forced expiratory volumes are not altered in pregnancy.[13]
  - The function of the diaphragm and chest wall musculature is unaffected.
- ***Hormonal changes:***
  - Progesterone stimulates the respiratory centre centrally, leading to increased tidal volume and minute ventilation. **The respiratory rate is unaffected**.
  - Progesterone, human chorionic gonadotropin (hCG), alpha-fetoprotein, and cortisol are all inhibitors of cell-mediated immunity.
- ***Changes in maternal immune status:*** The major factor predisposing pregnant women to severe pneumonic infections is an alteration in immune status, especially in cell-mediated immunity. This makes viral, fungal, and tuberculous infections particularly pathogenic in these women.

Diagnosis

- Presentation in a previously healthy patient without pre-existing cardiorespiratory disease usually involves symptoms of dyspnoea, fever, and cough. However, some symptoms such as dyspnoea may be attributed to physiological changes of pregnancy by patients themselves or by the healthcare professionals.[1,4]
- Because the respiratory rate remains normal during pregnancy, tachypnoea must be recognized as pathological. Incidence of tachypnoea may therefore be used to evaluate the severity of illness when pneumonia is present.
- Misdiagnosis or delay in diagnosis of pneumonia is not uncommon in pregnancy.
- Differential diagnosis includes exacerbation of asthma, pulmonary embolism, aspiration pneumonia, etc.
- In pneumonia, the dyspnoea is out of proportion with what normally expected in any pregnancy.
- Cough is not an usual accompaniment of dyspnoea in normal pregnancy and must raise the suspicion of pneumonia especially if fever is an added symptom.
- A firm diagnosis of pneumonia can only be made with a chest radiograph.
- In about one-third of cases where clinical symptoms are suggestive of pneumonia, this is not confirmed by chest radiograph[14] and other aetiology must be considered.
- The relative incidence of individual pathogens in the pregnant patient with pneumonia is similar to those reported in non-pregnant hosts of comparable age (see Table 2.5).
- Purulent sputum, chills, and a lobar infiltrate are classically considered suggestive of pneumococcal or *Haemophilus influenza* pneumonia.
- Even with extensive diagnostic testing, the etiological pathogen is not identified in 50–60% of cases.[4,15]
- An informed assessment of the risks from infection compared with any possible risks or adverse drug effects on the fetus or mother is essential before the initiation of any antimicrobial agent.

Table 2.5 Pathogens causing pneumonia and their relative frequency

Pathogen	*Relative frequency (%)*
Streptococcus pneumonia	17%
Haemophilus influenza	6%
Mycoplasma pneumonia	3%
Staphylococcus aureus	1%
Legionella sp.	1%
Influenza A virus	1%
Others	9%
Unknown	61%

Reproduced from *Thorax*, Lim WS et al., 'Pneumonia and pregnancy', 56, pp. 398–405, copyright 2001, with permission from BMJ Publishing Group Ltd.

Bacterial pneumonia

- Community-acquired pneumonia is the most common form of pneumonia in pregnancy with *Streptococcus pneumoniae*, *Haemophilus influenza*, and *Mycoplasma pneumonia* being the most common bacterial organisms.[9]
- Clinically, the features of acute bacterial pneumonia present no differently in pregnant and non-pregnant patients.[4] Symptoms include cough (>90%), phlegm (66%),dyspnoea (66%), and pleuritic chest pain (50%).[16]
- *S. pneumoniae* is the most common bacterial pathogen causing pneumonia in both pregnant and non-pregnant adult population.
- Multilobar pneumonia is a more serious condition than unilobar pneumonia.
- Maternal mortality has been greatly reduced due to antibiotics.
- Prompt admission is required for relevant investigations including FBC, electrolytes, measurement of oxygen saturation, blood cultures and chest radiograph (with shielding). While awaiting results, broad-spectrum IV antibiotics should be commenced.
  - Blood cultures are positive in only 7–15% of cases.[2,10]
  - Bacterial cultures of sputum with Gram staining are of some value, but have poor sensitivity and specificity.[15]
- Most patients with bacterial pneumonia will show a clinical response within 72 h of IV antibiotics being started, during which time, unless there is marked deterioration, therapy should preferably not be changed.
- ***Beta-lactam antibiotics (e.g. penicillins, ampicillin, amoxicillin) and macrolide antibiotics (e.g. erythromycin, clarithromycin) are generally safe and effective for community-acquired pneumonia in pregnancy.***
- **Co-amoxiclav is the preferred choice if anaerobic cover is required** e.g. for *Bacteroides* species.
- ***Most Gram-negative infections are treated with cephalosporins.***
- Quinolones, tetracycline, chloramphenicol, and sulpha compounds are contraindicated in pregnancy.
- Tetracyclines are contraindicated because of the risk of fulminant maternal hepatitis when given in the third trimester of pregnancy and also of staining and deformity of the fetal teeth when given at any time during the pregnancy. The neonate exposed to tetracyclines in utero may subsequently develop bony deformities.
- Sulfonamides administered shortly before delivery can cause fetal kernicterus, and the safety of trimethoprim is unknown.
- Chloramphenicol in the fetus, as in the adult, can lead to bone marrow suppression and even aplastic anaemia. Use of chloramphenicol near term produces an adverse drug reaction known as 'grey baby syndrome', characterized by ashen grey cyanosis, flaccidity, and cardiovascular collapse.
- *Pneumocystis jirovecii* pneumonia (PCP) is associated with HIV infection and carries a high mortality in pregnancy.[17] Treatment involves co-trimoxazole or pentamidine.[4] Prophylaxis is required in those with low CD4 counts (<200/μl).

Viral pneumonias

- Viral influenza is most commonly caused by **influenza virus** and **VZV**.
- Influenza viruses are of the myxovirus class, type A, B, or C. Most epidemics in humans are due to type A.
- VZV affects 0.7 per 1000 pregnancies and pneumonia occurs in 10% of cases.[18]
- Mortality rates have dropped to 14% compared with 35–40 % in the pre-antiviral therapy era.[19]
- Varicella pneumonia: The most serious maternal consequence of varicella infection is pneumonia. Varicella pneumonia carries a mortality of 35– 40% in pregnancy compared with 11–17% in the non-pregnant state.[18]
- Varicella pneumonia is most likely to complicate the final trimester, and infection is more serious if it occurs at this time.
- Pulmonary symptoms, including cough, haemoptysis, dyspnoea, tachypnoea, and pleuritic chest pain, begin 2–5 days after the appearance of fever and rash in VZV.
- Varicella zoster immunoglobulin given within 96 h of exposure to varicella can attenuate infection in susceptible women.
- Oral mucosal ulceration may also be present.
- The severity of illness ranges from coryza-like symptoms to life-threatening respiratory failure requiring mechanical ventilation and positive-end expiratory pressure (PEEP).[20]
- Classically, the chest radiograph shows localized miliary nodular infiltrates.
- Treatment is with IV aciclovir.
- **Severe acute respiratory syndrome (SARS)** is caused by a coronavirus, transmitted by respiratory droplets. High rates of morbidity and mortality are associated with SARS pneumonia due to respiratory failure, superimposed bacterial infections and disseminated intravascular coagulation (DIC). Intensive care is mandatory.

Fungal pneumonia

- Fungal pneumonia in pregnancy is mostly seen in those who are immunocompromised. Histoplasmosis, blastomycosis, cryptococci, or coccidiodomycosis are the unusual fungal infections and usually respond to amphotericin.[4] Other antifungal agents such as itraconazole and fluconazole are best avoided in pregnancy due to reported fetotoxicity and teratogenicity.[1]
- Dissemination can occur more rapidly, particularly when the infection is acquired in the third trimester.

General principles of medical management of pneumonia in pregnancy

- Regardless of the type of pneumonia, close monitoring and aggressive treatment are needed in the antenatal period.
- Oxygen supplementation to prevent fetal acidaemia and broad-spectrum antibiotics should be started before identification of the aetiologic agent.
- The antibiotics should be changed if required, as indicated once the culture and sensitivity results are back.
- The choice of antibiotic therapy in the pregnant patient with pneumonia is influenced by the presence or absence of coexisting illness and the severity of illness at presentation.
- Penicillins are only 50% protein-bound and can cross the placenta to achieve fetal concentrations that are 50% of maternal levels.
- The cephalosporins cross the placenta less effectively but also appear to have no adverse effect on the fetus.
- Most patients with community-acquired pneumonia may be adequately treated with ampicillin or a cephalosporin, which will cover pneumococcus, *H. influenzae*, and some non-pseudomonal Gram-negative bacteria (*M. catarrhalis*, *K. pneumoniae*, *H. influenzae*, and *E. coli*).
- If an atypical pathogen is strongly suspected, macrolides are the therapy of choice as they cover not only *S. pneumoniae* and *H. influenzae*, but also other atypical pathogens, namely *M. pneumoniae*, *C. pneumoniae*, and *L. pneumophila*.
- Supportive therapy of the pregnant patient with pneumonia is of paramount importance and follows the same principles as used in the non-gravid state.

- Hydration, antipyretic therapy, and supplemental oxygen are key. Maintenance of the arterial oxygen tension higher than 70 mmHg is critical because hypoxemia is less tolerated in the pregnant woman and also because respiratory alkalosis, a condition often associated with pulmonary disorders such as pneumonia, leads to reduction in uterine blood flow and results in fetal hypoxaemia.
- In viral pneumonias, aggressive therapy starting with early hospitalization is mandatory. Aciclovir has been extensively used and has been found safe in pregnancy.
- Treatment with amphotericin is required in fungal pneumonias.

Information for patients

Please see **Information for patients: Pneumonia and pregnancy** (p. 503)

References

1. Lim WS, et al. Pneumonia and pregnancy—review series: Respiratory diseases in pregnancy 2. Thorax 2001;56: 398–405.
2. Yost NP, et al. An appraisal of treatment guidelines for antepartum community-acquired pneumonia. Am J Obstet Gynecol 2000;183: 131–135.
3. Jin Y, et al. The effects of community-acquired pneumonia during pregnancy ending with a live birth. Am J Obstet Gynecol 2003;188: 800–806.
4. Laibl VR, Sheffield JS.Influenza and pneumonia in pregnancy. Clin Perinatol 2005;32: 727–738.
5. Chen Y-H., et al. Pneumonia and pregnancy outcomes: a nationwide population-based study. Am J Obstet Gynecol 2012;207: 288. e1–e7.
6. British Thoracic Society Standards of Care Committee. BTS guidelines for the management of community acquired pneumonia in adults. Thorax 2001;56: iv1–iv 64.
7. Saving Mothers' Lives: Reviewing maternal deaths to make motherhood safer: 2006–2008. The Eighth Report of the Confidential Enquiries into Maternal Deaths in the United Kingdom 2011. Centre for Maternal and Child Enquiries. BJOG 2011;118: 1–203.
8. Munn MB, et al. Pneumonia as a complication of pregnancy. J Matern Fetal Med 1999;8: 151–154.
9. Goodnight WH, Soper DE. Pneumonia in pregnancy. Crit Care Med 2005;33: S390–S397.
10. Berkowitz K, LaSala A. Risk factors associated with the increasing prevalence of pneumonia during pregnancy. Am J Obstet Gynecol 1990;163: 981–985.
11. Graves CR. Pneumonia in pregnancy. Clin Obstet Gynecol 2010;53: 329–336.
12. Nuorti JP, et al. Cigarette smoking and invasive pneumococcal disease. Active Bacterial Core Surveillance Team. N Engl J Med 2000;342: 681–689.
13. Bhatia P, Bhatia K. Pregnancy and the lungs. Postgrad Med J 2000;76: 683–689.
14. Woodhead MA, et al. Prospective study of the aetiology and outcome of pneumonia in the community. Lancet 1987; i: 671–674.
15. American Thoracic Society. Guidelines for the management of adults with community-acquired pneumonia. Am J Respir Crit Care Med 2001;163: 1730–1754.
16. Halm EA, Teirstein AS. Management of community-acquired pneumonia. N Engl J Med 2002;347: 2039–2045.
17. Ahmad H, et al. Pneumocystis carinii pneumonia in pregnancy. Chest 2001;120: 666–671.
18. Harger JH, et al. Risk factors and outcome of varicella-zoster virus pneumonia in pregnant women. J Infect Dis 2002;185: 422–427.
19. Smego RA, Asperilla MO. Use of acyclovir for varicella pneumonia during pregnancy. Obstet Gynecol 1991;78: 1112–1116.
20. Cole DE, et al. Acute respiratory distress syndrome in pregnancy. Crit Care Med 2005;33: S269–S278.

Community acquired pneumonia (CAP)

Community referral or self- referral to obstetric unit or acute medical admissions unit with symptoms of cough, dyspnoea, fever, pleuritic chest pain, phlegm: **admission mandatory**

Obtain detailed history
- Gestational age
- Duration of symptomatology
- Exposure to any recent infectious illness in other family members
- Any recent exposure to VZV or handling of sheep (Q-fever)
- Underlying comorbidities(e.g. asthma,anaemia, diabetes, HIV, cardiorespiratory disease)
- Smoking
- Substance abuse
- Any recent prescribed medication
- Any history of haemoptysis, orthopnoea

Immediate examination and investigations
- General clinical examination—temperature, pulse, BP, respiratory auscultation, respiratory rate, SOS score
- Antenatal assessment
- FBC, blood gases, electrolytes
- **Chest radiograph** with fetal shielding
- ECG
- Blood and sputum culture
- MRSA swabs

Chest radiograph highly suggestive of pneumonia

Localized infiltrate
Viral aetiology likely

Diffuse infiltrate
- Bacterial or fungal pneumonia likely
- ***Also consider ARDS***

Management
Immediate multidisciplinary input from respiratory physicians, obstetrician, anaesthetist, intensivists and midwife
- Oxygenation, hydration, antipyretics, and other supportive measures
- Seek urgent advice from **microbiologist** and start broad-spectrum IV antibiotics
- Once aetiology of CAP identified by microbiological tests, antimicrobial therapy should be targeted at that pathogen, ideally within 12 h of when empirical therapy was commenced
- Choice of antimicrobials influence by severity of condition at presentation; any comorbidities such as HIV, asthma, etc.; absence of fetotoxic or teratogenic potential
- Response to antimicrobials usually seen within 72 h
- Fetal well-being assessments to continue as fetal distress could result from intrauterine hypoxaemia
- Decisions regarding delivery to be based on obstetric indications only
- ***Caution before giving prophylactic steroids to accelerate fetal lung maturity if pre-term delivery anticipated—this can cause acute worsening of pneumonia, therefore maternal respiratory compromise***

Good response seen within 72 h
- Do not change type of antimicrobial
- After discussion with microbiologist, consider conversion to oral antimicrobials as relevant
- Supportive care to continue
- Fetal assessments to continue

No improvement or actual deterioration within first 72 h
- Review and joint discussions with microbiologist, respiratory physician, intensivists, and anaesthetist
- Differential diagnosis to be reviewed with further laboratory investigations
- Antimicrobial may need to be changed or a further medication added to current regime
- Admission to intensive care unit may need to be considered for mechanical ventilation, PEEP, etc.
- Atypical pathogens for pneumonia to be considered including SARS, ARDS due to other causes, MRSA pneumonia, etc. Appropriate antimicrobial therapy to be instituted
- Supportive care to continue
- Fetal assessments to continue

2.19 Bacterial Sepsis

FACT FILE

Sepsis may arise in pregnancy at any time—antepartum, intrapartum, and postpartum. In addition sepsis may arise may arise from extra-genital sources as well and involve a variety of pathogens including bacteria, viruses, and fungi.

The scope of this chapter is **antepartum sepsis caused by bacterial organisms**, which is a serious life-threatening condition in pregnancy.

Epidemiology

- Bacteraemia is not uncommon during pregnancy, occurring in about 8–9%,[1] but progression to severe sepsis and septic shock is relatively less frequent.[2]
- The severe mortality and morbidity from sepsis is, however, significant.
- Severe sepsis carries a maternal mortality of 20–40%, rising to 60% if septic shock sets in.[3]
- One-third of early maternal mortality is due to refractory hypotension while late maternal mortality is due to multiorgan failure.[4]
- Up to 20–30% of ICU admissions of obstetric patients result from sepsis in pregnancy.[4]
- Sepsis in pregnancy is an important cause of maternal death in the UK.[5,6] In fact, in the 2006–2008 report of CEMACE sepsis was identified as the leading cause of direct maternal deaths in the UK. Sepsis resulted in 29 maternal deaths. One-third of these deaths occurred before 24 weeks of gestation. Associated factors included minority ethnic origin and the presence of sickle cell disease or trait. Infant mortality in affected pregnancies was 45%. **Group A streptococcal (GAS) infection was the principal pathogen, causing nearly 50% of deaths.**

Definitions

- **Systemic inflammatory response syndrome:** More than one of the following clinical signs:
  - temperature more than 38 °C or less than 36 °C
  - tachycardia more than 100/min
  - hyperventilation (respiratory rate more than 20/min or Pco_2 less than 32 mmHg.
  - white cell count of more than 12 × 10^9 or less than 4 × 10^9.
- **Sepsis** is defined as infection plus systemic manifestations of inflammatory response syndrome.
- **Severe sepsis** may be defined as sepsis plus sepsis-induced organ dysfunction or developing tissue hypoperfusion.
- **Septic shock** is defined as persistence of hypoperfusion (hypotension) in a septic patient, despite adequate fluid replacement therapy.[5]
- **Hypotension** is defined as systolic BP less than 90 mmHg or mean arterial pressure (MAP) less than 60 mmHg, or a reduction of systolic BP of more than 40 mmHg from baseline.

Clinical presentation

- The onset of sepsis may be insidious and the woman may appear deceptively well but collapse suddenly.
- Four specific infectious conditions are most common in pregnancy:
  - pyelonephritis
  - chorioamnionitis
  - pneumonia
  - postpartum endometritis, infection of surgical sites, and genital tract infection.
- Other causes also include septic abortion or miscarriage, acute appendicitis, acute pancreatitis, or cholecystitis.

Risk factors for sepsis

- Obesity, diabetes, immunosuppressant conditions and medication, anaemia, prolonged rupture of membranes, amniocentesis, cervical cerclage, history of pelvic infection, GBS infection, or close contact with someone with GAS infection.

Clinical signs of sepsis

- Clinical signs of sepsis include one or more of the following: pyrexia, hypothermia, tachycardia, tachypnoea, hypoxia, hypotension, oliguria, decreased capillary refill and mottling, impaired consciousness, and failure to respond to treatment.[7]
- Constant severe abdominal pain and tenderness in sepsis warrants urgent medical assessment.
- Toxic shock syndrome due to staphyloccal or streptococcal exotoxins can result in nausea, vomiting, diarrhoea, a watery vaginal discharge (streptococcal infection), productive cough, urinary symptoms, generalized rash (purpura fulminans), or severe pain due to necrotizing fasciitis.
- These signs, including pyrexia, may not always be present or be as distinctive as in the non-pregnant. In severe sepsis, the temperature may be less than 36 °C. In addition, the signs are not necessarily related to the severity of sepsis.
- Early identification of severe sepsis allows prompt multidisciplinary management in secondary or tertiary care.
- All healthcare professionals should be aware of the symptoms and signs of maternal sepsis and septic shock and of the rapid, potentially lethal progression.
- ***The Modified Early Obstetric Warning Score (MEOWS) chart should be used in all maternity inpatients to identify seriously ill pregnant women. The MEOWS score can also prompt immediate coordinated multidisciplinary management by involvement of consultants in obstetrics, anaesthetics, microbiology, infectious disease, intensive care etc., as well as midwives and intensive care nurses.***
- Apart from the immediate risk to the fetus secondary to severe maternal sepsis and acidosis, there is an increased risk of neonatal encephalopathy and cerebral palsy developing due to the effect of intrauterine infection.[8]

Investigations

See Tables 2.6 and 2.7.[9,10]

- Blood cultures should be sent before antibiotics are started (IV antibiotics should not be delayed while awaiting microbiological results). Similarly a MSU, throat swabs, HVS, etc. as directed by individual symptomatology should be taken and sent for microbiological analysis before antibiotic therapy is commenced.
- Urgent serum lactate level within 6 h of the suspicion of severe sepsis. **If the serum lactate level is 4 mmol/litre or higher, this is indicative of tissue hypoperfusion.**
- Relevant imaging (e.g. chest radiograph or CT scan) in suspected abdominal necrotizing fasciitis.
- If MRSA (meticillin-resistant *Staphyloccus aureus*) status is unknown, rapid MRSA testing with a nose swab should be sent.

Commonly identified bacterial organisms

- Lancefield group A beta-haemolytic streptococcus (GAS)
- *Escherichia coli*
- Group B streptococcus
- Coliforms (especially associated with UTIs, PPROM, cerclage, etc.)
- *Staphylococcus aureus*
- Mixed infections with Gram-positive and Gram-negative organisms (particularly with chorioamnionitis)
- Anaerobes such as *Clostridium perfringens*, *Bacteroides* spp., peptococci.

Table 2.6 Assessment for end-organ dysfunction: some parameters to measure

End-organ dysfunction	*Parameters to measure*
Acute circulatory failure	Cardiovascular assessment, pulse, BP, peripheral perfusion, BP, CVP including signs of high or low cardiac output
Metabolic acidosis	pH, bicarbonate (HCO_3), partial pressure of carbon dioxide ($PaCO_2$), lactate
Acute hypoxaemia	Oxygen saturation measured by pulse oximetry(S_pO_2), partial pressure of oxygen
Acute renal failure	Urine output, urea, creatinine, electrolytes, fluid overload
Liver dysfunction	LFTs
Coagulopathy	FBC, coagulation profile
CNS disturbance	AVPU (alert, verbal, pain, unresponsive), Glasgow coma score (GCS), encephalopathy
Overall metabolism	Hypercatabolic state indicated by negative nitrogen balance (e.g. low albumin) or raised glucose levels in a non-diabetic

Data from Funk D et al., A systems approach to the early recognition and rapid administration of best practice therapy in sepsis and septic shock, *Current Opinion in Critical Care*, 2009, 15, pp. 301–307.

Table 2.7 Diagnostic criteria for sepsis (clinical variables and investigations)

Fever (>38 °C) or hypothermia (core temp <36 °C) Tachycardia (>100 bpm) Tachypnoea (>20/min) Significant oedema or positive fluid balance >20 ml/kg in 24 h Ileus Oliguria (<0.5 ml/kg per hour for at least 2 h, despite adequate fluid resuscitation)	
FBC	WBC >12 × 10^9 *or* < 4 × 10^9 *or* normal count with >10% immature forms. Thrombocytopenia: platelets <100 × 10^9
Plasma C-reactive protein	>7 mg/litre
Urea, electrolytes, creatinine	Creatinine rise of > 44.2 micromol/litre Severe sepsis if creatinine >176 micromol/litre
Plasma glucose and albumin (indicators of hypercatabolic metabolism)	Hyperglycaemia (plasma glucose >7.7 mmol/litre) in the absence of diabetes Low albumin (indicates negative nitrogen balance)
LFT	Hyperbilirubinaemia (plasma total bilirubin >70 micromol/litre
Coagulation profile	Coagulation defects: INR > 1.5 or APPT > 60 s Thrombocytopenia: platelets <100 × 10^9
Blood gases	Raised serum lactate ≥4 mmol/litre Arterial hypoxaemia (PaO_2:FiO_2 ratio <40 kPa) Severe sepsis if <33.3 kPa in absence of pneumonia or if <26.7 kPa in presence of pneumonia

Data from: RCOG Green-top Guideline No. 64a, *Bacterial sepsis in pregnancy*, 2012, Royal College of Obstetricians and Gynaecologists; and Levy MM et al., 2001 SCCM/ESICM/ACCP/ATS/SIS International Sepsis Definitions Conference, *Critical Care Medicine*, 2003, 31, pp. 1250–1256.

Staphylococcal and streptococcal toxic shock syndrome

Immediate management

See Table 2.8.[10,11,12]

- Blood cultures, urine MSU, other swabs as indicated to be taken without any delay, as well as blood for serum lactate levels, blood gas levels, electrolytes, LFTs, kidney function tests, FBC, etc.
- Immediate imaging, e.g. chest radiograph if pneumonia suspected.
- Urgent referral to the critical care team.
- Early institution of the Modified Survival Sepsis Campaign Resuscitation 'Bundle'.[3,7]
- **A combination of broad-spectrum antibiotics to be administered IV, within 1 h of recognition of severe sepsis** and after culture samples and swabs have been sent.

Table 2.8 Staphylococcal and streptococcal toxic shock syndrome: clinical presentation

Staphylococcal toxic shock	*Streptococcal toxic shock syndrome*
Fever ≥ 39.9 °C Rash—diffuse macular erythroderma Desquamation—10–14 days after onset of illness, especially palms and soles Hypotension—systolic BP <90 mmHg (adults)	Isolation of beta-haemolytic GAS from: • normally sterile site—blood, CSF, peritoneal fluid, tissue biopsy • non-sterile site—throat, vagina, sputum
Multisystem involvement	Clinical case definition
Three or more of the following systems affected: **Gastrointestinal**—vomiting or diarrhoea at onset of illness **Muscular**—severe myalgia or elevated creatinine phosphokinase **Mucous membranes**—vaginal, oropharyngeal, or conjunctival hyperaemia **Renal**—creatinine twice the upper limit of normal **Hepatic**—total bilirubin twice the upper limit of normal **Haematological**—platelets ≤100 × 10^9 **Central nervous system**—disorientation or alterations in consciousness without focal neurological signs	Multiorgan involvement characterized by hypotension **plus two or more** of the following: **Renal impairment**—creatinine >176 µmol/litre **Coagulopathy**—platelets <100 × 10^9/litre or disseminated intravascular coagulation **Liver involvement**—alanine transaminase or aspartame transaminase or bilirubin levels twice the normal upper limit for age **Acute respiratory distress syndrome** **Generalized erythematous macular rash** (present in 10%)—may desquamate **Soft tissue necrosis** including necrotizing fasciitis, myositis, or gangrene
Case Classification	Case Classification
Probable—four of the five clinical findings positive	*Probable*—meets clinical case definition plus isolation from non-sterile site
Confirmed—case with all five clinical findings	*Definite*—meets clinical case definition plus isolation of GAS from a normally sterile site

Reproduced from: Royal College of Obstetricians and Gynaecologists. Bacterial sepsis in pregnancy. Green-top Guideline No. 64a. London: RCOG; 2012, with the permission of the Royal College of Obstetricians and Gynaecologists

- **Early goal-directed resuscitation**[13,14,15,16] taking the physiological changes of pregnancy into account and adjusting the goals accordingly.[17]
- Aim to achieve and maintain a central venous pressure (which normally remains unaltered in pregnancy) of **at least 8 mmHg**.
- Venous oxygen saturation (SvO_2) progressively decreases in later gestation in normal pregnancies. Aim is to achieve and maintain the central venous oxygen saturation **at least 70%** or mixed venous oxygen saturation **at least 65%**.
- Once a causative organism (s) is identified the IV antibiotic therapy can be targeted to the sensitivity of that organism.
- IV immunoglobulin (IVIG) may be needed after discussion with the infection control physician and senior microbiologist in cases of severe invasive streptococcal or staphylococcal infection if other therapies fail.[7,18]
- In a critically ill pregnant woman, birth of the baby may be considered if it would be beneficial to the mother or the baby or to both.
- A decision about the timing and mode of delivery should be made by the Critical care team and the consultant obstetrician following discussion with the woman if her condition allows. Attempting delivery in the setting of maternal instability increases the maternal and fetal mortality rates unless the source of infection is intrauterine.[19] The decision on mode of delivery should be individualized taking into account the severity of maternal illness, gestational age, viability, feasibility, and anticipated duration of labour, etc.[7]
- If preterm delivery is anticipated, cautious consideration should be given to the use of antenatal corticosteroids for fetal lung maturity in the woman with sepsis.
- During the intrapartum period, continuous electronic fetal monitoring is recommended. Changes in cardiotocography (CTG), such as changes in baseline variability or new onset decelerations, must prompt reassessment of maternal MAP, hypoxia, and acidaemia.[7]
- **Epidural/spinal anaesthesia should be avoided** in women with sepsis and a general anaesthetic will usually be required for Caesarean section.
- If invasive GAS has been isolated in the mother, inform the neonatologist as the baby will need prophylactic antibiotics.
- For close family members and staff who have been exposed to respiratory secretions of a woman with GAS, prophylactic antibiotics may need to be considered according to guidelines.[20]
- Local infection control guidelines, including isolation in a single en-suite room, should be followed for hospital-specific isolation after advice has been sought from the hospital infection control team.[7]
- **Invasive GAS infection is a notifiable condition** and the infection control team and consultant for communicable diseases should be informed.

General guide for antimicrobial therapy

- **Co-amoxiclav:** Does not cover MRSA or *Pseudomonas*, and there is concern about an increase in the risk of necrotizing enterocolitis in neonates exposed to co-amoxiclav in utero.
- **Metronidazole:** Only covers anaerobes.
- **Clindamycin:** Covers most streptococci and staphylococci, including many MRSA, and switches off exotoxin production with significantly decreased mortality. Not nephrotoxic.
- **Piperacillin–tazobactam and carbapenems:** Cover all except MRSA and are renal sparing (in contrast to aminoglycosides).
- **Gentamicin** (as a single dose of 3–5 mg/kg): Poses no problem in normal renal function but if doses are to be given regularly serum levels must be monitored.
- ***Local antibiotic guidelines, which may differ between hospitals, have to be consulted and advice sought from the senior microbiologist.***[7]

Information for patients

Please see Information for patients: Sepsis and pregnancy (p. 503)

References

1. Bryan CS, et al. Bacteremia in obstetrics and gynecology. Obstet Gynecol 1984;64: 155–158.
2. Kankuri E, et al. Incidence, treatment and outcome of peripartum sepsis. Acta Obstet Gynecol Scand 2003;82: 730–735.
3. Dellinger RP, et al. Surviving Sepsis Campaign: International guidelines for management of severe sepsis and septic shock. Crit Care Med 2008;36: 296–327 [correction in Crit Care Med 2008;36:394–1396].
4. Prasad BGR, Sunanda GV. In:Johanson R, etal., ed., Managing obstetric emergencies and trauma. The MOET course manual. London: RCOG Press, 2003, pp 231–234.
5. Saving Mother's Lives: reviewing maternal deaths to make motherhood safer: 2006–2008. Centre for Maternal and Child Enquiries (CMACE). BJOG 2011; 118 Suppl. 1: 1–203.
6. Lewis G, ed. Saving Mothers' Lives: reviewing maternal deaths to make motherhood safer - 2003–2005. The Seventh Report on Confidential enquiries into Maternal Deaths in the United Kingdom. London: RCOG Press, 2007.
7. RCOG Green-top Guideline No. 64a. Bacterial sepsis in pregnancy. London: Royal College of Obstetricians and Gynaecologists, 2012.
8. Yoon BH, et al. Fetal exposure to an intra-amniotic inflammation and the development of cerebral palsy at the age of three years. Am J Obstet Gynecol 2000;182: 675–681.
9. Funk D, et al. A systems approach to the early recognition and rapid administration of best practice therapy in sepsis and septic shock. Curr Opin CritCare 2009;15: 301–307.
10. Levy MM C et al. , 2001 SCCM/ESICM/ACCP/ATS/SIS International Sepsis Definitions Conference. Crit Care Med 2003;31: 1250–1256.
11. Stevens DL. Streptococcal toxic-shock syndrome: spectrum of disease, pathogenesis and new concepts in treatment. Emerg Infect Dis 1995;1: 69–78.
12. Lappin E, Ferguson AJ. Gram-positive toxic shock syndromes. Lancet Infect Dis 2009: 9: 281–290.
13. Neligan PJ, Laffey JG. Special populations—critical illness and pregnancy. Clinical review. Crit Care 2011;15: 227.
14. Rivers E, et al. Early goal-directed therapy in the treatment of severe sepsis and septic shock. N Engl J Med 2001;345: 1368–1377.
15. Joseph J, et al. Sepsis in pregnancy and early goal-directed therapy. Obstet Med 2009;2: 93–99.
16. Otero RM, et al. Early goal-directed therapy in severe sepsis and septic shock revisited concepts, controversies and contemporary findings. Chest 2006;130: 1579–1595.
17. Norwitz ER, et al. Pregnancy-induced physiologic alterations. In: Dildy GA III, et al., ed., Critical care obstetrics 4th ed. Malden, MA: Blackwell Science, 2004, pp. 19–42.
18. Department of Health. Clinical guidelines for immunoglobulin use, 2nd ed. 2008 <http://www.dh.gov.uk/en/Publicationsandstatistics/Publications/PublicationsPolicyAndGuidance/DH_085235>
19. Sheffield JS. Sepsis and septic shock in pregnancy. Crit Care Clin 2004;20: 651–660.
20. Health Protection Agency, Group A Streptococcus Working Group. Interim UK guidelines for management of close community contacts of invasive group A streptococcal disease. Commun Dis Public Health 2004;7: 354–361.

CARE PATHWAY

Early goal-directed therapy (EGDT) for sepsis during pregnancy

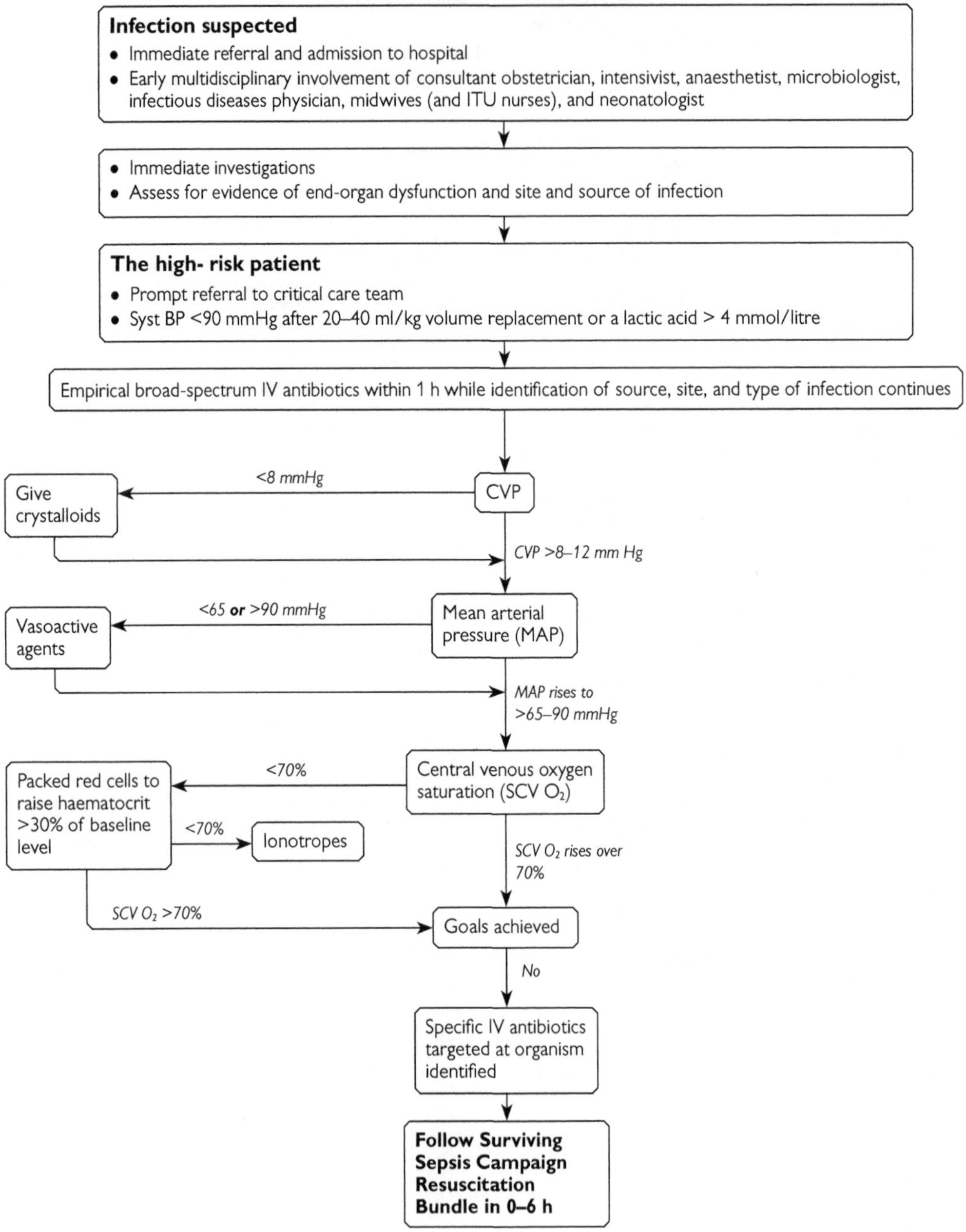

Infection suspected
• Immediate referral and admission to hospital
• Early multidisciplinary involvement of consultant obstetrician, intensivist, anaesthetist, microbiologist, infectious diseases physician, midwives (and ITU nurses), and neonatologist
• Immediate investigations
• Assess for evidence of end-organ dysfunction and site and source of infection
The high- risk patient
• Prompt referral to critical care team
• Syst BP <90 mmHg after 20–40 ml/kg volume replacement or a lactic acid > 4 mmol/litre
Empirical broad-spectrum IV antibiotics within 1 h while identification of source, site, and type of infection continues
CVP
<8 mmHg
Give crystalloids
CVP >8–12 mm Hg
Mean arterial pressure (MAP)
<65 or >90 mmHg
Vasoactive agents
MAP rises to >65–90 mmHg
Central venous oxygen saturation (SCV O2)
<70%
Packed red cells to raise haematocrit >30% of baseline level
<70%
Ionotropes
SCV O2 rises over 70%
SCV O2 >70%
Goals achieved
No
Specific IV antibiotics targeted at organism identified
Follow Surviving Sepsis Campaign Resuscitation Bundle in 0–6 h

Early goal-directed therapy: goals and normal values in pregnancy

Measures	*Resuscitation goals*	*Normal physiological levels in 3rd trimester*
Central venous pressure	8–12 mmHg	4–10 mmHg
Mean arterial pressure	≥65 mmHg	84–96 mmHg
Urine output	> 0.5 ml/kg/h	Minimum 0.5 ml/kg/h
Mixed venous oxygen saturation	>70%	>80%
Heart rate	Decreasing in response to treatment	83 ± 10 beats/min

Steps involved in Surviving Sepsis Campaign Resuscitation Bundle (0–6 h)

Diagnosis based on history, symptoms, and physical examination

- History: Diabetes, asthma, anaemia, amniocentesis, cervical cerclage, prolonged SROM, GAS infection in close contacts, GBS infection, obesity, black/ethnic minority women, IV drug users, recent TOP/miscarriage, etc.
- Symptoms: Fever, rigors, diarrhoea, vomiting, rash, abdominal /pelvic pain, offensive vaginal discharge, productive cough, urinary symptoms
- ***Multidisciplinary input, involve critical care team***

Signs

One or more of the following:

- Pyrexia (>38 °C) or hypothermia (<36 °C)
- Tachypnoea (> 20 breaths/min)
- Tachycardia (>90 bpm)
- Hypoxia
- Arterial hypotension (systolic BP <90 mmHg, MAP <70 mmHg or systolic BP drop >40 mmHg)
- Decreased capillary refill or mottling
- Oliguria: output < 0.5 ml/kg/h for at least 2 h despite adequate fluids
- Oedema or positive fluid balance(>20 ml/kg over 24 h)
- Ileus
- Impaired mental state, impaired consciousness
- Hyperglycaemia (in absence of diabetes) >7.7 mmol/litre
- Failure to respond to treatment
- Fetal distress secondary to maternal acidosis

- Investigations for potential sources and site of Infection, attempt to identify pathogen
  - Obtain blood cultures, HVS, throat swab
  - FBC, serum lactate, urea, electrolytes, creatinine, blood gases
- Broad-spectrum IV antibiotics within 1 h of suspecting sepsis
- Once pathogen is identified, targeted choice of IV antibiotics to be substituted
- If hypotension and/or serum lactate >4 mmol/litre, give minimum of 20 ml/kg of cystalloids or equivalent
- Rest of steps as in EGDT pathway (see p. 122)
- Multidisciplinary assessments to continue; if indicated, transfer to ITU
- IVIG for severe invasive streptococcal or staphylococcal infection if other therapies fail
- Obstetric consultant with the critical care team to individualize decision re delivery of baby—time and mode of delivery, great caution re prophylactic steroids
- Neonatologists to be made aware if mother found to have invasive GAS infection for prophylactic antibiotics for neonate

3 Maternal Respiratory Conditions

3.1 Severe Asthma

FACT FILE

Incidence

- At least 4% of pregnant women are affected with **asthma**; a small minority have severe asthma.
- The course of asthma in pregnancy is very variable. About 30% of asthmatic women improve symptomatically during pregnancy while it worsens in a third and remains unchanged during pregnancy in a further third.[1]
- The risk of deterioration is highest in those with severe asthma. Pregnancy is well tolerated if asthma is well-controlled.
- 11–18% of pregnant women with asthma will have at least one emergency department visit for an attack of acute asthma and of these 62% will require hospitalization.[2]
- **Pre-pregnancy** management is to optimize control and emphasize the importance of continuing medication in pregnancy. Women with asthma should be counselled regarding the importance and safety of continuing their asthma medications during pregnancy to ensure good asthma control. Poorly controlled asthma may lead to adverse pregnancy outcomes for both the mother and her baby.
- When a woman with asthma deteriorates in pregnancy, the usual reason is a mistaken belief that treatment for asthma is harmful to the fetus.
- ***Smoking cessation is particularly important in asthmatic women and women must be offered support to stop.***

Effects of poorly controlled asthma in pregnancy

- ***Uncontrolled asthma is associated with many maternal and fetal complications, including hyperemesis, hypertension, pre-eclampsia, fetal growth restriction, low birth weight, preterm birth, increased perinatal mortality, and neonatal hypoxia.***[1,3]
- Deterioration of asthma is mostly experienced between the 24th and 36th week of pregnancy, after which spontaneous improvement is usually seen with minimal symptoms in the last 4 weeks of gestation. Asthma symptoms do not occur in nearly 90% of women during labour or delivery.[4,5]

Asthma management

- Controlling the condition should enable a woman to maintain a healthy pregnancy with little risk to her or the baby. Complications may be minimized by effective asthma management strategies and it is important that this group of women and their developing babies are monitored regularly.
- Whenever possible, treatment should be by inhalation rather than oral agents, since this reduces systemic effects and any possible effects on the fetus.
- Monitor pregnant asthmatics closely so that appropriate changes to their treatment can be quickly implemented in response to changed symptoms.

Management of acute attacks during pregnancy

- ***Management of acute asthma in pregnancy should follow a stepwise approach as recommended by the British Thoracic Society/Scottish Intercollegiate Guidelines Network Guidelines.***[2]
- Acute severe asthma in pregnancy is an emergency and should be treated vigorously in hospital.
- Exacerbations should be treated vigorously with drug therapy given as for a non-pregnant patient with acute asthma.
- High-flow oxygen should be delivered to maintain 94–98% saturation in order to prevent maternal and fetal hypoxia.[6,7]
- In severe cases, intravenous β_2 agonists, aminophylline, or intravenous bolus magnesium sulphate can be used according to the stepwise approach recommended by British Thoracic Society/ Scottish Intercollegiate Guidelines Network Guidelines.[2]
- During an acute exacerbation when asthma is uncontrolled or severe, continuous fetal monitoring should be commenced on admission.
- Consideration should be given to early referral to an intensive care specialist in such cases.

Drug therapy in pregnancy

- The evidence to date suggests that conventional asthma medications, such as inhaled corticosteroids (ICS) and inhaled short-acting beta-agonists do not increase perinatal risk, and ICS treatment may actually be protective against outcomes such as low birth weight.[8]
- **ICS** are the most important pharmacological agent in maintaining asthma control in and out of pregnancy
- Beclometasone and budesonide are the most widely used ICS used in pregnancy and the safest for use, with no teratogenic effects on the fetus and safe in breastfeeding.
- **Systemic steroids** do not represent a significant teratogenic risk in human pregnancy. In doses equivalent to prednisolone 25 mg per day they do not cross the placenta (unlike beta-or dexamethasone). Even in higher doses, the effect of hydrocortisone or prednisolone on the fetus in terms of suppression of the hypothalamic–pituitary–adrenal axis is minimal.
- High doses of systemic steroids in the first trimester may be associated with cleft palate[9,10,11] though this has been refuted by other studies. The aim is to use the lowest dose that will provide adequate control.
- Women on long-term systemic steroids should have screening for corticosteroid-induced hyperglycaemia (GTT) which is reversible on cessation or reduction of the dose of steroids.
- There is **no evidence of an increased risk** of miscarriage, stillbirth, or neonatal death associated with maternal steroid therapy.
- **Leukotriene receptor antagonists** should not be commenced in pregnancy as the safety data are too limited. Leukotriene antagonists (LTRA) may, however, be continued in women who have demonstrated significant improvement in asthma control with these agents prior to pregnancy not achievable with other medications.[2,3]
- **Chromones:** No significant association has been demonstrated between major congenital malformations or adverse perinatal outcome and exposure to chromones which can be used as normal during pregnancy.[12]

Management of labour

- Plans should be discussed with the mother and documented.
- Reassure the mother that asthma exacerbations during labour are relatively rare due to the natural outpouring of endogenous steroids and adrenaline (epinephrine) associated with the stress of labour and delivery.
- In severe or brittle asthmatics, the use of beta-blocker antihypertensives such as labetalol during pregnancy or

antiinflammatories such as diclofenac after delivery is contraindicated.

- ***An asthma exacerbation is not an indication for elective delivery, although if there are other maternal and fetal indications, an asthmatic exacerbation is not a reason to delay delivery.***
- Prostaglandin F_2-alpha (Carboprost) can cause severe bronchoconstriction and great care must be taken before its use in postpartum haemorrhage (PPH). However, its use to treat life-threatening PPH may be unavoidable; the anaesthetist should be made aware.
- Prostaglandin E_2 can be used with safety.
- **Document in the notes that oxytocin/ergometrine (Syntometrine®) should only be used with caution in severe asthmatics** as it can cause bronchospasm, particularly in association with general anaesthetic.
- **Caution needs to be used in the use of morphine and pethidine in severe asthmatics**, although it is not generally a problem.
- Epidural anaesthesia is a preferred analgesic, particularly as triggers for asthma attacks such as pain or anxiety can be significantly reduced.
- Any patient who has been on more than 7.5 mg prednisolone per day for any more than 2 weeks prior to labour, in the preceding year, should have bolus doses of 100 mg IV hydrocortisone every 6–8 h during labour and for delivery.
- Women whose symptoms improve during the last trimester may experience postnatal deterioration.

During lactation

- Drugs used to treat asthma, including steroid tablets, have been shown to be safe to use during lactation. Systemic prednisolone/methylprednisolone is compatible with breastfeeding and although secreted in breast milk, the concentrations of prednisolone are only 5–25% of those in serum. Even with doses of 20 mg once or twice daily the infant is exposed to minimal amounts (<0.1%) of steroid with no clinically significant risk.
- Maternal asthma has been found to double the risk of asthma in her offspring. Advise the patient to breastfeed, as this has been shown to help prevent the onset of atopy and asthma in the child.
- No disease-specific recommendations for contraception in patients with asthma.
- ***Low-dose aspirin, which may otherwise have been used in pregnancy as prophylaxis against early onset pre-eclampsia, or in lupus and antiphospholipid syndromes, must be used with caution in brittle asthmatics due to the possibility of aspirin sensitivity and bronchospasm in a minority of asthmatics.***
- ***Pregnant women with asthma should be asked about a history of aspirin sensitivity before being advised to take low-dose aspirin.***

Information for patients

Please see Information for patients: Moderate/severe asthma and pregnancy (p. 503)

References

1. Dombrowski MP, et al. Asthma during pregnancy. Obstet Gynecol 2004;103: 5–12.
2. British Guideline on the Management of Asthma. British Thoracic Society Scottish Intercollegiate Guidelines Network 2008, revised 2011.
3. VE Murphy et al. A meta-analysis of adverse perinatal outcomes in women with asthma. BJOG 2011; 118: 1314–1323.
4. British Guidelines in Asthma Management: a national guideline. British Thoracic Society, Scottish Intercollegiate Guideline Network. Thorax 2003;58 suppl: S1–94.
5. Gluck JC, Gluck PA. The effect of pregnancy on the course of asthma. Immunol Allergy Clin North Am 2006;26: 63–80.
6. Murphy VE, et al. Asthma exacerbations during pregnancy: incidence and association with adverse pregnancy outcomes. Thorax 2006;61: 169–176.
7. Schatz M, et al. Spirometry is related to perinatal outcomes in pregnant women with asthma. Am J Obstet Gynecol 2006;194: 120–126.
8. Chambers C. Safety of asthma and allergy medications in pregnancy. Immunol Allergy Clin North Am 2006;26: 13–28.
9. Carmichael SL, et al. Maternal corticosteroid use and orofacial clefts. Am J Obstet Gynecol 2007;197: 585 e1–7
10. Kallen B. Maternal drug use and infant cleft lip/palate with special reference to corticoids. Cleft Palate Craniofac J 2003;40: 624–628.
11. Czeizel AE, Rockenbauer M. Population-based case-control study of teratogenic potential of corticosteroids. Teratology 1997;56: 335–340.
12. Bakhireva LN, et al. Effect of maternal asthma and gestational asthma therapy on fetal growth. J Asthma 2007;44: 71–76.

Further reading

1. Powrie R. Pulmonary disease in pregnancy. In: Greer IA, et al, ed., Medical problems in pregnancy. Edinburgh: Churchill Livingstone Elsevier, 2007, pp. 102–133.

CARE PATHWAY

Pregnant patient with severe/brittle asthma

Community midwife ± GP advises patient not to stop or decrease **asthma** medications once pregnant and to **stop smoking**

↓

Referral to maternal medicine clinic or specialist antenatal clinic

↓

First visit before 16 weeks

- Multidisciplinary management with obstetrician, respiratory physician, GP, midwife, asthma specialist nurse
- Review pregnancy, asthma symptoms, and medications. Advise not to stop or decrease asthma medications as all, except leukotriene, are safe during all trimesters of pregnancy, during labour, and while breastfeeding
- No increased risk of miscarriages or teratogenicity with commonly used asthma medications
- Inform patient that inadequate/poor control of asthma during pregnancy increases risks to both mother and baby (e.g. increased risk of preterm delivery, pre-eclampsia, IUGR, etc.)
- Reiterate smoking cessation—offer support and help resource
- Arrange GTT screening if on long-term steroids: inform patient that steroid-induced hyperglycaemia is reversible
- Arrange early referral for respiratory physician review
- Referral to anaesthetic high-risk clinic
- Labetalol is not an antihypertensive of choice in such cases: document in notes
- In severe asthma, arrange serial scans for growth and liquor at 28, 32, and 36 weeks gestation with specialist antenatal clinic review on same day
- Further follow-up in specialist antenatal clinic at 28, 32, 36 and 40 weeks, earlier if clinically indicated
- Discuss pregnancy, labour management, reassure patient that asthma exacerbation is not an indication for early IOL or Caesarean section, that exacerbations are rare during labour, and breastfeeding is to be encouraged
- **Ensure patient has asthma helpline/nurse contact** in case of exacerbation

↓

Vigilance for pre-eclampsia

Community midwife visits at 24, 26, 30, 34, and 38 weeks (suggested schedule—variable according to local protocol and resources)

↓

Further visits to maternal medicine or specialist antenatal clinic

- Vigilance for signs of pre-eclampsia, enquire about any asthma exacerbation, and note fetal growth scan findings
- Check that patient has had recent reviews by respiratory physician and anaesthetist
- Clear documentation in notes: to avoid ergometrine if possible, labetalol, diclofenac during/after labour and delivery, also opiate analgesia though these are not usually a problem. Caution if PGF2α (Carboprost) used for PPH
- Document that if on long-term or recent steroid use, hydrocortisone bolus doses 100 mg IV every 6–8 h during labour and to cover delivery
- ***IOL at 40^{+10} (or according to individual unit's protocol for post-date IOL). Asthma exacerbation not an indication for earlier IOL/ LSCS***
- Encourage breastfeeding to reduce infant/childhood atopy/ asthma—reassure mother regarding safety of conventional drugs to treat asthma

3.2 Cystic Fibrosis

FACT FILE

Incidence

- **Cystic fibrosis (CF)** is the most common inherited potentially fatal disease in the UK.
- CF is the commonest autosomal recessive disorder in the UK, with a carrier rate of 1 in 25 white Europeans.
- Female fertility, though impaired in CF, is not excluded.
- Increasing survival has been seen in those with CF due to a combination of early diagnosis, early and aggressive management of nutrition and respiratory infections, and early interventions to reduce other complications such as diabetes or liver disease.[1]
- In the UK, the pregnancy rate for women with CF over the age of 16 is 80/1000.
- This means more young women with well-managed CF want to have babies and pregnancy is becoming increasingly common with the expectation of generally good outcomes for the mother and baby. 70–80% of these pregnancies in CF patients will result in a live birth.
- However, in some women pregnancy is less well tolerated and serious adverse effects of CF could complicate pregnancy and pregnancy could adversely affect CF.

Clinical features

- Early, repeated, and persistent lung infection, bronchiectasis, and respiratory failure.
- Pancreatic insufficiency leading to malnutrition and diabetes.
- Pulmonary hypertension, cor pulmonale in severe cases.

Effects of CF on pregnancy and vice versa

- Maternal mortality, though significantly increased compared with that of normal pregnant women, is not different compared with that of age-matched non-pregnant women with CF.[1,2,3]
- Pregnancy does not significantly shorten survival in CF patients.
- Pregnancy is better tolerated by those with the less severe forms of the disease.
- Women with good pre-pregnancy lung function (FEV_1 >70% predicted) tolerate pregnancy well and have the lowest maternal and perinatal mortality.
- Maternal mortality increases when there is moderate to severe lung disease at the onset of pregnancy (<60% predicted FEV_1).
- ***Pulmonary hypertension and cor pulmonale are absolute contraindications for pregnancy in view of the very high probability of maternal death during pregnancy or delivery*.**
- Infection with the organism *Burkholderia cepacia*, associated with rapid deterioration in lung function, is also an indicator of poor maternal survival and may be a contraindication for pregnancy
- The main maternal morbidity in CF pregnancy is due to:
  - poor maternal weight gain, even emaciation
  - deterioration of lung function, worsening dyspnoea, and oxygen saturation
  - diabetes or impaired glucose tolerance unmasked during pregnancy

Fetal risks in a CF pregnancy

- **Prematurity (20–50%):** Some are delivered early due to concerns regarding deteriorating maternal condition.[1,2,3,4,5] Women with poorer lung function have a higher rate of spontaneous preterm birth.
- **IUGR:** due to chronic maternal hypoxia. Birth weight is positively correlated with pre-pregnancy lung function.
- **Sequelae of pre-existing or gestational diabetes** can result in increased fetal and neonatal morbidity and mortality including **stillbirth**.
- There is no increase in spontaneous miscarriage rates or in congenital malformations in CF pregnancies when compared with the general population.
- Poor pre-pregnancy BMI (<18) as well as poor maternal weight gain in pregnancy are associated with increased risks of both prematurity and **stillbirth**.

Pre-pregnancy counselling

- Pre-pregnancy counselling in a multidisciplinary tertiary CF unit will have taken place in most, if not all, cases, with the goal being optimization of pre-pregnancy health and therapy.[1,6,7,8]
- Accurate counselling with assessment of severity and rate of progression of CF is required.
- Stabilization and optimizing lung function and nutrition have a direct relationship to good maternal and fetal outcomes.
- Genetic counselling with partner testing should be offered: In general:
  - if the partner **does not** carry any of the common mutations for CF, the chance of an affected child is less than 1:250
  - if the partner **does** carry one of these genes, the risk is 1:2.
- Since all women with CF are homozygous, all offspring will be carriers of the CF gene although there is considerable heterogeneity of the CF gene.
- Pre-pregnancy GTT if glycaemic state has not been established as yet. Optimizing glycaemic control pre-pregnancy will reduce risks of congenital malformations and other pregnancy complications
- Review of medication is essential. Although most drugs used for CF are safe in pregnancy/ lactation, some are contraindicated and must be stopped under medical supervision only. Safe alternatives need to be substituted. The patient must be advised **not** to stop medications on her own volition, fearing any effect on the developing baby
- Patients with a FEV_1 of less than 50–60% of predicted should be counselled regarding the increased risks of maternal death and fetal loss. A FEV_1 of less than 30–40% of predicted is a contraindication for pregnancy. If an ECHO in such patients shows pulmonary hypertension, these patients should be strongly advised **not** to embark on a pregnancy.
- The realities of CF must be outlined to the patient and partner/ family. There are considerable implications around practical, psychological, and financial support as well as the issue of long-term child care.[1] These discussions need to be raised with sensitivity as the 10-year mortality rate for those with CF is about 20%.
- Folic acid supplementation (high-dose 5 mg/day) pre-pregnancy and during the first trimester should be recommended and prescribed.
- Vitamin D supplementation in doses greater than the usual 10 micrograms/day should be considered.[1,6]

Management during pregnancy

- Care of a pregnancy in a woman with CF must be multidisciplinary with close involvement of the regional/national specialist CF units. In severe cases, antenatal care and delivery should take place in a tertiary specialist CF unit.
- Coordination of appointments should be attempted, especially later in pregnancy.
- The involvement of and good communication between various healthcare professionals in both primary care and hospital-based services is mandatory. In addition to the CF team who have been responsible for the woman's care, once a pregnancy is planned and established, the team needs to expand to include respiratory physician, maternal medicine obstetrician, midwives, genetic counsellor, obstetric anaesthetist, etc.
- In certain severe cases of CF, a sensitive discussion regarding termination of pregnancy(TOP) may need to be considered such as if there is pre-existent pulmonary hypertension or cor pulmonale.[1]
- The method of TOP is no different than in those without CF but avoiding general anaesthesia wherever possible.

- Once a decision has been made to continue with the pregnancy, the woman should receive proactive and positive support at each stage.
- Monthly visits till about 24 weeks gestation, then bimonthly or more frequent visits till delivery are required for CF pregnant women in the tertiary CF unit. At each visit, physical examination including weight recording, measurement of pulmonary function and oxygen saturation, sputum culture, and evaluation of treatment are necessary.[1]
- Regular adjustments to the individualized treatment regime are vital.

General principles of antenatal management

- If not previously done, **genotyping of the pregnant woman and her partner** is important as soon as possible.[1,2,3,4] If the partner is negative, no further tests are required. If the partner is positive or if he is unavailable, antenatal testing of the fetal status by chorionic villus sampling (**CVS**) or **amniocentesis** must be offered.
- **Adequate maternal nutrition:** Specialist dietary advice with additional energy supplements, even parenterally delivered, are required. Admission may be required on several occasions. Nutritional supplements of vitamin D (usually more than the standard 10 micrograms/day, with serum levels monitored) should be advised as well as folic acid 5 mg/day till the end of the first trimester at least. Increased dietary consumption of iron- and folate-rich foods or of iron and folic acid supplementation during pregnancy are essential.
- **Control of pulmonary infection:** Infective exacerbation to be treated aggressively by admission and IV penicillin and aminoglycoside (with regular monitoring of drug levels) or cephalosporins in cases of resistant pseudomonas.
- ***Avoidance of prolonged hypoxia due to acute respiratory exacerbations and resultant loss of lung function. Antibiotics and intensified airway clearance strategies as well as supplemental oxygen therapy need to be considered if oxygen saturation measured by pulse oximetry is less than 90%.***
- **Regular assessment of fetal growth:** Routine anomaly scan followed by serial growth scans at 26–30–34 weeks gestation. Doppler monitoring with cardiotocograpy (CTG) is also usually necessary at regular intervals in later gestation.
- Great care should be taken to ensure adherence to physiotherapy regimes.
- GTT screening at 16 weeks, or if normal, repeated at 28 weeks in all CF pregnancies. Women with established CF related diabetes, those with known impaired glucose tolerance prior to pregnancy, or those newly diagnosed must be referred to the specialist diabetes/obstetric team to optimize the diabetes control.[9]
- Early referral to the obstetric anaesthetist should be arranged soon after booking and a planning meeting at about 26 weeks where the anaesthetic plan is discussed with the CF team and disseminated.[10]

Planning for delivery

- The majority of CF pregnancies result in spontaneous vaginal deliveries, although the rate of spontaneous or therapeutic preterm delivery is as high as 26–46%, mainly due to deteriorating maternal health.[5]
- In some, symptom deterioration will necessitate early delivery. Prophylactic steroids for acceleration of fetal lung maturity must be considered if delivery is planned before 34–35 weeks gestation.
- In some cases of maternal or fetal compromise, Caesarean section under spinal anaesthetic is preferable.
- Epidural is to be encouraged. Assisted vaginal delivery to cut short a prolonged second stage may be considered. A vaginal delivery is preferred to a Caesarean section.
- **Mode and timing of delivery**[3,5,7] in CF pregnancies need to be individualized, depending on state of maternal health and gestation age. Caesarean section rates in some studies[3,4] were up to 35%, two-thirds of which were for preterm deliveries and the rest for other obstetric complications at term. Of women who had vaginal deliveries, more than 40% required assisted instrumental deliveries.
- If a Caesarean section is needed, a general anaesthetic should be avoided,if possible. If a general anaesthetic is unavoidable, as in severely compromised patients, close liaison with intensivists is required.
- Peripartum care is usually in the obstetric high-dependency unit setting.

Postnatal care

- The new mother with CF will require a lot of extra help and support, which should ideally have been identified and organized in the antenatal period.
- She should be advised not to neglect CF treatment. Any chest infection must be treated aggressively.
- Nutrition and hydration are particularly important if breastfeeding.
- Analysis of breast milk in women with CF has shown normal content of sodium and protein, therefore breastfeeding may be encouraged but counsel the patient that this can be exhausting and uses up calories. She will need further additional nutritional supplement in the puerperium. Most CF patients find that exclusive breastfeeding is too difficult and alternative methods of feeding should be discussed.
- Infants of mothers with CF should be screened by paediatricians for CF.
- CF home care can be arranged through tertiary/regional CF centres.
- Effective contraception must be advised before discharge; the methods of contraception need not differ from those for women without CF.

Information for patients

Please see Information for patients: Cystic fibrosis and pregnancy (p. 504)

References

1. Edenborough FP, et al. On behalf of European Cystic Fibrosis Society. Guidelines for the management of pregnancy in women with cystic fibrosis. J Cystic Fibrosis 2008;7: S2–S32.
2. Goss CH, et al. The effect of pregnancy on survival in women with cystic fibrosis. Chest 2003;124: 1460–1468.
3. Goddard J, Bourke SJ. Cystic fibrosis and pregnancy. Obstetrician and Gynaecologist 2009;11: 19–24.
4. Dodge JA, et al. Cystic fibrosis mortality and survival in the UK: 1947–2003. Eur Respir J 2007;29: 522–526.
5. Edenborough FP, et al. The outcome of 72 pregnancies in 55 women with cystic fibrosis in the UK 1977–1996. BJOG 2000;107: 254–261.
6. Heaney RP, et al. Human serum 25-hydroxycholecalciferol response to extended oral dosing with cholecalciferol. Am J Clin Nutr 2003;77: 204–210.
7. Kotloff RM, et al. Fertility and pregnancy in patients with cystic fibrosis. Clin Chest Med 1992;13: 623–635.
8. McArdle JR. Pregnancy in cystic fibrosis. Clin Chest Med 2011;32: 111–120.
9. UK Cystic Fibrosis Trust Diabetes Working Group. Management of cystic fibrosis related diabetes mellitus. London: Cystic Fibrosis Trust, 2004.
10. Della Rocca G. Anaesthesia in patients with cystic fibrosis. Curr Opin Anaesth 2002;15: 95–101.

CARE PATHWAY

Pregnant patient with cystic fibrosis (CF)

Joint care and close multidisciplinary input with regional/national tertiary CF centre mandatory, with a coordinated, individualized, multidisciplinary plan of care

↓

Pre-pregnancy counselling, assessment, and advice will have been provided by specialist CF centre, including genetic counselling, phenotype check of partner, nutrition, pulmonary function, pre-pregnancy diabetes check, discussion of psycho-social issues, optimization of health, and medication review

↓

Patient referred asap in 1st trimester from community to maternal medicine antenatal clinic

- Discuss pregnancy options, genotype testing of partner and CVS/amniocentesis offered as appropriate
- Establish close liaison with CF team and GP
- Discussions with couple of practicalities of CF, possible deterioration of health during pregnancy, long-term support for infant/child care, need for repeated admissions in some cases, risk of preterm delivery, fetal growth problems
- If patient chooses to continue pregnancy, offer proactive and positive support
- High-dose folic acid (5 mg/day) in 1st trimester, vitamin D supplementation along with dietary advice about iron- and folate-rich foods
- If pre-existing CF-linked diabetes, refer to combined diabetes/obstetrics clinic

↓

Next visit to maternal medicine or specialist antenatal clinic at about 12–14 weeks

- Refer to obstetric anaesthetist asap
- Refer to local physiotherapist, specialist CF dietitian
- Close liaison with respiratory physicians in local DGH and regional CF centre
- GTT at 16 weeks if not previously known to be diabetic. If results normal at 16 weeks, repeat GTT at 26–28 weeks. If abnormal, refer to combined diabetes/obstetrics clinic
- **Discuss proposed schedule of antenatal appointments**, coordinated with scans and respiratory medicine appointments as far as possible
    - Monthly antenatal clinic appointments till 26 weeks with routine scans (1st trimester and anomaly scan at about 20 weeks), then every fortnight till planned delivery
    - Multidisciplinary interim planning meeting of the CF team, obstetric anaesthetist, specialist obstetrician with patient + partner/family at 26–28 weeks
    - Arrange for serial growth scans with Doppler studies at 3–4 week intervals from 26 weeks onwards with antenatal clinic visits on same day

(From pre-pregnancy counselling →) Specialist CF centre

↓

Monthly or bimonthly visits for physical examination, weight, oxygen saturation, pulmonary function, review of nutritional and pulmonary status, sputum cultures, review of medications, treatment adjustments, etc. to continue (↔ Next visit to maternal medicine or specialist antenatal clinic)

↓

Further visits to specialist antenatal clinic

- Close monitoring of maternal health, with particular attention to nutrition, control of any pulmonary infection, FEV1, etc. to be maintained throughout pregnancy
- GTT repeat at 26–28 weeks and refer to combined diabetes/obstetric clinic as indicated
- Repeated admission may be required during pregnancy if chest infections, signs of maternal compromise
- Ensure strict adherence to physiotherapy
- Serial fetal growth scans + Doppler studies from 26 weeks at regular intervals to check fetal growth and well-being
- Prophylactic steroids if preterm delivery <35 weeks planned in event of concerns about maternal/fetal status
- Close communication with regional CF unit, wide dispersal of jointly produced plans for obstetric, anaesthetic, and CF management for labour, delivery, and postpartum
    - Discussion and planning regarding place and timing of delivery to be individualized based on maternal and fetal condition
    - Encourage epidural and if term, aim for vaginal delivery if no other problems
    - Discuss breastfeeding and support available as well as alternative feeding
    - Postnatal physiotherapy, nutrition supplements, infection prophylaxis
    - Baby to be screened for CF by paediatricians
    - Confirm has help and support at home, if needed arrange CF Home Care via CF team
    - Contraception advice before discharge
    - Community team and family to be aware of chances of postnatal depression

3.3 Sarcoidosis

FACT FILE

Epidemiology

- **Sarcoidosis** is a multisystem granulomatous disorder of unknown etiology, most frequently affecting in women in their reproductive years.
- Incidence in pregnancy is about 0.02–0.05%.[1,2] It is 3–4 times more common in black women.
- Usually has a benign course, may occasionally result in severe organ injury.
- Sarcoidosis is **not** an inheritable condition.

Manifestations

- Sarcoidosis may affect the lungs, mediastinal lymph nodes, skin, liver, central nervous system, heart, and eyes.[1] Extrapulmonary manifestations include skin (maculopapular eruptions, skin nodules, and erythema nodosum), lymphatic system (lymphadenopathy), and eye (iriditis, uveitis, etc).
- Pulmonary lesions are typical with bilateral hilar adenopathy and/or infiltrates.
- Sarcoidosis may present with cough, dyspnoea, chest pain, fatigue, malaise, weakness, weight loss, and fever.
- 50% of cases are asymptomatic and are only incidentally detected on a routine chest radiograph.
- Problems with calcium metabolism leading to hypercalcuria and hypercalcaemia can be found with sarcoidosis.[3,4]
- Treatment is indicated for those with pulmonary symptoms or eye conditions.[5]

Prognosis

- Sarcoidosis can regress spontaneously.
- ***Pregnancy does not affect the course of the disease in those in whom sarcoidosis has been stable or inactive.[3–7] Women with active disease may improve both clinically and radiologically during pregnancy. Postpartum exacerbation can, however, occur 3–6 months after delivery.[1–3]***
- Sarcoidosis, being a T1 immune response mediated disease, follows a course similar to rheumatoid arthritis, with improvement during pregnancy and relapses within 3 months postpartum.[1] Improvement during pregnancy is also attributed to the effect of increased levels of oestrogen, progesterone, cortisol, and ACTH.
- Even those with inactive disease can present with symptomatic sarcoidosis for the first time postpartum.[1]
- In a few cases, sarcoidosis can progress during pregnancy. Risk factors for such progression include advanced radiographic staging, multiple pulmonary infiltrates, and parenchymal lesions or extrapulmonary sarcoidosis.[2,4,7] In the presence of one or more of these factors, specific plans for management in pregnancy and puerperium need to be drawn up with respiratory physicians in the local hospital and tertiary centre.
- ***Sarcoidosis, however, does not appear to affect pregnancy outcomes.[1,3] No increase has been noted in miscarriages, obstetric complications, or congenital abnormalities. The obstetric management of pregnancy, labour, and delivery does not differ except where there is severe respiratory compromise.[1,2]***

Treatment

- **Systemic corticosteroid therapy** is the mainstay of treatment. Remission can usually be achieved with a daily dose of 20–40 mg prednisolone.[1,8] Prednisolone is found in negligible amounts in breast milk with doses of 20 mg/day or less.
- Second-line agents like hydroxychloroquine, azathioprine, and ciclosporin have also been used to treat steroid-unresponsive sarcoidosis or as adjuvant therapy to reduce the dosage of steroids required.[8,9,10,11,12.]
- **Methotrexate and cyclophosphamide are contraindicated** in pregnancy.
- There is currently not enough safety information on the use of infliximab in pregnancy.

Fetal risks of sarcoidosis

- Apart from extreme cases of pulmonary fibrosis, hypoxaemia, and pulmonary hypertension, sarcoidosis does not appear to have any significant risk for the fetus.
- Sarcoid granulomas have been reported in the placenta but not in the fetus.

Pre-pregnancy counselling

- Pre-pregnancy counselling is particularly important in those with severe pulmonary fibrosis causing cor pulmonale, neurosarcoidosis, myocardial sarcoidosis, or pulmonary hypertension, because of the significant maternal mortality. Pregnancy should be avoided in such cases.
- Baseline chest radiograph and pulmonary function tests are recommended prior to pregnancy.
- The patient must be reassured that sarcoidosis (except in extreme cases) does not have an adverse effect on pregnancy outcomes.
- Corticosteroids[8] are to be continued if necessary during pregnancy, at doses less than 20–40 mg/day. Second-line drugs such as azathioprine can be used with safety during pregnancy.[9,10,11,12]
- Untreated maternal hypercalcaemia from sarcoidosis could lead to neonatal hypoglycaemia and tetany.
- **Pregnant patients with sarcoidosis should therefore generally avoid both vitamin D and calcium supplementation, and the ingredients of any antenatal vitamin preparation should be critically reviewed.** If needed, ferrous sulfate and folic acid replacements can be instituted instead of a generic vitamin preparation.

Antenatal care

- **Referral to the respiratory physician and to the anaesthetic high risk clinic are essential during pregnancy.**
- Regular oxygen saturation measurements (at rest and with exercise) if breathlessness is significant.
- Chest radiograph as recommended by respiratory physician.
- Pulmonary function tests, especially close to term, as advised by the respiratory physician. These results must be compared with the patient's pre-pregnancy values.
- Avoidance of vitamin D or calcium supplementation during pregnancy is essential in such patients due to the risk of hypercalcaemia or nephrocalcinosis.
- If on systemic steroids, a GTT needs to be performed at about 26–28 weeks.
- Serial growth scans in addition to the routine anomaly scan may be required in sarcoidosis at about 28 and 34 weeks.

Labour and delivery

- An epidural block is preferable to a general anaesthetic in women with pulmonary disease.
- ***If the patient has received prednisolone for more than 2 weeks in the year prior to delivery, she should receive 100 mg hydrocortisone IV every 6–8 h during labour and delivery or just before a Caesarean section.***
- Sarcoidosis with any degree of parenchymatous lung disease with restriction of pulmonary capacity is an indication for elective Caesarean section. Advice regarding lung capacity and degree of pulmonary compromise after near-term reassessment by the respiratory physician is a valuable guide in such cases

Postnatal care

- Prophylactic increase of steroid dosage postpartum may be required.
- Prednisolone or azathioprine can be used during breastfeeding as the amount transferred in breast milk is negligible.
- In such cases, breastfeeding is recommended just before the day's dose of medication is taken.
- Although there is little data about the most suitable contraceptive advisable in sarcoidosis, extrapolation from studies into erythema nodosum suggest avoidance of the combined pill in favour of progesterone implant or LNG-IUS.[9]

Information for patients

Please see **Information for patients: Sarcoidosis and pregnancy** (p. 505)

References

1. Vahid B, et al. Sarcoidosis in pregnancy and postpartum period. Curr Resp Med Rev 2007; 3: 79–83.
2. Sweiss NJ, et al. Rheumatologic manifestations of sarcoidosis. Semin Respir Crit Care Med 2010;31: 463–473.
3. Subramanian P, et al Pregnancy and sarcoidosis: an insight into the pathogenesis of hypercalciuria. Chest 2004;126: 995–998.
4. Burke RR, et al. Calcium and vitamin D in sarcoidosis: how to assess and manage. Semin Respir Crit Care Med 2010;31: 474–484.
5. Iannuzzi MC, et al. Sarcoidosis. N Engl J Med 2007;357: 2153–2165.
6. Abarquez C, et al. Sarcoidosis and pregnancy: clinical observation. Sarcoidosis 1990;7: 63–66.
7. Statement on Sarcoidosis. Joint statement of the American Thoracic Society (ATS), European Respiratory Society (ERS) and the World Association of Sarcoidosis and Other Granulomatous Diseases (WASOG) adopted by the ATS Board of Directors and by the ERS Executive Committee, February 1999. Am J Respir Crit Care Med 1999;160: 736–755.
8. Grutters JC, van den Bosch JM. Corticosteroid treatment in sarcoidosis. Eur Respir J 2006;28: 627–636.
9. Temprano KK, et al. Antirheumatic drugs in pregnancy and lactation. Semin Arthritis Rheum 2005;35: 112–121.
10. Oz BB, et al. Pregnancy outcome after cyclosporine therapy during pregnancy: A metal analysis. Transplantation 2001;71: 1051–1055.
11. Costedoat-Chalumeau N, et al. Safety of hydroxychloroquine in pregnant patients with connective tissue diseases: a study of one hundred thirty-three cases compared with a control group. Arthritis Rheum 2003;48: 3207–3211.
12. Judson MA. The treatment of pulmonary sarcoidosis. Respir Med. 2012;106: 1351–1361.

CARE PATHWAY

Pregnant patient with known sarcoidosis

Patient referred by GP or community midwife to specialist antenatal clinic before 14 weeks gestation

↓

First visit to specialist antenatal clinic at approximately 12–14 weeks

- Detailed history, including history of any recent pulmonary assessments, any extrapulmonary sites involved, current or recent medication/s, etc.
- Confirm dates, viability
- Urgent referral to respiratory physician
- Assessment of symptoms, drug doses to maintain symptom control
- Discussion of any medication—reassure patient regarding safety of systemic steroids, azathioprine, hydroxychloroquine in pregnancy
- Reassure patient that sarcoidosis is not an inheritable condition and she will not pass it on to the baby
- Reassure patient that except in extreme cases, sarcoidosis has little adverse effect on pregnancy outcomes
- Sarcoidosis symptoms generally improve during pregnancy but can relapse in the 3 months following delivery.
- Arrange detailed anomaly scan and serial growth scans at about 28 and 34 weeks followed by antenatal clinic review.
- Advise to avoid any multivitamin supplementation with vitamin D or calcium during pregnancy. Iron ± folic acid supplementation can be prescribed separately if indicated
- Refer to anaesthetic high-risk clinic

↓

Further visits to specialist antenatal clinic at about 28, 34, and 40 weeks or as indicated

- ***Multidisciplinary team input in antenatal care essential***
- Check progress of pregnancy, maternal symptoms, any current medications and dosage
- Serial growth scans
- If on systemic steroids, GTT at about 26–28 weeks
- Confirm patient has had pulmonary function tests and assessments by respiratory physician
- Confirm she has had anaesthetic review
- In the absence of significant respiratory symptoms or signs, aim for vaginal delivery
- If no respiratory compromise, early IOL or Caesarean section reserved for other obstetric indications only
- Reassure patient that breastfeeding is not contraindicated while on prednisolone/ azathioprine
- If pulmonary compromise is significant, after joint consultation with Respiratory physician and anaesthetist, an elective LSCS at 38–39 weeks under regional block is a reasonable option. Bolus doses of 100 mg IV hydrocortisone for Caesarean section or every 6–8 h during labour and for delivery if patient has been on long-term prednisolone during pregnancy

↓

Community midwife visits to continue according to usual NICE guidelines

↓

Postnatal

- **Breastfeeding not contraindicated** as negligible amounts of steroids or azathioprine found in breast milk: advise feeding baby just before taking that day's medication
- Advise pre-pregnancy assessment and counselling before next pregnancy

4 Maternal Cardiac Disease

4.1 Maternal Cardiac Disease: General Points

FACT FILE

The remit of this fact file is to highlight the general principles involved in the antenatal care of women with a **history of cardiac disease**, making only brief mention of individual cardiac conditions. All such cases need joint cardiology–obstetric care based either in the local hospital or in a tertiary unit. It is beyond the scope of this chapter to address management of every cardiac condition in depth and the reader is recommended to consult reference books for further reading.

- About 7–8 in every 1000 babies is born with a congenital heart defect and with advances in cardiac surgery and medication, the majority now survive to adulthood.[1,2,3]
- ***Cardiac disease, including cardiac arrhythmias, stroke, and heart failure, is a leading cause of maternal mortality and morbidity.***
- Fetal morbidity and mortality are related to intrauterine growth retardation (IUGR) and prematurity.
- ***Incidence of cardiac disease in pregnancy in the UK has remained constant at 0.9% for some decades.***[4]
- Pregnancy carries increased risks for women with congenital heart disease and particular efforts should be made to prevent any unwanted pregnancies.[1]
- In particular, teenage girls with congenital heart disease should have access to a specialist who can advise on contraception and, later in life, pre-conception counselling.

Pre-conception counselling and assessment

- Pre-conception counselling and assessment with the cardiologist and specialist obstetrician is highly recommended.[1,2,3,4]
- The approach to pre-conception counselling should be proactive, including advice about safe and effective contraception.
- Every effort should be made to obtain details of the cardiac diagnosis and any surgery or other interventions
- All women of reproductive age with either congenital or acquired heart disease should have access to specialized multidisciplinary pre-conceptual counselling, so as to help them make choices about pregnancy. Women with congenital cardiac disease should be informed of the risks of congenital heart disease in the offspring and the need for increased monitoring while pregnant.[1]
- All those with significant heart disease should have received regular cardiology review to ensure that there has been a recent assessment prior to pregnancy.
- The majority of women who die in pregnancy of heart disease have **not been previously identified as 'at risk'**. Maternal death from cardiac disease has risen from 1.01 per 100 000 maternities in the triennium 1985–1987 to 2.27 per 100 000 maternities in the triennium 2003–2005.[5]

During pregnancy

- Once pregnant, any patient with a previously known cardiac condition, either congenital or acquired, should be referred by the GP and/or community midwife as soon as possible to the maternal medicine antenatal clinic or to the joint cardiology–obstetric clinic in those units where such facilities are available.
- This includes patients who have had cardiac surgery of any kind, coarctation of the aorta (both corrected/uncorrected), Marfan's, hypertrophic cardiomyopathy, previous infective or peripartum cardiomyopathies, and those who have or have had supraventricular tachycardia (SVT).
- If a patient gives a non-specific history of 'having been told she has/had a murmur', community healthcare professionals should refer her to a specialist/maternal medicine clinic **only if**
  - she is currently under the care of cardiologists
  - she has had heart problems investigated recently and is awaiting results/follow-up
  - she has had cardiac-related problems /investigations in a previous pregnancy.
- A pregnant woman with a history of flow murmur that has been previously investigated and deemed as 'benign' or of 'little clinical significance' can continue her care in the community according to the NICE antenatal schedule for low-risk women. More than 93% of healthy pregnant women have benign systolic murmurs at some time during their pregnancy, some with a diastolic component as well.
- Pregnant women with a non-specific murmur detected by the GP during a clinical examination that has hitherto not been investigated should have an ECG performed and reviewed in the community. If there are continuing concerns, an urgent and direct referral needs to be initiated by the GP directing her to Cardiology, not to a general obstetrics clinic.
- The patient can **then** be referred to the Maternal Medicine antenatal clinic by the community midwife.
- **The care of a pregnancy with maternal cardiac disease must be multidisciplinary,[1,2,3] including the specialist obstetrician, cardiologist, midwives, anaesthetist, radiologist, and neonatologist** (especially if fetal problems such as IUGR or an ultrasound-detected cardiac abnormality are found).
- **The patient may need referral to a tertiary centre for further investigations and/or management.** Such multidisciplinary referrals should be initiated as soon as possible from the maternal medicine clinic. In units where there is a joint cardiology–obstetrics clinic, this is the ideal setting for continued antenatal care and a joint plan for labour and delivery to be formulated. Such a plan must be shared with the patient after her views are taken into account.

Risk stratification

- Risk stratification is of paramount importance.[1,2,3]
- Depending on assessment of the complexity and severity of maternal cardiac disease by the cardiology and obstetric specialists at the local hospital, further antenatal care is to be continued either in the local hospital or directed to a tertiary referral centre. The risk stratification and locally available services and facilities, especially for out-of-hours cardiology cover, should help inform the decision.
- Tertiary centres will be able to provide combined obstetric, cardiological and surgical expertise in the care of pregnant women with significant heart disease.
- **Pregnant women with heart disease should have a risk stratification performed by a multidisciplinary team** to determine the frequency and content of each of their antenatal follow-up visits.
- Depending on the severity of the condition, women may need to be seen every 2–4 weeks until 20 weeks gestation, then every 2 weeks until 24 weeks gestation and then weekly.[1]
- Early referral to the high-risk anaesthetic clinic is necessary.

- Women with congenital heart disease are at a relatively increased risk of having a baby affected by congenital cardiac disease (3%, vs 1% population incidence). While up to 90% of congenital heart disease is of unknown aetiology, around 3% of cases follow Mendelian inheritance patterns (autosomal dominant or recessive). Referral for genetic counselling in such cases is advisable.
- Fetal cardiac scan in addition to the routine fetal anomaly scan at 20 weeks ± fetal ECHO, if appropriate, is indicated.
- Serial fetal growth and liquor scans may be indicated especially if the patient is on beta-blockers.
- Low threshold for thromboprophylaxis during pregnancy.
- Low-dose aspirin (75 mg/day) is a safe and effective adjunct to LMWH (low molecular weight heparin) in those with mechanical valves or at increased risk of intracardiac thrombosis.
- Plans regarding timing, mode, and place of delivery must preferably be discussed by 28 weeks gestation
- A detailed management plan of labour, delivery, and puerperium including intrapartum and postnatal analgesia requirements should be formulated in advance and clearly documented. This should be distributed to all key areas as well as shared with the patient.
- Plans must be put in place and clearly documented regarding transfer or delivery in the local hospital for a patient who has been booked to deliver in a tertiary centre but goes into labour before her planned admission there. This should involve discussions ahead of time with the patient and her partner, local cardiologists, anaesthetist, and midwifery lead of labour ward.
- Vaginal delivery is the preferred mode for most cases. A Caesarean section is required only for obstetric indications or in certain very specific cardiac conditions.
- Spontaneous onset of labour is to be anticipated, although a planned induction may be required if patient is either on anticoagulants in cases of valvular disease or if there is a deterioration of maternal cardiac function. Induction of labour may be appropriate to optimize the timing of delivery and the availability of specific medical staff.
- Pain relief such as an epidural is important as this will limit the demands on the heart.
- Assisted vaginal delivery, preferably with the ventouse (vacuum), may be required to cut short or even avoid maternal pushing in some cases, depending on severity of the cardiac disease and an third-trimester assessment of cardiac function by the cardiologist.
- **Document 'no syntometrine/ergometrine for third stage'.** Ergometrine can cause a sudden and significant increase in circulating blood volume,which in turn puts on additional load on the heart. Also, boluses of high-dose oxytocin when repeated can cause hypotension and should be avoided.
- Oxytocin infusion (40 units in 1 litre over 4–6 h) after the initial IM injection of oxytocin IM 5 mg is the safer option. The safety of misoprostol in those with pre-existing significant cardiac disease is as yet unconfirmed.
- **Discuss and document** plans for postnatal cardiac surveillance and contraceptive advice. Reiterate need for pre-conceptual assessment and counselling for future pregnancy.
- **Postnatal cardiac surveillance:** Cardiac follow-up usually takes place about 6 weeks after delivery and, if there are any continuing concerns, 6 months after delivery. Beyond this time, the woman can return to her periodic cardiac outpatient care.
- **Appropriate contraceptive advice before discharge** is vitally important, taking into account risks of thrombosis or infection with some methods of contraception. Mirena® IUS or etonogestrel implants are the safest and most efficacious methods of contraception.

Additional information for care of women with cardiac disease in pregnancy

- All pregnant women whose cardiac condition puts them at increased risk of aortopathy (eg, those with repaired aortic coarctation, Marfan's syndrome, or aortopathy with bicuspid aortic valve) should be made aware of the symptoms of acute dissection and be advised to seek urgent help.
- A recent NICE guideline[6] advises against the use of routine antibiotic prophylaxis against infective endocarditis in those women with cardiac disease either for obstetric interventions or for childbirth.
- However, prophylactic antibiotics may be required in cases of operative delivery in women at increased risk, such as those with mechanical valves or a history of previous endocarditis. Prophylactic antibiotic cover should also be given before any intervention likely to be associated with significant or recurrent bacteraemia. The possibility of endocarditis should also be considered in any woman with a cardiac defect who has positive blood cultures.[3]
- ***If there are any doubts regarding the use of prophylactic antibiotics, particularly for Caesarean section in women at increased risk, consult with the cardiologists and document the advice clearly in the maternity notes.***
- Angiotensin converting enzyme (ACE) inhibitors which are contraindicated in pregnancy are safe to use in breastfeeding mothers.

Acquired cardiac disease

- ***This includes cardiomyopathies, ischaemic heart disease (acute myocardial infarction), aortic root dissection, valvular heart disease, and cardiac arrhythmias.***

Puerperal cardiomyopathy and cardiomyositis

- See also fact file on cardiomyopathies (Chapter 4.3).
- Also known as **peripartum cardiomyopathy**, it can present one month before as well as 5 months after delivery.
- The incidence is 1 in 1500 to 1 in 4000 live births.
- Risk factors include older maternal age, greater parity, black ethnicity, and multiple gestations.
- Viral myositis has been implicated in aetiology.
- Dyspnoea, fatigue, and ankle oedema can present in both late pregnancy and with cardiomyopathy, but nocturnal dyspnoea, nocturnal cough, and chest pain are symptoms that should raise suspicion.
- Signs may include new regurgitant murmurs, pulmonary crackles, elevated jugular venous pressure, and hepatomegaly.

Investigations

- ECG may show left ventricular hypertrophy and chest radiograph invariably shows cardiomegaly.
- Echocardiography demonstrates recent left ventricular dysfunction.

Treatment

- Salt restriction should be instituted and diuretics prescribed to relieve pulmonary oedema.
- Vasodilators such as hydralazine, nitrates, or amlodipine should be given to reduce afterload in the presence of ventricular dysfunction. ACE inhibitors are fetotoxic, but are the mainstay of treatment postpartum.
- The timing of delivery should be based on obstetric considerations.

Ischaemic heart disease (myocardial infarction)

Incidence and presentation

- The incidence is 1 in 10 000 pregnancies.[7]
- Maternal mortality of acute myocardial infarction (MI) is 5–7%; most deaths occur at the time of infarction.[8]
- The condition occurs more commonly in the later stages of pregnancy, peri- and postpartum.
- Risk factors include smoking, increasing maternal age, obesity and diabetes, hypertension, hypercholesterolaemia, family history of ischaemic heart disease, and cocaine abuse.
- The causative mechanism is often coronary artery dissection, involving a mechanism similar to aortic dissection.
- The presenting symptom is chest pain but symptoms may be atypical with epigastric pain and nausea.

Investigations

- ECG may be normal or equivocal.
- Troponin levels are usually raised.

- Early coronary angiography is indicated. Nearly 20% of women have intracoronary thrombus or arteriosclerosis on angiography.

Management

- Treatment of MI in pregnancy is identical to that in the non-pregnant state.[7]
- Nitrates, heparin, and beta-blockers are the mainstay of treatment.
- Aspirin in doses of 150–300 mg may be needed in acute MI.
- Treatment involves coronary artery stenting and percutaneous catheter intervention employed as first-line treatment.[7] Aspirin or clopidogrel is recommended after stenting, but must be discontinued for delivery and immediately after because of the increased risk of bleeding.
- Tissue plasminogen activator (TPA) is another option. It does not cross the placental barrier so does not cause fetal problems, but should be avoided for delivery or in the early puerperium as it increases the risk of haemorrhage.
- In women with a history of previous MI, prognosis for a future pregnancy is poor if there is residual left ventricular dysfunction and continuing ischaemia.

Aortic dissection

See also fact file for Marfan's syndrome (Chapter 14.2).

- Marfan's is rare, but accounts for 50% of aortic dissection in women under 40. It occurs in association with severe hypertension secondary to pre-eclampsia, coarctation of the aorta, or **connective tissue disease such as Marfan's** where the risk of thoracic aorta aneurysm resulting in aortic dissection or rupture is increased during pregnancy. The presenting symptoms are chest pain or interscapular pain associated with end-organ ischaemia, acute heart failure, aortic incompetence, or haemopericardium with tamponade.
- All pregnant women whose condition places them at risk of aortopathy (such as those with repaired coarctation or Marfan's syndrome) should be made aware of the symptoms of acute dissection and be advised to seek urgent help if they experience any of them.[3] **Their antenatal, intrapartum, and immediate postnatal care are best conducted in a tertiary unit with ready access to emergency cardiovascular surgery.**

Investigations

- The condition is diagnosed by CT or transoesophageal echocardiography (TOE). Aortic root diameter will need to be monitored closely throughout pregnancy and if there are any signs of dilatation, aggressive hypertension management as well as prophylactic beta-blockers.
- If the aortic root diameter is less than 4 cm the maternal mortality rate is about 1% but if this increases to more than 25% if the aortic root diameter is more than 4 cm.[4]
- The patient should be advised not to get pregnant till postsurgical repair is complete. In the event of an unplanned pregnancy, termination may be advisable.[4]

Treatment

- If aortic root dilatation is more than 4 cm, beta-blockers, aggressive management of hypertension, and monthly ECGs may be required[3] and delivery considered if there is progressive aortic root dilatation.
- The safest mode of delivery may be by elective Caesarean section under regional block, with aortic repair performed postnatally as there is a continued risk of dissection.

Valvular heart disease

- Immigrant women[3] who have not had health screening in childhood are a high-risk group for undiagnosed cardiac disease, especially of the acquired variety (e.g. mitral stenosis after childhood rheumatic fever). Therefore, any cardiovascular or respiratory symptoms should warrant careful clinical and echocardiographic assessment.
- Valvular heart disease may come to light only during pregnancy due to the increased demands on the cardiovascular system.

Mitral stenosis

- Mitral stenosis of rheumatic fever aetiology is the most common acquired heart disease with a maternal mortality in mild cases being less than 1%, but high neonatal mortality rates.
- In severe cases (NYHA class III–IV) or with mitral valve diameter less than 1 cm the maternal mortality rate is very high.[8]
- ***Pre-pregnancy assessment and advice:***
  - This is essential and should include thorough cardiological evaluation, both clinical and ECHO based.
  - Advise about deferring pregnancy until after valve correction by balloon valvostomy or replacement and discuss the use of potentially teratogenic drugs during the first trimester.
  - In certain situations, such as the presence of pulmonary hypertension, pregnancy is contraindicated because maternal mortality is as high as 30–60%.
  - Pre-pregnancy advice should emphasize smoking cessation and peri-pregnancy folic acid.
- In mitral stenosis, increased left atrial pressure occurs due to narrowing of the mitral valve. Symptoms can deteriorate during pregnancy and immediately after delivery. Tachycardia due to pain, anxiety, or maternal effort during labour and delivery could also cause acute deterioration. Symptoms include dyspnoea, increasing exercise intolerance, orthopnoea, paroxysmal nocturnal dyspnoea and pulmonary oedema, atrial fibrillation, and heart failure.
- After initial combined assessment at booking with the cardiologist and maternal medicine obstetrician, such assessments should continue at least once in each trimester and more frequently if indicated.
- Treatment is mainly aimed at reducing volume overload with bed rest, diuretics, and beta-blockers to improve ventricular filling. The benefits of beta-blockers in this instance outweigh the small risk of IUGR.
- If medical management does not work, balloon mitral valvuloplasty, which is safe and effective in pregnancy, is used.
- If atrial fibrillation develops, prompt DC cardioversion, beta-blockers or digoxin, and full anticoagulation with treatment doses of LMWH are required.
- Serial fetal growth scans are recommended.
- Referral to and assessment by senior anaesthetist is mandatory.
- Mode of delivery is usually vaginal, with Caesarean section for obstetric indications.
- Document:
  - Avoid lithotomy or supine position in labour.
  - Second stage to be cut short with assisted instrumental delivery.
  - Epidural recommended with precautions to avoid volume overload.
  - Third-stage management: Avoid ergometrine /syntometrine.

Mitral regurgitation

- Usually as a result of rheumatic heart disease or accompanies mitral valve prolapse.
- Often well tolerated in pregnancy; asymptomatic women do not require treatment during pregnancy and the patient must be reassured.
- If signs of heart failure develop, treatment is with nitrates, digoxin, diuretics, and hydralazine.[8]

Mitral valve prolapse

- This benign condition is the most common cardiac abnormality in pregnancy, seen in about 15% of women of childbearing age.[8]
- If associated mitral regurgitation is excluded on ECHO, it is of little clinical significance.

Aortic stenosis

- Usually congenital in origin. The degree of narrowing of the aortic valve effects pregnancy outcomes.
- Angina, hypertension, and arrhythmias can result in cardiac failure.
- Aortic balloon valvulostomy as an interim procedure while awaiting valve replacement after delivery should be considered.[8]

Prosthetic heart valves

- Pregnancies in women who have had heart valve replacement with mechanical heart valves pose special challenges in terms of the anticoagulation therapy that is critical to prevent valve thrombosis.
- Bioprosthetic (grafted tissue) heart valves do not usually require anticoagulation unlike mechanical (metal) heart valves where there is a high risk (45%) of thromboses and full anticoagulation is therefore required throughout pregnancy.[7,9] In those with mechanical heart valves the risk of maternal mortality is 1–4%.
- **Warfarin** is the mainstay of anticoagulation in patients with mechanical heart valves. In pregnancy, however, there is a conflicting issue of its effect on the fetus.
- While continuation of warfarin gives the maximum protection against thromboses, it carries an increased risk of teratogenicity, embryotoxicity, miscarriages, microcephaly, congenital cataracts, stillbirths, and intracerebral bleeding, especially when the dose required to maintain therapeutic levels is more than 5 mg/day.[9]
- High-dose LMWH, while safe for the fetus as it does not cross the placenta, is less effective than warfarin in preventing valve thromboses.
- ***Three regime choices[7,10] have been reported:***
  - Warfarin throughout pregnancy, stop at 38 weeks, followed by full anticoagulation doses of SC LMWH or IV unfractionated heparin for elective delivery and immediate postpartum. Warfarin can be recommenced about 3 days after delivery. **This regime carries a lower rate of maternal thromboembolism (4%) but a high rate of fetal abnormality (6%).**
  - Replace warfarin with LMWH from 6 weeks until the end of 12 weeks gestation, after which warfarin is restarted. Warfarin is then continued till 38 weeks then substituted by therapeutic doses of SC LMWH or IV unfractionated heparin for elective delivery. Warfarin is resumed postpartum. **This carries a low risk of teratogenicity but a doubling of the risk of valve thromboembolism (to 9%).**
  - LMWH throughout pregnancy with low-dose aspirin as an adjunct. **This has no risk of fetal teratogenicity or embryo toxicity but has a high risk of valve thromboses (25%).**
- **Note: With all three regimes a fetal loss rate of 30% has been reported. The patient must be advised of this and an informed choice made.**
- Warfarin requires close monitoring to maintain INR in the range 2.5–3.5.
- Warfarin is associated with small for gestational age babies,[11] therefore fetal growth must be monitored with serial scans.
- LMWH doses should be adjusted according to factor Xa levels,[9,11] to maintain a 4-h peak of 0.8–1.2 U/ml.
- LMWH needs to be stopped for labour and delivery. If IV unfractionated heparin is used, the dosage should be reduced to prophylactic levels of approximately 1000 U/h.[9] Full anticoagulant doses of heparin can be recommenced after delivery once the risk of excess bleeding has passed.

Cardiac arrhthythmias

- Pregnancy can increase the incidence of cardiac arrhythmias, the risk being highest during labour and delivery.[7]
- **Investigations** of arrhythmias start with ECG. 24-h Holter monitoring and ECHO may also be required. Thyroid status must be checked.
- **Atrial and ventricular premature beats** are common and of little significance for the mother or the baby. Once diagnosed, no further investigations or monitoring is required.
- **Persistent sinus tachycardia** needs investigations to exclude other pathology such as hyperthyroidism, cardiorespiratory pathology, or sepsis.[9]
- **Atrial flutter and fibrillation** are rare, usually associated with mitral valve disease or sepsis.
- **Paroxysmal SVT:**
  - Both pre-existing and de-novo episodes increase during pregnancy.
  - Treatment is necessary during pregnancy for life-threatening arrhythmias, atrial fibrillation or flutter and if SVT is frequent and symptomatic.
  - Initial treatment of SVT in a haemodynamically stable pregnant woman is vagal manoeuvres and if this does not work, IV adenosine which is safe in pregnancy. Second-line treatment of persistent SVT may include digoxin, beta-blockers, or calcium channel blockers[7]
- **Ventricular tachycardia** is rare. Initial treatment is with lidocaine or procainamide if haemodynamically stable.
- Rate control in **atrial fibrillation** can be achieved with digoxin.
- **Pharmacological management** of arrhythmias in pregnancy includes verapamil and beta-blockers such as propranolol, metoprolol, sotalol or atenolol.
- **DC cardioversion** is safe in pregnancy and is required in all women who are haemodynamically unstable.

Information for patients

Please see Information for patients: Heart disease and pregnancy (p. 505)

References

1. RCOG Good Practice No. 13. Cardiac disease and pregnancy. London: Royal College of Obstericians and Gynaecologists, 2011. <https://www.rcog.org.uk/globalassets/documents/guidelines/goodpractice13cardiacdiseaseandpregnancy.pdf>
2. ESC Guidelines on the management of cardiovascular diseases during pregnancy: the Task Force on the Management of Cardiovascular Diseases during Pregnancy of the European Society of Cardiology (ESC). Eur Heart J 2011; 32: 3147–3197.
3. RCOG Consensus Views Arising from the 51st Study Group: Heart disease and pregnancy. London: Royal College of Obstetricians and Gynaecologists, 2006.
4. Gelson E, et al. Cardiac disease in pregnancy. Part 1: Congenital heart disease. Obstetrician and Gynaecologist 2007; 9: 15–20.
5. Lewis G (ed.) CEMACH. Saving mothers' lives: reviewing maternal deaths to make motherhood safer—2003-2005. The Seventh Report on Confidential Enquiries into Maternal Deaths in the United Kingdom. London: Confidential Enquiry into Maternal and Child Health, 2007.
6. NICE Guideline. Prophylaxis against infective endocarditis. CG64. London: National Institute for Health and Clinical Excellence, 2008.
7. Gelson E, et al. Cardiac disease in pregnancy. Part 2: Acquired heart disease. Obstetrician and Gynaecologist 2007; 9: 83–87.
8. Ladner H, et al. Acute myocardial infarction in pregnancy and the puerperium: a population-based study. Obstet Gynecol 2005; 105: 480–484.
9. Nelson-Piercy C. Heart disease. In: Handbook of obstetric medicine, 4th ed. London: Informa Health Care, 2010, pp. 32–33.
10. Chan WS, et al. Anticoagulation of pregnant women with mechanical heart valves: a systematic review of the literature. Arch Intern Med 2000; 160: 191–196.
11. McLintock C, et al. Maternal complications and pregnancy outcome in women with mechanical prosthetic heart valves treated with enoxaparin. BJOG 2009; 116: 1585–1592.

Further reading

Steer PJ, et al. Heart disease in pregnancy. London: RCOG Press, 2006.

CARE PATHWAY

- Any patient with a history of **significant cardiac disease** of any kind (see fact files in Chapters 4.1, 4.2, and 4.3) must be referred to the maternal medicine antenatal clinic as soon as pregnancy is reported to primary care
- Using the general principles of care of cardiac disease in pregnancy as specified in the preceding fact file, ***individualized joint care pathways*** need to be designed depending on the particular cardiac condition and its severity
- Such care pathways will often need to be designed jointly with the tertiary cardiac centre
- Ideally these care pathways would commence with **pre-pregnancy assessment and counselling**, progressing to early risk stratification jointly by the local DGH cardiologist, specialist obstetrician, and anaesthetist
- Such care pathways must be circulated to all concerned in the patient's care in both the DGH and tertiary centre and a copy given to the patient
- Depending on how the pregnancy progresses, including any possible worsening of the patient's cardiovascular status or development of complications, care pathways may need updating during the course of pregnancy. These dynamic changes must be promptly documented and communicated to all areas
- Prompt referral to a tertiary cardiac centre, as indicated by the type and severity of the cardiac disease, must be initiated by both/either the cardiologist and/or specialist obstetrician at the DGH
- The ideal place, timing, and mode of delivery will need to be discussed in conjunction with the tertiary centre and clearly documented and communicated to all involved, including the local neonatologist, particularly if severe IUGR is suspected or pre-term delivery is likely or if the baby is suspected to have an inherited cardiac lesion as well
- Care pathways should always include plans for **postnatal cardiac follow-up**, appropriate advice regarding **contraception**, and reiteration of the importance to seek **pre-pregnancy counselling and assessment**

4.2 Congenital Cardiac Disease (Maternal and Fetal)

FACT FILE

Epidemiology

- **Congenital heart disease (CHD)** is the most common congenital condition, diagnosed in 1% of newborns.
- Only about 3% of all CHD follows a Mendelian mode of inheritance. In over 90% the aetiology is largely unknown.[1]
- Congenital cardiac defects are also prominent in chromosomal disorders, especially autosomal trisomies and Turner's syndrome.
- Cardiac lesions may also be present in addition to other abnormalities as part of a Mendelian syndrome (e.g. Marfan's, supravalvular aortic stenosis syndrome, Kartagener, Holt–Oram syndrome).
- Likewise, cardiac abnormalities can occur as part of a non-Mendelian syndrome complex as in VATER, DiGeorge, or Goldenhar syndromes.

Genetic counselling

- Genetic counselling[2,3,4,5,6,7] is essential for pregnancies where
  - either partner has a congenital cardiac defect
  - a previous fetus or baby with a congenital cardiac defect
  - there is a strong family history of congenital cardiac defects (suggesting an autosomal dominant inheritance) especially on the maternal side.
- Rubella infection in the first trimester, maternal diabetes, and maternal age over 40 are other risk factors for fetal cardiac lesions.

Risk

- Risk of congenital cardiac defect in a child of a mother with congenital heart defect is higher than the risk if it is the father.
- However, in most studies, fewer pregnancies are screened for CHD where the father is the index case, compared with the mother as the index case. It is likely that the paternal history of CHD has not been identified or elicited in the assessment of the pregnancy.
- Certain very rare congenital heart defects are not represented by enough cases to offer secure recurrence risks.
- The risk of recurrence of congenital heart defects in a subsequent fetus is three times greater if two children (siblings) have heart defects compared with only one affected sibling (Table 4.1).
- ***This gives a risk recurrence of about 5% for the rare defects and 10% for the more common ones like ventricular septal defect or VSD.***
- Where recurrence does occur in a sibling, in only 50% is the defect the same as the previous one. Complete exact concordance of the type of CHD has been reported in about 21% and partial concordance in 20%[3,4]

Table 4.1 Recurrence risk (%) for congenital heart defects (CHD)

Single or multiple risk with family member(s) affected with CHD	*Overall CHD recurrence risk in index fetus*
One affected member of family:	4.0%
One previous sibling affected	3.5%
If mother affected	5.2%
If father affected	3–7.5%*
One second and third degree relative	3.5%
Two affected first-degree relatives:	3.0%
Two siblings affected	4.5%
Mother and one sibling affected	11.1%
Father and one sibling affected	8.3%

Type of CHD	*If mother affected*	*If father affected*	*One sibling affected*	*Two siblings affected*
Aortic stenosis	12–18%	3%	2%	6%
Atrial septal defect	4–5%	1.5%	2.5%	8%
Ventricular septal defect	6–10%	2%	3%	10%
Tetralogy of Fallot	2.5–4%	1.5%	2.5%	6–8%
Coarctation of aorta	4%	2%	2%	6%
Patent ductus arteriosus	3.5–4%	2.5%	3%	10%
Pulmonary stenosis	4–7%	2%	2%	6%
Transposition of great arteries			1–2%	5%
Hypoplastic left heart syndrome			2–3%	6–10%
Tricuspid atresia			1%	3%
Pulmonary atresia			1%	3%
Ebstein anomaly	6%		1%	6%

* The higher figure of 7.5% quoted in the paper by Fesslova et al.[3] is probably explained by the fact that far fewer pregnancies were screened prenatally for CHD where the father was the index case, compared with the mother being the index case. In general, the risk of CHD for the offspring is 2% lower when the father is the affected parent rather than the mother.

Data from: Nora JJ and Nora AH, Update on counselling the family with a first degree relative with congenital heart defect, *American Journal of Medical Genetics*, 1988, 29, pp. 137–142; Nora JJ, From generational studies to a multilevel genetic-environmental interaction, *Journal of the American College of Cardiology*, 1994, 23, 6, pp. 1459–1467; Fesslova V et al., Recurrence of congenital heart disease in cases with familial risk screened prenatally by echocardiography, *Journal of Pregnancy*, 2011, Article ID 368067, doi:10.1155/2011/368067; Blue GM et al., Congenital heart disease: current knowledge about causes inheritance, *Medical Journal of Australia*, 2012, 197, 3, pp. 155–159; Roos-Hesselink JW et al., Inheritance of congenital heart disease, *Netherlands Heart Journal*, 2005, 13, pp. 88–91; and Calcagni G et al., Familial recurrence of congenital heart disease: an overview and review of the literature, *European Journal of Pediatrics*, 2007, 166, pp. 111–116.

- The risk to more distant relatives of an isolated case of congenital cardiac lesion is less than 1%.[1]
- In high-risk families, especially those in which there is an affected parent (usually the mother), the recurrence risk in an offspring varies from 50% (autosomal dominant inheritance) to 100% (maternal cytoplasmic inheritance pattern where all the offspring of an affected mother are also affected).[3]
- A careful history of exposure to any teratogens (e.g. lithium, dexamfetamine) is also essential before quoting recur risks.
- In all cases where either parent or a sibling is known to have any CHD, fetal cardiac scans at 20–22 weeks and fetal ECHO (as recommended by consultant radiologist) are essential.[4]

Management after CHD has been diagnosed

- Management must be individualized.
- Depending on the type of congenital cardiac lesion detected in the index fetus, prompt referral must be made to a tertiary centre with neonatal cardiology/fetal medicine with paediatric cardiothoracic surgery services.
- The place of delivery (either local hospital or tertiary referral centre) must be discussed well ahead of time and appropriate arrangements made and discussed with the patient and partner/family.
- When a congenital cardiac defect is detected in the fetus, the neonatologists of the local unit must be informed without delay. Clearly document an agreed plan in the event of the pregnant woman, who has been booked to deliver in the tertiary unit, presenting to the local hospital in active labour which does not permit a safe transfer to the tertiary centre.

Information for patients

Please see **Information for patients: Congenital heart disease and pregnancy** (p. 505)

References

1. Gill HK, et al. Patterns of recurrence of congenital heart disease. An analysis of 6,640 consecutive pregnancies evaluated by detailed fetal echocardiography. J Am Coll Cardiol 2003; 42: 923–929.
2. Nora JJ and Nora AH, 'Update on Counselling the Family with a First Degree Relative with Congenital Heart Defect', American Journal of Medical Genetics, 1988, 29, pp. 137–142
3. Nora JJ, 'From generational studies to a multilevel genetic-environmental interaction', Journal of the American College of Cardiology, 1994, 23, 6, pp. 1459–1467
4. Fesslova V et al., 'Recurrence of Congenital Heart Disease in Cases with Familial Risk Screened Prenatally by Echocardiography', Journal of Pregnancy, 2011, Article ID 368067, doi:10.1155/2011/368067
5. Blue GM et al., 'Congenital heart disease: current knowledge about causes inheritance', Medical Journal of Australia, 2012, 197, 3, pp. 155–159
6. Roos-Hesselink JW et al., 'Inheritance of congenital heart disease', Netherlands Heart Journal, 2005, 13, pp. 88–91
7. Calcagni G et al., 'Familial recurrence of congenital heart disease: an overview and review of the literature, European Journal of Pediatrics, 2007, 166, pp. 111–116.

CARE PATHWAY

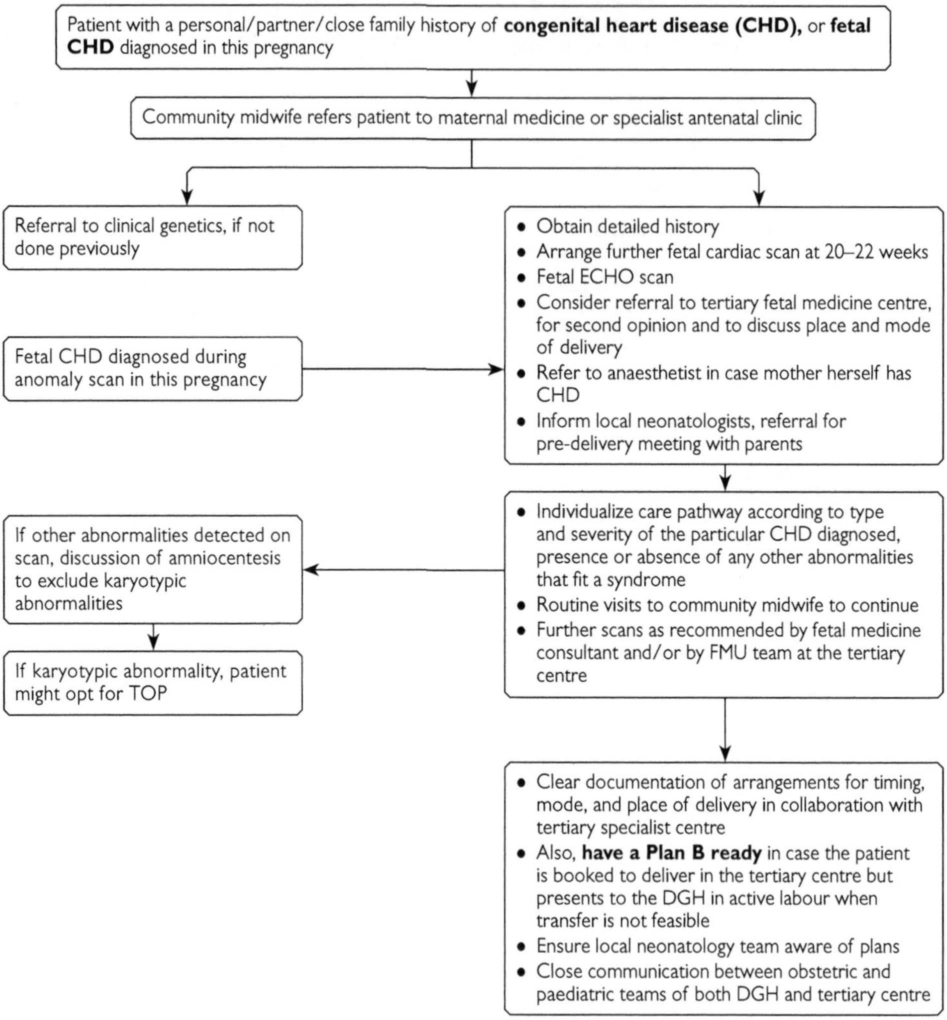

4.3 Hypertrophic Cardiomyopathy

FACT FILE

- **Cardiomyopathy** is a weakening or alteration in the heart muscle that impedes normal cardiac function.[1,2,3]
- **Cardiomyopathies can be either of the hypertrophic or the dilated type** (Figure 4.1).
- **Hypertrophic cardiomyopathy (HCM)** is where the heart muscle becomes thick and hardened. It can be either **hypertrophic obstructive cardiomyopathy (HOCM)** or **non-obstructive hypertrophic cardiomyopathy**.
- **Dilated cardiomyopathy** is a condition in which the heart becomes enlarged. Causative agents include bacteria, viruses, neuromuscular, immunological, endocrine and haematological aetiologies as well as certain connective tissue disorders.
- **Peripartum cardiomyopathy** is a rare pregnancy-specific cardiomyopathy that is similar in presentation to the dilated cardiomyopathies.
- Both hypertrophic and dilated cardiomyopathies impose a strain on the heart and can cause serious complications, such as heart failure, blood clots, heart attack, and sudden cardiac death.
- **HCM** is a mainly autosomal dominant, inherited genetic disorder with variable penetrance and expression.
- The symptoms are complex and HCM can carry a high incidence of sudden death. HCM is the leading cause of sudden cardiac death in preadolescent and adolescent children.
- The classic feature of the disorder is abnormal and asymmetrical myocardial hypertrophy in the absence of an obvious causative factor and resulting in an obstruction of flow through the left ventricular outflow tract.
- Overall prevalence of HCM is low; it is estimated to occur in 2 in 1000 of the population.
- *HCM is a familial disease.* Familial HCM occurs as an autosomal dominant Mendelian-inherited disease in approximately 70% of cases. Some of the sporadic forms may be caused by spontaneous mutations.
- Approximately 25% of first-degree relatives of a patient with HCM are found by echocardiography to have evidence of disease.
- HCM occurs in both men and women.
- In adults, the peak incidence is in the third decade of life, with the vast majority of cases occurring in the age range between the third and sixth decades of life.
- Most patients with HCM are asymptomatic.[1,2] Unfortunately, the first clinical manifestation of the disease in such individuals may be sudden death. Investigations of a heart murmur may reveal the condition.
- **Complications of HCM** may include:
  - congestive heart failure
  - ventricular and supraventricular arrhythmias
  - infective mitral endocarditis
  - atrial fibrillation with mural thrombus formation
  - sudden death.
- Annual mortality rate in patients with HCM ranges from less than 1% to 2%.[1,2]
- ***HCM is a progressive condition that worsens over time.***
- **The most common symptoms** include:
  - dyspnoea on exertion, orthopnoea, nocturnal dyspnoea
  - chest pain, which may be caused or worsened by exertion
  - syncope and presyncope
  - palpitations
  - fatigue
  - swelling of the legs and feet (oedema).
- Patients with no or only minor symptoms generally have a better prognosis than those with more severe symptoms.
- ***However the severity of symptoms does not necessarily correlate with the extent of cardiac involvement or the risk of sudden death.***
- Early diagnosis is crucial in order to advise an appropriate level of safe activity for the patient

Figure 4.1 Types of cardiomyopathies.

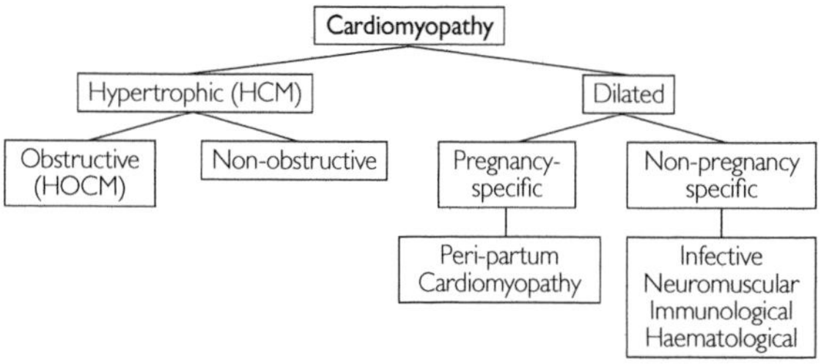

HCM in pregnancy

- In the first trimester, the natural decrease in peripheral resistance can be deleterious in HCM, whereas the increased circulating blood volume is beneficial. The balance between these two influences determines the condition of the patient.
- Towards the end of pregnancy, aortocaval compression causing a decrease in venous return could compromise cardiac output.
- The pain and stress of labour and delivery is often associated with sympathetic stimulation and tachycardia, which can cause deteriorating cardiac function.

Pre-pregnancy assessment and counselling in HCM

- A thorough cardiovascular examination and assessment of HCM by the cardiologist must ideally precede conception. This should include a careful history and physical examination, an ECHO and ECG.
- The patient with HCM must be offered pre-pregnancy counselling[1] with respect to inheritance pattern. The risk of inheritance in familial forms is 50%. This must be compared with the background risk of any congenital cardiac disease (around 1%). As signs of HCM are usually not detectable in the fetus or even at birth, antepartum investigations such as ultrasound cannot be used for antenatal prediction of HCM in the baby.
- Maternal risks during a future pregnancy must be discussed. Pregnancy itself in asymptomatic women is mostly well tolerated but worsening of symptoms would require repeated hospital admissions.
- Women who have symptoms prior to pregnancy are at higher risk of complications during pregnancy.
- Women with clinical heart failure should be advised against pregnancy as they may be unable to tolerate the increased haemodynamic load even in the early stages of pregnancy.
- Decisions regarding internal placement of a cardioverter defibrillator or surgical procedures to decrease symptoms should be made prior to any pregnancy.
- Contraception must be discussed. Women with HCM are not candidates for combined oral contraceptives. The levonorgestrel intrauterine system (Mirena®) or etonogestrel implant are the safest contraceptive choices.
- Current medications should be reviewed if a woman is planning a pregnancy.

Information for patients

Please see Information for patients: Cardiomyopathy and pregnancy (p. 505)

References

1. Thaman R, et al. Pregnancy related complications in women with hypertrophic cardiomyopathy. Heart 2003; 89: 752–756.
2. Adamson DL, et al. Cardiac disease in pregnancy. In:Greer I, et al., ed., Maternal medicine. London: Churchill Livingstone Elsevier, 2007.
3. Stergiopoulos K, et al. Pregnancy in patients with pre-existing cardiomyopathies. J Am Coll Cardiol 2011; 58: 337–350.

CARE PATHWAY

Multidisciplinary, coordinated care should be planned on the following general principles with the cardiologist, maternal medicine obstetrician, anaesthetist, midwife, and neonatologist on a case-by case basis

- ***Prompt referral to a tertiary centre for further cardiology assessments or for ongoing management of the pregnancy and for delivery in high-risk cases of HCM***
- Frequent cardiovascular monitoring and checks are warranted during pregnancy and puerperium
- The frequency of obstetric and cardiology assessments must be determined on a case-to-case basis depending on maternal cardiac functional status during each stage of pregnancy
- As pregnancy itself can induce symptoms such as dyspnoea, palpitations, and dizziness, echocardiography may need to be repeated to establish whether or not these phenomena are related to progression of the HCM
- If necessary, beta-blockers to reduce cardiac contractility and sympathetic stimulation can be prescribed and vigilance for IUGR must be maintained
- Diuretics and digitalis should be reserved for women who develop congestive cardiac failure
- Beta-mimetic drugs for tocolysis are contraindicated
- Atrial fibrillation can be treated with medication or with DC conversion, if there is no response to medical therapy
- Fetal cardiac scan at 20 weeks, repeated at about 24 weeks
- Serial fetal growth scans from 26–28 weeks at monthly intervals, more frequently if signs of IUGR are detected
- The patient should be advised to avoid lying on her back
- Referral to the anaesthetic obstetric clinic is vital for assessment and discussions regarding analgesia for labour, delivery, or a Caesarean section
- Antenatal referral to neonatologist/paediatrician due to the 50% inheritance risk in familial HCM
- Plans for labour and delivery should be planned with a multidisciplinary team well in advance. This plan should be documented, shared with the patient and all involved in the patient's care in the DGH and tertiary centre, as relevant. **Clear documentation of the plans for delivery must be readily available in the main notes as well in the maternity hand-held notes**
- Endocarditis prophylaxis at the time of labour and delivery may not be recommended in women with HCM according to NICE guidelines; however, some experts continue to advice antibiotics because the risk of developing endocarditis has major health consequences
- Vaginal delivery is generally recommended unless there are obstetric indications for a Caesarean section
- Effective analgesia for labour and delivery is essential to minimize maternal cardiac stress. Epidural anaesthesia should be very carefully managed with adequate volume expansion to avoid hypotension as vasodilatation is poorly tolerated
- Most women with HCM do not require invasive monitoring. Basic cardiac monitoring with continuous ECG may be necessary in some instances for early detection of arrhythmias
- The second stage can be cut short with ventouse or forceps
- Oxytocin can induce vasodilation and arterial hypotension and should be administered with great care
- Hypovolemia or blood loss should be aggressively corrected
- If the mother has been on large doses of beta-blockers, the neonatologist should be alerted to the possibility of bradycardia and hypoglycaemia
- Paediatric consultation and follow-up is advised for the presence of HCM in the newborn

Postpartum care:

- Effective contraception (levonorgestrel intrauterine system (Mirena®) or etonogestrel implant) should be advised
- The haemodynamic changes of pregnancy may take up to 6 months to normalize. Women should be seen early after pregnancy (usually within 6–8 weeks). The frequency of further follow-up visits depends on the clinical status

4.4 Peripartum Cardiomyopathy

FACT FILE

- **Peripartum cardiomyopathy (PPCM)** is a rare cause of pregnancy-related heart failure.
- Maternal mortality rate can be as high as 20%.
- PPCM is defined[1] as an idiopathic cardiomyopathy presenting with heart failure secondary to left ventricular systolic dysfunction towards the end of pregnancy or in the months following delivery. No other cause of heart failure is found and there is no history of previous heart disease.

Symptoms

- Symptoms may include fatigue, dyspnoea, orthopnoea, persistent cough, paroxysmal nocturnal dyspnoea, peripheral oedema, chest pain, palpitations, or abdominal discomfort.
- Early signs and symptoms of PPCM could mimic normal physiological changes of pregnancy and puerperium.[2]

Diagnosis

- The diagnosis is one of exclusion,[2,3] made on clinical presentation and non-invasive imaging.[3]
- Postulated **risk factors** include inflammatory aetiology (myocarditis), viral infections, immunological responses, or genetic susceptibility. A greater incidence is seen in older mothers, multiple pregnancy, PIH, and those of Afro-Caribbean descent.
- Cardiac decompensation in a hitherto normal patient may be brought on by beta-agonists given for tocolysis, steroids for fetal lung maturation, or IV fluids or syntocinon infusion.[4] PPCM must be suspected in such cases.
- Finding left ventricular systolic dysfunction by echocardiography is an important diagnostic criterion. Chest radiograph will show an enlarged heart and pulmonary oedema.
- Intracardiac thrombus may develop with subsequent risk of thromboembolism to any site. This can occur in 25–40% of patients without anticoagulation and could result in acute MI, stroke (in 5%), pulmonary embolism, or lower limb ischaemia.
- Ventricular arrhythmias develop in 20% of PPCM.

Prognosis

- Outcome of patients with PPCM is highly variable.
  - Some deteriorate rapidly, developing endstage cardiac heart failure with poor response to medical therapy.
  - Others show swift improvement in both clinically and on ECHO imaging.
  - Still others have persistent evidence of cardiac dysfunction with slow return to normal cardiac function, taking several years.
- Patients with PPCM can show a reduction in cardiac function during subsequent pregnancies.[3]
- Symptoms of cardiac failure develop in 20% of women whose cardiac function was normal at the start of a subsequent pregnancy as well as in 50% of those who start a subsequent pregnancy with residual left ventricular dysfunction.[2,3]
- Frequency of premature birth and maternal mortality are higher in this group.

Management

- Treatment of pregnant women with PPCM is along the same lines as in other patients with heart failure.
- Treatment includes oxygen, adopting a sitting position, diamorphine, salt restriction, diuretics to reduce pulmonary oedema, and vasodilators such as hydralazine to reduce afterload.
- Iatrogenic preterm delivery may be required due to rapid cardiac decompensation. **Great care is required with steroids for acceleration of fetal lung maturity as they can cause further fluid overload.**
- ACE inhibitors are contraindicated in pregnancy but can be used postpartum for vasodilatation.
- PPCM poses increased risks for thromboembolism and anticoagulation prophylaxis is required with LMWH during pregnancy, switched to warfarin postpartum.
- Follow-up ECHO at 6 and 12 months after delivery is mandatory.

Contraception and subsequent pregnancy

- If cardiac dysfunction persists 6–12 months after the initial diagnosis of PPCM, this indicates irreversible damage **contraindicating subsequent pregnancy**. The patient must be advised not to consider another pregnancy and effective contraception or tubal ligation considered.
- Any subsequent pregnancy in women with a past history of PPCM is associated with significant deterioration of cardiac function, leading to clinical deterioration and even death.
- Effective contraception with levonorgestrel intrauterine system (Mirena®) or etonogestrel implant should be advised. Tubal ligation as a permanent method should also be discussed with the patient.

Information for patients

Please see Information for patients: Peripartum cardiomyopathy (p. 506)

References

1. Sliwa K, et al . Current state of knowledge on aetiology, diagnosis, management and therapy of peripartum cardiomyopathy: a position statement from the Heart Failure Association of the European Society of Cardiology working group on peripartum cardiomyopathy. Eur J Heart Fail 2010; 12: 767–768.
2. Blauwet LA, Sliwa K. Peripartum cardiomyopathy. Obstet Med 2011; 4: 44–52.
3. Elkayam U, et al. Maternal and fetal outcomes of subsequent pregnancies in women with peripartum cardiomyopathy. N Engl J Med 2001; 344: 1567–1571.
4. Adamson DL, et al. Cardiac disease in pregnancy. In:Greer I, et al., ed., Maternal medicine. London: Churchill Livingstone Elsevier, 2007.

CARE PATHWAY

- Given the rarity of **peripartum cardiomyopathy (PPCM)** and its variable clinical course, it is crucial that **a multidisciplinary care pathway is devised for an individual patient on a case-to-case basis**
- General pointers in the development of such an individualized care pathway should include not only immediate cardiac and pregnancy management but also clear documentation regarding plans for delivery, postpartum, and subsequent arrangements for cardiac follow-up
- Such care pathways should include advice about contraception and advance counselling before considering a future pregnancy. Such care plans must be easily accessible and shared with the patient and all concerned in the care of the woman in the hospital (DGH ± tertiary centre) and subsequently in primary care. This would include the cardiologist, maternal medicine obstetrician, intensive care specialist, anaesthetist, midwives, and neonatologist

↓

- By definition, pregnant patients who develop PPCM have no previous history of cardiac disease. Therefore, a high level of suspicion must be maintained if any pregnant woman unexpectedly develops any symptoms or signs of cardiac failure. Early diagnosis is essential to decrease maternal and resulting fetal mortality
- Signs of acute cardiac failure may be provoked in such patients by beta-mimetics (for tocolysis) or antenatal steroids used for fetal lung maturation
- Those at higher risk of PPCM are multips, multiple pregnancies, older mothers, or those of Afro-Caribbean origin
- Diagnosis is achieved by a process of exclusion
- Characteristic ECHO features of left ventricular dysfunction and dilatation of the heart are also accompanied by chest radiograph signs of cardiac enlargement and pulmonary oedema

↓

Immediate management

- Prompt multidisciplinary involvement by physicians (as listed above) and midwife
- Includes oxygen administration, sitting up the patient, diamorphine, diuretics, and hydralazine to achieve vasodilatation
- Hydralazine and nitrates to be used in combination to achieve vasodilatation instead of ACE inhibitors during pregnancy
- LMWH prophylaxis, weight-adjusted dosage, as well as digoxin for atrial fibrillation or flutter
- Preterm delivery may be necessary in the face of deteriorating cardiac function
- Great care with steroid prophylaxis as this can tip patient into further overload

↓

Planning for labour and delivery

- Antenatal anaesthetic review prior to time of delivery is highly advisable
- Labour and delivery best conducted in units with expertise in managing pregnancies with maternal cardiac disease
- Timing and mode of delivery depend on the haemodynamic state of the patient
- If the pregnant woman is clinically stable, no need for early delivery
- In such situations, awaiting spontaneous onset of labour is acceptable. **However, continuous cardiac monitoring, haemodynamic and fluid management may be easier to arrange with planned induction with the requisite senior personnel available on site**

↓

Intrapartum care

- Vaginal delivery with ventouse or forceps to cut short the second stage may be advisable
- Planned Caesarean section is the preferred mode of delivery in patients with haemodynamic instability to prevent further deterioration of cardiovascular status
- Spinal or epidural have been safely used for both labour and for Caesarean section
- Careful fluid volume management to prevent pulmonary oedema
- During a Caesarean section, sequential compression devices for the lower limbs must be applied
- **No ergometrine or syntometrine for third-stage management.** Oxytocin infusion following standard IM dose of 5 mg

↓

Post delivery and puerperium

- Thromboprophylaxis to be recommenced after delivery
- After delivery, ACE inhibitors can be used for afterload reduction and LMWH converted to warfarin
- To prevent the sudden significant pre-load expected after delivery, a diuretic such as furosemide given IV is advisable
- Post-delivery careful monitoring in ICU for a minimum of 24 h is highly advisable because of high risk for severe acute cardiopulmonary failure
- Breastfeeding is not advisable due to potential detrimental cardiac effects

↓

Follow-up and contraception

- Cardiology follow-up is essential, 1–2 weeks after delivery
- Good contraception, either Mirena® or etonogestrel implant, should be advised. COCP is contraindicated
- Postnatal follow-up in 8–12 weeks after delivery should involve further discussions regarding tubal ligation, Mirena®, or etonogestrel implant

↓

Pre-pregnancy advice before patient considers another pregnancy

- Even in women whose cardiac function has returned to normal within 6–12 months after delivery, 20% will still develop cardiac failure in a subsequent pregnancy
- In women whose left ventricular dysfunction has not returned to normal in 6–12 months, 50% will develop cardiac failure in a subsequent pregnancy with a 25% mortality rate. Pregnancy is to be strongly discouraged in such women

5 Maternal Hypertension

5.1 Hypertension in Pregnancy

FACT FILE

The scope of this chapter is mainly the **antenatal** management of **hypertensive diseases in pregnancy**, but as there is a continuum involved, reference has also been made to postnatal management and pre-pregnancy advice before a subsequent pregnancy.

Epidemiology and effects on pregnancy

- Hypertensive disorders affect 10–22%[1,2] of pregnancies and have been classified into four conditions to reflect potential aetiological differences and pregnancy outcomes:
  - chronic hypertension
  - gestational hypertension
  - pre-eclampsia–eclampsia
  - pre-eclampsia superimposed on chronic hypertension.
- Although the rate of eclampsia in the UK appears to have fallen, hypertension in pregnancy remains one of the leading causes of maternal death in the UK.[3]
- Hypertensive diseases during pregnancy are also associated with considerable maternal morbidity, particularly chronic hypertension and its consequences, as well as an increase in lifetime cardiovascular risk.[4,5,6]
- Pre-eclampsia affects about 5–8% of pregnancies. Chronic hypertension accounts for approximately 20% of the cases of high blood pressure seen in pregnancy.[1,2]
- Hypertensive disorders also carry significant risks for the baby. In the most recent UK perinatal mortality report, 1 in 20 (5%) **stillbirths** in infants without congenital abnormality occurred in women with pre-eclampsia.[7]
- The contribution of pre-eclampsia to the overall **preterm birth rate** is substantial.[4]
- 1 in 250 (0.4%) women in their first pregnancy will give birth before 34 weeks as a consequence of pre-eclampsia and 8–10% of all preterm births result from hypertensive disorders. Half of women with severe pre-eclampsia give birth preterm.
- Small-for-gestational-age (SGA) babies are common, mainly because of fetal growth restriction arising from placental disease. About 20–25% of preterm births and 14–19% of term babies in women with pre-eclampsia weigh less than the tenth centile of birth weight for gestation.

Reducing the risk of hypertensive disorders in pregnancy[4]

Aspirin prophylaxis

- Advise women at *high risk* of pre-eclampsia to take 75 mg of aspirin daily from 12 weeks until the birth of the baby.
  - **Women at high risk:**
  - hypertensive disease during a previous pregnancy
  - chronic kidney disease
  - autoimmune disease such as systemic lupus erythematosus or antiphospholipid syndrome
  - type 1 or type 2 diabetes
  - chronic hypertension
- Advise women with **more than one moderate risk factor** for pre-eclampsia to take 75 mg of aspirin daily from 12 weeks until the birth of the baby.
  - **Women at moderate risk:**
  - first pregnancy
  - age 40 years or older
  - pregnancy interval of more than 10 years
  - body mass index (BMI) of 35 kg/m^2 or more at first visit
  - family history of pre-eclampsia
  - multiple pregnancy.

Highlighting awareness of symptoms

- Pregnant women should be made aware of the need to seek immediate advice from a healthcare professional if they experience symptoms of pre-eclampsia. Symptoms include:
  - severe headache
  - problems with vision, such as blurring or flashing before the eyes
  - severe pain just below the ribs
  - vomiting
  - sudden swelling of the face, hands, or feet.

Lifestyle interventions

- Advice regarding rest, exercise, healthy diet, etc.

Unnecessary interventions

- There is no evidence for the use of nitric oxide donors, progesterone, diuretics, or low molecular weight heparin to prevent hypertensive disorders in pregnancy.
- There is no evidence that any of the following nutritional supplements can prevent hypertensive disorders in pregnancy.
  - magnesium
  - folic acid
  - anti-oxidants (vitamins C and E)
  - fish or algal oil
  - garlic.

Assessment of proteinuria

- Use an automated reagent-strip reading device or a spot urinary protein:creatinine ratio to estimate proteinuria in secondary care.[4]
- If an automated reagent-strip reading device shows proteinuria 1+ or more, use a spot urinary protein:creatinine ratio or 24-h urine collection to quantify proteinuria.
- Diagnose significant proteinuria if urinary protein:creatinine ratio greater than 30 mg/mmol or a validated 24-hour urine collection result shows more than 300 mg protein.
- Where 24-h urine collection is used to quantify proteinuria, there should be a recognized method of evaluating completeness of the sample.

Chronic hypertension

- Chronic hypertension is diagnosed when hypertension is confirmed before pregnancy or before 20 weeks gestation (blood pressure >140 mmHg systolic and/or >90 mmHg diastolic).[8]
- However, chronic hypertension is frequently diagnosed when high blood pressure fails to resolve postpartum.
- Women with chronic hypertension require careful monitoring during pregnancy as they have an increased risk of adverse events, including superimposed pre-eclampsia, placental abruption, fetal growth restriction, premature delivery, and stillbirth.[8]
- Pre-pregnancy counselling and management of chronic hypertension is essential. Some commonly prescribed antihypertensive drugs are contraindicated or best avoided during pregnancy (Table 5.1). These include angiotensin converting enzyme (ACE) inhibitors, angiotensin receptor antagonists (ARBs), diuretics, and most beta-blockers.

Table 5.1 Antihypertensive drugs to avoid pre-conception and in pregnancy

Antihypertensive	*Advice*	*Potential adverse effects*
ACE inhibitors	Contraindicated	Teratogenic in 1st trimester Fetal renal dysfunction, skull hypoplasia, oligohydramnios, etc. in 2nd and 3rd trimesters
Angiotensin receptor blockers	Contraindicated	Teratogenic in 1st trimester Fetal renal dysfunction and oligohydramnios in 2nd and 3rd trimester
Diuretics	Avoid, if possible	Fetal electrolyte disturbances, reduction in maternal blood volume
Beta-blockers (except labetalol)	Avoid	Fetal bradycardia; also long-term use of atenolol associated with fetal growth restriction
Calcium channel antagonists (except nifedipine)	Avoid	Maternal hypotension and fetal hypoxia

Management of pregnancy with chronic hypertension

- Before starting a pregnancy, women with chronic hypertension on ACE inhibitors, angiotensin II receptor blockers (ARBs) or chlorothiazide, must be advised to have their antihypertensive agents changed to those that are safe during pregnancy (Table 5.2).
- Antihypertensive treatment in women taking ACE inhibitors, ARBs and/or chlorothiazide diuretics must be changed to alternatives such as methyldopa or labetalol, if they become pregnant (preferably within 2 working days of notification of pregnancy).[4]
- If ACE inhibitors are used at any gestation during pregnancy there are increased rates of congenital malformations, IUGR, hypoglycaemia, kidney disease, and preterm birth.
- Studies of the use of ARBs in pregnancy also showed unfavourable outcomes (mainly congenital malformations) and fetal renal damage.
- Chlorothiazide may carry the risk of congenital abnormality, neonatal thrombocytopenia, hypoglycaemia, and hypovolaemia.
- Antihypertensive treatments other than ACE inhibitors, ARBs, or chlorothiazide have not shown an increased risk of congenital malformation with such treatments.
- The aim in the management of pregnant women with chronic hypertension is to keep the blood pressure consistently lower than 150/100 mmHg.
- While there is no direct evidence that continued treatment of chronic hypertension leads to a reduction in the risk of adverse pregnancy events,[3] there is much benefit in reducing severe hypertension to 160 mmHg systolic and/or 100 mmHg diastolic or less on more than one occasion.[8]
- Blood pressure reduction to 140–160 mmHg systolic and 90–100 mmHg diastolic is an acceptable treatment goal in the management of chronic hypertension in pregnant women with uncomplicated chronic hypertension.
- Stricter blood pressure control may be associated with fetal growth restriction, presumed to be related to relative placental hypoperfusion. Treatment to lower the diastolic blood pressure to below 80 mmHg is not necessary.
- If there is target-organ damage secondary to chronic hypertension, however (e.g. kidney disease). treatment should aim to keep the blood pressure lower than 140/90 mmHg.
- In those with secondary chronic hypertension need to be referred to a specialist in hypertensive disorders (nephrologist or endocrinologist, if relevant).
- There is insufficient evidence to support the practical value of uterine artery Dopplers at 24 weeks gestation in women with chronic hypertension, who are already advised to take aspirin during pregnancy.
- Encourage women with chronic hypertension to keep their dietary sodium intake low, either by reducing or substituting sodium salt, because this can reduce blood pressure.
- Offer low-dose aspirin 75 mg/day to women with chronic hypertension who are pregnant, starting from about 12 weeks gestation, continued till the end of pregnancy.
- The frequency of antenatal clinic visits for women with chronic hypertension needs to be adapted with additional antenatal consultations scheduled based on the individual needs of the woman and her baby.
- Importantly, women need to be carefully monitored for any signs of pre-eclampsia which may include worsening hypertension and new or worsening proteinuria.
- Serial assessment of fetal well-being and growth should be performed; the frequency of monitoring should be individualized and influenced by the common association of intrauterine growth restriction in such cases.

Fetal monitoring in chronic hypertension

- In women with chronic hypertension, ultrasound fetal growth and amniotic fluid volume assessment and umbilical artery Doppler velocimetry is recommended between 28 and 30 weeks and between 32 and 34 weeks. If these are normal, there is no need to repeat scanning later than 34 weeks, unless otherwise clinically indicated.
- In women with chronic hypertension, cardiotocography is indicated only if fetal activity is abnormal.
- For women with chronic hypertension whose blood pressure has remained lower than 160/110 mmHg with or without antihypertensive treatment, delivery must be considered after 37 weeks with input from the senior obstetrician.
- In women with refractory severe chronic hypertension, delivery before 37 weeks may be required after prophylactic steroids have been given.

Postnatal management in women with chronic hypertension

- Measure blood pressure:
  - daily for the first 2 days after birth
  - at least once between day 3 and day 5 after birth
  - as clinically indicated if antihypertensive treatment is changed after birth.
- In women with chronic hypertension who have given birth, aim to keep blood pressure lower than 140/90 mmHg.

Table 5.2 Relatively safe antihypertensives to use in pregnancy

Antihypertensive	*Class*	*Starting dose*	*Maximum dose*	*Important adverse effects*
Labetalol	Beta-blocker	100–200 mg twice a day	400 mg three times a day	Bradycardia, bronchospasm
Methyldopa	Centrally acting	250 mg twice a day	500 mg four times a day	Headache, lethargy, sedation, light-headedness, dry mouth, nasal congestion, haemolytic anaemia, depression
Nifedipine	Calcium channel antagonist	10 mg twice a day 30 mg daily controlled release	20–40 mg twice a day 120 mg daily controlled release	Severe headache, peripheral oedema
Hydralazine	Vasodilator	25 mg twice a day	50–200 mg total daily dose	Flushing, headache, lupus-like syndrome
Oxprenolol	Beta-blocker	40–80 mg twice daily	80–160 mg twice daily	Bradycardia, bronchospasm

- In women with chronic hypertension who have given birth:
  - Continue antenatal antihypertensive treatment if on labetalol or nifedipine.
  - If a woman has taken methyldopa to treat chronic hypertension during pregnancy, stop within 2 days of birth and restart the antihypertensive treatment the woman was taking before she planned the pregnancy.
  - Review long-term antihypertensive treatment 2 weeks after the birth, usually in primary care.
- Ideally, a medical review (postnatal review) 6–8 weeks after the birth must be performed in primary care by the GP. This also provides also an opportunity to discuss pre-pregnancy BP control before the next pregnancy and long-term implications and monitoring of chronic hypertension.

Gestational hypertension

- Gestational hypertension is defined as:
  - new onset of hypertension after 20 weeks gestation
  - no other features to suggest pre-eclampsia
  - normalization of blood pressure within 3 months postpartum.

Management of pregnancy with gestational hypertension

- In women with gestational hypertension, full assessment should be carried out in a secondary care setting by a healthcare professional who is trained in the management of hypertensive disorders.
- In women with gestational hypertension, the following risk factors require additional assessment and follow-up:
  - nulliparity
  - age 40 years or older
  - pregnancy interval of more than 10 years
  - family history of pre-eclampsia
  - multiple pregnancy
  - BMI of 35 kg/m^2 or more
  - gestational age at presentation
  - previous history of pre-eclampsia or gestational hypertension
  - pre-existing vascular disease
  - pre-existing kidney disease
- *Gestational hypertension is associated with adverse pregnancy outcomes*. These are more common if it presents earlier in the pregnancy, if it progresses to pre-eclampsia, or if hypertension is severe (≥170/110 mmHg).[8]
- In women with gestational hypertension, the antihypertensive of choice is labetalol, followed by methyldopa and nifedipine.
- In women with **severe** gestational hypertension, stabilization has to be achieved as an in-patient in hospital; outpatient monitoring can then continue with blood pressure and urine examination twice weekly with weekly blood tests.
- In women with mild hypertension presenting before 32 weeks, or at high risk of pre-eclampsia, measure blood pressure and test urine twice weekly.
- Bed rest in hospital as a treatment for gestational hypertension has been proven to be unnecessary and ineffective.[1]
- The benefits of treating mild to moderate hypertension are limited to the prevention of severe hypertension and appear to have no effect on the potential for adverse pregnancy outcomes.
- The indications for treatment with antihypertensive drugs, goals of therapy, and the choice of drug are similar to the treatment of chronic hypertension in pregnancy (discussed earlier in the chapter).
- Up to 25% of women who develop hypertension in pregnancy will eventually be diagnosed with pre-eclampsia, even if no other manifestations are present initially.
- Regular monitoring of blood pressure, and investigation for proteinuria and other features of pre-eclampsia (up to once or twice per week) is reasonable.

Fetal monitoring in gestational hypertension

Mild or moderate gestational hypertension

- Ultrasound scan for fetal growth and amniotic fluid volume assessment and umbilical artery Doppler velocimetry if gestation is less than 34 weeks. If results are normal, there is no need to repeat after 34 weeks, unless otherwise clinically indicated.[4]
- Do not carry out ultrasound fetal growth and amniotic fluid volume assessment and umbilical artery Doppler velocimetry if diagnosis is confirmed after 34 weeks, unless otherwise clinically indicated.
- Only carry out cardiotocography if fetal activity is abnormal.

Severe gestational hypertension or pre-eclampsia

- Cardiotocography at diagnosis of severe gestational hypertension or pre-eclampsia
- If conservative management of severe gestational hypertension or pre-eclampsia is planned, ultrasound fetal growth and amniotic fluid volume assessment as well as umbilical artery Doppler velocimetry are to be performed at diagnosis.
- If the results of all fetal monitoring are normal in women with severe gestational hypertension or pre-eclampsia, there is no need to repeat cardiotocography more than weekly.
- In women with severe gestational hypertension or pre-eclampsia, repeat cardiotocography if any of the following occur:
  - the woman reports a change in fetal movement
  - vaginal bleeding
  - abdominal pain
  - deterioration in maternal condition.
- In women with severe gestational hypertension or pre-eclampsia, do not routinely repeat ultrasound fetal growth and amniotic fluid volume assessment or umbilical artery Doppler velocimetry more than every 2 weeks.
- If the results of any fetal monitoring in women with severe gestational hypertension or pre-eclampsia are abnormal, the consultant obstetrician needs to be informed without delay.
- For women with severe gestational hypertension or pre-eclampsia, **a care plan that includes all of the following** needs to be documented by the senior obstetrician:
  - the timing and nature of further fetal monitoring
  - indications for delivery and if and when corticosteroids should be given
  - when discussion with neonatal paediatricians and obstetric anaesthetists should take place and what decisions should be made.

Timing of birth

- For women with gestational hypertension whose blood pressure is lower than 160/110 mmHg with or without antihypertensive treatment delivery needs to be organized after 37 weeks.
- For those with severe refractory gestational hypertension, delivery may be required after a course of prophylactic steroids—delivery must be offered.[8]
- By definition, gestational hypertension should resolve within 3 months postpartum.
- The patient can generally be weaned off antihypertensive drugs within weeks. If hypertension has not resolved within 3 months, an alternative diagnosis such as chronic (essential or potentially secondary) hypertension needs to be considered.
- There is a risk of recurrence in subsequent pregnancies, so increased monitoring will be required.
- For women with gestational hypertension who did not take antenatal antihypertensive treatment and have given birth, start antihypertensive treatment if their blood pressure is higher than 149/99 mmHg.
- **Document a care plan** for women with gestational hypertension who have given birth and are being transferred to community care that includes all of the following:
  - who will provide follow-up care, including medical review if needed
  - frequency of blood pressure monitoring needed
  - thresholds for reducing or stopping treatment
  - indications for referral to primary care for blood pressure review.

Pre-eclampsia

For features of pre-eclampsia, see *Box 5.1*.

- The aetiology of pre-eclampsia is unclear. It is a disorder with many manifestations.

Box 5.1 Features of pre-eclampsia

- Hypertension, with onset after 20 weeks gestation
- Renal manifestations
- Significant proteinuria
- Serum creatinine >90 micromol/litre (or renal failure)
- Oliguria
- Haematological manifestations
- Disseminated intravascular coagulation
- Thrombocytopenia
- Haemolysis
- Hepatic manifestations
- Raised serum transaminases
- Severe right upper quadrant or epigastric pain
- Neurological manifestations
- Eclamptic seizure
- Hyperreflexia with sustained clonus
- Severe headache
- Persistent visual disturbances
- Stroke
- Pulmonary oedema
- Fetal growth restriction
- Abruptio placenta

- Pre-eclampsia can be associated with fetal growth restriction, preterm delivery, placental abruption, and perinatal death.[7] Severe pre-eclampsia has the potential for progression to eclampsia, multiorgan failure, severe haemorrhage, and rarely maternal mortality.
- New-onset hypertension after 20 weeks gestation and proteinuria are the most common presenting features. A urine dipstick for proteinuria can be a useful screening test, but is confounded by high false-positive and false-negative rates. If there is any uncertainty, assessment of the urine protein:creatinine ratio is advised.
- Peripheral oedema is no longer considered a diagnostic feature of pre-eclampsia as it is neither a sensitive nor a specific sign. Other clinical manifestations are outlined in Box 5.1, with their presence suggesting severe pre-eclampsia.
- The **presence of severe pre-eclampsia mandates urgent review**.
- A multidisciplinary team approach (obstetrician, midwife, anaesthetist, and neonatologist) is often required.
- ***Delivery is the only definitive management for pre-eclampsia.***
- Although pre-eclampsia progressively worsens while the pregnancy continues, outpatient management may be considered in selected cases.
- The timing of delivery is dependent on the gestational age and well-being of the fetus and the severity of the pre-eclampsia. The pregnancy is rarely allowed to go to term.
- Severe hypertension may require parenteral antihypertensive drugs (such as hydralazine), which should only be given in a suitably monitored environment (birth suite or high-dependency unit).
- IV magnesium sulfate is given for the prevention of eclampsia in severe cases.[9]
- The antihypertensive drugs used in pre-eclampsia are the same as those used to treat chronic and gestational hypertension (see *Table 5.2*).
- The treatment goals for blood pressure control are also the same (140–160 mmHg systolic and 90–100 mmHg diastolic).
- Although it was widely advised in the past, there is little evidence to support bed rest. Given the potential for venous thromboembolism from immobilization, bed rest is generally only advised with severe, uncontrolled hypertension.[10]
- Only offer women with pre-eclampsia antihypertensive treatment other than labetalol after considering side-effect profiles for the woman, fetus, and newborn baby. Alternatives include methyldopa and nifedipine.

Fetal monitoring in pre-eclampsia or women at high risk of pre-eclampsia

- Ultrasound fetal growth and amniotic fluid volume assessment, and umbilical artery Doppler velocimetry starting at between 28 and 30 weeks (or at least 2 weeks before previous gestational age of onset if earlier than 28 weeks) and repeating 4 weeks later in women with previous:
  - severe pre-eclampsia
  - pre-eclampsia that needed birth before 34 weeks
  - pre-eclampsia with a baby whose birth weight was less than the 10th centile
  - intrauterine death
  - placental abruption.
- In women who are at high risk of pre-eclampsia only carry out cardiotocography if fetal activity is abnormal.

Timing of birth

- Manage pregnancy in women with pre-eclampsia conservatively (that is, do not plan same-day delivery of the baby) until 34 weeks.[4,11]
- Consultant obstetrician should document maternal (biochemical, haematological, and clinical) and fetal thresholds for elective delivery before 34 weeks in women with pre-eclampsia.
- The consultant obstetrician should document a plan for antenatal and intrapartum fetal monitoring during birth.
- Plan delivery before 34 weeks, after discussion with the mother, neonatal and anaesthetic teams and a course of corticosteroids has been given if:
  - severe hypertension develops refractory to treatment
  - maternal or fetal indications develop as specified in the consultant plan.
- In women with pre-eclampsia and severe hypertension after 34 weeks, plan delivery when the blood pressure has been controlled and a course of corticosteroids has been completed (if appropriate).
- Plan delivery in women who have pre-eclampsia with mild or moderate hypertension at 34+0 to 36+6 weeks depending on maternal and fetal condition, risk factors, and availability of neonatal intensive care.
- Plan delivery within 24–48 h for women who have pre-eclampsia with mild or moderate hypertension after 37+0 weeks.

Postpartum management and secondary prevention

- Most of the manifestations of pre-eclampsia resolve within the first few days or weeks postpartum.
- Rarely, the first manifestations occur postpartum. Frequent review of blood pressure during this period is essential, for example once to twice weekly.[12]
- Blood pressure In women with pre-eclampsia who did not take antihypertensive treatment and have given birth, measure blood pressure:
  - at least four times a day while the woman is an in-patient
  - at least once between day 3 and day 5 after birth
  - on alternate days until normal if blood pressure was abnormal on days 3–5.
- In women with pre-eclampsia who have not received antihypertensive treatment and have now delivered, start antihypertensive treatment if blood pressure is 150/100 mmHg or higher.
- Enquire about severe headache and epigastric pain each time blood pressure is measured.
- In women with pre-eclampsia who have received antihypertensive treatment and have now delivered, measure blood pressure:
  - at least four times a day while the woman is an in-patient
  - every 1–2 days for up to 2 weeks after transfer to community care until the woman is off treatment and has no hypertension.
- Continue antenatal antihypertensive treatment if on labetalol.
- If she has been on methyldopa to treat pre-eclampsia, change antihypertensive within 2 postnatal days

- Reduce antihypertensive treatment if blood pressure falls below 130–140/80–90 mmHg
- Discharge a post natal woman who has had severe pre-eclampsia to community care if all of the following criteria have been met:
  - there are no symptoms of pre-eclampsia
  - blood pressure, with or without treatment, is 149/99 mm Hg or lower
  - blood test results are stable or improving.
- A **postnatal discharge care plan** should include all of the following:
  - who will provide follow-up care, including medical review if needed
  - frequency of blood pressure monitoring
  - thresholds for reducing or stopping treatment
  - indications for referral to primary care for blood pressure review
  - self-monitoring for symptoms
- Those still on antihypertensive treatment 2 weeks after transfer to community care need medical review by the GP.
- Offer all women who have had severe pre-eclampsia/eclampsia a medical review at the postnatal review (6–8 weeks post-delivery). If the blood pressure does not normalize within 6–8 weeks and antihypertensive treatment is still required at the postnatal review, consider an alternative diagnosis. It is also important to confirm that proteinuria has resolved.
- Referral to a hypertension specialist for reconsideration of the original diagnosis may be necessary in some instances.

Pre-pregnancy advice before a subsequent pregnancy

- Advise the women that that their risk of developing gestational hypertension in a future pregnancy ranges from about 1 in 8 (13%) to about 1 in 2 (53%).
- In otherwise uncomplicated mild to moderate pre-eclampsia, the risk of recurrence in a future pregnancy is up to about 1 in 6 (16%).
- If the previous pregnancy was complicated by severe pre-eclampsia, HELLP syndrome, or eclampsia and led to birth before 34 weeks, the risk of recurrence in a future pregnancy is about 1 in 4 (25%).
- If their pre-eclampsia was complicated by severe pre-eclampsia, and if it led to birth before 28 weeks, the risk of recurrence is as high as 1 in 2 (55%).
- Advise weight loss if obese.
- Remind women on ACE inhibitors, ARBs, statins, or diuretics that these medications need to be changed while planning a pregnancy or as soon as a pregnancy is established.
- Low-dose aspirin from 12 weeks of a future pregnancy up to delivery.

Long-term follow-up

- Pre-eclampsia and gestational hypertension appear to be associated with an increased long-term risk of cardiovascular disease, including hypertension, ischaemic heart disease, stroke, and venous thromboembolism. There may also be a small increased risk of chronic renal failure and thyroid dysfunction after pre-eclampsia.[5,6]
- Annual assessments of blood pressure and at least 5-yearly assessments for other cardiovascular risk factors are advisable.[8]
- Thyroid and renal function should also be measured intermittently.
- **For further details, refer to the NICE guidelines.**[13,14]

Information for patients

Please see Information for patients: High blood pressure (hypertension) and pregnancy (p. 506)

References

1. ACOG Committee on Obstetric Practice. Clinical management guidelines for obstetrician-gynecologists. Diagnosis and management of preeclampsia and eclampsia. ACOG Practice Bulletin 2002; 33: 1–9. <http://mail.ny.acog.org/website/SMIPodcast/DiagnosisMgt.pdf> [cited 2012 Mar 6]
2. Brown MA, et al. The classification and diagnosis of the hypertensive disorders of pregnancy: statement from the International Society for the Study of Hypertension in Pregnancy (ISSHP). Hypertens Pregnancy 2001; 20: IX–XIV.
3. Cantwell R, et al. Saving mothers' lives: reviewing maternal deaths to make motherhood safer: 2006-2008. The Eighth Report of the Confidential Enquiries into Maternal Deaths in the United Kingdom. BJOG 2011; 118 Suppl 1: 1–203.
4. National Collaborating Centre for Women's and Children's Health. Hypertension in pregnancy: the management of hypertensive disorders during pregnancy. NICE Clinical Guideline 2010 (revised reprint January 2011). London: Royal College of Obstetricians and Gynaecologists.
5. Bellamy L, et al. Pre-eclampsia and risk of cardiovascular disease and cancer in later life: systematic review and meta-analysis. BMJ 2007; 335: 974.
6. Vikse BE, et al. Preeclampsia and the risk of end-stage renal disease. N Engl J Med 2008; 359: 800–809.
7. Centre for Maternal and Child Enquiries (CMACE). Perinatal Mortality 2009: United Kingdom. London: CMACE, 2011.
8. Lowe SA, et al. Guidelines for the management of hypertensive disorders of pregnancy 2008. Aust N Z J Obstet Gynaecol 2009; 49: 242–246.
9. Sibai BM. Magnesium sulfate prophylaxis in preeclampsia: evidence from randomized trials. Clin Obstet Gynecol 2005; 48: 478–488.
10. Meher S, et al. Bed rest with or without hospitalisation for hypertension during pregnancy. Cochrane Database Syst Rev 2005; 19: CD003514.
11. Ferguson S, et al. Timing of indicated delivery after antenatal steroids in preterm pregnancies with severe hypertension. Hypertens Pregnancy 2009; 28: 63–75.
12. Milne F, et al. The pre-eclampsia community guideline (PRECOG): how to screen for and detect onset of pre-eclampsia in the community. BMJ 2005; 330: 576–580.
13. National Institute for Health and Care Excellence (NICE). Hypertension in pregnancy: the management of hypertensive disorders during pregnancy. CG 107. London: NICE, 2010. Revised reprint 2011.
14. National Institute for Health and Care Excellence (NICE). Hypertension in pregnancy overview <http://pathways.nice.org.uk/pathways/hypertension-in-pregnancy>.

CARE PATHWAY

Management of chronic hypertension in pregnancy

Pre-pregnancy advice

Antihypertensive treatment

- Inform women who are taking ACE inhibitors, ARBs or chlorothiazide:
  - ***There is an increased risk of congenital abnormalities and neonatal complications if ACE inhibitors, ARBs, or chlorothiazides are taken during pregnancy***
  - Limited evidence shows no increased risk of congenital abnormalities with other antihypertensive treatments
  - To discuss alternative antihypertensive medications with the healthcare professional responsible for managing their hypertension, if they are planning pregnancy
- **Dietary sodium:** Encourage the woman to lower dietary sodium intake or use a sodium substitute

Antenatal care

- Early referral from community in 1st trimester
- Prescribe low-dose aspirin from 12 weeks gestation till end of pregnancy
- Arrange regular BP monitoring and urine analysis in the community and hospital, at individualized frequencies as directed by response to medication
- Schedule additional appointments based on individual needs of mother and fetus

Timing of delivery

- If BP <160/110 mmHg with or without antihypertensive treatment, defer delivery till after 37 weeks, if no additional complications
- After 37 weeks, plan timing of delivery after discussion with patient depending on maternal and fetal indications
- If refractory severe chronic hypertension or development of complications before 37 weeks, offer delivery after course of corticosteroids (if required) has been completed.

Antihypertensive management

- Stop ACE inhibitors and ARBs within 2 days of notification of pregnancy and offer alternatives
- Offer antihypertensive treatment based on pre-existing treatment, side-effect profile, and teratogenicity
- Aim for BP <150/100 mmHg
- If target organ damage, aim for BP <140/90 mmHg
- Avoid treatment to lower DBP to < 80 mmHg
- If secondary chronic hypertension, offer referral to specialist in hypertensive disorders

Fetal monitoring

- *At 28–30 and 32–34 weeks:*
  - ultrasound fetal growth and amniotic fluid volume assessment
  - umbilical artery Doppler velocimetry
- **If these results normal**, no need to repeat after 34 weeks unless clinically indicated
- **If fetal movements are abnormal**, carry out cardiotocography

Postnatal care for chronic hypertension

Antihypertensive treatment

- Aim to keep BP <140/90 mmHg
- Measure BP:
  - daily for first 2 days after birth
  - at least once 3–5 days after birth
  - as clinically indicated if antihypertensive treatment has been changed
- If methyldopa was used during pregnancy, stop within 2 days of birth and restart pre-pregnancy antihypertensive treatment
- Continue antenatal hypertensive treatment

Breastfeeding

- ***Avoid diuretics***
- Inform women that the following drugs have no known adverse effects on babies receiving breast milk:
  - labetalol
  - nifedipine
  - enalapril
  - captopril
  - atenolol
  - metoprolol
- Inform women that there is insufficient evidence on the safety of the following drugs in babies receiving breast milk:
  - ARBs
  - amlodipine
  - ACE inhibitors other than enalapril and captopril
- Assess clinical wellbeing of baby, especially adequacy of feeding, at least daily for first 2 days after birth

Follow-up care

- Review long-term treatment 2 weeks after birth
- A medical review at 6–8 week postnatal review with GP or hospital physician who was supervising anti-hypertensive control before her pregnancy

Reproduced from: National Collaborating Centre for Women and Children's Health/NICE. Hypertension in Pregnancy. Clinical Guideline No. 107. London: RCOG; 2010, with the permission of the Royal College of Obstetricians and Gynaecologists

Antenatal management of gestational hypertension

Referral from primary care or gestational hypertension detected in hospital

- Carry out full assessment in secondary care. A healthcare professional trained in the management of hypertensive disorders should carry out the assessment
- Take into account previous history of pre-eclampsia or gestational hypertension, pre-existing vascular or kidney disease, moderate risk factors for pre-eclampsia, and gestational age at presentation

Mild hypertension (BP 140/90–149/99 mmHg)

- Do not admit to hospital routinely
- No need to treat hypertension (decision to be made at senior level)
- Measure BP once a week: more frequently if proteinuria develops
- Test for proteinuria at each visit using an automated reagent-strip reading device or urinary protein:creatinine ratio
- Carry out routine antenatal blood tests
- If presenting before 32 weeks or at high risk of pre-eclampsia, test for proteinuria and measure BP 2 times a week

Moderate hypertension (BP 150/100–159/109 mmHg)

- Senior review needed to admit to hospital, do not admit routinely
- Treat with first-line oral labetalol to keep BP <150/80–100 mmHg
- Measure BP at least 2 times a week
- Test for proteinuria at each visit using an automated reagent-strip reading device or urinary protein:creatinine ratio
- Test kidney function, electrolytes, FBC, transaminases, bilirubin
- No further blood tests if no subsequent proteinuria

Severe hypertension (BP ≥160/110 mmHg)

- Admit to hospital for BP control
- Advice against total bed rest while in hospital
- Treat with first-line oral labetalol to keep BP <150/80–100 mmHg
- Measure BP at least 4 times a day.
- Test for proteinuria every day using an automated reagent strip reading device or urinary protein:creatinine ratio
- Test kidney function, electrolytes, FBC, transaminases, bilirubin at presentation and then monitor weekly in Day Assessment Unit

Fetal monitoring

If diagnosis of mild/moderate gestational hypertension confirmed before 34 weeks:

- Ultrasound fetal growth and amniotic fluid volume assessment
- Umbilical artery Doppler velocimetry
- If these results are normal, no need to repeat after 34 weeks, unless complications develop
- If fetal activity abnormal, perform cardiotocography

In women receiving outpatient care after severe hypertension has been effectively controlled in hospital:

- Measure BP and test for proteinuria 2 times a week
- Carry out blood tests weekly

Timing of birth

- Routine induction/ delivery unnecessary before 37 weeks
- After 37 weeks, timing of delivery, depending on maternal and fetal indications, discussed with patient by senior obstetrician
- If refractory severe gestational hypertension, offer delivery after course of corticosteroids (if required) is completed

Fetal monitoring in severe gestational hypertension

At diagnosis

- **Ultrasound fetal growth+ amniotic fluid volume + umbilical artery Doppler velocimetry** (if conservative management planned).
- No need to repeat more than every 2 weeks.
- **Cardiotocography**: Repeat if any:
  - change in fetal movement
  - vaginal bleeding
  - abdominal pain
  - deterioration in maternal condition.
- Do not repeat more than weekly if results of all fetal monitoring normal.

Document clear care plan

- Timing and nature of future fetal monitoring
- Fetal indications for birth if and when antenatal steroids should be given
- When discussion with neonatologists and obstetric anaesthetists should take place and what decisions should be made

- If results of any fetal monitoring are abnormal, **inform consultant obstetrician without delay**

Postnatal care for gestational hypertension

- Continue antenatal antihypertensive treatment **except** if methyldopa was used during pregnancy, stop within 2 days of birth and change to alternative antihypertensive
- If no antenatal antihypertensive treatment, start antihypertensive treatment if BP ≥150/100 mmHg.
- Measure BP:
  - daily for first 2 days after birth
  - at least once 3–5 days after birth
  - as clinically indicated if antihypertensive treatment has been changed
- If BP falls to <140/90 mmHg, consider reducing antihypertensive treatment
- If BP falls to <130/80 mmHg, reduce antihypertensive treatment

↓

If the mother is breastfeeding:

- Avoid diuretics
- Inform her that the following drugs have no known adverse effects on babies receiving breast milk:
  - labetalol
  - nifedipine
  - enalapril
  - captopril
  - atenolol
  - metoprolol
- Inform her that there is insufficient evidence on the safety of the following drugs in babies receiving breast milk:
  - ARBs
  - amlodipine
  - ACE inhibitors other than enalapril and captopril
- Assess clinical wellbeing of baby, especially adequacy of feeding, at least daily for first 2 days after birth

↓

Follow-up care

- At transfer to community care, clear documentation of a care plan that includes:
  - who will provide follow-up care, including medical review if needed
  - frequency of BP monitoring
  - thresholds for reducing or stopping treatment
  - indications for referral to primary care for BP review
- If antihypertensive treatment is to be continued, GP medical review 2 weeks after transfer to community care
- GP medical review at 6–8 week postnatal review
- If antihypertensive treatment is to be continued after 6–8 week postnatal review, referral from primary care for specialist assessment of hypertension may be required

Antenatal management of pre-eclampsia

- Referral from community or self- referral to the hospital; a healthcare professional trained and experienced in management of hypertensive disorders of pregnancy should assess the woman at each consultation
- Admit the woman to hospital
- Do not repeat quantification of proteinuria
- Carry out fetal monitoring

Mild hypertension (BP 140/90–149/99 mmHg)
- Do not treat hypertension
- Measure BP at least 4 times a day
- Test kidney function, electrolytes, FBC, transaminases, bilirubin twice a week

Moderate hypertension (BP 150/100–159/109 mmHg)
- Treat with first-line oral labetalol to keep BP <150 /80–100 mmHg.
- Measure BP at least 4 times a day
- Test kidney function, electrolytes, FBC, transaminases, bilirubin 3 times a week

Severe hypertension (BP ≥160/110 mmHg)

Is referral to level 2 critical care required?

- Yes: Multidisciplinary input—admit to level 2 critical care

- No:
- Treat with first-line oral labetalol to keep BP <150 /80–100 mmHg
- Measure BP more than 4 times a day depending on clinical circumstances
- Test kidney function, electrolytes, FBC, transaminases, bilirubin 3 times a week.

Fetal monitoring

Ultrasound
- Fetal growth and amniotic fluid volume assessment + umbilical artery Doppler velocimetry
- Perform initially when pre-eclampsia diagnosed and if conservative management is planned
- Do not repeat more than every 2 weeks unless complications develop

- If any results of fetal monitoring are abnormal, the consultant obstetrician needs to be informed

Cardiotocography
- Perform when pre-eclampsia first diagnosed
- Repeat if any:
  - change in fetal movements
  - vaginal bleeding
  - abdominal pain
  - deterioration in maternal condition

- CTG needs to be repeated only once a week if results of all fetal monitoring are normal

Care plan

Document a care plan that includes:
- Timing and nature of future fetal monitoring
- Fetal indications for birth
- If and when antenatal steroids should be given
- When discussions with neonatal paediatricians and obstetric anaesthetists should take place and what decisions should be made

Timing of birth

Before 34 weeks
- Manage conservatively (do not routinely plan same-day delivery of baby)
- Consultant obstetrician to:
  - document maternal (biochemical, haematological, and clinical) and fetal indications for elective birth before 34 weeks
  - write plan for antenatal fetal monitoring
- Plan delivery, after discussion with woman, neonatal and anaesthetic teams and, if required, after course of corticosteroids, if:
  - severe refractory hypertension
  - maternal or fetal clinical indication develops as defined in plan

34^{+0}–36^{+6} weeks
- Advise delivery after 34 weeks if pre-eclampsia with severe hypertension, BP controlled and, if required, course of antenatal steroids completed.
- Plan delivery at 34^{+0}–36^{+6} weeks if pre-eclampsia with mild or moderate hypertension, depending on maternal and fetal condition, risk factors and availability of neonatal intensive care.

After 37^{+0} weeks
- Recommend birth within 24–48 h if pre-eclampsia with mild or moderate hypertension.

Reproduced from: National Collaborating Centre for Women and Children's Health/NICE. Hypertension in Pregnancy. Clinical Guideline No. 107. London: RCOG; 2010, with the permission of the Royal College of Obstetricians and Gynaecologists

Postnatal care and follow-up in pre-eclampsia

- If methyldopa used to treat pre-eclampsia, stop within 2 days of birth
- Ask the woman about severe headache and epigastric pain each time BP measured
- If mild or moderate pre-eclampsia or after stepdown from critical care, measure platelet count, transaminases, and serum creatinine 48–72 h after birth or stepdown. Repeat as clinically indicated
- Do not repeat if results normal
- Do not measure fluid balance if creatinine within normal range after stepdown from critical care level 2
- Offer transfer to community midwifery care if BP <150/100 mmHg, blood test results stable or improving, and no symptoms of preeclampsia
- Discuss and document suitable contraception before discharge

If the patient has not required antenatal antihypertensive treatment

- Measure BP:
  - at least 4 times a day while inpatient
  - at least once 3–5 days after birth
  - on alternate days If BP abnormal 3–5 days after birth
- If BP ≥150/100 mmHg, start antihypertensive treatment

If antenatal antihypertensive treatment has been required:

- Continue antenatal antihypertensive treatment
- Reduce antihypertensive treatment if BP falls to <130/80 mmHg; consider reducing if BP falls to <140/90 mmHg
- Measure BP at least 4 times a day while inpatient

If woman is breastfeeding:

- Avoid diuretics
- Inform her that the following drugs have no known adverse effects on babies receiving breast milk:
  - labetalol
  - nifedipine
  - enalapril
  - captopril
  - atenolol
  - metoprolol
- Inform her that there is insufficient evidence on the safety of the following drugs in babies receiving breast milk:
  - ARBs
  - amlodipine
  - ACE inhibitors other than enalapril and captopril
- Assess clinical wellbeing of baby, especially adequacy of feeding, at least daily for first 2 days after birth.

Follow-up care and postnatal review

At transfer to community care:

- Document a detailed care plan that includes:
  - who will provide follow-up care, including medical review if needed
  - frequency of blood pressure monitoring
  - thresholds for reducing or stopping treatment
  - indications for referral to primary care for BP reviews
  - self-monitoring for symptoms.
- Measure BP every 1–2 days for up to 2 weeks after transfer to community care, until antihypertensive treatment stopped and no hypertension
- Offer medical review if still taking antihypertensive treatment 2 weeks after transfer to community care
- If biochemical and haematological indices improving but within abnormal range, or not improving relative to pregnancy ranges, repeat platelet count, transaminases, and serum creatinine measurements as clinically indicated

At postnatal review (6–8 weeks after birth):

- Discuss suitable contraception with advice to avoid combined OCP.
- Offer medical review
- Offer referral for specialist assessment if antihypertensive treatment still needed
- Repeat platelet count, transaminases, and serum creatinine measurements if indicated
- Carry out urine dipstick test
- If proteinuria still ≥1+:
  - offer further review at 3 months to assess kidney function
  - consider offering referral for specialist kidney assessment

CARE PATHWAY

Antenatal care in women at moderate and high risk of pre-eclampsia

If previous history of:
- severe eclampsia
- pre-eclampsia needing birth <34 weeks
- pre-eclampsia with baby's birth weight <10th centile
- intrauterine death
- placental abruption

↓

- Discuss and document advice regarding symptoms which may signify pre-eclampsia
- Uterine artery Doppler at 20 weeks
- Serial ultrasound fetal growth and amniotic fluid volume assessment + umbilical artery Doppler velocimetry
- Ultrasound scans to start at 28–30 weeks, or at least 2 weeks before previous gestational age of onset of hypertensive disorder if <28 weeks
- Repeat every 4 weeks, earlier if any concerns
- Continued vigilance for development of symptoms ± signs of pre-eclampsia

Risk factors for pre-eclampsia

Moderate
- First pregnancy
- Age ≥40 years
- Pregnancy interval >10 years
- BMI ≥35 kg/m^2 at first visit
- Family history of pre-eclampsia
- Multiple pregnancy

High
- Hypertensive disease during previous pregnancy
- Chronic kidney disease
- Autoimmune disease such as systemic lupus erythematosus or antiphospholipid syndrome
- Type 1 or type 2 diabetes
- Chronic hypertension

↓

If *at least two moderate risk factors,*

or

at least one high risk factor for pre-eclampsia:

↓

Advise woman to take aspirin 75 mg/day from 12 weeks until birth,

and

Refer to individual care pathways for each of the above-mentioned risk conditions

6 Maternal Renal Disease

6.1 Chronic Renal Disease

FACT FILE

- **Chronic renal diseases (CKD)** encompass a wide range of conditions that ultimately lead to various degrees of renal impairment.
- These include conditions such as reflux nephropathy, diabetic nephropathy, chronic glomerulonephritis, SLE, polycystic kidney disease, pyelonephritis, IgA nephropathy, previous urinary tract surgery, polyarteritis nodosa, and scleroderma.
- The impact of CKD on fertility and pregnancy is determined by two factors irrespective of the original condition causing renal damage:
  - the degree of renal impairment
  - the presence or absence of hypertension.

Definitions of pre-pregnancy renal impairment

- **Mild renal impairment: serum creatinine levels of ≤125 µmol/litre or less** with absent/minimal hypertension, is associated with a generally good pregnancy outcome in about 96%. Perinatal mortality is low, and pregnancy does not, in general, impair the mother's long-term prognosis except in rare cases such as scleroderma or polyarteritis nodosa.
- **Moderate renal impairment:** a **serum creatinine of 125–250 µmol/litre** where there is moderate hypertension often needing medication with a generally good pregnancy outcome of nearly 90%.
- **Severe renal impairment:** a **serum creatinine of more than 250 µmol/litre** with severe, difficult to control hypertension, and a successful pregnancy outcome of no more than 75%.
- If, during pregnancy there is a deterioration of renal function in a woman with CKD, reversible causes such as urinary tract infection (UTI) should first be excluded.
- Significant proteinuria is not uncommon in CKD, but as long as there is no hypertension or severe hypoalbuminaemia (<20 g/litre) and renal function remains satisfactory, without additional signs of superimposed pre-eclampsia (such as altered liver function tests or haemolysis) the outcome is generally good and pregnancy can continue.
- ***Hypertension is a main factor in increasing perinatal loss associated with CKD.*** If CKD is associated with hypertension that is either resistant or poorly controlled at the start of pregnancy, the risk of fetal loss is increased by at least 10-fold compared with the risk in normotensive or well-controlled hypertensive women with CKD.
- ***Pregnancy management in CKD should start before pregnancy with pre-conceptual assessment and advice from both the nephrologist and maternal medicine specialist obstetrician.***

Pre-pregnancy assessment

- Pre-pregnancy assessment of renal function can indicate possible outcomes of a pregnancy as well as long-term maternal outcomes.[1] It should include:
- Baseline renal function tests:
  - presence of any hypertension and its control
  - baseline quantitative measurement of proteinuria.
- Discussion about the expected course of the underlying renal disease during pregnancy and long-term prognosis:
  - possible impact of CKD on pregnancy outcomes
  - possible impact of pregnancy on CKD prognosis.
- Angiotensin converting enzyme (ACE) inhibitors and angiotensin receptor blockers (ARBs) are usually continued along with statins to achieve renal protection, **but need to stopped before pregnancy with conversion to methyldopa or labetalol as first-line antihypertensives.**
- Folic acid is advised, starting from before pregnancy and continued till the end of the first trimester. In those who have diabetes and CKD, high-dose folic acid 5 mg/day needs to be prescribed instead of the usual 400 micrograms available as an over-the-counter pregnancy supplement.
- **Low-dose aspirin** is advised as a means of reducing the risk of superadded pre-eclampsia as well as an antiplatelet aggregating agent initiated from the start of pregnancy and continued throughout.
- For a diabetic woman, optimal glycaemic control needs to be achieved prior to and during the pregnancy.

Principles of management during pregnancy and puerperium

A suggested schedule of antenatal and renal assessments would be monthly checks till 28 weeks, alternating between nephrology and maternal medicine antenatal clinics. This allows fortnightly surveillance to be maintained. After 28 weeks this is increased to fortnightly checks alternating between nephrology and maternal medicine clinics.[2]

- Confirm the woman has stopped ACE inhibitors, ARBs, and/or statins when pregnancy test is positive. Ensure she is on pregnancy-compatible antihypertensive management.
- If she is diabetic:
  - Aim for optimal glucose control,
  - Check fundi for any retinopathy in the first trimester and repeat in each trimester. Prompt treatment of significant retinopathy if found.
- Baseline renal function tests in the first trimester along with routine booking blood tests and liver function tests.
- Renal function tests to be repeated in each trimester
- Monthly midstream urine (MSU) for culture and sensitivity (C&S)
- 24-hour urine collection for total protein and creatinine clearance along with serum creatinine levels around the time of booking and repeated in each trimester.
- Check for other comorbidity risks, e.g. cardiovascular disease, thromboembolism, obesity, smoking, family history of coronary or thromboembolic disease.
- Viability and dating scan before 13 weeks gestation.
- Careful BP monitoring and control with antihypertensives appropriate for pregnancy.
- Continuation of folic acid till end of 12 weeks gestation.
- Low-dose aspirin throughout pregnancy.
- If there is dehydration due to hyperemesis and significant proteinuria, consider thromboprophylaxis.
- If heavy proteinuria is present, consider thromboprophylaxis with low molecular weight heparin (LMWH) and below knee compression stockings.
- Routine screening tests to be offered.
- If abnormal glomerular filtration rate is found in baseline renal function tests, repeat **monthly** full blood count, serum creatinine, electrolytes, liver function tests, and polymerase chain reaction (PCR).
- Correction of anaemia which is commonly associated with CKD.

- Serial ultrasound scans from about 26 weeks gestation along with Doppler flow studies at monthly intervals.
- If there is a history of maternal reflux nephropathy, antenatal scans for evidence of fetal hydronephrosis/hydroureter, followed by neonatal and infancy review if detected.
- Close vigilance for superadded pre-eclampsia which could be very difficult to distinguish from signs of worsening CKD. Liver enzymes and platelet counts usually remain within normal limits in CKD.
- If preterm delivery is indicated before 35 weeks gestation, both magnesium sulphate for fetal neuroprotection and, prophylactic steroids for acceleration of fetal lung maturity to be given.
- Preterm delivery may need to be considered if:
  - signs of significant growth restriction or fetal compromise.
  - presence of superadded severe pre-eclampsia or eclampsia
  - uncontrollable hypertension
  - significant deterioration of renal function.
- Restart ACE inhibitors after delivery; statins, if indicated, after the baby has been weaned.
- Postnatal review in the renal clinic is required within the first 4 weeks after delivery and an obstetric postnatal visit can be organized for 6 weeks after birth.
- In about 50% of women who start out with moderate to severe renal impairment, pregnancy causes a worsening of their long-term prognosis.
- In 10%, there is rapid progression towards endstage renal failure postnatally.

Conditions leading to chronic renal disease

Reflux nephropathy

- Previously known as chronic pyelonephritis.
- Reflux nephropathy describes the unilateral or bilateral scarring found in those with **vesicoureteric reflux (VUR)**.
- VUR is the most common form of congenital abnormalities of the kidney and urinary tract, with an incidence in the general population of about 0.4–1.8%
- Not all children with VUR go on to develop reflux nephropathy, however about 8% of those with VUR progress to **endstage renal disease (ESRD)**.
- Reflux nephropathy accounts for 10% of all ESRD.[3]
- Severe bilateral renal scarring leads to progressive renal compromise and finally to ESRD, even if the VUR has resolved and in the absence of infection.[4]
- Hypertension is a common feature.
- Reflux nephropathy is often detected during investigations for complex UTIs, proteinuria and hypertension in children and adults or screening undertaken for a strong family history.
- **During pregnancy**, reflux nephropathy in some asymptomatic women may be detected when investigations for recurrent UTIs, hypertension, or proteinuria are performed.[5]
- Those with previously diagnosed reflux nephropathy often give a history of recurrent or persistent UTIs and some are already on long-term suppressive low-dose antimicrobials.
- Any UTI, whether symptomatic or asymptomatic bacteriuria, needs to be vigorously treated during pregnancy so as to prevent further renal scarring.
- In those with reflux nephropathy, regular screening of MSU samples must be maintained throughout pregnancy. Some advocate this at a frequency of once in each trimester, but more frequently if there was a previous tendency for recurrent UTIs.
- Reflux nephropathy increases the risk of both maternal and perinatal complications, depending on the severity of renal scarring and presence of hypertension.
- Preterm rupture of membranes, preterm delivery, low birthweight, pre-eclampsia, maternal pyelonephritis, and sepsis may result. A fetal loss rate of 18% has been noted in women with reflux nephropathy when the serum creatinine level at the start of pregnancy was more than 110 μmol/litre, vs 8% when these levels were less than 110 μmol/litre.[6]
- **VUR has a distinct familial component**, thought to be of a polygenic pattern of inheritance affecting both sexes equally. The maternal history must be provided when scans are requested. The fetal anomaly scan and subsequent serial scans may reveal fetal hydronephrosis or hydroureter. Postnatal screening of these infants for prompt detection and active treatment is recommended.

Diabetic nephropathy

- ***Diabetes is now the most common cause of ESRD.***
- Approximately 20–30% of all diabetics develop nephropathy within 10 years of diagnosis of diabetes and 5–10% of pregnancies in diabetics are complicated with nephropathy.
- In the CEMACH enquiry,[7] 8% of pregnant women with type 1 diabetes and 5% of those with type 2 diabetes had developed nephropathy.
- Microalbuminuria (30–300 mg in 24 h) or incipient nephropathy develops into overt proteinuria with progressive nephropathy in these patients.
- Hypertension usually develops at the same time as microalbuminuria in those with type 1 diabetes.
- Optimal **pre-pregnancy** glycaemic control as well as active ACE inhibition has shown distinct and sustained benefits[8,9] during pregnancy although ACE inhibitors are stopped with the first missed period or a positive pregnancy test.
- Comorbidities are not uncommon with diabetic nephropathy including retinopathy, cardiovascular disease, especially coronary artery disease, as well as an increased risk of thromboembolism in pregnancy.
- Diabetic nephropathy is also associated with increased risks of superadded pre-eclampsia, IUGR, abruption, preterm delivery, and perinatal loss due to the combined effects of diabetes, hypertension, nephropathy, and associated vascular disease.
- The effect of pregnancy on the long-term prognosis in diabetics with nephropathy is difficult to predict because of studies using different time periods for follow-up, differences used as end points, etc. Some studies have shown a worsening[10,11] while others have not seen a significant adverse impact of pregnancy on the progress of renal disease in diabetic women.[9]
- **Pre-pregnancy counselling is highly advisable** in such patients. Women with untreated coronary disease, ESRD (creatinine clearance <30 ml/min),[12] uncontrolled hypertension, and proliferative retinopathy not in remission need to be counselled about the significant risks and therefore advised to avoid a pregnancy.[13]

Nephrotic syndrome (non-pre-eclamptic)

- During any normal pregnancy, there is a physiological degree of proteinuria that does not, however, exceed 300 mg in 24 h. This represents an increase compared with the upper limit for proteinuria outside of pregnancy in a normal woman. The increase is attributed to increased renal blood flow and glomerular filtration rate during pregnancy.[14]
- **Protein loss exceeding 3 g /day is generally regarded as being in the nephrotic range**, the most common cause of which during pregnancy is pre-eclampsia. **It is imperative that pre-eclampsia is first considered if such proteinuria occurs after 20 weeks gestation.**[15]
- Spot protein/creatinine above 230 mg/mmol may indicate that the 24-h protein loss is likely to be 3 g/24 h or more.
- Causes of non-pre-eclamptic proteinuria in pregnancy include diabetes, lupus nephritis, IgA nephropathy, renal diseases such as reflux nephropathy, polycystic kidney disease, interstitial nephritis, and drug- or infection-related glomerulonephritis.
- Increased proteinuria per se, even if severe, in the absence of hypertension or renal impairment does not seem to cause adverse fetal and maternal outcomes.
- When associated with intrinsic renal disease, proteinuria in the nephrotic syndrome range can lead to fetal growth restriction, preterm labour, or stillbirth most likely due to reduced utero-placental blood flow.

Pre-pregnancy counselling

- The best pregnancy outcomes associated with nephrotic syndrome are seen when the underlying renal disease is well controlled before starting a pregnancy.
- Drugs such as ACE inhibitors or ARBs are usually advised to be continued till a positive pregnancy test is obtained. These

antiproteinuric drugs must be stopped, however, as soon as a pregnancy is established due to their teratogenic potential.[16]

- Statins must be stopped before or at conception.
- Immunosuppressive drugs such as azathioprine, ciclosporin, and tacrolimus can be continued during pregnancy with the addition of high-dose folic acid (5 mg/day). Others such as mycophenolate mofetil need to be stopped prior to pregnancy.
- Low-dose aspirin is recommended to attempt to decrease the incidence of superadded pre-eclampsia in this patient population.
- Pre-pregnancy renal function assessments and investigations serve as a guide to the current status of the underlying renal conditions, the optimal control that ideally needs to be achieved before initiating a pregnancy as well as acting as a baseline for subsequent renal function tests during pregnancy.

Management of nephrotic syndrome during pregnancy

- Management of nephrotic syndrome during pregnancy requires a multidisciplinary team including the nephrologist, maternal medicine obstetrician, midwives, dietician, and nephrology nurses in close communication. Frequency of clinical visits and laboratory monitoring need to be individualized on a case-by-case basis.
- **Oedema:** Most cases of oedema associated with nephrotic syndrome respond to conservative management such as the use of pressure stockings, reduction of dietary salt to no more than 100 mmol/day (2.3 g of sodium) and fluid restriction to about 1.5 litres/day. Some patients will require daily diuretics, at small doses of 5–10 mg to start with.
  - A loop diuretic such as furosemide is often the diuretic of choice to start with.
  - Careful monitoring of weight, electrolytes (sodium, potassium, calcium, and magnesium) and bicarbonates (to avoid diuretic-induced alkalosis), fluid balance, and blood pressure checks may be required on a daily basis till stable BP and electrolyte and fluid balance are achieved with diuretics.
  - *Serial fetal growth scans are essential if any diuretic is used in pregnancy.*
- **Control of blood pressure:** Depending on the underlying cause of nephrotic syndrome, BP may be high, normal, or low. When treating hypertension, if present, a balance must be achieved between lowering the BP to a level sufficient to protect the kidneys, yet not to compromise uteroplacental blood flow.[17] Usually BP levels not below 110–120/80 mmHg are aimed for in nephrotic syndrome, individualized to the clinical condition and fetal well-being. Methyldopa and labetalol are the first-line antihypertensives of choice in pregnancy.
- **Thromboprophylaxis** needs to be considered as nephrotic syndrome increases the thromboembolic risk during pregnancy, due to not only increased urinary loss due to anticoagulant proteins but also additional risk factors such as obesity, decreased mobility due to peripheral oedema, or as a result of underlying lupus or known thrombophilia.[18] Different thresholds are suggested for initiation of prophylactic LMWH—some use proteinuria levels above 3–3.5 g/day; others use serum albumin levels below 20–25 g/litre. Dosages will depend on the body mass index (BMI) and total perceived risk of thromboembolism. Thromboprophylaxis must be continued postpartum.
- **Anaemia:** Supplements of iron, folic acid, and vitamin B_{12} may be required to correct deficiencies and promote reticulocytosis. Intravenous iron therapy may be required due to decreased absorption of oral preparations secondary to intestinal wall oedema in nephrotic syndrome.
- **Vitamin D** levels in such pregnancies may be significantly low due to increased urinary loss of vitamin D. In severe deficiency, high doses of vitamin D are needed to achieve rapid correction followed by daily maintenance doses of about 1000 i.u. supplements with monthly serum and calcium checks are often required.
- **Malnutrition** is not uncommon in nephrotic syndrome, especially of proteins, and the involvement of a dietitian in the on-going management is recommended.
- **Infections:** secondary to the increased urinary loss of gamma-globulins—vigilance for prompt detection and treatment. Influenza vaccine must be advised.
- **Delivery:** the timing and mode of delivery have to be individualized depending on both maternal and fetal conditions. Early delivery may be needed in the presence of deteriorating renal function, superadded pre-eclampsia, or signs of impending fetal compromise. The presence of severe uncontrollable oedema (anasarca) which can compromise clinical management, such as inability to take blood pressure readings or gain intravenous access, may be an indication for delivery, if after 37 weeks gestation.
- **Postpartum:** Spontaneous diuresis often occurs, sometimes amounting to several litres/day, with swift improvement of oedema. Salt and fluid restrictions or need for diuretics must therefore be re-evaluated on a daily basis in the first few days following delivery.
  - Diuretics, though not contraindicated in breastfeeding, may interfere with milk production.
  - Antihypertensives such as ACE inhibitors or ARBs can be reintroduced after delivery and most are compatible with breastfeeding.
  - Vigilance must be maintained for infections.
  - Thromboprophylaxis must be continued.
  - NSAIDs are contraindicated

Information for patients

Please see Information for patients: Chronic kidney disease and pregnancy (p. 507)

References

1. Davison JM. Chronic renal disease in pregnancy. Obstetrician and Gynaecologist 1999; 1: 29–32.
2. Brown MA. Chronic renal disease in pregnancy: patterns of care and general principles of management. In:Davison et al., ed., Renal disease in pregnancy. London: RCOG Press, 2008, pp. 31–44.
3. Bailey R. Vesicoureteric reflux and reflux nephropathy. In:Schrier RW, Gottschalk CW, ed, Diseases of the kidney, 4th ed. Boston. MA: Little, Brown, 1988, pp. 747–783.
4. Lynn K. Vesicoureteral reflux and reflux nephropathy. In:Feehaly et al, ed., Comprehensive clinical nephrology. Oxford: Elsevier Health Sciences, 2007, pp. 691–702.
5. Brunskill NJ. Reflux nephropathy in pregnancy. In:Davison et al., ed., Renal disease in pregnancy. London: RCOG Press, 2008, pp. 89–93.
6. El-Khatib M, et al. Pregnancy-related complications in women with reflux nephropathy. Clin Nephrol 1994; 41: 50–55.
7. CEMACH. Diabetes in pregnancy: are we providing the best care? Findings of a National Enquiry: England, Wales and Northern Ireland. London: Confidential Enquiry into Maternal and Child Health, 2007.
8. Hod M, et al. Diabetic nephropathy and pregnancy: the effect of ACE inhibitors prior to pregnancy on feto-maternal outcome. Nephrol Dial Transplant 1995; 10: 2328–2383.
9. Bar J, et al. Pregnancy outcomes inpatients with insulin dependent diabetes mellitus and diabetic nephropathy treated with ACE inhibitors before pregnancy. J Pediatr Endocrinol Metab 1999; 12: 659–665.
10. Biesenbach G, et al. How pregnancy influences renal function in nephropathic type 1 diabetic women depends on their pre-conceptual creatinine clearance. J Nephrol 1999; 12: 41–46.
11. Gordon M, et al. Perinatal outcome and long term follow-up associated with modern management of diabetic nephropathy. Obstet Gynecol 1996; 87: 401–409.
12. Kitzmiller JL, Combs A. Diabetic nephropathy and pregnancy. Obstet Gynecol Clin North Am 1996; 23: 173–203.
13. McCarthy A. Diabetic nephropathy in pregnancy. In:Davison et al., ed., Renal disease in pregnancy. London: RCOG Press, 2008, 111–125.
14. Cote AM, Sauvé N. The management challenges of non-preeclampsia-related nephrotic syndrome in pregnancy. Obstet Med 2011; 4: 133–139.
15. Moran P, et al. The renal response to pre-eclampsia. Semin Nephrol 2004; 24: 588–595.
16. Cooper WO, et al. Major congenital malformations after first trimester exposure to ACE inhibitors. N Engl J Med 2006; 354: 2443–2451
17. Von Dadelszen P, Magee L. A fall in mean arterial blood pressure and fetal growth restriction in pregnancy hypertension: an updated metaregression analysis. J Obstet Gynaecol Can 2002; 24: 941–945.
18. RCOG Green-top Guideline No.37a. Reducing the risk of thrombosis and embolism during pregnancy, the puerperium. London: Royal College of Obstetricians and Gynaecologists, 2009.

Chronic renal disease and pregnancy

Pre-pregnancy assessment and counselling

- Baseline renal function tests including quantitative measurement of proteinuria, serum creatinine, creatinine clearance
- Hypertension and degree of control
- Assessment of any signs of nephropathy, retinopathy, cardiovascular disease
- If diabetic, aim for optimal glycaemic control: advice and support.
- Advice regarding smoking cessation, if applicable.
- If anaemic, correction advice and prescription of iron/folate/vitamin B_{12} as relevant
- If on ACE inhibitors or ARB ± statins can continue before pregnancy **but** stop as soon as first missed period/positive pregnancy test
- If hypertension, labetalol or methyldopa first-line antihypertensive medication in pregnancy—communicate this to GP as switch needs to be initiated in primary care even before booking
- Folic acid starting pre-pregnancy and continued till end of 1st trimester, high-dose (5 mg/day) if diabetic
- Low-dose aspirin especially in the presence of multiple risk factors: advise continuation throughout pregnancy
- Discuss possible pregnancy complications and perinatal outcomes, based on pre-pregnancy investigations and assessment
- Outline multidisciplinary management in future pregnancy
- Discuss possible accelerated deterioration of CKD as a result of pregnancy, especially if hypertension, coronary disease, and ESRD present
- If pregnancy inadvisable or patient decides against it, discuss effective contraception. COCP contraindicated

↓

Positive pregnancy test, urgent referral from primary care to maternal medicine or specialist antenatal clinic or to a joint obstetrics–renal clinic

↓

First visit to maternal medicine and nephrology clinics (early 1st trimester)

- Confirm has stopped ACE inhibitors, ARBs, and statins. If hypertensive, check is on pregnancy-compatible antihypertensives. Close monitoring of BP control to continue
- Folic acid till end of first trimester. If diabetic, ensure high-dose folic acid (5 mg/day)
- Low-dose aspirin throughout pregnancy
- In diabetics, aim for optimal control. Ensure has fundi examination for retinopathy, to be repeated in each trimester
- Baseline renal function tests, routine booking bloods, liver function tests, MSU for C&S
- Check for other comorbidies (e.g. if vascular/coronary disease, ECG in 1st trimester)
- Assess thromboprophylaxis risk—if diabetic, obese, smoker, hyperemesis, family history
- Active thromboprophylaxis to be considered in those with dense proteinuric CKD
- Viability and dating scan, other routine pregnancy screening tests to be offered
- Discuss multidisciplinary team management, plan schedule of visits to maternal medicine/nephrology clinics and regular BP checks: frequency individualized on a case-by –case basis
- Good communication between different specialities: nephrologist, diabetologist, maternal medicine obstetrician, ophthalmologist, community midwife, and GP

↓

Further visits to maternal medicine and nephrology clinics

- **To be individualized—usually monthly till 26–28 weeks, then fortnightly**
- More frequent assessments may be required if significant comorbidities (e.g. diabetes)
- Assess hypertension, diabetes control as applicable. Tight control essential
- Medication review
- Renal function tests in each trimester including 24-h urine for total protein, creatinine clearance, serum creatinine, LFTs, FBC
- Fetal anomaly scan at approx. 20 weeks gestation; serial fetal scans at monthly intervals from 26 weeks with Doppler flow studies as indicated. If maternal reflux nephropathy, check fetal renal system for hydronephrosis, hydroureter
- Exclude UTI at each visit
- Ensure patient is continuing low-dose aspirin, advise to continue till end of pregnancy
- Continued assessment for risk of thromboembolism; if such increased risks identified, LMWH thromboprophylaxis
- Correction of anaemia, if present
- Close vigilance for superadded pre-eclampsia

↓

Delivery and postpartum

- Preterm delivery to be considered if: signs of fetal compromise, superadded pre-eclampsia, uncontrolled hypertension, significant deterioration of renal function
- If preterm delivery is considered necessary, prophylactic steroids if <36 weeks gestation
- After delivery, restart ACE inhibitors, reassure patient that she can breast feed while on these
- Neonatology review if fetal hydronephrosis identified, long-term follow-up and treatment if vesicoureteric reflux suspected
- Nephrology follow-up for mother within 4 weeks post-delivery.
- Postnatal follow-up by obstetrician in 6–8 weeks, advice about contraception: avoid COCP - inform GP

6.2 Renal Calculi

FACT FILE

Epidemiology

- **Renal calculi (urolithiasis) or 'kidney stones'** present infrequently in pregnancy, with an incidence of about 0.1–0.5% of all pregnancies,[1] but are one of the most common non-obstetrical causes of abdominal pain warranting hospitalization.
- The incidence is similar to that in the non-pregnant population, about 1:1500.
- Risk factors that are associated with renal calculi include decreased water intake, hot and dry climate, a diet with high calcium and sodium, and the rare hereditary condition of cystinuria. The role of these in pregnancy is unclear, whereas physiological hydroureteronephrosis of pregnancy or frequent infections may increase the risks.
- Most are diagnosed after the first trimester[2] as spontaneous passage of the calculus becomes more difficult in the second and third trimesters due to increasing compression by the gravid uterus[3] and pain is experienced.
- Renal stones occur with the same frequency on either side, with ureteric stones twice as common as kidney stones in pregnancy.
- There may be an associated history of frequent UTIs, or history of renal stones in a previous pregnancy or in the non-pregnant state.
- Most renal stones in pregnancy are of calcium oxalate or phosphate.

Diagnosis in pregnancy

- Diagnosis in pregnancy can pose a challenge not only because of its rarity but also due to symptoms mimicking other intra-abdominal pathology such as appendicitis, placental abruption, or pyelonephritis. Delay in diagnosis may lead to permanent renal impairment.
- Renal ultrasonography (with or without Doppler) is the most commonly used as the first-line screening tool in pregnancy, with vaginal ultrasonography used to diagnose stones in the distal ureter. Ultrasonography has been quoted to have a specificity of 86% and a sensitivity of 34% for detection of renal calculi in pregnancy.
- MRI, although it provides poor visualization of renal calculi, may be indicated to gain a differential diagnosis if the scan findings are equivocal.[4]
- Excretory urography in the form of a limited IVU (intravenous urography) may be required in the second or third trimester if ultrasonography results are equivocal. Due consultation with the radiologists is highly advisable in such cases.
- CT scanning is to be avoided in pregnancy due to the risk of ionizing radiation.

Symptoms, signs, and management

- The majority of renal calculi are asymptomatic and detected only as incidental findings, especially if they are located in the renal pelvis rather than in the ureter.
- Most calculi (65–85%) are passed spontaneously with conservative management, including bed rest, hydration and analgesia and antibiotics where indicated,[3,5] especially if they are less than 4 mm in diameter.
- Those calculi that are not passed spontaneously, usually 7 mm or more in diameter, can cause severe intractable pain, obstruction, infection, sepsis, and pyonephrosis triggering premature uterine contractions, miscarriage, or preterm delivery and/or hypertension.
- Flank pain and macroscopic haematuria are the most common symptoms, occurring in about 90% of all cases.[6] Painless haematuria is not often seen with renal calculi and alternative diagnoses must be considered.
- Symptomatology may include restlessness, costovertebral angle or generalized flank tenderness radiating along the path of the ureter into the groin, pyrexia, and rigors if infection is a feature as well as nausea, vomiting, guarding, dysuria, and frequency.
- Occasionally invasive interventions such as percutaneous nephrostomy, double-J stent placement, or basket stone extraction, which have superseded open pyelolithotomy, may be required.[3,7] If a stent is chosen, it may need changing every 2 months because of the more rapid rate of stent encrustations seen during pregnancy. A percutaneous nephrostomy tube, placed through the skin directly into the kidney, does not need changing during pregnancy but requires an external drainage bag.
- ***Ureteroscopy with laser lithotripsy is the usual intervention during pregnancy.***
- ***Percutaneous nephrostomy or stenting may be sufficient as temporary measures if the pregnancy is close to term, with stent removal after delivery.***[8,9]
- ***Smooth muscle relaxant drugs such as tamsulosin (an alpha-blocker) and nifedipine (a calcium channel blocker) have undergone early testing for enabling spontaneous passage of calculi.***[10] ***Alpha-blockers are avoided in pregnancy, but nifedipine is widely used for other health problems with a good safety profile and can be taken as once-daily capsules.***
- ***Preliminary results are encouraging, appearing to increase the chance of passing the stone by 50% and accelerating the process by 4 days.***

Follow-up

- If pregnancy has been managed conservatively, follow-up after delivery should include IVU, metabolic evaluation, and dietary advice as relevant.

Information for patients

Please see Information for patients: Kidney stones and pregnancy (p. 507)

References

1. Fligelstone LJ, et al . Problematic renal calculi presenting during pregnancy. Ann R Coll Surg Engl 1996; 78: 142–145.
2. Biyani CS, Joyce AD. Urolithiasis in pregnancy. II: management. BJU Int 2002; 89: 819–823.
3. Burgess KL, et al. Diagnosis of urolithiasis and rate of spontaneous passage during pregnancy. J Urol 2011; 186: 2280–2284.
4. Srirangam SJ, et al. Management of urinary calculi in pregnancy: a review. J Endourol 2008; 22: 867–875.
5. Parulkar BG, et al. Renal colic during pregnancy: a case for conservative treatment. J Urol 1998; 159: 365–368.
6. Stothers L, Lee LM. Renal colic in pregnancy. J Urol 1992; 148: 1383–1387.
7. Loughlin KR, Ker LA. The current management of urolithiasis during pregnancy. Urol Clin North Am 2002; 29: 701–704.
8. Denstedt JD, Razvi H. Management of urinary calculi in pregnancy. J Urol 1992; 148: 1072–1075.
9. Kavoussi LRC et al. Percutaneous management of urolithiasis in pregnancy. Urology 1992; 148: 1069–1071.
10. McClinton S, et al. Use of drug therapy in the management of symptomatic ureteric stones in hospitalized adults (SUSPEND), a multicentre, placebo-controlled, randomized trial of a calcium channel blocker (nifedipine) and an α-blocker (tamsulosin): study protocol for a randomized controlled trial. Trials 2014; 15: 238.

CARE PATHWAY

Presentation suggestive of renal calculi in pregnancy

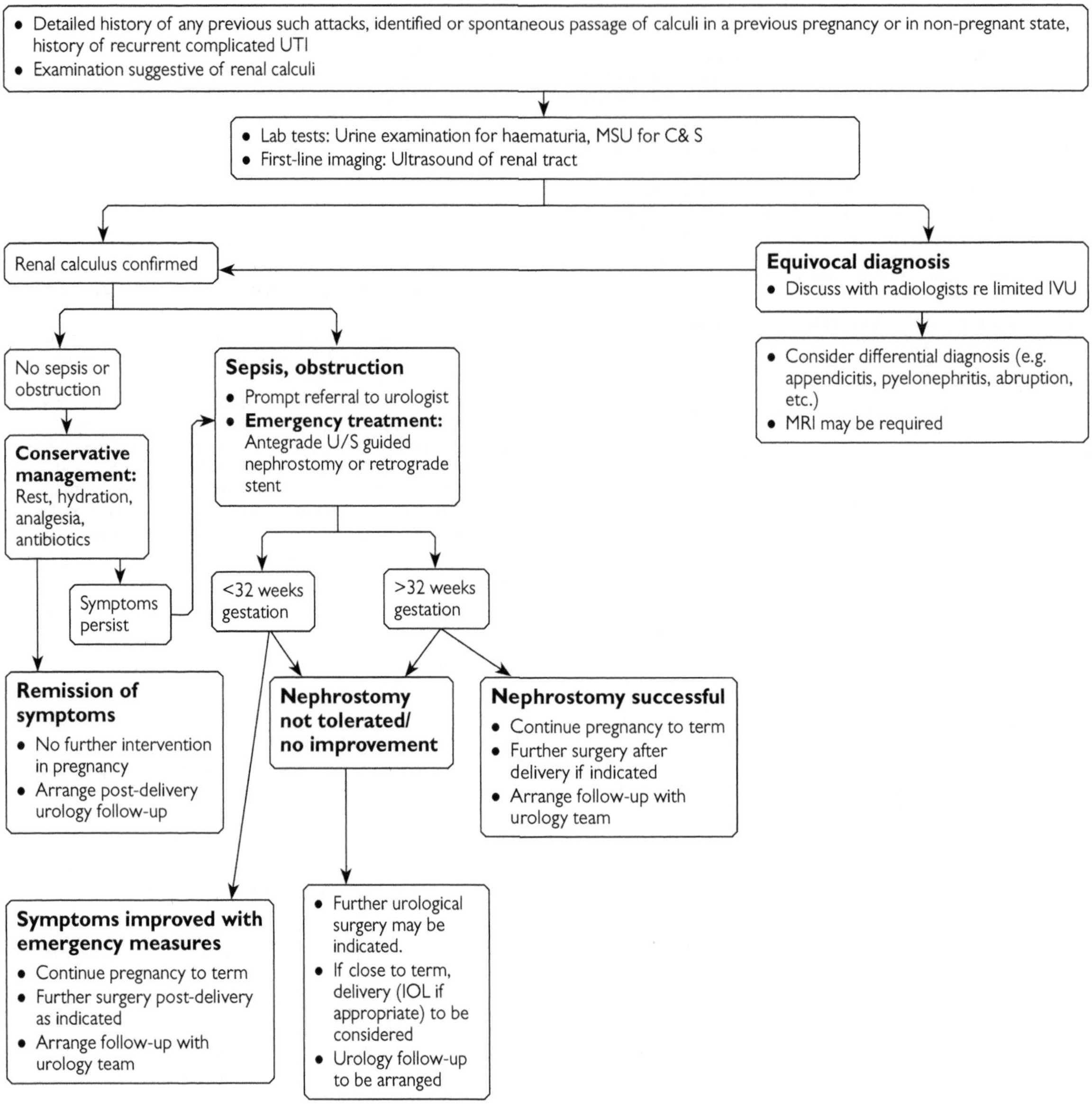
• Detailed history of any previous such attacks, identified or spontaneous passage of calculi in a previous pregnancy or in non-pregnant state, history of recurrent complicated UTI
• Examination suggestive of renal calculi
• Lab tests: Urine examination for haematuria, MSU for C& S
• First-line imaging: Ultrasound of renal tract
Renal calculus confirmed
Equivocal diagnosis
• Discuss with radiologists re limited IVU
• Consider differential diagnosis (e.g. appendicitis, pyelonephritis, abruption, etc.)
• MRI may be required
No sepsis or obstruction
Sepsis, obstruction
• Prompt referral to urologist
• Emergency treatment: Antegrade U/S guided nephrostomy or retrograde stent
Conservative management: Rest, hydration, analgesia, antibiotics
Symptoms persist
<32 weeks gestation
>32 weeks gestation
Remission of symptoms
• No further intervention in pregnancy
• Arrange post-delivery urology follow-up
Nephrostomy not tolerated/ no improvement
Nephrostomy successful
• Continue pregnancy to term
• Further surgery after delivery if indicated
• Arrange follow-up with urology team
Symptoms improved with emergency measures
• Continue pregnancy to term
• Further surgery post-delivery as indicated
• Arrange follow-up with urology team
• Further urological surgery may be indicated.
• If close to term, delivery (IOL if appropriate) to be considered
• Urology follow-up to be arranged

Adapted from Fligelstone LJ et al., Problematic renal calculi presenting during pregnancy, *Annals of the Royal College of Surgeons of England*, 78, pp. 142–145.

6.3 IgA Nephropathy

FACT FILE

Epidemiology

- **IgA nephropathy (also known as Berger's disease)** is the most common form of chronic glomerulonephritis affecting women of childbearing age.
- It is a condition where the immune complexes of IgA are deposited in the glomeruli thereby activating complement fixation.
- It affects white and Asian people more than those of African descent.
- It is twice as common in males as in females.
- It is most often diagnosed between 16 and 35 years of age.
- IgA nephropathy can coexist with a number of other conditions such as systemic lupus erythematosus, Henoch–Schönlein purpura, hepatitis, dermatitis herpetiformis, and coeliac disease.
- Though the disease usually runs a slow course, with signs of renal damage visible in 10–20 years post-diagnosis, about 25% of adults with IgA nephropathy will develop endstage renal failure.[1,2]
- The condition is not considered to have a genetic basis.

Clinical features

- In the early stages, patients are either asymptomatic or have haematuria. The urine may show red cells, leukocytes, casts, and proteinuria. The disease runs a very variable course, from microscopic haematuria to rapidly progressive glomerulonephritis.
- Frank haematuria is often associated with an upper respiratory tract infection. The symptoms include loin pain and red-brown coloured urine.
- Between episodes of frank haematuria, microscopic haematuria may persist.
- The presence of persistent unexplained haematuria with the presence of renal casts gives the first clue to the condition.
- Occasionally hypertension and in later stages when glomerular damage results in nephrotic syndrome, heavy proteinuria and oedema can appear outside of pregnancy.

Investigations

- Other investigations include 24-h urine for total protein, serum urea and electrolytes and 24-h urine for creatinine clearance with a matched serum creatinine level.
- Plasma IgA is raised in 50%, but this is not specific to nephropathy.
- Diagnosis can be made only by renal biopsy which during pregnancy can have increased risks and is therefore best performed pre-pregnancy.
- Hypertension needs early and aggressive treatment as sustained hypertension carries a poor prognosis.

Effect of pregnancy on IgA nephropathy

- In women with normal or near normal renal function before conception, pregnancy does not worsen the course of IgA nephropathy.[1,3,4,5,6]
- Moderate to severe renal impairment (high creatinine levels >125 μmol/litre) and proteinuria (>500 mg loss/24 h) along with poorly controlled hypertension at the time of conception are indicators of rapid deterioration of renal function during pregnancy.
- If there is evidence of rapidly worsening renal function towards the last few weeks of pregnancy, consideration must be given to early delivery.

Effect of IgA nephropathy on fetal/maternal outcomes

- Pregnancy outcomes are largely determined by:
  - extent of pre-existent renal impairment
  - presence or absence of pre-existent hypertension
  - amount of proteinuria
  - significant tubulo-interstitial damage found on renal biopsy.
- Impaired renal function and hypertension are associated with increased rates of miscarriage, preterm delivery, IUGR, IUD, and perinatal mortality.
- Higher incidence of pre-eclampsia,[7] eclampsia and abruption, and deteriorating renal function, which sometimes is irreversible, seen in among women with IgA nephropathy.
- ACE inhibitors and ARBs for control of hypertension are contraindicated in pregnancy and need to have been changed pre-pregnancy to methyldopa or labetalol ± nifedipine.
- Low-dose aspirin should be considered from about 12 weeks gestation onwards, continued till the end of pregnancy.
- Immunosuppressive therapy with prednisolone and azathioprine may be required in those with heavy proteinuria.[4]
- Serial fetal growth scans from 26 weeks gestation at monthly intervals.
- Thromboprophylaxis with LMWH to be considered in those with dense proteinuria, both during pregnancy and in the first 6 weeks after delivery.

Information for patients

Please see Information for patients: IgA nephropathy and pregnancy (p. 507)

References

1. Kim YJ, et al. Fetal and maternal outcomes of pregnancy in women with IgA nephropathy. Korean J Nephrol 2010; 29: 224–231.
2. D'Amico G. Natural history of idiopathic IgA nephropathy and factors predictive of disease outcome. Semin Nephrol 2004; 24: 179–196.
3. Abe S. The influence of pregnancy on the long-term renal prognosis of IgA nephropathy. Clin Nephrol 1994; 41: 61–64.
4. Harmankaya O, et al. Efficacy of immunosuppressive therapy in IgA nephropathy presenting with isolated hematuria. Int Urol Nephrol 2002; 33: 167–171.
5. Limardo M, et al. Pregnancy and progression of IgA nephropathy: results of an Italian multicenter study. Am J Kidney Dis 2010; 56: 506–512.
6. Kincaid-Smith P, Fairley KF. Renal disease in pregnancy. Three controversial areas: mesangial IgA nephropathy, focal glomerular sclerosis (focal and segmental hyalinosis and sclerosis), and reflux nephropathy. Am J Kidney Dis 1987; 9: 328–333.
7. Singh M, et al. Early pre-eclampsia unmasks underlying IgA nephropathy. Pathol Lab Med Int 2011; 3: 1–5.

CARE PATHWAY

Pre-pregnancy assessment in IgA nephropathy

- Check baseline renal function including 24 h urine total protein, urate, 24 h urine creatinine clearance matched to serum creatinine
- Assess BP. If on antihypertensives, review medication. If on ACE inhibitors or ARBs, change asap to methyldopa or labetalol ± nifedipine
- Prescribe low-dose aspirin, advise to continue throughout pregnancy
- If on immunosuppressants such as prednisolone and/or azathioprine, advise high-dose folic acid (5 mg/day) for the first trimester
- Discuss how outcomes of pregnancy depend on pre-pregnancy levels of serum creatinine, renal impairment and hypertension. If pre-pregnancy renal function is unimpaired, good pregnancy outcomes can be expected
- Discuss possible pregnancy complications including worsening hypertension, further impairment of renal function, superadded pre-eclampsia, preterm labour, IUGR, and increased perinatal mortality

↓

Community midwife/GP refers patient with known IgA nephropathy to maternal medicine antenatal clinic as soon as possible in 1st trimester

↓

First visit to maternal medicine clinic

- Confirm viability and dates. Check BP and assess antihypertensive medication. If has not stopped ACE inhibitors or ARBs, advise change to methyldopa or labetalol
- Arrange BP series checks at regular intervals in day assessment unit
- Check is on folic acid.
- Prescribe low-dose aspirin to continue throughout pregnancy
- Baseline renal function tests including serum creatinine, 24-h urine for protein and 24 h urine for creatinine clearance, FBC
- Urine check for haematuria, casts, leukocytes, and protein
- MSU at each visit both in the hospital and in the community
- Serial growth, liquor, and Doppler scan to be arranged from 26 weeks gestation
- Routine checks with community midwife to continue

↓

Further visits to maternal medicine or specialist antenatal clinic

- Check fetal growth, liquor, and Dopplers
- Close collaboration with nephrologist for care throughout pregnancy
- Vigilance for worsening hypertension, PIH or superadded pre-eclampsia, preterm labour. Symptoms and examination should assist in differential diagnosis
- Ensure is continuing low-dose aspirin, antihypertensives as required
- If on prednisolone, GTT at 28 weeks. If GTT in diabetes range, refer to joint diabetes–obstetric clinic
- Consider LMWH thromboprophylaxis in those with dense proteinuria

↓

Delivery and postpartum

- Early delivery to be planned if complications such as worsening renal function, severe PIH, pre-eclampsia, IUGR, etc.
- Encourage breastfeeding, reassure patient regarding safety of azathioprine or prednisolone during breastfeeding
- ACE inhibitors can be used after delivery and during breast-feeding. ARBs after baby is weaned
- Ensure has renal follow-up appointments in place before discharge
- Contraception advice (see Chronic renal disease Care pathway, p. 162) before discharge. Not for COCP

6.4 Autosomal Dominant (Adult) Polycystic Kidney Disease

FACT FILE

The terms 'adult 'or 'infantile' polycystic kidney disease (PKD) are no longer used because they are inaccurate descriptions: both can involve the presence of renal cysts at any time during an affected person's life, from the prenatal period to adolescence or later in life.

Epidemiology and inheritance

- **Autosomal dominant PKD (APKD)** is the most common inherited disorder of the kidneys.[1,2,3]
- AKPD occurs in 1 in 400 to 1 in 1000 of the population and both sexes can be affected.
- In 90% of cases APKD is **autosomal dominant**, in 10% it is due to a spontaneous mutation. APKD is due to two abnormal genes: *PKD1* (in 90%) on the short arm of chromosome 16, and *PKD2* (in 10%) on chromosome 4.
- If one parent is affected, there is a 50% chance of transmission to offspring.
- If both parents affected there is a 50% chance that the fetus is a heterozygous carrier, a 25% chance of an unaffected fetus, and a 25% chance that the offspring is homozygous for the condition.
- Homozygosity usually leads to death in utero of the affected fetus.
- Cysts need not be confined to the kidneys, but considerable variation is seen within families. Extrarenal manifestations of ADPKD include polycystic liver disease (seen in 75% by age of 50 years) and intracranial aneurysms (10%).
- **Women with a family history of intracranial aneurysms must be screened for these before pregnancy**.

Clinical presentation

- Onset of symptoms is usually in early adult life.[4] Approximately one-half of individuals with APKD develop endstage renal disease (ESRD) by 60 years of age. As APKD is the common inherited disorder of the kidneys, it accounts for approximately 10% of the patient population with ESRD.
- Some individuals are asymptomatic and the condition is found only due to family screening.
- Macroscopic haematuria in APKD results mainly from rupture of some cysts into the renal pelvis. Kidney stones and UTIs can also cause haematuria.
- The current management for individuals with ADPKD is aimed at reducing both the morbidity and mortality from the renal and extra renal complications of the disease.[5,6]
- **In pregnancy, APKD may present with loin pain (in 50% of patients, especially if kidneys exceed 15 cm in length), hypertension (in 50%), recurrent UTIs and pyelonephritis, renal calculi, haematuria (in 30–50%), or some degree of renal impairment**. Macroscopic haematuria is a common complication that is usually related to the PKD.
- On examination, there may be hepatomegaly or splenomegaly as well as enlarged palpable kidneys.
- Hypertension is likely to occur early in pregnancy.[1,2]
- Main risks during pregnancy are of UTIs and pre-eclampsia, especially if there is pre-existing hypertension.
- Pregnancy itself does not worsen APKD either in the short or long term.

Management

- Management must be multidisciplinary with the involvement of renal physician, obstetric specialist in high-risk pregnancies and midwife. Genetic input, if not obtained already, must be arranged.
- **Pre- or early pregnancy baseline** BP, renal function tests including measurement of 24-h urine total protein and creatinine, serum creatinine, electrolytes, uric acid, liver function tests, and MSU are essential to compare later trends.[1,2]
- Due to the significant risk of pre-eclampsia, low-dose aspirin (75 mg/day) must be advised, starting from the first trimester and continued till the end of pregnancy.
- A suggested schedule for women with APKD is monthly antenatal checks till 28 weeks, then fortnightly specialist antenatal clinic visits alternating with community midwife or the GP till delivery.
- Careful monitoring of BP is essential, with a low threshold to start anti-hypertension medication. The aim is to keep BP below 140/90.[1,2]
- Treatment of hypertension outside of pregnancy is usually with ACE inhibitors or angiotensin receptor antagonists, both of which are contraindicated in pregnancy.
- BP control in pregnancy is usually achieved with first-line antihypertensive agents[1] such as **methyldopa** (500 mg to 3 g/day in 2–3 divided doses), **labetalol** (200–2400 mg/day in 2–3 divided doses), or **nifedipine** (20–120 mg/day as slow-release preparation). Sometimes a combination of two drugs or all three may be required.
- New drugs such as sirolimus (similar to tacrolimus) are being introduced for treatment of APKD following trials.[3]
- **Renal function tests including serum creatinine and 24-h total protein or PCR** must be performed as a minimum once in each trimester, more frequently depending on the severity of hypertension ± proteinuria.
- An increase in the degree of microalbuminuria is not uncommon in pregnancy without necessarily implying that there is superadded pre-eclampsia or worsening renal disease.[2] Along with serum creatinine measurements, serum albumin, bicarbonates, calcium, and full blood count for haemoglobin and platelets must be monitored. In APKD, the kidneys could produce excess erythropoietin and therefore high haemoglobin levels.
- ***Vigilance for UTIs: pregnant women are more prone to developing urinary infections and require active management for UTIs. MSUs, after the booking sample should be repeated at about 24, 28, 32–34 weeks.***
- Apart from the routine anomaly scan at 20 weeks, regular growth scans with measurement of the amniotic fluid should be arranged from 24–26 weeks onwards at monthly intervals

Fetal anomaly scans and subsequent scans

- Fetal anomaly scans and subsequent scans for growth may show cysts in the fetal kidneys which may suggest that the baby is also affected by the same inherited APKD as the mother. Sonographic appearances may help identify the type of PKD.
- APKD in the fetus should be suspected when cystic enlarged kidneys are detected in association with a normal amount of amniotic fluid. The anomaly can be found as late as the third trimester, with normal-looking kidneys in the second trimester.
- Unlike infantile polycystic kidneys, where there is a loss of the corticomedullary junction, in APKD there is accentuation of this junction. If the fetus has inherited APKD, the amniotic fluid volume is either normal or reduced. The kidney size is usually smaller than the infant polycystic kidneys.[3]
- Parents at risk should be counselled about the possibility of first-trimester prenatal diagnosis. Prenatal diagnosis is possible, by chorionic villus sampling, using a DNA probe linked to the locus of the mutant gene.
- If the diagnosis is made before viability, the option of pregnancy termination may be discussed to the parents. If the diagnosis of APKD is made after the stage of viability has been reached, this should probably not alter standard obstetrical management.

Information for patients

Please see Information for patients: Autosomal dominant polycystic kidney disease (adult polycystic kidney disease) and pregnancy (p. 508)

References

1. Davison JM, et al., ed. Renal disease in pregnancy. London: RCOG Press, 2008.
2. Nelson-Piercy C. Renal disease. In: Handbook of obstetric medicine, 4th ed. London: Informa Healthcare, 2010.
3. Serra AL, et al. Sirolimus and kidney growth in autosomal dominant polycystic kidney disease. N Engl J Med 2010; 363: 820–829.
4. Watnick S, Morrison G. Cystic diseases of the kidney. In: McPhee SJ, Papadakis MA, ed., Current medical diagnosis and treatment, 49th ed. New York: McGraw-Hill, 2010, pp. 846–848.
5. Torres VE, Harris PC. Autosomal dominant polycystic kidney disease: the last 3 years. Kidney Int 2009; 76: 149–168.
6. Patel V, et al. Advances in the pathogenesis and treatment of polycystic kidney disease. Curr Opin Nephrol Hypertens 2009; 18: 99–106.

CARE PATHWAY

Note: this care pathway refers to only Autosomal Dominant PKD and not to the autosomal recessive or infantile variety.

Pre-pregnancy assessment and advice in known APKD

- Detailed history of any family history of intracranial aneurysm, screening before pregnancy highly recommended
- Referral for genetic counselling as 90% are autosomal dominant
- Assessment of baseline BP, renal function tests (serum creatinine, electrolytes, bicarbonate, uric acid, 24 h urine for both total protein and creatinine clearance) liver scan (if not done recently) and liver function tests
- Examination for any hepato/splenomegaly, renal enlargement.
- If on ACE inhibitors or angiotensin receptor antagonists, these should be changed to pregnancy-compatible first-line antihypertensives (e.g. methyldopa or labetalol). Sometimes large doses or a combination of these are required. Follow up in primary care till control is stable and BP averages not more than about 130/85–140/90
- Reassure that pregnancy does not adversely affect long-term prognosis of APKD
- Reassure that with appropriate management, good outcomes for mother and baby in general
- Inform patient that management in pregnancy will be multidisciplinary and involve more visits for both renal and obstetric assessments, growth scans, etc.
- Inform patient and partner that prenatal diagnosis with CVS is available, explaining invasive test-related risk of miscarriage
- If BP well controlled and no fetal growth issues management of pregnancy, labour, delivery as normal

↓

Community midwife or GP refers patient with known APKD to maternal medicine clinic asap in first trimester

↓

First visit to maternal medicine or specialist antenatal clinic

- Confirm viability and dates
- Assess BP, review medications, change to pregnancy-safe antihypertensives (methyldopa, labetalol ± nifedipine) if on ACE inhibitors, or ARBs
- Advise to start low-dose aspirin, to continue throughout pregnancy
- All other NSAIDs contraindicated
- Check most recent pre-pregnancy renal function test results
- Regular BP checks at 2–4 week intervals. Aim for levels <140/90 mmHg
- Arrange 1st-trimester/pre-pregnancy renal function tests (serum creatinine, electrolytes, bicarbonate, uric acid, FBC (for Hb and platelet counts in particular) with rest of booking bloods, 24-h urine for both total protein and creatinine clearance)
- These tests are to be repeated in each trimester as a minimum
- Kidney and liver ultrasound scan and liver function tests. Repeated later in pregnancy, if indicated
- Arrange MSU for C & S and ensure that MSU is performed at 24, 28, 32–34 weeks
- Discuss prenatal diagnosis with CVS, explaining invasive test-related risk of miscarriage
- Joint renal and obstetric care to continue: monthly antenatal checks till 28 weeks alternating with community midwife, then fortnightly specialist clinic checks till end of pregnancy

↓

Further visits to specialist antenatal clinic

- Monthly till 28 weeks then every fortnight, shared with renal specialist team and community midwife
- Check progress of pregnancy, BP control, and medication compliance
- Close communication with renal specialist
- Check results of renal and liver function tests in each trimester.
- Check serial fetal scans for growth and liquor, any signs of fetal renal cysts
- ***If good fetal growth, normal maternal renal function tests and no hypertension or proteinuria, anticipate spontaneous onset of labour and normal delivery. No need for elective LSCS or early IOL except for other obstetric reasons***
- If onset of complications such as hypertension, pre-eclampsia, IUGR, increasing renal impairment, consider early IOL

↓

Postpartum

- Before discharge from hospital, ensure patient has renal follow-up within 4–6 weeks.
- Advise effective contraception, avoid COCP
- Further BP follow-up to continue in primary care
- If antenatal scans have suggested fetal renal cysts, alert paediatricians to maintain longer-term follow-up
- Ensure nephrology follow-up is organized before hospital discharge

7 Maternal Adrenal Disease

7.1 Congenital Adrenal Hyperplasia

FACT FILE

Epidemiology and inheritance

- **Congenital adrenal hyperplasia (CAH)** is a group of autosomal recessive disorders characterized by impaired cortisol synthesis.
- Most types of CAH are autosomal recessive disorders. Both parents need to be carriers of the disease for a child to have classic CAH.
- In a small proportion of people, CAH is caused by a de-novo gene mutation.
- If a woman has previously had a child with CAH and becomes pregnant with the same partner, her fetus will have a one in four chance of having CAH.
- Incidence in the white population is 1:10 000–1:20 000 live births.[1,2,3,4]
- The most common form of CAH is caused by mutations in *CYP21* A2.
- Most cases (95%) of CAH are due to deficiency of the enzyme 21-hydroxylase. This enzyme converts 17-hydroxyprogesterone (17-OHP) to 11-deoxycortisol and progesterone to deoxycorticosterone precursors for cortisol and aldosterone.
- The cardinal feature of the **classic or severe virilizing CAH** seen in 3 out of 4 **newborn females is genital ambiguity** caused by excessive fetal adrenal androgen secretion in utero.
- An affected female child will need reconstructive surgery at several stages during childhood and adolescence.
- The birth of a baby with ambiguous genitals causes deep anxiety and emotional trauma for the parents.
- ***In severe enzyme deficiency, neonatal salt loss and death can occur in babies of either sex.***
- About 75% of classic CAH babies of either sex suffer aldosterone deficiency with salt-wasting, failure to thrive, and potentially fatal hypovolaemia and shock. The neonatal death rate in unrecognized salt-wasting CAH is between 4% and 10%.[2]
- If the disorder is not recognized and treated, both girls and boys undergo rapid postnatal growth and sexual precocity.
- In addition to the so-called classic salt-wasting and simple virilizing forms of CAH, there is also a mild non-classic form, which may show variable degrees of postnatal androgen excess but is sometimes asymptomatic.[2,5] The mild subclinical impairment of cortisol synthesis in non-classic CAH (nC-CAH) generally does not lead to Addisonian crises.

Inheritance patterns

- If both parents are carriers, there is a 25% chance that an offspring will have classic CAH, 50% of offspring will be carriers, and 25% will be unaffected.
- If one parent has CAH and the other is a carrier, there is a 50% chance that a child will be affected and a 50% chance that a child will be a carrier. It is certain that all children will either have CAH or be carriers.
- If one parent has CAH and the other is unaffected, none of their offspring will have CAH but all will be carriers.
- If both parents have CAH, all children will have CAH.
- If one parent is a carrier and the other is unaffected, none of their offspring will be affected, but there is a 25% chance that that an offspring is a carrier.

Genetic counselling and antenatal diagnosis

- Genetic counselling must be offered to parents of a CAH child irrespective of whether further pregnancies are planned. Similarly, genetic counselling would benefit adolescents at the transition to adult care.[2]
- CAH is mostly **autosomal recessive**. The genotype and phenotype correlate well; siblings with CAH generally, but not always, have similar symptoms and degrees of female virilization.
- There is a 25% probability that siblings of the index case will have CAH and a 50% probability that they are asymptomatic carriers. Based on a classic CAH incidence of 1:10 000–1:20 000, the incidence of carriers in the general population is 1:50–1:71.[2]
- Due to the rarity of the condition, genetic counselling and prenatal testing of the couple and index case is best conducted in referral centres and DNA sent for analysis to a central reference laboratory (e.g. London or Manchester, in the UK).
- Antenatal management of a subsequent pregnancy in a secondary care unit (DGH) would benefit from additional genetic and endocrinological input from tertiary referral centres.
- Antenatal diagnosis of the condition is now possible with the identification of CYP21 deficiency.
- Genetic diagnosis for both fetal sex and for CAH is possible using by chorionic villus sampling (CVS), but is feasible only after 9–10 weeks gestation. Glucocorticoid (GC) treatment, however must be started at 6–7 weeks gestation, therefore all pregnancies at risk for CAH need to have initial GC treatment, even though only 1 in 4 is affected. Furthermore, only half of the affected fetuses will be female; hence, prenatal treatment is potentially beneficial for only 1 in 8 fetuses.[1,2]

Prenatal treatment with dexamethasone

- Suppression of fetal adrenal cortex in a female fetus, thereby reducing the levels of adrenal androgens, is a strategy to help prevent severe virilization in CAH.[1,2]
- The mechanism of action of dexamethasone in the fetus is incompletely understood. Nevertheless, suppression of fetal adrenal androgens in CAH is feasible by administering GCs to the mother.[6,7,8]
- Dexamethasone is used because it is not inactivated by placental 11β-hydroxysteroid dehydrogenase type 2 and is therefore accessible to the fetus.
- Because the period during which the genitalia of a female fetus may become virilized begins can be as early as 6 weeks after conception, treatment must be instituted essentially as soon as the woman knows she is pregnant.
- ***Prenatal treatment with dexamethasone is still debatable because only 1 in 8 pregnancies results in an affected female fetus. If treatment were administered during each pregnancy, 7 out of 8 fetuses would have been exposed to supra-physiological doses of dexamethasone for at least 6 weeks before a CVS-derived diagnosis can be made.***[2]
- ***Fetal sex determination from the identification of fetal Y-chromosomal DNA in maternal blood is now possible in specialist centres and this technique has been used in conjunction with prenatal treatment of CAH. This can reduce the number of fetuses that need to be exposed to antenatal dexamethasone.***[8,9,10,11]

- Prenatal treatment aims to reduce female genital virilization, the need for reconstructive surgery, and the emotional distress associated with the birth of a child with ambiguous genitalia.
- Prenatal treatment does not, however, change the need for lifelong hormonal replacement therapy, the need for careful medical monitoring, or the risk of life-threatening salt-losing crises if therapy is interrupted.
- Although a single short course of dexamethasone is widely used to induce fetal lung development in the third trimester of pregnancy, this is not entirely comparable to the effects of administration of long-term maternal dexamethasone to minimize virilization of a CAH female fetus.
- Certain important factors should be considered in considering antenatal GC treatment of CAH: efficacy, safety for the mother, safety for the fetus including any long-term effects on neuro-behaviour.
- Antenatal dexamethasone therapy has been shown to be **effective** in reducing and often eliminating virilization of female fetal genitalia in about 80–85%.[2,12]

Safety issues

Maternal effects

- Exposure to dexamethasone **in this context** is contraindicated in pregnant women with pre-existent diabetes, hypertension, etc.
- Several studies indicate that prenatal treatment is associated with modest but manageable maternal complications that do not appear to pose a major risk to the mother. These include maternal weight gain exceeding average for normal pregnancy, oedema, mood swings, depression, striae with Cushingoid effects, and gastric irritation.[1,2,13,14,15]
- Dexamethasone has not been reported to increase the incidence of maternal gestational diabetes or hypertension during pregnancy.[15]
- In adolescent and adult women with CAH, overtreatment with glucocorticoid may cause Cushingoid symptoms, whereas undertreatment may cause Addisonian symptoms. Overtreatment with mineralocorticoids may cause hypertension; undertreatment may lead to low blood pressure, salt loss, fatigue, and increased requirements for GC replacement.

Fetal safety

- **Teratogenic effects**, especially orofacial clefts, produced by high doses of dexamethasone administered have been reported in animal and human studies.[16,17,18,19]
- **Low birth weight:** Follow-up reports of prenatally treated children have reported birth weights reduced by about 0.4–0.6 kg in the largest studies.[2,14] The magnitude of this change in birth weight has been calculated as equivalent to or greater than that seen with maternal cigarette smoking.[2]
- Long-term effects on **neuro-behaviour** as a result of antenatal exposure of the developing hippocampus to glucocorticoids are as yet unclear.

Pregnancy in women affected by CAH

- Women with CAH are often overweight, with high blood pressure, diabetes, and risk factors for cardiovascular disease.
- Despite an apparent normal pregnancy rate of about 90%, **classic CAH women** have low fecundity (0.25 live births per woman vs 1.8 in the general population).[20]
- Women who have had reconstructive genital surgery will in most cases need an elective Caesarean section as mode of delivery.
- In women with CAH, bolus 'stress doses' of IV hydrocortisone must be given every 6–8 h to cover labour and delivery, including operative delivery .This is rapidly tapered after delivery to reach the previous maintenance dose.

Information for patients

Please see **Information for patients: Congenital adrenal hyperplasia (CAH) and pregnancy** (p. 509)

References

1. Levine LS, Pang S. Prenatal diagnosis and treatment of congenital adrenal hyperplasia. J Pediatr Endocrinol Metab 1994; 7: 193–200.
2. Speiser PW, et al. Congenital adrenal hyperplasia due to steroid 21-hydroxylase deficiency. J Clin Endocrinol Metab 2010; 95: 4133–4160.
3. White PC, Speiser PW. Congenital adrenal hyperplasia due to 21-hydroxylase deficiency. Endocr Rev 2000; 21: 245–291.
4. Lo JC, Grumbach MM. Pregnancy outcomes in women with congenital virilizing adrenal hyperplasia. Endocrinol Metab Clin North Am 2001; 30: 207–229.
5. Kohn B. Late-onset steroid 21-hydroxylase deficiency: a variant of classical congenital adrenal hyperplasia. J Clin Endocrinol Metab 1982; 55: 817–827
6. David M, Forest MG. Prenatal treatment of congenital adrenal hyperplasia resulting from 21-hydroxylase deficiency. J Pediatr 1984; 105: 799–803.
7. Evans M, et al. Pharmacologic suppression of the fetal adrenal gland in utero attempted prevention of abnormal external genital masculinization in suspected congenital adrenal hyperplasia. JAMA 1985; 253: 1015–1020.
8. Forest MG, et al. Prenatal diagnosis and treatment of 21-hydroxylase deficiency. J Steroid Biochem Mol Biol 1993; 45: 75–82.
9. Lo YM, et al. Presence of fetal DNA in maternal plasma and serum. Lancet 1997; 350: 485–487.
10. Lo YM, et al. Quantitative analysis of fetal DNA in maternal plasma and serum: implications for non-invasive prenatal diagnosis. Am J Hum Genet 1998; 62: 768–775.
11. Bartha JL. Fetal sex determination from maternal blood at 6 weeks of gestation when at risk for 21-hydroxylase deficiency. Obstet Gynecol 2003; 101: 1135–1136.
12. Forest MG. Recent advances in the diagnosis and management of congenital adrenal hyperplasia due to 21-hydroxylase deficiency. Hum Reprod Update 2004; 10: 469–485.
13. Forest MG. Prenatal treatment of congenital adrenal hyperplasia. Trends Endocrinol Metab 1998; 9: 284–289.
14. New MI, et al. Prenatal diagnosis for congenital adrenal hyperplasia in 532 pregnancies. J Clin Endocrinol Metab 2001; 86: 5651–5657.
15. Pang S, et al. Maternal side effects of prenatal dexamethasone therapy for fetal congenital adrenal hyperplasia. J Clin Endocrinol Metab 1992; 75: 249–253.
16. Czeizel AE, et al. Population-based case control study of teratogenic potential of corticosteroids. Teratology 1997; 56: 335–340.
17. Robert E, et al. Malformation surveillance and maternal drug exposure: the MadReproject. Int J Risk Safety Med 1994; 6: 78–118.
18. Rodríguez-Pinilla E, et al. Corticosteroids during pregnancy and oral clefts: a case-control study. Teratology 1998; 58: 2–5.
19. Carmichael SL, Shaw GM. Maternal corticosteroid: use and risk of selected congenital anomalies. Am J Med Genet 1999; 86: 242–244.
20. Casteras A, et al. Reassessing fecundity in women with classical congenital adrenal hyperplasia (CAH):normal pregnancy rate but reduced fertility rate. Clin Endocrinol (Oxf) 2009; 70: 833–837.

Antenatal care for a woman with a previous child with congenital adrenal hyperplasia (CAH)

Prenatal care

- Prenatal genetic testing and counselling for parents of previous child with CAH: co-ordinated with tertiary centre. Confirmation of *CYP21* gene mutation
- Establish any contraindications for maternal dexamethasone in a future pregnancy, as applicable in this context (e.g. diabetes, hypertension, etc.)
- ***Establish parents' views regarding future pregnancy:***
  - Whether they would wish CVS diagnosis of fetal sex and CAH in future pregnancy, having received information about procedure-associated risks of miscarriage
  - Whether they would consider antenatal treatment with dexamethasone in a future pregnancy before CVS after having received detailed information regarding maternal and fetal risks, efficacy, and that 7 out of 8 fetuses might be unaffected by CAH but be exposed to high-dose dexamethasone for at least 6 weeks in early pregnancy before CVS diagnosis is possible

↓

In a subsequent pregnancy

- Multidisciplinary management with tertiary referral centre input recommended
- ***If parents wish to commence treatment and no contraindications for maternal dexamethasone exist:***
  - Pre-pregnancy information for GP/community midwife/obstetrician/geneticist so that early plans and management are in place
  - Pregnancy confirmed by pregnancy test as soon as period missed
  - Dexamethasone treatment as soon as pregnancy confirmed: 20–25 micrograms/kg/day in 3 divided doses
  - CVS at 9–11 weeks, one sample to local cytogenetics lab for fetal sex and any karyotype abnormalities (rapid result in 48–72 h) and another sample to central lab (London, Manchester) for mutational analysis for CAH (results in 2 weeks)

↓

Karyotype XX
Continue dexamethasone treatment till mutational analysis for *CYP21* available

- Negative for *CYP21* mutation → Stop treatment
- Positive for *CYP21* mutation →
  - Continue dexamethasone till term
  - Stop/reduce dexamethasone at any stage if unacceptable maternal side effects

Karyotype XY
Stop dexamethasone

↓

Multidisciplinary care with obstetrician, endocrinologist, midwife, and neonatologist

- After first trimester, review monthly till 28 weeks gestation, then 2-weekly till term
- At each visit, assess pregnancy, monitor:
  - maternal weight, striaie
  - blood pressure
  - urine: glycosuria, proteinuria
  - signs of pre-eclampsia
  - maternal plasma unconjugated oestriol levels (for fetal adrenal suppression): levels to be maintained between 100–200 nmol/litre—samples to reference labs
  - enquiry regarding depression, emotional lability, insomnia: appropriate referral
- Oral GTT at 26–28 weeks
- Fetal scans (anomaly scan ~ 20 weeks, serial growth scans ≈ 28, 32, 36 weeks)
- Local and tertiary unit neonatologists to be kept informed about pregnancy, plans regarding delivery
- Careful neonatal monitoring and continued follow-up by paediatricians

Data from British Society for Paediatric Endocrinology and Diabetes Protocol, Jan 2002, with reference to research protocol in Tertiary Centre setting.

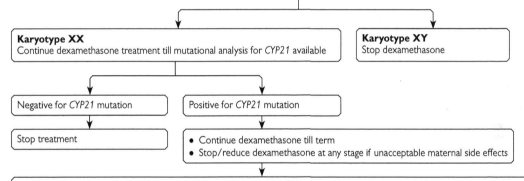

Antenatal Care for a Woman with CAH

Special points of obstetric management

- Pre-pregnancy genetic testing of partners, and counselling
- Prenatal fetal diagnosis for fetal sex and CAH offered.
- Continued adult management of CAH by endocrinologist. Glucocorticoids (GC) (hydrocortisone) ± mineralocorticoids (MC) (fludrocortisone). Dosage may need increase if symptoms of adrenal insufficiency, including postural hypotension
- Avoid GC overtreatment (may cause Cushingoid symptoms) or under treatment (may cause Addisonian symptoms). Overtreatment with MCs may cause hypertension; undertreatment may lead to low blood pressure, salt loss, fatigue, and increased requirements for GC replacement
- Dexamethasone to be avoided in pregnancy in women with CAH. Glucocorticoid of choice is hydrocortisone
- During pregnancy the dose of hydrocortisone needs to be monitored by measuring androstenedione as 17-hydroxyprogesterone is always elevated in pregnant women and cannot be used to monitor CAH
- Careful BP monitoring, early detection of signs of pre-eclampsia
- Oral GTT at 16 weeks, if normal repeat at 28 weeks (20% incidence of gestational diabetes)
- Serial growth scans of fetus
- Referral for senior anaesthetic assessment during pregnancy
- If previous reconstructive genital surgery, plan delivery by elective LSCS
- 'Stress doses' of hydrocortisone boluses IV every 6–8 h during labour and for delivery, either vaginal or for Caesarean section
- Rapid reduction to usual maintenance doses of hydrocortisone after delivery

7.2 Phaeochromocytoma

FACT FILE

- **Phaeochromocytoma** is a rare catecholamine-producing endocrine tumour derived from adrenal chromaffin cells.
- Phaeochromocytoma and paragangliomas are neuroendocrine tumours that can cause secondary hypertension.
- Heightened sympathetic nervous system activity due to excess release of catecholamines (adrenaline and noradrenaline) causes the typical symptomatology of phaeochromocytoma.
- Noradrenaline (norepinephrine) causes α-1 adrenoreceptor-mediated peripheral vasoconstriction with elevation of peripheral vascular resistance and a rise in both systolic and diastolic BP. Noradrenaline-producing tumours cause sustained symptomatology with hypertension, sweating, and headaches.
- Adrenaline (epinephrine) causes increased cardiac output and systolic BP, leading to episodic or paroxysmic symptoms and signs such as palpitations, syncope, and hyperglycaemia.

Incidence

- Phaeochromocytoma is found in about 0.05–0.1% of patients with sustained hypertension.[1,2]
- Reported incidence of phaeochromocytoma in pregnancy is 1 in 54 000 pregnancies[1] or less than 0.2 per 10 000 pregnancies.[3]
- Though extremely rare in pregnancy, phaeochromocytoma carries a maternal and fetal mortality as high as 58%,[3] mainly due to failure or delay in diagnosis.[1,2,3,4,5,6,7,8]

Maternal mortality and morbidity

- With earlier diagnosis and appropriate management, maternal mortality rates are now about 2–5%[1,2,3,4,5,6,7,8] with fetal mortality of 11–15%,[3,7] levels which could be further reduced with early clinical suspicion, prompt diagnosis and effective treatment.
- Even today, diagnosis might only be made post-mortem in up to 10%.[7]
- Delayed diagnosis is attributable to the rarity of phaeochromocytoma, its ability to mimic pre-eclampsia/PIH features (see Table 7.1 for differentiation), and limitations of certain imaging modalities due to pregnancy.[2,4]
- Pregnancy itself could create a catecholamine crisis in those with undiagnosed phaeochromocytoma due to compression effects on the tumour brought about by uterine expansion, fetal movements, contractions, increased intra-abdominal pressure at delivery, any abdominal surgery, or general anaesthetics.[1,2,3,4,5]
- Unrecognized phaeochromocytoma could lead to severe cardiac manifestations especially peripartum,[8,9] such as arrhythmias, angina, dilated cardiomyopathy, acute cardiac failure, and cardiogenic shock.[3,6,7] This accounts for the maternal (and therefore fetal) mortality rates in undiagnosed cases.
- Labile BP resistant to conventional antihypertensives used in pregnancy, sustained headaches, sweating, and palpitations should alert the clinicians to a possible diagnosis of phaeochromocytoma.
- Usually it is only when there is a persistence of the classic symptoms (paroxysmal hypertension with headache, sweating, and palpitations) despite maximal doses of a combination of antihypertensives such as methyldopa, labetalol ± nifedipine, is phaeochromocytoma suspected.
- **Gestational diabetes**, seen in 1 in 3 patients, caused by excess catecholamines, is reversible once the phaeochromocytoma is treated.[10]
- Maternal catecholamines do not readily cross the placental barrier, thus protecting the fetus from the excessive maternal levels.
- The paroxysmal surges of very high maternal catecholamines can however cause adverse effects on the uteroplacental circulation. Extreme vasoconstriction in the uteroplacental vessels can cause placental abruption, growth restriction, acute and chronic fetal hypoxia.[1,2,11]
- Vaginal delivery has a higher maternal mortality rate (31%) than Caesarean section (19%).[2,12,13]

Diagnosis

- The ***24-h urinary catecholamines measurement*** is an essential test, particularly because pregnancy does not cause any significant elevation of these levels, even in pre-eclampsia, thus narrowing the differential diagnosis.[1,2,3,4,5]
- ***Free metanephrine in plasma or urinary fractionated metanephrine*** can also be used in the diagnosis of phaeochromocytoma. **However, both have a false-positive rate of 10–15%, especially with the confounding effect**

Table 7.1 Differential diagnosis: pre-eclampsia and phaeochromocytoma

Features	*Pre-eclampsia*	*Phaeochromocytoma*
Signs and symptoms		
Time of presentation	Usually >24 weeks gestation	Any time during pregnancy
Hypertension	Usually sustained	Paroxysmal
Orthostatic hypotension	Absent	Present
Oedema	Present	Absent
Headaches	Present in more severe cases	Present, almost constant
Flushing and palpitations	Absent	Present
Weight changes	Weight may increase due to oedema	Weight loss may be present
Reflexes	Hyper-reflexia in severe pre-eclampsia	Usually normal
Abdominal pain	Upper right quadrant pain may be present	Absent
Lab findings		
Proteinuria	Present	Often absent
Glucose	Normal	Elevated
Liver transaminases	Elevated	Normal
Catecholamines	Normal	Elevated
Platelets	May be reduced	Normal

Reproduced from Oliva R et al., Pheochromocytoma in pregnancy: a case series and review, *Hypertension*, 55, 3, pp. 600–606. © 2010 American Heart Association, Inc, with permission.

of drugs such as methyldopa or labetalol. In this situation, following the finding of elevated urine/plasma metanephrine levels, MRI should be promptly used to reach a conclusive diagnosis.

- Other tests such as urinary vanillylmandelic acid (VMA) or plasma catecholamines are less accurate than plasma or urinary metanephrine. Tests such as glucagon stimulation test or clonidine suppression test are contraindicated in pregnancy.
- **MRI is the imaging modality of choice** during pregnancy to establish a diagnosis of phaeochromocytoma. Ultrasound may be employed, but is less effective in the presence of small tumours, especially with the enlarged uterus in late second and in the third trimesters.

Management

- The principal goal of management is prevention of a hypertensive crisis that may lead to maternal and fetal fatality.
- Multidisciplinary management with the maternal medicine obstetrician, endocrinologist, anaesthetist, radiologist, endocrine surgeon, midwives, and neonatologist is mandatory in such cases.[12]
- Medical management with alpha-blockers such as phenoxybenzamine should be commenced immediately for such a life-threatening condition.[2,7] Phenoxybenzamine is usually commenced upon advice from the endocrine specialist at doses of 10 mg twice a day with an increase every 2–3 days by 20 mg till a maximum of 1 mg/kg per day is reached.[1] To reach haemodynamic stability, the duration of treatment proposed is about 10–14 days[1,2] and management is usually on an in-patient basis.
- ***Doxazocin*** is another adrenoceptor blocking agent that can be used instead of phenoxybenzamine with similar clinical outcomes.
- **Beta-adrenergic blockers needed to control or prevent tachyarrhythmias should be commenced only after a few days of appropriate alpha-adrenergic blockade and never before alpha-blockers have been commenced**. Propranolol, atenolol, or labetalol are suitable in these circumstances.
- **Methyldopa should not be used,** because of possible worsening of symptoms of phaeochromocytoma.[7,10] If the patient has been treated as for PIH or pre-eclampsia, with methyldopa or labetalol used to control hypertension, these should be withdrawn as soon as the definitive diagnosis of phaeochromocytoma has been made. Ideally they should have been withdrawn even before the 24-h urinary catecholamine test or plasma fractionated metanephrine tests are performed as these drugs can interfere with the quantification of the catecholamines.[1]
- Labetalol can be reintroduced if necessary to control tachycardia a few days after alpha-adrenergic blockade has been achieved.
- ***Surgical adrenalectomy is the definitive treatment for phaeochromocytoma after achieving effective alpha-adrenergic blockade***.
- Timing of the surgery depends on many factors, including gestational age, clinical response to medical treatment, tumour accessibility, and any evidence of acute fetal compromise.[2,11]
- The surgical procedure most preferred is laparoscopic tumour removal which has a complication rate of less than 8%.[1]
- Before 24 weeks gestation, laparoscopic adrenalectomy is recommended if the tumour mass is less than 7 cm.
- If the diagnosis has been made after 24 weeks gestation, continuation of the medical management with alpha-adrenergic blockade as well as beta-blockers to control tachyarrhythmias till mid–late third trimester is advisable. This can be followed by elective Caesarean section and adrenalectomy either under the same anaesthetic or laparoscopic adrenalectomy a few days following the Caesarean section.[1,2,6]
- Elective Caesarean section before the onset of contractions is the preferred mode of delivery.[1,2,3,4,5,12,13]
- **Anaesthetic management** is crucial because some agents (e.g. halothane and desflurane) can trigger a hypertensive crisis.
- Alpha-blockers such as phenoxybenzamine can cross the placenta and cause transient hypotension in the neonate, while beta-blockers may have an effect on neonatal renal function as well as an impact on fetal growth in utero. The neonatalogists must be informed of the mother's condition and treatment well ahead of the time of delivery.
- Long-term follow-up is mandatory for patients with phaeochromocytoma because of the recurrence risk (14%) seen for up to 10–20 years post-surgery, due to incomplete tumour excision.
- A third of young women with the condition have a hereditary predisposition and genetic screening for hereditary phaeochromocytoma is advisable.[1]
- Patients with phaeochromocytoma must also be tested for other conditions such as multiple endocrine neoplasia, von Hippel–Lindau syndrome, retinal angiomatosis and neurofibromatosis.[14,15]

Information for patients

Please see Information for patients: Phaeochromocytoma and pregnancy (p. 509)

References

1. Lenders JW. Pheochromocytoma and pregnancy: a deceptive connection. Eur J Endocrinol 2012; 166: 143–150.
2. Oliva R, et al. Pheochromocytoma in pregnancy: a case series and review. Hypertension 2010; 55: 600–606.
3. Harrington JL, et al. Adrenal tumours and pregnancy . World J Surg 1999; 23: 182–186.
4. Kondziella D, et al. A diagnosis not to miss: pheochromocytoma during pregnancy. J Neurol 2007; 254: 1612–1613.
5. Manger WM. An overview of pheochromocytoma: history, current concepts, vagaries, and diagnostic challenges. Ann N Y Acad Sci 2006; 1073: 1–20.
6. Ahlawat SK. Pheochromocytoma associated with pregnancy: case report and review of the literature. Obstet Gynecol Survey 1999; 54: 728–737.
7. Reisch N, et al. Pheochromocytoma: presentation, diagnosis and treatment. J Hypertens 2006; 24: 2331–2339.
8. Sarathi V, et al. Phaeochromocytoma and pregnancy: a rare but dangerous combination. Endocr Pract 2010; 16: 300–309.
9. Schenker JG, Granat M. Phaeochromocytoma and pregnancy -an updated appraisal. Aust N Z J Obstet Gynaecol 1982; 22: 1–10.
10. Tong C, et al. Diabetes mellitus as the only manifestation of occult phaeochromocytoma prior to acute haemorrhage in pregnancy. Aust N Z J Obstet Gynaecol 2005; 45: 91–92.
11. Griffin JB, et al. Pheochromocytoma in pregnancy: diagnosis and collaborative management. South Med J 1984; 77: 1325–1327.
12. Junglee N, et al. Pheochromocytoma in Pregnancy: when is operative intervention indicated? J Womens Health 2007; 16: 1362–1365.
13. Kariya N, et al. Cesarean section at 28 weeks gestation with resection of pheochromocytoma: perioperative antihypertensive management. Clin Anesth 200; 17: 296–299.
14. Lenders JMW, et al. Pheochromocytoma. Lancet 2005; 366: 665–675.
15. George J, Tan JYL. Pheochromocytoma in pregnancy: a case report and review of literature. Obstet Med 2010; 3: 83–85.

CARE PATHWAY

Symptomatic patient with hypertension resistant to conventional antihypertensives as well as headaches, palpitations, sweating but without signs and laboratory evidence of pre-eclampsia

↓

Suspect **phaeochromocytoma**, undertake screening

↓

24-h urinary catecholamines or plasma metanephrines

↓

MRI, if elevated catecholamines found

↓

Positive for phaeochromocytoma

- ***Prompt multidisciplinary management essential***
- Start immediate medical treatment with alpha-adrenergic blocker (e.g. phenoxybenzamine) for at least 10–14 days till haemodynamically stable
- Stop methyldopa and labetalol as soon as diagnosis made
- Add beta-blocker (e.g. propranolol) to prevent or reduce tachycardia only after alpha-adrenergic blockade for a few days
- Maternal ECHO, ECG to exclude arrhythmias or phaeochromocytoma-induced cardiomyopathy

Negative for phaeochromocytoma

- Multidisciplinary care, input essential
- Seek other causes for hypertension (e.g. extra-adrenal paragliomas, multiple endocrine neoplasias, renal artery stenosis)
- Additional investigations may include serum renin, aldosterone, ECG, ECHO, renal ultrasound, Doppler

Pregnancy <24 weeks gestation, tumour size <7 cm

- Senior anaesthetic assessment, multidisciplinary review, and joint planning
- Laparoscopic removal of tumour by endocrine surgeon after achieving effective control with alpha-adrenergic blockade ± beta-blocker
- Watch for post-op maternal hypotension, fetal bradycardia
- Later in pregnancy, delivery by elective Caesarean section—timing individualized according to fetal condition, IUGR, etc.
- Neonatologists to check for sustained neonatal hypotension (maternal alpha-blocker)
- Long-term endocrine follow-up and BP monitoring
- COCP contraindicated
- Genetic testing for hereditary phaeochromocytoma

Pregnancy >24 weeks gestation, large tumour, no signs of immediate fetal compromise

- Continue medical management with alpha- and beta-blockers
- Continue careful monitoring of materno-fetal condition
- Senior anaesthetic assessment
- Regular multidisciplinary review and joint planning
- Plan delivery by Caesarean under GA—timing individualized depending on maternal response and fetal condition
- Surgical removal of adrenal tumour by endocrine surgeon either as combined procedure with Caesarean section performed by consultant obstetrician or after LSCS delivery as a delayed procedure
- Neonatologists to check for sustained neonatal hypotension (maternal alpha-blocker)
- Long-term endocrine follow-up and BP monitoring.
- COCP contraindicated
- Genetic testing for hereditary phaeochromocytoma

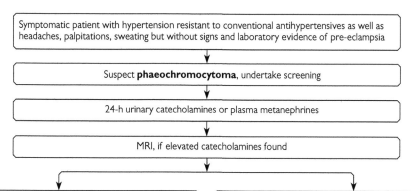

8 Maternal Hepatobiliary Conditions

8.1 Obstetric Cholestasis

FACT FILE

- **Obstetric cholestasis (OC) or intrahepatic cholestasis** is an as yet incompletely understood multifactorial condition of pregnancy **characterized by pruritus in the absence of skin rash, and abnormal liver function tests.**[1]
- OC affects 0.7% of all pregnancies and up to 1.5% of pregnant women of Indo-Asian origin.[2,3]
- OC is a diagnosis of exclusion. Relevant investigations must be performed (and proven negative) for other conditions that might cause pruritus and abnormal liver function tests before a definitive diagnosis of OC is made.
- **Diagnosis of OC** is based on:
  - a typical history of pruritus **without rash**
  - abnormal liver function tests (LFTs)[4]
  - exclusion of other causes of itching and abnormal liver function
- The pathophysiology, extent of associated effects, type of fetal monitoring required and any benefits of it, and indications for and timing of planned delivery are incompletely understood aspects of OC at present.
- The **clinical significance** of OC lies in the associated potential fetal risks such as sudden intrauterine death (IUD), iatrogenic or spontaneous preterm delivery. Maternal morbidity is associated with intense and often round-the-clock pruritus which can lead to significant sleep deprivation. Iatrogenic interventions such as induction of labour (IOL) ± Caesarean section can also contribute to maternal morbidity.
- **Pruritus** may occur for several days or weeks in some women, before any derangement of LFTs is detected. Serial LFTs, including bile acid measurements, are therefore advised in women with persistent itching without rash.
- Pruritus is not an uncommon symptom in pregnancy, affecting 23% of all pregnancies, of which only a small proportion have OC.
- In OC, pruritus is widespread but particularly affects the palms and soles and is worse at night.[2] Differential diagnosis of pruritus in pregnancy includes eczema, atopic dermatitis, or pruritic folliculitis. If it is accompanied by a rash, pemphigoid gestations and polymorphic eruptions of pregnancy must be considered.[5,6]
- ***Abnormal LFTs:***
  - moderate (less than threefold) increase in aspartate transaminase (AST)
  - raised gamma-glutamyl transferase (GGT)
  - ***increased serum bile acid concentration***
  - primary bile acids (cholic acid and chenodeoxycholic acid) may increase 10-to 100-fold
  - raised alkaline phosphatase, usually placental in origin, **does not reflect liver disease**[1]
  - rarely, a mild elevation of bilirubin.
- ***In some instances, an increased concentration of bile acids may be the only biochemical abnormality or raised bile acids may precede other liver function abnormalities.***
- Also, normal bile acids do not always exclude the condition and in those with unexplained and persistent pruritus with initially normal LFTs, these should be repeated along with bile acids once in 1–2 weeks.[4]
- The patient should be asked whether she has noticed pale stools, dark-coloured urine, etc. Hepatitis C carrier status, jaundice, and gallstones must also be excluded.[1]
- Other investigations including liver ultrasound and viral serology (for hepatitis A, B, C, Epstein–Barr virus, and cytomegalovirus), liver autoimmune screen (antinuclear and antimitochondrial antibody) for chronic active hepatitis or primary biliary cirrhosis may help narrow the differential diagnosis in atypical cases, but these tests are not routinely indicated.
- Abnormal LFTs as seen in pre-eclampsia or acute fatty infiltration of the liver must also be considered taking the overall clinical picture into account.[1,5]

Maternal risks

- Vitamin K deficiency (malabsorption of fat-soluble vitamins) and therefore increased risk of postpartum haemorrhage (PPH) is associated with OC.

Fetal monitoring for well-being

- This remains the most difficult aspect in the management of OC. No specific method of fetal monitoring can be used to predict IUD.[1]
- No difference has been demonstrated on Doppler blood flow analysis of the uterine, umbilical, or fetal mid-cerebral arteries even in severe cases of OC with high levels of bile acids.
- Ultrasound and cardiotocography (CTG) are not reliable methods for predicting fetal compromise in OC as there is no evidence of any associated placental insufficiency, intrauterine growth restriction (IUGR), oligohydramnios, or of poor uterine artery Doppler results.
- Continuous intrapartum CTG must be offered.
- Risk of any particular complication of OC is higher if a woman has suffered that complication in a previous pregnancy.

Fetal considerations

- Intrapartum fetal distress (12–22%).[5]
- Preterm delivery (12–44%): Iatrogenic prematurity accounts for much of the prematurity.
- Intrauterine fetal death (from 11%[7] in earlier studies to 0.5–1% in more recent studies[8,9,10]).
- Passage of meconium: Some studies show this is more common in preterm (25%) rather than term cholestasis (12%).[8] Meconium is also more commonly seen in severe cholestasis (>40 micromoles/litre).[10]
- Risk of IUD increases towards term, but does not correlate with maternal symptoms or transaminase levels.
- Fetal risk may be related to the severe concentration of maternal bile acids, though this remains controversial at present.
- A significant increase in fetal risk has been demonstrated **in women with bile acid levels in excess of 40 micromol/litre.** The risk of fetal complications (spontaneous preterm deliveries, asphyxia, and meconium staining) is increased by 1–2% per additional micromol/litre of serum bile acids above 10 micromol/litre.[9]
- ***Bile acids cause a concentration-dependent vasoconstrictive effect on placental chorionic veins. An abrupt reduction of oxygenated blood flow leading to fetal asphyxia may explain acute fetal anoxia and demise.***

Management

- No specific treatment has been shown to improve perinatal outcomes. This must be explained to the patient and this discussion must be documented.

- **Topical emollients:** Safe, though of uncertain efficacy.
- **Vitamin K**: In OC, there is reduced absorption of dietary fats due to impaired excretion of bile salts into the GI tract. This in turn, causes reduced absorption of fat-soluble vitamin K which is necessary for the manufacture of coagulation factors such as II, VII, IX, and X. Therefore water-soluble vitamin K (phytomenadione), 10 mg oral, is recommended in women with OC to reduce the risk of PPH and fetal or neonatal bleeding. This is commenced from 32 weeks or from when a definitive diagnosis of OC is made if this is after 34 weeks until delivery. Vitamin K needs to be started from about this stage because of the increased risk of preterm delivery in OC.
- **Antihistamines**: Chlorphenamine 4 mg or promethazine 25 mg at night to relieve symptoms to a certain extent..
- **Ursodeoxycholic acid (URSO):** A hydrophilic bile acid and a choleretic agent that reduces proportion of hepatotoxic bile acids.
  - Doses of 1000–1500 mg daily in 2–3 divided doses can result in relief of symptoms and reduction of total bile acid and live enzyme levels in most patients (80–90%).
  - ***There is, however, lack of robust evidence that URSO makes any difference as far as rates of fetal compromise or perinatal death are concerned.***[1]
- **Dexamethasone:** Should not be used as first-line therapy.[1]
  - When used as a second-line therapy in women who have not responded to URSO, dexamethasone (12 mg/day oral) may lead to a partial clinical/biochemical improvement.
  - ***However, it is important to consider the potential fetal and maternal side effects from such prolonged use of high doses of corticosteroid. Also, just as with URSO, dexamethasone does not change the risk of underlying perinatal morbidity or of sudden fetal demise. There is some evidence that such doses might even provoke preterm pre-labour rupture of membranes (PPROM).***

Management principles

- ***Once OC is diagnosed, it is reasonable to measure LFTs with bile acids till delivery.***
- **Postnatal resolution of both symptomatology and biochemical abnormalities** should be demonstrated to achieve a definitive diagnosis of OC, which in turn is important in counselling women regarding recurrence risks in future pregnancies. Postnatal LFTs must be deferred for at least 10–14 days [1] and are ideally done at the 6 weeks postnatal check in the community.

Discussions with the patient

These should include:

- Role of induction of labour after 37 weeks gestation, pointing out that there may be increased perinatal morbidity (especially of respiratory distress) as well as maternal morbidity (failed IOL resulting in Caesarean section) as a consequence of such intervention.
- There may be greater place for IOL after 37 weeks in those with severe OC (bile acid levels >40 micromol/litre).
- There is no secure method of predicting IUD in OC.
- Close monitoring during labour due to a higher risk of fetal distress.
- The neonate should preferably receive vitamin K orally rather than IM.
- Postnatal resolution of abnormal LFTs should be confirmed about 6 weeks after delivery. The community midwife, GP, and patient must be so informed.
- Oral contraceptives with oestrogen are contraindicated. Even if progesterone-only-pill is used, LFTs should be monitored on a regular basis.
- Hormone replacement therapy (HRT) need not be avoided as this provides only physiological levels of oestrogen.
- Recurrence risk of OC in future pregnancies is about 45–90%.[11]
- There is an increased incidence of OC in family members.

Information for patients

Please see Information for patients: Obstetric cholestasis (itching liver disorder of pregnancy) (p. 510)

References

1. RCOG Green-top Guideline No. 43. Obstetric cholestasis. London: Royal College of Obstetricians and Gynaecologists, 2011.
2. Kenyon AP, et al. Pruritus in pregnancy: a study of anatomical distribution and prevalence in relation to the development of obstetric cholestasis. Obstet Med 2010; 3: 25–29.
3. Abedin P, et al. Intrahepatic cholestasis of pregnancy: prevalence and ethnic distribution. Ethn Health 1999;4: 35–37.
4. Kenyon AP, et al. Pruritus may precede abnormal liver function tests in pregnant women with obstetric cholestasis: a longitudinal analysis. BJOG 2001;108: 190–192.
5. Kenyon AP, Girling JC. Obstetric cholestasis. In: Studd J, ed., Progress in obstetrics and gynaecology vol. 16. Edinburgh: Churchill Livingstone, 2004, pp. 37–56.
6. Ambros-Rudolph CM, et al. The specific dermatoses of pregnancy revisited and reclassified: results of a retrospective two-center study on 505 pregnant patients. J Am Acad Dermatol 2006;54: 395–404.
7. Reid R, et al. Fetal complications of obstetric cholestasis. Br Med J 1976; i: 870–872.
8. Kenyon A, et al. Obstetric cholestasis, outcome with active management: a series of 70 cases. BJOG 2002;109: 282–288.
9. Glantz A, et al. Intrahepatic cholestasis of pregnancy: relationships between bile acid levels and fetal complication rates. Hepatology 2004;40: 467–474.
10. Lee RH, et al. Pregnancy outcomes during an era of aggressive management for intrahepatic cholestasis of pregnancy. Am J Perinatol 2008;25: 341–345.
11. Shaw D, et al. A prospective study of 18 patients with cholestasis of pregnancy. Am J Obstet Gynecol 1982;142: 621–625.

CARE PATHWAY

Community midwife when booking patients who have had a **past history** of **obstetric cholestasis (OC):**
- Discusses risk of recurrence of about 45–90%
- Advises patients to report any pruritus especially after 26 weeks gestation
- Advise patient to promptly report any decrease in fetal movements
- Routine visits for antenatal checks with community midwife to continue according to NICE protocol, if no other risk factors
- Await spontaneous labour or post-dates IOL as per individual unit's policy as per unit policy if no recurrence of OC

Community midwife or GP refers patient who has developed symptoms suggestive of obstetric cholestasis during this pregnancy to maternity day assessment unit or to specialist antenatal clinic as appropriate, explaining reasons to patient

↓

Day assessment unit/specialist antenatal clinic
- Careful history-taking: any previous history of OC, drug history, any close family history of OC, colour of urine, stools
- Examination: BP, urine analysis, any associated rash, jaundice, right upper quadrant tenderness
- Investigations to exclude other causes (e.g. gallstones), viral screen for Hep A, B, C, CMV, ultrasound of gallbladder and liver, etc.
- Send blood for LFTs and bile acids
- CTG if appropriate (>28 weeks gestation) mainly for maternal reassurance
- Topical emollients, chlorphenamine nocte can be prescribed if pruritus is severe and interferes with sleep
- ***Recall within 24–48 h if bile acids ± LFT results abnormal***

←

- If a rash is present—**this is not OC; refer to dermatology**
- If gallstones—symptomatic management, refer to surgeons
- Appropriate management (see relevant care pathways) if Hep A, B, C or CMV positive
- Topical emollients, chlorphenamine nocte can be continued if pruritus interferes with sleep
- If pruritus spontaneously resolves in absence of rash/ gallstones, etc. and LFTs normal, no further tests/ interventions required

No rash, no other causes found, but severe pruritus continues, repeat LFTs and bile acids in 1–2 weeks. If abnormal results, recall to day assessment unit or specialist antenatal clinic

↓

Counselling and antenatal care
- Explain incidence of OC is about 1% of all pregnancies, what the condition of OC is, the associated small risk of IUD, preterm birth, meconium passage, need for continuous fetal monitoring in labour
- Explain that only limited evidence exists regarding pathophysiology, risk associations, pregnancy management, type and value of fetal monitoring, drug treatment to reduce fetal risks, etc. **Give information leaflets and web addresses**
- Discuss delivery (IOL) at /just after 37 weeks gestation, especially if severe OC (bile acids >40 micromoles/litre). Explain risks versus benefits of early IOL
- Explain no risk of maternal liver damage either in short-or long term and that pruritus will resolve after delivery.
- Arrange repeat LFTs and bile acids weekly.
- If severe pruritus, prescribe URSO but explain and document that this is for symptom relief; **it may reduce bile acid concentration but does not change any perinatal risk**
- Prescribe oral water-soluble vitamin K (phytomenadione) 10 mg od from 32–34 weeks or from when diagnosis of OC is made, if after 32 weeks
- Document need for continuous CTG monitoring in labour
- If patient agrees, arrange IOL at about 37 weeks.

↓

Postnatal: before hospital discharge
- Discuss contraception—avoid COCP
- Discuss risk of recurrence in subsequent pregnancies of 45–90%
- Reassure patient that no long-term sequelae for her or baby if delivered in good condition
- Resolution of abnormal LFTs should be confirmed by repeat bloods sent at least 4–6 weeks after delivery. Best done at 4–6 weeks post-delivery and results reviewed at routine 6-week visit by GP. The patient, her GP, and midwife must be informed before hospital discharge that this is to be performed and followed up in primary care.
- Inform patient that other women in the immediate family may have an increased incidence of OC in pregnancy

8.2 Gilbert's Syndrome

FACT FILE

Epidemiology and inheritance

- **Gilbert's syndrome**, also referred to as **constitutional hepatic dysfunction** or **familial non-haemolytic jaundice**, is a chronic benign disease clinically manifested as jaundice and characterized by mild increase in unconjugated bilirubin.
- The condition arises due to a genetic mutation of the gene for the enzyme UGT glucuronosyltransferase, located on chromosome 2. **In pregnancy, because there is induction of liver enzymes including glucuronosyltransferases, there is less jaundice.**[1,2,3]
- The condition is caused by relative deficiency of glucuronyl transferase and poor uptake of unconjugated bilirubin by hepatocytes[4]
- Those with Gilbert's syndrome are otherwise entirely normal with no other signs or symptoms.
- Gilbert's syndrome is most often recognized in the second or third decade of life and is rarely diagnosed before puberty.
- Situations that are associated with elevated blood bilirubin levels (such as stress, exercise, surgery, menstruation, fasting, destruction of red blood cells, or illnesses) may aggravate hyperbilirubinaemia which is when jaundice becomes evident.[5] Serum bilirubin levels are mildly elevated at less than 60 micromol/litre (<6 mg/dl) in most cases. In a third of patients, bilirubin levels are normal.
- Gilbert's syndrome occurs in about 3–7% of the population, and men are more commonly affected than women.[1]
- Other types of mutations in the same gene cause the Crigler–Najjar syndrome, which is a more severe form of hyperbilirubinemia.
- The mode of inheritance is autosomal recessive so that both parents must have the gene for the offspring to express the abnormality.[6]

Diagnosis

- The diagnosis is often made following routine screening blood tests or when a period of fasting such as associated with surgery or intercurrent illness unmasks the hyperbilirubinemia.
- Symptoms can range from clinical jaundice to nausea, malaise, and discomfort in the right hypochondrium and diffuse abdominal pain.
- Gilbert's syndrome has been recognized as an important cause of postoperative jaundice.
- ***Gilbert's syndrome may come to light for the first time during pregnancy. In such cases:***
  - obtain a family history
  - exclude other disorders of the liver or blood.
- ***A presumptive diagnosis of Gilbert's syndrome can be made if:***
  - the essentially healthy and asymptomatic woman is found to have elevated levels of unconjugated serum bilirubin on repeated occasions
  - normal results of complete blood cell counts, blood film, and reticulocyte count
  - normal liver enzyme tests
  - other disease processes have been excluded.
- Once the diagnosis is established, further management should involve reassuring the patient with regard to the benign nature of the disorder and that the prognosis is excellent.

Prognosis and management

- **Paracetamol and morphine need to be avoided in patients with Gilbert's syndrome.** Although paracetamol is not metabolized by glucuronyl transferase, it is metabolized by another enzyme that is also deficient in some cases of Gilbert's syndrome,[7,8] making these patients susceptible to the potential risk of paracetamol toxicity.[9] Morphine can also exert a prolonged effect in Gilbert's syndrome as its metabolism in the liver is dependent on the deficient enzyme.[10]
- There are significant risks of anaesthetic toxicity with agents such as halothane in those with Gilbert's syndrome; therefore **antenatal referral to the anaesthetic high-risk clinic is mandatory.** Varying degrees of hepatic impairment may result if volatile inhalational agents, especially halothane, are used; similarly, agents such as thiopentone, ketamine, and etomidate may exert an adverse effect.[11]
- Many drugs are metabolized in the liver by enzymes including glucuronyl transferase. Gilbert's syndrome can potentially cause the accumulation of drugs that utilize these enzymes for their metabolism and excretion, leading to adverse outcomes.[11]
- Diclofenac sodium can be safely used for postoperative analgesia.[11]
- Apart from symptomatic management of any dehydration or calorie replacement,[12] no treatment is required for Gilbert's syndrome and the prognosis for the mother and baby is excellent.
- No additional ultrasound scans for fetal growth are required in maternal Gilbert's syndrome. Obstetric management need not be changed and there is no call for interventions such as Caesarean section or early IOL unless for other indications.

Information for patients

Please see Information for patients: Gilbert's syndrome and pregnancy (p. 510)

References

1. Taylor S. Gilbert's syndrome as a cause of post-operative jaundice. Anaesthesia 1984;39: 1222–1224.
2. Chapman RW, et al. Liver and biliary tract disease. In: Boon NA, Colledge NR, Walker BR, ed., Davidson's principles and practice of medicine 20th ed. Philadelphia, PA: Churchill Livingstone Elsevier, 2008, pp. 925–926.
3. Bosma PJ, et al. The genetic basis of the reduced expression of bilirubin UDP-glucuronosyltransferase 1 in Gilbert's syndrome. N Engl J Med 1995;333: 1171–1175.
4. Strassburg CP. Hyperbilirubinemia syndromes (Gilbert-Meulengracht, Crigler-Najjar, Dubin-Johnson, and rotor syndrome). Best Pract Res Clin Gastroenterol 2010;24: 555–571.
5. Radu P, Atsmon J. Gilbert's syndrome—clinical and pharmacological implications. Isr Med Assoc J 2001;3: 593–598.
6. Borlak J, et al. Molecular diagnosis of a familial non hemolytic hyperbilirubinemia (Gilbert's syndrome) in healthy subjects. Hepatology 2000;32: 792–795.
7. Rauchschwalbe SK, et al. Glucuronidation of acetaminophen is independent of UGT1A1 promotor genotype. Int J Clin Pharmacol Ther 2004;42: 73–77.
8. de Morais SM, et al. Decreased glucuronidation and increased bioactivation of acetaminophen in Gilbert's syndrome. Gastroenterology 1992;102: 577–586.
9. Esteban A, Pérez-Mateo M. Heterogeneity of paracetamol metabolism in Gilbert's syndrome. Eur J Drug Metab Pharmacokinet 1999;24: 9–13.
10. Nishimura TG, et al. Prolongation of morphine anaesthesia in a patient with Gilbert's disease: Report of a case. Can Anaesth Soc J 1973;20: 709–712.
11. Nag S, et al. General anesthesia in a patient with Gilbert's syndrome. J Anaesthesiol Clin Pharmacol 2011;27: 253–255.
12. Felsher BF, et al. The reciprocal relation between caloric intake and the degree of hyperbilirubinemia in Gilbert's syndrome. N Engl J Med 1970;283: 170–172.

CARE PATHWAY

Patient already known to have Gilbert's syndrome before pregnancy

- Reassure patient that it is a benign condition with no adverse effects on her health or on fetal outcome
- Good prognosis to be expected

Patient not known to have Gilbert's syndrome

Jaundice in a hitherto asymptomatic pregnant woman or a chance finding of mildly elevated levels (<60 μmol/dl) of unconjugated bilirubin detected in repeated tests

- Obtain family history—Gilbert's is of autosomal recessive inheritance
- FBC, blood film, LFTs, reticulocyte count—NAD
- Other disease processes (e.g. gallstones, hepatitis) excluded
- Ultrasound scan, negative for any liver enlargement, gallstones, etc.

↓

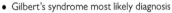

- Gilbert's syndrome most likely diagnosis
- Reassure patient that it is benign condition with no adverse effects on her health or on fetal outcome
- Good prognosis to be expected

↓

- Advise to avoid paracetamol, dehydration, fasting, exhaustion, stress, etc.
- Refer to anaesthetic–obstetric high-risk clinic
- Correct of dehydration, caloric replacement as relevant
- ***Document in notes: No paracetamol or morphine. Avoid dehydration in labour***
- Epidural safe, but risks with certain general anaesthetic agents
- Diclofenac safe for post-op pain relief

↓

- No further investigations or monitoring required specifically directed towards Gilbert's syndrome
- No indication for extra fetal scanning in Gilbert's syndrome
- No change in management otherwise required during pregnancy, labour, delivery, and puerperium
- No indication for early IOL or Caesarean section except for usual obstetric reasons

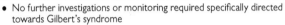

8.3 Gallstones and Pancreatitis

FACT FILE

Epidemiology and aetiology

- Biliary disorders in pregnancy can range from asymptomatic gall stones to acute necrotizing pancreatitis.
- ***The three most common gastrointestinal emergencies encountered in pregnancy are cholecystitis, appendicitis, and intestinal obstruction.***
- Incidence of gallstone-related diseases including acute cholecystitis and biliary pancreatitis complicating pregnancy is 0.05–0.8%.[1,2]
- The reported incidence of acute pancreatitis (AP) in pregnancy varies from 1 in 1000 to 1 in 12 000 in studies spanning different countries and ethnic populations.[3,4]
- Although older reports quoted significant maternal mortality (4–37%)[5] and perinatal mortality rates associated with AP in pregnancy, these have been reduced dramatically with advances in the management of maternal disease and improved neonatal care. More recent series report no maternal mortality and a perinatal loss rate of 2–4.7%.[6,7,8,9,10,11]
- As in the general population, pancreatitis in pregnancy is most often due to gallstone disease and/or hyperlipidaemia **with gallstones responsible for more than 70% of cases of AP in pregnancy.**[11]
- The symptoms of gallbladder disease can be currently present or precede the clinical presentation of AP.[12]
- Hypertriglyceridaemia is most often seen in the third trimester of pregnancy when there is an oestrogen-driven threefold increase in serum triglyceride levels (>1000 mg/dl).[4,8] This is responsible for 4–6% of cases of AP during pregnancy and can be associated with pregnancy complications such as preterm labour.[8,13,14,15]
- Other aetiologies for AP in pregnancy are, as in the general population, obesity, chronic alcoholism, viral infections, drug-induced, or idiopathic.

Gallstone disease in pregnancy

- Incidence of cholesterol gallstone disease in women varies from 5% to 20% between the ages of 20–55 years depending on age, parity, ethnicity, obesity, genetic prevalence, etc. Increased prevalence has been noted in women from Scandinavian countries, Latin American countries, and northern India.[4,16]
- Obesity, sudden weight loss, higher parity, and pregnancy itself are risk factors for cholelithiasis (gallstones) and biliary sludge formation. Oestrogen induces an increase in the hepatic biliary cholesterol levels (lithogenicity) while progesterone induces relaxation of the gallbladder, thus impairing its emptying. Together they are responsible for an increased incidence (3–31%) of gallstones and of biliary sludge during pregnancy.[1,17]. These changes disappear in the puerperium.

Symptomatology of acute biliary pancreatitis

- Impaction of gallstones or microlithiasis in the ampulla of Vater can lead to obstruction of the secretion of pancreatic juices, resulting in dilatation of the biliary duct, pancreatitis, and cholangitis. Cholangitis is diagnosed when the patient is pyrexial, jaundiced, and has abdominal pain due to obstruction of the common bile duct and infection.
- Most patients with gallstones in pregnancy are asymptomatic and require no therapy.
- Symptomatic gallstones can occur at any stage in pregnancy, but are most common in the third trimester (19% in the first trimester, 26% in the second, and >50% in the third trimester).[4]
- Establishment of a biliary cause is essential because of the high recurrence rate of AP in about a third to two-thirds of patients, unless the gallstones are removed.[4]
- Recurrence of repeated episodes of AP within the course of the same pregnancy have been reported in 50–70%.[6,18]
- Biliary pancreatitis is associated with an increased risk of preterm delivery (15–19%).[6,11,18]
- Non-gallstone-related pancreatitis has an overall worse outcome in pregnancy than simple gallstone pancreatitis.[8]
- Similar to the symptoms seen in the non-pregnant state, AP in pregnancy presents as sudden, severe epigastric pain radiating to the right flank, the scapular region, and the back. Postprandial nausea, vomiting, and dyspepsia are often noted as well as low-grade pyrexia. The patients often adopts the fetal position with knees drawn up.
- Maximal intensity of pain is usually reached in about 15–20 min with band-like radiation to the back in about one-half of the cases.[12]
- Signs of tachycardia, hypotension, decreased bowel sounds due to paralytic ileus, and diffuse abdominal tenderness are often found.
- Pyrexia is due to the retroperitoneal inflammatory process.
- In severe cases, maternal dyspnoea, tachypnoea, and hypoxaemia can occur.
- Altered maternal acid–base status can, in turn, lead to adverse fetal acid–base levels with resultant hypoxia, hypoxaemia, decompensation, and even fetal death.[7,19]
- Pregnancy can pose challenges for both the diagnosis and treatment options.

Investigations and diagnosis of biliary acute pancreatitis

- Initial blood tests should include serum amylase and lipase, both being elevated and reliable markers of AP during pregnancy although serum lipase is more specific than serum amylase.[12,20]
  - ***Total serum amylase level rises within 6–12 h of onset of symptoms and remains elevated for some 3–5 days.***
  - ***Serum lipase is elevated on the first day of the illness and remains elevated for longer than the serum amylase.***
- **Elevated serum alanine aminotransferase level** (≥3 times normal) is another sensitive marker of biliary pancreatitis.[21]
- Abdominal **ultrasound** is the imaging technique of choice during pregnancy for the detection of gallstones, although it is insensitive in detection of biliary sludge or in imaging the pancreas.
- Other imaging techniques used include MRI and magnetic cholangio-pancreatography (MRCP) which are non-invasive and without exposure to radiation, though MRCP is less efficient in visualizing small ductal stones in the distal common bile duct.
- The role of the semi-invasive technique of endoscopic ultrasonography (EU) has not been clearly defined in pregnancy.
- Endoscopic retrograde cholangiopancreatography (ERCP) carries a radiation risk and its use is limited in pregnancy as a diagnostic tool.

Management of acute pancreatitis

- ***This must necessarily be by a team approach involving the obstetrician, gastroenterologist, radiologist, surgeon, and midwives.***
- Early evaluation of the severity of AP by gastroenterological and surgical teams is mandatory, with admission of severe cases to intensive care.
- For pregnant women with mild AP, without evidence of cholangitis, antibiotics are not usually indicated; those with cholangitis, however, need appropriate antibiotic therapy.
- In pregnant women with gallstone-associated AP, further management decisions need to be based on the gestational age, presence or absence of dilatation of the common bile duct, and severity of the AP.
- The management in mild cases is mainly supportive with in-patient admission, rehydration with IV fluids, analgesia, antiemetics, and bowel rest by advising the patient to remain nil by mouth for the initial 3–5 days while providing IV nutritional support. A low-fat diet can usually recommence after this time.

- ***Fetal assessment should be part of the management plan, with the modalities of such assessment depending on the stage of pregnancy.***
- The pregnant woman with AP due to gallstones must be evaluated for cholecystectomy to prevent even more severe attacks of AP later in pregnancy which can cause significant maternal and fetal risks.[15]
- When surgical intervention is indicated, **laparoscopic cholecystectomy** has been shown to be safe in pregnancy at any stage, but preferably in the second trimester.
- The laparoscopic approach has all the benefits as in non-pregnant patients with quicker recovery, less immobilization, less postoperative pain, and less uterine manipulation being required.
- Laparoscopic techniques have to be modified during pregnancy. For example: adopting the open technique for the insertion of the umbilical port; avoiding high intraperitoneal CO_2 pressures for pneumoperitoneum (≤10–12 mmHg) in order to prevent fetal acidosis; using electrocautery with care, away from the uterus; placing the patient in the left lateral position to prevent aorto-caval compression; and total avoidance of any uterine manipulation.[12,22]
- In those pregnant women who are not suitable for cholecystectomy, endoscopic sphincterotomy of the biliary duct may prevent further episodes of biliary pancreatitis.[23]
- Cholecystectomy is the most common laparoscopic procedure performed during pregnancy.[22,24,25]

Information for patients

Please see Information for patients: Gallstones and pancreatitis in pregnancy (p. 510)

References

1. Ko CW. Risk factors for gallstone-related hospitalization during pregnancy and the postpartum. Am J Gastroenterol 2006;101: 2263–2268.
2. Ramin K.D., Ramsey P.S. Disease of the gallbladder and pancreas in pregnancy. Obstet Gynecol Clin North Am 2001;28: 571–580.
3. McKay AJ, et al. Pancreatitis, pregnancy and gallstones. Br J Obstet Gynaecol 1980;87: 47–50.
4. Jain V, et al. Biliary pancreatitis in pregnancy. Pract Gastroenterol 2009; XXXIII(3): 16–30.
5. Cortlett RC, Mishell DR. Pancreatitis in pregnancy. Am J Obstet Gyncol 1972;113: 281–290.
6. Hernandez A, et al. Acute pancreatitis and pregnancy: a 10-year single center experience. J Gastrointest Surg 2007;11: 1623–1627.
7. Date RS, et al. A review of the management of gallstone disease and its complications in pregnancy. Am J Surg 2008;196: 599–608.
8. Eddy JJ, et al. Pancreatitis in pregnancy: a 10 year retrospective of 15 Midwest hospitals. Obstet Gynecol 2008;112: 1075–1081.
9. Legro RS, Laifer SA. First trimester pancreatitis: maternal and neonatal outcome. J Reprod Med. 1995;1: 689–695.
10. Chen CP, et al. Acute pancreatitis in pregnancy. Acta Obstet Gynecol Scand 1995;74: 607–610.
11. Ramin SM, et al. Acute pancreatitis in pregnancy. Am J Obstet Gynecol 1995;173: 187–191.
12. Štimac T, Štimac D. Acute pancreatitis during pregnancy. In: , ed., Rodrigo L, ed., Acute pancreatitis. Rijeka: InTech 2012. <http://www.intechopen.com/books/acute-pancreatitis/acute-pancreatitis-during-pregnancy>
13. Neill AM, et al. Active management of acute hyperlipidaemic pancreatitis in pregnancy. J Obstet Gynaecol 1998;18: 174–175.
14. Abu Musa AA, et al. Recurrent hypertriglyceridemia-induced pancreatitis in pregnancy. Pancreas 2006;32: 227.
15. Bank S. Evaluation of factors that have reduced mortality from acute pancreatitis over the past 20 years. J Clin Gastroenterol 2002;35: 50–60.
16. Shaffer EA. Epidemiology and risk factors for gallstone disease: has the paradigm changed in the 21st century? Curr Gastroenterol Rep 2005;7: 132–140.
17. Valdivieso V, et al. Pregnancy and cholelithiasis: pathogenesis and natural course of gallstones diagnosed in early puerperium. Hepatology 1993;17: 1–4.
18. Swisher SG, et al. Management of pancreatitis complicating pregnancy. Am Surg 1994;60: 759–792.
19. Crisan LS, et al. Acute hyperlipidemic pancreatitis in pregnancy. Am J Obstet Gynecol 2008;198: e57–59.
20. Karsenti D, et al. Serum amylase and lipase activities in normal pregnancy: a prospective case control study. Am J Gastroenterol 2001;96: 697–699.
21. Wang SS, et al. Clinical significance of ultrasonography, computed tomography, and biochemical tests in the rapid diagnosis of gallstone-related pancreatitis: a prospective study. Pancreas 1988;3: 153–158.
22. Society of American Gastrointestinal and Endoscopic Surgeons (SAGES). Guidelines for diagnosis, treatment, and use of laparoscopy for surgical problems during pregnancy. Surg Endosc 2008;22: 849–861.
23. Baillie J, et al. Endoscopic management of choledocholithiasis during pregnancy. Surg Gynecol Obstet 1990;171: 1–4.
24. Cosenza CA, et al. Surgical management of biliary gallstone disease during pregnancy. Am J Surg 1999;178: 545–548.
25. Andreoli MJ, et al. Laparoscopic surgery during pregnancy. Am Assoc Gynecol Laparosc 1999;6: 229–233.

CARE PATHWAY

Pregnant patient previously known to have **gallstones** presents with acute upper abdominal symptoms

Pregnant patient self-refers or is referred from primary care with upper abdominal symptoms

Diagnosis

Symptoms

- Acute symptoms—severe epigastric pain radiating to right flank, scapula, and back—maximum intensity in 15–50 min, band-like pain radiating to back
- Nausea, vomiting, pyrexia

Signs

Tachycardia, hypotension, diffuse abdominal tenderness, decreased bowel sounds in severe cases, dyspnoea, tachypnoea, hypoxaemia

Diagnosis

Blood tests:

- Total amylase: increases in 6–12 h of symptoms onset, remains elevated for 3–5 days
- Serum lipase also increased

Imaging

- Ultrasound—gallstones
- MRI if any ambiguity

Admission

- Multidisciplinary management essential. Early involvement of gastroenterologist, GI surgeon, radiologist, senior obstetricians, midwives
- Management options depend on gestational age, severity of acute pancreatitis, presence of cholangitis, etc.

Mild cases

- Conservative, supportive management, fluids, analgesia, antiemetics, nil by mouth for 3–5 days, fetal monitoring—frequency and modality of which depends on gestational age
- If pyrexial, cholangitis needs treatment with appropriate antibiotics
- If apyrexial, acute pancreatitis—no antibiotics required
- After recovery from acute bout, patient must be warned of recurrence of attacks during rest of pregnancy (seen in 50% of cases) and to report symptoms immediately
- Warn about increased risks of preterm delivery, signs and symptoms to be aware of and to report without delay
- No change in obstetric management in most cases unless signs of fetal distress associated with maternal acid–base imbalance seen in severe cases
- Definitive treatment after postnatal stage
- **Ensure has follow-up appointment with GI medical and surgical team before discharge**

Severe cases of biliary acute pancreatitis (AP)

- Admission mandatory, may need to be in ITU
- Urgent assessment by GI surgical team with view to evaluate for cholecystectomy to prevent even more severe attacks of AP later in pregnancy which can cause significant maternal and fetal risks
- IV antibiotics, IV fluids, analgesia, nil by mouth, antiemetics, fetal monitoring by most appropriate modality for the gestation
- Laparoscopic cholecystectomy, safest when done in 2nd trimester, avoiding any uterine manipulation or fetal hypercarbia or acidosis. Techniques used to be modified for pregnancy
- If not suitable for laparoscopic cholecystectomy, endoscopic sphincterotomy of the biliary duct may prevent further episodes of biliary pancreatitis
- Risks of preterm birth, perinatal mortality, and/or morbidity depend on degree of severity of maternal hypoxaemia in severe cases which may lead to adverse fetal acid–base levels with resultant fetal hypoxia, hypoxaemia, decompensation, and even fetal death

8.4 Autoimmune Hepatitis

FACT FILE

- **Autoimmune hepatitis (AIH)** is a disorder of unknown aetiology in which hepatic parenchyma is progressively destroyed, leading to cirrhosis.[1] It is more common in women than in men.
- If untreated, severe cases carry a high morbidity and mortality rate.
- Fertility is decreased in women with untreated AIH.
- AIH is a rare condition in pregnancy.
- In women with AIH and compensated cirrhosis, close adherence to the immunosuppressive and disease-modifying drug regime during pregnancy can result in good control and favourable perinatal outcomes.[2]

AIH and pregnancy complications

- AIH may sometimes be diagnosed for the first time during pregnancy in previously unsuspected cases. Pregnant patients may present with severely abnormal LFTs, ascites, and decompensated liver disease. The high fetal loss rate is mainly related to this.
- Multidisciplinary management is essential in pregnancy and after, to reduce the risk of complications, both maternal and fetal/neonatal.
- Older studies reported increased pregnancy complications in women with AIH including pre-eclampsia, premature delivery, low birth weight, and a high Caesarean section rate.[3]
- Fetal loss rate in untreated AIH has been quoted as 14–24%,[1,3] with most occurring before 20 weeks gestation.[4]
- Increased rates of early and late miscarriages as well as of preterm birth (10–17%)[3,5] have been reported.
- Exacerbations of AIH during pregnancy occur in about 12–20%.[1,5,6]
- Careful surveillance and disease control during pregnancy are recommended given that there is at present no way to identify those patients likely to suffer reactivation of AIH.[7,8]
- Exacerbations can occur postpartum in about 12% of women with AIH, even if AIH was well controlled during pregnancy, probably due to the disappearance after childbirth of the natural immunosuppression seen during pregnancy.[1,4,9]

Management of AIH in pregnancy

- ***Immunosuppressive therapy with steroids (prednisolone) and/or azathioprine forms the mainstay of treatment.***
- Azathioprine has been widely used in a variety of conditions in pregnancy, e.g. systemic lupus or inflammatory bowel disease, or in transplant recipients. There is little evidence that it causes congenital malformations when used in usual doses in humans, neither is there evidence of any defective immune systems in the children.
- The safety of azathioprine in pregnancy is mainly due to the fetal liver lacking the enzymes that convert azathioprine to its active metabolites.
- In AIH patients hitherto controlled with azathioprine[1] there is little evidence to suggest that there should be a reduction of dose or drug withdrawal at any stage of pregnancy.
- In case of a relapse of maternal AIH during pregnancy the risk to the fetus is certainly greater than any theoretical risk due to azathioprine, when taken at the therapeutic dose of 1–2 mg/kg per day orally.
- If the patient has been on and is continuing azathioprine, it is prudent to advise high-dose folic acid (5 mg/day), at least till the end of 12 weeks gestation.
- Steroids such as prednisolone are often required in addition to azathioprine to maintain remission during pregnancy.
- Those who are on steroids during pregnancy need to have diabetes excluded during pregnancy. A glucose tolerance test (GTT) is recommended at about 16 weeks if the patient has been on steroids since before the pregnancy. If the results are normal the GTT should be repeated at 26–28 weeks gestation.
- If gestational diabetes is detected, referral to the joint endocrine–obstetric clinic must be initiated.

Precautions during labour

- Those on steroids during pregnancy need to receive bolus doses of IV hydrocortisone 100 mg every 6–8 h during labour and in the immediate postpartum as well as steroid cover for any Caesarean section.
- Particular care must be taken while prescribing any other medications during pregnancy for those with AIH. For example, labetalol is not advised in those with chronic/persisting derangement of liver enzymes.

Breastfeeding

- Women on AIH have been traditionally advised not to breastfeed because of a theoretical risk of immunosuppression in the neonate. The amount of active metabolites of azathioprine found in breast milk is so low (1–2%) that it could be argued that the benefits of breastfeeding outweigh this small theoretical risk.
- Recent evidence[10] suggests that breastfeeding is relatively safe with azathioprine, with no adverse effects noted for the baby. The patient should be advised accordingly, and advised to breastfeed just before taking that day's dose of azathioprine.

Contraception

- ***The combined oral contraceptive pill is contraindicated.***

Information for patients

Please see Information for patients: Autoimmune hepatitis and pregnancy (p. 511)

References

1. Heneghan MA, et al. Management and outcome of pregnancy in autoimmune hepatitis. Gut 2001;48: 97–102.
2. Levine AB. Autoimmune hepatitis in pregnancy. Obstet Gynecol 2000;95: 1033.
3. Steven MM, et al. Pregnancy in chronic active hepatitis. Q J Med 1979;192: 519–531.
4. Candia L, et al. Autoimmune hepatitis and pregnancy: a rheumatologist's dilemma. Semin Arthritis Rheum 2005;35: 49–56.
5. Schramm C, et al. Pregnancy in autoimmune hepatitis: outcome and risk factors. Am J Gastroenterol 2006;101: 556–560.
6. Colle I, Hautekeete M. Remission of autoimmune hepatitis during pregnancy: A report of two cases. Liver 1999;19: 55–57.
7. Uribe M, et al. Pregnancy and autoimmune hepatitis. Ann Hepatol 2006;5: 187–189.
8. Terrabuio DR, et al. Follow up of pregnant women with auto-immune hepatitis: disease behavior along with maternal and fetal outcomes. J Clin Gastroenterol 2009;43: 350–356.
9. Izumi Y, et al. Development of liver dysfunction after delivery is possibly due to postpartum autoimmune hepatitis. A report of three cases. J Intern Med 2002;252: 361–367.
10. Buchel E, et al. Improvement of autoimmune hepatitis during pregnancy followed by flare-up after delivery. Am J Gastroenterol 2002;97: 3160–3165.

CARE PATHWAY

GP/community midwife refers woman known to have **autoimmune hepatitis (AIH)** to maternal medicine/specialist antenatal clinic in first trimester

↓

First visit to maternal medicine clinic

- Ideally, **pre-pregnancy counselling** including assessment of risk factors (e.g. oesophageal varices, portal hypertension, etc.) by gastroenterologist
- Advise to continue immunosuppressive medication
- Reassure regarding safety of azathioprine and prednisolone in pregnancy
- Advise 5 mg/day folic acid if on azathioprine
- Advise regarding close adherence to immunosuppressives in order to reduce complications and improve perinatal outcomes
- Discuss risk of relapse and greater fetal risk if immunosuppressive drugs are stopped in pregnancy
- Discuss fetal loss rate (14–24%) and prematurity (6–10%) especially with severe exacerbations during pregnancy
- Caution regarding other medications during pregnancy which might worsen liver function (e.g. labetalol)
- Referral and close communication with gastroenterologist/hepatologist during pregnancy and postpartum
- Referral for anaesthetic high-risk clinic review
- Baseline liver function tests with booking bloods
- Routine 20 week anomaly scan
- Arrange serial growth scans at 28, 32 and 36 weeks (or according to individual unit's policy on frequency of serial scans)
- If on long-term steroids, arrange GTT at 16 weeks gestation; if normal results, repeat at 26 weeks gestation
- Routine antenatal care in community to continue avoiding overlap

↓

Subsequent follow-up in maternal medicine or specialist antenatal clinic

At about monthly intervals from 28 weeks gestation (suggested visits at 28, 32, 36, and 40 weeks gestation)

↓

- Assess pregnancy, fetal growth trend on serial growth scans, maternal symptoms, etc.
- If abnormal GTT, refer to joint endocrine–obstetric clinic
- LFTs to be repeated in each trimester
- Labetalol is contraindicated in those with hepatic impairment. If hypertensive, methyldopa to be prescribed
- Coagulation profile in the 3rd trimester at 34–36 weeks
- Ensure patient is continuing immunosuppressive medications
- Ensure she has had anaesthetic and hepatology review
- Discuss any fresh developments with gastroenterologist/hepatologist
- Discuss risk of postpartum recurrence of AIH with mother
- Discuss relative safety of breastfeeding while on most immunosuppressive drugs
- If patient is on steroids, document need for hydrocortisone 100 mg IM bolus 6–8 hourly for labour and delivery
- Routine antenatal care in community (according to NICE guidelines) to continue unless specifically indicated in hand-held notes
- Consider oral vitamin K 10 mg/day for last 3–4 weeks of pregnancy if LFTs are very impaired
- ***AIH is not an indication for early IOL or for Caesarean section except when indicated for other obstetric reasons***
- Discuss contraception before discharge—**not COCP**.
- Ensure hepatic follow-up is in place before discharge.

8.5 Acute Intermittent Porphyria

FACT FILE

Epidemiology and pathophysiology

- **Porphyrias** are a group of genetically well-defined inborn errors of **haem** biosynthesis.[1,2,3,4,5,6,7,8,9] The liver produces about 15% of the body's haem and the bone marrow the rest.
- The overall prevalence of porphyria in the population is estimated as 1.5–5 per 100 000.[1,2]
- Porphyria results from accumulation of porphyrins either in the skin or in the liver.
- Normally, porphyrins are converted from one type to another through a series of enzymatic reactions to synthesize the final product, haem. If any one of these enzymes is deficient or defective, the process stops and there is a build-up of the porphyrin produced up to that point.
- In all acute porphyrias, there is overproduction and accumulation of the porphyrin precursor 5-aminolaevulinic acid (ALA), and of porphobilinogen, a pyrrhole.
- Depending on the major site of expression and the predominant symptoms, porphyrias are classified as hepatic (acute) and cutaneous (erythropoietic) forms.
- Cutaneous or erythropoietic porphyrias cause photosensitive lesions on the skin.
- Porphyria cutana tarda is the most common variety of porphyria and causes photosensitive skin blisters usually presenting in middle age. Unlike the other types of porphyria, this form is rarely inherited, but acquired secondary to other conditions such as alcoholism, haemochromatoses, hepatitis C or HIV.
- Hepatic porphyrias are divided into five types of which four are the acute hepatic porphyrias. Each represents a particular enzyme deficiency in the haem biosynthetic pathway. The acute porphyrias are: **acute intermittent porphyria (AIP)**, hereditary coproporphyria (HCP), variegate porphyria (VP), and ALA-dehydratase deficiency porphyria.[3]
- About 80% of carriers of AIP, HCP, and VP are asymptomatic and others may have only one or two attacks during life.[3]
- In each of these types there is at least a 50% deficiency of the normal level of the particular enzyme.

Manifestations of porphyria

- ***All acute porphyrias have characteristic neurological manifestations such as peripheral neuropathy, neuropathic severe abdominal pain, and psychiatric disturbances.***
- These manifest mainly in adult life and are more common in women (male:female ratio 3:2).[7]
- In AIP, which is the most common form seen in the West and the most severe form of acute porphyria, porphobilinogen deaminase is the deficient enzyme (decreased by nearly 50% of normal values).[7]
- The disease remains latent but symptoms can be triggered by drugs, dietary factors, endogenous or exogenous hormones (as in pregnancy or with progesterone-only contraception respectively).[3,7]
- Severe neuropathic abdominal pain is the most common symptom found in 85–95% of patients. The pain is often diffuse rather than localized and is often associated with nausea, vomiting, abdominal distension, constipation, or diarrhoea.
- Peripheral neuropathy, primarily motor neuropathy, can cause pain in the extremities and symmetrical paresis. In severe cases, respiratory and bulbar paralysis can lead to mortality, often when there is delayed diagnosis.[3]
- Other symptoms include insomnia, palpitations, convulsions, hallucinations, anxiety, disorganization, paranoia, and other acute psychiatric symptoms.
- Hyponatraemia, systemic arterial hypertension, and cardiac arrhythmias are also seen especially during phases of acute attacks.
- Long-term complications include chronic arterial hypertension, chronic liver and renal failure, and hepatocellular cancer.[10,11]
- Common exacerbating factors, sometimes acting in unison, include:
  - drugs that increase the demand for hepatic haem (particularly for cytochrome P450 enzymes) and induce ALA synthase
  - smoking (which also increases hepatic cytochrome P450 enzymes)
  - crash dieting or hyperemesis gravidarum where there is significant reduction of caloric and carbohydrate intake
  - endogenous hormones of pregnancy
  - metabolic stress as seen in infections, after surgery, during and after delivery, etc.

Porphyria presentations in pregnancy and pregnancy outcomes in porphyric patients

- Flare-ups during pregnancy were seen in about 95% in older studies, which also reported maternal mortality rates of 27%.[8]
- In more recent reports, a 24% incidence of exacerbations during pregnancy, maximal in in early weeks of gestation and in the puerperium, and a maternal mortality rate of 0.5%[9] were found. In this study the spontaneous miscarriage rate was 6%, perinatal mortality rate was 7%, hypertension was seen in 16%, and significant IUGR was also noted.
- In hyperemesis gravidarum as well as during and after labour and delivery, the caloric and carbohydrate loss or restriction can provoke an attack of porphyria.
- Signs associated with a flare-up of porphyria may mimic those of eclampsia with common features of hypertension, convulsions (10–20% in AIP), abdominal pain, tachycardia, etc. A delay in making the right diagnosis can lead to inappropriate administration of certain drugs which can themselves aggravate the attack of porphyria.[7]
- Some pregnant women may have had porphyria previously diagnosed and be aware of precipitating factors. Those with an established diagnosis of porphyria should be encouraged to wear a Medi-Alert bracelet and carry an Alert card at all times.
- In such women where the diagnosis is already known, recurrent attacks are similar and diagnosed on clinical grounds, without repeat biochemical confirmation being needed. Treatment should be commenced immediately after exclusion of other causes such as placental abruption or appendicitis.
- It is not uncommon, however, for the first attack to occur during pregnancy, if porphyria has remained dormant. It may come to light only during pregnancy in hitherto asymptomatic women due to a combination of dietary factors, the hormone milieu of pregnancy, and first-time exposure to certain drugs.
- In such women, presentation is often with severe unexplained and generalized abdominal pain, pain in the extremities, new-onset hypertension, proximal muscle weakness, tachycardia, and acute psychiatric manifestations.
- The urine is dark reddish brown and the colour becomes more pronounced if it is left standing for a while. Urine should be sent as an urgent request to the laboratory and a preliminary test for the presence of porphobilinogen in the urine (production of a violet colour when urine is mixed with Ehrlich's reagent) can quickly confirm the diagnosis. Urinary porphobilinogen is significantly elevated in those with acute attacks of AIP, HCD, or VP.[3]
- Second-line biochemical tests and investigations to measure enzyme activity can be performed later to identify the type of acute porphyria.[3]
- ***Once the preliminary test confirms acute porphyria, immediate treatment should commence.***

Management of acute attack

- An acute attack can be life-threatening and requires immediate multidisciplinary team management involving acute medicine physicians, senior anaesthetist, high-risk obstetrician, midwives, haematologist, cardiologist, ITU/HDU physicians, etc.

- Immediate steps should be taken to ensure adequate carbohydrate intake. In mild cases this can be by oral intake of glucose polymer drinks.
- In more severe cases either constant slow infusion of carbohydrate solution through a nasogastric tube or IV administration of dextrose (usually 10% glucose) and correction of electrolyte imbalances (hypernatremia in particular).[7]
- Once the patient is able to tolerate oral feeding, a high-carbohydrate diet (300–500 g daily) should be instituted.[7]
- Urgent review of medications that the patient has been exposed to; any that are identified as harmful in porphyrics should be withdrawn.
- **Symptomatic therapy** is required for control of pain, nausea, vomiting, tachycardia, hypertension, and convulsions. Great care must be taken to avoid drugs known to cause an exacerbation of symptoms in acute porphyria.
  - **Pain control:** Paracetamol, dihydrocodeine, pethidine, morphine, and diamorphine or PCAS for more constant pain relief.
  - **Nausea, vomiting:** Chlorpromazine, promazine, or prochlorperazine can be used, but **not metoclopramide**.
  - **Tachycardia and acute hypertension:** Sympathetic overactivity may need to be controlled with great care by beta-blockers such as propranolol, but only after correction of any hypovolaemia. Paroxysmal cardiac arrhythmias may also occur. Continuous ECG monitoring and full resuscitative facilities are necessary and immediate cardiology input in management must be obtained.
  - **Convulsions: phenobarbital, primidone, phenytoin, carbamazepine, are all strictly contraindicated in porphyria**, but benzodiazepines and sodium valproate are relatively safe. IV diazepam[3] has been used to control status epilepticus in such cases.
- **Specific therapy** of the underlying disease involves administering IV haematin (haem arginate). Its safety in pregnancy has not been fully established. Multidisciplinary consultation and advice sought from national porphyria centres are recommended.
- Most attacks of porphyria in pregnancy settle with adequate supportive therapy with good maternal and fetal outcomes. As there is, at present, insufficient information about fetal safety with the use of **haematin**, this should be reserved for only severe cases when the mother's condition warrants it.

Pre-pregnancy counselling

- The patient is often aware of exacerbating factors.
- Advise her not to smoke or drink alcohol. She needs to avoid any drugs contraindicated in porphyria from the list supplied and to report symptoms promptly so that early treatment can be initiated.
- Genetic counselling must be offered as this is an autosomal dominant disease with each offspring carrying a 50% chance of inheriting the trait. The patient must be informed that, despite this risk of inheritance, the majority of porphyrics remain clinically latent throughout life.
- There may be a family history of porphyria and because 80% of carriers could be asymptomatic, genetic screening needs to be offered to asymptomatic members of the family.
- If the woman has had repeated clinical attacks and has increased porphyrins and its precursors in urine, she is more likely to suffer exacerbations during pregnancy. In these circumstances, consider advising that pregnancy be deferred till she has been free of symptomatic attacks for about 12–18 months, depending on individual circumstances.
- Discuss the possible effects of pregnancy on the underlying disease. Exacerbations can be expected in the early part of gestation, associated with hyperemesis, or at the time of labour and delivery. Preventive measures involve ensuring adequate carbohydrate and caloric intake, control of nausea and vomiting, IV glucose, analgesia, etc. The patient must be made aware of this and have written information given to her.
- Discuss possible effects of porphyria on pregnancy outcome. Increased risks of miscarriages, hypertension, and IUGR have been reported in those who have experienced attacks during pregnancy.[7,9]
- Reassure patient that a referral will be made during pregnancy for discussion with a senior anaesthetist regarding analgesia during labour and delivery, or analgesia for Caesarean section as well as postoperatively. Regional anaesthesia in the form of spinal or epidural anaesthesia using bupivacaine has been used with safety.[12]
- If discussion regarding contraception is relevant, advise not using either the combined pill or the progesterone-only pill as these can trigger acute porphyria reaction in up to 15% of patients. Depo-Provera® and Norplant® implant are in particular best avoided.[12] There is not enough information regarding the levonorgestrel-loaded IUS (Mirena®), which is likely to be safe given the minimal systemic absorption of progesterone.

Information for patients

Please see Information for patients: Acute porphyria and pregnancy (p. 511)

References

1. Anderson KE, et al. Disorders of heme biosynthesis: X-linked sideroblastic anemia and the porphyrias. In: Scriver C, et al., ed., Metabolic and molecular bases of inherited disease, vol. 1. New York: McGraw-Hill, 2001, pp. 2991–3062.
2. Tollånes MC, et al. Excess risk of adverse pregnancy outcomes in women with porphyria: a population-based cohort study. J Inherit Metab Dis 2011;34: 217–223.
3. Anderson KE, et al. Recommendations for the diagnosis and treatment of the acute porphyrias. Ann Intern Med 2005;142: 439–450.
4. Kauppinen R, Mustajoki P. Prognosis of acute porphyria: occurrence of acute attacks, precipitating factors, and associated diseases. Medicine (Baltimore) 1992;71: 1–13.
5. Milo R, et al. Acute intermittent porphyria in pregnancy. Obstet Gynecol 1989;73: 450–452.
6. Shenhav S, et al. Acute intermittent porphyria precipitated by hyperemesis and metoclopramide treatment in pregnancy. Acta Obstet Gynecol Scand 1997;76: 484–485.
7. Kanaan C, et al. Pregnancy and acute intermittent porphyria. Obstet Gynecol Surv 1989;44: 244–249.
8. Hunter DJS. Acute intermittent porphyria and pregnancy. BJOG 1971;78: 746–750.
9. Brodie MJ, et al. Pregnancy and the acute porphyrias. BJOG 1977;84: 726–731.
10. Church SE. Hypertension and renal impairment as complications of acute porphyria. Nephrol Dial Transplant 1992;7: 986–990.
11. Kauppinen R, Mustajoki P. Acute hepatic porphyria and hepatocellular carcinoma. Br J Cancer 1988;57: 117–120.
12. UK Medicines Information Wales. Porphyria—a medicines information bulletin. Cardiff and Vale NHS Trust, 2008.

CARE PATHWAY

- **Porphyria is a rare diagnosis**, but must be suspected in women presenting with severe acute abdominal pain, peripheral muscle weakness, acute psychiatric symptoms, hyponatraemia, and reddish dark urine where other pathologies such as acute appendicitis, pancreatitis, cholecystitis, torsion of ovarian cyst or uterine scar rupture, abruption, etc. have been excluded
- Establish diagnosis promptly by checking for increased porphobilinogen in urine
- If increased porphobilinogen, immediate treatment to be started. Obtain input from haematologist, metabolic physician, and nutritionist

↓

Treatment of acute attack

- Hospitalize patient for acute symptom control
- Withdraw any unsafe medication or other precipitating factors
- Nutritional support, correction of caloric/carbohydrate loss if nausea and vomiting
- Symptomatic treatment, IV fluids, restore electrolyte balance especially hyponatraemia
- Seizure control with medication safe to use in porphyria (slow IV diazepam infusion for status epilepticus)
- Narcotic analgesics for pain control
- Phenothiazine to control nausea and vomiting
- Beta-adrenergic blockers for acute hypertension, symptomatic tachycardia, or arrhythmias.
- IV glucose (10% glucose, at least 300 mg daily)
- Haematin treatment as directed by consultant haematologist
- Close monitoring to continue, monitoring vital capacity (if impaired, may need ICU admission); neurological status, including proximal muscle strength, check daily serum electrolytes, creatinine, magnesium levels
- Vigilance for urinary retention, bladder distension
- Fetal surveillance—mode of surveillance dependent on gestational age

↓

Follow-up

- Discuss porphyria, explain disease, aggravating factors such as certain drugs, smoking, alcohol, carbohydrate or caloric loss, inheritance pattern (autosomal dominant, therefore 50% risk of inheritance for any offspring), and important preventive measures, further tests to establish type of acute porphyria
- Offer referral for genetic testing for family members who might be asymptomatic carriers.
- Advise patient to wear a MedicAlert bracelet; give list of unsafe medications for patient to keep with her
- Give emergency contact numbers to access advice or help during pregnancy
- Arrange further antenatal checks, continue fetal surveillance, serial growth scans
- Arrange review by senior anaesthetist for analgesia plans for labour and delivery, and anaesthetic for emergency or elective LSCS should one become necessary
- **Early IOL or LSCS only for obstetric indications**
- Ensure documentation in notes regarding adequate caloric and carbohydrate replacement during labour, delivery, and post-delivery to prevent porphyria attack. Glucose 10% IV in postoperative period, exclude hyponatraemia
- Advice regarding contraception: Not to use OCP, either combined pill, progesterone-only pill, or depot progesterone or implant. Mirena® may be safe but little information available at present
- Ensure has adequate support and help at home

8.6 Wilson's Disease

FACT FILE

- **Wilson's disease (WD)**, also known as **hepatolenticular degeneration**, is an autosomal recessive genetic disorder where, due to excessive copper accumulation in the body, particularly in the liver and brain, hepatic impairment and neurological and behavioural abnormalities can result.
- The condition is due to an inherited defect in the biliary excretion of copper.
- The build-up of copper damages certain organs including the liver, nervous system, brain, kidneys, and eyes. In around half of cases, only the liver is affected.
- The copper begins to accumulate at birth, but symptoms usually appear during the teenage years.

Incidence

- Around 1 in 30 000 people have the disorder,[1] with southern Italians and eastern Europeans at slightly increased risk. Sometimes, the disorder is caused by a spontaneous gene mutation.
- Unlike many genetic disorders, WD is treatable. Without treatment, however, it is fatal. There is no cure, but the condition can be managed.
- WD can present as chronic active hepatitis, cirrhosis, fulminant hepatic failure, and haemolytic anaemia and persistently elevated serum aminotransferases

Symptoms

- The earliest symptom to appear is an asymmetrical tremor usually followed by excessive salivation, ataxia, clumsiness, gait disturbances, dystonia, etc.
- 10–20% have psychiatric problems that may be behavioural, affective, cognitive, or schizophrenic.
- Neuropsychiatric, ophthalmologic signs (Kayser–Fleisher rings at the junction of cornea and sclera), renal disease, arthropathy, and haemolytic anaemia (in 10–15%) have also been described in those with WD.

Clinical manifestations

- The clinical spectrum of liver disease varies widely. The clinical manifestations can present from childhood to adulthood.
- Younger patients in the presymptomatic stage of WD may be diagnosed by a chance finding of isolated liver function abnormalities or as part of family screening.

Pre-pregnancy counselling

Pre-pregnancy counselling is vital in women with WD and should include the following points:

- Fertility is reduced in women with untreated WD. Similarly, multiple miscarriages can occur in untreated WD.[2]
- Inheritance risk for the baby: In a woman with WD, the chances of producing a homozygote child is 0.5%; partner testing can therefore be justified.
- The woman's copper status must be optimized before starting a pregnancy.[4]
- She must be advised to continue penicillamine if this has kept her WD under stable control. Her fears regarding possible teratogenicity must be allayed. She should be informed that the risks of withdrawing treatment are far greater to her and the baby than the small probability of teratogenesis.
- Contraception:[4] **The oestrogen-containing combined pill and any copper-containing IUCD are contraindicated in WD**. The progesterone-only minipill or progesterone implant or levonorgestrel IUS (Mirena®) can be safely prescribed.

Diagnosis

- Diagnostic tests for WD include finding low serum caeruloplasmin levels, raised serum free copper levels, and excessive amounts of copper in 24-h urine collection.

Management

- **Treatment[2,3] for WD is with chelating agents such as D-penicillamine and trientine**, which chelate excess tissue copper that is then excreted in the urine.
- D-penicillamine in high dose is associated with congenital abnormalities such as micrognathia, low-set ears, or cutis laxa syndrome. Such high doses are, however, not used for maintenance therapy for WD.[3]
- **Zinc** is also an important treatment modality and acts by inhibiting intestinal absorption of copper. Zinc is particularly used as first-line therapy in those who are at a presymptomatic stage of WD or are intolerant of chelating agents. Zinc is also used as an adjuvant to chelating agents. Zinc therapy is also used in pregnancy.
- Successful management of pregnancy requires close assessment and collaboration with the gastroenterologist/hepatologist.
- Referral to a tertiary centre for further advice and input is also recommended.
- Fetal and maternal outcomes are good if the disease is adequately treated.
- ***If the disease is stable on treatment, the patient should be advised to continue her current medication with penicillamine as there are reports of haemolysis, hepatic deterioration, and death in women who have stopped treatment for fear of teratogenicity.***[1,2]
- Mothers and babies tolerate pregnancy safely, provided compliance with the prescribed regime is maintained.[2]
- The aim is to achieve and maintain disease control with relatively low doses of chelating agents. Chelating agents also reduce serum iron and have antipyridine effects. **Supplemental iron should not be used with chelating agents but vitamin B_6 (pyridoxine) should be given.**
- ***The dose of chelating agents is generally advised to be reduced during the first trimester to reduce the risk of malformations and again in the last couple of months of the third trimester as well as for about a month after delivery. This is to increase the maternal tissue copper levels, which is required for proper healing of any wounds.***
- Babies of mothers with WD have normal copper and ceruloplasmin levels.
- There are several reports[2,5] of the safety of breastfeeding with the mother on chelating agents, but the recent EASL guideline does not recommend breast feeding while on chelating agents.[4]

Information for patients

Please see Information for patients: Wilson's disease and pregnancy (p. 512)

References

1. Tavill AS, Schilsky ML. Wilson's disease. Curr Treat Options Gastroenterol 1999;2: 68–71.
2. Sternlieb I. Wilson's disease and pregnancy. Hepatology 2000:31; 531–532.
3. Williamson C. Hepatic disorders. In: Greer I et al., ed., Maternal medicine. London: Churchill Livingstone Elsevier, 2007.
4. European Association for the Study of the Liver. EASL Clinical Practice Guidelines: Wilson's Disease. J Hepatol 2012;56: 671–685.
5. Messner U, et al. Wilson disease and pregnancy. Review of the literature and case report. Z. Geburtshilfe Neonatol 1998;202: 77–79.

CARE PATHWAY

Pre-pregnancy assessment and counselling by hepatologist and/or maternal medicine obstetrician

- Aim for optimal copper status before pregnancy
- Discuss inheritance risk in offspring: chance of producing homozygous affected offspring is 0.5%, therefore partner testing, may be justified
- Advise that penicillamine or other chelating agents ± zinc must be continued throughout pregnancy to keep **Wilson's disease (WD)** well controlled. Withdrawal of treatment can have worse consequences compared to very small risk of teratogenicity
- Advise that dosage of chelating agents will be maintained at lowest dose to ensure effective WD control during 1st trimester to further reduce risk of teratogenicity
- Contraception advised while achieving good copper levels before a pregnancy: COCP or copper-containing IUCDs contraindicated; Progesterone implant or Mirena® advisable
- Advise peri-pregnancy folic acid

↓

Community midwife/GP refers pregnant woman with known WD to maternal medicine or specialist antenatal clinic in early first trimester

↓

First visit to maternal medicine or specialist antenatal clinic

- Check viability, dates, maternal well-being
- Ensure patient is on folic acid, continue till end of 13 weeks
- Close communication with gastroenterologist/hepatologist in DGH and tertiary centre as relevant
- Advise compliance with prescribed medication and doses; point out that stopping medication can be dangerous, even fatal, for the mother and fetus
- If dose of penicillamine has been reduced on hepatologist's advice during first trimester, it can be restored to normal doses after 14 weeks gestation. Close collaboration with hepatologist essential
- For those on chelating agents, do not prescribe supplemental iron but prescribe vitamin B6 (pyridoxine), to continue throughout pregnancy
- Arrange serial growth scans at around 28, 32, and 36 weeks with maternal medicine or specialist antenatal clinic follow-up on same days
- Routine antenatal care according to NICE protocol to continue in community
- Referral to or additional advice from tertiary centre as required.
- Refer to anaesthetic high-risk clinic

↓

Further visits to maternal medicine clinic

- Assess pregnancy progress, fetal growth, movements, continue vitamin B6
- Ensure that patient continues to have routine monitoring of serum copper, caeruloplasmin, liver enzymes as directed by hepatologists
- Ensure has had anaesthetic and hepatology review and hepatology follow-up has been arranged
- In last 4–6 weeks of pregnancy, some would advise reducing levels of chelating agents to allow increase in tissue/serum copper essential for healing of any tissue trauma
- Breastfeeding to be discussed. Generally contraindicated while mother is on chelating agents, but benefits may outweigh risks of tiny doses of chelating agents lowering baby's copper levels; breastfed babies reported to have normal copper and caeruloplasmin levels
- Continue routine antenatal checks with community midwife according to NICE protocol

↓

Delivery and postpartim

- No change in obstetric management, no indication for early IOL or Caesarean section except for other obstetric reasons
- IOL at 40 + 10 or according to individual unit's post-date IOL policy
- If delivery involves perineal tears, episiotomy, or is by Caesarean section, **remember tissues may have impaired healing ability. Therefore, careful suturing techniques and prevention of infection.**
- Inform neonatologist that mother has WD and is on chelating agents
- Remind patient about which contraception to be used, which types to be avoided
- Ensure she has long-term haematology/hepatology follow-up in place before hospital discharge

8.7 Haemochromatosis

FACT FILE

Epidemiology and inheritance

- **Haemochromotosis** may be **hereditary** or **acquired** (due to other medical conditions such as thalassaemia, haemolytic anaemia, sideroblastic anaemia, or over-transfusion).
- **Hereditary haemochromatosis (HH)** is one of the most common heritable genetic conditions in people of northern European descent, with a prevalence of 1 in 200 to 1 in 500.[1,2,3]
- About 10% of people of white European descent carry one of the gene defects linked to haemochromatosis. Most affected individuals by HH will have two copies of a variant called *C282Y*. Some will have one copy of *C282Y* and one of *H63D*. People with two copies of *H63D* do not seem to be at particular risk of iron overload themselves.
- Haemochromatosis has an autosomal recessive pattern of inheritance.

Pathophysiology and clinical manifestations

- Haemochromatosis is caused by excessive absorption of iron from the duodenum and upper intestine, with increased accumulation and deposition of iron in the reticuloendothelial system and in various parenchymal organs, notably the liver, pancreas, joints, heart, pituitary gland, and skin, with resultant end-organ damage.[4] Hepatomegaly, elevation of liver enzymes, and progressive development of fibrosis and cirrhosis result.
- The classic description of HH is of cutaneous hyperpigmentation, diabetes mellitus, and hepatomegaly. Diabetes mellitus develops in 30–60% of patients, and may result from a hereditary predisposition, cirrhosis, or deposition of iron in the pancreas.[5]
- Other clinical manifestations include fatigue (the commonest symptom), abdominal pain, abnormal liver tests, hepatocellular carcinoma, cardiomyopathy, cardiac conduction defects, hypogonadism, hypothyroidism, impotence, and arthropathy.
- Hepatomegaly is present in 95% of symptomatic patients, and abdominal pain of a dull, aching character with hepatic tenderness may be noted in 56% of patients.[6]
- Arthropathy is seen in 20–70% of patients, and may even be the presenting feature.[5]
- Clinical features may be non-specific and include lethargy and malaise, or reflect target organ damage and present with abnormal liver tests, cirrhosis, diabetes mellitus, arthropathy, cardiomyopathy, skin pigmentation, and gonadal failure.
- HH is due to mutations in the gene *HFE*.[1] In those with haemochromatosis both copies of the *HFE* gene on chromosome 6 are faulty.
- Transmission of the full disease to an offspring is rare, but siblings of the affected individual have a 1 in 4 risk. Each sib of an affected individual has a 25% chance of being affected, a 50% chance of being an asymptomatic carrier, and a 25% chance of being unaffected and not a carrier.
- Heterozygotes (carriers) are asymptomatic and do not have abnormalities of iron levels.
- Carrier testing for at-risk family members and prenatal testing for pregnancies at increased risk are possible if disease-causing mutations have been identified in the family.
- Nowadays about 75% of people with haemochromatosis are diagnosed as a result of routine blood tests or family testing.
- A large proportion of patients will be asymptomatic and may be identified by serum iron studies as part of screening studies or screening of family members of affected individual.[7]
- A normal adult has about 4 g of iron in the body, mostly as part of haemoglobin. In haemochromatosis, there is a gradual build-up of iron in various organs such as the liver, pancreas, brain, and heart. If untreated, the amount of iron in the body could be up to 5–10 times as much as usual, i.e. about 20–40 g.

Symptomatology

- Before the stage where symptoms develop, the only clue may be a 'healthy tan' all-year round and an increased tendency to develop bacterial infections.
- Early symptoms include fatigue, weakness, weight loss, muscle tenderness, and cramps.
- Untreated haemochromatosis can lead to arthritis, cirrhosis of the liver, hepatomegaly, dilated cardiomyopathy, hypothyroidism, and diabetes along with skin pigmentation, leading to the term 'bronzed diabetes'.[8] Alcohol worsens the cirrhosis and increases the risk of hepatocellular cancer.
- Symptoms usually develop later in women than in men. Iron levels in the body are reduced to near-normal values due to the blood loss associated with menstruation or childbirth, as well as the active transport of iron across the placenta during pregnancy.

Diagnosis

- The diagnosis must be considered in any patient with unexplained hepatomegaly, abnormal skin pigmentation, idiopathic cardiomyopathy, arthritis, diabetes, etc. Diagnosis is usually made by finding elevated transferrin saturation (>45%) and high serum iron and ferritin levels.[4,9,10]
- Laboratory investigations for HH usually start with two blood tests, **transferrin saturation** and **serum ferritin**, which are measures of the body's iron metabolism and the amount of iron stored. Confirmatory tests may include a genetic test and in a few case a liver biopsy outside of pregnancy. The latter can be used to find out if fibrotic or cirrhotic changes have occurred.

Treatment in the non-pregnant patient

- Treatment is aimed at removing excess iron from the system. This is done by **weekly phlebotomy** initially. Institution of phlebotomy before the onset of cirrhosis reduces the morbidity and mortality from HH.
- Phlebotomy of 500 ml of whole blood can be carried out in most patients once a week and although some patients may tolerate a twice-weekly regimen, this can be tedious. A venesection of 500 ml of whole blood removes 250 mg of iron. Each venesection should be preceded by measurement of the haematocrit, aiming for a drop of no more than 20% of the starting level.
- Serum ferritin levels are checked every 10–12 phlebotomies.
- Stop frequent phlebotomy when serum ferritin falls below 50 ng/mL.
- Continue phlebotomy at intervals to keep serum ferritin to between 25 and 50 ng/ml.
- Some clinical manifestations such as malaise, fatigue, skin pigmentation, insulin requirements in diabetics, and abdominal pain are ameliorated by phlebotomy, but others, such as arthropathy, hypogonadism, and cirrhosis, are not affected.[11]
- End-organ damage should also be assessed and managed appropriately, e.g. diabetes control with insulin or oral hypoglycaemics as well as treatment of macrovascular and microvascular complications. Arthritis should be managed with simple analgesia as far as possible.[12]
- Patients need to be closely followed for the development of complications such as cirrhosis and hepatocellular carcinoma, which may develop in one-third of patients and will not respond to phlebotomy.
- Survival in patients who have had liver transplants for haemochromatosis is lower than those transplanted for other liver diseases.[13]
- A normal balanced diet is usually sufficient, although reduced intake of iron-containing and iron-fortified foods can avoid excessive dietary iron. Tannin in tea may inhibit iron absorption (blocking agent), but it is not a substitute for phlebotomy.[14]

- Treatment usually consists of repeated phlebotomy at periodic intervals required throughout life, **though discontinued during pregnancy**.

Treatment during pregnancy

- Phlebotomy is to be discontinued for the duration of pregnancy and the puerperium.
- **Iron and vitamin C supplements should be avoided**, including during pregnancy.[15] Peri-pregnancy folic acid (400 micrograms/day) without additional iron must be prescribed for women with haemochromatosis.[1]
- **Iron-chelating agents such as desferrioxamine**[1,2] may be required in addition.
- The perinatal inheritance of haemochromotosis can present as hydrops fetalis in recurrent pregnancies and successful outcome has been reported[3] with maternal immunodilution with antenatal weekly IV immunoglobulin administration from 18 weeks gestation till delivery.
- Serial LFTs during pregnancy are recommended.[15]
- During pregnancy, liver scans might reveal hepatomegaly or fibrotic or cirrhotic changes.
- Serial fetal growth scans are advisable.

Information for patients

Please see Information for patients: Hereditary haemochromatosis and pregnancy (p. 512)

References

1. Merryweather-Clarke AT, et al. Geography of HFE C282Y and H63D mutations. Genet Test 2000;4: 183–198.
2. Bacon BR, et al. Molecular medicine and haemochromatosis: at the crossroads. Gastroenterology 1999;116: 193–207.
3. Ryan E, et al. Hemochromatosis in Ireland and HFE. Blood Cells Mol Dis 1998;24: 428–432.
4. Adams P, et al. EASL International Consensus Conference on Haemochromatosis. J Hepatol 2000;33: 485–504.
5. Powell LW, Yapp TR. Hemochromatosis. Clin Liver Dis 2000;4: 211–228.
6. Niederau C, et al. Long term survival in patients with hereditary haemochromatosis. Gastroenterology 1996;110: 1107.
7. Bacon BR, Sadiq S. Hereditary haemochromatosis: diagnosis in the 1990s. Am J Gastroenterol 1997;92: 784–789.
8. Limdi JK, Crampton JR. Hereditary haemochromatosis. Q J Med 2004;97: 315–324.
9. McCullen MA, et al. Screening for haemochromatosis. Clin Chim Acta 2002;315: 169–186.
10. Bassett ML, et al. Diagnosis of haemochromatosis in young subjects: Predictive accuracy of biochemical screening tests. Gastroenterology 1984;87: 628–633.
12. Tavill AS. Diagnosis and management of haemochromatosis. AASLD Practice Guidelines. Hepatology 2001;33: 1321–1328
13. Farrell FJ, et al. Outcome of liver transplantation in patients with haemochromatosis. Hepatology 1994;20: 404–410.
14. Cunningham E. Is there a role for diet in the treatment of haemochromatosis? J Am Diet Assoc 2003;103: 593.
15. Aslam MF, et al. Unusual case of postpartum hepatitis due to hereditary haemochromatosis. BJOG 2010; 117: 620–622.

- Diagnosis of **haemochromatosis** already established before pregnancy in most cases
- GP/midwife to refer patient asap in first trimester to maternal medicine/joint haematology–obstetric, or a specialist antenatal clinic

↓

First visit to specialist antenatal clinic or combined obstetric–haematology antenatal clinic

- If patient has been taking over-the-counter 'pregnancy multivitamin' with iron content, advise to stop. Prescribe 400 micrograms folic acid till end of 13 weeks gestation and vitamin D 10 micrograms/day till end of pregnancy
- Detailed family and personal history to differentiate between acquired and hereditary disease
- Enquire whether being assessed for or under treatment for diabetes or any cardiac problems.
- If she has not received genetic counselling previously, refer—autosomal recessive pattern in most cases
- Confirm she has had recent follow-up with haematologist, whether on phlebotomy programme before pregnancy, as well as checking pre-pregnancy levels of erum iron, ferritin, and transferrin saturation
- Confirm viability and dates. Liver ultrasound scan for any evidence of hepatomegaly, changes of fibrosis, etc.
- Routine booking bloods to include the above tests as well as baseline LFTs, thyroid function tests, diabetes screening (early 2nd trimester GTT may be considered) if not known to have pre-existing diabetes
- Advise **not** to take supplemental iron or vitamin C.
- Confirm that patient attends regular haematology follow-up
- Refer to hepatologist if abnormal liver enzymes or if hepatomegaly is suspected
- Regular phlebotomy will be suspended during pregnancy and iron chelators (desferrioxamine) may be prescribed instead, as advised by haematologists
- Arrange regular serial growth scans to be arranged at 28, 32, and 36 weeks; specialist antenatal clinic appointments to be scheduled after scans on the same day
- Routine antenatal community midwife care to continue

↓

Further visits to specialist antenatal clinic or combined obstetric–haematology antenatal clinic

- Check progress of pregnancy and any maternal symptoms
- Regular LFTs, serum iron, ferritin, and transferrin saturation in each trimester
- Ensure fetal growth is satisfactory on serial scans
- If any suspicion of hydrops fetalis, after excluding other causes, antenatal haemachromatosis may be suspected. In this instance, with haematologist's input, weekly IV maternal immunoglobulin to achieve immunodilution may be required

↓

Delivery and postpartum

- Anticipate normal vaginal delivery
- In the absence of IUGR, hydrops, etc., **no indication for early IOL or elective LSCS except if other standard obstetric indications**
- Further neonatal management if hydrops has been due to antenatal haemachromatosis in offspring

9 Maternal Endocrine Disorders

9.1 Diabetes

FACT FILE

The remit of this chapter is to give a thumbnail sketch of pre-pregnancy and pregnancy management of women with **type 1 and type 2 diabetes** as well as of those diagnosed to have developed **gestational diabetes** in pregnancy. The reader is referred to the NICE clinical guideline[1] and its updates for further detailed information.

Introduction

- Diabetes is the most common pre-existing maternal medical disorder complicating pregnancy in the UK, with significantly increased maternal complications and fetal and neonatal risks.[5,6]
- **Type 1, type 2, and gestational diabetes affect 5% of pregnancies in the UK.** This rate is rapidly rising, reflecting the global trend.[1,2,3,4]
- **Of women who have diabetes during pregnancy, it is estimated that approximately 87.5% have gestational diabetes (which may or may not resolve after pregnancy), 7.5% have type 1 diabetes and the remaining 5% have type 2 diabetes.**[1]

Possible pregnancy complications in women with pre-existing diabetes

Increased risk of diabetic complications

- Ketoacidosis.
- Hypoglycaemia and unawareness of the same.
- Progression of **microvascular complications including retinopathy and nephropathy.**
- Poor glycaemic control in the first trimester as well as pregnancy-induced or chronic hypertension are independently associated with a worsening of retinopathy.
- Worsening nephropathy can affect maternal blood pressure, and nephropathy with superimposed pre-eclampsia is the most common cause for preterm delivery in women with diabetes.

Increased risk of obstetric complications

- Spontaneous miscarriage.
- Pregnancy-induced hypertension.
- Pre-eclampsia.
- Thromboembolism.
- Intrauterine death (IUD).
- Premature labour: babies are five times more likely to be born before 37 weeks.[5,6]
- **Fetal macrosomia:** Twice as many babies weigh more than 4 kg in diabetics than in the general maternity population, and 8% of babies of diabetic mothers have shoulder dystocia compared with 3% of the general population. Obstructed labour is another consequence of macrosomia, thereby increase in Caesarean sections.
- ***Caesarean section:*** *The 2007 CEMACH survey found a 67% lower segment Caesarean section (LSCS) rate in diabetics compared with 22% in the general maternity population.*
- Increased maternal infection rate.

Increased risk of fetal and neonatal complications

- Congenital malformations (twofold increased risk), especially neurological or cardiac abnormalities.[5,6]
- Late IUD/stillbirth (fivefold increased risk).
- Fetal distress in labour.
- Hypoglycaemia.
- Respiratory distress syndrome.
- Jaundice.
- Increased perinatal mortality rate (threefold increased risk).
- Erb's palsy due to shoulder dystocia at birth is 10 times more likely in babies of diabetic mothers.

Pre-conception assessment and counselling

Pre-conception assessment and counselling of women with pre-pregnancy diabetes should include[1]:

- Counselling either in a specially designated pre-pregnancy diabetic clinic or as part of endocrinologist-led diabetes clinics, with the additional availability of diabetes specialist nurses and dietitian.
- The aim of pre-conception care is to help reduce the risks of adverse pregnancy outcomes for the mother and the baby.
- Women with diabetes who are planning a pregnancy should be informed that establishing good glycaemic control from before conception and continuing this throughout the pregnancy is vital for improved pregnancy outcomes. This will reduce (but not eliminate) the risks of miscarriage, congenital malformations, macrosomia, intrapartum problems such as shoulder dystocia, stillbirth, and neonatal death.
- Role of diet, body weight, and exercise, especially weight loss for women with a body mass index (BMI) greater than 30.
- High-dose folic acid (5 mg/day) should be prescribed from pre-conception until end of 12 weeks gestation.
- Need for assessment of diabetic retinopathy before and during pregnancy. Retinal assessment must be offered to women with diabetes seeking preconception care at their first appointment (unless they have had an annual retinal assessment in the last 6 months) and then annually if no diabetic retinopathy is found.[1]
- Need for assessment of diabetic nephropathy before and during pregnancy.
- ***Review of medication and possible changes to it: For example, changing antihypertensive medication from angiotensin-II receptor antagonists (ARBs) and angiotensin converting enzyme (ACE) inhibitors to either methyldopa or labetalol.***
- Similarly if patient is on **beta-blockers (other than labetalol)** or **diuretics**, these should be stopped and methyldopa or labetalol commenced instead.
- Statins should be discontinued either before or as soon as pregnancy is confirmed.
- The importance of planning pregnancy, the role of contraception, and when to stop contraception should be discussed.
- Explain to women with diabetes that their choice of contraception should be based on their own preferences and any risk factors. Advise women with diabetes that they can use oral contraceptives (if there are no standard contraindications to their use).[1]
- Referral to a nephrologist if the serum creatinine is 120 micromol/litre or more.
- Low-dose aspirin (75 mg) should be considered in this high-risk group of women, especially those with either chronic or diabetes-related hypertension or nephropathy. The low-dose aspirin can be continued throughout pregnancy.
- Review of glycaemic targets and glucose monitoring.

Table 9.1 Conversion of old (NGSP) HbA_{1c} (%) to new (IFCC) HbA_{1c} (mmol/mol)

%	4.0	4.1	4.2	4.3	4.4	4.5	4.6	4.7	4.8	4.9
mmol/mol	20	21	22	23	25	26	27	28	29	30
%	5.0	5.1	5.2	5.3	5.4	5.5	5.6	5.7	5.8	5.9
mmol/mol	31	32	33	34	36	37	38	39	40	41
%	6.0	6.1	6.2	6.3	6.4	6.5	6.6	6.7	6.8	6.9
mmol/mol	42	43	44	45	46	48	49	50	51	52
%	7.0	7.1	7.2	7.3	7.4	7.5	7.6	7.7	7.8	7.9
mmol/mol	53	54	55	56	57	58	60	61	62	63
%	8.0	8.1	8.2	8.3	8.4	8.5	8.6	8.7	8.8	8.9
mmol/mol	64	65	66	67	68	69	70	72	73	74
%	9.0	9.1	9.2	9.3	9.4	9.5	9.6	9.7	9.8	9.9
mmol/mol	75	76	77	78	79	80	81	83	84	85
%	10.0	10.1	10.2	10.3	10.4	10.5	10.6	10.7	10.8	10.9
mmol/mol	86	87	88	89	90	91	92	93	95	96
%	11.0	11.1	11.2	11.3	11.4	11.5	11.6	11.7	11.8	11.9
mmol/mol	97	98	99	100	101	102	103	104	105	107
%	12.0	12.1	12.2	12.3	12.4	12.5	12.6	12.7	12.8	12.9
mmol/mol	108	109	110	111	112	113	114	115	116	117
%	13.0	13.1	13.2	13.3	13.4	13.5	13.6	13.7	13.8	13.9
mmol/mol	119	120	121	122	123	124	125	126	127	128

- Monthly HbA_{1c} monitoring should be offered in those planning to get pregnant. Inform women that any reduction in HbA_{1c} may reduce risks in a subsequent pregnancy with the target aimed for being less than 48 mmol/mol (<6.5%) if safe. **Women with HbA_{1c} 86 mmol/mol or more (≥10%) should be advised to avoid a pregnancy till better control is established.**
- The way in which HbA_{1c} results expressed in the UK changed in 2011. Results are now reported in the IFCC reference method of mmol/mol, rather than the DCCT units as a percentage. **Clinicians need to be familiar with these ranges**. (Table 9.1).

Antenatal care of diabetes in pregnancy (pre-existing and gestational diabetes)

See the **NICE guideline**[1] with particular attention to:

- Regular monitoring of weight, BP, urine for protein ± ketones, retinal screening, assessment of renal function if known diabetic nephropathy, vigilance for pre-eclampsia, PIH.
- Screening for trisomy 21 based on nuchal fold thickness measurement.
- Regular serial fetal growth and liquor scans from 26–28 weeks onwards
- Timing and mode of delivery would depend on the above factors, previous obstetric history, whether hypoglycaemics have been required or not during pregnancy, etc.
- Encourage breastfeeding.
- Discuss suitable family planning measures, including appropriate contraceptive advice or permanent sterilization.
- Advise longer-term dietary and exercise regime, weight loss management, etc.

Gestational diabetes (GDM)

- The NICE clinical guideline[1] recommends **targeted screening** of women with risk factors for developing gestational diabetes.
- Independent risk factors for screening for gestational diabetes (which, in effect, cover about 30–50% of the pregnant population) include:
  - BMI ≥30 kg/m^2
  - previous macrosomic baby ≥4.5 kg
  - previous gestational diabetes
  - first-degree relative with diabetes
  - minority ethnic family origin with a high prevalence of diabetes, including but not exclusive to South Asian (Indian, Pakistani, Bangladeshi, Sri Lankan, Nepali), African Caribbean, Middle Eastern etc.,
- In addition to the above-mentioned categories of women at greater risk of developing gestational diabetes, **by local consensus some units have also included women in the following groups as eligible for screening:**
  - previous history of polycystic ovarian syndrome (PCOS)
  - recurrent miscarriages (>3) if glucose tolerance test (GTT) not done previously
  - glycosuria: -(See Below)
  - polyhydramnios.
- **Diagnose gestational diabetes[1] if the woman has either: - a fasting plasma glucose level of 5.6 mmol/litre or above or a 2-hour plasma glucose level of 7.8 mmol/litre or above.**
- Most of these risk factors are identifiable at the booking visit and GTTs are to be booked at the appropriate gestation by the community midwife.
- If there is a history of previous gestational diabetes, a 2-h 75-g oral GTT should be performed at 16–18 weeks gestation followed by another oral GTT at 28 weeks if the first test is normal.
- For all other risk factors (except polyhydramnios and consecutive episodes of glycosuria, which may occur at any stage of pregnancy), an oral GTT should be done at around 26–28 weeks gestation.
- **Screening for gestational diabetes using HbA1c, plasma glucose or by a random blood glucose is not to be offered**. Only **the oral GTT (2 h, 75 g oral glucose)** is to be used for screening.
- ***Note:* Glycosuria of 2+ or above on 1 occasion or of 1+ or above on 2 or more occasions(usually testing within a week of each other) detected by reagent strip testing during routine antenatal care may indicate undiagnosed gestational diabetes.[1] An oral GTT (OGTT) must, in such instances, be performed as soon as possible**.

- Most gestational diabetics will respond to exercise such as walking briskly for 30 minutes after a meal, and diet control. **Refer all women with gestational diabetes to a dietitian.** Lifestyle advice including dietary modification is the primary intervention in all women diagnosed with gestational diabetes.
- **A trial of changes in diet and exercise should be offered to women with gestational diabetes who have a fasting plasma glucose level below 7 mmol/litre at diagnosis.**[1]
- **Offer immediate treatment with insulin, with or without metformin, as well as changes in diet and exercise, to women with gestational diabetes who have a fasting plasma glucose level of 7.0 mmol/litre or above at diagnosis.**[1]
- **Immediate treatment with insulin, with or without metformin, as well as changes in diet and exercise, must be considered for women with gestational diabetes who have a fasting plasma glucose level of between 6.0 and 6.9 mmol/litre if there are complications such as macrosomia or hydramnios.**[1]
- Women with gestational diabetes should be instructed in self-monitoring of blood glucose and targets for blood glucose control specified.
- However, 7–20% of women fail to achieve adequate glycaemic control with diet and exercise alone and will require hypoglycaemic therapy with oral metformin and/or SC insulin injections. In these women, if the exercise and diet control do not maintain blood glucose targets over a period of 1–2 weeks or if the ultrasound scan already shows signs suggestive of fetal macrosomia (AC >90th percentile) at the time of diagnosis of gestational diabetes, hypoglycaemic therapy is recommended without delay.
- Before starting metformin, the pregnant woman and her family members need to be made aware that though the product information says 'Not to be used in pregnancy' and the drug is not licensed for use in pregnancy, the safety of metformin in pregnancy has been well established. Metformin has been used for several years in tens of thousands of pregnant women worldwide. The discussion should also include a description of possible side effects such as tummy upsets, nausea, vomiting, loose motions, etc. for the first 7–10 days of starting medication. It is therefore advisable for pregnant woman to take metformin with meals and not on an empty stomach.
- **The same capillary plasma glucose target levels should be used for women with gestational diabetes as for women with pre-existing diabetes.**[1]
- Women with gestational diabetes should be informed that good glycaemic control throughout the pregnancy will reduce the risk of fetal macrosomia, birth trauma, Caesarean section, neonatal hypoglycaemia, and perinatal death.
- In women with gestational diabetes, the incidence of large-for-gestational age babies and birth trauma have been shown to be reduced by up to 50% with treatment and rigorous glycaemic control.
- The combination of obesity and gestational diabetes exerts a synergistic effect on short-term complications in pregnancy.
- The management of women who are on metformin is identical to those on insulin for induction of labour, active labour, or emergency Caesarean section. Once active labour sets in, a sliding scale of glucose and insulin is commenced and titrated according to hourly blood sugar monitoring. Similarly, the preoperative admission schedule and protocol for an elective Caesarean section is identical to that of insulin-managed diabetics.
- Women with gestational diabetes can be instructed to stop metformin and insulin after the delivery.
- An oral GTT should be arranged for these women at 6–8 weeks post-delivery.
- ***Note:* With the publication of the HAPO Study[6,7], the previous NICE guidelines (2008) have been updated and published in Feb 2015.**[1] It is essential for the reader to refer to the new NICE guidelines for the detailed management of **Diabetes in Pregnancy**.

Information for patients

Please see Information for patients: Diabetes and pregnancy (p. 513)

References

1. NICE Clinical Guideline. Diabetes in pregnancy: management of diabetes and its complication from pre-conception to the postnatal period. NG3. National Collaborating Centre for Women's and Children's Health. London: RCOG Press, 2015.
2. Diabetes UK. State of the nation 2012 report. <http://www.diabetes.org.uk/Documents/.../State-of-the-Nation-2012.pdf>
3. Scottish Diabetes Survey Monitoring Group. Scottish Diabetes Survey 2011, NHS Scotland. <http://www.diabetesinscotland.org.uk/Publications/SDS%202011.pdf>
4. Hunt KJ, Schuller KL The increasing prevalence of diabetes in pregnancy. Obstet Gynecol Clin 2007; 34: 173–199.
5. RCOG Scientific Advisory Committee Opinion Paper 23. Diagnosis and treatment of gestational diabetes. London: Royal College of Obstetricians and Gynaecologists, 2011.
6. Coustan DR, et al. The Hyperglycemia and Adverse Pregnancy Outcome (HAPO) study: paving the way for new diagnostic criteria for gestational diabetes mellitus. Am J Obstet Gynecol 2010; 202: 654.e1–654.e6.
7. Metzger BE, et al. Hyperglycemia and Adverse Pregnancy Outcome (HAPO) Study Cooperative Research Group. N Engl J Med 2008; 358: 1991–2002.
8. Metzer BE, et al. International Association of Diabetes and Pregnancy Study Groups Consensus Study Groups. Recommendations on the diagnosis and classification of hyperglycaemia in pregnancy. Diabetes Care 2010; 33: 676–682.

- Immediate referral to joint obstetrics–diabetes clinic of **women with diabetes** who are pregnant.
- Contact with diabetes care team every 1–2 weeks throughout pregnancy to assess glycaemic control
- Advice on where to have the birth, which should be in a hospital with advanced neonatal resuscitation skills available 24 h/day
- Information and education at each appointment
- Care specifically for women with diabetes, **in addition to routine antenatal care**

First appointment: joint diabetic antenatal clinic (joint clinic), as early as possible in 1st trimester, ideally by 10 weeks

- Midwife to have arranged scan to confirm viability and dates and, if opted for, trisomy 21 screening at about 11 weeks gestation by measurement of nuchal fold thickness
- Offer information, advice and support on glycaemic control. (see Boxes 9.1–9.3) **If the woman has not attended for preconception care and advice, give information, education and advice for the first time.**
- Take a clinical history to establish the extent of diabetes-related complications (including neuropathy and vascular disease)
- Review medications for diabetes and its complications. (see Box 9.4)
- Offer retinal and renal assessment if these have not been done in previous 3 months (see Boxes 5–6)
- Measure HbA1c levels for women with pre-existing diabetes to determine the level of risk for the pregnancy.
- Advise 5 mg/day folic acid to continue till end of 13 weeks gestation
- Prescribe low-dose aspirin if diabetic, overweight, ± hypertensive, advise to continue till end of pregnancy

↓

10–11 weeks (ideally): joint clinic appointment

- Check viability with scan.
- Discuss information, education, and advice about how diabetes will affect pregnancy, birth, and early parenting (such as breastfeeding and initial care of the baby)
- Arrange all subsequent scans (routine 20+ week anomaly scan, and serial growth scans 28, 32, 36 weeks)
- Offer a 75 g 2-hour OGTT as soon as possible for women with a history of gestational diabetes who book in the first trimester.

↓

16 weeks: joint clinic

- Glycaemic control review
- Offer retinal assessment at 16–20 weeks to women with pre-existing diabetes who had signs of diabetic retinopathy at the first antenatal appointment (see Box 9.5)
- Offer a 75 g 2-hour OGTT as soon as possible for women with a history of gestational diabetes who book in the second trimester.

↓

20 weeks: joint clinic appointment, with detailed anomaly scan on same day if possible

- ***Detailed anomaly scan including examination of the fetal heart (4 chambers, outflow tracts and 3 vessels).***
- Review glycaemic control and advise
- Referral to anaesthetists if comorbidities (e.g. gross obesity, autonomic neuropathies etc.)
- Patient to maintain contact with DSN meanwhile

↓

24 weeks: diabetes specialist nurse or diabetes—only clinic

- Review of glycaemic control and advise patient to maintain weekly contact with DSN
- Ensure has a routine antenatal check with the community midwife around this time.

↓

26 weeks: community midwife care

- Routine antenatal check, vigilance for pre-eclampsia

↓

28 weeks: joint clinic appointment with growth and liquor scan on same day

- Routine antenatal check and blood tests, Anti D if Rh(D) −ve
- Review of growth and liquor volume scan (see Box 9.7)
- Offer retinal assessment to women with pre-existing diabetes
- **Women diagnosed with gestational diabetes as a result of routine antenatal testing at 24–28 weeks enter the care pathway.**

↓

30 weeks: community midwife visit at 28–32 weeks

- Vigilance for pre-eclampsia, advice regarding fetal movement awareness

↓

32 weeks: joint clinic appointment with growth and liquor scan on same day

- Routine antenatal check
- Review ultrasound scan of fetal growth and amniotic fluid volume
- Plan for delivery at approximately 38 weeks
- Patient to maintain weekly contact with DSN

↓

34 weeks: community midwife visit

- Routine antenatal check, maintain vigilance for pre-eclampsia, fetal movements
- Patient to maintain weekly contact with diabetes nurse

↓

36 weeks: joint clinic appointment with growth and liquor scan on same day

- Review scan for fetal growth and amniotic fluid volume
- Offer information and advice about:
  - timing, mode, and management of birth
  - analgesia and anaesthesia
  - changes to hypoglycaemic therapy during and after birth
  - initial care of the baby
  - initiation of breastfeeding and the effect of breastfeeding on glycaemic control
  - contraception and follow-up
- Plan for delivery **between 37–38^{+6} weeks for women with Type 1 or 2 diabetes or those gestational diabetics on medication but where control has been suboptimal or macrosomia/polhydramnios suspected.** Give relevant information leaflets and book the first slot of the day for either IOL or Caesarean section, as relevant
- If Caesarean section is planned, give consent information form

↓

38 weeks–40 weeks

- IOL, or Caesarean section if indicated, at 38 weeks gestation for diabetic women and those gestational diabetic women who have needed metformin and/or insulin in this pregnancy
- For **women with gestational diabetes who are only diet-controlled** during pregnancy, IOL/Caesarean section as relevant at about 40 weeks. Book the first slot of the day, if possible
- ***Close monitoring for development of pre-eclampsia essential in diabetic women***
- Offer ***additional tests*** for fetal well being ***such as more frequent scans for Dopplers, biometry,*** **CTG etc., for those with GDM who decline IOL at between 39–40^{+6} weeks. Advise women with uncomplicated gestational diabetes to give birth no later than 40^{+6} weeks.**

Box 9.1 Blood glucose targets and monitoring

- Advise pregnant women with type 1 diabetes to test their fasting, pre-meal, 1-hour post-meal and bedtime blood glucose levels daily during pregnancy.
- Advise pregnant women with type 2 diabetes or gestational diabetes who are on a multiple daily insulin injection regimen to test their fasting, pre-meal, 1-hour post-meal and bedtime blood glucose levels daily during pregnancy.
- Advise pregnant women with type 2 diabetes or gestational diabetes to test their fasting and 1-hour post-meal blood glucose levels daily during pregnancy if they are: on diet and exercise therapy or taking oral therapy (with or without diet and exercise therapy) or single-dose intermediate-acting or long-acting insulin.
- Agree individual targets for self-monitoring
- Advise women to aim for a fasting blood glucose of between 4 and 5.9 mmol/litre and 1-h postprandial blood glucose <7.8 mmol/litre or 2-h postprandial <6.8 mmol/litre
- ***Use the same capillary plasma glucose target levels for women with gestational diabetes as for women with pre-existing diabetes***
- Do not use HbA1c routinely to assess blood glucose control in the 2nd and 3rd trimesters

Box 9.2 Additional care for women taking insulin-and risks of hypoglycaemia.

Offer:
- Concentrated oral glucose solution to all women taking insulin
- Glucagon to women with type 1 diabetes and instruct the woman and her partner or other family members in its use.
- Continuous subcutaneous insulin infusion (CSII) also known as insulin pump therapy if glycaemic control using multiple injections is not adequate and the woman experiences significant disabling hypoglycaemia

Advise:
- Women to test their blood glucose before going to bed at night
- On the risks of hypoglycaemia and hypoglycaemia unawareness, especially in the first trimester
- **Advise pregnant women with insulin-treated diabetes to always have available a fast-acting form of glucose (for example, glucose tablets or glucose-containing drinks)**

Box 9.3 Detecting and managing diabetic ketoacidosis

- If diabetic ketoacidosis is suspected during pregnancy, admit women immediately for level 2 critical care, where both medical and obstetric care are available
- For women with type 1 diabetes:
  - Offer ketone testing strips and a meter, and advise women to test their ketone levels if they are hyperglycaemic or unwell
  - Test urgently for ketonaemia if a pregnant woman with any form of diabetes(including GDM) presents with hyperglycaemia or becomes unwell.

Box 9.4 Safety of medications before and during pregnancy

- Women with diabetes may be advised to use metformin as an adjunct or alternative to insulin in the preconception period and during pregnancy. All other oral blood glucose-lowering agents should be discontinued before pregnancy and insulin substituted.
- Data from clinical trials and other sources do not suggest that the rapid-acting insulin analogues (aspart and lispro) adversely affect pregnancy or the health of the fetus or newborn baby
- Use isophane insulin (NPH insulin) as the first choice for long-acting insulin during pregnancy. Consider continuing treatment with long-acting insulin analogues (insulin detemir or insulin glargine) in women with diabetes who have established good blood glucose control before pregnancy
- Before or as soon as pregnancy is confirmed:
  - Stop oral hypoglycaemic agents, apart from metformin, and commence insulin if required
  - Stop ACE inhibitors and ARBs and consider antihypertensives compatible with pregnancy
  - Stop statins

Box 9.5 Retinal assessment for women and pre-existing diabetes

- Offer retinal assessment:
  - As soon as possible after the first contact in pregnancy if it has not been performed in the past 3 months
  - Following the first antenatal clinic appointment
  - At 28 weeks if the first assessment is normal
  - At 16–20 weeks if any diabetic retinopathy is present
- Retinal assessment should be carried out with mydriasis using tropicamide
- Diabetic retinopathy is not a contraindication to rapid optimisation of blood glucose control in women who present with a high HbA1c in early pregnancy

Box 9.6 Renal assessment for women with pre-existing diabetes

- Offer renal assessment at the first contact in pregnancy if it has not been done in the past 3 months
- Consider referral to a nephrologist if serum creatinine is abnormal (≥120 micromole/litre) or total protein excretion >2 g/day or the urinary albumin: creatinine ratio is greater than 30 mg/mmol.
- Consider thromboprophylaxis if proteinuria >5 g/day

Box 9.7 Monitoring and screening

Offer:
- The detailed anomaly scan at around 20wk should include examination of the fetal heart (4 chambers, outflow tracts and 3 vessels)
- Ultrasound monitoring of fetal growth and amniotic fluid volume every 4 weeks from 28 to 36 weeks
- Individualized monitoring of fetal well-being to women at risk of IUGR (those with microvascular disease or nephropathy)

National Institute for Health and Care Excellence 2015 Adapted from NG3 *Diabetes in pregnancy: management of diabetes and its complications from preconception to the postnatal period.* Manchester: NICE. Available from www.nice.org.uk/NG3. This information was accurate at the time of press. For any further updates to this information, please visit the NICE website.

9.2 Hypothyroidism

FACT FILE

- Management of thyroid diseases during pregnancy requires particular consideration not only because pregnancy itself induces major changes in thyroid function, but also because maternal thyroid disease can have adverse effects on the pregnancy and fetus.[1]
- Pregnancy may affect the course of these thyroid disorders and, conversely, thyroid diseases may affect the outcomes of pregnancy.

Incidence

- **Hypothyroidism** occurs in 1–2%[2] of all pregnancies; the prevalence is estimated to be 0.3–0.5% for overt hypothyroidism and 2–3% for subclinical hypothyroidism.[3]

Aetiology of hypothyroidism during pregnancy

- Chronic autoimmune thyroiditis is the main cause in developed countries.
- Previous treatment of Graves's disease with radioactive iodine, antithyroid medication, or surgical thyroidectomy; hyperthyroidism (with radioiodine ablation or surgery); or surgery for thyroid tumours.
- Inadequate iodine intake or iodine deficiency prevalent in certain areas of the world is the most important cause of thyroid insufficiency due to iodine deficiency (ID) and is known to affect over 1.2 billion individuals.[1]

Physiology

- Thyroid stimulating hormone (TSH) is an indicator for the adequacy of T_4 and T_3.
- Maternal thyroxine requirements are increased during pregnancy, sometimes by as much as 50% during the first half of pregnancy from as early as the fifth week of gestation.
- Normal maternal thyroid levels need to be normal for fetal neural development. Thyroid hormone and specific nuclear receptors are found in fetal brain at 8 weeks after conception.[4]

Pathophysiology and pregnancy outcomes

- ***Untreated or inadequately corrected hypothyroidism in pregnancy can result in significant detriment to the child's IQ and neurodevelopment.***
- ***Uncorrected hypothyroidism can be associated with increased risk of miscarriage, abruption, preterm delivery, anaemia, IUGR, pre-eclampsia, and PPH. These complications, including neonatal problems such as premature birth, low birth weight, and neonatal respiratory distress, are more frequent with overt than with subclinical hypothyroidism. Adequate thyroxine treatment greatly decreases the risk of a poorer obstetric outcome.***

Diagnosis

- **Hypothyroidism may remain undetected or subclinical.** Hitherto undetected hypothyroidism can present in pregnancy with non-specific signs such as weight increase due to excess fluid retention early in pregnancy, persistent maternal bradycardia, oversensitivity to cold, dry skin, significant cold intolerance, drowsiness, or constipation.
- Diagnosis of primary hypothyroidism is **elevation of serum TSH**. Serum free T_4 levels further distinguish subclinical from overt hypothyroidism, depending on whether free T_4 is normal or below normal for gestational age respectively.
- **Hypothyroidism may coexist with insulin-dependent diabetes, lupus, etc.** It is worth screening such high-risk women for hypothyroidism with the booking bloods at the start of pregnancy.

Management in pregnancy

- Multidisciplinary care is essential with involvement of obstetricians, endocrinologists, midwives, GPs, and paediatricians.
- Levothyroxine is the treatment of choice for maternal hypothyroidism, if the iodine nutritional status is adequate, as it is in general in the UK.
- Hypothyroid pregnant women require larger thyroxine replacement doses than when not pregnant.
- In women who are already on thyroxine before conception, the need to adjust the pre-conception thyroxine daily dosage becomes important as early as 4–6 weeks gestation, hence the need for adequate thyroxine replacement to ensures that maternal euthyroidism is maintained during early pregnancy.
- Women already on thyroxine replacement may require an increase from the first trimester. This is why women who are hypothyroid need to have TSH levels included with booking bloods to allow appropriate increase in the thyroxine as soon as possible.
- By **anticipating the expected increase in serum TSH, an alternative approach is to advise that all women who already take levothyroxine before pregnancy need to increase their daily dosage** by, on average, 30–50% above pre-conception dosage or, as a clinical guide, **by 25 micrograms/day as soon as a pregnancy is confirmed.**
- Advise the patient to take thyroxine on an empty stomach
- Hypothyroidism in pregnancy is treated with a larger dose of thyroxine than in a non-pregnant state. A slight overcorrection is better than inadequate thyroxine replacement in pregnancy.
- ***Thyroid function tests (TSH) should be repeated every 6–8 weeks during pregnancy and the dosage of levothyroxine adjusted by 25 micrograms in order to maintain the TSH level in the range 0.5–2.5 μIU/ml.***
- ***Note: This TSH reference range is pregnancy specific and is narrower than ranges used outside of pregnancy. Midwives and GPs in primary care need to be aware of this pregnancy-specific range and make any adjustment of dosage as indicated by the TSH checks every 6–8 weeks during pregnancy.***
- The thyroxine requirements increase further later in pregnancy due to increased binding of the free drug molecules by the oestrogen-driven increase in thyroxine-binding globulins, the increased distribution volume of thyroid hormones (vascular, hepatic, fetal-placental unit), and the increased placental transport and metabolism of maternal T_4.[5,6,7]
- Thyroxine absorption can be inhibited by oral iron and/or calcium. The patient may be advised to avoid taking thyroxine at the same time as oral iron or calcium. Otherwise, an increase in thyroxine dosage as indicated by TSH levels may be required.
- Women without residual functional thyroid tissue (after radioiodine ablation or total thyroidectomy, or due to congenital agenesis of the gland) require a greater increment in thyroxine dosage than women with Hashimoto's thyroiditis, who usually have some residual thyroid tissue.[1]
- The thyroxine requirement usually falls after delivery in women whose dose had increased during pregnancy.
- After delivery, most patients need to decrease the thyroxine dosage to pre-pregnancy levels, over a period of approximately 4 weeks postpartum.
- Breastfeeding is entirely safe while on thyroxine.

Information for patients

Please see Information for patients: Hypothyroidism (undereractive thyroid) and pregnancy (p. 513)

References

1. Abalovich M, et al. Management of thyroid dysfunction during pregnancy and postpartum: An Endocrine Society Clinical Practice Guideline. J Clin Endocrinol Metab 2007; 92: S1–S47.
2. Girling J. Thyroid disease in pregnancy. Obstetrician and Gynaecologist 2008: 10: 237–243.
3. Abalovich M, et al. Overt and subclinical hypothyroidism complicating pregnancy. Thyroid 2002; 12: 63–68.
4. Morreale de Escobar G, et al. Maternal thyroid hormones early in pregnancy and fetal brain development. Best Pract Res Clin Endocrinol Metab 2004; 18: 225–248.
5. Brent GA. Maternal hypothyroidism: recognition and management. Thyroid 1999; 9: 661–665.
6. Glinoer D. The regulation of thyroid function in pregnancy: pathways of endocrine adaptation from physiology to pathology. Endocrinol Rev 1997; 18: 404–433.
7. Mandel SJ, et al. Increased need for thyroxine during pregnancy in women with primary hypothyroidism. N Engl J Med 1990; 323: 91–96.

CARE PATHWAY

- GP advises increase of levothyroxine dosage by 25 micrograms in women already on thyroxine supplements, once pregnancy is confirmed with a positive pregnancy test
- Community midwife includes TSH in the booking bloods request and refers **hypothyroid** patient within the 1st trimester to joint obstetric–endocrine or maternal medicine clinic

Detailed history taken in specialist clinic

Previous treated thyrotoxicosis, now hypothyroid

First visit to specialist antenatal clinic

- Detailed history of previous treatment for Grave's
- Patient and pregnancy assessed
- TSH result checked, if not already done, blood for TSH check the same day
- Clear documentation and communication to primary care regarding pregnancy-specific range of TSH and thyroxine adjustment as indicated by TSH checks 6–8 weeks during pregnancy
- Reassure patient that thyroxine supplementation safe during pregnancy and breastfeeding. Advise thyroxine taken on an empty stomach and not within 2 hours of oral iron supplement.
- Arrange for TFTs every 6–8 weeks in pregnancy with thyroxine doses adjusted in community by 25 microgram increments aiming to maintain **TSH range between 0.5 and 2.5**
- Advise patient to continue routine community midwife antenatal checks

Subsequent maternal medicine visits at 28, 32, and 36 weeks

- TBII or TRAb check at 28 weeks if previously treated Grave's disease
- Inform Paediatricians if TBII or TRAb is elevated, with documentation to perform a 6 h neonatal check
- Serial growth scans at 28, 32, 36 weeks, with antenatal clinic visit on same day
- Weekly CTGs after 34 weeks may be indicated if TBII or TRAb raised to detect persistent fetal tachycardia may be indicative of fetal hyperthyroidism
- No need for early IOL or LSCS unless indicated by other obstetric reasons

Delivery and postpartum

- Cord bloods at birth for fetal thyroid levels
- Neonatal thyroid check by paediatrician
- Mother can revert to pre-pregnancy thyroxine dosage after delivery
- Maternal thyroid check by GP about 4 weeks after delivery

Primary uncomplicated hypothyroidism

First visit to specialist antenatal clinic

- Check TSH result at first visit
- If not already done, request TSH check the same day, with communication to GP and community midwife to advise patient to adjust thyroxine dosage by increment of 25 micrograms/day, aiming to maintain TSH levels between 0.5 and 2.5 during pregnancy (**Note: Pregnancy-specific range is different from non-pregnant range.**)
- Repeat TSH every 6–8 weeks in primary care
- Clear documentation and communication to primary care regarding pregnancy-specific range of TSH and thyroxine adjustment as indicated by TSH checks 6–8 weeks during pregnancy with incremental changes of 25 micrograms thyroxine at any one time if required
- Reassure patient that thyroxine supplementation is safe during pregnancy and breastfeeding and advise her to take thyroxine on an empty stomach and not within 2 hours of oral iron supplement.

Subsequent visits to maternal medicine clinic at 28–34 weeks

- Check most recent TSH results, and adjust dose of thyroxine if necessary
- Assess pregnancy, if all well, transfer back to routine midwifery-led care
- No change in obstetric management for rest of pregnancy, labour, or delivery on basis of hypothyroidism

Delivery and postpartum

- Routine post-dates IOL arranged by community midwife according to individual unit policy between 40^{+10-14} days
- Neonatal thyroid check as in standard practice
- Mother can revert to pre-pregnancy thyroxine dosage after delivery
- Maternal thyroid check (by GP) 4–6 weeks postpartum.

9.3 Hyperthyroidism

FACT FILE

Incidence

- **Hyperthyroidism** in pregnancy is not uncommon, with a reported prevalence of 0.1–0.4%, with Graves' disease (autoimmune thyrotoxicosis) accounting for 85% of cases.
- The most common cause of hyperthyroidism is Graves' disease, which is 5- to 10-fold more common in women, with a peak incidence during the reproductive age.[1]
- Graves' disease has an incidence of 2 in 1000 pregnancies.
- Transient gestational hyperthyroidism, single toxic adenoma, toxic multinodular goitre, subacute thyroiditis, or gestational trophoblastic tumours comprise most of the remaining cases of hyperthyroidism in pregnancy.[2]

Pathophysiology and presentation

- The activity level of Graves' disease, like that of other autoimmune conditions, may fluctuate during gestation, with exacerbation during the first trimester and a gradual remission during the latter half.[3,4]
- An exacerbation may occur postpartum. Rarely, labour, Caesarean section, or infections may aggravate hyperthyroidism and even trigger a thyroid storm.[5,6]
- Non-specific symptoms of hyperthyroidism such as tachycardia, warm moist skin, tremors, heat intolerance, and systolic murmur may be mimicked by symptoms of normal pregnancy. The presence of classic thyroid eye changes, or a significant goitre, may indicate true Graves' disease. A careful physical examination should be performed.
- Hyperthyroidism does not often present for the first time in early pregnancy, but awareness of signs and symptoms is essential, particularly as it could be mistaken for severe hyperemesis gravidarum.
- A woman who is found to have Graves' disease before pregnancy and has been treated with antithyroid drugs, goes into remission, and is euthyroid after stopping medication, has a low risk of recurrent hyperthyroidism during pregnancy. However, the risk of relapse (as well as the risk of postpartum thyroiditis) during the postpartum period is relatively high.

Diagnosis

- Patients suspected of having hyperthyroidism require measurement of serum TSH, free T_4 and T_3 levels, as well as thyroid receptor antibodies. High levels of free T_4 and T_3 and suppressed TSH levels are diagnostic.
- A key point is that reference ranges for thyroid function tests are different during various stages of pregnancy.
- ***Serum TSH levels may be below the non-pregnant reference range in the first half of a normal pregnancy due the result of stimulation of the normal thyroid by high levels of serum hCG. Therefore, low serum TSH levels with normal free T_4 values in early pregnancy do not indicate abnormal thyroid function.***[7]
- Serum total T_4 and T_3 normally increase in early pregnancy. From the late first trimester, they remain stable, with reference ranges close to 1.5 times non-pregnancy ranges during the second and third trimesters.[7]
- ***Transient hCG-mediated thyrotrophin suppression in early pregnancy should not be treated with antithyroid drug therapy.***
- In **the non-pregnant state**, a radioactive iodine uptake (RAIU) is indicated when the diagnosis is in question; **however, this is contraindicated in pregnancy or in breastfeeding women**.
- Ultrasonography does not generally contribute to the differential diagnosis of thyrotoxicosis. When radioactive iodine is contraindicated, such as during pregnancy or breastfeeding, ultrasound showing increased colour Doppler flow may be helpful in confirming a diagnosis of thyroid hyperactivity.[7]

Management during pregnancy

- Newly diagnosed hyperthyroidism needs prompt and aggressive treatment.
- Pregnant patients with Graves' disease or past history of Graves' disease, transient gestational hyperthyroidism, or toxic multinodular goitre, should be referred by the community midwife and/or GP to the joint obstetric–endocrine clinic. Ideally such a patient would have been assessed before conception by the GP/endocrinologist.
- The primary object of management in pregnancy is to ensure that euthyroidism is achieved as early as possible during pregnancy, ideally even before conception, to minimize chances of maternal and/or fetal complications.[8,9]
- Graves' disease during pregnancy should be treated with the lowest possible dose of antithyroid drugs needed to keep the mother's thyroid hormone levels slightly above the normal range for total T_4 and T_3 values in pregnancy and the TSH suppressed.
- Free T_4 estimates should be slightly above the upper limit of the non-pregnant reference range. Thyroid function should be assessed monthly, and the antithyroid drug dose adjusted as required.[3]
- ***The risk of complications for both mother and fetus is related to the duration and control of maternal hyperthyroidism.***[3]
- In poorly controlled or untreated maternal hyperthyroidism, there is an increased incidence of **maternal problems**, e.g.[2,10,11]
  - subfertility
  - miscarriage
  - pre-eclampsia
  - 'thyroid storm'
  - maternal cardiac failure.
- Poorly controlled or untreated maternal hyperthyroidism can also lead to an increased incidence of **fetal and neonatal problems**, e.g.:[12,13]
  - congenital anomalies such as oesophageal atresia, aplasia cutis
  - fetal goitre
  - fetal growth restriction
  - low birth weight
  - fetal tachycardia
  - fetal cardiac failure and hydrops
  - preterm delivery
  - intrauterine death
  - neonatal death.
- Overtreatment of the mother with antithyroid drugs during the second and third trimesters, when the fetal thyroid has begun to function, can result in iatrogenic hypothyroidism.[14]
- With prompt and adequate treatment and appropriate maternal and fetal monitoring, the outcomes for the mother and baby are excellent.
- **Smoking** is a well-established risk factor for the development Graves' ophthalmopathy: the risk is proportional to the number of cigarettes smoked per day. **Robust advice and support for smoking cessation must be offered.**
- ***Treatment with radioiodine iodine (I^{131}) is absolutely contraindicated in pregnancy as well as in women planning a pregnancy in the future (within 4–6 months).***
- **Thyroid surgery** may be indicated if there is a large goitre producing symptoms of tracheal compression and radioiodine therapy is contraindicated, as in women planning a pregnancy within 4–6 months.
- **Pregnancy is a relative contraindication** for thyroid surgery and should only be used when rapid control of hyperthyroidism is required and antithyroid medications cannot be used.
- Thyroidectomy is best avoided in the first and third trimesters of pregnancy because of teratogenic effects associated with anaesthetic agents, the increased risk of miscarriage in the first trimester, and the increased risk of preterm labour in the third. Thyroidectomy, if strictly indicated, is therefore best performed in the latter part of the second trimester. Although this is the safest time, thyroid surgery even at this gestation is not without risk (4.5–5.5% risk of preterm labour).[7]

- **Antithyroid drugs** such as carbimazole or propylthiouracil (PTU) are used to achieve euthyroidism.
- Both drugs cross the placenta in similar amounts.
- Traditionally, PTU has been the drug of choice in pregnancy as it is more protein bound and therefore thought less likely to cross the placenta.
- The advice has been that any woman taking carbimazole who is found to be pregnant should have her medication promptly changed to PTU. ***50 mg PTU is equivalent to 5 mg carbimazole.***
- ***PTU, unlike carbimazole, needs to be given on a twice-daily regime***. For example, if a patient has been euthyroid on 20 mg od of carbimazole, this should be changed to 100 mg bd of PTU.
- Some reports linked carbimazole to a rare congenital fetal defect called aplasia cutis congenita of the scalp as well as choanal or oesophageal atresia. This association has been challenged more recently.[8]
- Both PTU and carbimazole can produce agranulocytosis and the pregnant patient must be warned to report a sore throat immediately.
- Recent reports have raised concerns about the association of PTU with a rare but potentially fatal PTU hepatotoxicity.[12] Liver function tests may therefore need to be considered while the patient remains on PTU, at the same time that thyroid function is assessed.[3]
- To prevent overtreatment which may lead to fetal hypothyroidism especially in the second and third trimesters, when the fetal thyroid has itself begun to function, treatment regimens should aim to keep maternal free thyroxine within the upper third of normal reference range for non-pregnant women.[3]
- Similarly, **block replacement therapy, consisting of antithyroid medication plus levothyroxine, should not be used in pregnancy**. If a woman receiving such therapy becomes pregnant, treatment should be changed to antithyroid medication alone.[3]
- **Beta-blockers** such as propranolol should be used for control of severe symptoms, as the benefits outweigh the any concerns of later fetal growth.

Fetal hyperthyroidism

- ***In women with a current or past history of treated Graves' disease, there is a continued circulation of thyroid receptor antibodies and therefore a risk of neonatal hyperthyroidism.***
- TSH itself does not cross the placenta. However, clinically significant amounts of maternal T_4 do cross the placenta.
- ***The likelihood of developing fetal hyperthyroidism requiring treatment is related to the level of maternal TSH receptor stimulating antibodies (TRAb) as these cross the placenta.***
- ***Fetal hyperthyroidism requiring treatment is rare (<0.01% of all pregnancies), but occurs in 1–5% of neonates of mothers with Graves' disease due to transplacental passage of stimulating maternal TRAb.***
- All antibodies that can compete with TSH for binding to the TSH receptor are identified as TSH-binding inhibitory immunoglobulins (TBII)
- ***TBII measurements are often used as surrogate for an assay of TRAb. TRAb should be measured by the level of TBII at 26–28 weeks gestation.***
- ***TBII levels of in excess of 1 i.u. are regarded as high with a potential for causing neonatal hyperthyroidism.***
- If high TBII levels are detected, further monitoring needs to be considered for signs of fetal thyrotoxicosis including **persistent fetal tachycardia ± excessive movements detected by weekly CTGs after about 34 weeks**, ultrasound scan findings of IUGR, hydrops, fetal goitre, fused skull bones, signs of fetal cardiac failure, poly- or oligohydramnios.
- Rarely, early delivery may need to be considered in the case of fetal thyroid dysfunction, depending on the gestation at diagnosis and severity of indicative signs.
- TRAb (TBII or TSI) measurement is also useful to assist in the evaluation of disease activity in a woman being treated with antithyroid drugs for Graves' disease during pregnancy.[3]
- In many patients, Graves' disease gradually remits during pregnancy. If TRAb has been tested for and found to positive in the first trimester, subsequent disappearance of TRAb when tested for at the start of the third trimester is an indication that antithyroid drug therapy may no longer be necessary. Continuation of antithyroid drugs in this situation may put the fetus at risk for hypothyroidism.[3]
- At birth, umbilical cord blood sampling for fetal thyroid function is essential.

The neonate

- **Symptomatic neonatal hyperthyroidism** should be considered an emergency and treated appropriately.
- Paediatricians need to be alerted to check the baby after 6 h of birth for any signs of neonatal hyperthyroidism. Ensure adequate documentation of this in both handheld and main notes in the 'baby' page
- Any overactivity of the thyroid in the neonate is usually self-limiting to about 3 months because of the disappearance of the circulating maternal antibody during this time. Parents must be instructed before discharge to watch for changes such as weight loss or poor feeding and advised to contact paediatricians according to local procedures.

Postpartum and breastfeeding

- PTU is safer for breastfeeding than carbimazole as the latter in larger doses can cause fetal hypothyroidism.
- The amount of PTU transmitted in breast milk is negligible provided the maternal daily dose is not greater than 250 mg/day. Also, the mother should be advised to take her PTU medication for the day just **after** an episode of breastfeeding.
- Because of the potential for hepatic necrosis in either mother or child from maternal PTU use, methimazole (MMI) is the preferred antithyroid drug in nursing mothers.
- In women with symptomatic postpartum thyrotoxicosis, use of beta-adrenergic blocking agents should be considered. Beta-blockers are secreted in very low levels into breast milk, therefore no special monitoring is needed for breastfed infants of mothers on these medications.[3]

Maternal follow-up and pre-pregnancy assessment

- There is a significant risk of exacerbation of hyperthyroidism postpartum. The mother's thyroid function tests must be followed up by the GP at 6 weeks and 3 months after delivery.[4]
- Any woman who is on carbimazole for hyperthyroidism, or whose hyperthyroidism is not well controlled, should ideally have been referred before pregnancy to the endocrinologist.
- **Graves' ophthalmopathy** (GO) is a debilitating, sight-threatening inflammatory eye disease that develops in association with autoimmune thyroid disorders. Approximately 50% of those with Graves' disease have signs and/or symptoms of GO, and 5% suffer from severe disease.[3]
- **Smoking** is a well-established risk factor for the development of GO; the risk is proportional to the number of cigarettes smoked per day.[15] **Robust advice and support, including referral to a structured smoking cessation programme, is mandatory. Patients exposed to second-hand smoke must also be identified and appropriate advice offered.**

Postpartum thyroiditis

- Autoimmune thyroiditis occurs in up to 10% of women of reproductive age. Generally, the result is hypothyroidism, although a hyperthyroid phase of Hashimoto's thyroiditis and silent thyroiditis may both occur. Postpartum thyroiditis occurs after up to 10% of all pregnancies and may have a hyperthyroid phase, usually within the first month or two.[16]
- It can occur in 50% of patients who have had Graves' disease in the past. The hypothyroid phase is usually symptomatic and needs thyroxine replacements.
- These patients usually present with recurrent thyrotoxicosis; some have a recurrence of Graves' disease while others develope postpartum thyroiditis.
- Such patients should be referred to a specialist endocrinologist.

Hyperemesis gravidarum

See also Chapter 24.8.

- Severe vomiting in early pregnancy that causes more than 5% weight loss, dehydration, and ketonuria is defined as hyperemesis gravidarum and occurs in 0.5–10 cases per 1000 pregnancies.[17]
- Patients with gestational thyrotoxicosis present in the mid to late first trimester, often with hyperemesis. Usually classic hyperthyroid symptoms are absent or minimal, except for weight loss, which may be a result of vomiting and poor nutrition.[18]
- In about 60% of cases of severe hyperemesis, abnormal thyroid function tests can be found with suppressed TSH and high or very high free T_4 levels. This is due to the TSH-like effects of beta-hCG which is usually transient. Nearly 50% have an elevated free T_4 concentration.[18]
- **It is essential to differentiate between this transient state and genuine Graves' disease occurring for the first time in the first trimester.** A detailed history of symptoms occurring only after diagnosis of pregnancy, absence of eye signs, tachycardia corrected by rehydration, and return of TFTs to normal once there is resolution of hyperemesis and absence of thyroid antibodies are indicative of hyperemesis gravidarum.
- In hyperemesis gravidarum, the transient hCG-linked hyperthyroidism does not require antithyroid medication. Subclinical hyperthyroidism (TSH below normal limits with free T_4 and total T_4 in the normal pregnancy range) is seen in hyperemesis gravidarum syndrome. Treatment of maternal subclinical hyperthyroidism has not been found to improve pregnancy outcome and may risk unnecessary exposure of the fetus to antithyroid drugs.[18,19,20]

Information for patients

Please see **Information for patients: Hyperthyroidism(overactive thyroid) and pregnancy** (p. 514)

References

1. Mandel SJ, Cooper DS. The use of antithyroid drugs in pregnancy and lactation. J Clin Endocrinol Metab 2001: 86: 2354–2359.
2. Mestman JH. Hyperthyroidism in pregnancy. Best Pract Res Clin Endocrinol Metab 2004; 18: 267–288.
3. Abalovich M. Management of thyroid dysfunction during pregnancy and postpartum. An Endocrine Society Clinical Practice Guideline. J Clin Endocrinol Metab 2007; 92: S1–S47.
4. Amino N, et al. Aggravation of thyrotoxicosis in early pregnancy and after delivery in Graves' disease. J Clin Endocrinol Metab 1982; 55: 108–112.
5. Mestman JH, et al. Thyroid disorders of pregnancy. Endocrinol Metab Clin North Am 1995; 24: 41–71.
6. Sheffield JS, Cunningham FG. Thyrotoxicosis and heart failure that complicate pregnancy. Am J Obstet Gynecol 2004; 190: 211–217.
7. Stagnaro-Green A, et al. Guidelines of the American Thyroid Association for the diagnosis and management of thyroid disease during pregnancy and postpartum. Thyroid 2011; 21: 1081–1125.
8. Girling J. Thyroid disease in pregnancy. Obstetrician and Gynaecologist 2008; 10: 237–243.
9. Thangaratinam S, et al. Association between thyroid autoantibodies and miscarriage and preterm birth: meta-analysis of evidence. BMJ 2011; 342: d2616.
10. Millar LK, et al. Low birth weight and preeclampsia in pregnancies complicated by hyperthyroidism. Obstet Gynecol 1994; 84: 946–949.
11. Davis LE, et al. Thyrotoxicosis complicating pregnancy. Am J Obstet Gynecol 1989; 160: 63–70.
12. Bahn RS, et al. The role of propylthiouracil in the management of Graves' disease in adults: report of a meeting jointly sponsored by the American Thyroid Association and the Food and Drug Administration. Thyroid 2009; 19: 673–674.
13. Peleg D, et al. The relationship between maternal serum thyroid-stimulating immunoglobulin and fetal and neonatal thyrotoxicosis. Obstet Gynecol 2002; 99: 1040–1043.
14. Glinoer D. Regulation of maternal thyroid during pregnancy. J Clin Endocrinol Metab 1990; 71: 276–287
15. Pfeilschifter J, Ziegler R. Smoking and endocrine ophthalmopathy: impact of smoking severity and current vs lifetime cigarette consumption. Clin Endocrinol (Oxf) 1996; 45: 477–481.
16. Stagnaro-Green A, et al. Detection of at risk pregnancy by means of highly sensitive assays for thyroid autoantibodies. JAMA 1990; 264: 1422–1142.
17. Verberg MF, et al. Hyperemesis gravidarum, a literature review. Hum Reprod Update 2005; 11: 527–539.
18. Goodwin TM, et al. The role of chorionic gonadotropin in transient hyperthyroidism of hyperemesis gravidarum. J Clin Endocrinol Metab 1992; 75: 1333–1337.
19. Casey BM, et al. Subclinical hyperthyroidism and pregnancy outcomes. Obstet Gynecol 2006; 107: 337–341
20. Tan JY, et al. Transient hyperthyroidism of hyperemesis gravidarum. BJOG 2002; 109: 683–688.

- Pre-pregnancy referral to and assessment by endocrinologist
- GP/community midwife refers pregnant patients with either a past or present history of **hyperthyroidism** to the joint obstetric–endocrine clinic in 1st trimester

↓

First visit to joint obstetric–endocrine clinic

- Confirm dates and viability by 1st-trimester scan
- Diagnosis confirmed, thyroid status assessed by endocrinologist
- Carbimazole may need to be changed to PTU
- TSH, free T4, free T3 to be sent with booking bloods
- Discuss effects of hyperthyroidism on pregnancy and vice versa; **advise smoking cessation, if relevant**.
- Discuss treatment effect on mother, on fetus, need for TFT blood tests every 6–8 weeks, check TRAb/TBII at 28 weeks, serial growth scans from about 28 weeks
- Discuss and document cord bloods, baby checks, safety of breastfeeding while on PTU
- Arrange routine anomaly scan at 20+ weeks
- Arrange serial growth scans at 28, 32, 36 weeks (or according to individual unit's protocol) with joint clinic appointments on same day
- Advise patient to continue routine antenatal checks with community midwife

↓

Subsequent visits to joint obstetric–endocrine clinic at about 28, 32, and 36 weeks

- Check TSH every 6–8 weeks
- Serial fetal scans for growth, liquor, any hydrops, or fetal goitre
- TBII or TRAb check at about 28 weeks along with routine bloods (remember it can take up to 10–14 days to get results of TBII or TRAb in some units)
- If TBII or TRAb significantly raised:
  - discuss possible transplacental transfer of antibodies that may cause transient fetal/ neonatal hyperthyroidism
  - CTGs weekly from about 34 weeks gestation for signs of persistent fetal tachycardia
  - Alert mother to report excessive fetal movements
  - Alert paediatricians for vigilance for signs of neonatal hyperthyroidism
- Breastfeeding not contraindicated if dosage of PTU is <250 mg/day. Advise patient to take the day's dose of PTU medication after a breastfeed.

↓

Postnatal management

- Cord bloods for fetal thyroid status
- Baby check for thyroid levels
- If high TBII or TRAb found during pregnancy, paediatricians should be alerted to check baby after 6 h of birth and follow up for first 3 months
- Paediatrician to advise parents to report any undue loss of weight or poor feeding
- Postnatal endocrinology follow up for mother
- Routine Guthrie test at 6 weeks

9.4 Hashimoto's Thyroiditis, Postpartum/Subclinical Thyroiditis, Thyroid Nodules

FACT FILE

Hashimoto's thyroiditis

- **Hashimoto's thyroiditis (HT)**, a form of autoimmune thyroiditis, is the most common cause of hypothyroidism.[1] It describes a combination of autoimmune thyroiditis and goitre.

Epidemiology and effects on pregnancy

- HT results from autoimmune destruction of the thyroid gland associated with microsomal antibodies.
- The two main causes of hypothyroidism in pregnancy are HT and previously treated Graves' disease.
- HT is 10–20 times more common in women than in men.
- Unrecognized hypothyroidism is deleterious, therefore early diagnosis of HT and prompt treatment will improve fetal outcomes and neuropsychological developmental of the newborn.[2]
- While an overall HT prevalence of 0.8% has been reported in the general population,[3] based on abnormally elevated TSH, low thyroid hormones, and the confirmatory presence of thyroid autoantibodies,[4] **the prevalence of cytology-proven HT has been reported to be more than 10% in patients with thyroid nodules.**[5]
- In the early stages of the HT autoimmune process, the patient is generally euthyroid and the diagnosis might be clinically missed.[6,7]
- The risk of poor obstetric outcomes[8] is increased with relative thyroxine deficiency.
- Pregnancy complications such as pregnancy-induced hypertension, anaemia, placental abruption, preterm labour, or IUGR is greater in women with overt, rather than subclinical, hypothyroidism.[9,10,11]

Investigations and diagnosis

- The sonographic appearance of HT is that of a diffusely enlarged, heterogeneous, and hypervascular thyroid with micronodules, echogenic septations, and decreased echogenicity.[12,13]
- **The hallmark in the diagnosis of HT is the presence of thyroid peroxidase (TPO) autoantibodies.**

Management

- Women with HT have, in general, some residual thyroid tissue, unlike in conditions such as previous radioiodine ablation or extensive thyroid surgery with very little residual tissue and where greater increments of thyroxine replacement are required.
- Both benign and malignant nodules can coexist within diffuse HT;[14] there is a reported incidence of cancer of 9–13% in the general population of patients with thyroid nodules selected for fine-needle aspiration.[15,16]
- Since women with hypothyroidism during pregnancy, especially of the autoimmune variety, might have a flare up of the disorder postpartum, or might continue to require thyroxine replacement postpartum, adequate follow-up is mandatory.
- Following delivery, in most women, the dose of thyroxine received during pregnancy can be tapered down over a period of approximately 4 weeks to pre-pregnancy values.

Postpartum thyroiditis

- Reported incidence of postpartum thyroiditis (PPT) is about 1–7%.
- Usually presents within 3–6 months of delivery.
- More common in those with a family history of thyroid dysfunction (25% have such a history).
- In those with thyroid peroxidase antibodies, 50% can develop postpartum thyroiditis.
- A small and painless goitre is present in about 50% of PPT.
- In PPT, two patterns of thyroid dysfunction have been described:
  1. Postpartum thyroiditis can characterized by a phase of transient hyperthyroidism (in 40%) or transient hypothyroidism (in 40%) with spontaneous return to euthyroidism, **or**
  2. Biphasic (in 20%): Transient hyperthyroidism followed by temporary or rarely longer-term hypothyroidism which may last for 4–8 months postpartum and may even be permanent.
- The hyperthyroid phase of postpartum thyroiditis often presents with excess fatigue and palpitations. Treatment is with beta-adrenergic antagonists rather than antithyroid medication, unlike in Graves' disease.
- Transient hypothyroidism can present with tiredness, depression, etc. Treatment is with T_4, which may be continued till 6–8 months and then tapered to determine if the hypothyroidism is permanent (in 3–4%) or whether spontaneous recovery has taken place. If the woman becomes pregnant once again during the 6–8 month period while on replacement thyroxine, it should not be withdrawn during the course of the pregnancy.
- The symptoms of PPT are therefore often attributed to the general symptoms experience post-partum and the condition missed.
- Similar to HT, PPT results from a slow depletion of thyroid reserve due to autoimmune thyroiditis.
- Routine screening for PPT is recommended in those with type 1 diabetes.
- Risk of recurrence of PPT in future pregnancies is about 10–25%.
- A quarter of women with TPO antibodies who have developed PPT will progress within 4 years to becoming permanently hypothyroid.
- Long term follow-up with yearly thyroid function tests is therefore essential and both the patient and GP must be so informed before hospital discharge.

Subclinical hypothyroidism

- Subclinical hypothyroidism is defined as an increased TSH with normal levels of FT_4 and FT_3, but no specific signs or symptoms of clinical hypothyroidism.
- The prevalence of subclinical hypothyroidism during pregnancy is estimated to be 2% to 5%.[17] It is almost always asymptomatic. Women with subclinical hypothyroidism are more likely than euthyroid women to be TPO antibody positive.
- Subclinical hypothyroidism may be a stage in the continuum of reducing thyroid reserve.
- The aetiology of subclinical hypothyroidism is similar to that of overt hypothyroidism and the general recommendation is for treatment with thyroxine replacement if there is a previous history of pregnancy complications suggestive of thyroid hypofunction including spontaneous miscarriages, pre-eclampsia, gestational hypertension, gestational diabetes, preterm delivery, and decreased IQ in a previous offspring.[18,20]
- Routine thyroxine supplementation is therefore not required, based on the available data for asymptomatic pregnant women who are euthyroid but are thyroid antibody positive and have no previous history of poor obstetric outcomes. Prospective trials are however, ongoing to evaluate the impact of levothyroxine therapy in women with subclinical hypothyroidism and subsequent pregnancy outcomes.[20]

Thyroid nodules

- Present in 1–2 % of pregnant women.[19]
- Nearly 40% can be malignant, especially if the lesion is large, solid, and fixed. Lymphadenopathy, voice changes, and rapid growth of a painless tumour are sinister signs.
- In benign subacute thyroiditis (de Quervain's), before the appearance of the tender nodule, there is a history of systemic illness, usually due to a viral aetiology, and sore throat.

Investigations

- TFTs and TPO antibodies to exclude a toxic nodule or HT.
- A raised thyroglobulin level indicates malignancy.

- Ultrasound to distinguish solid from cystic lesion.
- Cytology of fluid aspirate from nodule and/or fine-needle biopsy.

Treatment

- Surgery can be performed in the second or third trimesters. and sufficient thyroxine given postoperatively to ensure suppression of TSH (any residual tumour being TSH dependent).

Information for patients

Please see **Information for patients: Hashimoto's thyroiditis and pregnancy** (p. 515)

References

1. Klein RZ, et al. Prevalence of thyroid deficiency in pregnant women. Clin Endocrinol (Oxf) 1991; 35: 41–46.
2. Brent GA: Diagnosing thyroid dysfunction in pregnant women: is case finding enough? J Clin Endocrinol Metab 2007; 92: 39–41.
3. Tunbridge WM, et al. The spectrum of thyroid disease in a community: the Whickham survey. Clin Endocrinol (Oxf) 1977; 7: 481–493.
4. Weetman AP. Thyroid disease. In:Rose NR, Mackay IR, ed., The autoimmune diseases. St. Louis, MO: Elsevier Academic Press, 2006, pp. 467–482.
5. Staii A, et al. Hashimoto thyroiditis is more frequent than expected when diagnosed by cytology which uncovers a pre-clinical state. Thyroid Res 2010; 3: 11.
6. Surks MI, Ocampo E. Subclinical thyroid disease. Am J Med 1986; 100: 217–223.
7. Cooper DS. Subclinical thyroid disease: a clinician's perspective. Ann Intern Med 1998; 129: 135–137.
8. Allan WC, et al. Maternal thyroid deficiency and pregnancy complications: implications for population screening. J Med Screen 2000; 7: 127–130.
9. Benhadi N, et al. Higher maternal TSH levels in pregnancy are associated with increased risk for miscarriage, fetal or neonatal death. Eur J Endocrinol 2009; 160: 985–991.
10. Negro R, et al. Thyroid antibody positivity during pregnancy. J Clin Endocrinol Metab 2011; 96: E920–E924.
11. Abalovich M, et al. Overt and subclinical hypothyroidism complicating pregnancy. Thyroid 2002; 12: 63–66.
12. Anderson L, et al. Hashimoto thyroiditis: Part 1, Sonographic analysis of the nodular form of Hashimoto thyroiditis. AJR 2010; 195: 208–215.
13. Yeh HC, et al. Micronodulation: ultrasonographic sign of Hashimoto thyroiditis. J Ultrasound Med 1996; 15: 813–819.
14. Takashima S, et al. Thyroid nodules associated with Hashimoto's thyroiditis: assessment with US. Radiology 1992; 185: 125–130.
15. Frates MC, et al. Management of thyroid nodules detected at US: Society of Radiologists in Ultrasound consensus conference statement. Radiology 2005; 237: 794–800.
16. F Boi, et al. High prevalence of suspicious cytology in thyroid nodules associated with positive thyroid autoantibodies. Eur J Endocrinol 2005; 153: 637–642.
17. Woeber KA. Subclinical thyroid dysfunction. Arch Intern Med 1997; 157: 1065–1068.
18. Negro R, et al. Levothyroxine treatment in euthyroid pregnant women with autoimmune thyroid disease: effects on obstetric complications. J Clin Endocrinol Metab 2006; 91: 2587–2591.
19. Nelson-Piercy C. In: Handbook of obstetric medicine, 4th ed. London: Informa Healthcare, 2010.
20. Negro R, Stagnaro-Green A. Diagnosis and management of subclinical hypothyroidism in pregnancy. BMJ 2014;349: g4929.

9.5 Prolactinomas, Pituitary Tumours

FACT FILE

Epidemiology

- **Pituitary adenomas (prolactinomas)** are the most common pituitary tumours in pregnancy,[1] accounting for some 30%.
- Prolactinomas are rare and complicate approximately 1 in 4500 pregnancies.
- Hyperprolactinaemia can be caused by
  - normal pregnancy
  - pituitary adenomas (prolactinomas)
  - hypothalamic and pituitary stalk lesions
  - hypothyroidism (rare)
  - drugs (e.g. metoclopramide)
  - chronic renal failure.

Pathophysiology and effects in pregnancy

- Prolactinomas are **macroadenomas** if greater than 1 cm and **microadenomas** if less than 1 cm in size. Macroprolactinomas are benign tumours of the pituitary.
- Ninety per cent of pituitary tumours are intrasellar adenomas that rarely increase in size, while the rest are macroadenomas.
- Pituitary tumours that secrete excess hormones may be associated with higher incidence of mortality and morbidity. Cushing's disease and acromegaly are associated with higher incidence of hypertension, potentially leading to pre-eclampsia, diabetes, cardiac failure, spontaneous miscarriage, prematurity (43%), and stillbirths (6%).[2]
- Normally, there is a progressive increase in the volume of the anterior pituitary during pregnancy, by up to 35%. This expansion of prolactin-secreting lactotrophs is a direct result of increasing oestrogen secretion and action during pregnancy. This expansion is not accompanied by local pressure effects.
- However, pre-existing pituitary tumours like macroadenomas or craniopharyngiomas can also increase in size, causing pressure on the optic chiasma and bitemporal hemianopia, symptoms of raised intracranial pressure, and visual disturbances.
- The risk of tumour expansion is highest with untreated macroprolactinomas (26%) and to a lesser extent microprolactinomas (1.6%), especially in the third trimester.
- In untreated macroadenomas, the risk of enlargement is approximately 26% compared with 3% in women previously treated with surgery and/or radiation.

Diagnosis

- Prolactin levels are greatly raised (more than 10-fold) in normal pregnancy and cannot be used for either the diagnosis or assessment of progression of hyperprolactinomas in pregnancy.
- In pregnancy, diagnosis relies on pituitary MRI or CT imaging.
- Women with microadenomas and intrasellar macroadenomas do not require serial MRI or visual field testing as required in macroadenomas with extrasellar extension,[3] with vigilance maintained in each trimester for any clinical signs and symptoms related to tumour.
- If tumour enlargement is suspected, MRI of the pituitary is indicated. CT is not usually employed in pregnancy because of the associated radiation risk. Serial scans may also be performed to document temporal progressions of any lesion.
- Visual fields should be measured regularly if symptoms develop during pregnancy or in women with macroprolactinomas.
- A CT or MRI scan may be performed postpartum, if indicated, to detect tumour enlargement and if detected, repeat scans at 6–12 month intervals are warranted.[3]

Management during pregnancy

- The medication of choice is cabergoline,[4,5] despite licensing guidance that it should not be used in pregnancy due to the possible association of high doses of dopamine receptor agonists and the development of fibrotic valvular heart disease found in non-pregnant patients (MHRA guidance).
- Cabergoline has not been reported to cause any fetal congenital malformations or cardiac fibrosis in either the pregnant woman or the fetus.
- Dopamine receptor agonists,[4,5,6] like bromocriptine or cabergoline, that have been used to treat hyperprolactinaemia result in amenorrhoea, and are usually discontinued once pregnancy is diagnosed.
- There is, however, no evidence of any teratogenic effect, miscarriages, malformations, multiple gestation, or any other adverse effects on pregnancy even with continuation of these drugs in pregnancy.[7]
- Termination of pregnancy is not necessary just because the patient inadvertently becomes pregnant while taking cabergoline or bromocriptine.
- Cabergoline has a better side-effect profile than bromocriptine, in particular causing less nausea. Pregnant women with large macroadenomas should continue taking cabergoline according to the advice of the endocrinologist.[7]
- Shrinkage of prolactinomas with dopamine receptor agonists is associated with a reduced risk of symptomatic growth during pregnancy, even after the medication has been discontinued.
- Dopamine receptor agonists may need to be reintroduced during pregnancy if symptoms suggestive of tumour expansion occur, according to the advice of endocrinologists.
- During pregnancy, pituitary adenomas can present with frontal headaches, visual disturbances and visual field defects, and rarely with diabetes insipidus. These are also symptoms of tumour expansion.
- Breastfeeding is safe and does not lead to growth of underlying prolactinomas.[6,7]

Information for patients

Please see **Information for patients: Prolactinomas and pregnancy** (p. 515)

References

1. Kredentser JV, et al. Hyperprolactinoma—a significant factor in female infertility. Am J Obstet Gynecol 1981; 139: 264–267.
2. Bronstein MD, et al. Medical management of pituitary adenomas: the special case of management of the pregnant woman. Pituitary 2002; 5: 99–107.
3. Bajwa SK, et al. Management of prolactinoma with cabergoline treatment in a pregnant woman during her entire pregnancy. Indian J Endocrinol Metab 2011; 15: S267–S270.
4. Webster J, et al. A comparison of cabergoline and bromocriptine in the treatment of hyperprolactinemic amenorrhea. N Engl J Med 1994; 331: 904–909.
5. Stalldecker G, et al. Effects of cabergoline on pregnancy and embryo-fetal development: Retrospective study on 103 pregnancies and a review of the literature. Pituitary 2010; 13: 345–350.
6. Holmgren U, et al. Women with prolactinomas: effect of pregnancy and lactation on serum prolactin and on tumour growth. Acta Endocrinol (Copenh) 1986; 111: 452–459.
7. Hoffman AR, et al. Patient guide to hyperprolactinemia diagnosis and treatment. J Clin Endocrinol Metab 2011; 96: 35–36.

CARE PATHWAY

- Patient known to have a pituitary tumour, hyperprolactinaemia, microadenoma, or macroadenoma
- GP/community midwife refers patient to joint obstetric–endocrine antenatal clinic

↓

Joint assessment by consultant endocrinologist/obstetrician

- Visual fields checks, routine pregnancy assessments
- Advice regarding bromocriptine/cabergoline, reassure that if she has taken either drug during 1st trimester, no increased risk of teratogenicity
- Regular reviews in joint clinic with visual field checks in each trimester (e.g. 13, 26, and 34–36 weeks), especially in macroadenomas
- Raise patient awareness of any relevant symptoms
- If symptoms suggestive of tumour expansion occur, urgent review in joint clinic, urgent MRI, and immediate referral to consultant neurologist
- Decision to reintroduce dopamine agonists such as bromocriptine on endocrinologist's/neurologist's advice
- Referral to anaesthetic high-risk clinic
- Advise patient to continue routine visits to community midwife
- Reassure regarding breastfeeding, no enlargement of prolactinomas seen despite high prolactin levels

↓

- If no problems during pregnancy, routine antenatal management
- Early IOL or LSCS only for obstetric indications or if rapid tumour expansion warrants urgent delivery to allow any further maternal treatment such as trans-sphenoidal surgery

9.6 Hyperparathyroidism

FACT FILE

Epidemiology

- Parathyroid glands secrete parathyroid hormone, an amino-acid polypeptide, the main function of which is to maintain calcium levels through a parathyroid-calcium negative feedback loop.
- **Primary hyperparathyroidism (PHP)** is the most common cause for hypercalcaemia in the general population, with a prevalence of about 1.5 in 1000.[1,2]
- PHP is the third most common endocrine disorder after diabetes and thyroid disease.
- PHP is more common in women with a female to male ratio of 3:1.[1]
- About a quarter of PHP is diagnosed in women during their reproductive years.
- Although PHP is rare in pregnancy, with an incidence of about 8 per 100 000 of the population per year,[2] it can lead to life-threatening hypercalcaemia, with significant morbidity and even mortality of the mother and the baby.[3]
- Maternal complications occur in nearly 70% of cases of PHP in pregnancy,[4] with fetal complication rates of at least 80%.
- It is only with prompt recognition and treatment that the maternal, fetal, and neonatal morbidity and mortality can be reduced.
- Diagnosis of PHP is challenging during pregnancy because of the normal physiological changes that take place.

Normal physiology of calcium metabolism during pregnancy

- During pregnancy calcium is required by the developing baby, with about 25–30 g of calcium needed by term gestation for mineralization of fetal bones. Nearly 80% of this process occurs in the third trimester.[5]
- Fetal demands for calcium are met by increased (doubled) calcium absorption from the gut, in keeping with the doubled production of 1,25-dihydroxyvitamin D (calcitriol)[6,7] as well as mobilization of calcium from the maternal skeleton.
- In normal pregnancy, physiological changes including haemodilution because of intravascular volume expansion, increased glomerular filtration rate, active transfer of maternal calcium across the placenta, and a decrease in serum albumin levels, can all lead to normal or even low serum calcium levels. Other hormonal effects of human placental lactogen, oestriol, etc. also increase the production and activity of vitamin D.

Pathophysiology involved in PHP

- The most common cause of PHP in pregnancy is a single adenoma (in 85%), followed by primary parathyroid hyperplasia (10%), multiple adenomas (3%), and parathyroid malignancy (2%).[2,7]
- In PHP, the very changes in calcium homeostasis that affect calcium and parathyroid hormone metabolism may mask concurrent PHP.
- This can lead to delayed diagnosis and treatment, further worsening the maternal hypercalcaemia.
- The normal gestational hypoalbuminaemia leads to a fall in total serum calcium giving a falsely reassuring level, if appropriate corrections for the low albumin levels are not made. In actual fact, with less albumin-binding, there is more free ionized calcium present in the maternal circulation.
- In PHP, with more maternal calcium reaching the fetus because of the elevated calcium transfer gradient across the placenta, a state of severe suppression of the fetal parathyroid gland occurs. This results in fetal hypocalcaemia-related complications during pregnancy as well as to neonatal tetany.[8,9]
- The lowest level of neonatal calcium is seen 6–12 h after birth, due to parathyroid gland suppression as well as cessation of placental calcium transport after birth.[2]

Presentation and pregnancy complications of maternal PHP

- In both the non-pregnant state and during pregnancy, **23–80% of women with PHP may be asymptomatic.**[1,2,10,11]
- Generalized non-specific symptoms such as fatigue, arthralgia, myalgia, loss of appetite, nausea, vomiting, depression, constipation, or blurred vision, usually relate to mild PHP when the serum calcium levels are increased, but remain below 11 mg/dl.
- More profound problems occur with calcium levels increasing beyond a threshold of 11.4 mg/dl:
  - repeated pregnancy losses[1,3,9,12,] usually in the late first trimester or early second trimester; a sixfold second-trimester pregnancy loss rate has been reported with maternal PHP, rising with increasing maternal serum calcium levels
  - nephrolithiasis (kidney stones) seen in 24–36%[11,13]
  - pancreatitis in 7–13%[13]
  - fractures[14]
  - dehydration due to polyuria.
- Once calcium levels exceed 13 mg/dl, end-organ calcifications manifest as renal failure, cardiac arrhythmias, peptic ulcers, osteopenia, muscle atrophy, psychiatric changes, etc.
- Rarely the most severe form of presentation of PHP, **hypercalcaemic crisis, is encountered with serum calcium levels above 14–15 mg/dL, resulting invariably in ureamia, coma, cardiac arrest, and death.**[1,11,15,16]

Pregnancy complications

- Pregnancy complications may include the following maternal or fetal and neonatal complications.

Maternal complications

- Recurrent miscarriages, especially in the early part of the second trimester.
- Pre-eclampsia, including HELLP syndrome: a 25% incidence of pre-eclampsia has been reported with PHP.[1,11,16,17]
- Polyhydramnios due to fetal polyuria
- Maternal dehydration due to hypercalcaemia induced nephrogenic diabetes insipidus.
- Fractures
- ***Abdominal pain, which may be due to pancreatitis or renal stones.***
- Arrhythmias, cardiac arrest, renal damage, and hypercalcaemic crisis.
- Hypercalcaemic crisis can occur very quickly after delivery due to a combination of dehydration during labour as well as absence of transplacental transfer of calcium.

Fetal and neonatal complications

In untreated cases, the fetal complications can be as high as 80% and include:

- ***Preterm labour.***
- ***Intrauterine fetal growth restriction, small for gestational age.***[18]
- **Intrauterine death:** With appropriate maternal management of PHP, intrauterine and neonatal mortality rates have reduced from 27–31% to less than 5%.[16,18]
- **Neonatal tetany:**[1,9,11] Up to 50% of babies born to women with untreated PHP will have hypocalcaemia[9] and can develop tetany due to suppressed parathyroid gland development. **Often, it is neonatal tetany that raises the first suspicion that the mother might have PHP.**

- Although neonatal hypocalcaemia secondary to maternal PHP can be corrected with calcium supplementation and is thought to be a transient condition, in some cases neonatal hypoparathyroidism can persist for several months or is permanent.[1,11]
- ***With appropriate treatment of maternal PHP, a fourfold reduction of fetal complications can be achieved.***[3,16,18]

Laboratory confirmation of PHP

- With the clinical presentation suggesting PHP, the diagnostic work-up that confirms hyperparathyroidism is the finding of simultaneously elevated levels of serum calcium (> 9.5 mg/dl, correcting for the physiological albuminaemia of pregnancy) or ionized calcium, as well as hypophosphatemia and elevated serum parathyroid hormone levels.[1,7]
- Other causes for hypercalcaemia must have been excluded for the diagnosis of **primary** hyperparathyroidism to be established.

Localization of parathyroid adenoma

- During pregnancy, ultrasonography of the neck is the investigation of choice for localization of parathyroid adenomas. MRI of the neck can also be safely used.
- CT scan or sestamibi scintigraphy is contraindicated in pregnancy.[3]

Treatment

- A multidisciplinary team approach involving the obstetrician, endocrinologist, midwife, neonatologist, anaesthetist, and endocrine surgeon is necessary to ensure prompt recognition and therapy to improve maternal and fetal outcomes.
- Management of hyperparathyroidism during pregnancy needs to be individualized and is influenced by the severity of the patient's symptoms and level of hypercalcaemia as well as the gestational age of the fetus.
- Management of PHP in pregnancy may require a two-step approach.
- The **first step is the treatment of the acute phase**, aimed at lowering serum calcium with vigorous IV hydration.
  - A eucalcaemic diet, oral phosphate, loop diuretics such as furosemide, and calcitonin have also been used with limited success in the treatment of the acute phase.
  - The complication rates for medical management continued for a prolonged period are still considerable.
  - The risks of obstetric complications with medical management are significantly higher than with surgery.
  - Neonatal complication rates of 23–37% have been reported with medical management vs 3–11% with maternal parathyroidectomy.[11,18]
  - Similarly, the rate of maternal complications was as high as 25% in those receiving management alone, vs 12.5% in surgically managed patients.[11,18]
  - During the time of stabilization, close fetal and maternal monitoring should be continued with particular attention to detecting pre-eclampsia, HELLP, renal impairment, hypercalcaemic crisis during pregnancy and postpartum, and IUGR.
- **Once the acute phase has been stabilized, definitive therapy must to be considered.** If, during this time, despite medical management, the patient becomes symptomatic, surgical intervention becomes necessary, irrespective of gestational age.
  - ***Surgery is the definitive treatment for PHP.*** A minimally invasive parathyroidectomy during the second trimester is considered the optimum management when organogenesis is complete and the risk of preterm delivery provoked by the surgery or anaesthetic is low.[11,18]
  - Others, however, recommend that surgery must be offered to all women with PHP irrespective of gestational age.[11]
  - Some recommend that even in the third trimester, parathyroidectomy must be considered if the benefits outweigh the risks. Clinically significant maternal complications from surgery have been reported as less than 6% and 0%.[11]
  - With minimal-access surgery guided by ultrasound localization, the time of exposure to anaesthetic agents is significantly reduced.

Information for patients

Please see Information for patients: Hyperparathyroidism and pregnancy (p. 516)

References

1. Schnatz PF, Curry SL. Primary hyperparathyroidism in pregnancy: evidence-based management. Obstet Gynecol Surv 2002; 57: 365–376.
2. Kohlmeier L, Marcus R. Calcium disorders of pregnancy. Endocrinol Metabol Clin North Am 1995; 24: 15–39.
3. Malekar-Raikar S, Sinnott BP. Primary hyperparathyroidism in pregnancy-a rare cause of life-threatening hypercalcaemia: case report and literature review. Case Rep Endocrinol 2011; 2011: 520516.
4. Kort KC, et al. Hyperparathyroidism and pregnancy. Am J Surg 1999; 177: 66–68.
5. Kovacs CS, Kronenberg HM. Maternal-fetal calcium and bone metabolism during pregnancy, puerperium, and lactation. Endocrine Rev 1997; 18: 832–872.
6. Hosking DJ. Calcium homeostasis in pregnancy. Clin Endocrinol 1996; 45: 1–6.
7. Armson BA. Parathyroid function and calcium homeostasis. Infert Reprod Med Clin North Am 1994; 5: 709–727.
8. Ip P. Neonatal convulsion revealing maternal hyperparathyroidism: an unusual case of late neonatal hypoparathyroidism. Arch Gynecol Obst 2003; 268: 227–229.
9. Norman J, et al. Hyperparathyroidism during pregnancy and the effect of rising calcium on pregnancy loss: a call for earlier intervention. Clin Endocrinol 2009; 71: 104–109.
10. Kokrdova Z. Pregnancy and primary hyperparathyroidism. J Obstet Gynaecol 2010; 30: 57–59.
11. Schnatz PF, Thaxton S. Parathyroidectomy in the third trimester of pregnancy. Obstet Gynecol Surv 2005; 60: 672–682.
12. Perin E, et al. Primary hyperparathyroidism in pregnancy. Fertil Steril 2008; 90: 2014. e13–e15.
13. Hong MK, et al. Primary hyperparathyroidism and acute pancreatitis during the third trimester of pregnancy. J Matern Fetal Med 2001; 10: 214–218.
14. Negishi H, et al. Primary hyperparathyroidism and simultaneous bilateral fracture of the femoral neck during pregnancy. J Trauma 2002; 52: 367–369.
15. Clark D, et al. Hyperparathyroid crisis and pregnancy. Am J Obstet Gynecol 1981; 140: 840–842.
16. Baron YM, et al. Primary hyperparathyroidism in pregnancy—case report and review. Malta Med J 2010; 22: 37–39
17. Hultin H, et al. Association of parathyroid adenoma and pregnancy with preeclampsia. J Clin Endocrinol Metab 2009; 94: 3394–3399.
18. Jaafar R, et al. Neonatal seizures due to maternal hyperparathyroidism. J Paediatr Child Health 2004; 40: 329.

CARE PATHWAY

Those already found to have primary hyperparathyroidism (PHP) identified during investigations for mild non-specific symptoms before pregnancy or during investigations for recurrent miscarriages, especially early 2nd-trimester pregnancy losses: Current advice is that parathyroidectomy is best done before a pregnancy is commenced

↓

PHP diagnosed during pregnancy based on correlation of clinical features to maternal serum hypercalcaemia (corrected values), high parathyroid hormone, and hypophosphataemia.:
- Ultrasound scan ± MRI of the neck for localization of adenoma.
- Multidisciplinary management involving endocrinologist, obstetrician, midwife, GP, endocrine surgeon, anaesthetist and neonatologist

↓

Management directed through joint endocrinology–obstetrics antenatal clinic, guided by severity of hypercalcaemia, symptomatic/ asymptomatic, gestational age, presence or absence of features of end-organ damage: Frequency of visits to specialist antenatal clinic individualized on a case-to-case basis

Asymptomatic

Mild PHP, hypercalcaemia <11 mg/dl, no features of end-organ damage

Conservative management
- Adequate hydration, aggressive IV fluid replacement if persistent vomiting
- Intermittent parenteral loop diuretic (e.g. furosemide) to promote calciuresis may be required
- Low-calcium diet
- Endocrinologist may consider SC calcitonin—but risk of tachyphylaxis to be considered
- Close maternal serum calcium level monitoring as directed by endocrinologist
- Frequency of antenatal clinic visits to be individualized.
- Close maternal surveillance for development of pre-eclampsia, polyhydramnios, preterm labour, dehydration
- Careful fetal surveillance: serial scans for assessment of fetal growth, exclusion of polyhydramnios
- Alert mother to recognize signs of preterm labour, premature rupture of membranes, close daily vigilance for fetal movements, headaches, abdominal pain, visual disturbances. Give information on how to seek urgent help
- Refer to anaesthetic high risk antenatal clinic, neonatologist, and endocrine surgeon
- If mother becomes symptomatic or serum corrected calcium levels increase to ≥11.4 mg/dl, **admit** for stabilization and to consider definitive surgical treatment (i.e. parathyroidectomy)

Symptomatic

Calcium levels >11.4 mg/dl with or without other signs of end-organ impairment—**admit**

1st and 3rd trimesters
- Initial stabilization with aggressive hydration, intermittent diuretic, etc.
- Endocrinologist, anaesthetist, neonatologist, and surgeon to be involved
- Discuss benefits and risks of surgery to prevent hypercalcaemic crisis, neonatal tetany
- If worsening hypercalcaemia levels—parathyroidectomy by minimal access surgery is strongly advisable at any gestation

2nd trimester
- After initial stabilization, on advice from endocrinologist, anaesthetist, and endocrinology surgeon, surgical management by parathyroidectomy recommended to reduce risk of later maternal hypercalcaemia especially postnatal, as well as of pre-eclampsia, preterm delivery, 2nd-trimester miscarriage, IUGR, IUD, neonatal tetany, etc.

10 Maternal Neurological Conditions

10.1 Epilepsy

FACT FILE

Epidemiology

- **Epilepsy** is seen in about 0.5% of all pregnancies (1 in 200) and 1 in 250 pregnancies are exposed to antiepileptic drugs (AEDs).
- There is a 10-fold increase in mortality as a direct result of seizures among pregnant women with epilepsy, compared with the 2–3-fold increased mortality rate associated with epilepsy in the general population.[1]
- Most women whose epilepsy is optimally controlled will have uncomplicated pregnancies and deliveries and give birth to normal children.[1,2]
- Most patients with epilepsy do not experience an increase in seizures during pregnancy.
- In up to one-third of women with epilepsy, especially in those who have had poor epilepsy control pre-conception or those with multiple seizure types, seizure frequency worsens during pregnancy. This may also be due to poor adherence with treatment, vomiting, sleep deprivation,[2,3,4] and importantly, altered AED pharmacokinetics.
- Certain physiological changes during pregnancy affect the pharmacokinetics of AEDs. The increased plasma volume and renal clearance during pregnancy affect the AED concentration as well as increased protein (globulin) binding especially in the third trimester. This increased protein binding in turn, reduces the amount of free active drug molecules available to maintain optimal epilepsy control.
- The risk of seizures is at its peak in the intrapartum period: 1–2% of women with active epilepsy will have a tonic-clonic seizure during labour and a further 1–2% in the 24 h after delivery.[1,2]
- Status epilepticus (a seizure that lasts 30 min or longer or a series of seizures without consciousness being regained in between) has been reported in less than 1% of pregnancies.

Obstetric complications

- Obstetric complications associated with epilepsy include:
  - spontaneous miscarriages
  - fetal congenital malformation
  - placental abruption
  - pre-eclampsia (A recent study[5] has shown an increased incidence of pre-eclampsia in pregnant women on AEDs compared with epileptic pregnant women not on AEDs. The mechanism involved is still unclear.)
  - preterm labour
  - stillbirth and perinatal mortality.
- There is a significant increase of obstetric interventions with associated problems, including failed labour induction, prolonged labour, and Caesarean sections being approximately twice as likely in women with epilepsy.[6,7]
- AED exposure in utero is associated with increased risks of congenital abnormalities[8] and possible long-term neurological effects[9] on the fetus. These risks are related to the type of drug, whether a single or multiple AEDs are used, and on the dose of some of the older AEDs.
- There is uniform consensus that the risk of uncontrolled seizures outweighs the possible teratogenic risks of AEDs.[10,11]
- The prime objective is to achieve freedom from seizures before conception and during pregnancy (particularly for those with generalized tonic–clonic seizures) as well as to consider the risk of adverse effects of AEDs. There are limited data on risks to the unborn child associated with newer drugs.
- Women may stop taking their medication as soon as they realize they are pregnant, fearing the potential teratogenic effects of AEDs. Many epileptic women are unaware that uncontrolled epilepsy, especially generalized tonic–clonic seizures, can cause miscarriages, fetal hypoxia and acidosis, and intrauterine death.
- A substantial number of women, being unaware that fetal organogenesis is complete by the end of the first trimester, tend not to take AEDs regularly even at later stages of pregnancy.
- Caesarean sections seem to be approximately twice as likely in women with epilepsy.[12,13]

Pre-conceptual care

- Pre-pregnancy assessment and advice by the consultant neurologist and/or a maternal medicine obstetrician are essential for women with epilepsy planning a pregnancy in order to review the control of seizures and of the AED regimen. Unfortunately however, most pregnancies in epileptic women are unplanned.
- Women with epilepsy as well as their partners/carers, must be given accurate information and counselling to help make informed decisions and choices. This should include information about the type of AEDs, contraception, pregnancy, and care of a baby.[1,14]
- Some women may have had no seizures for several years, maintained with just small doses of AED. In addition, their EEG or MRI scan might not have shown any abnormalities. In women who have been seizure-free for more than 2 years, **neurologist-supervised withdrawal of AEDs** over a 3–6-month period may be appropriate.
- All women and girls on AEDs should be offered high-dose folic acid (5 mg/day) before any possibility of pregnancy.[14] Unless this is emphasized in the pre-pregnancy stage, a significant number of pregnant women on AEDs, especially the older AEDs, assume that the pregnancy supplements they can purchase over the counter have sufficient folic acid for their requirements.
- Specific information regarding the need for high-dose folic acid must ideally be provided from before pregnancy by the neurology nurse, GP, neurologist, obstetrician, or midwife. A prescription should be supplied pre-pregnancy by the GP, neurologist, or obstetrician with advice to start the high-dose folic acid from at least 3 months before a pregnancy.
- Many pregnancies in women with epilepsy are unplanned; very few women take the correct dose of folic acid at the appropriate time, and advice about malformation risk and folate is often forgotten. Every opportunity to discuss contraception, and pre-pregnancy counselling including high-dose folic acid from at least 3 months before conception, must be sought in primary care, neurology clinics, gynaecology clinics, postnatal wards, and family planning centres for any woman of childbearing age with epilepsy.
- Pre-pregnancy education and information is therefore vital in the care of all women with epilepsy who are of childbearing age.
- For women on antifolate AEDs such as sodium valproate, carbamazepine, or phenytoin, which can lead to maternal folic acid deficiency (megaloblastic anaemia) it is advisable to continue high-dose folic acid for the duration of pregnancy.
- ***The potential teratogenic risks of AEDs should be discussed and an assessment made of the risks and benefits of treatment. The patient should be advised not to stop AEDs abruptly due to a fear of fetal teratogenicity but to discuss their medication regimen with the GP and neurologist. This allows assessment of their AED(s) which can be***

changed to one more suitable in a future pregnancy or the dosage reduced to keep any potential teratogenic risk to a minimum.

- The basic principle is that if the epilepsy has remained under good control with effective medication, it is best not to tamper with it. Any substantive change must be made only on the neurologist's advice.
- Encouraged by the data from epilepsy pregnancy registers, and the Study of Standard versus New Antiepileptic Drugs (SANAD), there is an increased preference among clinicians to prescribe the newer AEDs such as lamotrigine, topiramate, or levetiracetam, with ***lamotrigine being the AED of first choice in women of childbearing age***.[15]
- The overall rate of major congenital malformations in women on AEDs during the first trimester is 4.2%, compared with 3.5% for women with epilepsy who are not on AEDs. Given that the overall risk of major fetal malformation in any pregnancy in the general population is approximately 2%, this represents an increase of 2–3-fold in women taking a single AED.
- Sodium valproate is associated with the greatest risk of malformations. Higher doses of sodium valproate (>800 mg/day), polytherapy with more than one AED especially including sodium valproate,[1] a previous pregnancy with a major malformation, and low folate levels are all linked to an increased risk of congenital malformations.
- Of the older AEDs, carbamazepine is associated with the lowest frequency of major congenital malformation (2.2% for monotherapy).
- The most common major malformations associated with AEDs are neural tube, orofacial, and cardiac defects.
- The minor malformations include hyperteleorism, epicanthic folds, and digital hypoplasia.
- If more than one AED is used, there is a significantly higher incidence of major malformations than monotherapy (e.g. up to 24% in those taking four AEDs).
- Recent registries have shown an increased risk of oral clefts with newer AEDs like lamotrigine and topiramate.
- **Pre-pregnancy genetic counselling may be required if both parents have epilepsy or if the disease is of an inherited variety**. If the mother has idiopathic generalized epilepsy (IGE), the risk of seizure in the child is 4–8%; in a child of a father with IGE the risk is only slightly higher than that of the general population. When more than one first-degree relative is affected, the risk of the baby being affected will be higher, sometimes as high as 30%.

Antenatal care

- Epilepsy remains an important indirect cause of death in the United Kingdom. In the 2011 Confidential Enquiry report, 14 out of the 154 indirect deaths were related to epilepsy[16] and in the MBBRACE report 2009–12, 14 maternal deaths during pregnancy or up to 42 days postpartum were attributable to epilepsy or seizures, a rate of 0.40 per 100,000 maternities.[17]
- The need for specialist advice in pregnancy, and the risk of sudden unexpected death in epilepsy (SUDEP) should be discussed with all women who plan to stop AED therapy.[17]
- Care of all pregnant women should be shared between the specialist obstetrician and the neurologist.[14]
- Although the risk of seizures during labour is low, it is essential that an early discussion is held with the patient to recommend that delivery takes place in an obstetric unit with facilities for treating maternal seizures and for maternal and neonatal resuscitation.[14]
- For women who first present already pregnant with no pre-conceptual care, modification of a hitherto effective AED regime may be unnecessary, as the pregnancy may have already passed the period of fetal organogenesis (13 weeks gestation).
- There may be an increase in seizure frequency in early pregnancy linked to hyperemesis. Women should be advised not to discontinue medication without consulting the neurologist.
- Women should be reassured that there is no evidence that focal, absence, and myoclonic seizures affect the pregnancy or developing fetus adversely unless they fall and sustain an injury.[1,14]
- Routine monitoring of AED levels in pregnancy is not recommended at present unless control is erratic or non-compliance is suspected.[1,14]
- In addition to the routine 20+ weeks scan, patients on AEDs are also offered a scan at 16 weeks for fetal neural tube defects, cleft lip, palate, etc. Clear mention of the AED medication must be documented in all scan request forms.
- Serial growth scans at 28, 32, and 36 weeks are recommended if the mother is on any type of anti-convulsant medication.
- All children born to mothers taking enzyme-inducing AEDs (e.g. carbamazepine, phenytoin, primidone, and phenobarbital), are at increased risk of haemorrhagic disease of the newborn, caused by deficiency of vitamin K dependent clotting factors. These babies should be given 1 mg of vitamin K parenterally at delivery.[14]
- It is also recommended that women taking these drugs should be given prophylactic **oral vitamin K 10 mg daily from 36 weeks gestation until delivery**.
- Information should be given to all parents about safety precautions to be taken when caring for the baby.[14]
- In some epileptic patients, factors such as pain, stress, sleep deprivation, hyperventilation, and dehydration increase the risk of seizures during labour, delivery, and postpartum. An epidural is advisable as the most appropriate method of analgesia and an antenatal referral to the high-risk anaesthetic clinic is advisable.
- ***Interventions such as early induction of labour or Caesarean section are indicated only if there are other obstetric complications and not just on the basis of epilepsy***.[2]
- Pethidine may sometimes have a convulsive effect on some women and should be used with caution.
- The woman's normal AED medication should be continued throughout labour.
- The AED dosage should be reviewed postnatally and the dosage returned gradually to what it was at the start of pregnancy.

Postnatal care

- It is generally safe for women taking AEDs to breastfeed as only a small fraction is transmitted in breast milk is (3–5%), far less than what the fetus has been exposed to in utero.
- Lamotrigine and phenobarbital cross into the breast milk in significant amounts. Unless the patient has already been on either of these AEDs during pregnancy, initiating these drugs for the first time during breastfeeding is not recommended.
- Help with baby care to assist the mother to get maximum rest will be helpful in the immediate postpartum period.
- Parents should be advised that risk of injury to the infant caused by a maternal seizure is low with appropriate support to reduce risk of accidents. Simple measures such as never bathing the baby while alone, minimizing carrying of the baby, and sitting on the floor or at a low level to breastfeed or to change nappies, should be advised.
- Women who have had a recent increase of AEDs towards the end of pregnancy will need to have the dosage decreased gradually over a period of 1 week after delivery, on the advice of the neurologist.
- An appointment with the consultant neurologist 3–4 months after delivery should be organized before the patient's discharge.
- Advice about appropriate contraception is mandatory.[1,14] **Mirena® IUS** is the preferred contraceptive, followed by progesterone implant. If the patient is on enzyme-inducing AEDs and chooses to have **Depo-Provera®, repeat injections must be administered at 10-week intervals (not the usual 12 weeks**) and the patient and primary care professionals informed accordingly. If the patient is on enzyme-inducing AEDs, oral contraception is more likely to fail (Table 10.1). **Enzyme induction persists up to 4 weeks after the AED is withdrawn**.
- The importance of pre-conceptual counselling before any subsequent pregnancy must always be emphasized.

Information for patients

Please see Information for patients: Epilepsy and pregnancy (p. 516)

Table 10.1 AEDs and their effect on hepatic enzymes

Hepatic enzyme-inducing[a] *AEDs*	*Non-enzyme-inducing AEDs*
Carbamazepine	Acetazolamide
Phenobarbital	Benzodiazepine
Phenytoin	Lamotrigine
Primidone	Gabapentin
Topiramate	levetiracetam

[a] Enzyme-inducing AEDs make oral contraception less effective and interfere with the metabolism of vitamin K, Depo-Provera®, etc.

References

1. NICE Clinical Guideline. The diagnosis and management of the epilepsies in adults and children in primary and secondary care. CG137. London: National Institute for Health and Clinical Excellence, 2012.
2. Bardy AH. Incidence of seizures during pregnancy, labor and puerperium in epileptic women: a prospective study. Acta Neurol Scand 1987;75: 356–360.
3. Gjerde IO, et al. The course of epilepsy during pregnancy: a study of 78 cases. Acta Neurol Scand 1988;78: 198–205.
4. Schmidt D, et al. Change of seizure frequency in pregnant epileptic women. J Neurol Neurosurg Psychiatry 1983;46: 751–755.
5. Borthen I, et al. Obstetric outcome in women with epilepsy: a hospital-based, retrospective study. BJOG 2011;118: 956–965.
6. Tanganelli P, Regesta G. Epilepsy, pregnancy, and major birth anomalies: an Italian prospective, controlled study. Neurology 1992;42 (4 Suppl 5): 89–93.
7. Olafsson E, et al. Pregnancies of women with epilepsy: a population-based study in Iceland. Epilepsia 1998;39: 887–892.
8. Meador K, et al. Pregnancy outcomes in women with epilepsy: a systematic review and meta-analysis of published pregnancy registries and cohorts. Epilepsy Res 2008;81: 1–13.
9. Adab N, et al. Common antiepileptic drugs in pregnancy in women with epilepsy. Cochrane Database Syst Rev 2004;3: CD004848.
10. CEMACH. Saving mothers lives: reviewing maternal deaths to make motherhood safer (2003-2005). London: Confidential Enquiry into Maternal and Child Health, 2007.
11. NICE Clinical Guideline. The epilepsies: diagnosis and management of the epilepsies in adults and children in primary and secondary care. CG20. London: National Institute for Health and Clinical Excellence, 2004.
12. Yerby MS. Management issues for women with epilepsy: neural tube defects and folic acid supplementation. Neurology 2003;61 (6 Suppl 2): S23–S26.
13. Why mothers die 1997–1999. The Confidential Enquiries into Maternal Deaths in the United Kingdom. London: Department of Health, 2000.
14. SIGN Guideline No 70. Diagnosis and management of epilepsy in adults. Edinburgh: Scottish Intercollegiate Guidelines Network, 2003; updated October 2005.
15. Marson AG, et al. The SANAD study of effectiveness of valproate, lamotrigine, or topiramate for generalised and unclassifiable epilepsy: an unblinded randomised controlled trial. Lancet 2007;369 (9566): 1016–1026.
16. Cantwell R, et al. Saving mothers' lives: reviewing maternal deaths to make motherhood safer: 2006–2008. The Eighth Report on Confidential Enquiries into Maternal Deaths in the United Kingdom. BJOG 2011;118 Suppl 1: 1–203.
17. Kelso A on behalf of the MBBRACE-UK Learning from neurological complications chapter writing group. Caring for women with epilepsy. In Knight M, et al (Eds.) on behalf of MBRRACE-UK. Saving Lives, Improving Mothers' Care—Lessons learned to inform future maternity care from the UK and Ireland Confidential Enquiries into Maternal Deaths and Morbidity 2009–12. Oxford: National Perinatal Epidemiology Unit, University of Oxford 2014:73–77.

CARE PATHWAY

Pre-conceptual assessment of epilepsy, seizure control, review of medications

- If the woman planning a pregnancy has been seizure-free for several years with no EEG or MRI abnormalities, a gradual withdrawal of antiepileptic drug (AED) over 6 months under neurologist's supervision to be considered
- Advise patient not to stop AED on her own volition without consultation with the neurologist as the risk of uncontrolled seizures can be more dangerous to mother and fetus
- Neurologist may advise change of AED if required, e.g. monotherapy rather than polytherapy, or change from sodium valproate to carbamazepine or lamotrigine.
- Oral folic acid 5 mg/day from at least 3 months prior to conception to be continued throughout any future pregnancy if on antifolate AEDs
- Confirm patient is on lowest effective dose of single AED
- Refer for genetic counselling if strong family history of epilepsy
- Exclude lupus, antiphospholipid syndrome (APS): Idiopathic epilepsy can be a manifestation of lupus or APS
- If seizure control poor or unstable, review type of contraception and other medications being used and arrange urgent referral to neurologist. Advise patient not to attempt to get pregnant until stable epilepsy control is achieved
- Discuss type of AED-linked malformations, lower incidence with monotherapy and supplemental high-dose folic acid. Explain extra scans at 16 and 22–24 weeks and serial growth scans from 28 weeks
- Explain that in the latter part of a future pregnancy, there may be a need to increase dose of AED to maintain stable control of epilepsy
- Advise patient about multidisciplinary care during a future pregnancy
- Advise patient that for reasons of safety, delivery needs to take place in a hospital unit with all facilities and personnel available for managing an emergency, although most pregnancies and deliveries proceed uneventfully with good fetal and maternal outcomes

During pregnancy

Community midwife/GP refers patient to a specialist antenatal clinic or maternal medicine clinic, ideally before 12 weeks gestation

↓

First visit to maternal medicine clinic

- Detailed history, confirm fetal viability
- Check seizure control and current AED medication, current dose of folic acid
- If on anti-folate AEDs, check is on high-dose 5 mg folic acid ; if not, prescribe and advise continuation throughout pregnancy if on enzyme-inducing AEDs, or at least to end of first trimester if on non-enzyme-inducing AEDs
- Confirm has had recent neurologist follow-up—if not, arrange
- Advise not to stop AEDs abruptly on her own volition, as poor seizure control more damaging to mother and fetus
- If on AEDs, arrange extra scan at about 16 weeks to exclude neural tube defects or orofacial clefts. Specify that patient is on AED medication in all scan request forms
- Arrange detailed anomaly scan at about 20 weeks gestation, if on AED also arrange further fetal cardiac scan at 22–24 weeks, and serial growth scans at 28, 32, and 36 weeks.(this can be modified according to protocol of individual units.)
- Advise to maintain compliance with AED medication
- Advise patient and carers about extra precautions needed for safe care of the baby
- Refer to high-risk anaesthetic clinic, especially if brittle seizure control
- Arrange further follow-up visits to maternal medicine clinic on same day as serial scans at 28, 32, and 36 weeks gestation(or according to individual unit's protocol for serial growth and liquor scans)
- Continued community midwife antenatal visits, vigilance for signs of pre-eclampsia
- Advise patient that for reasons of safety, delivery needs to take place in the hospital unit with all facilities and personnel available for managing an emergency
- Check patient and partner have emergency epilepsy helpline number

↓

Further visits to maternal medicine clinic

At 28, 32, and 36 weeks with growth scans on same day (modified according to individual unit's protocols for serial scans):

- Assess pregnancy, **vigilance for pre-eclampsia**
- Check seizure control; urgent referral to neurologist for medication review if the seizure control has been poor or erratic
- Confirm compliance with prescribed medication, advise to continue folic acid 5 mg if on enzyme-inducing AEDs
- Prescribe 10 mg/day oral vitamin K for mother for 4 weeks from about 37 weeks onwards if on enzyme-inducing AEDs
- **No indication for early IOL or LSCS other than for other obstetric indications such as pre-eclampsia or IUGR**
- Routine post-dates IOL at 40^{+11} or according to individual unit's policy for post-dates IOL
- Check patient has had anaesthetic review in the anaesthetic high-risk clinic
- Encourage epidural to avoid triggers for seizure (e.g. stress, anxiety, pain. or exhaustion)

↓

Postnatal

- Encourage breastfeeding: most AEDs transferred only in insignificant amounts in breast milk
- Check home support available, advise safety procedures with baby care
- Before discharge, recommend appropriate contraception: If patients elects Depo-Provera® injections and is on enzyme-inducing AEDs, advise she needs injections once in 10 weeks (not the usual 12 weeks) and inform GP. Mirena® IUS or progesterone implants are ideal
- Remind patient to seek pre-pregnancy assessment and counselling before next pregnancy and to commence 5 mg folic acid from at least 3 months prior to next pregnancy

10.2 Idiopathic Intracranial Hypertension

FACT FILE

- Previously used terms such as benign intracranial hypertension (BIH) or pseudotumour cerebrii have been replaced by **idiopathic intracranial hypertension (IIH)**.

Epidemiology

- Female to male preponderance is 8:3, and IIH is most common in in obese young women.
- Incidence of IIH is 1 per 100 000 general population and it occurs in 10–20/100 000 obese women.[1]
- IIH is usually self-limiting and generally does not adversely affect reproductive outcome. There is no increased risk of spontaneous miscarriage or fetal loss and it is **not** an indication to terminate pregnancy.

Symptomatology

- Symptoms include nausea, vomiting, retro-orbital headaches, diplopia, and, in severe cases, even visual impairment.[1,2,3]
- Symptoms may worsen during pregnancy and resolve after delivery.
- Risk of recurrence in subsequent pregnancies is about 10%; a risk of permanent visual impairment is 10%.[2,3]
- Symptoms of IIH can present in any trimester of pregnancy.

Diagnosis

- Diagnosis[4] is made by finding a combination of papilloedema and raised intracranial pressure with exclusion of hydrocephalus or a space-occupying lesion by CT (before a pregnancy) or MRI during pregnancy.

Management

- Referral to **neurologist** for ongoing review is essential during pregnancy.
- Almost all treatment regimens for IIH can be used during pregnancy, as in the non-pregnant.
- Glucocorticoids, acetazolamide, diuretics, and even serial lumbar puncture[1,2] are used to lower intracranial pressure and to prevent permanent visual loss.
- Thiazide diuretics like furosemide are to be used with great care in pregnancy due to the risk of decreased placental blood flow and neonatal thrombocytopenia.
- Acetazolamide[5] is the preferred therapy. Like other sulphonamides, acetazolamide acts as a competitive inhibitor of dihydropteroate synthetase (DHPS), an enzyme involved in **folate** synthesis. High-dose folic acid (5 mg/day) must be prescribed, especially in the first trimester, due to the antifolate effect of acetazolamide.
- Use of acetazolamide in late pregnancy has been associated with neonatal electrolyte imbalance and metabolic acidosis.[6,7] Following in-utero exposure, monitoring of the neonatal electrolytes is recommended. Inform paediatricians if the mother has been on acetazolamide in late pregnancy as neonatal electrolyte check is required.[7]
- Visual acuity and fields should be carefully monitored every 2 months during pregnancy in IIH. Any impairment of visual acuity or visual fields should be treated promptly with corticosteroids.
- Except in severe or untreated cases of IIH, labour and normal vaginal delivery are to be aimed for, with Caesarean section reserved for obstetric indications. **The obstetric management should remain unchanged if there are no signs of progressively worsening papilloedema and/or visual loss.**
- ***Referral to the anaesthetic high-risk clinic during pregnancy is essential.***
- Appropriate and adequate analgesia in labour and for delivery are essential. **Epidural is the safe and preferred option.**[8] Narcotic analgesics (pethidine/morphine) are **not generally recommended** as they increase PCO_2 via respiratory depression and thereby increase cerebral blood flow and possible increase in cerebrospinal fluid (CSF) pressure. A general anaesthetic may lead to increased CSF pressure. **Regional block is safer even if an emergency Caesarean section is required.**
- There is not enough literature about the safety of acetazolamide in breastfeeding although the amount transferred in breast milk is minimal. The benefits vs possible risks[5] must be weighed when advising women about breastfeeding.

Information for patients

Please see Information for patients: Idiopathic intracranial hypertension and pregnancy (p. 517)

References

1. Digre KB. Not so benign intracranial hypertension. BMJ 2003;326 (7390): 613–614.
2. Huna-Baron R, Kupersmith MJ. Idiopathic intracranial hypertension in pregnancy. J Neurol 2002;249(8): 1078–1081.
3. Badve M, McConnell MJ. Idiopathic intracranial hypertension in pregnancy treated with serial lumbar punctures. Int J Clini Med 2011;2: 9–12.
4. Friedman DI, Jacobson MD. Diagnostic criteria for idiopathic intracranial hypertension. Neurology 2002;59: 1492–1495.
5. Lee AG, et al. The use of acetazolamide in idiopathic intracranial hypertension during pregnancy. Am J Ophthalmol 2005;139: 855–859.
6. Use of acetazolamide in pregnancy, 2011. <http://www.toxbase.org>
7. Ozawa H, et al. Transient renal tubular acidosis in a neonate following transplacental acetazolamide. Eur J Pediatr 2001;160: 321–322.
8. Yun EM, et al. Neurological and muscular disease. In: Datta S, ed., Anesthetic and obstetric management of high-risk pregnancy, 2nd ed. St. Louis: Mosby, 1996, pp. 137–139.

CARE PATHWAY

Community midwife refers patient with idiopathic **intracranial hypertension (IIH)** to maternal medicine clinic within the 1st trimester

↓

First visit to maternal medicine clinic

- Assess pregnancy
- Enquire about any recent symptoms of IIH
- Check current medications
- If on acetazolamide, reassure safety in pregnancy and prescribe high-dose folic acid (5 mg/day) to be continued throughout pregnancy
- Check when last visual field and retinal examination was done
- Ensure visual field checks are done at 2–3 month intervals during pregnancy—refer to ophthalmologist
- Early referral for neurology review
- Refer to anaesthetic high-risk clinic
- If on medication with acetazolamide, steroids or furosemide, arrange serial growth and liquor volume scans at 28, 32, and 36 weeks
- Reassure patient that if IIH is stable without any progressive worsening of vision, spontaneous vaginal delivery would be suitable in the absence of any other problems
- Continue routine community midwife antenatal checks according to NICE schedule

↓

Further visits to maternal medicine clinic

At 28, 32, and 36 weeks:

- Assess pregnancy progress and growth scans, the latter organized if on current medications for IIH
- Check on IIH symptomatology and recent reviews by neurologist and ophthalmologist
- Check has had anaesthetic high-risk clinic review
- If all well, advise to aim for vaginal delivery, no indication for early IOL
- If progressive worsening vision and IIH symptoms hard to control, an earlier IOL or even elective delivery by a planned LSCS under spinal block may become necessary
- At 36 weeks, if asymptomatic or stable on treatment, give date for routine post-dates IOL at 40^{+10} or according to individual unit's policy for post-dates IOL
- If worsening vision problems, steroids required to save vision. Also an elective Caesarean section or early (<40 wks) IOL may be required
- If on long-term or recent steroids, will need hydrocortisone IM injections 100 mg 6–8 hourly during labour and for delivery
- If patient has been on furosemide, cord bloods to exclude fetal thrombocytopenia

↓

Postpartum

- Low-dose steroids safe for breastfeeding. Acetazolamide to be avoided during breastfeeding as little is known regarding its passage through breast milk
- Before hospital discharge, advise weight loss before starting a new pregnancy to reduce risk of recurrence of IIH symptoms

10.3 Multiple Sclerosis

FACT FILE

- **Multiple sclerosis (MS)** is a demyelinating disorder characterized by recurrent or chronically progressive neurological dysfunction. Lesions may be found in the brain, optic nerves, or spinal cord.

Epidemiology

- Women are more commonly affected and the disease onset is often in their childbearing years.
- This disease is relatively common (0.6–0.1%) in the UK.

Clinical presentation

- Common presentations include optic neuritis, diplopia, and weakness of the limbs or sensory symptoms.
- Progress of MS may be highly variable, with some patients remaining asymptomatic for years between attacks while others develop cumulative and steadily progressive neurological disability.
- Most pregnant patients are aware of their condition, with the diagnosis having been made before pregnancy.

Effect of MS on pregnancy outcomes

- There is little effect of MS on pregnancy outcomes - the patient needs to be reassured about this.

Effect of pregnancy on MS

- MS is less likely to present for the first time and less likely to relapse during pregnancy.[1,2,3]
- Remission is most marked in the third trimester.
- The MS relapse rate increases after birth and remains exacerbated for about 3 months postnatally, with a return to the pre-pregnancy state by about 10 months after delivery.
- Exacerbation during 3–6 months after delivery occurs in 30–40% of patients.
- There is an increased rate of postpartum relapse if the patient has had relapses in the year preceding pregnancy or during pregnancy.
- Neither breastfeeding nor epidural has any adverse effect on postpartum relapse rates.[1,2]
- The occurrence of postpartum relapse is not related to age at onset of MS, age at time of pregnancy, disease duration, total number of relapses during pregnancy, parity, or gender of the offspring.[1]
- MRI shows cessation of disease activity during the remission phase in pregnancy.

Management in pregnancy

- The overall rate of progression of disability is not altered by pregnancy or breastfeeding.[1,2,3]
- ***Multidisciplinary care should be provided by neurologist, physician, GP, community midwife, obstetrician, hospital midwives, and health visitors.***
- The management of acute severe relapse is with high-dose steroids, as in the non-pregnant. In such cases, hydrocortisone must also be given to cover labour and delivery as IM bolus doses of 100 mg every 6–8 h.
- Steroids used in cases of acute severe relapses are not contraindicated during pregnancy, neither are drugs like imipramine for urinary urgency or bethanechol for urinary retention.
- Prophylactic treatment with disease-modifying or immunosuppressive agents such as interferon beta and glatiramer are contraindicated in pregnancy and during breastfeeding.
- Women with neuropathic bladders may have increased problems with urinary tract infection (UTI) during pregnancy. Vigilance for urinary retention and UTIs must be maintained in those with a neuropathic bladder. Drugs like imipramine for urinary urgency or bethanechol for urinary retention can be used if required during pregnancy.
- The patient should also be advised regarding safety of use of drugs like gabapentin/carbamazepine for short periods of time for any paroxysmal pain that might occur in pregnancy.
- Early referrals to neurologist and anaesthetist in pregnancy are indicated.
- There is no contraindication for epidural but careful documentation of pre-existing neurological deficit in the legs is necessary to avoid any postpartum exacerbation of MS being wrongly attributed to the regional block.
- Mode of delivery and anaesthetic choices are similar to those for women without MS.
- **MS is not an indication for Caesarean section or for early IOL and a normal delivery can be anticipated.**
- ***Fatigue and depression can be managed with support and medication. Common antidepressants are used with relative safety during pregnancy and in the puerperium.***
- Breastfeeding should be encouraged and there is no increased risk of relapse associated with this. However, if drugs such as high-dose steroids, certain antidepressants, interferon beta, or glatiramer are required in the puerperium to modify the disease,[4] the advice is not to breastfeed.
- Postnatal depression (PND) can be a feature associated with MS and it is important that women have access to support systems. The family and healthcare professionals involved must be made aware of this risk and maintain vigilance for early detection of signs of PND.
- Relapse rates are increased for up to 6 months in the postpartum period with an increased risk of re-hospitalization. The woman and her partner and family should be encouraged to have strong support systems in place.
- All hormonal contraception can be used by women with MS. Some studies suggest that oestrogen may have protective effects against disease progression.

Pre-pregnancy counselling

- Recent studies have found an association between low vitamin D levels and increased risks of developing MS, increased risk of new MS attacks ('relapses'), new lesions on MRI, and disability compared with patients with higher vitamin D levels.[5,6,7,8,9]
- The results of the first published randomized double-blind placebo-controlled trial of vitamin D supplementation in patients with MS suggest that **it may be beneficial for patients with MS who have vitamin D insufficiency or deficiency to take vitamin D supplementation.**[10]
- Further research is ongoing to determine the ideal doses required in these individuals. **In the meantime, the recent DH recommendation that all pregnant and breastfeeding women should take a daily supplement containing 10 micrograms of vitamin D should be rigorously followed in women with MS.**[10]
- Women should be advised that there is no increased risk of ectopic, miscarriage, preterm birth, IUD, IUGR, or malformations associated with MS.
- There is no contraindication to pregnancy in women with MS as long as their level of disability has been assessed and a management plan is made once pregnancy is established.
- If the women is on medication and is planning a pregnancy, pre-pregnancy consultation with the neurologist ± maternal medicine obstetrician is vital. **Women should be advised NOT to stop their medication suddenly.**
- Some drugs used in the management of MS in the non-pregnant are contraindicated in pregnancy (e.g. interferon beta, glatiramer acetate).[4] Referral to the neurologist before pregnancy is therefore essential.

- Women are generally advised to gradually taper and then stop disease-modifying drugs like interferon beta or glatiramer at least 3 months before pregnancy. However, in the event of conception having taken place while she is still on these agents, the patient must be advised to gradually taper down doses before stopping these medications rather than trying to stop abruptly.
- The risk of the child developing MS in future needs to be discussed, although MS is not directly inherited.
- The risk in the general white population is for 1 in every 800 children to develope MS. If one parent has MS, there is a 1 in 50 risk of the child developing MS in the future. The absolute risk is still relatively small, although having a parent with MS does increase the risk,.

Information for patients

Please see **Information for patients: Multiple sclerosis and pregnancy** (p. 517)

References

1. Vukusic S, et al. Pregnancy and multiple sclerosis (the PRIMS study):clinical predictors of post-partum relapse. Brain 2004;127: 1353–1360.
2. Stuart M, Bergstrom L Pregnancy and multiple sclerosis. J Midwifery Womens Health 2011;56: 41–47.
3. Houtchens MK. Pregnancy and multiple sclerosis. Semin Neurol 2007;27: 341–434.
4. Alex T, Lee M. Multiple sclerosis and pregnancy. Curr Opin Obstet Gynecol 2011;23: 435–439.
5. Ascherio A, et al. Vitamin D and multiple sclerosis. Lancet Neurol 2010;9: 599–612.
5. Burton JM, et al. A phase I/II dose escalation trial of vitamin D3 and calcium in multiple sclerosis. Neurology 2010;74: 1852–1859.
6. Mowry EM. Vitamin D: evidence for its role as a prognostic factor in multiple sclerosis. J Neurol Sci 2011;311: 19–22.
7. Pierrot-Deseilligny C, Souberbielle JC. Is hypovitaminosis D one of the environmental risk factors for multiple sclerosis? Brain 2010;133: 1869–1888.
8. Solomon AJ, Whitham RH. Multiple sclerosis and vitamin D: a review and recommendations. Curr Neurol Neurosci Rep 2010;10: 389–396.
9. Solomon AJ. Multiple sclerosis and vitamin D. Neurology 2011;77; e99–100.
10. Department of Health. Vitamin D—advice on supplements for at risk groups, 2012. <http://www.dh.gov.uk/prod_consum_dh/groups/dh_digitalassets/@dh/@en/documents/digitalasset/dh_132508.pdf> and <http://www.scotland.gov.uk/Topics/Health/health/Health/EatingHealth/vitaminD/CMOletter>.

CARE PATHWAY

Multidisciplinary care along with family support is mandatory for pregnant women with **multiple sclerosis (MS)**

Early referral by GP/community midwife to maternal medicine/specialist antenatal clinic

Maternal medicine or specialist antenatal clinic

- Multidisciplinary care essential
- Reassure patient and partner/family that disease relapse decreases during pregnancy and no adverse effect of MS on pregnancy and vice versa
- Refer for neurology review in pregnancy
- Ensure has support from partner, family, and friends
- Folic acid—routine prophylaxis during 1st trimester
- Vitamin D 10 micrograms/day throughout pregnancy and lactation
- Aggressive treatment of UTIs if neuropathic bladder—regular checks of MSU during pregnancy
- Early referral to anaesthetic high-risk clinic
- No indication for extra scans unless has had exposure to disease-modifying agents such as beta-interferon or glatiramer in early pregnancy
- Epidural/spinal not contraindicated
- Discuss safety of steroids for management of sudden severe relapse during pregnancy and puerperium
- If steroids used in pregnancy, bolus hydrocortisone cover for labour and delivery
- MS not an indication of either early IOL or for Caesarean section
- Appropriate advice regarding backache, fatigue, shift of centre of gravity during later pregnancy, and use of walking aids to ensure balance
- Watch for signs of depression in pregnancy—may need antidepressants

Neurologist

- Disease assessment by neurologist—multidisciplinary care provision with good communication to be maintained
- Disease-modifying drugs such as beta-interferon and glatiramer are contraindicated in pregnancy and breastfeeding
- Advise gradual cessation 3 months before conception
- Advise regarding symptom management and treatment of relapses during pregnancy and puerperium
- Follow-up appointments as appropriate
- In case of severe relapse, no contraindication for use of steroids during pregnancy

Postpartum

- Encourage breastfeeding (unless on certain disease-modifying drugs)
- Watch for postnatal depression—low threshold for use of antidepressants

Remember: Give contact details of MS support groups

10.4 Stroke

FACT FILE

This fact file deals with general background information about stroke and pregnancy, as well as recurrence risk during pregnancy in women who have suffered a previous stroke. Immediate multidisciplinary stroke management in pregnancy or the puerperium, ideally in centralized units, is outside the remit of this fact file.

- **Stroke (cerebrovascular accident)** is a significant cause of maternal morbidity and mortality.[1,2,3,4,5,6,7,8,9,10]
- Fortunately, **pregnancy-related stroke** is relatively rare.
- Stroke contributes to about 12% of all maternal deaths.[1,2]
- Estimates of the incidence of stroke vary widely. Incidence of pregnancy-related stroke is about 26–34 per 100 000 deliveries,[1,2,3,4,5,10] compared with the incidence among non-pregnant women which is about 10.7 per 100 000.[5]
- An average maternity unit in the UK with about 3300 deliveries per year could expect to see a pregnancy-related stroke every 9 months to 2 years, which makes the case for their management to take place in centralized units with a specialist multidisciplinary team (neurologist, obstetrician, midwives, neurosurgeon and senior anaesthetic input) available round the clock. Follow-up with rehabilitation services based in the same specialist unit would be ideal.[2]
- The recent UKOSS study, however, found a lower incidence of antenatal stroke than previous studies. An estimated incidence of 1.5 cases per 100 000 maternities were reported with a haemorrhagic stroke incidence of 0.6 and non-haemorrhagic stroke of 0.9 per 100 000 maternities.[7]
- **Arterial and venous strokes** are classified as **ischaemic**, while **subarachnoid** or **intracerebral strokes** are **haemorrhagic**.
- The risk of both ischaemic and haemorrhagic strokes increases in the third trimester and in the puerperium (particularly in the 6 weeks after delivery).[1,2,8,7,10,11]
- Subarachnoid haemorrhage can occur at any stage of pregnancy and in the puerperium, while intracerebral bleeding or bleeding from arteriovenous malformation or aneurysm usually takes place in late pregnancy and puerperium.[1,11]
- Mortality rate associated with pregnancy-related stroke is about 10–20%.[2,7,10]
- In the recent MBBRACE-UK report[4] twenty-six women died of haemorrhagic stroke in the UK and Ireland between 2009 and 2012 (0.75 per 100 000 maternities overall) while death from ischaemic stroke in pregnancy was uncommon, with a mortality rate of 0.03 per 100 000 maternities.

Risk factors for pregnancy-related stroke

- The prothrombotic states of normal pregnancy and puerperium when there is a combination of the triad of hypercoagulability, venous stasis, and vascular endothelial damage.[1,2,7,11,12,13,14]
- Maternal age greater than 35 years.
- Obesity—a significant risk factor for both vascular and thrombotic stokes.
- Multiparity
- Smoking
- History of migraine[7]
- Afro-Caribbean ethnicity
- Hypertension, pre-eclampsia,[7] eclampsia, HELLP
- Diabetes—gestational or preceding pregnancy.
- Multiple gestation
- Heart conditions such as patent foramen ovale, peripartum cardiomyopathy, prosthetic mechanical heart valve
- Alcohol and substance abuse (esp. cocaine)
- Autoimmune conditions such as lupus, antiphospholipid syndrome (APS)
- Thrombophilias
- Sickle cell disease
- Dehydration, electrolyte imbalances
- Postpartum infection
- Thrombotic thrombocytopenic purpura

Specific stroke-provoking syndromes in pregnancy/puerperium

Pre-eclampsia, eclampsia, HELLP

- Associated with 25–45% of pregnancy-associated stroke.[1,2,7,8,10]
- Widespread endothelial dysfunction, vasospasm, and hypertension.
- Imaging may show intracerebral haemorrhage or arterial ischaemic events.
- Cerebral haemorrhage is the most common cause of death in patients with eclampsia.[15]
- Risk of ischaemic stroke persists beyond pregnancy and puerperium as women with a history of pre-eclampsia are 60% more likely to suffer a non-pregnancy-related stroke later in life.[16]
- Stroke is the most common cause of death seen in HELLP.[17]

Peri- or postpartum angiopathy

- Thought to be due to reversible cerebral vasoconstriction affecting large and medium-sized cerebral vessels.
- Usually occurs a few days after delivery.[1,2]
- Most patients have had uncomplicated pregnancy and delivery.
- Presenting features include sudden severe 'thunderclap' headache, vomiting, photosensitivity, altered consciousness, even seizures and temporary or permanent focal neurological deficit.
- Migraine can be a risk factor.[2,7]
- Process is usually self-limiting, with spontaneous and complete resolution of symptoms although can recur in subsequent pregnancies.

Subarachnoid haemorrhage and rupture of cerebral aneurysm

- Subarachnoid haemorrhage (SAH), mostly from aneurysm rupture, accounts for about 3% of all strokes.[2]
- Most cases of SAH are due to rupture of cerebral aneurysm.
- Incidence of cerebral aneurysms in the general population is about 4–6%.[2]
- Risk of SAH during pregnancy and puerperium is nearly six times more than in non-pregnant women.[8]
- About 1 in 10 000 pregnancies complicated by rupture of cerebral aneurysm, usually in the second or third trimesters[2] and up to 6 weeks after delivery.[8]
- Nearly 50% of all aneurysm ruptures in women under 40 years of age are pregnancy related.
- Greater mortality when aneurysms rupture during pregnancy than in non-pregnant state.[1]
- Non-aneurysm-related SAH usually associated with pregnancy-induced hypertension and eclampsia.
- Surgical treatment for aneurysmal SAH that has occurred during pregnancy can improve maternal and fetal outcomes. Treatment of choice during pregnancy appears to be endovascular coiling and is recommended prior to delivery.[2]
- Once surgically corrected, the mode of delivery does not seem to have any effect on maternal or fetal outcomes.[1,2] These pregnancies can generally progress to term unless there are obstetric complications warranting earlier delivery.
- Caesarean sections are indicated if the aneurysm has been detected only at term or if the neurosurgical intervention has taken place within the week before delivery, otherwise Caesarean sections for purely obstetric indications.
- Epidural insertion in such patients must be performed only by an experienced anaesthetist as there are some risks of intracranial haemorrhage or SAH if a dural tap occurs.

- It may be reasonable to use instrumental-assisted vaginal delivery to cut short the second stage, preferably with an epidural on board
- Oxytocin/ergometrine must be avoided and oxytocin alone (without ergometrine) is the drug of choice for the routine active management of the third stage of labour.[4]

Cerebral venous thrombosis

- Cerebral venous thrombosis **(CVT)** accounts for about 2% of pregnancy-related stroke.[2]
- Increased risk of CVT in pregnancy, particularly in the puerperium.
- CVT carries a high fatality rate ranging from 4–36%,[18,19] mainly due to secondary intracranial haemorrhage which is seen in up to 40% of these women.[2,5]
- Risks for CVT include hypertension, older mothers, Caesarean sections, associated infections, dehydration.
- Occlusion of major venous sinuses leads to intracranial hypertension.
- In most patients symptoms commence within 3 weeks after delivery.
- Typically the patient presents with headache, vomiting, disturbance of consciousness, focal neurological symptoms, and seizures.
- Antithrombotic agents as well as low-dose aspirin are used for treatment of CVT in pregnancy and puerperium.[18,19,20] Presence of secondary intracranial haemorrhage does not seem to be a contraindication for the use of use of low molecular weight heparin (LMWH) therapy.
- During pregnancy, treatment regimes can consist of LMWH for the first 13 weeks gestation, followed by oral warfarin until mid-third trimester and switching back to LMWH till delivery and immediately after. The alternative is to continue LMWH with factor Xa monitoring throughout pregnancy and postnatally for about 12 weeks.[1,2]

Paradoxical embolism

- Well-recognized link between pregnancy-related stroke and patent foramen ovale (PFO).[1]
- PFO found in over half the patients with paradoxical embolism.
- Medical therapy includes low-dose aspirin, warfarin, or antiplatelet agents.
- If, despite optimum medical therapy, recurrent cryptogenic stroke, percutaneous transcatheter PFO closure under ECHO guidance can be performed.

Management of stroke in pregnancy

- ***The role of the obstetrician is to have a high index of suspicion and, having made a presumptive diagnosis, to obtain urgent neurology and neurosurgical input. Appropriate imaging studies and their interpretation and institution of treatment which may be lifesaving can then be instituted by the neurologist and neurosurgeon.***[12]
- Apart from pregnancy-related causes, other factors for stroke in pregnancy must also be considered.
- Assessment and treatment are generally along the same lines as in non-pregnant patients.
- CT head, which uses ionizing radiation, exposes the fetus to a maximum of 50 mrad and cerebral angiography to 10 mrad, whereas MRI does not involve ionizing radiation.
- Thrombolytic treatment is relatively contraindicated due to maternal and fetal complications such preterm labour, placental abruption, fetal death, postpartum haemorrhage.
- However, there are encouraging results of the use of thrombolytic therapy in pregnancy in recent studies.[21] **In the absence of any definitive studies of the fetal effects of thrombolytic treatments, potentially lifesaving medications should not be withheld because of theoretical harm to the fetus.**[12]

Prognosis

- Mortality from pregnancy-related stroke results from intracranial haemorrhage or malignant hypertension.[1,3]
- Ischaemic stroke is less likely to result in mortality unless accompanied by secondary haemorrhage.
- Approximately 50% of patients who survive a pregnancy-related stroke are left with a residual neurological deficit.[1,21]

Recurrence risk

- In a large study of women who had a stroke in pregnancy, no recurrences were found in subsequent pregnancies.[20]
- Therefore, previous ischaemic stroke should not be a contraindication to further pregnancies.[20] However, the risk of recurrent stroke (in non-pregnant state) in these women is about 1% in the following 12 months and 2.3% within 5 years.
- After acute treatment for stroke the patient needs to be thoroughly evaluated for underlying predisposing factors.
- Thrombophilias and autoimmune conditions[1] might be responsible for both arterial and venous strokes. Screening for these conditions needs to take place about 4–6 weeks after stopping anticoagulation therapy and no earlier than 8–12 weeks after delivery. Lupus anticoagulant, cardiolipin antibodies, and anti-β2-glycoprotein are best repeated some 12 weeks after the first test to reach a definitive diagnosis.
- **Effective contraception** needs to be discussed and documented before discharge from the hospital. Any oestrogen-containing oral contraception is contraindicated.
- Before discharge, advice and support to help stop smoking, alcohol, or illicit drug usage, as relevant to each patient, must be provided. If the patient has been on drugs such as methylergonovine or bromocriptine, these must be stopped forthwith.
- Pre-pregnancy assessment and advice is highly recommended for this group of patients.

Pre-pregnancy assessment and advice: important factors

- If autoimmune conditions or thrombophilias, cardiac abnormalities, or diabetes have been detected on screening, **for management of the next pregnancy refer to the specific Care Pathways suggested in this Compendium for these conditions.**
- If autoimmune conditions or thrombophilias, cardiac abnormalities, and diabetes have been excluded, care should be taken during the next pregnancy to avoid risk factors such as smoking, alcohol, or illicit drug use, and dehydration through excessive hyperemesis. Robust management of hypertension, if present, and prophylactic low-dose aspirin is recommended from the first trimester till the end of pregnancy and puerperium.
- Thromboprophylaxis with LMWH and low-dose aspirin during any future pregnancy and in the puerperium is recommended.[2]

Information for patients

Please see Information for patients: Stroke and pregnancy (p. 518)

References

1. Davie CA, O'Brien P Stroke and pregnancy. J Neurol Neurosurg Psychiatry 2008;79: 240–245.
2. Treadwell SD, et al. Stroke in pregnancy and the puerperium. Postgrad Med J 2008;84: 238–245.
3. Sharshar T, et al. Incidence and causes of strokes associated with pregnancy and puerperium. A study in public hospitals of Ile de France. Stroke 1995;26: 930–936.
4. Wills A on behalf of the MBBRACE-UK Learning from neurological complications chapter writing group on behalf of the MBBRACE-UK Learning from neurological complications chapter writing group. Messages for stroke care. In Knight M, et al (Eds.) on behalf of MBRRACE-UK. Saving Lives, Improving Mothers' Care—Lessons learned to inform future maternity care from the UK and Ireland Confidential Enquiries into Maternal Deaths and Morbidity 2009–12. Oxford: National Perinatal Epidemiology Unit, University of Oxford 2014:77–79
5. Pettiti DB, et al. Incidence of stroke and myocardial infarction in women of reproductive age Stroke 1997;28: 280–283.
6. Lanska DJ, Kryscio RJ Risk factors for peripartum and postpartum stroke and intracranial venous thrombosis. Stroke 2000;31: 1274–1282.
7. Scott CA, et al. Stroke in pregnancy: incidence, risk factors, management, and outcomes. Obstet Gynecol 2012;120 (2 Pt 1): 318–324.
8. James AH, et al. Incidence and risk factors for stroke in pregnancy and the puerperium. Obstet Gynecol 2005;106: 509–516.

9. Ros HS, et al. Increased risks of circulatory diseases in late pregnancy and puerperium. . Epidemiology 2001;12: 456–460.
10. Jaigobin C, Silver FL Stroke and pregnancy. Stroke 2000;31: 2948–2951.
11. Cantu C, Barinagarrementaria F Cerebral venous thrombosis associated with pregnancy and the puerperium: a review of 67 cases. Stroke 1993;24: 1880–1884.
12. Walsh J, et al. Maternal cerebrovascular accidents in pregnancy: incidence and outcomes. Obstet Med 2010;3: 152–155.
13. Okanloma KA, Moodley J Neurological complications associated with the pre-eclampsia/eclampsia syndrome. Int J Gynaecol Obstet 2000;71: 223–225.
14. Brown DW, et al. Preeclampsia and the risk of ischemic stroke among young women. Stroke 2006;37: 1055–1059.
15. Isler CM, et al. Maternal mortality associated with HELLP (hemolysis, elevated liver enzymes, and low platelets) syndrome. Am J Obstet Gynecol 1999;181: 924–928.
16. Bogousslavsky J, et al. Postpartum cerebral angiopathy: reversible vasoconstriction assessed by transcranial Doppler ultrasounds. Eur Neurol 1989;29: 102–105.
17. Calado S, et al. Postpartum cerebral angiopathy: vasospasm, vasculitis or both? Cerebrovasc Dis 2004;18: 340–341.
18. Bates SM, et al. Use of antithrombotic agents during pregnancy. The seventh ACCP conference on antithrombotic and thrombolytic therapy. Chest 2004;126: 627S–644S.
19. Turan TN, Stern BJ Stroke in pregnancy. Neurol Clin 2004;22: 821–840.
20. Lamy C, et al. Ischaemic stroke in young women: risk of recurrence in subsequent pregnancies. Neurology 2000;55: 269–274.
21. Murugappan A, et al. Thrombolytic therapy of acute ischaemic stroke during pregnancy. Neurology 2006;66: 770.

CARE PATHWAY

Pre-pregnancy counselling of patient with history of previous stroke (pregnancy-related or outside of pregnancy)

- **Obtain history** including previous details of stroke, whether any provoking factors for stroke, investigations, continued treatment following CVA, duration of treatment, any residual neurological sequelae, etc. Attempt to get further information from previous hospital if treated elsewhere
- **Identify pre-disposing risk factors for recurrence of stroke,** e.g. smoking,diabetes, hypertension, thrombophilic or autoimmune conditions (APS, lupus, antithrombin variant, protein C and S deficiency), sickle cell disease, alcohol/substance abuse, uncorrected patent foramen ovale, drugs such as bromocriptine
- Screen for APS, lupus, inherited thrombophilias if not already done. If positive, follow relevant care pathways during future pregnancy
- Advise smoking cessation and/or alcohol or substance abuse if relevant
- Enquire regarding medications: anticoagulation, aspirin, antihypertensives, contraception used (must not use COCP). If on ACE inhibitors or beta-blockers, change to methyldopa or labetalol before pregnancy and to continue during. If on warfarin pre-pregnancy, advise change to LMWH SC injections once pregnancy established
- Check she has had recent neurology appointment and neurologist's assessment regarding any residual neurological deficit
- In absence of ongoing risk factors, reassure patient regarding low risk for stroke recurrence during a future pregnancy
- Ensure she is on low-dose aspirin indefinitely, advise to continue during pregnancy and after
- Discuss thromboprophylaxis during future pregnancy and puerperium, anticoagulation regime options

↓

Antenatal care for patient with history of previous stroke

- Early referral from community to specialist antenatal clinic
- Multidisciplinary team management with neurologist, obstetrician, midwife, and anaesthetist

↓

First visit to maternal medicine antenatal clinic

- Check viability, dates
- Ascertain if any residual neurological deficits and check she has had recent neurology assessment
- If pre-existing conditions such as lupus, APS, diabetes, sickle cell, hypertension, etc., refer to relevant care pathways. Close monitoring and control of diabetes and hypertension essential
- Ensure she is on continuous low-dose aspirin throughout pregnancy and thromboprophylaxis during pregnancy and puerperium
- Refer to anaesthetic high-risk clinic
- Advise to avoid dehydration if vomiting in early pregnancy
- Advise to continue routine antenatal visits to community midwife

↓

Subsequent visits to specialist antenatal clinic

- If pre-existing conditions such as diabetes, hypertension, lupus, APS, etc., serial growth and liquor scans
- Assess pregnancy, ensure continuing low-dose aspirin, thromboprophylaxis
- Multidisciplinary team management liaising with neurological and anaesthetic assessments
- If previously repaired cerebral aneurysm, vaginal delivery not contraindicated
- Unless other obstetric indications, no need for routine early IOL or LSCS
- Oxytocin alone (without ergometrine) is the drug of choice for the routine active management of the third stage of labour.

↓

Postpartum

- Before discharge, advise about contraception. **COCP contraindicated,** Mirena® or etonogestrel implant ideal

10.5 Bell's Palsy

FACT FILE

- **Bell's palsy or idiopathic unilateral facial nerve (cranial nerve VII) paralysis,** is an acute, benign, and common idiopathic neurological disorder.
- Usually a mononeuritis with the common symptoms of acute facial palsy, posterior auricular pain on the affected side, altered taste sensation, and incomplete hyperasthesia over the trigeminal nerve distribution.

Prevalence

- Prevalence in pregnancy is estimated to be about 4–5 per 10 000, about 10 times more frequent than in the non-pregnant population.[1]
- It is common in the third trimester and immediate postpartum period.[2] Most women who develop Bell's palsy have no risk factors before pregnancy, including diabetes or chronic hypertension

Prognosis

- Prognosis in the long-term is generally good.

Aetiology

- Several studies have suggested that Bell's palsy in pregnancy is due to similar causes as in non-pregnancy, such as altered susceptibility to herpes simplex viral reactivation, Epstein–Barr virus, or cytomegalovirus during the third trimester of pregnancy.[3,4] Bell's palsy may be secondary to latent herpes simplex infection.
- Other studies have shown an association of Bell's palsy with pregnancy-induced hypertension and pre-eclampsia, more than 4–5 times in the general obstetric population.[5,6]
- Various theories have been proposed to establish a link between Bell's palsy and pre-eclampsia including an increase in the extracellular fluid volume in the third trimester[7] or thrombosis of the vasa nervorum, leading to nerve ischaemia and paralysis.[8]
- Increased perineural oedema, as seen in carpal tunnel syndrome, may be involved in impingement of the facial nerve leading to facial nerve palsy.
- Some studies report 100% recovery in those with incomplete Bell's palsy or only a 52% improvement in those with complete palsy, which is significantly worse than in the general population.[9]
- Bell's palsy can recur in more than one pregnancy in the same woman.[10]
- ***Ramsay–Hunt syndrome is herpes zoster (shingles) infection of the geniculate ganglion. This can cause unilateral facial nerve palsy that mimics Bell's palsy, except that there are ear vesicles present.***

Management

- Bell's palsy usually recovers in 85–95% of cases, but can take several months to do so.
- If seen within 48–72 h of developing symptoms, a short 2-week course of high-dose prednisolone 40 mg/day gradually tapered down after the first week may achieve a speedier recovery. However, if herpetic infection is suspected, steroids should be either avoided or combined with aciclovir.[11,12]
- Physiotherapy and eye care may become necessary.
- **Steroids must not be used in Ramsay–Hunt syndrome,** therefore before prescribing steroids in what is assumed to be Bell's palsy, **examination of the ear for any vesicles is mandatory**.
- **Bell's palsy is itself not a reason for earlier induction of labour or for Caesarean section.**

Information for patients

Please see **Information for patients: Bell's palsy and pregnancy** (p. 519)

References

1. Hilsinger REL Jr Idiopathic facial paralysis, pregnancy, and the menstrual cycle. Ann Otol 1975;84: 433–442.
2. Shapiro L, et al. Bell's palsy and tinnitus during pregnancy: predictors of pre-eclampsia. Acta Otolaryngol 1999;19: 647–651.
3. Murakami S, et al. Bell's palsy and herpes simplex virus: identification of viral DNA in endoneurial fluid and muscle. Ann Intern Med 1996;124: 27–30.
4. Dorsey DL, Camann WR Obstetric anesthesia in patients with idiopathic facial paralysis (Bell's palsy): a 10-year survey. Anesth Analg 1993;77: 81–83.
5. Sibai BM., et al. Prevention of preeclampsia with low-dose aspirin in low dose healthy, nulliparous pregnant women. National Institute of Child Health and Human Development Network of Maternal-Fetal Medicine Units. N Engl J Med 1993;329: 1213–1218.
6. Shmorgun D, et al. Association between Bell's palsy in pregnancy and pre-eclampsia. Q J Med 2002;95: 359–362.
7. Davison JM Edema in pregnancy. Kidney Int 1997;59Suppl:
8. Falco NA, Eriksson E Idiopathic facial palsy in pregnancy and the puerperium. Surg Gynecol Obstet 1989;169: 337–340.
9. Gilman GS, et al. Bell's palsy in pregnancy: a study of recovery outcomes. Otolaryngol Head Neck Surg 2002;126: 26–30.
10. English JB, et al. Recurrent Bell's palsy. Neurology 1996;47: 604–605.
11. Sullivan FM, et al. Early treatment with prednisolone or acyclovir in Bell's palsy. N Engl J Med 2007;357: 1598–1607.
12. Sullivan FM, et al. A randomised controlled trial of the use of aciclovir and/or prednisolone for the early treatment of Bell's palsy: the BELLS study. Health Technol Assess 2009;13 (47): iii-iv, ix-xi, 1–130.

CARE PATHWAY

GP or community midwife refers patient with **Bell's palsy** to a specialist antenatal clinic within 48 h of symptom onset

If seen within 72 h of onset of symptoms:

- Check that there are no ear vesicles, then start 2-week course of prednisolone 40 mg/day: taper after first week
- If ear vesicles seen, **do not use prednisolone**. Refer promptly to ENT
- If herpes infection suspected, **avoid prednisolone** or combine with aciclovir
- Reassure patient that 85–95% recover, though may take some months
- Refer for physiotherapy and eye care
- Vigilance for pre-eclampsia
- Early IOL or LSCS only for obstetric reasons, not for Bell's palsy per se

If seen after 72 h of onset of symptoms:

- Steroids of little benefit
- If ear vesicles seen, urgent referral to ENT
- If herpetic infection suspected, treat with aciclovir
- Reassure patient that 85–95% recover, though may take some months
- Refer for physiotherapy and eye care
- Vigilance for pre-eclampsia
- Early IOL or LSCS for obstetric reasons only, not for Bell's palsy per se

10.6 Myasthenia Gravis

FACT FILE

Aetiology and pathogenesis

- **Myasthenia gravis (MG)** is an autoimmune disorder affecting the neuromuscular junction, characterized by muscle fatigability and weakness.
- MG is caused by IgG antibodies directed against nicotinic acetylcholine receptors which leads to insufficient nerve impulse transmission to striated muscle fibres.[1,2,3]
- ***This results in weakness and fatigue of skeletal muscle, but not of smooth muscle.***
- MG is rare: 1 in 10 000 to 1 in 50 000. Female to male preponderance of 2:1.
- Onset is usually in second or third decades.

Clinical features

- There may be exacerbations and remissions.[2]
- Symptoms and signs include:
  - diplopia (double vision)
  - ptosis (droopy eyelids)
  - dysphagia
  - respiratory muscle weakness in severe cases.

Effect of pregnancy on MG

- MG patients can have normal pregnancy and delivery but the course is unpredictable.
- About 40% of patients have an exacerbation during pregnancy, in 30% remissions occur, and there is no change in the remainder.[3]
- Exacerbations can occur at any stage of pregnancy but are mostly seen in the first trimester and in the first month postpartum.[4,5] An improvement is seen in 20–40% of women in the second and third trimesters of pregnancy,[4] coinciding with the physiological relative immunosuppression which normally takes place during this stage of gestation.
- With reactivation of normal immune response at the time of delivery and in puerperium, an exacerbation and deterioration of MG are more likely peripartum.
- Postpartum exacerbation occurs in 30% of women and this may require higher doses of medications.
- One pregnancy can vary from the next. The clinical course of MG in a first pregnancy does not predict the symptoms and outcomes of subsequent pregnancies.[6]
- Exacerbations are less likely if the woman has undergone previous thymectomy.
- Physiological changes of pregnancy (e.g. hyperemesis, delayed gastric emptying, increased volume of drug distribution, and renal clearance) may all lead to subtherapeutic levels of medication.
- Pregnant women with MG can get more tired simply because of the extra weight carried, changing centre of gravity, and extra strains on some muscles.
- There are no definite predictive factors that identify the mother at risk for peripartum exacerbation of MG or the infant at risk for neonatal MG. It has been suggested that a shorter disease history and the occurrence of infections may predispose to puerperal exacerbation.[1]
- Pregnancy does not worsen the long-term prognosis of MG.[6,7,8]
- Maximum maternal morbidity seen in MG is inversely related to the duration of the disease, highest in the first year and lowest after 7 years of the disease.[9]
- Thymectomy, outside of pregnancy, is the primary disease-controlling measure.[10]
- Exacerbations are seen less commonly in those who have had previous thymectomy than in those who have not. There is no difference in the incidence of neonatal MG in either group; therefore thymectomy, if not already performed pre-pregnancy, can be postponed to after childbirth.

Effect of MG on pregnancy

- ***The course of MG in pregnancy as well as its influence on pregnancy outcomes can be variable.***
- There is a high incidence of preterm rupture of membranes, preterm delivery, and growth restriction (40%).[3,7,8] There is no increased risk of miscarriage.
- In MG, maternal antibodies directed against nicotinic acetylcholine receptors. These antibodies belong to the IgG immunoglobulin group which may cross the placenta and cause transitory neonatal MG.
- Transplacental passage of antibodies may rarely cause **neonatal arthrogryposis multiplex congenita**—a syndrome of non-progressive congenital contractures resulting from lack of fetal movements in utero (fetal dyskinesia).[11]
- More commonly, transient signs of myasthenia are seen in the neonate (10–30%).
- The first stage of labour is unaffected by MG. Maternal effort using voluntary striated muscles that is required in the active phase of the second stage may be impaired. Assisted instrumental assistance for delivery may be required.

Management in pregnancy

- Pre-pregnancy assessment and advice based on the severity of the disease is essential.
- Pre-pregnancy advice should include discussions about possible fetal and maternal risks.
- Optimal pregnancy care in women is achieved with a multidisciplinary team approach involving the obstetrician, neurologist, anaesthetist, midwife, and paediatrician.
- There is no change in the medical management of MG during pregnancy compared with pre-pregnancy except that certain immunosuppressants such as methotrexate, ciclosporin, cyclophosphamide, or mycophenolate mofetil are contraindicated in pregnancy and breastfeeding and need to be stopped before pregnancy.
- **Long-acting anticholinesterase drugs like pyridostigmine** used to treat MG should be continued in pregnancy.
  - Increased doses may be required as pregnancy advances. This may be more appropriately achieved by decreasing the dosage interval rather than simply increasing each dose.
  - Anticholinesterases should be given parenterally during labour to avoid erratic absorption due to delayed gastric emptying.
  - Overdose of anticholinesterase drugs may result in paraesthesia, weakness, and respiratory failure.
- Azathioprine can be used safely during pregnancy with vigilance for fetal growth restriction.
- Referral to the anaesthetic high-risk clinic before 24 weeks gestation is highly advisable.

Fetal monitoring

- Serial growth scans must be arranged from 26–28 weeks onwards at frequencies according to the individual unit's policy regarding serial growth scans.
- A biophysical profile at weekly intervals from 34 weeks may be required if decreased fetal movements are reported. The rare condition of arthrogryposis congenita or fetal dyskinesia can manifest by a reduction in fetal body and breathing movements and associated hydramnios.[10]

Labour and delivery

- Pregnancy can lead to exacerbation of maternal respiratory problems, particularly hypoventilation, especially in late pregnancy. Respiratory crisis is a serious emergency and warrants immediate multidisciplinary measures.[8]

- Vaginal delivery should be the aim, although assisted instrumental vaginal delivery is often required to prevent the woman from becoming exhausted.
- Early induction of labour or Caesarean section for obstetric indications only.

Analgesia and use of other drugs in MG

Analgesia and use of other drugs in MG need careful consideration.[12]

- Epidural and spinal are safe.
- Local anaesthetics like lidocaine and those of the amide type are safe for labour and delivery
- **Local anaesthetics of the ester type (e.g. chloroprocaine, tetracaine) should not be used** if the mother is on anticholinesterases.
- If inhalational anaesthesia is used, **ether and halothane should be avoided. Suxamethonium and curare** may have an exaggerated or prolonged effect.
- Other drugs such as **gentamicin (aminoglycoside), ritodrine, salbutamol (beta-adrenergics), and narcotics (pethidine, morphine)** may exacerbate MG and are best avoided.
- ***Magnesium sulfate should not be used in patients with MG as it may precipitate a crisis.***
- **Diazepam (benzodiazepine) should instead be used for eclampsia control.** Clear documentation to this effect needs to be made antenatally irrespective of whether the pre-eclampsia is mild, moderate, or severe.

Postpartum

- MG can worsen after delivery.
- It is important to avoid infections.

Breastfeeding

- Breastfeeding is not contraindicated if the mother is on low–medium doses of steroids or azathioprine.
- It is probably advisable to avoid breastfeeding if high doses of prednisolone are needed for maternal MG control (e.g. >40 mg prednisolone daily, or 80 mg on alternate days).
- Breastfeeding is not advisable if any other immunosuppressant (e.g. methotrexate, ciclosporin, cyclophosphamide, or mycophenolate mofetil) is used for maternal symptom control.
- If the baby shows signs of neonatal MG, the patient must be advised **not** to breastfeed as the baby might have poor sucking and/or impaired swallowing.

Neonatal MG

- 12–20% of neonates born to myasthenic mothers may be affected by transient neonatal myasthenia due to transplacental passage of IgG antibodies.[13]
- Neuromuscular symptoms usually manifest within the first 12–48 h postpartum. Close monitoring of the neonate is therefore essential.
- There is little correlation in general between severity of maternal MG and occurrence of neonatal MG.[8]
- Mothers must be informed that though their MG may have been stable during pregnancy, there is still a 1 in 5 to 1 in 10 chance that the baby may show signs of transient neonatal MG.
- Antenatal referral to neonatologist and ensuring the presence of a paediatrician at delivery are recommended.
- Vigilance for neonatal MG to detect characteristic signs (e.g. difficulty in feeding, floppiness, weak cry, poor sucking, or breathing problems).
- Neonatal MG is transient and resolves within 4–8 weeks, which corresponds to the disappearance of maternal antibodies from the baby
- Neonatal MG responds to anticholinesterases given to the baby.
- Pyridostigmine (Mestinon) is usually given to the baby just before a feed. Tube feeding, suction of mouth/throat fluids or respiratory assistance, or treatment with IVIG or plasmapheresis are only rarely required.

Information for patients

Please see Information for patients: Myasthenia gravis and pregnancy (p. 520)

References

1. Djelmis J, et al. Myasthenia gravis in pregnancy: report on 69 cases. Eur J Obstet Gynecol Reprod Biol 2002;104: 21–25.
2. Nelson-Piercy C. Myasthenia gravis. In: Handbook of obstetric medicine, 4th ed. London: Informa Healthcare, 2010, pp. 163–166.
3. Plauche WC. Myasthenia gravis. Clin Obstet Gynecol 1983;26: 592–604.
4. Mitchell PJ, Bebbington M. Myasthenia gravis in pregnancy. Obstet Gynecol 1992;80: 178–181.
5. Plauche WC. Myasthenia gravis in mothers and their newborns. Clin Obstet Gynecol 1991;34: 82–99.
6. Batocchi AP, et al. Course and treatment of myasthenia gravis during pregnancy. Neurology 1999;52: 447–452.
7. Hoff JM, et al. Myasthenia gravis: consequences for pregnancy, delivery, and the newborn. Neurology 2003;61: 1362–1366.
8. Berlit S, et al. Myasthenia gravis in pregnancy: a case report. Case Rep Obstet Gynecol 2012;2012: 36024.
9. Scott JS. Immunological diseases in pregnancy Scott JS. Immunologic diseases in pregnancy. Prog Allergy 1977;23: 371–375.
10. Gronseth GS, Barohn RJ. Thymectomy for autoimmune myasthenia gravis: an evidence-based review. Neurology 2000;55: 7–15.
11. Stoll C., et al. Prenatal diagnosis of congenital myasthenia with arthrogryposis in a myasthenic mother. Prenat Diagn 1991;11: 17–22.
12. Almeida C, et al. Myasthenia gravis and pregnancy: anaesthetic management—a series of cases. Eur J Anaesthesiol 2010;27: 985–990.
13. Morel E, et al. Neonatal myasthenia gravis: a new clinical and immunologic appraisal on 30 cases. Neurology 1988;38: 138–142.

CARE PATHWAY

GP or community midwife refers patient with **myasthenia gravis (MG)** to maternal medicine or specialist antenatal clinic early in 1st trimester

↓

First visit to maternal medicine or specialist antenatal clinic

- Check what medication(s) patient is on
- Remind patient that anticholinesterase inhibitors can continue to be used safely in pregnancy. If she is on pyridostigmine or azathioprine these should be continued throughout pregnancy
- Check symptom control, history of pre-pregnancy or early pregnancy exacerbations
- Refer to neurologist, offer contact number for neurology nurse helpline
- Refer to senior anaesthetist in high-risk anaesthetic clinic
- Arrange for serial growth scans from approx. 26–28 weeks onwards (28, 32, and 36 weeks or according to individual unit's policy)
- Reassure patient that outcome of pregnancy good in most cases for both mother and baby
- Reassure patient that pregnancy does not affect the long-term course or prognosis of MG
- Discuss small increase in risk of preterm labour, PPROM, fetal akinesia, IUGR, etc.; recognition of symptoms of any such complications
- Discuss unpredictable course of MG in pregnancy, exacerbation in 40%, remission in 30%, and no change in 30%
- Exacerbations most common in 1st trimester or in first month postpartum—increased dosage of medication may be required
- Discuss plan of management of pregnancy including advice regarding prompt treatment of any infection that may otherwise exacerbate MG symptoms, 1 in 5–10 chance of transient neonatal MG, etc.
- If on prednisolone for symptoms control, document need for hydrocortisone bolus doses 100 mg IV for labour and delivery
- Continue routine community antenatal checks according to NICE low-risk schedule, avoiding overlap with hospital appointments

↓

Further visits to maternal medicine or specialist antenatal clinic

At about 28, 32, 36, and 38 weeks gestation:

- Review pregnancy, maternal symptoms, scan biometry and fetal movements
- Vigilance for pre-eclampsia, IUGR
- Biophysical profile may be required if patient reports reduced fetal movements
- Ensure patient has had anaesthetic and neurology review
- **Document in hand-held and main notes: 'Following drugs to be avoided: gentamicin, narcotics, magnesium sulfate, ritodrine, salbutamol, inhalational GA agents (e.g. ether, halothane), ester type of local anaesthetics (e.g. chloroprocaine)'**
- Document: that spinal/epidural are safe according to anaesthetic advice
- Inform neonatologist
- **Document in delivery and baby page of maternity notes:' Paediatrician to be present at delivery and close neonatal checks for possible transient neonatal MG'**

↓

Labour and delivery

- Aim for vaginal delivery
- **Caesarean section or early IOL for obstetric reasons only**
- **Document that assisted instrumental vaginal delivery usually required with ventouse or forceps to avoid maternal muscle fatigue during active second stage**
- If patient has required steroids for control of MG during pregnancy, prophylactic IM or IV hydrocortisone 100 mg 6–8 hourly to cover labour and vaginal delivery or Caesarean section
- Pyridostigmine to be given parenterally during labour to avoid erratic absorption

↓

Postpartum

- Advise regarding **breastfeeding** (see Fact File) on an individualized basis, weighing pros and cons, and depending on maternal medication, evidence of neonatal MG, etc.
- Warn about **puerperal exacerbation of MG (in 30%),** also chance of transient neonatal MG

10.7 Charcot–Marie–Tooth Disease

FACT FILE

Epidemiology

- **Charcot–Marie–Tooth disease (CMTD)** is one of the most common inherited neurological disorders, affecting approximately 1 in 2500 people.
- CMTD, also known as **hereditary motor and sensory neuropathy** or **peroneal muscular atrophy**, causes peripheral neuropathy as it affects peripheral nerves that supply the muscles and sensory organs in the limbs.
- People with most forms of CMTD have a normal life expectancy.
- The neuropathy of CMTD affects both motor and sensory nerves.

Symptoms and signs

- In CMTD, peripheral nerves gradually degenerate. This results in muscle weakness and atrophy in the extremities (arms, legs, hands, or feet), leading to weakness of the feet and lower leg muscles, scoliosis, foot drop, and a high-stepped gait with frequent trips and falls.
- In some cases, the degeneration involves sensory nerves, resulting in a reduced ability to feel heat, cold, and pain.
- The lower legs may acquire an **'inverted champagne bottle' appearance** due to the loss of muscle bulk.
- Later in the disease, weakness and atrophy may occur in the muscles of the hands and tongue, resulting respectively in difficulty in carrying out fine motor skills and in slurred speech and swallowing difficulties.
- In severe cases, respiratory muscles and vertebral anatomy can be affected, both of which may have significant impact on any planned or unplanned anaesthetic.
- Onset of symptoms is most often in adolescence or early adulthood, but in some individuals may not present till the fifth or sixth decade.
- The severity of symptoms varies greatly among individuals and even among family members with the disease.
- Pain is a feature and can range from mild to severe.
- Progression of symptoms is gradual.

Inheritance

- CMTD disease is usually inherited as autosomal dominant, sometimes as autosomal recessive, X-linked, or as a de-novo mutation.
- There are many forms of CMTD, including CMT1, CMT2, CMT3, CMT4, and CMTX.

Treatment

- There is no 'cure' for CMTD, but physiotherapy, braces, and other orthopaedic devices, and even orthopaedic surgery can help.
- Analgesia may be required.

Specific management in pregnancy

- **Genetic counselling is advisable**, given that most cases have an autosomal inheritance pattern.
- **Prenatal diagnosis** can be offered. chorionic villus sampling (CVS) or amniocentesis using fluorescent in situ hybridization can detect duplication of 17p12, which is found in the majority of type 1 CMTD (98%).[1]
- Most pregnancies proceed without problems. In those who have had early onset of symptoms and disabilities from childhood or early adolescence, an exacerbation of CMTD symptoms, especially increasing weakness, can occur during pregnancy.[2]
- Such exacerbations can be limited to the duration of pregnancy or persist long term.
- Exacerbations can recur in subsequent pregnancies. There is a 50% chance of such deterioration in at least one pregnancy in women who have had early-onset CMTD. If pain is a symptom, analgesics avoiding NSAIDs can be used.
- In contrast, in those whose CMTD symptomatology appeared only in adulthood, pregnancy does not seem to affect the course of the disease.[2]
- Physiotherapy involving muscle-strengthening exercises and muscle and ligament stretching can continue during pregnancy and no-impact exercises, such as swimming, are particularly recommended.
- No deleterious effects have been noted with fetal outcomes in women with CMTD.
- Multidisciplinary care must be available to these patients during pregnancy, involving the neurologist, specialist obstetrician, midwife, anaesthetist, geneticist, and physiotherapist.
- Referral during pregnancy to the high-risk anaesthetic clinic is strongly recommended in order for discussions regarding analgesia in labour and delivery.
- Severe scoliosis and respiratory compromise are major risks in severe cases and may have a significant impact on any planned or unplanned anaesthetic intervention.
- Timely assessment by a senior anaesthetist and a clear plan for analgesia during labour and delivery should be documented in the notes covering both planned and emergency situations. This must be widely communicated to all those involved in the patient's care.
- Malpresentations have been reported to be more common in women with CMTD.[3]
- There is a theoretical risk that the muscle relaxant succinylcholine could have a prolonged effect on some women with CMTD. This has not, however, been confirmed in other studies.[4] Regional block is safe as is the use of other muscle relaxants such as atracurium in the case of a general anaesthetic being required.
- In women with muscle weakness and fatigue, an epidural is advisable to provide analgesia during labour and to avoid the patient getting overtired by premature efforts at bearing down.
- Assisted vaginal instrumental delivery is more common in this group of parturients as muscle fatigue and exhaustion are common.
- Increased incidence of atonicity of the uterus and resulting postpartum haemorrhage (PPH) have also been reported[4] and **active management of the third stage is recommended. This must be documented in the notes.**
- There is no contraindication for breastfeeding.

Information for patients

Please see Information for patients: Charcot–Marie–Tooth disease and pregnancy (p. 521)

References

1. Kashork CD, et al. Prenatal diagnosis of Charcot-Marie-Tooth disease type1A by interphase fluorescence in situ hybridization Prenat Diagn 1999;19: 446–449.
2. Rudnik-Schoneborn S, et al. Pregnancy and delivery in Charcot-Marie-Tooth disease type 1. Neurology 1993;43: 2011–2016.
3. Hoff JM, et al. Pregnancies and deliveries in patients with Charcot-Marie-Tooth disease. Neurology 2005;64: 459–462.
4. Antognini JF. Anaesthesia for Charcot-Marie-Tooth disease: a review of 86 cases. Can J Anaesth 1992;39: 398–400.

GP or community midwife refers patient with **Charcot–Marie–Tooth disease (CMTD)** to maternal medicine or a specialist antenatal clinic in the first trimester

↓

First visit to maternal medicine clinic

- Detailed history, assess patient, confirm viability and dates
- Refer for genetic counselling if not previously offered
- Discuss prenatal diagnosis for CMTD, arrange if patient opts for this
- Refer to physiotherapist
- Refer to high-risk anaesthetic clinic
- Refer to neurologist if not reviewed within the last year and if symptoms have worsened
- Advise continued non-impact exercises, e.g. swimming
- Reassure that most pregnancies are uncomplicated in CMTD
- Continued antenatal checks with community midwife according to routine NICE low-risk schedule

↓

Further visits to maternal medicine clinic (e.g. 32 and 37 weeks)

- Enquire regarding symptomatology
- Confirm has had anaesthetic review, patient's view on epidural
- Confirm presentation at 37 weeks
- No indication for interventions such as early IOL or LSCS except for other obstetric indications
- ***Document in notes:***
  - Active management of third stage with high-dose syntocinon infusion in addition to initial bolus dose: atonic PPH to be anticipated
  - Epidural recommended, if patient willing
  - Avoid prolonged pushing by assisted vaginal instrumental delivery, if signs of muscle fatigue and maternal exhaustion

↓

Postpartum

- Encourage breastfeeding

10.8 Muscular and Myotonic Dystrophy

FACT FILE

- 'Muscle disease' is a term which includes primary disorders of muscle and the neuromuscular junction
- The primary symptom for most muscle dystrophies is muscle weakness, while some dystrophies can also cause heart disease or mental impairment. The type of symptoms and the pattern of the genetic abnormality differentiates the various muscle dystrophies
- With advances in molecular genetics, significant changes have taken place in gene localization, screening techniques, and therefore genetic counselling.
- Any patient suspected of having a genetic muscle disease should be referred to a neuromuscular physician and for prenatal genetic counselling.

Muscular dystrophy

- Muscular dystrophy is an inherited disorder that causes progressive muscle weakness and atrophy. Several forms of inherited muscular dystrophy have been described. All are progressive diseases caused by defects in one or more genes (some of which have been identified) that are required for normal muscle function.
- The **most common forms** of muscular dystrophy include:
  - Duchenne and Becker muscular dystrophy
  - Emery–Dreifuss muscular dystrophy
  - myotonic dystrophy
  - limb-girdle muscular dystrophy
  - facioscapulohumeral muscular dystrophy (FSHD)
  - congenital muscular dystrophy.

Inheritance

- Most often as an **autosomal dominant trait** (myotonic dystrophy, facioscapulohumeral dystrophy, oculopharyngeal dystrophy) where one parent passes on the defective gene.
- Some are **autosomal recessive** (limb-girdle muscular dystrophy, congenital muscular dystrophy) where both the mother and father pass a defective chromosome to their infant.
- Some are **X-linked recessive** (e.g. Duchenne and Becker muscular dystrophy, Emery–Driefuss muscular dystrophy) where mutations are found on one of the X chromosomes carried by the mother. These muscular dystrophies will affect 50% of all male infants of mothers who carry the genetic defect. Female progeny who inherit their mother's defective X chromosome (carrier females) are usually not significantly affected, although mild symptoms can occasionally occur.
- Chromosomal loci have been identified for these muscular dystrophies although at present accurate and relatively simple gene testing is available only for some (e.g. Duchenne and Becker dystrophy).

Diagnosis

- Diagnostic tools include genetic testing, blood tests (e.g. for creatinine kinase) that can identify the signs of muscle damage, electromyography (EMG), muscle biopsy, electrocardiogram (ECG), and/or echocardiogram (ECHO). Diagnostic tests should be based on the clinical presentation and the type of disease suspected.
- In most cases, muscle dystrophies will have been diagnosed before a pregnancy.

Myotonic dystrophy

- Myotonic dystrophy is a clinically and genetically heterogeneous disorder with two major forms: type 1 and a milder form, type 2. The abnormal gene which codes for myotonin is localized to chromosome 19.
- Life expectancy appears to be reduced in myotonic dystrophy, with respiratory and cardiac diseases being the most common causes of death.
- The prevalence is 1 in 8000 in the general population. Symptoms typically occur in adolescence or adulthood, although a neonatal form does occur.
- Myotonic dystrophies are autosomal dominant conditions that are among the most common forms of adult-onset muscular dystrophy, especially of the facial muscles, arms, and legs.
- Myotonia, muscle wasting, and weakness can become symptomatic or dramatically worsen during pregnancy: usually, but not exclusively, this occurs during the third trimester.[1,2,3] The worsened clinical state is temporary, and return to baseline is usual after delivery.
- Myotonic dystrophies can cause smooth-muscle weakness of the oesophagus, stomach, bowel, and the **uterine myometrium**. Apart from muscle weakness especially of the facial muscles, arms, and legs, myotonic dystrophies can also display multisystem manifestations such as cataracts, cardiac conduction abnormalities, dysphagia, infertility, insulin resistance, and even severe developmental delay. Excessive daytime sleepiness is found in about one-third of patients with myotonic dystrophy.
- In myotonic dystrophy, complications in pregnancy can have significant effects on both the mother and fetus/neonate.[1,3,4,5,6,7,8]
  - ***Dystrophy of uterine myometrium can cause problems such as miscarriages, polyhydramnios, preterm birth, protracted labour, and atonic postpartum haemorrhage (PPH).***[9,10,11,12]
  - Atonic PPH is due to failure of sustained uterine contraction after delivery. Labour can be prolonged in both the first stage because of poor uterine contraction from myometrial involvement[3,7] and in the second stage due to poor bearing-down efforts because of voluntary muscle weakness.
- Extended bed rest should be avoided because disuse of muscles will further weaken any patient with myotonic dystrophy.
- General anaesthetics have special risks in patients with myotonic dystrophy as depolarizing neuromuscular blocking agents, such as succinylcholine, can cause myotonic spasm[10,11,12] in which muscles contract and cannot be relaxed. This is temporary and without permanent sequelae; however, it may be impossible to ventilate the patient during the spasm.
- 50% of children of an affected parent may have the disease; 20% of them are asymptomatic at birth. Fetal involvement may be manifested by polyhydramnios,[6] arthrogryposis multiplex in utero, hydrops fetalis, etc.
- Severely affected newborns have a recognizable disorder unrelated to the severity of the maternal disease. The affected neonate may display severe hypotonia, floppiness at birth, and respiratory distress. The clinical diagnosis can be confirmed by direct DNA analysis in serum.
- Prenatal diagnosis is possible from CVS. Preimplantation genetic diagnosis for myotonic dystrophy type 1 is also available in the UK.[13]

Duchenne muscular dystrophy

- Duchenne muscular dystrophy (DMD) is caused by a defective dystrophin gene located on the X chromosome. A protein called dystrophin normally functions to protect muscle fibres and when the gene responsible for producing it is defective, muscles are broken down by enzymes thereby causing dystrophy.
- DMD occurs in 1 in 3500 of all males. It is mainly inherited as a X-linked recessive condition although up to a third can occur as de-novo mutations.[13] It is a condition primarily seen in boys, and occurs in all ethnic groups.
- On average, affected boys develop symptoms for DMD at around 5 years of age, become wheelchair bound by about age 10–12, and die by their early 20s.[14] Survival appears to be improving with advances in gene therapies in respiratory and cardiac care.[15] Individuals may develop symptoms earlier or later in life.
- **Becker dystrophy** is milder than DMD, with the same milestones reached about a decade later.

- Weakness starts near the trunk, and spreads to the extremities, affecting the legs before the arms. A child may have difficulty running, jumping, and walking up steps, and may use their hands to push upright from squatting or sitting (Gower's sign).
- DMD may also cause dilated cardiomyopathy, arrhythmias, and scoliosis. Fractures, caused by falling over, are common
- Most female DMD carriers have few or no symptoms. Mild muscle weakness may develop in a small proportion.
- Because of the devastating effect of DMD and the lack of a cure, any woman with a family history of muscular dystrophy should be offered pre-pregnancy genetic counselling to discuss carrier status detection and the probability of having an affected child.
- In families with such dystrophies, prenatal diagnosis of an affected fetus and preimplantation genetic diagnosis are available and must be offered.[16]

Congenital myotonic dystrophy

- Congenital muscular dystrophy (CMD) refers to cases of muscular dystrophy that display symptoms that are apparent at birth.[17]
- Symptoms of CMD are usually seen at birth, and include lack of muscle strength ('floppy baby') and multiple joint contractures (arthrogryposis). No definitive treatment is available for CMD.
- CMD occurs only when the mother is the affected parent and can present in utero, at birth, or in early childhood.[17]
- The risk of an affected woman having a congenitally affected child is 10%, but this risk increases to about 40% if she has already had a congenitally affected offspring.[17]
- It appears that the older the mother, the greater the severity of the offspring's disease.
- ***Congenital myotonic dystrophy can be associated with polyhydramnios and reduced fetal movements and arthrogryposis multiplex congenita at birth.***[18]
- Neonatal onset of myotonic dystrophy is frequently fatal as a result of respiratory failure. In any neonate with respiratory failure and poor feeding, CMD must be suspected, especially as the condition may not yet have been diagnosed in the mother.[18]
- Affected children without the fetal or neonatal presentation can display signs such as talipes, developmental delay, mental retardation, facial diplegia, weakness,[18] clumsiness, or dysarthria.
- Prenatal testing is possible with CVS or amniocentesis.[19]

Limb-girdle muscular dystrophy

- Limb-girdle muscular dystrophy (LGMD) includes a group of autosomal recessive disorders that have a slow progressive effect on the shoulder or the pelvic girdle, or both.[20,21]
- Type 2A LGMD is the most common and is characterized by symmetrical proximal dystrophy with no facial muscle disturbance.
- Elevated creatinine kinase and features of myopathy may provide a clue to the diagnosis, which is usually confirmed by muscle biopsy or by genetic testing.[20]
- The age of onset of LGMD varies from early childhood to adulthood although it usually manifests in the first or second decade of life,[20,21] progressing steadily to loss of independent movement without 10 years. This is worsened by pregnancy-related changes in weightbearing.
- Low back pain may be a prominent symptom, and severe pelvic girdle and trunk weakness may be associated with restrictive respiratory impairment, hypoventilation, and pulmonary hypertension.
- Caesarean section under regional anaesthetic or assisted vaginal delivery is generally required, although successful spontaneous unassisted vaginal delivery has been reported.[22,23]
- General anaesthetic agents such as suxamethonium and volatile gases may cause life-threatening complications such as malignant hyperthermia, postoperative atelectasis, and chest infections.[24]
- Cognitive function is usually normal, although cardiac involvement may occur in certain forms of LGMD.
- Treatment of LGMD involves prevention of contractures. Stretching exercises and calf tendon release by surgery are often recommended.

Information for patients

Please see **Information for patients: Muscular dystrophy and pregnancy** (p. 521)

References

1. Norwooda F, Rudnik-Schönebornb S 179th ENMC international workshop: Pregnancy in women with neuromuscular disorders, 5–7 November 2010, Naarden, The Netherlands. Neuromusc Disord 2012;22: 183–190.
2. Awater C, et al. Pregnancy course and outcome in women with hereditary neuromuscular disorders: comparison of obstetric risks in 178 patients. Eur J Obstet Gynecol Reprod Biol 2012;162: 153–159.
3. Jaffe R, et al. Myotonic dystrophy and pregnancy: a review. Obstet Gynecol Surv 1986;41: 272–278.
4. O'Brien TA, Harper PS Reproductive problems and neonatal loss in women with myotonic dystrophy. J Obstet Gynecol 1984;4: 170–173.
5. Rudnik-Schöneborn S, Zerres K Outcome in pregnancies complicated by myotonic dystrophy: a study of 31 patients and review of the literature. Eur J Obstet Gynecol Reprod Biol 2004;114: 44–45.
6. Esplin MS, et al. Myotonic dystrophy is a significant cause of idiopathic polyhydramnios. Am J Obstet Gynecol 1998;179: 974–977.
7. Webb D, et al. Myotonia dystrophica: obstetric complications. Am J Obstet Gynecol 1978;132: 265–270.
8. Argov Z, de Visser M What we do not know about pregnancy in hereditary neuromuscular disorders: review article. Neuromusc Disord 2009;19: 675–679.
9. Cope I Myotonic dystrophy and pregnancy. Aust N Z J Obstet Gynaecol 1981;21: 240–241.
10. Yun EM, et al. Neurologic and muscular diseases. In:Datta S, ed., Anesthetic and obstetric management of high-risk pregnancy 2nd edn. St. Louis: Mosby 1996.
11. Kumar R, Hirsch NP Neuromuscular disorders: relevance to anaesthesia and intensive care. Review article. Anesth Intens Care Med 2011;12: 229–232.
12. Bader AM Neurologic and neuromuscular disease in the obstetric patient. Anesth Clin N Am 1998;16: 459–476.
13. Kakouroua G, et al. Preimplantation genetic diagnosis for myotonic dystrophy type 1 in the UK. Neuromusc Disord 2008;18: 131–136.
14. Sussman M Duchenne muscular dystrophy . J Am Acad Orthop Surg 2002;10: 138–151.
15. Fairclough RJ, et al. Progress in therapy for Duchenne muscular dystrophy. Exp Physiol 2011;96: 1101–1113.
16. Malcov M, et al. Preimplantation genetic diagnosis (PGD) for Duchenne muscular dystrophy (DMD) by triplex-nested PCR. Prenat Diagn 2005;25: 1200–1205.
17. Koch MC, et al. Genetic risks for children of women with myotonic dystrophy. Am J Hum Genet 1991;48: 1084–1091.
18. Campbell C Congenital myotonic dystrophy. J Neurol Neurophysiol 2012, S7.
19. Martorell L, et al. Prenatal diagnosis in myotonic dystrophy type 1. Thirteen years of experience: implications for reproductive counselling in DM1 families. Prenat Diagn 2007;27: 68–72.
20. Bushby K Diagnosis and management of the limb girdle muscular dystrophies . Pract Neurol 2009;9: 314–323.
21. Zatz M, et al. The 10 autosomal recessive limb-girdle muscular dystrophies. Neuromusc Disord 2003;9: 314–323.
22. Black C, Said J Normal vaginal delivery in a patient with autosomal recessive limb-girdle muscular dystrophy. Obstet Med 2010;3: 81–82.
23. Ayoubi J, et al . Vaginal delivery in a woman with limb-girdle muscular dystrophy: a case report. Reprod Med 2000;45: 498–500.
24. Allen T, Maguire S Anaesthetic management of a woman with autosomal recessive limb-girdle muscular dystrophy for emergency caesarean section. Int J Obstetr Anaesth 2007;16: 370–374.

11 Maternal Uterine, Cervical, and Vulvovaginal Conditions

11.1 Previous Excisional Treatment of Cervix

FACT FILE

- Cervical cancer is caused by human papillomavirus (HPV) infection and is a leading cause of death from cancer in women.
- **Cervical intraepithelial neoplasia (CIN)** represents early cellular changes of the cervical epithelium.
- Premalignant cervical lesions found on screening are often treated with **excision or ablation**.
- **Most women with high-grade CIN are of the reproductive age group,**[1,2] therefore the treatment they receive is most likely to have an impact on subsequent pregnancy outcomes.
- ***Excision techniques:***
  - cold knife conization (knife cone biopsy)
  - laser conization
  - large loop excision of transformation zone (LLETZ).
- ***Ablative techniques:***
  - laser ablation
  - cryotherapy.
- CIN itself can slightly increase the risk of preterm delivery even without treatment.[3]
- All excisional treatments are associated with an increased risk of preterm premature rupture of membranes and/or preterm delivery.[4,5]
- A large meta-analysis has demonstrated a relative risk of 2.61 for preterm delivery with a core depth of cone specimen greater than 10 mm (95% CI).[5]
- A LLETZ with removal of no more than 10 mm depth of cervix is safer than knife cone biopsy.
- The more cervical tissue is excised, as in knife cone biopsy, the greater the risk of adverse pregnancy outcomes such as preterm premature rupture of membranes (PPROM), late miscarriage, preterm birth, small for gestational age, neonatal death due to extreme prematurity, or extremely low birth weight.
- Depth of conization and the **volume of cervical tissue removed** have been evaluated as risk factors for adverse pregnancy outcome and infertility. The proportion of the **total cervical volume** or endocervical canal removed has been shown in some studies to be more important than the actual depth of excision.[6]
- These risks are significantly increased if the patient has had more than one cervical excisional procedure, e.g. cone biopsy plus LLETZ or two LLETZ or two cone biopsies.
- When less cervical tissue is removed, as in LLETZ, the risks are reduced in comparable to those associated with ablative techniques.
- **Ablative techniques** such as laser ablation or cold coagulation (cryotherapy) are associated with fewer adverse pregnancy outcomes than excisional treatments.[5,7]
- Gynaecologists are increasingly using LLETZ no deeper than 10 mm, and cold coagulation techniques in younger women with CIN to minimize possible adverse obstetric outcomes in subsequent pregnancies.[1]
- The timing of pregnancy following cervical excisional procedure is also important in considering outcomes. **The shorter this interval the greater the incidence of subsequent PPROM, mid-trimester pregnancy loss, and preterm delivery**.[8]
- Women of reproductive age who need to have a conization procedure or LLETZ should be advised that conceiving within 2–3 months of the procedure may be associated with an increased risk of preterm birth.[9]
- ***Women who have had either knife cone biopsy or deep LLETZ (>10 mm depth of cervix excised) need greater surveillance during subsequent pregnancy following the procedure.***

Antenatal management

- At the time of booking in the community, specific query about any excisional procedure or cone biopsy or laser treatment of the cervix must be made. If such a history is obtained, the pregnant woman must be referred to a specialist obstetric clinic before 13 weeks pregnancy.
- The details of the type of cervical procedure and the depth of cervix excised needs to be established as the first step of further antenatal care planning. **Every effort must be made to get the details of the previous histology report which will contain the specific depth of the excised cervical tissue**.
- If the patient has had a shallow LLETZ (<10 mm depth) she must be reassured that she does not have a significantly increased risk compared with someone who has not had a cervical excisional biopsy for pregnancy complications such as PPROM, miscarriage due to cervical incompetence, or preterm birth, provided there has been a reasonable interval between the cervical excision and conception.
- If there are no other high-risk factors, she can remain under midwifery-led care during the pregnancy.
- **Only if the patient has had a deeper LLETZ (>10 mm depth) or a knife cone biopsy** does she need to continue hospital-based specialist antenatal care, shared however, with primary care.
- Serial cervical length scans may then be considered in such cases at approximately 14–16 weeks gestation, repeated at 19–20 weeks and the third at 22–24 weeks.
- If signs of full-length cervical canal funnelling or progressive pathological shortening of the cervix to 2.5 cm or less are identified in any of these scans, this should prompt clinical examination of the cervix to assess possible incompetence and further management.[7]
- This might involve elective or emergency cervical cerclage or in some centres insertion of the Arabin cervical pessary.[10,11] The cervical cerclage or pessary needs to be removed at 37 weeks gestation.
- Prophylactic cervical cerclage might be required as early as 14–15 weeks in those who have had more than one cervical excisional procedure and have been left with a very short cervix as identified in a follow-up colposcopy check even before the pregnancy
- Progesterone 400 mg od vaginal or rectal pessaries/suppositories may also be used[9,12] in addition to cervical cerclage, if the cervix shows pathological shortening (≥2.5 cm). Progesterone can be safely continued for several weeks and it is usual to stop this at about 35–36 weeks gestation.
- Infrequently, the previous cervical procedure could leave a fibrosed and stenosed[9,13,14] cervix which fails to dilate in labour. This is an indication for emergency Caesarean section.

Information for patients

Please see **Information for patients: Pregnancy following any cervical surgical procedure (excision biopsy, laser, cone, loop, etc.)** (p. 522)

References

1. Simoens C, et al. Adverse obstetrical outcomes after treatment of precancerous cervical lesions: a Belgian multicentre study. BJOG 2012;119: 1247–1255.
2. Arbyn M, et al. Analysis of 13 million patient records pertaining to Pap smears, colposcopies, biopsies and surgery on the uterine cervix (Belgium 1996-2000). Prev Med 2009;48: 438–443.
3. Albrechtsen S, et al. Pregnancy outcome in women before and after cervical conisation: population based cohort study. BMJ 2008;337: 803–805.
4. Editorial: adverse pregnancy outcomes after treatment for cervical intraepithelial neoplasia. BMJ 2008;337: 769–770
5. Arbyn M, et al. Perinatal mortality and other severe adverse pregnancy outcomes associated with treatment of cervical intraepithelial neoplasia: meta-analysis. BMJ 2008;337: 798–803.
6. Khalid S, et al. Risk of premature labor after LLETZ: does size matter? Paper presented at: British Society for Colposcopy and Cervical Pathology Annual Meeting 2009, Dublin, Ireland.
7. Kyrgiou M, et al. Obstetric outcomes after conservative treatment for intra-epithelial or early invasive cervical lesions: a systematic review and meta-analysis of the literature. Lancet 2006;367: 489–498.
8. Himes KP, Simhan HN. Time from cervical conization to pregnancy and preterm birth. Obstet Gynecol 2007;109: 314–319.
9. Chase DM, et al. Fertility and pregnancy after cervical procedures: the challenge of achieving good outcomes. Sex Reprod Menopause 2011;9: 1–9.
10. Sieroszewski P, et al. The Arabin pessary for the treatment of threatened mid-trimester miscarriage or premature labour and miscarriage: a case series. J Matern Fetal Neonatal Med 2009;22: 469–472.
11. Goya M, et al. on behalf of the Pesario Cervical para Evitar Prematuridad (PECEP) Trial Group. Cervical pessary in pregnant women with a short cervix (PECEP): an open-label randomised controlled trial. Lancet 2012;379: 1800–1806.
12. Jolley JA, Wing DA. Pregnancy management after cervical surgery. Curr Opin Obstet Gynecol. 2008;20 (6): 528–533
13. Baldauf JJ, et al. Risk of cervical stenosis after large loop excision or laser conization. Obstet Gynecol 1996;88: 933–938.
14. Santos C, et al. One-session management of cervical intraepithelial neoplasia: a solution for developing countries. A prospective, randomized trial of LEEP versus laser excisional conization. Gynecol Oncol 1996;61: 11–15.

CARE PATHWAY

If this is the woman's first pregnancy following any cervical procedure such as **laser treatment for pre-cancer cells**, or **cone biopsy**, **LLETZ**, or **laser biopsy**, the community midwife obtains a history at the booking visit

↓

Referral to specialist antenatal clinic before 13 weeks of pregnancy

- Confirm viability of pregnancy. Explain reason for antenatal clinic visit due to possible effects of previous cervical procedure affecting pregnancy outcomes
- Obtain details of type of cervical procedure performed from hospital notes/request details
- If previous cervical excisional procedure, obtain details from histology report of maximal depth of cervix excised by cone biopsy or LLETZ procedure. Details to be requested from another hospital if procedure performed there

↓ (left branch)

LLETZ/cone biopsy ≤10 mm cervical depth or cold coagulation (cryotherapy) of cervix-reassure patient.

↓

Routine midwifery-led care according to NICE guidelines for low-risk women

↓ (right branch)

Deep LLETZ (>10 mm cervical depth) or knife cone biopsy with depth >10 mm

↓

- Discuss increased risks of preterm labour, late miscarriage, PPROM, SGA
- Inform patient about warning signs to be aware of
- Arrange 3 cervical length serial scans at 14–16 weeks, repeat at 20 and 23–24 weeks. Explain that these might be TVS scans
- Consider progesterone 400 mg PV or PR daily from about 14–16 weeks to 35–36 weeks gestation

↓

- If abnormal shortening of ≤ 2.5 cm with cervical canal funnelling: Speculum examination ± VE to assess cervix, explain scan and clinical findings
- Discuss cervical cerclage (and Arabin pessary, if available as in some units), pros and cons and rate of effectiveness in well selected cases.
- Arabin pessary (perforated variety) can be inserted in antenatal clinic on the same day after due explanation-to expect increased vaginal discharge (non-infective, perforations in pessary rim will allow spontaneous drainage)
- For cervical cerclage, book for theatre asap, explain spinal anaesthetic, procedure, and post-op stay of 24 h
- Discuss and document risks including inadvertent rupture of membranes, miscarriage, cervical trauma, infection, and success rates of cervical cerclage procedure
- Explain suture removal at 37 weeks, earlier as emergency if PPROM/preterm contractions
- Progesterone self-insertion PR or PV, 400 mg od from 14–16 weeks and continued till 35–36 weeks

↓

- Further ANC visits at about 24, 30 and, 36/37 weeks gestation
- Assess pregnancy , symptomatology if any.
- Cyclogest can be stopped at about 35-36 weeks
- Serial growth scans if any suspicion of IUGR
- Arrange cervical suture removal in Delivery Suite at 37 weeks.
- Cervical ARABIN pessary can be removed in antenatal clinic
- If all well, give date for routine post-dates IOL at 40^{+10} (or as per individual unit's post-dates IOL policy)

11.2 Previous Radical Trachelectomy

FACT FILE

- CIN is commonly diagnosed in women of childbearing age.
- Over the past decade or so, treatment for early cervical cancer has evolved with a greater focus on fertility preservation without compromising overall survival.[1]
- **Trachelectomy** is a safe and feasible fertility-retaining surgical procedure, intended to preserve the uterus in women who wish to become pregnant in future.[2,3,4]
- Trachelectomy can be either:
  - **simple**, involving a supravaginal amputation of the cervix, or
  - **radical**, involving removal of the cervix along with the parametrium and vaginal cuff. Radical trachelectomy is recommended for stage 1b1 cervical cancer.
- Radical trachelectomy has disease-free survival and overall cervical rates comparable to those of radical hysterectomy.[5]
- ***Prophylactic placement of transabdominal cervical cerclage can be performed at the time of the trachelectomy.***[3,6,7,8,9,10]
- Approximately 10% of those undergoing radical trachelectomy for fertility preservation will go on to require adjuvant radiation therapy to the pelvis, usually because positive lymph nodes are found on further pathology examination. Such adjuvant treatment usually leads to permanent sterility due to the effect on the ovaries and/or endometrial lining.[11]
- In those who have received adjuvant radiotherapy after radical trachelectomy, additional problems may arise during a subsequent pregnancy. These include poor vascularization and IUGR, abnormal placentation resulting in either abruption or abnormally adherent placenta, and postpartum haemorrhage (PPH). Radiation can also result in the myometrium being less elastic and able to stretch to accommodate the growing fetus, resulting in miscarriage or preterm labour.[11]
- Infertility (voluntary or involuntary) rates of 25–57% have been reported after radical trachelectomy. While some patients had fertility problems prior to radical trachelectomy, of those who attempted without success to conceive, absence of cervical mucus, cervical stenosis, subclinical salpingitis, and adhesions[7,12] may be contributory factors.
- Pregnancy rates following radical trachelectomy range between 41% and 79% and term deliveries are achieved in about a third of these.[1,12]
- Obstetric morbidity and pregnancy loss rates in pregnancies conceived after radical trachelectomy are mainly due to second-trimester miscarriages (10%), preterm delivery (20%), cervical incompetence, PPROM, and chorioamnionitis.[1]
- As radical trachelectomy involves amputation of the cervix below the cervical isthmus, pregnancy outcomes are worse than those after conization procedures of the cervix.[13]
- Overall, the preterm delivery rate (<37 weeks) is twice that of the general population.[12,14]
- Pregnancy after radical trachelectomy has been reported in about 400 cases worldwide.[1,12]
- **No standardized management protocols are available at present for the care of such pregnancies**, as highlighted in recent literature.[11,12,13,14]
- An attempt has been made to define certain empirical investigations and interventions for the antenatal management of such pregnancies in this fact file, extrapolated from experience with pregnancy management following deep cone or LLETZ procedures of the cervix.

Pre-pregnancy evaluation and counselling

- An interval of at least 6 months from radical trachelectomy to pregnancy is advisable.
- If the IVF route being taken, preferably avoid multiple-embryo transfers as preterm delivery rate is significantly higher with multiple pregnancies.
- Ascertain whether a transabdominal cervicoisthmic cerclage has been placed at time of radical trachelectomy.
- Discuss increased complication rates associated with such high-risk pregnancies including second-trimester pregnancy loss, preterm delivery, PPROM, and chorioamnionitis. Women who have had radical trachelectomy must be informed that the **term (>37 weeks) live birth rate is about 30–40%.**
- Discussions should include monitoring by transvaginal scans in the second trimester, consideration of progesterone during pregnancy, prophylactic antibiotics, and elective Caesarean section delivery.

Management options during pregnancy

- ***These pregnancies pose such challenges that multidisciplinary management and expertise are mandatory, with close networking between the gynaecological oncologist, reproductive medicine specialist, obstetrician specialized in high-risk pregnancies, midwife, and neonatologist.***
- **Serial transvaginal scans** from approximately 14 weeks gestation at 3–4-week intervals till about 24–26 weeks gestation to measure any residual cervical length.
  - Following trachelectomy, there is often insufficient cervical tissue to attempt vaginal cerclage.
  - Transabdominal cervicoisthmic cerclage is an option to be considered in early second trimester of pregnancy for the women after radical trachelectomy where there is insufficient cervical tissue for vaginal cerclage.[13]
- **Prevention of infection:** Loss of the protective mucus plug after radical trachelectomy may facilitate ascending infection leading to PPROM and chorioamnionitis. Prophylactic vaginal clindamycin cream may be considered for a 7-day application at about 16 weeks and repeated between 22–24 weeks.
- **Progesterone**: A significant reduction in the incidence of preterm delivery before 34 weeks in those with cervical shortening has been shown in a systematic meta- analysis with the use of intravaginal progesterone.[15] In practice, a daily self-inserted progesterone pessary (400 mg) is recommended from about 13 weeks onwards till 34 weeks.
- If preterm or term contractions, rupture of membranes, or an intrauterine death occur with a transabdominal cerclage in situ, urgent delivery by Caesarean section or hysterotomy must be performed. Similarly, if signs of ascending infection are detected during conservative management of PPROM, urgent laparotomy and Caesarean section or hysterotomy under antibiotic cover is indicated. Rupture of the uterus, catastrophic bleeding, or overwhelming sepsis could otherwise cause maternal mortality or severe morbidity.
- Randomized clinical trials are needed to confirm the efficacy of management strategies in pregnancies after radical trachelectomy including the role of cerclage, prophylactic antibiotics, and progesterone.

Information for patients

Please see Information for patients: Radical trachelectomy and pregnancy (p. 523)

References

1. Beiner ME, Covens A. Surgery Insight: radical vaginal trachelectomy as a method of fertility preservation for cervical cancer. Nature Clin Prac Oncology 2007;4: 353–361.
2. Plante M, et al. The vaginal radical trachelectomy: an update of a series of 125 cases and 106 pregnancies. Gynecol Oncol 2011;121: 290–297.
3. Roman LD. Pregnancy after radical vaginal trachelectomy: maybe not such a risky undertaking after all. Gynecol Oncol 2005; 98: 1–2.

4. Hertel H, et al. Radical vaginal trachelectomy (RVT) combined with laparoscopic pelvic lymphadenectomy: prospective multicenter study of 100 patients with early cervical cancer. Gynecol Oncol 2006;103: 506–511.
5. Rob L. Fertility-sparing surgery in patients with cervical cancer. Lancet Oncol 2011;12: 192–200.
6. Song J-E., et al. Successful term pregnancy after transabdominal cerclage with previous second trimester loss following vaginal radical trachelectomy. Korean J Obstet Gynecol 2012;55: 332–334.
7. Plante M, et al. Vaginal radical trachelectomy: a valuable fertility-preserving option in the management of early-stage cervical cancer. A series of 50 pregnancies and review of the literature. Gynecol Oncol 2005; 98: 3–10.
8. Lotgering FK, et al. Outcome after transabdominal cervicoisthmic cerclage. Obstet Gynecol 2006;107: 779–784.
9. Lee KY, et al. Successful twin pregnancy after vaginal radical trachelectomy using transabdominal cervicoisthmic cerclage. Am J Obstet Gynecol 2007;197: 5–6.
10. Roy M, Plante M. Pregnancies after radical vaginal trachelectomy for early-stage cervical cancer. Am J Obstet Gynecol 1998;179: 1491–1496.
11. Plante M, et al. The case of a viable pregnancy post vaginal trachelectomy followed by combined chemo-radiation therapy. Gynecol Oncol 2011;123: 421–423.
12. Boss EA, et al. Pregnancy after radical trachelectomy: a real option. Gynecol Oncol 2005;99 Suppl 1: S152–S156.
13. Lee K-Y., Song J-E. Management of pregnancy after conization and radical trachelectomy. In: Al-Hendy A, Sabry M, ed., Hysterectomy. Rijeka: InTech, pp. 325–331.
14. Jolley JA, et al. Management of pregnancy after radical trachelectomy: case reports and systematic review of the literature. Am J Perinatol 2007;24: 531–540.
15. Dodd JM, et al. Progesterone for the prevention of preterm birth: a systematic review. Obstet Gynecol 2008;112: 127–134.

CARE PATHWAY

Pre-pregnancy evaluation and advice

- Encourage patient to avoid pregnancy for the first 6 months following **radical trachelectomy (RT),** to ensure healing and no persistence or recurrence of disease
- If she is considering IVF, encourage single embryo transfer to try to avoid multiple pregnancy
- Ascertain whether transabdominal cervicoisthmic cerclage was applied at time of RT
- Ascertain whether she has received adjuvant radiotherapy
- Discuss possible complications of pregnancy including miscarriage rate of nearly 30% (1st and 2nd trimester), preterm delivery of <37 weeks (20%), PPROM, chorioamnionitis, IUGR, etc.
- Discuss multidisciplinary team care during pregnancy, serial transvaginal scans, prophylactic antibiotics, progesterone pessaries from early 2nd trimester to 36 weeks gestation as well as to anticipate delivery by Caesarean section

↓

Referral to specialist antenatal clinic before 13 weeks gestation by community team

↓

First visit to specialist antenatal clinic

- Detailed history: Time interval from RT to pregnancy, whether cervicoisthmic cerclage inserted at time of RT, whether has had radiotherapy as adjuvant, follow-up cytology
- Confirm viability and dates
- Discuss risks of pregnancy, outline plans for management during pregnancy
- Transvaginal scans for residual cervical length or any signs of funnelling of internal os at 3–4 week intervals from 14 weeks
- Prophylactic PV clindamycin cream for 1 week at about 16 weeks and repeated at approximately 22–24 weeks
- Consider progesterone pessaries (Cyclogest) 400 mg od from approximately 14–36 weeks pregnancy
- If patient has had adjuvant radiotherapy, arrange serial growth scans with same-day antenatal clinic follow-up at approximately 26, 30, 34 weeks gestation
- Discuss delivery by elective Caesarean section at about 37 weeks
- Advise to continue routine antenatal checks with community midwife
- Multidisciplinary team network with gynaecological oncology team

↓

Further visits to specialist antenatal clinic

- Check serial cervical length scans if any residual cervix. If patient has not had a previous transabdominal cervicoisthmic suture inserted at time of RT, it may need to be considered in early 2nd trimester in specialist centres
- Check consistent fetal growth is maintained
- Consider prophylactic steroids
- Advise patient to report immediately to delivery suite if any contractions or PPROM as she will need urgent Caesarean section if she has had transabdominal cervicoisthmic cerclage at any stage
- If all well till 37 weeks, plan elective Caesarean section at approximately 37+ weeks. At Caesarean section the transabdominal cervicoisthmic cerclage should be left intact

Empirical care pathway extrapolated from pregnancy management in women with previous deep cone/LLETZ

11.3 Uterine Malformations

FACT FILE

Epidemiology and types of malformations

- The normal development of the female genital tract is a result of complex steps during embryogenesis in the first trimester, involving differentiation, migration, and fusion followed by canalization of the Müllerian system. Uterine anomalies can result if any of these processes is interrupted.
- The spectrum of uterine malformation ranges from Müllerian agenesis due to complete failure of Müllerian ducts to develop, resulting in an absent uterus, to just a slight dimpling of the uterine contour in mild cases of an arcuate uterus.
- The types of uterine abnormalities can be classified depending on whether it a **fusion (unification) defect** (resulting in unicornuate or bicornuate uteri, or uterine didelphys) or a **canalization defect**, due to incomplete resorption of the midline septum, leading to septate or subseptate uteri[1] (see Figure 11.1).
- These several types of uterine anomalies have different effects and degrees of impact on the subsequent reproductive outcomes in such women.

Incidence

- Uterine malformations are estimated to be present in about 3–4% of any unselected population, but a higher incidence ranging from 5–10% in those with recurrent early pregnancy losses, to as high as 25% in those with recurrent late first-trimester and second-trimester pregnancy losses or preterm deliveries.[2,3,4,5,6,7]

Impact on pregnancy

- In general, uterine malformations are associated with difficulty in maintaining a pregnancy rather than impairment of fertility,[6,7,8] although some studies report a greater representation in those with subfertility or infertility.[3,9]
- Canalization defects such as septate or subseptate uteri appear to be associated with worse pregnancy outcomes than unification defects such as unicornuate or bicornuate uteri or uterine didelphys.
- **The detection and identification of the type of uterine malformations** is achieved by various imaging modalities[10,11,12,13] such as transabdominal and/or transvaginal ultrasound scans, by three-dimensional ultrasonography, or by the gold standard MRI technique.
- Hysterosalpingography (HSG) though still in common use, cannot define the external uterine contour and has been superseded by other imaging modalities. While HSG can diagnose up to 55% of septate and subseptate uteri, for example, the rate of detection is improved to over 90% when it is combined with ultrasound.[14]
- Congenital uterine anomalies are implicated in adverse pregnancy outcomes, although the mechanisms involved can be multiple, such as:
  - reduced cavity size
  - impaired ability to distend
  - abnormal endometrial bed for implantation to occur[15,16]
  - insufficient myometrium relative to fibrous tissue in the region of a septum

Figure 11.1 Uterine Malformations

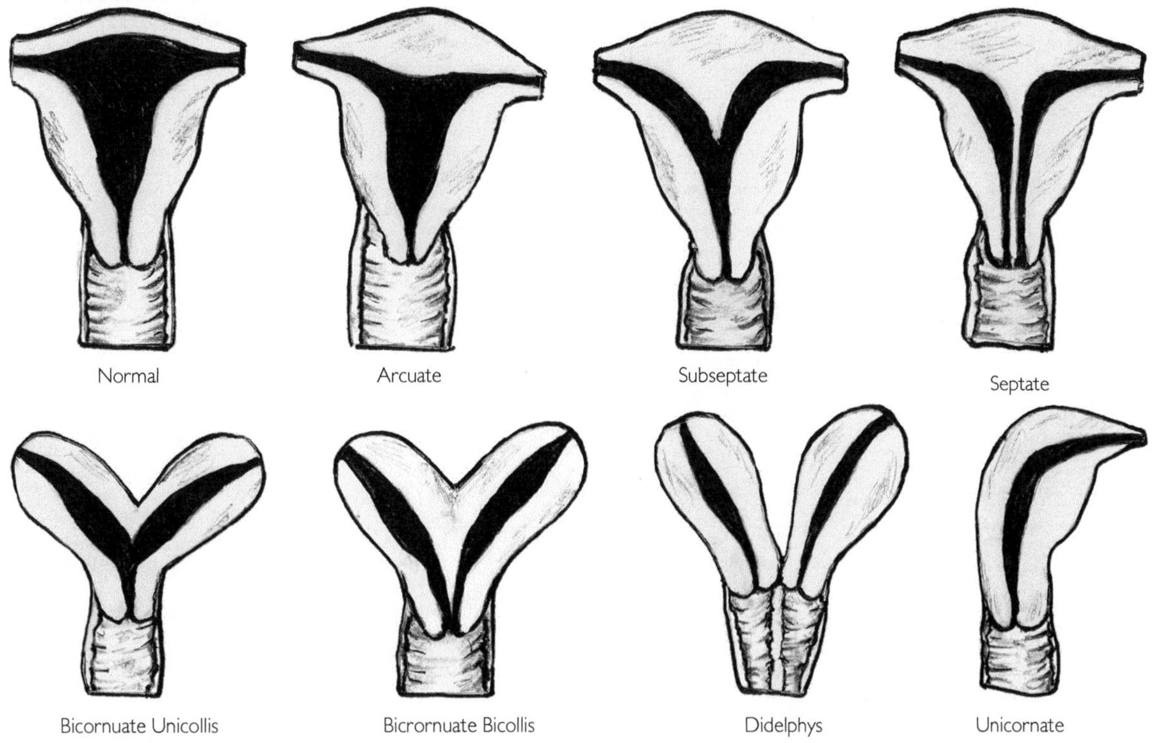

- abnormal or reduced vascular supply
- abnormal myometrial and cervical function.
- Uterine malformations are associated with increased rates of recurrent pregnancy loss (21–33%), preterm delivery, malpresentations, IUGR, higher Caesarean section rates, abruption, and postpartum haemorrhage (see Table 11.1).
- Compared with women with normal uteri, women with significant uterine malformations can have poorer reproductive outcomes and lower pregnancy rates whether conception has been spontaneous or with assisted reproductive techniques,.
- Anomalies of the renal tract are seen to coexist with uterine anomalies in up to 30% of cases.[7] Upper urinary tract anomalies such as horseshoe-shaped kidney, pelvic kidney, ectopic ureters, renal agenesis, or duplicated collecting system are detected by imaging techniques such as intravenous pyelogram or CT scan.

Fusion (unification) defects

Unicornuate uterus

- This occurs where one Müllerian duct fails to develop in whole or partially, resulting in a functional uterus with a normal cervix and fallopian tube as well as a rudimentary horn on the other side which might be either communicating or non-communicating (70–90%) with the main unicornuate uterus.[7,9]
- Adverse pregnancy outcomes include:
  - spontaneous miscarriage rate of about 37%
  - ectopic pregnancy rate of 50%
  - preterm delivery rate of about 16%
  - term delivery rate of about 54%
  - live birth baby rate of only 38–75%.
- A surgical procedure such as removal of the rudimentary horn will not change pregnancy complications, but has a role in gynaecological symptoms such as pelvic pain, dysmenorrhoea, or to prevent pregnancy in the obstructed horn.
- Prophylactic cervical cerclage is only for standard indications and not to be a routine procedure in those with unification defects.

Uterus didelphys

- This arises from failure of fusion of the two Müllerian ducts,[8,17] therefore duplication of uterus, two uterine cavities, two cervices, and a longitudinal vaginal septum are found in 75% of cases.[7]
- Adverse pregnancy outcomes include:
  - high spontaneous miscarriage rate of about 32%
  - preterm birth rate of 28%
  - term delivery rate of 36%
  - live birth rate of 19–64%.
- Not associated with cervical incompetence.
- Only in selected cases of recurrent pregnancy losses or preterm delivery is metroplasty (unification of the uterine cavities by surgery) worth considering. This has been shown to improve the live birth rate from 55% prior to metroplasty to 80% after surgery.
- Excision of longitudinal vaginal septum recommended to prevent dysmenorrhoea, haematocolpos, etc.

Bicornuate uterus

- This occurs due to failure of fusion at the fundal end of the two Müllerian ducts, therefore two uterine cavities but one cervix and normal vagina.[9] External contour of uterus is usually indented by more than 1 cm.[18,19]
- Adverse pregnancy outcomes include:
  - spontaneous miscarriage rate of about 36%
  - preterm delivery rate of about 23–66% depending on degree of cavity separation
  - term delivery rate of about 38–41%.
  - live birth rate of 52–58%.
- ***High incidence of associated cervical incompetence in more than one-third of cases.***
- Metroplasty should be reserved for those with no other cause found for recurrent pregnancy loss or preterm labours.
- Cervical cerclage not routinely applied, but to be considered if history of previous pregnancy loss attributable to cervical incompetence.

Canalization defects

- These result from incomplete resorption of the midline septum between the two Müllerian ducts.[20,21,22]

Septate uterus (including complete septum and subseptate)

- Most common type of uterine malformation, occurs in about 1% of all females.[7,22]
- Septal tissue composed of more fibrous, less vascular tissue with abnormal overlying endometrium.

Table 11.1 Summary of uterine malformations, pregnancy complications and surgical correction, if appropriate

Type of uterine anomaly	*1st and 2nd trimester pregnancy loss (%)*	*Ectopic pregnancy or associated cervical incompetence*	*Preterm delivery rate (%)*	*Term delivery rate (%)*	*Live birth rate (%)*	*Surgery (if indicated)*
Unicornuate	37%	Ectopic pregnancy rate up to 50% Associated with renal tract anomaly rate of up to 40%	16%	54%	38–75%	Removal of rudimentary horn only if gynaecological problems, not for improvement of pregnancy outcomes
Didelphys (vaginal septum in up to 75%)	32%	No increased association	28%	36%	19–64%	Metroplasty only in selected cases, improves live birth outcome to 80% Vaginal septum excision indicated
Bicornuate	36%	Cervical incompetence in 33%	23–66%	38–41%	52–58%	Metroplasty in those with previous pregnancy loss Cervical cerclage not routinely indicated
Septate (most common type of uterine anomaly and poorest pregnancy outcomes; vaginal septum a frequent association)	27–44% (25% in 1st trimester: 6% in 2nd trimester	No increased association	12–22%	33–61%	53%	Hysteroscopic metroplasty indicated in those with previous poor obstetric outcomes
Arcuate (associated with fewer pregnancy complications)	Increased		Increased		80%	Not indicated

Data from: Edmonds DK, Congenital malformations of the genital tract and their management, *Best Practice & Research Clinical Obstetrics & Gynaecology*, 2003, 17, 1, pp. 19–40; Mollo A et al., Hysteroscopic resection of the septum improves the pregnancy rate of women with unexplained infertility: a prospective controlled trial, *Fertility and Sterility*, 2009, 91, pp. 2628–2631; and Patton PE et al., The diagnosis and reproductive outcome after surgical treatment of the complete septate uterus, duplicated cervix and vaginal septum, *American Journal of Obstetrics and Gynecology*, 2004, 190, pp. 1669–1675.

- Despite the abnormality within the endometrial cavity, the external contour of the uterus appears normal.
- A longitudinal vaginal septum is frequently associated with a complete septated uterus.
- **Associated with the worst reproductive outcomes:**
  - pregnancy loss rate of 27– 44% (first-trimester loss rate of 25%, second-trimester loss rate of about 6%)
  - preterm delivery rate of around 12–22%
  - term delivery rate of about 33–61%
  - live birth rate of 53%.
- Hysteroscopic metroplasty[21] with excision of the septum has significantly improved subsequent pregnancy outcomes in those with previous poor pregnancy outcomes (post-metroplasty miscarriage rate of 15% and term delivery rate of nearly 80%).

Arcuate uterus

- A slight midline septum with a broad fundus and little more than fundal cavity indentation.[6,7]
  - Associated with the fewest obstetric complications, with term birth rates of nearly 80%.
  - Compared with women with normal uteri, higher rates of second-trimester pregnancy loss, preterm labour, and fetal malpresentations are seen.
  - Surgical procedures such as metroplasty are not indicated.

Counselling and management

- In those with a previously diagnosed uterine anomaly, pre-pregnancy or early pregnancy counselling should include a discussion about potential obstetric complications, need for serial fetal scans, awareness of risks of malpresentations, cord prolapse, and increased Caesarean section rates.
- Management of women with either uncorrected or corrected Müllerian duct anomalies should be managed on a case-by-case basis.
- During pregnancy in those with Müllerian abnormalities, vigilance needs to be maintained for signs of second-trimester cervical incompetence, IUGR, abruption, malpresentations, preterm labour, PPROM, cord or arm prolapse, UTIs if renal tract anomalies coexist, retained or morbidly adherent placenta, PPH, etc.
- Routine insertion of cervical cerclage is not recommended though an increased incidence of coexisting cervical incompetence has been reported. Prophylactic cervical cerclage is to be considered only if there is a previous history of second-trimester pregnancy loss (some guidelines suggest recurrent second-trimester pregnancy losses) with suspected cervical incompetence as aetiology.
- If there are no concerns with fetal growth and no malpresentation seen at term, a vaginal delivery is to be anticipated and Caesarean section performed only when there is some other obstetric indication.
- If not previously performed, women with Müllerian duct anomalies must be advised to have an intravenous urethrogram/pyelogram about 3 months after delivery to exclude or confirm associated renal tract anomalies seen in 30–40%.
- Those with double cervix as in uterine didelphys must be reminded (as should their GPs) that they need to have cervical smears taken from both cervices on each occasion.
- Similarly, if a woman with uterine didelphys is considering the intrauterine contraceptive device such as the IUCD (coil), either inert or levonorgestrel-loaded (Mirena®), one device needs to be inserted into each horn of the uterus and the position of each checked by ultrasound about 6–8 weeks later.
- Surgical interventions such as hysteroscopic metroplasty or excision of vaginal septum need to be scheduled, if indicated, for when the woman is at least 12 weeks postpartum.

Information for patients

Please see **Information for patients: Abnormal shape of the uterus (womb)** (p. 524)

References

1. Chan YY, et al. Reproductive outcomes in women with congenital uterine anomalies: a systematic review. Ultrasound Obstet Gynecol 2011;38: 371–382.
2. Jurkovic D, et al. Ultrasound screening for congenital uterine anomalies. Br J Obstet Gynaecol 1997;104: 1320–1321.
3. Raga F, et al. Reproductive impact of congenital Mullerian anomalies. Hum Reprod 1997;12: 227–228. Mullerian defects in women with normal reproductive outcome. Fertil Steril 1991;56: 1192-1193.
4. Lin PC, et al. Female genital anomalies affecting reproduction. Fertil Steril 2002;78: 899–915.
5. Lin PC. Reproductive outcomes in women with uterine anomalies. J Women's Health 2004;13: 33–39.
6. Rackow BW, Arici A. Reproductive performance of women with Mullerian anomalies. Curr Opin Obstet Gynecol 2007;19: 229–237.
7. Grimbizis GF, et al. Clinical implications of uterine malformations and hysteroscopic treatment results. Hum Reprod Update 2001;7: 161–174.
8. Tulandi T, et al. Arcuate and bicornuate uterine anomalies and infertility. Fertil Steril 1980;34: 362–364.
9. Kupesic S. Clinical implications of sonographic detection of uterine anomalies for reproductive outcome. Ultrasound Obstet Gynecol 2001;18: 387–400.
10. Pellerito JS, et al. Diagnosis of uterine anomalies: relative accuracy of MR imaging, endovaginal sonography, and hysterosalpingography. Radiology 1992;183: 795–800.
11. Andreotti RFJ. Three-dimensional sonography of the endometrium and adjacent myometrium: Preliminary observations. Ultrasound Med 2006;25: 1313–1319.
12. Olpin J.D., Heilbrun M. Imaging of Mullerian duct anomalies. Clin Obstet Gynaecol 2009;52: 40–56.
13. Reuter KL, et al. Septate versus non-septate uteri: errors in imaging diagnosis. Radiology 1989;172: 749–752.
14. Candiani GB, et al. Endometrial patterns in malformed uteri. Acta Eur Fertil 1983;14: 311–318.
15. Fedele L, et al. Ultrastructural aspects of endometrium in infertile women with septate uterus. Fertil Steril 1996;65: 750–752.
16. Gholoum S, et al. Management and outcome of patients with combined vaginal septum, bifid uterus, and ipsilateral renal agenesis (Herlyn-Werner-Wunderlich syndrome). J Pediatr Surg 2006;41: 987–992.
17. Troiano RN, McCarthy SM. Mullerian duct anomalies: imaging and clinical issues. Radiology 2004;233: 19–34.
18. Fedele L, et al. Ultrasonography in the differential diagnosis of 'double' uteri. Fertil Steril 1988;50: 361–364.
19. Fedele L, et al. Septums and synechiae: approaches to surgical correction. Clin Obstet Gynecol 2006;49: 767–788.
20. Mollo A., et al. Hysteroscopic resection of the septum improves the pregnancy rate of women with unexplained infertility: a prospective controlled trial. Fertility and Sterility 2009;91: 2628–2631
21. Patton PE., et al. The diagnosis and reproductive outcome after surgical treatment of the complete septate uterus, duplicated cervix and vaginal septum. American Journal of Obstetrics and Gynecology 2004;190: 1669–1675.
22. Edmonds DK. Congenital malformations of the genital tract and their management. Best Pract Res Clin Obstet Gynaecol 2003;17: 19–40.

CARE PATHWAY

GP or community midwife refers woman with known **uterine anomaly** to specialist antenatal clinic in 1st trimester

Incidental finding of **uterine malformation** noted in 1st trimester or at the 20 week anomaly scan

↓

First visit to specialist antenatal clinic

- Confirm type of uterine malformation. Further discussions need to be individualized according to type of anomaly
- Discuss increased risks of pregnancy complications such as 2nd-trimester miscarriages, preterm labour, IUGR, abruption, malpresentations, etc.
- In a woman with previous 2nd-trimester miscarriages with history suggestive of cervical incompetence, serial cervical length scans from 14 weeks: cervical cerclage only for standard indications
- Serial fetal growth scans from 26–28 weeks onwards with clinic follow-up on same day if possible
- Continue routine antenatal checks with community midwife
- Advise patient to report any bleeding, pain, PPROM without delay to maternity unit

↓

Further visits to specialist antenatal clinic

- Check consistent growth and liquor scans
- If cephalic presentation and longitudinal lie with no evidence of IUGR, aim for spontaneous onset of labour at term and vaginal delivery with Caesarean section only for obstetric reasons
- If broad-based, thick, longitudinal vaginal septum likely to obstruct delivery is identified antenatally, an elective Caesarean section may be indicated
- If a thin longitudinal vaginal septum is present, avoid excision during pregnancy or during labour/delivery as such a septum usually flattens itself onto the lateral wall of vagina during delivery

↓

Postnatal: before discharge

- If not done previously, advise IVU after 3 months post-delivery to exclude coexistent renal tract abnormalities
- Appropriate contraception advice: In cases of uterine didelphys, GP and patient to be informed that if inert IUCD or Mirena opted for, dual insertion required
- In uterine didelphys, cervical smears from both cervices mandatory
- Hysteroscopic metroplasty and/or vaginal septum excision, if indicated, needs to be scheduled only after 3 months after delivery and after due counselling

11.4 Female Genital Mutilation

FACT FILE

This fact file deals only with the antenatal management of **female genital mutilation (FGM)**. For a wider overview, see <http://www.who.int/mediacentre/factsheets/fs241/en/>

- FGM, also referred to as female circumcision, infibulation or 'cutting' is defined as all procedures involving partial or total removal of the external female genitalia or other injury to the female genital organs, whether for cultural or other non-therapeutic reasons.
- Female mutilation is prohibited by law in England, Scotland, and Wales, whether committed against a UK national or a permanent UK resident in the UK or abroad. According to the Female Genital Mutilation Act 2003, the penalty for a person guilty of such an offence is a prison sentence of up to 14 years.[1]
- WHO estimates show that more than 130 million women worldwide have suffered FGM and a further 2 million are at risk. More than 6000 FGMs are estimated to take place per day, with one child/young woman dying every 10 min from the sequelae of the procedure.[2]
- Although a deeply rooted tradition mainly in Africa and the Middle East, FGM is practised in some form, to a lesser extent, in some Asian countries.
- With increased immigration, however, FGM is a true global problem. It is estimated that more than 20 000 girls in the UK are at risk,[3] with the the single most important risk factor being a country of initial origin where there is a high prevalence of the practice: for example, Somalia, Sudan, and Egypt.
- The most common age range for FGM varies between a few days after birth to 15 years of age.[4]
- It is estimated that 90% of FGM worldwide are of categories I, II, III, and IV with 10% involving type III[5](see Table 11.2).
- It is imperative that any woman who has had FGM is treated with kindness and genuine sympathy. She did not choose to have FGM which was carried out in childhood and under restraint. The healthcare professionals should also ensure that their non-verbal body language and expressions do not reveal disgust or disapproval in any way.

Antenatal care

- In catchment areas that include a large population of women with FGM, a nominated specialist team of an experienced midwife and obstetrician can help disseminate a greater understanding of FGM and the potential complications during childbirth to the other staff.
- Community midwives must, very sensitively, ask all pregnant women originating from countries where it is widely practised, whether they have had FGM.

Table 11.2 WHO classification of types of female genital mutilation procedures

Type	*Definition*
I	Partial or total removal of the clitoris and/or the prepuce (clitoridectomy)
II	Partial or total removal of the clitoris and the labia minora, with or without excision of the labia majora (excision)
III	Narrowing of the vaginal orifice with creation of a covering seal by cutting and appositioning the labia minora and/or the labia majora, with or without excision of the clitoris (infibulation)
IV	All other harmful procedures to the female genitalia for non-medical purposes, e.g. pricking, piercing,[a] incising, scraping and cauterizing

[a] Although piercing is part of this WHO classification, its legal status in the UK is unclear.

Reproduced with kind permission from the World Health Organization. <http://www.who.int/reproductivehealth/topics/fgm/overview/en/>.

- As there is often a large cultural/traditional barrier in most cases as well as psychological issues and language difficulties involved, these factors must all be taken into consideration when offering appropriate antenatal care for such patients.
- To enable the patient to overcome obvious barriers, it is highly beneficial if a senior obstetrician and midwife with prior experience in caring for FGM patients, can meet and examine the patient during the first antenatal visit to the hospital antenatal clinic.
- During this first visit, after due explanations (with a non-related translator, if one is required), physical examination of the external genitalia is very helpful in planning further management during pregnancy, particularly whether antenatal defibulation would be beneficial.
- If the urethral meatus can be seen, or if two fingers can be inserted into the vagina without causing discomfort, the extent of FGM is unlikely to cause problems during delivery. Women with a tight introitus are more likely to suffer major perineal trauma at the time of delivery.
- As indicated in the **RCOG Green-top guideline**,[6] a proforma with a predrawn diagram outline of the external genitalia is invaluable in assessing the degree of the FGM, to plan antenatal or intrapartum interventions.

Defibulation

- Ideally, defibulation should take place pre-pregnancy.
- Women should be offered elective defibulation around 20 weeks gestation, aiming to restore as much as normal anatomy as possible while allowing sufficient time for recovery and healing before delivery.
- Counselling regarding defibulation should recognize that a significant number will decline antenatal defibulation, preferring to wait until the onset of labour.
- The obstetrician should discuss problems that could be encountered antenatally if antenatal defibulation is declined, such as recurrent UTIs, retention of urine, and vaginal infections.
- In those with type III infibulation, urine is always contaminated with vaginal secretions giving a false positivity for protein. Interpretation of routine antenatal urine tests is therefore likely to be less reliable.
- If examination is declined during the antenatal period, discussions must point out that the inability to perform vaginal examinations, to adequately empty the bladder, or to apply a fetal scalp electrode or to take a fetal blood sample, could all result in higher chances of needing a Caesarean section.
- Antenatal defibulation, ideally at 20 weeks gestation, can be performed either under local anaesthetic or a spinal. Because of the psychological trauma that the woman is likely to have suffered at the time of the original FGM, a general anaesthetic may be required to avoid causing the patient distress and flashbacks.
- Defibulation is performed by anterior excision exactly in the midline with a probe or dilator inserted into the undersurface of the 'hood' or scar of the FGM. Once the urethral meatus is revealed, the excision is complete and the raw edges on either side are oversewn with rapidly absorbed sutures such as Vicryl Rapide.
- Post defibulation, adequate analgesia must be offered (in accordance with the Female Genital Mutilation Act) to try to prevent traumatic flashbacks.
- An epidural anaesthetic is recommended for labour if defibulation needs to be performed during labour.
- A Caesarean section is required only in severe forms of FGM which has caused such anatomical distortion that precludes defibulation.
- An episiotomy being required during delivery must be discussed antenatally.
- The patient and partner must be reminded that re-infibulation is prohibited by law in the UK.[6,7,8]

Information for patients

Please see **Information for patients: Female genital mutilation** (p. 525)

References

1. Female Genital Mutilation Act 2003 <http://www.hmso.gov.uk/acts/acts2003/20030031.htm>.
2. WHO. Eliminating female genital mutilation. An interagency statement. Geneva: World Health Organization, 2008.
3. Dorkenoo E, et al. A statistical study to estimate the prevalence of female genital mutilation in England and Wales. Summary report. London: Foundation for Women's Health, Research and Development (FORWARD), 2007
4. WHO. Female genital mutilation—new knowledge spurs optimism. Progr Sex Reprod Health Res 2006;72: 1.
5. DHS Working Papers No. 39. Numbers of women circumcised in Africa. The production of a total. USAID Contract No. GPO-C-00-03-00002-00. Calverton: Micro International Inc., 2008.
6. RCOG Green-top Guideline No.53. Female genital mutilation and its management. London: Royal College of Obstetricians and Gynaecologists, 2009.
7. BMA. Female genital mutilation: caring for patients and child protection. London: British Medical Association, 2006 http://www.bma.org.uk/health_promotion_ethics/human_rights/FGM.jsp>.
8. RCM Position Paper 21. Female genital mutilation (female circumcision). London: Royal College of Midwives, 1998.

CARE PATHWAY

Booking visit by community midwife for woman with female genital mutilation (FGM)

- Must be conducted in private, with a sensitive approach. If there is any language barrier arrange for an interpreter to be present, if acceptable to the woman. Friends or relatives should not be used for interpretation. Language Line facilities may be used. An information leaflet about FGM can be given
- To classify the type of FGM a previously prepared diagram can be used which reduces the woman's embarrassment at this first midwifery visit and also limits the need for repeated examinations
- A psychological assessment is useful, and referral to a psychologist may be made if deemed necessary and agreed to by the woman
- After the assessment, if the woman is a primigravida with extensive type II or type III FGM, or a multigravida who has been reinfibulated, where it is felt that vaginal examination or delivery will be difficult or impossible, a referral must be made to the antenatal clinic for a female consultant or senior obstetrician

↓

Assessment in hospital antenatal clinic by a female consultant or senior obstetrician

- Enquire about any previous problems passing urine, urinary infections, dyspareunia, difficulties during a previous childbirth, whether has been 'opened before', etc.
- Examination should be conducted with sensitivity and professionalism

↓

- If type III or extensive type II FGM confirmed, and vaginal access deemed very limited, discuss benefits of defibulation during pregnancy or during active labour (either late first stage or second stage)
- Inform woman about legal implications of FGM in the UK

↓

- Antenatal defibulation accepted
- Ideally done at around 20 weeks gestation (allows time for healing to be complete before term)
- Book for gynaecology theatre
- Follow-up appointment in antenatal clinic 1–2 weeks after procedure, then transfer back to midwifery-led care if no other risk factors

- Antenatal defibulation declined
- Reversal recommended in first or second stage of labour
- Defibulation in labour with consent

↓

- Follow-up postnatal appointment, check healing is complete
- Health visitor and GP informed
- Remind woman about legal implications of FGM in the UK

↓

- Type I or II infibulation identified— no further action
- Inform woman about legal implications of FGM in the UK

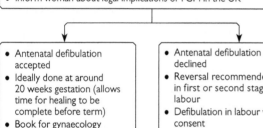

11.5 Uterine Fibroids

FACT FILE

- **Fibroids or leiomyoma** are very common smooth muscle benign tumours found in 20–40% of women during their reproductive years.
- Afro-Caribbean women are three times more likely than white women to develop fibroids.
- Increasing maternal age and nulliparity are strong associations for fibroids in pregnancy.
- Estimates of the incidence of fibroids in pregnancy vary from about 2.7% found at routine second-trimester ultrasound scans to 12–25% in older women undergoing fertility treatment.[1]
- With more women delaying childbearing, fibroids are more likely encountered in the pregnant population.
- Only about 40% of large fibroids (>5 cm) can be diagnosed during pregnancy on physical examination and that too depending on their location. Due to the difficulty in differentiating between physiological gestational thickening of the myometrium and fibroids, detection by ultrasound is also limited.[2,3]
- Most fibroids are asymptomatic in pregnancy and are incidental findings on clinical or ultrasound examinations or seen at Caesarean section.
- However, 10 -30 % of women with fibroids can develop complications during pregnancy.[4,5]

Effects of pregnancy on fibroids

- The majority (60–70%) show no change in size during pregnancy.[6]
- Those fibroids that increase in size are likely to do so in the first trimester, with little growth in the second and third trimesters. Fibroids do not change significantly during the puerperium.[1,5,6]
- Fibroids can undergo 'red degeneration' or impaction during pregnancy. Rarely, torsion of a pedunculated subserosal fibroid may be encountered.
- Pain is the most common complication especially with large fibroids (> 5 cm) often in the second and third trimesters due to the process of red degeneration. Pain is postulated to be due to the rapid growth of the fibroid outstripping the vascular supply leading to necrosis and infarction.[4] However, as red degeneration can also occur without an increase in the size of the fibroid, the necrosis and infarction could be due to kinking of the vascular supply by the growing uterus.
- Release of prostaglandins from the surface of the fibroid due to cellular damage can also produce pain.

Management of fibroid pain

- Usually managed conservatively by bed rest, hydration, and analgesics.
- NSAIDs which are effective for fibroid-related pain relief are, however, contraindicated during pregnancy due to risk of premature closure of the fetal ductus arteriosus, pulmonary hypertension, necrotizing enterocolitis, intracranial haemorrhage, or oligohydramnios..
- In **very** rare cases, intractable pain from a torted degenerating fibroid, only if pedunculated, may require myomectomy in the first or second trimesters of pregnancy if conservative management fails.[1,5]

Effects of fibroids on pregnancy outcomes

In early pregnancy

- A doubling of spontaneous miscarriage rate, related more to the presence of multiple fibroids than to the size of a fibroid. Submucosal and intramural fibroids are implicated as well in causing miscarriages.[1,4]
- Bleeding in early pregnancy is more common if the placenta is implanted close to the fibroid.

In late pregnancy and labour

- **Preterm labour and delivery** are twice as likely in women with fibroids than those without (16.1 % vs 8.7%).[1].If there are multiple fibroids or if the placental implantation impinges on or is close to the fibroid(s), the risks of preterm labour and delivery are greater. Fibroids are, however, not associated with an increased risk of PPROM.
- **Placental abruption:** Threefold increased risk of abruption in pregnant women with fibroids, especially with submucosal or retroplacental fibroids or if the fibroids are large.[7]
- **Fetal growth restriction:** Only a few studies have shown an association with IUGR.
- **Fetal compression** due to distortion of the uterine cavity by large fibroids can cause fetal dolicocephaly, torticollis, etc.[1,5]
- **Malpresentations** are more common with large fibroids and contribute to an increased Caesarean section rate.
- The rate of **dysfunctional labour** has been reported as doubled.[8] However, as a high successful vaginal delivery rate is reported in women with fibroids, even large fibroids, a **trial of vaginal delivery** in labour-eligible cases is **not** contraindicated.[9,10]
- **Caesarean section rates** are nearly four times greater than controls.[1]
- There is a significant risk of **atonic postpartum haemorrhage** (double the risk of controls) as well as of peripartum hysterectomy.[1] Uterine atony is attributed to poor contractility of the myometrium achieved by the distortion of the uterus due to large or multiple fibroids.
- **Retained placenta** is more common in women with fibroids, irrespective of where the fibroids are located in the uterus.
- Increased incidence of **uterine rupture** is associated with **previous abdominal myomectomy where the uterine cavity is breached.**
- Likewise, there is an increased risk of **intrapartum and pre-labour uterine rupture** (0.5–1%) with previous **laparoscopic myomectomies.**[11,12,13,14,15,16]
- Elective Caesarean delivery is therefore recommended in the case of previous laparoscopic myomectomies as well as with a history of open laparotomy and myomectomy where the uterine cavity has been breached.
- Uterine artery embolization (UAE) for fibroids is contraindicated in pregnancy and in women desiring future fertility.

Information for patients

Please see Information for patients: Fibroids and pregnancy (p. 525)

References

1. Katsky PC, et al. Fibroids and reproductive outcomes: a systematic literature review from conception to delivery. Am J Obstet Gynecol 2008;198: 357–366.
2. Muram D, et al. Myomas of the uterus in pregnancy: ultrasonographic follow-up. Am J Obstet Gynecol 1980;138: 16–19.
3. Rice JP, et al. The clinical significance of uterine leiomyomas in pregnancy. Am J Obstet Gynecol 1989;160: 1212–1216.
4. Katz VL, et al. Complications of uterine leiomyomas in pregnancy. Obstet Gynecol 1989;73: 593–596.
5. Lee HJ, et al. Contemporary management of fibroids in pregnancy. Reviews in Obstetrics and Gynecology 2010;3: 20–27.
6. Rosati P, et al. Longitudinal evaluation of uterine myoma growth during pregnancy: a sonographic study. J Ultrasound Med 1992;11: 511–515.
7. Exacoustos C, Rosati P. Ultrasound diagnosis of uterine myomas and complications in pregnancy. Obstet Gynecol 1993;82: 97–101.
8. Coronado GD, et al. Complications in pregnancy, labor and delivery with uterine leiomyomas: a population based study. Obstet Gynecol 2000: 95: 764–769.

9. Qidwai IG, et al. Obstetric outcomes in women with sonographically identified uterine leiomyomata. Obstet Gynecol 2006;107: 376–382.
10. Vergani P, et al. Large uterine leiomyomata and risk of caesarean delivery. Obstet Gynecol 2007;109: 410–414.
11. Harris WJ. Uterine dehiscence following laparoscopic myomectomy. Obstet Gynecol 1992;80: 545–546.
12. Dubuisson JB, et al. Uterine rupture during pregnancy after laparoscopic myomectomy. Hum Reprod 1995;10: 1475–1477.
13. Dubuisson JB, et al. Pregnancy outcome and deliveries following laparoscopic myomectomy. Hum Reprod 2000;15: 869–873.
14. Lieng M, et al. Uterine rupture after laparoscopic myomectomy. J Am Assoc Gynecol Laparosc 2004;11: 92–93.
15. Goldberg J, Pereira L. Pregnancy outcomes following treatment for fibroids: uterine fibroid embolization versus laparoscopic myomectomy. Curr Opin Obstet Gynecol 2006;18: 402–406.
16. Dubuisson JB, et al. Laparoscopic myomectomy: a current view. Hum Reprod Update 2000;6: 588–594.

CARE PATHWAY

- Community midwife refers patient known to have **fibroids** to specialist antenatal clinic
- When large (> 5 cm) fibroids are found incidentally by clinical or ultrasound examination patient directed to the specialist antenatal clinic

↓

First visit to specialist antenatal clinic

- Confirm viability, dates, assess any symptoms such as pain, bleeding
- Ultrasound assessment of size, single or multiple, location, type of fibroids (submucous, intramural, or subserous)
- Obtain more information if available, from previous gynaecological investigations, any operative notes (e.g. myomectomy/hysterocopy/laparoscopy), previous ultrasound, etc.
- If has had previous myomectomy, ascertain whether open or laparoscopic; if open procedure (not laparoscopic) myomectomy, was the uterine cavity breached? Time interval between myomectomy and conception? Try to obtain operation details if performed elsewhere
- Explain possible symptomatology of complications during pregnancy ; provide urgent contact details to report symptoms such as:
  - Pain: Conservative management of red degeneration with bed rest, hydration, and analgesia (avoiding NSAIDs)
  - Bleeding: explain increased risks of miscarriage
  - Urinary retention: Especially if incarceration develops with large anterior cervical fibroids
  - Preterm labour
  - Placental abruption
  - Advise patient that if SROM occurs, she should attend delivery suite immediately to exclude cord or arm prolapse exclusion, especially with large lower segment fibroids
- Arrange anomaly and serial growth/liquor volume scans
- Advise to continue antenatal checks with community midwife meanwhile

↓

Further visits to specialist antenatal clinic

At approx. 28, 32, 36, and 40 weeks:

- Check serial fetal growth and liquor volume on ultrasound scans, and whether any further increase in size of fibroids on scans, any scan appearance of red degeneration?
- Assess pregnancy progress, any fibroid-related symptoms?
- At >36 weeks, identify fetal presentation to advise mode of delivery. If any malpresentation, elective Caesarean section delivery. ECV contraindicated in large fibroids
- If previous laparoscopic myomectomy or open procedure with breach of uterine cavity, advise elective LSCS preferably at 38 weeks
- ***If large fibroids are present, warn patient about atonic PPH that might require peripartum hysterectomy. Document this discussion***
- Keep a minimum of 6–8 units blood cross-matched and where available UAE facilities on the standby as an alternative to hysterectomy. Inform interventional radiologist if service available
- Refer to anaesthetist and inform blood bank if large submucous/intramural fibroids, fibroids on the lower segment, or multiple fibroids are present
- ***Document above in notes and ensure senior obstetrician performs the potentially complex Caesarean section***
- **Document active management of third stage with PPH prophylaxis** including misoprostol, carboprost, etc. and not to attempt a myomectomy at the time of Caesarean section

12 Maternal Dermatological Conditions

12.1 Pruritic Urticarial Papules and Plaques of Pregnancy (PUPPP)

FACT FILE

- **Pruritic urticarial papules and plaques of pregnancy (PUPPP)**, also known as **polymorphic eruption of pregnancy**, toxaemic rash of pregnancy, toxaemic erythema of pregnancy, and late-onset prurigo of pregnancy
- It is one of the two most common dermatoses of pregnancy, the other being atopic eruption of pregnancy seen earlier in gestation.
- PUPPP occurs in about 1 in 160 pregnancies (about 0.5–1%). It may be less common in black populations.
- It is almost invariably limited to a first pregnancy; recurrence in subsequent pregnancies is very rare.
- PUPPP is a **benign dermatosis** that typically arises in the late third trimester of pregnancy.[1] The clinical appearance may provoke anxiety for the patient, therefore reassurance is required as to the nature of the skin eruption.
- **It is not associated with any fetal or maternal risks.** Prognosis for both the mother and baby is excellent and no additional fetal monitoring is required.
- PUPPP is more common in **multiple gestations**: meta-analyses have shown that 11.7% of PUPPP cases are seen in multiple pregnancies.[2] The greater the distension of the abdomen the higher the chances of PUPPP: with twins the incidence is nearly 3% but with triplets it is 14%.[3]
- Its appearance in late gestation (usually in the last 5 weeks) when maximal skin distension is seen and its association with excess weight gain in pregnancy lends further support to the theory that **PUPPP is caused by damage to connective tissue that triggers an allergic-type reaction.**
- Interestingly, there is a **preponderance of male babies** in mothers affected by PUPPP, with a male: female ratio of 2:1,[4,5] suggesting that male fetal DNA found in the circulation of mothers could have a role in the pathogenesis.
- Symptoms are mainly of severe itching leading to disturbed sleep pattern in late pregnancy.
- PUPPP usually resolves within 4–6 weeks postpartum, whatever the mode of delivery.[6] One study has found that about 15% may occur in the immediate postpartum period.[7]
- PUPPP does not reappear with subsequent use of oral contraception.

Clinical presentation

- Classically, intensely pruritic papules arise within the striae gravidarum, late in the third trimester usually of a first pregnancy.
- The eruption soon spreads to the back, buttocks, and upper thighs, also general spread over the trunk and limbs. The neck, face, palms, and soles are not affected in PUPPP.
- Small vesicles that coalesce to form plaques are seen, but not blisters or bullae.
- Characteristically, the periumbilical area is not involved and has a halo-like appearance of uninvolved normal skin. This is an important distinction from pemphigoid gestationis where the lesions start from the umbilical area and spread centrifugally.(Table 12.1).

Differential diagnosis

This includes:

- Atopic eruptions of pregnancy, including eczema of pregnancy and prurigo
- Pemphigoid gestationis (PG)
- Intrahepatic cholestasis
- Erythema multiforme
- Drug allergies, acute or chronic urticaria, scabies, contact or allergic dermatitis, viral rashes.

Investigations

- A clear distinction must be made between pruritus without a rash (when OC must be considered) and pruritus with a rash (as in PUPPP), where unneccessary LFTs, CTGs, early IOL must be avoided
- No blood or urine tests are diagnostic in PUPPP, which is essentially a clinical diagnosis. Serum immunosorbent assays or direct immunoflourescent studies of skin punch biopsy are indicated only to differentiate PUPPP from PG in equivocal cases.
- Histological examination of punch skin biopsy reveals normal epidermis in PUPPP, with some spongiosis and parakeratosis. Some dermal oedema may be seen.[8]

Management

- The primary aim is to relieve the pruritus associated with PUPPP. Topical corticosteroids are the mainstay of treatment. **High-potency topical corticosteroids used 2–3 times a day usually alleviate the itching after 2–3 days.** In some cases **systemic steroids (prednisolone) may be required.**
- Other measures include **cool baths, emollients**, loose cotton garments.
- **Oral antihistamines** such as diphenhydramine are mildly effective but may help the patient sleep better.
- If systemic steroids have been required during the last few weeks of pregnancy, bolus doses of hydrocortisone may be required to cover labour and delivery.

Information for patients

Please see Information for patients: Pruritic urticarial papules and plaques of pregnancy (p. 526)

References

1. Lawley TJ., et al. Pruritic urticarial papules and plaques of pregnancy. J Am Med Assoc 1979; 241: 1696–1699.
2. Kroumpouzos G, Cohen LM. Specific dermatoses of pregnancy: an evidence-based systematic review. Am J Obstet Gynecol 2003;188: 1083–1092.
3. Elling SV, et al. Pruritic urticarial papules and plaques of pregnancy in twin and triplet pregnancies. J Eur Acad Dermatol Venereol 2000;14: 378–381.
4. Vaughan Jones SA, et al. A prospective study of 200 women with dermatoses of pregnancy correlating clinical findings with hormonal and immunopathological profiles. Br J Dermatol. 1999;141: 71–81.
5. Aractingi S, et al. Fetal DNA in skin of polymorphic eruptions of pregnancy. Lancet 1998;352 (9144): 1898–1901.
6. Rudolph CM, et al. Polymorphic eruption of pregnancy: clinicopathology and potential trigger factors in 181 patients. Br J Dermatol 2006;154: 54–60.

Table 12.1 Essential differences between pemphigoid gestationis (PG) and PUPPP

	PG	*PUPPP*
Distinguishing feature		
Incidence	Rare, 1:50 000	Relatively common, 1:160; almost entirely limited to first pregnancies
Trimester	Usually 2nd/3rd or immediate postpartum, brief respite in last few weeks of 3rd trimester	Usually in last 5 weeks of 3rd trimester, about 15% immediate postpartum
Lesions	Papules, vesicles, bullae and blisters, urticarial plaques starting from umbilicus spreading outwards to torso, extremities. Face palms, soles, mucous membranes spared	Papules, plaques starting within striae gravidarum, spreading to thorax, upper thighs, buttocks. Periumbilical area spared. No involvement of skin breast upwards, face, palms, or soles
Pruritus	Severe, unremitting, can last for several weeks and months after delivery	Severe, usually resolves within 4–6 weeks after delivery
Breastfeeding	Seems to limit duration of PG in postpartum	No difference
Recurrence	High recurrence rate in subsequent pregnancies but can skip pregnancies	Highly unlikely to recur in future pregnancies, PUPPP usually limited to primigravidae
Other triggers	OCP within 1–5 months of delivery of affected pregnancy, menstruation	No association with OCP or subsequent menstrual cycles
Maternal risks	None reported	None reported
Fetal/neonatal risks	Prematurity (20%), growth restriction, signs of placental insufficiency; 5–10% neonates may have transient skin lesions lasting for up to 2 months until maternal antibodies cleared	None
Additional fetal surveillance (serial growth scans, AFI, Doppler, etc.)	Indicated if any suspicion of placental insufficiency, surveillance escalated if IUGR suspected	None indicated
Antibodies	Majority have circulating anti-HLA antibodies esp. HLA-DR3 /DR4	No associated circulating anti-HLA antibodies
DIF of perilesional skin	Characteristic linear band of complement at the basement membrane zone	No such feature on DIF examination
Histology of skin biopsy	Inflammatory exudate in dermal-epidermal junction and perivascular spaces	Normal epidermis with some spongiosis, parakeratosis, some dermal oedema
Other autoimmune conditions	Associated with other conditions, e.g. Grave's, Hashimoto's thyroiditis, pernicious anaemia	No association
Management		
Primary aim	To suppress new blister formation, alleviate intense pruritus	Alleviation of intense pruritus
Medication	**Mainstay of treatment: systemic (oral) steroids** Topical steroids only of limited help. Antihistamines to aid sleep. In steroid-resistant cases, rarely plasmapheresis/immunoadsorption may be indicated	**Mainstay of management: potent topical steroids applied 2–3 times a day.** In very severe cases systemic steroids (Prednisolone) may be indicated. Antihistamines to aid sleep, of limited benefit otherwise
Other measures	If on systemic steroids for prolonged period, screen for drug-induced gestational diabetes	Cool baths, emollients. GTT screening not required when only topical steroids used
Labour, delivery	Mode of delivery has no impact on course of PG postpartum. If IUGR identified, close monitoring in labour. If on systemic steroids, bolus IM/IV 100 mg hydrocortisone 6–8-hourly during labour and delivery and 6 h postpartum	Mode of delivery has no impact on course of PUPPP postpartum. No need for hydrocortisone bolus when only potent topical steroids used. If on systemic steroids for a few weeks, consider bolus IM/IV 100 mg hydrocortisone 6–8-hourly during labour, delivery and 6 h postpartum
Breastfeeding	Encouraged, may curtail duration of PG in postpartum	Encouraged, but no impact on duration of postpartum PUPPP which spontaneously resolves in 4–6 weeks
Before postnatal discharge	Continuation of systemic steroids at minimal levels to alleviate symptoms. Recovery may take several weeks, months, sometimes even longer. Advise not to use OCP for contraception for 5–6 months as PG can recur. Warn patient that occasionally PG may recur with resumption of menstruation Inform patient about high risk of recurrence in future pregnancies	Reassure patient regarding spontaneous recovery within 4–6 weeks after delivery. Advise continuation of low-dose topical steroids during this time, emollients, cool baths, etc. No need to avoid OCP. Very little risk of recurrence in any future pregnancy

DIF, direct immunofluorescence; GTT, glucose tolerance test; IUGR, intrauterine growth retardation; OCP, oral contraceptive pill.

7. Ambros-Rudolph CM, et al. The specific dermatoses of pregnancy revisited and reclassified: results of a retrospective two-center study on 505 pregnant patients. J Am Acad Dermatol. 2006;54: 395–404.
8. Ahmadi S, Powell FC. Pruritic urticarial papules and plaques of pregnancy: current status. Australas J Dermatol 2005;46: 53–58.

12.2 Pemphigoid Gestationis

FACT FILE

- Rare autoimmune blistering skin condition unique to pregnancy or postpartum period.[1,2]
- Not caused by or linked to herpesvirus, so old name of herpes gestationis is misleading and now replaced by **pemphigoid gestationis (PG)**.
- PG causes intensely pruritic papular, vesicular, bullous skin eruptions or urticarial plaques with tense vesicles or bullae within the plaques.
- Occurs in about 1 in 2000 to 1 in 50 000 pregnancies; rare in black populations, reflecting the association with specific HLA haplotypes.
- Circulating IgG antibodies against hemidesmosomal proteins **BP 180** and **BP 230** have been identified in the majority of patients with PG. The binding of the IgG to the basement membrane between the epidermis and dermis triggers an immune response resulting in the formation of subepidermal vesicles and blisters.
- Almost all patients with PG have demonstrable anti-HLA antibodies. HLA-DR3/DR4 is present in 45–85%[3] with PG, vs 3–25% in the general population. The placenta is the main source of paternal HLA against which the anti-HLA antibodies are directed, triggering PG.

Clinical presentation and course

- Usually begins in second or third trimester, but may occasionally occur in the first trimester or in the immediate postpartum period.
- Abrupt onset of intense pruritus followed by erythematous lesions usually starting from the umbilical area, spreading outwards to involve the trunk and limbs.
- Characteristically, the umbilical region is invariably involved, while the face, soles, palms, and mucous membranes are usually spared.
- In 75% of cases, a relative remission is seen in in the last few weeks of pregnancy, but invariably flares up at the time of delivery and postpartum. Spontaneous regression is seen.
- About 25% of cases are reported in the immediate postpartum period and can be severe, lasting for weeks to months.[4,5]
- Recurrences can occur with menstruation, or with the use of the oral contraceptive pill, usually if started within 1–5 months after delivery of the affected pregnancy.[5,6]
- Breastfeeding appears to curtail the postpartum course of PG[6] with average time for resolution of both bullous and urticarial lesions being 5–24 weeks in breastfeeding mothers compared with 24–68 weeks for those who do not breastfeed.
- ***PG does not pose any maternal risk.***
- ***The impact of PG on the fetus*** is still debated. While some studies did not find any increased risk,[7] others[8,9,10] found a link between PG and small for gestational age (SGA) and prematurity (20%) especially if PG had appeared in the first or early second trimester. At present, an association between PG and potential placental insufficiency cannot be excluded and fetal surveillance may need to be stepped up, especially in the third trimester.[11,12]
- Such surveillance can include serial growth and amniotic fluid volume scans with Doppler; if growth restriction is suspected, weekly. Doppler studies, AFI and CTG may be considered.[1]
- In up to 10% of maternal PG, transient skin lesions are seen in the neonate as a result of passive transplacental transfer of maternal IgG antibodies. These lesions are usually mild and resolve within 3 months as maternal antibodies are cleared.[2]
- **Recurrence risk** in a subsequent pregnancy can be as high as 95% and may be more severe and of earlier onset, irrespective of whether the father is the same partner or a new one.[13,14] In 5–8% of cases, however, the subsequent pregnancy may be unaffected, only to recur in a third pregnancy.[14,15]
- PG has also been reported with molar pregnancies and choriocarcinoma.[16]
- In 5–10% of cases PG may be associated with other autoimmune conditions such as Grave's disease, Hashimoto's thyroiditis and pernicious anaemia.[14,15]

Differential diagnosis

See Table 12.1 in 'Pruritic papules and plaques of pregnancy' Fact File.

- PUPPP
- Bullous pemphigoid
- Linear IgA dermatosis
- Cicatricial pemphigoid

Diagnosis

- The initial diagnosis is based on the characteristic appearance of the affected areas and the abrupt onset of symptoms. The lesions usually begin in the periumbilical area, which is invariably uninvolved in PUPPP.
- Laboratory investigations are non-specific and may only show eosinophilia and elevated ESR.
- Skin biopsy needs to be taken from the skin around the actual blister (perilesional skin). If taken directly from the vesicle or bullae, necrosis from the blister can obscure the picture.
- Histology findings show inflammatory infiltrate is localized to the dermal–epidermal junction and perivascular areas.
- Direct immunofluorescence (DIF) examination of the perilesional skin detects a characteristic linear band of complement C3 at the basement membrane zone.

Treatment

- ***The primary goal of treatment is the suppression of new blisters, relief of symptoms, and prevention of secondary infection.***
- **Multidisciplinary involvement** of dermatology, obstetrics, and midwifery is required. The neonatologists must also be alerted as 5–10% of babies can be born with transient PG lesions, due to passive transfer of maternal antibodies.
- While **topical steroids** such as triamcinolone acetonide cream (0.1% up to 6 times/day) may help mild symptoms, **systemic oral steroids** are the mainstay of symptom control in PG. Prednisolone may be started at a dose of about 40 mg oral per day or 0.3–0.5 mg/kg per day.
- Once there is alleviation of pruritus and blistering with this dose of prednisolone, the dosage can be reduced to the minimum required to control the disease. Sometimes addition of steroid-sparing drugs such as azathioprine may be required to allow reduction of dosage of steroids. In postpartum flares a temporary increase in steroid dose may be required.
- **Antihistamines** (diphenhydramine) may be added for symptom control.
- Screening for **steroid-induced transient diabetes** is recommended when steroids have been used for several weeks.
- **Bolus doses of 100 mg hydrocortisone** IV/IM are required just before a Caesarean section as well as at 6–8 h intervals during labour and at delivery as well as the first 6–12 h after delivery in those who have been on systemic steroids for control of PG symptoms during pregnancy.
- In some cases resistant to maximum safe doses of prednisolone, plasmapheresis[16] and immunopheresis[17,18] have also been used.

Information for patients

Please see Information for patients: Pemphigoid gestationis (p. 526)

References

1. Sherard G B III, Atkinson SM Jr. Pruritic dermatological conditions in pregnancy. Obst Gynecol Surv 2001;56: 427–432.
2. Shimanovich I, et al. Pemphigoid gestationis: new insights into the pathogenesis lead to novel diagnostic tools. BJOG 2002;109: 970–976.
3. Shornick J. Dermatoses of pregnancy. Semin Cutan Med Surg 1998;17: 172–181.
4. Shorrnik J. Herpes gestationis. Dermatol Clin 1993;11: 527–533.
5. Shornick J. Herpes gestationis. J Am Acad Dermatol 1987;17: 539–555.
6. Holmes R, et al. Clues to the aetiology and pathogenesis of herpes gestationis. Br J Dermatol 1983;109: 131–139.
7. Kolodny R. Herpes gestationis: A new assessment of incidence, diagnosis and fetal prognosis. Am J Obstet Gynecol 1969:104: 39–45.
8. Lawley TC et al. Fetal and maternal risk factors in herpes gestationis. Arch Dermatol 1978;114: 552–555.
9. Holmes R, et al. A comparative study of toxic erythema of pregnancy and herpes gestationis. Br J Dermatol 1982;106: 499–510.
10. Shornick J, Black M. Fetal risks in herpes gestationis. J Am Acad Dermatol 1992;26: 63–68.
11. Shornick J, Black M. Secondary autoimmune diseases in herpes gestationis. J Am Acad Dermatol 1992;26: 563–566.
12. Holmes R, Black M. The fetal prognosis in pemphigoid gestationis (herpes gestationis). Br J Dermatol 1984;110: 67–72.
13. Chen S, et al. Herpes gestationis in a mother and child. J Am Acad Dermatol 1999;40: 847–849.
14. Semkova K, Black M. Pemphigoid gestationis: current insights into pathogenesis and treatment. Eur J Obstet Gynecol Reprod Biol 2009;145: 138–144.
15. Jenkins RE, et al. Clinical features and management of 87 patients with pemphigoid gestationis. Clin Exp Dermatol 2006:24: 255–259.
16. Van de Wiel A, et al. Plasma exchange in herpes gestationis. Br Med J 1980;281 (6247): 1041–1042.
17. Wohrl S, et al. Pemphigoid gestationis:treatment with immunoapheresis. J Dtsch Dermatol Ges 2003;1: 126–130.
18. Westermann L, et al. Glucocorticosteroid-resistant pemphigoid gestationis: successful treatment with adjuvant immunoadsorption. J Dermatol 2012;39: 168–171.

12.3 Scleroderma and Systemic Sclerosis

FACT FILE

- **Scleroderma** is a rare autoimmune tissue disorder, more common in women than in men (5:1 ratio).[1]
- Scleroderma, especially systemic sclerosis, is a multisystem disease with increased complications during pregnancy. With careful antenatal evaluations, discussion of potential problems and multidisciplinary care, outcomes can be optimized.

Clinical manifestations

- Scleroderma can present as a:
  - **localized cutaneous** form: Thick, waxy skin, especially on the forearms and hands
  - **systemic sclerosis:** A multisystem autoimmune disease associated with Raynaud's phenomenon, renal or pulmonary disease, especially pulmonary hypertension
  - **CREST syndrome:** with calcinosis, Raynaud's phenomenon, oesophageal involvement, sclerodactyly.
- The skin in scleroderma is taut, bound down to produce sclerodactyly, beaking of the nose, fixed facial expression, limitation of mouth opening, skin ulceration, and partial digital amputation.
- Systemic involvement due to obliteration of the end arteries and collagen proliferation within tissues can produce progressive fibrosis, usually involving the oesophagus (80%), lungs (45%), heart (40%), and kidneys (35%).
- ***The most serious sequelae for the mother during pregnancy could be development of pulmonary hypertension or renal crisis.***

Effect of pregnancy on scleroderma/systemic sclerosis

- If only localized cutaneous scleroderma without any organ involvement, prognosis of pregnancy is good.[2,3]
- In those with diffuse systemic sclerosis and renal involvement, there is an increased risk of significant and rapid overall deterioration and renal crisis.
- Symptoms of Raynaud's disease may actually improve during pregnancy due to vasodilation and increased blood flow.
- Worsening of gastroesophageal reflux especially in the third trimester.[4,5]
- ***Those with severe pulmonary fibrosis/pulmonary hypertension have a significant risk of mortality during pregnancy or postpartum.***

Effect of scleroderma on pregnancy

- Previously, pregnant patients with systemic sclerosis were thought to be at high risk for poor fetal and maternal outcome. However, more recently, careful planning, close monitoring, and appropriate therapy can allow these patients to have a successful pregnancy.[3,4,5,6,7]
- In general, 70–80% have a good outcome if there is no systemic disease.
- In systemic disease, especially with hypertension, there is an increased risk of miscarriages, preterm delivery, pre-eclampsia, IUGR, and increased perinatal mortality.
- If there is the concomitant presence of anti-Ro or anti-La antibodies, **fetal and neonatal heart block** must be considered.
- These patients can pose significant **anaesthetic challenges**, ranging from difficult IV access to difficult endotracheal intubation or problems with regional anaesthesia.

Pre-pregnancy assessment and advice

- Pre-pregnancy assessment and advice is particularly important in those with systemic manifestation of scleroderma.
- ***Pregnancy outcome is directly associated with the state of disease at the time of conception.***
- Assessment for presence of organ complications which would pose risks during pregnancy.
- Those with pulmonary hypertension, extensive pulmonary fibrosis, or renal failure should be strongly advised not to embark on a pregnancy because of the high risk of maternal mortality.
- Pre-pregnancy advice must be based on:
  - Recent renal function tests
  - Autoimmune antibodies for lupus and antiphospholipid syndrome (APS) as well as anti-Ro antibodies
  - Echocardiography
  - Recent lung function tests
- In order to reduce complications, pregnancies in women with systemic sclerosis should be planned when the disease is stable, and should be avoided in rapidly progressing diffuse disease because such patients are at a greater risk for developing serious cardiopulmonary and renal problems.[3]
- In patients with systemic sclerosis and severe visceral involvement, the presence of significant cardiomyopathy (ejection fraction <30%), pulmonary hypertension, severe restrictive lung disease (forced vital capacity <50%), renal insufficiency, etc., adverse outcomes of pregnancy are to be expected and pre-pregnancy advice should be to avoid pregnancy in such circumstances.[8]
- In case of rapid worsening of disease activity, termination in the first trimester or induced preterm birth in the last trimester (see note below regarding avoiding steroids).... may need consideration.
- In order to minimize risks, a multidisciplinary team should be involved in the antenatal care of scleroderma patients.

Management during pregnancy

- Regular multidisciplinary assessments for disease activity, blood pressure monitoring, and serial scans for growth, liquor, and Doppler flow are essential.
- If lupus positive, low-dose aspirin needs to be started from early pregnancy and continued throughout pregnancy. If APS positive, LMWH and low-dose aspirin need to be advised. If anti-Ro positive, arrange fetal ECHO scan and inform paediatricians about the risk of possible neonatal heart block.
- Early assessment by a senior anaesthetist in the anaesthetic high-risk clinic should be arranged.
- The greatest danger in pregnant women with systemic sclerosis is the occurrence of renal crisis, secondary to acute-onset severe hypertension. This can be life-threatening for both mother and fetus.
- In contrast to pre-eclampsia, delivering the fetus does not affect the hypertension or renal dysfunction. Even mild hypertension should be considered potentially very serious in those with systemic sclerosis.
- Pre-eclampsia rate does not seem to be increased in those with systemic sclerosis.[7]
- Renal crises can present with acute-onset severe hypertension with deteriorating renal function. Close monitoring of renal function is therefore essential.
- ***ACE inhibitors are generally contraindicated in pregnancy due to the teratogenic risks and fetal renal dysfunction. However, if a renal crisis develops in pregnancy in those with systemic sclerosis, ACE inhibitors will have to be used for aggressive control of the blood pressure.***
- ***In those with severe renal involvement, steroids may precipitate a renal crisis[3] and must be avoided (including steroids used for acceleration of fetal lung maturity). However, this applies to only those patients with scleroderma with severe renal disease and not in those with non-renal manifestations.***
- The majority of patients need treatment for severe gastro-oesophageal reflux especially in the third trimester. Histamine

blockers and proton pump inhibitors may be used for the treatment of oesophageal reflux, nausea and vomiting.[9] Ranitidine and metoclopramide may be required.

- Timing and mode of delivery depend on obstetric indications, gestational age, and the presence of systemic organ complications.
- There is a high risk of rapid deterioration after delivery, and close monitoring should continue.

Information for patients

Please see **Information for patients: Scleroderma, systemic sclerosis, and pregnancy** (p. 527)

References

1. Mayes MD, et al. Prevalence, incidence, survival, and disease characteristics of systemic sclerosis in a large US population. Arthritis Rheum 2003;48: 2246–2255.
2. Miniati I, et al. Pregnancy in systemic sclerosis. Rheumatology 2008;47: iii16–iii18
3. Chakravarty EF. Vascular complications of systemic sclerosis during pregnancy. Int J Rheumatol 2010;2010: 287248.
4. Chin KA, et al. Mallory-Weiss syndrome complicating pregnancy in a patient with scleroderma: diagnosis and management;. Br J Obstet Gynaecol 1995;102: 498–500.
5. Cho KH, et al. A case of Mallory-Weiss syndrome complicating pregnancy in a patient with scleroderma. Korean J Intern Med 2003;18: 238–240.
6. Launay D, et al. Systemic sclerosis and pregnancy. Rev Med Interne 2002;23: 607–621
7. Jimenez FX, et al. Scleroderma and pregnancy: obstetrical complications and the impact of pregnancy on the course of the disease. Med Clin 1999;113: 761–764.
8. Steen VD. Pregnancy in scleroderma. Rheum Dis Clin North Am 2007;33: 345–358.
9. Diav-Citrin O, et al. The safety of proton pump inhibitors in pregnancy: a multicentre prospective controlled study Aliment. Pharmacol Ther 2005;21: 269–275.

Pre-pregnancy assessment and advice for patient with scleroderma/ systemic sclerosis

- Information from rheumatologist/immunologist, renal and/or respiratory physician with up-to-date assessments of disease severity and organ involvement before maternal medicine obstetrician meets patient for pre-pregnancy counselling based on:
  - renal function tests
  - presence/absence of autoimmune antibodies including lupus anticoagulant, antiphospholipid antibodies, anti-Ro antibodies, anti-La antibodies
  - lung function tests
  - echocardiography

GP or community midwife refers any patient with pre-existing scleroderma/systemic sclerosis as early as possible in first trimester to the maternal medicine or specialist antenatal clinic

↓

Maternal medicine or specialist antenatal clinic

- Baseline renal function tests
- Referral to respiratory physician, cardiologist, anaesthetic high-risk clinic, rheumatologist as necessary for assessments: may need further assessment later in pregnancy
- Close BP monitoring
- Gastro-oesophageal reflux treated with ranitidine ± metoclopramide
- Arrange serial scans 28, 32, and 36 weeks with Dopplers
- If lupus/APS or anti-Ro positive, see relevant care pathways. Inform Paeds regarding possible neonatal heart block
- If renal crisis develops, urgent multidisciplinary input, treatment with ACE inhibitors to be considered

↓

- Frequency of visits to maternal medicine/specialist antenatal clinic to be individualized according to disease severity
- Assess progress of pregnancy, fetal growth scans, Dopplers, vigilance for PIH, preeclampsia
- Advise re fetal movements
- Close monitoring of fetal well-being -consider BPP/Doppler studies + AFI and CTG once a week from about 32–34 weeks
- Renal function and lung function tests as planned with multidisciplinary specialists
- Confirm has had anaesthetic review

→ Routine antenatal visits to community midwife/GP continue according to NICE protocol with vigilance for PIH, pre-eclampsia, fetal activity

↓

Timing and mode of delivery depending on obstetric indications and any complications of disease

12.4 Neurofibromatosis

FACT FILE

Epidemiology and inheritance

- **Neurofibromatosis (NF)** is an autosomal dominant common genetic disorder. It can affect multiple organ systems that develop from the ectodermal and mesodermal tissues.
- Two distinct forms of NF are recognized on clinical and genetic grounds: **NF1** and **NF2**.
- **NF1** or **von Recklinghausen's neurofibromatosis** or **peripheral NF** comprises 90–95% of all cases of NF.
- The remaining 10% of cases are of **NF2**.
- The birth incidence of NF1 lies between 1 in 2500 and 1 in 3300, and its prevalence in the population is 1 in 5000.[1,2]
- The chance of inheritance from an affected parent is about 50%. In 30–50% cases, there is no family history and these are sporadic cases due to gene mutation.

Clinical manifestations

- The degree to which individuals with NF are affected can vary greatly.

NF1

Diagnostic features include:[1]

- Café-au-lait spots: Symmetrical flat areas of hyperpigmented skin seen in newborns and found in 95% of adults with NF1.
- Freckling of the intertriginous area of the armpit and groin.
- Cutaneous neurofibromas: Discrete benign, soft tissue lesions that are characteristic of the condition and develop in the dermis of the skin.
- Nodular neurofibromatosis arises in peripheral nerves.
- Plexiform NF occurs in NF1 with infiltration of long portions of the nerve and surrounding tissues causing disfigurement.
- Other tumours such as **phaeochromocytomas** or **malignant gliomas** may coexist.
- Macrocephaly, relatively short stature are often seen.
- ***Epilepsy and learning difficulties, deafness, vision problems.***
- ***Skeletal abnormalities*** such as thoracic spinal deformities causing kyphoscoliosis, bowed legs, flail chest, etc.
- ***Hypertension***[3,4,5] is found in 6% of NF1 patients. In 70% of these cases, essential hypertension coexists with NF but in about 30%, hypertension is secondary to renal artery stenosis, coarctation of the aorta or phaeochromocytoma.
- About 0.1–5.7% of patients with NF1 have phaeochromocytoma, but almost 25% of those with phaeochromocytoma have NF1.[3]

NF2

- NF2 is characterized by bilateral vestibular schwannomas—tumours arising from cranial nerve VIII leading to hearing loss.

Neurofibromatosis and pregnancy

- No effect on fertility, but **increased risk of complications such as spontaneous miscarriage (21%), preterm delivery, IUGR (13%), stillbirths (8.7%), pregnancy-induced hypertension/pre-eclampsia.**[6,7,8,9,10,11,12] **Caesarean section rates are increased in NF1 patients.**[9,10,11,12]
- Pregnancy can cause an increase in the size and number of the cutaneous neurofibromas,[1] which is of relevance if there are spinal plexiform neurofibromas or pelvic neurofibromas.
- ***Hypertension is often associated with pregnancy and is a major cause of morbidity, even mortality in those with NF1.***[13,14,15,16] ***Arterial blood pressure needs to be monitored with care throughout pregnancy.***
- Hypertension can be due to renal artery stenosis, coarctation of the aorta, or phaeochromocytoma. Pre-eclampsia and HELLP are more common, especially when renal–vascular hypertension exists.
- **NF manifestations can pose serious anaesthetic challenges**[1] due to **airway problems, chest wall and spine deformities, intrapulmonary neurofibromas, hypertension, presence of coarctation of the aorta, phaeochromocytoma, epilepsy**, or undiagnosed **CNS tumours**. Siting of regional anaesthetic may be technically difficult if scoliosis or spinal neurofibromas are present as well due to cutaneous lesions.
- Patients with NF may also have an increased sensitivity to non-depolarizing neuromuscular blocking anaesthetic drugs.[1]

Information for patients

Please see Information for patients: Neurofibromatosis and pregnancy (p. 528)

References

1. Hirsch NP, et al. Neurofibromatosis: clinical presentations and anaesthetic implications. Br J Anaesth 2001;86: 555–564.
2. Huson SMA, et al. Genetic study of von Recklinghausen neurofibromatosis in south east Wales. 1. Prevalence, fitness, mutation rate, and effect of parental transmission on severity. J Med Genet 1989;26: 704–711.
3. McClellan MW, et al. Von Recklinghausen's disease and phaeochromocytomas. J Urol 1999;162: 1582–1586.
4. Bourke E, Gatenby PBB Renal artery dysplasia with hypertension in neurofibromatosis. Br Med J 1971; ii: 681–682.
5. Sharma AK Renal artery aneurysm, hypertension and neurofibromatosis. J R Soc Med 1991;84: 373–374.
6. Dugoff L, Sujansky E Neurofibromatosis type 1 and pregnancy. Am J Med Genet 1996;66: 7–10.
7. Hadi HA Clinical significance of neurofibromatosis in pregnancy. Am J Perinatol 1995;12: 459–461.
8. Hagymasy L, et al. Neurofibromatosis type 1 with pregnancy-associated renovascular hypertension, and the syndrome of haemolysis, elevated liver enzymes, and low platelets. Am J Obstet Gynecol 1998;179: 272–274.
9. Huson SM Recent developments in the diagnosis and management of neurofibromatosis. Arch Dis Child 1989;64: 745–749.
10. Ferner RE, et al. Guidelines for the diagnosis and management of individuals with neurofibromatosis 1. J Med Genet 2007;44: 81–88.
11. Segal D, et al. Neurofibromatosis in pregnancy. Maternal and perinatal outcome. Eur J Obstet Gynecol Reprod Biol 1999;84: 59–61.
12. Weissman A, et al. Neurofibromatosis and pregnancy. An update. J Reprod Med 1993;38: 890–896.
13. Pilmore HL, et al. Neurofibromatosis and renovascular hypertension presenting in early pregnancy. Nephrol Dial Transplant 1997;12: 187–189.
14. Swapp GH, Main RA Neurofibromatosis in pregnancy. Br J Dermatol. 1973;80: 431–435.
15. Edwards JNT, et al. Neurofibromatosis and severe hypertension in pregnancy. Br J Obstet Gynaecol 1983;90: 528–531.
16. Sharma JB, et al. Maternal and perinatal complications in neurofibromatosis during pregnancy. Int J Gynaecol Obstet 1991;34: 221–227.

CARE PATHWAY

Pre-pregnancy multidisciplinary assessment and advice for patient with neurofibromatosis

- Genetic history and counselling—autosomal dominant, but 50% are random gene mutations. If one parent is affected, 50% chance of inheritance by offspring
- Confirm type of NF—NF1 or NF2: 90% are NF1
- Discuss availability of invasive prenatal testing by CVS or amniocentesis to identify defects in chromosome 17 q (NF1) or in chromosome 22 (NF2) if parents opt for it
- Multidisciplinary assessment of manifestations of condition and of comorbidities
- Comorbidities—hypertension, kyphoscoliosis, other CNS tumours, epilepsy, cardiovascular abnormalities (e.g. renal stenosis, coarctation of aorta)
- Imaging studies best done pre-pregnancy, may include CT/MRI
- Assess pre-pregnancy BP—if hypertensive, it is essential that hypertension due to phaeochromocytoma, renal stenosis, or coarctation of aorta is excluded. Appropriate endocrine and imaging studies to be organized
- Discuss possible enlargement of cutaneous neurofibromas, also of pelvic or spinal plexiform lesions if present
- Discuss increased pregnancy complications in NF patients including risks of spontaneous miscarriage, preterm birth, IUGR (~13%), stillbirth (~8–9%), pregnancy-induced hypertension, pre-eclampsia and HELLP, threefold increase of Caesarean delivery
- Discuss maternal and fetal assessment and monitoring for above pregnancy problems
- Change antihypertensive medication if on ACE inhibitors, to methyldopa or labetalol
- Advise peri-pregnancy folic acid. If on antiepileptic medications that have antifolate action, advise high-dose folic acid (5 mg/day) starting from before pregnancy
- Advise low-dose aspirin to reduce risk of pre-eclampsia, starting from first trimester to continue till end of pregnancy
- Reassure patient that though a future pregnancy is likely to be complex, with appropriate antenatal care and increased surveillance, most patients have a good outcome, especially if severe hypertension is not an issue

↓

First visit to maternal medicine antenatal clinic following early referral in first trimester from community midwife/GP

- Confirm viable pregnancy and dates
- Obtain detailed history of familial or sporadic variety, type of NF manifestations in individual patient, any known associated comorbidities, and current medications
- If patient has not had pre-pregnancy assessment/counselling, instigate urgent referrals to genetics, endocrinology, senior anaesthetic assessment, neurology, cardiology, urology, etc. as relevant
- Referral to tertiary unit highly advisable for further pregnancy, delivery, and postpartum management if phaeochromocytoma, renal artery stenosis, or coarctation of aorta
- Discuss NF diagnostic prenatal tests available (CVS/amnio), risks of procedure-related miscarriage rate
- BP check: If already on antihypertensives, check whether these are pregnancy compatible. If not, change to methyldopa ± labetalol
- Prescribe low-dose aspirin to start from now and to continue till end of pregnancy
- If on antifolate antiepileptics for epilepsy, ensure she is on high-dose folic acid (5 mg/day)
- Discuss increased risk of pregnancy complications and additional fetal and maternal surveillance required in NF patients. Risks of spontaneous miscarriage, preterm birth, IUGR (~13%), stillbirth (~8–9%), pregnancy induced hypertension, pre-eclampsia and HELLP, threefold increase of Caesarean delivery, etc. to be discussed and clear management plans to be documented
- Organize BP surveillance at least once in 2 weeks, aiming to maintain good control with BP medication. Renal function tests as relevant, once in each trimester
- Arrange uterine artery Doppler at ~20–22 weeks
- Arrange serial fetal growth scans ± Dopplers from 26 weeks onwards
- Further maternal medicine antenatal clinic follow-up visits to be individualized depending on maternal BP control, presence of pregnancy problems (e.g. IUGR) that might develop. Suggested model :Monthly appointments till 26 weeks, then fortnightly
- Community midwife visits for routine antenatal checks to continue in between clinic visits, avoiding overlap

↓

Further visits to maternal medicine antenatal clinic

- Assess progress of pregnancy, results of maternal and fetal surveillance to date
- Confirm patient has had reviews by other specialities—anaesthetics, neurology, endocrinology, cardiology, etc.—as relevant
- If epileptic and on antifolate AED medication, prescribe oral vitamin K 10 mg daily from about 37 weeks onwards
- If pelvic neurofibromas distort pelvic cavity or if severe kyphoscoliosis exists, elective Caesarean indicated after detailed anaesthetics work-up
- If IUGR, earlier delivery by either IOL or elective Caesarean section
- **Clear plans with multidisciplinary input for intrapartum management to be made and documented,** including discussions with patient regarding of mode of delivery, management of labour and delivery, analgesia for labour, delivery, anaesthetic for Caesarean section, etc.
- These plans must be shared with all professionals caring for the pregnant patient with NF and with the patient herself
- Neonatologist must be informed prior to delivery date as 50% chance of offspring inheriting NF—for neonatal and later assessments

↓

Postpartum

- Prior to discharge, contraception advice- to avoid COCP if hypertensive
- Advise patient to seek pre-pregnancy assessment/counselling before next pregnancy

12.5 Epidermolysis Bullosa

FACT FILE

Epidemiology

- **Epidermolysis bullosa (EB)** is a rare inherited group of heterogenous diseases characterized by the development of skin blisters produced by even minor degrees of friction, trauma, or heat.[1,2,3,4,5]
- These disorders are the result of a variety of inherited defects of the proteins that are required to maintain skin integrity.
- Incidence worldwide is about 1 in 50 000 births, irrespective of sex or ethnicity.
- Effects of EB can range from death in early infancy to increasing morbidity and disability but a near-normal life expectancy.[2]

Clinical manifestations

- EB subtypes are described according to the depth at which the resultant blister occurs.[1,2,3]
- Four main types of EB are described: **simplex**, **junctional**, **dystrophic**, and **Kindler syndrome**.
- **EB simplex** is the most common type of EB, characterized by blistering in the intradermal level of the skin. Blistering is most common at sites that are most exposed to friction. Permanent scarring is minimal and near-normal lifespan can be expected. Mild cases may not be diagnosed till adulthood.
- **Junctional EB** is an autosomal recessive variety with the **Herlitz subtype being lethal in early infancy**. In the non-Herlitz form, large blisters in the lamina lucida layer of the skin with granulation tissue and atrophic scarring are typical. Extracutaneous features of this subtype can include mucosal blistering, gastrointestinal (pyloric atresia or stenosis), urological (ureterovesicular obstruction, hydronephrosis), and laryngeal involvement (causing airway obstruction)
- **Dystrophic EB** results from abnormal production of collagen VII with very fragile skin and other epithelial surface blisters and extensive scarring. There is sometimes an overlap of clinical features in the subtypes of dystrophic EB.[4] The majority are of the less severe **autosomal dominant** form, with blisters seen mainly in areas most exposed to friction.
- Only a minority suffer the **recessive form of dystrophic EB** which causes severe effects with widespread blisters which are slow to heal, atrophic scarring leading to flexural contractures of various joints, debilitating hand and foot deformities ('mitten deformities', pseudosyndactyly), loss of nails, teeth, and hair. Severe oesophageal and mouth scarring and strictures can lead to malnutrition, anaemia, weight loss, and growth limitation.
- **Kindler EB** is an autosomal recessive form which manifests in infancy with photosensitivity and blistering. These seem to improve over time but some may develop oesophageal, urethral, vaginal, or anal stenosis later in life.[1,2]

Genetic counselling if either partner has EB

- Referral for specialist genetic counselling is an important part of pre-pregnancy preparation.[6]
- The carrier rate of the **recessive form of dystrophic EB** in the general population is thought to be about 1 in 350, so if either partner has this type of EB the chance of the offspring having EB is about 1 in 700.
- Carrier rate for autosomal **recessive non-Herlitz junctional** EB is about 1 in 300 of the general population. If either partner has this form of EB, the chances that the offspring will have EB is 1 in 600.
- ***If either parent has an autosomal dominant variety of EB (i.e. dominant dystrophic EB or EB simplex), there is often a strong family history. Very rarely there is no such family history as the EB may have resulted from a de-novo mutation.***
- In autosomal dominant conditions there is no carrier state and the chance of the offspring having EB is in the order of 1 in 2.
- **Prenatal testing for EB** is now available in specialist centres employing chorionic villus sampling (CVS).

Management of pregnancy, delivery, and puerperium when the mother has EB

- **Multidisciplinary management** with the midwife, obstetrician, dermatologist, geneticist, neonatologist, and anaesthetist is of vital importance in EB.
- **Antenatal management is often intensive throughout pregnancy** and plans and additional preparations required for delivery should be in place well ahead of time.
- As in all cases of EB, the basic objective of care is to **avoid blistering and secondary infection**.
- Patients with extracutaneous complications of EB need careful surveillance in addition to standard care.
- The limited literature available indicates that **pregnancy does not affect the underlying skin condition of EB and women with EB do not develop any non-dermatological antenatal complications compared with the general population.**[3,7,8]

Antenatal management

- Prenatal diagnosis by CVS is available in specialist centres and this must be discussed with the patient.
- Care should be taken to use adequate padding when using blood pressure cuffs or applying even slight pressure during palpation. Adequate lubrication and only minimal pressure is to be applied when ultrasound transducer or probes are placed on the skin surface. Cardiotocography belts must be very well padded and applied for as short a time as strictly necessary.
- Access to veins may be difficult in the presence of excessive blistering or atrophic scarring and contractures. Tourniquet application may need to be avoided and gentle manual pressure may be preferable. Care must be taken when using spirit swabs prior to drawing blood. The routine use of adhesive dressings must be avoided in EB.
- Nutritional deficiency and anaemia are particularly common in those with scarring and mucocutaneous blisters of the oropharyngeal area restricting mastication and swallowing as well as in those with oesophageal strictures. Symptomatic strictures may need repeated dilatation and in severe cases nutrient supplements may need to be given via a gastric tube or parenterally. Oral iron, folic acid, vitamin D, and calcium supplementation are required in many pregnant women with EB.
- Women with dystrophic EB or non-Herlitz junctional EB are particularly prone to gum and dentition problems. Periodontal problems can be causally associated with several pregnancy complications such as miscarriage, IUGR, preterm delivery, and bacterial meningitis.[9,10] Women with periodontal manifestations of EB must be encouraged to see their dentists and reminded that dental treatment is free during pregnancy and for 1 year after childbirth.
- Blisters and slow-healing lesions in the vulvovaginal, groin, or abdominal sites must be receive prompt treatment with appropriate antibiotics(oral ± topical) as guided by the sensitivity profile from wound swabs. If blisters require dressings, soft silicone dressings are to be used.
- While no increase is reported in gestational diabetes in women with EB,[3] it is recommended that renal function be monitored with care in pregnancy because of the not infrequent association between exacerbations of dystrophic EB and renal impairment.[3,8]
- There may be certain ultrasound abnormalities which, in the absence of prenatal diagnosis, could raise suspicion of the baby being possibly affected by EB as well.

- These signs include visualization of a distended stomach and polyhydramnios (suggestive of pyloric stenosis); fetal hydronephrosis (if urethral stenosis is present); ear, nose, or limb deformities; or a 'snowflake' sign seen in utero indicating fetal skin denudation.[5,11,12,13.]

Mode of delivery and anaesthetic considerations

- The most challenging decisions in any EB pregnancy are the **mode of delivery** and **anaesthetic/analgesia requirements**. Detailed discussions with the patient and the anaesthetist are necessary. Antenatal referral to and review by an experienced consultant anaesthetist is required. All such multidisciplinary plans need to be clearly recorded in the patient's hand-held notes as well as in the main hospital notes.
- Vaginal delivery may be the first choice in EB simplex. However, vaginal mucosal blistering and sloughing of the cervical and perineal epithelium are seen more often with dystrophic EB or non-Herlitz form of junctional EB, and Caesarean section may become necessary. Labouring in a dorsal position with direct pressure on the back, buttocks, and elbows can cause severe blistering. Application of vaginal instruments such as forceps and ventouse is also more likely to cause significant blistering and scarring.[3]
- A Caesarean section might provoke blisters, scarring, and secondary infection at the site of the incision, as well as problems of providing suitable anaesthetic for the procedure.
- Extensive antenatal anaesthetic assessment is required by a consultant anaesthetist, one preferably with experience with cases of EB.
- Regional analgesia for both elective and emergency Caesarean delivery, on balance, seems a more suitable option than a general anaesthetic especially in those cases of EB where scarring, contractures, or oesophageal strictures may restrict intubation and airway manipulation.[14,15,16,17]
- Sometimes, however, regional anaesthetic is precluded by the presence of infected bullae at the site.
- If epidural analgesia is administered for pain relief in labour, care must be taken to avoid frictional wiping of the skin surface with antiseptic lotion and the catheters should be secured in place only by a soft silicone dressing and not with adhesive tape.
- At Caesarean section, great care must be taken at each step, from cleaning the skin with antiseptic solution to avoiding the application of pressure on the skin surface on any part of the body by the surgeon and the assistant. Diathermy pads and adhesive tapes must be avoided and all monitoring devices must be specially padded.
- The above preparations and necessary equipment must be planned for during the antenatal period and availability checked well ahead of time. Clear documentation of multidisciplinary plans for both elective and emergency situations must be shared with all involved in the patient's care and with the patient herself.
- Compression stockings should, if possible be avoided because of the inevitable shearing force caused during application and removal.[7]
- The patient must be reassured that breastfeeding is not contraindicated unless there are infected bullae at the site of the nipples and areolae.[7] Well-lubricated nipple shields should be provided.

Information for patients

Please see **Information for patients: Epidermolysis bullosa and pregnancy** (p. 528)

References

1. Heymann WR. Classifying epidermolysis bullosa. J Am Acad Dermatol 2008:59: 1075–1076.
2. Horn H, Tidman M The clinical spectrum of dystrophic epidermolysis bullosa. Br J Dermatol 2002;146: 267–274.
3. Bolt LA, et al. A review of the obstetric management of patients with epidermolysis bullosa. Obstet Med 2010;3: 101–105.
4. Das BB, Sahoo S. Dystrophic epidermolysis bullosa. J Perinatol 2004;24: 41–47.
5. Katorza E, et al. Unusual prenatal sonographic findings of epidermolysis bullosa mimicking an amniotic band constriction ring. J Ultrasound Med 2009;28: 73–75.
6. Sybert VP. Genetic counselling in epidermolysis bullosa. Dermatol Clin 2010;28: 239–243.
7. Baloch MS, et al. Anaesthetic management of two different modes of delivery in patients with dystrophic epidermolysis bullosa. Int J Obstet Anesth 2008;17: 153–158.
8. Buscher U, et al. Pregnancy and delivery in a patient with mutilating dystrophic epidermolysis bullosa (Hallopeau-Siemens type). Obstet Gynecol 1997:89: 817–820.
9. Pirie M, et al. Dental manifestations of pregnancy. Obstetrician and Gynaecologist 2007;9: 21–26.
10. Jeffcoat MK, et al. Periodontal infection and preterm birth: results of a prospective study. J Am Dent Assoc 2001;132: 875–880.
11. Okoye BO, et al. Pyloric atresia: five new cases, a new association, and a review of the literature with guidelines. J Pediatr Surg 2000;35: 1242–1245.
12. de Jenlis Sicot B, et al. Prenatal findings in epidermolysis bullosa with pyloric atresia in a family not known to be at risk. Ultrasound Obstet Gynecol 2005;25: 607–609.
13. Meizner I, Carmi R. The snowflake sign: a sonographic marker for prenatal detection of fetal skin denudation. J Ultrasound Med 1990;9: 607–609.
14. Azizkhan RG, et al. Surgical management of epidermolysis bullosa: Proceedings of the IInd International Symposium on Epidermolysis Bullosa, Santiago, Chile, 2005. Int J Dermatol 2007;46: 801–808.
15. James I, Wark H. Airway management during anaesthesia in patients with epidermolysis bullosa dystrophica. Anaesthesiology 1982;56: 323–326.
16. Ames WA, et al. Anaesthetic management of epidermolysis bullosa. BrJ Anaesth 1999;82: 746–751.
17. Spielman FJ, Mann ES. Subarachnoid and epidural anaesthesia for patients with epidermolysis bullosa. Can J Anaesth 1984;31: 549–551.

CARE PATHWAY

Referral for genetic counselling is recommended when either partner has any form of **epidermolysis bullosa (EB)**

Pre-pregnancy counselling

If the woman has EB this counselling should preferably be at a specialist EB centre and include:

- Assessment of the type of EB and extent of its manifestations
- Assessment of nutritional state and of any anaemia
- If hand contractures or oesophageal strictures are severe, the patient may be advised to consider corrective hand surgery or oesophageal dilatation to improve nutritional state before embarking on a pregnancy
- Prenatal diagnosis is available for diagnosing fetal EB by performing CVS between 8–11 weeks gestation, mention procedure-related risk of miscarriage associated with CVS
- Nutritional supplements including iron, folic acid, vitamin D, and calcium must be prescribed before pregnancy and patient advised to continue throughout pregnancy
- Reassure patient that there are no additional problems, either antenatal or postnatal, and that pregnancy does not worsen the skin condition
- Outline the extra care that will be taken in the course of the routine management of pregnancy
- Advise that the most challenging decisions would be regarding mode of delivery and anaesthetic issues. Multidisciplinary care for the safest management of delivery will be offered and her preferences duly considered
- Advise that breastfeeding is not contraindicated
- Advise that following childbirth, she will need increased assistance to care for the baby and to consider sources of support
- Give DebRA UK EB link and leaflet
- Peri-pregnancy folic acid: If poor nutritional status, prescribe high-dose (5 mg/day) folic acid

↓

Antenatal care

Multidisciplinary team management is vital in the pregnancy care of patients with EB

Community referral to maternal medicine antenatal clinic in early first trimester

First visit to maternal medicine antenatal clinic

All examinations including palpation, checking BP, ultrasound scans, etc. must be performed taking care to avoid friction, and skin trauma

- Confirm viability, dates
- Ascertain type of EB and its manifestations to date. Record of any previous operative procedures or anaesthetic to be sought
- Routine pregnancy bloods by expert phlebotomist if limited venous access
- Discuss CVS for fetal prenatal EB diagnosis. Arrange if patient opts for it. Subsequent management depending on results and parent's choice
- Those with extracutaneous manifestations such as urethral or oesophageal strictures require additional surveillance such as monitoring renal function, dilatation of strictures, etc. with multispecialty involvement
- Early referral to **dermatology follow-up** and for **consultant anaesthetic assessment**
- Nutritional supplementation especially iron, folic acid, vitamin D, and calcium throughout pregnancy
- If periodontal or oral manifestations with poor gum/dentition health advice dental intervention—remind patient about it being free during pregnancy and for the first year after childbirth
- Arrange routine antenatal appointment at 24–28 weeks, advise community care meanwhile
- Similar precautions in the community for BP cuff, gentle palpation to avoid friction on skin surface

↓

Subsequent visits to maternal medicine clinic

- ***Frequency of visits to be decided on a case-by-case basis***
- Same precautions for palpation, BP cuff, phlebotomy, etc. to be observed
- Assess progress of pregnancy, nutritional state
- Ensure the patient is not anaemic and is continuing nutritional supplements
- Confirm she has had appointment to see dermatologist during course of pregnancy
- Confirm she has had detailed assessment by consultant anaesthetist and note opinion
- Note any blisters, bullae over lower abdomen, groin, back, any vulvovaginal lesions, etc. Swabs from bullae to be sent for C&S; if infection, active treatment with appropriate antibiotics
- Discuss options for mode of delivery and patient's preferences
- Arrange a multidisciplinary team meeting if possible, with patient and partner, anaesthetist, obstetrician, neonatologist, dermatologist, senior midwives from ward and delivery suite, specialist wound care nurse
- Detailed plans to be documented both for planned and emergency situations
- All precautions, special devices such as padded transducers of monitoring equipment, etc. required for delivery by either Caesarean section or vaginal route
- Compression stockings only if strictly necessary
- Special dressings required for wound care if Caesarean section and full course of antibiotic continued

↓

Postpartum

- Neonate to be examined and follow-up arranged
- Breastfeeding not contraindicated, but specially lubricated nipple shields to be provided to patient
- Before discharge, ensure patient has adequate additional support for care of the baby

13 Maternal Autoimmune Disorders

13.1 Lupus, Antiphospholipid Syndrome, and Anti-Ro Antibodies

FACT FILE

Lupus

Lupus (systemic lupus erythematosus, SLE) is an autoimmune disease where the immune system fails to distinguish between the body's own tissue 'self' antigens and 'non-self' foreign antigens (e.g. bacteria, viruses). Production of autoantibodies capable of harming some of the body's own tissues can ultimately lead to disease.

Epidemiology and clinical manifestations

- SLE is a systemic connective tissue disease characterized by periods of flares and remission.
- Incidence is 1:750 women in white populations, higher in Afro-Caribbean and Asian populations.
- Lupus is the classic multisystem syndrome.
- 90% of lupus patients are female, primarily of childbearing age.
- No two lupus patients need present alike: the spectrum of problems may range from skin rashes to kidney failure.
- Patients may have just a few or a multiplicity of symptoms.

Presentations of lupus

These may include:

- Heart and lungs:
  - hypertension
  - pericarditis
  - myocarditis
  - endocarditis
  - coronary artery disease
  - congenital complete heart block—in neonatal lupus syndrome (presence of maternal IgG anti-Ro antibodies)
  - pulmonary hypertension
- Kidneys:
  - lupus nephritis
  - mesangial proliferative glomerulonephritis
  - membranous nephropathy
- Skin and connective tissues:
  - malar rash
  - discoid rash
  - mucocutaneous ulceration
  - photosensitivity
  - inflammatory arthritis
  - serositis
  - vasculitis
  - Sjögren's syndrome
  - polymyositis, dermatomyositis
  - Raynaud's
  - scleroderma
- Haematological disorders:
  - thromboembolism
  - thrombocytopenia
  - leukopenia
  - haemolytic anaemia
- Neurological disorders (focal and diffuse neurological syndromes):
  - seizures (epilepsy of uncertain origin)
  - psychosis
  - meningitis
  - chorea, cerebella ataxia
- Gastrointestinal:
  - inflammatory bowel disease
  - pancreatitis
  - mesenteric vasculitis
- Eyes:
  - keratoconjunctivitis
  - scleritis
  - retinal disease—lupus retinopathy
  - hypertensive retinopathy
  - lupus choriodopathy.
- Lupus is presently 'incurable' but early diagnosis can make a significant difference in management.
- At times, certain environmental triggers such as chemical/infection exposure, smoking, or drugs like isoniazid and procainamide may trigger the SLE response.
- Immunopathology may begin years before clinical disease becomes evident

Possible obstetric complications

- Miscarriage, recurrent miscarriages—both first and second trimester[1,2,3]
- Prematurity
- Low birth weight
- Pre-eclampsia
- Intrauterine death (IUD) in second and third trimester
- Abruption
- DVT and pulmonary embolus (if antiphospholipid syndrome (APS) positive as well)

The risk of such complications is higher when any one or more of the following is present:

- Renal involvement:[4,5] - Increased risks of miscarriage, pre-eclampsia, intrauterine growth restriction (IUGR), preterm delivery and IUD are seen with lupus nephropathy, especially if serum creatinine levels are >180 µmol/litre, even if lupus itself is in a quiescent phase. Lupus nephropathy may manifest for the first time in pregnancy.
- Hypertension.
- Antiphospholipid antibodies in addition to lupus.
- Active disease at the time of conception or SLE presenting for the first time during a pregnancy is often associated with an increased risk of IUGR, preterm delivery, or pre-eclampsia.

Testing for lupus

Specific tests

- Lupus anticoagulant test (elevated DRVVT)
- Antiphospholipid (aPL) antibodies, otherwise called anticardiolipin (aCL) antibodies, because 30–40% of patients with lupus also have aPL antibodies. The risk of fetal loss is directly related to antibody titre, especially of aPL IgG.
- Both lupus and APS screening must show positive results when checked at least 12 weeks apart and ideally at least 12 weeks after a recent pregnancy
- If either or both of the lupus and APS screening is positive, anti-Ro and anti-La antibodies must also be performed.

Additional non-specific clues from 'routine' tests

- ***FBC*** (if disease active):
  - anaemia (normochromic, normocytic)
  - leucopoenia
  - thrombocytopenia
  - haemolytic anaemia
  - increased reticulocyte count
  - increased MCV.
- ***Urine*** (if disease active):
  - proteinuria (lupus nephropathy).

Others

- **Antinuclear antibodies (ANA):** Positive in up to 95–99% of patients with severe thrombocytopenia in untreated lupus.
- **Complement C3 and C4 assay:** Elevated levels in those with lupus nephropathy.

Maternal lupus: possible impact on neonate

- Apart from the neonatal problems of low birth weight and preterm birth which may be associated with maternal SLE, if anti-Ro antibodies are present as well, the risk of neonatal lupus is significantly increased.
- 1 in 3 of lupus-positive women have anti-Ro antibodies as well (also see later under 'Anti-Ro, neonatal lupus, congenital heart block')
- 1 in 20 of such women will have a baby with neonatal lupus,[6] usually presenting as a photosensitive transient red rash.
- Congenital cardiac block of the neonate is detected in 2% of all babies of anti-Ro positive mothers
- If anti-Ro antibodies are detected, fetal ECHO at about 20 weeks followed by a fetal heart scan at 32 weeks may be indicated.
- The baby may survive and may later need a pacemaker.
- Mothers who have had one baby with neonatal lupus run a greater chance (16% incidence of recurrence) in a subsequent pregnancy.

Management of pregnancy with maternal lupus

- Ideally, **pre-pregnancy counselling** (see 'Lupus and antiphospholipid syndrome: pre-pregnancy assessment and advice') and further investigations must be offered for women with previously identified lupus or if recently diagnosed during investigations following pregnancy complications (IUD, second-trimester pregnancy loss, recurrent miscarriages, severe early-onset pre-eclampsia, severe IUGR, etc.). Exclusion of coexistent APS and anti-Ro antibodies is best done pre-pregnancy.
- Low-dose aspirin is advisable from the first missed period till end of pregnancy. In those with lupus and APS, as placental damage begins early in gestation, low-dose aspirin is recommended from pre-conception or at least from the very start of pregnancy.
- Vigilance for hypertension must be maintained, especially for early-onset severe pre-eclampsia. Uterine artery Doppler scans at about 20–22 weeks may help identify those at increased risk.[7]
- Regular fetal surveillance with serial growth and Doppler scans.
- Timely delivery, usually at 38–40 weeks gestation, is advisable, decided on a case-to-case basis. Earlier delivery may be indicated by the development of significant problems such as IUGR, hypertension or pre-eclampsia.
- Disease flares, especially of lupus nephritis, arthritis, or inflammatory bowel disease, require multispeciality management: for example, active management with steroids after joint consultation with nephrology, rheumatology, gastroenterology, etc.
- ***In case of flares:***
  - Seek input from rheumatologist/haematologist without delay.
  - Make the diagnosis.
  - Prednisolone, azathioprine can be used; tacrolimus is useful in heavy proteinuria.
  - IV immunoglobulin may be considered.

Drugs used for lupus during pregnancy

- **Drugs that are safe to continue in pregnancy**: Prednisolone, aspirin, hydroxychloroquine, azathioprine, sulfasalazine, ciclosporin, or tacrolimus.
- **Drugs contraindicated** for lupus control or for the treatment of lupus-associated morbidities during pregnancy (these should have been stopped before conception): Mycophenolate mofetil, cyclophosphamide, rituximab, methotrexate, chlorambucil, ACE inhibitors, warfarin.
- If the patient is on sulfasalazine, hydroxychloroquine, or azathioprine, remember to prescribe high-dose folic acid (5 mg/day) due to the antifolate effect of these drugs.
- Low-dose aspirin: Aspirin inhibits thromboxane and thus reduces the risk of vascular thrombosis in both SLE and APS.
- As placental damage begins early in gestation in APS and lupus, aspirin from pre-conception is advised to reduce the risk of poor placentation.
- Antihypertensives such as labetalol and methyldopa for blood pressure control. ACE inhibitors and angiotensin II receptor blockers (ARBs) are contraindicated during pregnancy but may be suitable after delivery.
- Steroids: Usually used for short periods to control disease flares. **If the patient has been on long-term steroids, watch for gestational diabetes. A GTT might have to be done earlier than the routine 26–28 weeks gestation.**
- ***If the patient has been on steroids during the pregnancy, remember to document the need for bolus doses of hydrocortisone (100 mg IV 6–8 hourly) to cover labour and delivery.***

Relationship between lupus and APS in pregnancy

- 30–40% of lupus-positive women will also have APS.
- SLE mainly affects small vessels, whereas APS affects both large and small vessels, causing vasculitis.
- Those with APS plus SLE (secondary APS) have a greater incidence of valvular heart disease, neutropenia and haemolytic anaemia than those with primary APS.[7]
- 50% of SLE evolves to APS within 10 years.
- 50% of primary APS will also develop SLE after 10 years.
- In those with APS, lupus flares especially renal, skin, or joint lesions are more common in pregnancy and the puerperium.

Antiphospholipid syndrome (APS) or Hughes syndrome

- APS is an acquired autoimmune condition which leads to hypercoagulability of blood resulting in arterial or venous thrombosis and recurrent pregnancy loss as well as a range of clinical manifestations affecting organs such as the heart, kidneys, and skin.
- APS is termed **primary** where aPL antibodies are present but lupus anticoagulant is negative, or **secondary** when it exists against a background of other autoimmune conditions especially SLE. The clinical manifestations and outcomes of pregnancy are similar in both primary and secondary APS.
- aPL antibodies are found in 30% of all lupus-positive women.
- aPL antibodies are directed against plasma proteins that have an affinity for negatively charged phospholipids.
- The diagnostic serological markers are:
  - **persistent presence of aPL on at least two occasions 12 weeks apart, especially aPL IgG**
  - **anti-β2-glycoprotein or anti-apolipoprotein H.**
- **Maternal aPL antibodies may be downregulated during pregnancy,**[8] therefore diagnostic tests are best performed pre-conceptually or at least 12 weeks after the end of a pregnancy.
- As in lupus, patients may present with a wide range of clinical associations such as idiopathic epilepsy, rheumatoid and connective tissue disorders, Behçet's or Sjögren's syndromes, psoriatic arthropathy, venous or arterial thromboembolism, autoimmune thrombocytopenia, haemolytic anaemia, and myeloproliferative disorders (e.g. malignant lymphomas).

Obstetric complications with APS

- Previous obstetric history is the best predictor of pregnancy outcome in women with APS.

- A major feature of APS is pregnancy loss. Decidual vasculopathy and placental thrombosis are the most likely causes of inflammation-mediated placental damage, which seems to be prevented by heparin due to its effect in blocking activation of complement.[9]
- aPL has also been found to cause direct trophoblastic damage and inhibit trophoblast invasiveness, thus leading to early pregnancy loss.
- Miscarriage, especially late fetal loss and recurrent miscarriages. Prevalence of aPL antibodies among women with recurrent miscarriages is 15–20%.[10,11] In women with recurrent miscarriages due to APS, the prospective fetal loss rate may be as high as 90% if untreated.[12]
- Intrauterine death of a morphologically normal fetus in late second or in the third trimester.[14] Fetal death is usually preceded by IUGR and oligohydramnios.
- Significant risk of thromboembolism (70%), both arterial and venous. aPL antibodies are found in about 2% of those presenting with acute thromboembolism.
- Venous thromboembolism, especially DVT of the legs, occurs in 30–50% of those with APS.[15] An IgG aPL of more than 40 iu is associated with an increased thrombotic risk.
- Pre-eclampsia, especially severe and of early onset.[14]
- Gestational hypertension/pre-eclampsia occurs in 30–50% of untreated women with known APS.[10]
- IUGR due to placental insufficiency (30–40% increased risk).
- Preterm births, usually due to pre-eclampsia or IUGR (risk increased to 30–40%).[13,16]
- Abruption (placental histology often shows thromboses and infarction).
- When managed proactively, however, an 85% successful pregnancy outcome rate can be achieved.[13]

APS and lupus: association with other medical disorders

- Mild thrombocytopenia (found in 25% of APS) but increased tendency to form thrombi.
- There is a strong association between coronary heart disease in women between 35–44 years of age and APS/lupus.[14]
- Arterial thrombosis resulting in cerebrovascular events culminating in stroke, as well as myocardial infarction.
- There is also an increased association between hypertension, diabetes, and lupus/APS.
- There is a significant association between idiopathic epilepsy and APS as well as lupus.
- In each of the medical conditions listed above, it is worth screening for lupus and APS in pregnancy.
- In the rare condition of catastrophic APS, multiorgan failure due to widespread microvascular thrombi results in a high mortality rate.[14]

APS management in pregnancy and after

- A multidisciplinary approach to management is essential, with haematologist, obstetrician, and midwife. Depending on any systemic involvement, specialist input from rheumatology, dermatology, or nephrology may be needed during pregnancy.[14]
- Low-dose aspirin (from pre-pregnancy) and subcutaneous low molecular weight heparin (LMWH) commenced from 5–6 weeks of pregnancy after a positive pregnancy test. Pre-pregnancy information regarding this will facilitate prompt commencement of LMWH injections. Both low-dose aspirin and LMWH can be continued throughout pregnancy.[13]
- Once LMWH has been commenced, the platelet count should be monitored, weekly for the first 3 weeks, every 4–6 weeks thereafter.[14]
- Exclude anti-Ro antibodies and anti-La antibodies if not previously done.
- Plan antenatal, intrapartum and post-natal care with haematology, anaesthetic, and anticoagulation colleagues.
- Routine first-trimester scan for viability and dates; anomaly scan at about 20 weeks gestation.
- Uterine artery Doppler as discussed earlier.
- Serial growth scans ± Dopplers at regular intervals from 26 weeks gestation.
- If hypertension or renal disease: monitor progress and treat accordingly (see relevant care pathways).
- Below-knee elasticated compression stockings throughout pregnancy and puerperium are advised, due to the significantly high risk of thrombosis.
- If fetal growth and well-being are normal, delivery is advisable by 38 weeks gestation.
- Continue LMWH or warfarin for 6 weeks after delivery. LMWH injections may be changed to oral warfarin after delivery.
- Long-term thromboprophylaxis is required if there has been any thromboembolic episode.
- Continue low-dose aspirin in between pregnancies.
- Contraceptive advice: Combined oral contraceptives contraindicated due to the associated risk of thromboembolism (risk of thromboembolism increased by 50%). Give alternative family planning advice.
- Thromboprophylaxis advice for long-distance air travel, prolonged immobility, etc.
- Advise smoking cessation and weight reduction if overweight.
- In female offspring of a mother with APS, test for APS before starting oral contraceptives.

Primary seronegative APS

This is a condition where:

- Repeat immunological tests remain negative for APS.
- The patient may or may not have rheumatoid arthritis, Raynaud's, Sjögren's, etc.
- The clinical history is, however, highly suggestive of APS, e.g.:
  - vascular thrombosis (venous/arterial)
  - 3 or more consecutive miscarriages (<13 weeks)
  - 1 or more fetal loss (>13 weeks)
  - 1 or more premature births (>34 weeks) with severe pre-eclampsia, IUGR, abruption, etc.
- ***When one or more of these clinical criteria are present, think of seronegative APS.***
- In these rare cases, after joint discussion with haematologists, despite negative lab results, LMWH may be commenced based on the strength of the previous poor obstetric history and a presumptive diagnosis of primary seronegative APS.

Anti-Ro, neonatal lupus, congenital heart block

Anti-Ro antibodies

- Prevalence in the general population is less than 1%, although anti-Ro/LA is present in about 30% of patients with SLE, Sjögren's syndrome, etc.
- More than 90% of mothers of babies affected by neonatal lupus or congenital heart block have anti-Ro antibodies.
- In babies of anti-Ro positive mothers, risk of transient cutaneous lupus is only about 5% and the risk of congenital heart block is about 2%.
- Risk of neonatal lupus is increased if a previous child has been affected, rising to 16–18% with one affected child and to 50% if two children are affected.
- There is no correlation between the severity of maternal disease and incidence of neonatal lupus.

Cutaneous forms of neonatal lupus

- Usually manifest in the first 2 weeks after birth.
- Photosensitive erythematous skin lesions.
- Rash disappears within 4–6 months.
- Sunlight and phototherapy to be avoided.

Congenital heart block (CHB)

- Develops in utero, is permanent, and may be fatal (15–30% mortality).
- CHB not usually detected until 18–30 weeks gestation.

- Once fetal bradycardia is recognized, fetal ECHO at 18–26 weeks may show atrioventricular dissociation, confirming CHB.
- Heart block usually progresses through first and second-degrees before complete heart block (third degree) develops.
- There is no treatment that reverses CHB if the heart block is complete.
- Perinatal mortality is increased, 19% of affected children dying in the early neonatal period. However, most infants who survive this period do well, although 50–60% will require pacemaker placement in infancy and all will need pacemaker placement by their early teens.

Information for patients

Please see **Information for patients: Lupus, antiphospholipid syndrome, and pregnancy** (p. 529)

References

1. McKillop L, et al. SLE in pregnancy. BMJ 2007; 335: 933–936.
2. Nelson-Piercy C. Connective tissue disease. In: Handbook of obstetric medicine, 4th ed. London: Informa Healthcare, 2010.
3. RCOG Green-top Guideline No. 17. The investigation and treatment of couples with recurrent miscarriage. London: Royal College of Obstetricians and Gynaecologists, 2003.
4. Germain S, Nelson-Piercy C. Lupus nephritis and renal disease in pregnancy. Lupus 2006; 15: 148–155.
5. Imbasciati E, et al. Pregnancy in women with pre-existing lupus nephritis: predictors of fetal and maternal outcome. Nephrol Dial Transplant 2009; 24: 519–525.
6. Buyon JP, Clancy RM. Neonatal lupus syndromes. Curr Opin Rheumatol 2003; 15: 535–541.
7. Venkat-Raman N, et al. Uterine artery Doppler in predicting pregnancy outcome in women with antiphospholipid syndrome. Obstet Gynecol 2001; 98: 235–242.
8. Vianna JL, et al. Comparison of the primary and secondary antiphospholipid syndrome: a European Multicenter Study of 114 patients. Am J Med 1994; 96: 3–9.
9. Kwak JYH, et al. Down-regulation of maternal antiphospholipid antibodies during early pregnancy outcome. Am J Obstet Gynecol 1994; 171: 239–246.
10. Myers B, Pavord S. Diagnosis and management of antiphospholipid syndrome in pregnancy. Obstetrician and Gynaecologist 2011; 13: 15–21.
11. Yetman DL, Kutteh WH. Antiphospholipid antibody panels and recurrent pregnancy loss: prevalence of anticardiolipin antibodies compared with other antiphospholipid antibodies. Fertil Steril 1996; 66: 540–546.
12. Rai RS, et al. Antiphospholipid antibodies and beta2-glycoprotein-1 in 500 women with recurrent miscarriage: results of a comprehensive screening approach. Hum Reprod 1995; 10: 2001–2005.
13. Rai RS, et al. Randomised controlled trial of aspirin and aspirin plus heparin in pregnant women with recurrent miscarriage associated with phospholipid antibodies(or antiphospholipid antibodies). BMJ 1997; 314: 253–257.
14. Greaves M, et al. Guidelines on the investigation and management of the antiphospholipid syndrome. Br J Haematol 2000; 109: 704–715.
15. Asherson RA, et al. The 'primary' antiphospholipid syndrome: major clinical and serological features. Medicine (Baltimore) 1989; 68: 366–374.
16. Branch DW, et al. Outcome of treated pregnancies in women with antiphospholipid syndrome: an update of the Utah experience. Obstet Gynecol 1992; 80: 614–620.

LUPUS AND APS: PRE-PREGNANCY ASSESSMENT AND ADVICE

- ***Ideally patients who have suffered previous pregnancy losses (recurrent miscarriages,[1,2] IUD) or preterm births (more than one preterm birth not attributable to any other cause), severe early-onset pre-eclampsia, significant IUGR, abruption of the placenta, thromboembolic episode (whether during or out of a pregnancy), those with renal disease, unexplained persistent proteinuria, those with rheumatoid arthritis, Sjögren's or Behçet's syndromes, scleroderma, or epilepsy should have had pre-pregnancy investigations and counselling including screening for lupus and APS.***
- **Lupus** is diagnosed[3] by persistent positive lupus anticoagulant (raised DRVVT) on at least two occasions 12 weeks apart, best tested in the non-pregnant state and ideally at least 3 months after the end of any pregnancy.
- **APS:** According to the **International Consensus Statement** [4,5,6] updated in 2006, APS can be diagnosed **if at least one of the following clinical criteria and one of the laboratory criteria are met**, with the caveat that the interval between the clinical episode and the positive lab test is not shorter than 12 weeks or longer than 5 years.

Clinical criteria

- **Vascular thrombosis:** One or more clinical episodes of arterial, venous, or microvascular thrombosis occurring in any tissue or organ (excluding superficial thrombophlebitis).
- **Pregnancy complications:**
  - One or more unexplained deaths of a morphologically normal fetus at 10 weeks gestation or more.
  - Three or more unexplained consecutive spontaneous miscarriages before 10 weeks gestation when maternal and paternal chromosomal abnormalities have been excluded as have maternal hormonal or uterine abnormalities.
  - One or more preterm births of a morphologically normal neonate before 34 weeks gestation due to severe pre-eclampsia/eclampsia **or** recognized features of placental insufficiency.

Laboratory criteria

- **Lupus anticoagulant** present on two or more occasions at least 12 weeks apart (detected according to the guidelines of the International Society on Thrombosis and Haemostasis[3])
- **Anticardiolipin antibodies of IgG and/or IgM** isotype in serum or plasma, present in medium or high titre (>40 GPL or MPL or >99th percentile), on two or more occasions, at least 12 weeks apart, measured by standardized ELISA.
- **Anti-β2-glycoprotein 1 antibody of IgG and/or IgM isotype** in serum or plasma (in titre >99th percentile) on two or more occasions, at least 12 weeks apart, measured by standardized ELISA.
- In a few cases, despite very strong clinical manifestations and outcomes suggestive of APS, the lab tests may be negative. This has been described as **seronegative APS**. Management options in such situations are ideally planned pre-pregnancy after joint discussions with haematologists. Referral to a specialist centre for lupus and APS may be warranted in some cases.

Pre-pregnancy assessment and planning

- Detailed review of medical and obstetric history and of any current medication.
- Lab tests:
  - Confirm and document persistent aPL, lupus antibodies, and/or anti-β2-glycoprotein 1 antibody as described in the previous section.
  - If any of them are present, test for anti-Ro and anti-La antibodies (even if there is no evidence of active SLE).

- FBC to detect thrombocytopenia, anaemia.
- Baseline renal function tests.

- Advise the patient to plan a pregnancy during a period of disease quiescence as conception during a time of disease activity is associated with more complications and adverse outcomes of pregnancy.
- Advise deferring a pregnancy if a thromboembolic episode has occurred within the last 6 months.
- In cases of associated systemic disease such as hypertension, rheumatoid arthritis, epilepsy, inflammatory bowel disease, optimize management and review pharmacological agents for disease control.
- If there is a renal component to the autoimmune condition, pre-pregnancy assessment should include recent renal function tests, BP checks, and review of any antihypertensive drugs.
- If the patient is on ACE inhibitors or ARBs, change antihypertensives to methyldopa or/and labetalol. Advise continued BP monitoring in primary care to achieve stable control of BP prior to commencing a pregnancy.
- If lupus + APS has previously been diagnosed, the patient will have been advised to commence **low-dose aspirin even before pregnancy**.
- If the patient is found to be APS positive, advise **LMWH** sc injections from as early as 6 weeks gestation (in addition to the low-dose aspirin) to be continued throughout the pregnancy.
- If the patient is already on warfarin following a thromboembolic episode, advise a prompt change to sc LMWH as soon as a pregnancy is established. Ideally a prescription for the same and instructions regarding the injection technique should be provided during the pre-pregnancy visit or the patient given contact details to have LMWH started as soon as a pregnancy is diagnosed.
- If the patient is on drugs such as azathioprine, sulfasalazine, or hydroxychloroquine for symptom control of associated conditions such as rheumatoid arthritis or inflammatory bowel disease, prescribe **high-dose folic acid 5 mg/day** pre-pregnancy to be continued till the end of 13 weeks gestation.
- **Pre-pregnancy discussions** should include the possible effects of lupus ± APS on pregnancy and vice versa:
  - Advice must be provided regarding symptom control and medications that are safe in pregnancy, as well as how pregnancy outcomes could be improved with appropriate pre-pregnancy and pregnancy management/interventions.
  - The woman needs to be informed that the care of pregnancy is likely to be multidisciplinary depending on the comorbidities that may be involved in her case.
  - The patient must be provided with a pregnancy plan outlining how the pregnancy will be closely monitored for development of any problems such as pre-eclampsia, PIH, IUGR, preterm labour, etc.
  - If comorbidities such as smoking and obesity are involved, discuss how these further increase the risks of thrombosis and pregnancy complications associated with SLE/APS.
  - Reassure the patient regarding breastfeeding; there is no contraindication for breastfeeding in either lupus or APS, even if the patient is on sulfasalazine or hydroxychloroquine, LMWH or warfarin after delivery. The amount of azathioprine found in breast milk is very low and the advice is to breastfeed just before taking that day's dose of azathioprine.
- ***All these discussions should be documented and a detailed summary sent to the GP with a copy to the patient and any other specialists already involved in her care.***

References

1. RCOG Green-top Guideline No. 17. Recurrent miscarriage, investigation and treatment of couples. London: Royal College of Obstetricians and Gynaecologists, 2011.
2. RCOG SAC Opinion Paper 26. The use of antithrombotics in the prevention of recurrent pregnancy loss. London: Royal College of Obstetricians and Gynaecologists, 2011.
3. Brandt JT, et al. Criteria for the diagnosis of lupus anticoagulants: an update. On behalf of the subcommittee on Lupus Anticoagulant/Antiphospholipid Antibody of the Scientific and Standardisation Committee of the ISTH. Thromb Haemost 1995; 74: 1185–1190.
4. Wilson WA, et al. International consensus statement on preliminary classification criteria for definite antiphospholipid syndrome: report of an international workshop. Arthritis Rheum 1999; 42: 1309–1311.
5. Miyakis S, et al. International consensus statement on an update of the classification criteria for definite antiphospholipid syndrome (APS). J Thromb Haemost 2006; 4: 295–306.
6. Myers B, Pavord S. Diagnosis and management of antiphospholipid syndrome in pregnancy. Obstetrician and Gynaecologist 2011; 13: 15–21.

Lupus without antiphospholipid syndrome (APS)

Any patient with a pre-pregnancy diagnosis of lupus (and/or APS) must be referred to maternal medicine or specialist antenatal clinic for an early (within 8–10 weeks gestation) consultation

First visit to maternal medicine or specialist antenatal clinic (at 8–10 weeks)

- **Drugs safe to continue in pregnancy:** Prednisolone, aspirin, hydroxychloroquine, azathioprine, ciclosporin or tacrolimus
- **Drugs to have stopped before conception:** Mycophenolate mofetil, cyclophosphamide, rituximab
- Check patient is on low-dose aspirin. Advise continuation throughout pregnancy
- Advise smoking cessation
- If on antihypertensives like ACE inhibitors, change to methyldopa or labetalol
- Arrange for BP checks in primary care to ensure good BP control after changing type of antihypertensive
- If on drugs like sulfasalazine, hydroxychloroquine and azathioprine, ensure patient is on high-dose folic acid (5 mg/day) for the 1st trimester, but to continue throughout pregnancy if macrocytic anaemia with low serum folate
- Test for anti- Ro and anti-La antibodies, if not previously done
- Check baseline renal function tests and platelet count
- Advise to avoid NSAIDs for lupus flare during pregnancy, especially in 3rd trimester
- Discuss increased risks of miscarriage, abruption, preterm labour, DVT, pre-eclampsia, IUGR, and **document discussions**
- Arrange:
  - **BP series monitoring**, if hypertensive—monthly until 24 weeks then fortnightly
  - **Ultrasound Scans**—viability scan at about 12 weeks, anomaly at 20+ weeks (mention medication history when requesting scan), uterine artery Doppler at 20–24 weeks (usually in a research setting), serial growth and liquor ± Doppler from 24–26 weeks gestation, at 3–4 week intervals according to individual unit's policy
  - **Further specialist antenatal clinic appointments** at 24–26 weeks, then at 28, 32, and 36 weeks gestation timed with ultrasound scans as above
  - **Community midwife** antenatal visits at around 16, 20, 25, 30, 34, 38 weeks gestation, avoiding overlap of appointments with specialist antenatal clinic

Further visits to maternal medicine or specialist antenatal clinic (~24, 28, 32, 36 weeks)

- Treatment of lupus to continue in pregnancy, ensure hydroxychloroquine or other drugs are continued to avoid lupus flares
- In case of flares:
  - seek input from rheumatologist/haematologist without delay
  - make the diagnosis
  - prednisolone, azathioprine
  - tacrolimus useful in heavy proteinuria
  - IVIG may be considered
- Vigilance for development of pre-eclampsia
- Adjust dosage of antihypertensives as indicated by regular BP series monitoring
- Refer to high-risk anaesthetic clinic
- Refer to tertiary unit for fetal ECHO if anti-Ro +ve
- Inform neonatologists if mother is anti-Ro +ve as 2% risk of neonatal heart block; 5% risk of neonatal lupus
- FBC and renal function tests once in 6–8 weeks. Watch platelet count for thrombocytopenia
- If patient has been on long-term steroids, check for gestational diabetes. A GTT might have to be done earlier than the routine 26–28 weeks
- Fetal growth monitoring—watch trend for IUGR
- Discuss increased risks and symptoms of abruption, preterm labour, also placental failure and therefore advise delivery at about 38–39 weeks gestation. **Document discussion**.
- In addition, consider weekly Doppler and CTG from 34 weeks, in selected cases at particularly high risk
- Regular fetal heart rate monitoring if mother is anti-Ro positive
- Plan for delivery at about 38–39 weeks

Delivery and postpartum

- If patient has been on steroids, she will need bolus hydrocortisone cover for labour and delivery. **Document in notes**
- ***Discuss and document breastfeeding advice as well as future contraception—not to use COCP***
- Inform paediatricians and **document need for neonatal assessment** for neonatal lupus and congenital heart block if mother is positive for anti-Ro antibodies. **In some cases delivery may need to take place in a tertiary setting with neonatal cardiology facilities**

Primary or secondary APS

Any patient with a pre-pregnancy diagnosis of **APS** must be referred from community to the maternal medicine or joint obstetric/haematology clinic for an early (if possible, <8 week) consultation

First visit to specialist antenatal clinic (preferably at <8 weeks)

- Check patient is on low-dose aspirin—to continue throughout pregnancy
- LMWH (SC) prophylaxis from positive pregnancy test, continue throughout pregnancy and to continue after delivery or replace with postnatal warfarin for 6 weeks
- If history of previous TED, high dose (treatment range) of SC LMWH throughout pregnancy and puerperium with change to warfarin postnatally
- Inform anticoagulant team
- ***Urgent referral to haematologists***
- Advise below knee compression stockings to be used throughout pregnancy and puerperium
- Check if any comorbidities are present (eg, hypertension, lupus nephritis, etc.). Ensure is on medications appropriate for use in pregnancy
- Refer to anaesthetic high-risk clinic
- Rest of plan as for lupus (⬅ **see previous care pathway**)

- Community midwife antenatal checks continue meanwhile according to routine (NICE)
- Particular vigilance for pre-eclampsia

Further visits to Specialist antenatal clinic (at 24, 28, 32, 36 weeks)

- **As for lupus** (⬅ **see previous care pathway**)
- Careful vigilance for any thromboembolism
- Ensure continued use of below knee compression stockings, aspirin and LMWH SC injections
- Renal function tests in each trimester if renal component or hypertension
- Close fetal monitoring for growth, liquor, Doppler ± biophysical profile for fetal well-being
- Advice regarding awareness of regular fetal movements—provide contact details if reduced fetal movements
- Ensure patient has seen anaesthetist in high-risk clinic

Delivery and postpartum

- Reiterate advice about omitting dose of LMWH on day of IOL/LSCS or if labour starts spontaneously
- Interval of at least 12 h required between last dose of LMWH and insertion of spinal/epidural if on prophylactic dose of LMWH and up to 24 hours if on treatment doses
- Date for IOL/LSCS to be arranged for about 38 weeks, earlier as indicated if additional problems (e.g. pre-eclampsia, IUGR, renal impairment, etc.)
- Discuss safety of drugs in breastfeeding and provide contraceptive advice—**not for COCP**

In lupus and/or APS

- If maternal **anti-Ro antibodies are positive**, the risk of neonatal lupus (in 5%) and neonatal congenital heart block (in 2%) must be considered
- The consultant neonatologists must be alerted both during the antenatal period and when patient is in labour
- Fetal cardiac ECHO in a tertiary centre at 20–24 weeks should be arranged. In some cases delivery in a tertiary centre with neonatal cardiology facilities may be warranted

13.2 Rheumatoid Arthritis

FACT FILE

- Approximately one woman in every 1000–2000 pregnant women is affected by **rheumatoid arthritis (RA)**.
- RA is a chronic inflammatory systemic disease affecting primarily the synovial joints.
- About 80–90% of patients are positive for rheumatoid factor **(RhF)**.
- About 5–10% of patients with RA have aPL antibodies.[1]
- Anaemia in RA is normochromic, normocytic, and related to the degree of disease activity.
- About 75% of women with RA experience improvement during pregnancy with about 16% entering complete remission.[2,3] Improvement usually begins in the first trimester. This improvement is attributed to the relative immunological tolerance in the mother during pregnancy[1,2,3,4] due to the decrease in cell-mediated immunity, elevated levels of anti-inflammatory cytokines, and hormonal changes during pregnancy (e.g. increased cortisol, oestrogen, and progestin levels).
- Of those who experience remission, 90% suffer postpartum exacerbations.[1]
- ***Unlike SLE, RA has no adverse effect on pregnancy. No special obstetric monitoring is therefore indicated beyond what is performed for usual obstetric care.***
- ***Only if there is coexistence of anti-Ro antibodies in RA do babies have a risk of neonatal lupus.***
- Atlanto-axial subluxation is a rare complication restricting intubation if a GA is required for Caesarean section.
- Caesarean delivery does not appear to be performed more commonly in patients with RA.
- Rarely, the limitation of hip abduction may be severe enough to impede vaginal delivery.
- The obstetrician needs to work closely with the patient's rheumatologist, especially if the patient is taking disease-modifying antirheumatic drugs or steroids.[5]

Medications used in pregnancy and lactation

The safety of medications used to treat RA is the main concern during pregnancy and breastfeeding.[6,7,8,9,10,11,12,13,14,15,16,17]

- **Simple analgesics:** Paracetamol is the first-line agent.
- ***Non-steroidal anti-inflammatory drugs (NSAIDs):***
  - These should be avoided in pregnancy due to the increased risks of negative effects on blastocyst implantation, on the fetal kidneys leading to oligohydramnios, premature closure of the ductus arteriosus resulting in fetal pulmonary hypertension, as well as the risk of neonatal bleeding. NSAIDs must be avoided particularly in the last trimester. Aspirin (>150 mg/day) is contraindicated in pregnancy.
  - Occasionally, especially prior to 28 weeks gestation, NSAIDs may need to be used, after discussion with the rheumatologists, for control of arthritic pain if there are relative contraindications for steroids (e.g. women with osteoporosis) or if steroids are relatively ineffective (e.g. ankylosing spondylitis)
  - ***Note: Short-acting NSAIDs (e.g. ibuprofen) may be used during lactation, particularly if the day's medication dose is taken just after an episode of breastfeeding. NSAIDs should be used with caution, first ensuring that the newborn does not have jaundice.***[9]
- ***Corticosteroids:***
  - These potent anti-inflammatory agents are considered relatively safe in pregnancy when used in low doses and may be continued during pregnancy. Corticosteroids are preferable to NSAIDs if paracetamol is insufficient in controlling symptoms.
  - Pregnant women taking high doses of steroids are at increased risk of gestational diabetes and preterm rupture of membranes. A GTT is advisable in the late second trimester if on long-term steroids.
  - If on long-term maintenance steroids (>7.5 mg prednisolone for more than 2 weeks), bolus doses of IV or IM hydrocortisone 100 mg should be administered every 6–8 h to cover the stress of labour and delivery, regardless of the route of delivery.
  - The lowest possible steroid dose needed to control disease activity should be used in pregnancy
  - The neonate should be monitored for evidence of adrenal insufficiency and infection.
  - Prednisolone is secreted in milk at doses estimated at less than 0.1% of the maternal dose which corresponds to less than 10% of the infant's endogenous cortisol levels,[10] therefore prednisolone is not contraindicated in breastfeeding.
- ***Azathioprine (AZP):***
  - This is the most common cytotoxic drug used in treatment of RA and SLE and is safe for use in pregnancy, especially as a steroid-sparing agent. There is no increase in fetal anomalies because although azathioprine crosses the placenta, the fetal liver lacks the enzyme which converts AZP to its active metabolite, 6-mercaptopurine. The fetus is therefore protected from any potential teratogenic effects.[6]
  - The concentration in breast milk is very low and the benefits of breastfeeding may outweigh the risks, especially if the patient can be advised to breastfeed just before the day's dose of prednisolone.
- ***Hydroxychloroquine:***
  - This antimalarial, used in RA and to prevent flares in SLE, is safe both in pregnancy and for breastfeeding at the dosage used for RA and connective tissue disease (6.5 mg/kg body weight).[13,14]
  - Hydroxychloroquine is found in human breast milk, and the infant may be exposed to 2% of the maternal dose per kilogram per day. Although the elimination is slow, most experts believe that the drug may be continued during breastfeeding. The drug should be discontinued if the neonate has jaundice.[13,14]
- ***Sulfasalazine:***
  - This dihydrofolate reductase inhibitor[12,14] does not increase fetal morbidity or mortality and is considered safe in pregnancy and breastfeeding.
  - However, as it is a folate reductase inhibitor, **concomitant folic acid (high dose, 5 mg/day)** must be started **from pre-pregnancy and continued throughout pregnancy** in order to reduce fetal risk of NTDs as well as the risk of maternal megaloblastic anaemia.
  - Sulfasalazine is transferred in negligible amounts in breast milk and is safe during breastfeeding.

Drugs contraindicated in pregnancy and lactation

- **Cytotoxic drugs (e.g. cyclophosphamide, methotrexate, chlorambucil):**
  - **Methotrexate** is both embryotoxic and teratogenic. The active metabolites have a long half-life, therefore must be stopped at least 3–6 months before a pregnancy is established. Male partners should also discontinue methotrexate at least 3 months before attempting to conceive.
  - Although it is excreted in low concentrations into breast milk methotrexate can accumulate in the infant's tissues and is therefore contraindicated during lactation.[7]
- Mycophenolate mofetil (MMF)
- ***Penicillamine***
- **Leflunomide:** A pyrimidine synthesis inhibitor, is highly teratogenic and is an absolute contraindication in pregnancy and lactation. Its half-life is 14–15 days, but the active metabolite undergoes extensive and prolonged enterohepatic circulation; thus, the drug takes up to 2 years to become undetectable in plasma. The drug needs to be eliminated with the administration of cholestyramine.

- **TNF-alpha antagonists**: Antitumour necrosis factor (TNF)-alpha class of drugs such as **infliximab** are commonly used in the treatment of RA. Evidence regarding its safety in pregnancy and lactation is still fairly limited.[1]
  - Infliximab is a mouse human chimeric monoclonal antibody that blocks the action of proinflammatory TNF-alpha.
  - It has a half- life of 8–10 days.
  - Though it is not teratogenic in animal studies, its long-term effects on neonates have not been determined, therefore use in pregnancy is not generally recommended.
  - If use is required for control of maternal disease, it must be discontinued by 30–32 weeks at the latest.
  - It does not pass into breast milk, but until more data are available on TNF-alpha antagonists, breastfeeding should probably be avoided during therapy with these agents.[17]

Pre-pregnancy counselling

- If the woman has not been previously tested for lupus, APS or anti-Ro antibodies, these tests should be done pre-pregnancy. If any of them are positive, the management of the pregnancy will require significant modification compared with RA in isolation.
- If there is coexistence of anti-Ro antibodies in RA, babies have a small risk of neonatal lupus or heart block.
- Reassure the patient that RA on its own has no adverse effect on pregnancy and therefore no special obstetric interventions are required.
- Discuss multidisciplinary management with rheumatologist in a future pregnancy.
- Discuss fetal growth monitoring with serial growth scans if on prednisolone, hydroxychloroquine, sulfasalazine, or azathioprine.
- It is important to counsel women of childbearing age about the teratogenicity and other adverse effects of some of the drugs such as methotrexate, leflunomide, and cyclophosphamide used to treat RA.
- Patients must be advised about the importance of using effective contraception during therapy with disease-modifying antirheumatic drugs, especially methotrexate, leflunomide, and cyclophosphamide.
- If sulfasalazine, azathioprine, etc., are used, advise high-dose folic acid 5 mg/day from pre-pregnancy to be continued at least till the end of the first trimester.

Information for patients

Please see Information for patients: Rheumatoid arthritis and pregnancy (p. 529)

References

1. Quinn C, et al. Changes in levels of IgM RF and alpha 2 PAG correlate with increased disease activity in rheumatoid arthritis during the puerperium. Scand J Rheumatol 1993; 22: 273–279.
2. Hazes JMW, et al. Rheumatoid arthritis and pregnancy: evolution of disease activity and pathophysiological considerations for drug use. Rheumatology 2011; 11: 1955–1968.
3. de Man YA, et al. Disease activity of rheumatoid arthritis during pregnancy: results from a nationwide prospective study. Arthritis Rheum 2008; 59: 1241–1248.
4. Kitridou RC. Pregnancy in mixed connective tissue disease. Rheum Dis Clin North Am 2005; 31: 497–508.
5. Branch DW. Pregnancy in patients with rheumatic diseases: obstetric management and monitoring. Lupus 2004; 13: 696–698.
6. Ostensen M, Forger F. Management of RA medications in pregnant patients. Nat Rev Rheumatol. 2009; 5: 382–390.
7. Ostensen M, Motta M. Therapy insight: the use of antirheumatic drugs during nursing. Nat Clin Prac Rheumatol 2007; 3: 400–406.
8. Vermillion ST, et al. The effect of indomethacin tocolysis on fetal ductus arteriosus constriction with advancing gestational age. Am J Obstet Gynecol 1997; 177: 256–259.
9. Temprano KK, et al. Antirheumatic drugs in pregnancy and lactation. Semin Arthritis Rheum 2005; 35: 112–121.
10. Ost L, et al. Prednisolone excretion in human milk. J Pediatr 1985; 106: 1008–1011.
11. Francella A, et al. The safety of 6-mercaptopurine for childbearing patients with inflammatory bowel disease: a retrospective cohort study. Gastroenterology 2003; 124: 9–17.
12. Moskovitz DN, et al. The effect on the fetus of medications used to treat pregnant inflammatory bowel-disease patients. Am J Gastroenterol. 2004; 99: 656–661.
13. Costedoat-Chalumeau N, et al. Safety of hydroxychloroquine in pregnant patients with connective tissue diseases: a study of one hundred thirty-three cases compared with a control group. Arthritis Rheum 2003; 48: 3207–3211.
14. Parke A, West B. Hydroxychloroquine in pregnant patients with systemic lupus erythematosus. J Rheumatol 1996; 23: 1715–1718.
15. Herold M, et al. Efficacy and safety of a combined rituximab chemotherapy during pregnancy. J Clin Oncol 2001; 19: 3439.
16. Kimby E, et al. Safety of rituximab therapy during the first trimester of pregnancy: a case history. Eur J Haematol 2004; 72: 292–295.
17. Stengel JZ, Arnold HL. Is infliximab safe to use while breastfeeding? World J Gastroenterol 2008; 14: 3085–3087.

CARE PATHWAY

Pre-pregnancy counselling for patients with rheumatoid arthritis (RA)

- Condition and extent of disease assessed
- Drugs reviewed and changed as necessary
- Screening for lupus, APS, and anti-Ro antibodies
- Discuss improvement, possible remission during pregnancy in most cases, relapse in puerperium
- No specific increased risks for future pregnancy, no change in pregnancy, labour and delivery management because of RA without associated lupus/anti-Ro/APS
- If patient is on sulfasalazine, prescribe high-dose folic acid (5 mg/day) from 3 months before pregnancy and then advise continued use throughout future pregnancy to reduce risk of fetal neural tube and cardiac defects and then to prevent maternal folic acid deficiency megaloblastic anaemia
- If on methotrexate, advise to stop before pregnancy for at least 3–6 months before conception. Advise effective contraception for at least 3–6 months after stopping methotrexate
- Also see fact file

↓

Community midwife refers patient with RA to maternal medicine clinic within 1st trimester

↓

First visit to maternal medicine or specialist antenatal clinic

- Check current medication
- Add high-dose folic acid (5 mg/day) if on sulfasalazine: advise to continue till end of pregnancy
- Screening for anticardiolipin, lupus anticoagulant and anti-Ro antibodies if not previously done
- If history of previous miscarriages or pregnancy loss in addition to RA, start low-dose aspirin from 12 weeks pregnancy to end of gestation
- Refer to rheumatologist
- Refer to anaesthetic high-risk clinic (cervical subluxation must be considered in all patients)
- Arrange anomaly scan (mentioning drugs) at 20+ weeks
- Arrange serial growth scans 28, 32, 36 weeks (or according to individual unit's serial scan protocol)
- Next antenatal clinic appointment at 28 weeks
- Continue routine antenatal care
- Community midwife care continues according to NICE protocol **provided no lupus/APS/anti-Ro detected**

↓

If lupus, APS and anti- Ro excluded:

Further visits to maternal medicine or specialist antenatal clinic (at 28, 32, 36, and 40 weeks)

- Routine pregnancy checks
- Check growth and liquor serial scans
- GTT at 28 weeks if on long-term steroids
- Warn about increased chance of recurrence within 6–8 weeks after delivery
- **Document** need for bolus cover of IV hydrocortisone for labour and delivery if on long term steroids
- Discuss breastfeeding and drugs that can be used during breastfeeding
- Routine bloods according to current practice
- Confirm has had anaesthetic review
- Routine post-dates IOL according to unit protocol at 40^{+7-14} if undelivered by then and no fetal growth problems

↓

If lupus, APS and/or anti- Ro +ve:

➡ See lupus/APS, anti-Ro care pathway (pp. 272–273)

13.3 Sjögren's Syndrome

FACT FILE

- A common autoimmune disorder, **Sjögren's syndrome (SS)** may be primary or secondary.
- **Primary SS:** SS not associated with any other underlying rheumatic disease. Primary SS is the second most common autoimmune disease after rheumatoid arthritis(RA).
- When defined strictly according to the American European Consensus Criteria[1], the prevalence rate of **primary SS** is 0.3–0.6%,[2] with a female: male ratio of 9:1. It can affect all ethnic groups.
- **Secondary SS:** Coexists with other autoimmune diseases such as lupus or RA.[3]
- SS could be associated with lupus, and screening for lupus and APS is recommended, if not previously performed, before or as soon as possible during pregnancy.
- People with SS have a slightly increased risk of developing lymphomas.
- It is uncommon for children to inherit SS from their parents.

Symptoms

- SS usually affects only the lachrymal and salivary glands but may cause inflammation of joints or rarely affect the liver/kidneys.
- Common and uncomfortable symptoms can vary from person to person[4,5] They include:
  - a dry, gritty, or burning sensation in the eyes
  - dry mouth, increased dental decay
  - vaginal and skin dryness
  - dry nose, burning sensation in the throat
  - difficulty talking, chewing, or swallowing
  - a sore or cracked tongue
  - dry or peeling lips
  - a change in taste or smell
  - joint pains and fatigue.

SS and pregnancy

- Pregnancy complications in SS are mainly due to the occurrence of anti-Ro/SSA and anti-La/SSB autoantibodies in the maternal serum.
- Anti-Ro and anti-La antibodies are found more frequently in primary SS than in other conditions. Anti-Ro occurs in 75% of primary SS and anti-La in 60% of primary SS.
- These antibodies are well recognized as causing neonatal lupus and congenital heart block (CHB).[6]
- The incidence of neonatal lupus in an offspring of a mother with anti-Ro/SSA antibodies is estimated at 1–2%[7] but may be more than 20% if the mother has previously given birth to a child with neonatal lupus or CHB.[8]
- In the absence of anti-Ro or anti-La antibodies in maternal serum in those with primary SS, no serious adverse outcomes are seen in pregnancy or after.[9,10,11]
- In those with secondary SS-associated SLE, there is considerable overlap of mechanisms that can cause placental insufficiency, pre-eclampsia, IUGR, low birth weight, preterm delivery, or even IUD.
- Commonly encountered problems experienced by pregnant women with SS include dry mouth and eyes, mouth ulcers, and dry cough, for which symptomatic relief with topical preparations are advised.
- Arthralgia (painful joints) and myalgia (generalized muscle ache) are not uncommon. Paracetamol is the preferred analgesic: avoid NSAIDs.
- Rarely, a short course of steroids may be prescribed if the joints are inflamed. If oral prednisolone at a dose of 7.5 mg /day or more has been taken for more than 2 weeks during pregnancy, labour and delivery need to be covered with hydrocortisone 100 mg IM or IV, every 6–8 h.
- If the patient is on hydroxychloroquine for arthralgia symptoms, high-dose folic acid (5 mg/day) is to be advised to combat its anti-folate effect, especially till the end of the first trimester.
- Liver problems are uncommon, but there could be mild liver function abnormalities that usually do not require treatment. After pregnancy longer-term LFT surveillance can be maintained in primary care.
- Pulmonary fibrosis, requiring joint management with the respiratory physicians, is very rarely seen in SS and may require steroids.

Patients with positive anti-Ro and anti-La antibodies

- If positive anti-Ro and anti-La antibodies are detected in a patient with SS, referral to a fetomaternal unit/tertiary centre for fetal ECHO at about 20–22 weeks is recommended due to the potential for causing neonatal lupus and fetal CHBs.[12,13]
- A repeat fetal ECHO at 30–32 weeks may also be considered as heart block can develop between 18 and 30 weeks gestation.
- Serial growth scans, as well as regular fetal cardiotocography in the last few weeks of pregnancy, should be considered.
- Paediatricians must be made aware, ahead of time, about the possibility of neonatal lupus or CHB.
- If significant fetal heart block is suspected antenatally, delivery is best arranged in a tertiary centre where paediatric cardiology services are readily available.
- After delivery, increased vigilance for heart block must be maintained by the paediatricians.

Information for patients

Please see Information for patients: Sjögren's syndrome and pregnancy (p. 530)

References

1. Vitali C, et al. Classification criteria for Sjögren's syndrome: a revised version of the European criteria proposed by the American-European Consensus Group. Ann Rheum Dis 2002; 61: 554–558.
2. Bowman SJ, et al. Estimating the prevalence among Caucasian women of primary Sjögren's syndrome in two general practices in Birmingham, UK. Scand J Rheumatol 2004; 33: 39–43.
3. Theander E, Jacobsson LT. Relationship of Sjögren's syndrome to other connective tissue and autoimmune disorders. Rheum Dis Clin North Am 2008; 34: 935–947.
4. Goodchild CE, et al. Measuring fatigue among women with Sjögren's syndrome or rheumatoid arthritis: a comparison of the Profile of Fatigue (ProF) and the Multidimensional Fatigue Inventory (MFI). Musculoskeletal Care 2008; 6: 31–48.
5. Strömbeck B, et al. Health-related quality of life in primary Sjögren's syndrome, rheumatoid arthritis and fibromyalgia compared to normal population data using SF-36. Scand J Rheumatol 2000; 29: 20–28.
6. Lee LA. Transient autoimmunity related to maternal autoantibodies: neonatal lupus. Autoimmun Rev 2005; 4: 207–213.
7. Brucato A, et al. Risk of congenital complete heart block in newborns of mothers with anti-Ro/SSA antibodies detected by counterelectrophoresis. Arthritis Rheum 2001; 44: 1832–1835.
8. Buyon JP. Neonatal lupus: bedside to bench and back. Scand J Rheumatol 1996; 25: 271–276.
9. Takaya M, et al. Sjögren's syndrome and pregnancy. Tokai J Exp Clin Med 1991; 16: 83–88.
10. Haga HJ, et al. Pregnancy outcome in patients with primary Sjögren's syndrome. a case-control study: J Rheumatol 2005; 32: 1734–1736.
11. Mecacci F, et al. The impact of autoimmune disorders and adverse pregnancy outcome. Semin Perinatol 2007; 31: 223–226.
12. Moutasim KA, et al. Congenital heart block associated with Sjögren syndrome: case report. Int Arch Med 2009; 2: 21.
13. Brucato A, et al. Pregnancy outcome in 100 women with autoimmune diseases and anti-Ro/SSA antibodies: a prospective controlled study. Lupus 2002; 11: 716–721.

CARE PATHWAY

Pre-pregnancy referral of patient with **Sjögren's disease** to specialist maternal medicine obstetrician is highly recommended to enable detailed previous history, assessment, further investigations and management plans for future pregnancy

GP or community midwife refers patient early in 1st trimester to maternal medicine or specialist antenatal clinic

↓

First visit to maternal medicine or specialist antenatal clinic

- Identify whether patient has primary or secondary Sjögren's
- Lupus, APS, anti-Ro, anti-La screening, if not already done
- Check medications. If on antifolate medication such as hydroxychloroquine, advise continuation throughout pregnancy
- Reassure that generally, no increased problems during or after pregnancy, or for neonate, if lupus, APS, anti-Ro, and anti-La antibodies are negative
- **If lupus, APS, anti-Ro positive, (refer to relevant care pathways)** arrange serial growth scans, fetal ECHO, referral to tertiary centre's fetal medicine unit, etc.
- Topical preparations for dry eyes, mouth—safe to continue in pregnancy
- Advise to avoid NSAIDs for analgesia
- Steroids, hydroxychloroquine can be continued
- If other symptoms, multispeciality referral may be required
- Advise to maintain routine community midwife visits according to standard NICE schedule

↓

Further visits to maternal medicine or specialist antenatal clinic

Frequency of these visits will depend on whether or not Sjögren's is associated with lupus, APS, anti-Ro—**see relevant care pathways**

If uncomplicated primary Sjögren's alone, without anti-Ro/anti-La antibodies

- ***Reassure mother that good pregnancy outcomes can be expected***
- Next specialist clinic visits at approx. 28 and 36 weeks
- Continued community-based antenatal visits according to routine
- No indication for early IOL/investigations/interventions except for other obstetric indications
- Routine 40^{+7-14} date for IOL (according to individual unit's post-dates IOL protocol)

If anti-Ro/anti La antibodies in mother with Sjögren's syndrome

- ***If mother with Sjögren's syndrome tests positive for lupus, APS, and/or anti-Ro/Anti-La antibodies, see relevant care pathways***
- Discuss 1–2% chance of congenital heart block and of neonatal lupus
- Refer to tertiary unit for detailed fetal heart scans and ECHO—may also need repeating later in pregnancy (at 30–32 weeks)
- If significant heart block suspected, **delivery to be arranged in tertiary unit with access to neonatal cardiology services**
- Further fetal surveillance with close communication between tertiary unit and DGH
- Local neonatologists to be alerted to possibility of neonatal lupus and/or congenital heart block, well ahead of time of delivery
- When mother is admitted in labour, inform neonatologist without delay
- ***Frequency of further antenatal visits, serial scans, timing of delivery, DVT prophylaxis, etc. to be individualized on a case-to-case basis***

13.4 Dermatomyositis and Polymyositis

FACT FILE

- **Dermatomyositis (DM)** and **polymyositis (PM)** are acquired myopathies with an autoimmune basis. Both are inflammatory muscle diseases.
- **DM** is characterized by muscle weakness especially of symmetric proximal muscles, distinctive inflammatory and erythematous skin rashes on hands, feet, elbows, face, and/or upper body.
- **PM** has the same inflammatory muscle disease as seen in DM, but without skin involvement.
- Both DM and PM are rare disorders, with a prevalence of 2.4–10.7 cases per 100 000 people.[1,2,3] Both sexes can be affected with a female:male ratio of 2:1.
- Extreme muscle weakness, especially of the striated muscles of the neck, upper arms, and thighs, are characteristic but intercostal, diaphragmatic and pharyngeal muscles may also be affected. Respiratory or swallowing difficulties are found in about 20% of affected individuals.
- Though not life-threatening except in fulminant cases where respiratory or pharyngeal muscles are affected, these conditions can be debilitating.
- Plasma levels of muscle enzymes are invariably elevated, especially of **creatinine kinase (CK)**, levels of which are used to define disease activity. The normal levels of CK are 160–173 iu/ litre,[2,4] but in active DM or PM the levels are more than double this range and sometimes in the thousands.
- DM and PM can be associated with other autoimmune conditions such as SLE, SS, scleroderma, RA, etc. If so, DM and PM are referred to as the **overlap syndrome**.
- A bimodal age incidence pattern is seen with two peaks, the first at 10–15 years of age and a second at 40–60 years.[2]
- Average age of onset of inflammatory myopathies is about 47 years.
- Only 14% of all DM/PM cases reported are between 15–30 years of age, hence the relative rarity in pregnant women.[5]
- Diagnosis is made by abnormal electromyography of affected muscles, muscle biopsy showing inflammatory exudates, high CK, ESR, and lactic dehydrogenase in addition to the clinical picture.

DM/PM and pregnancy

- **These pregnancies are high-risk and multidisciplinary team management is crucial.**[2] Disease activity and assessments of fetal growth and well-being need to be closely monitored.
- DM/PM is usually diagnosed before the woman is pregnant or less frequently arises de novo during pregnancy or postpartum.
- The myopathies can cause maternal morbidity, significant perinatal mortality, and morbidity while pregnancy itself can affect the course of the disease.
- Fetal outcomes, in general, parallel maternal disease activity.
- Women who are in disease remission[2,4] at the time of conception have better pregnancy outcomes (see Table 13.1), and exacerbations are better controlled with corticosteroids. Some patients who are already on steroids ± immunosuppressants can see an improvement in their symptoms and the drug dosages could be reduced without causing disease flares.
- When conception occurs when the disease is active[2,4] fetal outcomes are poor, despite treatment, and maternal morbidity is increased.

Table 13.1 DM/PM disease activity and pregnancy outcomes

	Disease active at conception	*Disease in remission at conception*
Fetal loss (miscarriages, IUDs)	40%	21.5%
Prematurity rate	30%	21.5%
IUGR rates	32%	13.6 %
Live term birth rate	30%	nearly 60%

- In pre-existent DM/PM, as opposed to de novo presentation in pregnancy, exacerbations are generally more amenable to control and occur mostly in the third trimester and postpartum.
- When DM/PM occurs for the first time during pregnancy[2,6] the disease is active throughout pregnancy and less responsive to treatment. Exacerbations can be severe, despite steroids and immunosuppressants. Remission occurs soon after delivery.
- Steroids are the first-line therapy. Initial dosage,[1,2,3,4,5] gradual tapering off and discontinuation is managed exactly as in non-pregnant patients. **Oral steroids are relatively safe to use in pregnancy and the risks to the fetus are low because placental enzymes inactivate prednisolone to 10% of the levels in maternal blood concentration.**[7]
- If oral steroids (at a dose of ≥7.5 mg/day) have been used for longer than 2 weeks during pregnancy, bolus doses of hydrocortisone 100 mg IV or IM are needed every 6–8 h during labour and to cover delivery to prevent acute adrenal insufficiency.
- Immunosupressants[2,6] such as azathioprine, ciclosporin, or hydroxychloroquine can be added for disease control during pregnancy. **Methotrexate, however, is contraindicated** in pregnancy and during breastfeeding.
- More recently, IV immunoglobulin therapy[8] has been successfully used in control of exacerbations of DM during pregnancy.
- There are particular **anaesthetic risks** associated with myositis.[9] **It is imperative that any pregnant woman with DM/PM is referred for high-risk anaesthetic assessment and a clear management plan documented for analgesia for labour, delivery, and for Caesarean section, both elective and as an emergency.**
- DM/PM patients may be sensitive to non-depolarizing muscle relaxants, causing delayed recovery. Succinylcholine, veccuronium, and pancuronium must be avoided as they can produce prolonged neuromuscular paralysis and even trigger malignant hyperthermia. Similarly volatile anaesthetic agents could provoke malignant hyperthermia and hyperkalaemia. Regional block, spinal or epidural are safe as well as is combined epidural–spinal for Caesarean sections.

Information for patients

Please see Information for patients: Dermatomyositis or polymyositis and pregnancy (p. 530)

References

1. Targoff IN. Polymyositis and dermatomyositis in adults. In: Maddison PJ, et al., ed., Oxford textbook of rheumatology. Oxford: Oxford University Press, 1998, pp. 1249–1287.
2. Silva CA, et al. Pregnancy outcome in adult- onset idiopathic inflammatory myopathy. Rheumatology 2003; 42: 1168–1172.
3. Yassaea M, et al. Pregnancy-associated dermatomyositis. Arch Dermatol 2009; 145: 952–953.
4. Papapetropoulos T, et al. Polymyositis and pregnancy: report of a case with three pregnancies. J Neurol Neurosurg Psychiatry 1998; 64: 406.
5. Ishii N, et al. Dermatomyositis and pregnancy: case report and review of the literature. Dermatologica 1991; 183: 146–149.
6. King CR, Chow S. Dermatomyositis and pregnancy. Obstet Gynecol 1985; 66: 589–592.
7. Levitz M, et al. The transfer and metabolism of corticosteroids in the perfused human placenta. Am J Obstet Gynecol 1978; 132: 363–366.
8. Williams L, et al. Successful treatment of dermatomyositis during pregnancy with intravenous immunoglobulin monotherapy. Obstet Gynecol 2007; 109: 561–563.
9. Gunusen I, et al. Anesthetic management for cesarean delivery in a pregnant woman with polymyositis: a case report and review of literature. Cases J 2009; 2: 9107.

CARE PATHWAY

- GP or community midwife/refers patient known to have **dermatomyositis (DM) or polymyositis (PM)** to maternal medicine or specialist antenatal clinic
- Multidisciplinary input essential for management, involving GP, maternal medicine obstetrician, rheumatologist, neurologist, anaesthetist, midwife

First visit to maternal medicine or specialist antenatal clinic

- Confirm dates, viability
- Enquire regarding symptomatology outside of and during pregnancy and disease activity around time of conception. Establish which group of muscles most affected and extent of skin lesions in DM
- Any history of respiratory or swallowing difficulties needs urgent assessment by neurologist, rheumatologist, and anaesthetist
- Confirm that other autoimmune conditions (e.g. lupus, Sjögren's, rheumatoid arthritis, scleroderma, etc.) have been tested for and excluded. If unsure, arrange lupus and APS screening
- Check patient's current medications and their dosage: Steroids, immunosuppressants, etc. **Note : methotrexate contraindicated in pregnancy**
- Reassure regarding safety of steroids and most immunosuppressants used during pregnancy
- Consider high-dose folic acid (5 mg/day) if on hydroxychloroquine, azathioprine, etc.
- Confirm whether patient has had recent follow-up with rheumatologist/neurologist/dermatologist. If not, arrange these appointments
- Send bloods for ESR, creatinine kinase, lactic dehydrogenase
- Depending on state of disease activity or remission at time of conception, discuss with patient about possible risks, plans for close monitoring of both fetal growth and well-being as well as maternal condition throughout pregnancy
- Inform patient to be vigilant for symptoms which might suggest abruption, preterm labour, etc. Daily awareness of fetal movements recommended
- Refer to anaesthetic high-risk clinic and ensure review by consultant anaesthetist
- Arrange serial scans for fetal growth, liquor, and umbilical artery Dopplers every 3–4 weeks, from about 26 weeks gestation. BPP as indicated in individual cases
- Document clear plan of obstetric care, including scan follow-up
- Advise too continue routine antenatal care with community midwife between clinic appointments
- If on steroids, **document clearly in both hand-held and hospital notes that bolus doses of 100 mg IV/IM hydrocortisone needed every 6–8 h during labour and to cover delivery**, either vaginal or Caesarean

Further visits to maternal medicine or specialist antenatal clinic

- Check progress of pregnancy, maternal symptoms, any exacerbations
- Clinical and serial ultrasound assessments of fetal growth and liquor, Dopplers. BPP if indicated
- Confirm has had recent follow- up with rheumatologist, neurologist, dermatologist (if relevant)
- Confirm has had senior anaesthetic assessment and a clear plan included in notes

Delivery and postpartum

- Discuss mode of delivery, vaginal delivery entirely feasible, obtain patient's views
- If IUGR suspected, obstetric management as appropriate (according to IUGR care pathway)
- Due to increased risk of IUD, abruption etc., consider delivery by approx. 38–39 weeks
- Discuss breastfeeding and drugs: Steroids, azathioprine relatively safe if breastfeeding just before the day's dose.
- **Breastfeeding contraindicated with ciclosporin or methotrexate**
- Senior anaesthetist to be involved if either emergency or elective Caesarean section required
- Advise pre-pregnancy assessment before next pregnancy, which is best planned at time of disease remission

14 Maternal Connective Tissue Disorders

14.1 Ehlers–Danlos Syndrome

FACT FILE

Epidemiology and inheritance

- **Ehlers–Danlos syndrome (EDS)** is a rare heterogeneous group of inherited connective tissue disorders characterized by joint hypermobility, skin elasticity, tissue and blood vessel fragility and easy bruising.
- EDS is predominantly autosomal dominant.
- Incidence ranges from 1:5000 to 1:10 000 and EDS occurs in all ethnic groups.[1]
- There are different types of EDS (previously described as types I–X) with varying clinical manifestations and considerable overlap, making exact clinical diagnosis complex.[2] The I–X nomenclature has been replaced by more descriptive terminology, e.g.:
  - **classic**, which includes type I (severe classic type), and type II (mild classic type)
  - **hypermobility** (type III)
  - **vascular** (type IV)
  - **kyphoscoliosis** (type VI)
  - **arthrochalasia** (type VII A and B)
  - **dermatosparaxis** (type VII C).
- With the exception of the vascular variety of EDS (type IV), affected individuals have a normal life expectancy. In the vascular variety the average life expectancy is reduced to less than 50 years mainly due to mortality associated with arterial rupture.[1,3]

Diagnosis

- Not always easy due to considerable overlap of clinical manifestations.
- Diagnosis suspected if
  - thin, semi-translucent skin, hyperelasticity (except in type IV)
  - extensive bruising
  - facial dysmorphia
  - hypermobility of small joints, tendon/muscle rupture
  - history of arterial, uterine, or gastrointestinal fragility or rupture
  - talipes equinovarus
  - family history of EDS.
- Diagnosis confirmation by biochemical or molecular testing. Biochemical tests reveal a deficit of collagen III from skin fibroblasts while molecular tests show a mutation in the *COL3A1* gene.[1]
- In vascular EDS (type IV) there is no hyperelasticity of the skin.
- In vascular EDS (type IV), morbidity and mortality arise due to vascular rupture, organ perforation, cerebral haemorrhage, uterine rupture, etc.
- Differential diagnosis includes Marfan's syndrome and Loeys–Dietz syndrome (type II)

Pregnancy and EDS

- The incidence of EDS in pregnant women is about 1:15 000 with types I, II, and III each accounting for about 30% of all EDS cases. The vascular type (type IV) is the most severe form and accounts for about 10%.
- The type of EDS determines potential obstetric complications: not all types are associated with significant mortality and morbidity rates. In the vascular type (type IV), a subtype of collagen which is a structural component of arterial walls, gastrointestinal tract and the uterus, is defective. This can cause major obstetric complications.[1,4,5,6,7]
- The identification of the type of EDS is therefore crucial before pre-pregnancy discussions take place.
- Because of the pregnancy-associated risks, and the potential for genetic transmission, the optimal time to determine genetic risk is before pregnancy, especially if EDS has already been diagnosed in the family. Genetic counselling for affected adult females is essential.
- The severe classic type (type I) and vascular EDS (type IV) are the most severe forms, with up to a 25% maternal mortality rate in type IV due to arterial rupture.
- Potentially life-threatening complications unique to pregnancy, probably due to the hypervascular state of pregnancy, are not uncommon in vascular EDS. Pregnancy is therefore best avoided in a woman with this type of EDS. If she does become pregnant, she should be managed in a tertiary/regional high-risk perinatal referral centre.[4,5,8,9,10]
- The mild classic type (type II) causes relatively few problems in pregnancy, mainly associated with hypermobile joints. Pregnancy is usually well-tolerated with successful vaginal delivery achieved.
- In hypermobility EDS (type III), pregnant patients can experience severe pain should intervertebral disc prolapse or recurrent joint dislocation occur. In general, however, pregnancy outcomes for both the mother and baby are good.[11]
- **Early referral to the anaesthetic high-risk clinic** is essential for pregnant women with any type of EDS as there are substantial problems to be considered.[12] Anaesthetic complications during labour and delivery may present unique maternal risks for EDS women, especially in the vascular (type IV) variety.
  - Epidural anaesthesia may be technically difficult because of maternal skeletal abnormalities.
  - With general anaesthesia, there is an increased risk of injury to the cervical spine during intubation due to lax neck ligaments as well as an increased risk of pneumothorax associated with positive pressure ventilation.

Effects of EDS on pregnancy

- Problems during pregnancy involve pelvic instability, associated pelvic pain, cervical incompetence, and second-trimester pregnancy loss or preterm birth, and IUGR as well as the risk of preterm premature rupture of membranes (PPROM) due to connective tissue fragility.[10,13]
- Most problems in severe classic type I or type IV EDS can occur at the **time of delivery and postpartum**, including:[3,6,7,9,14]
  - great vessel rupture
  - uterine rupture
  - damage to the perineum, urethra, bladder, and rectum
  - Increased risk of premature rupture of membranes (PROM)[4,7]
  - preterm delivery (occurs in 50% severe classic EDS (type I)[4]
  - precipitate delivery
  - increased risk of malpresentation
  - increased risk of IUGR (serial growth scans are therefore essential)
  - severe PPH
  - skin fragility and poor healing, extension of episiotomy[3]
  - prolapse of uterus/bladder
  - spontaneous vaginal, perineal and other visceral tears
  - haematomas, wound dehiscence
  - serious anaesthetic risks
  - cerebral haemorrhage.

- ***In Type IV, the maternal mortality rate has been found to be as high as 20–30%,[4] which makes the case for counselling the woman not to get pregnant, but if she does and wishes to continue the pregnancy, her care should be transferred to a tertiary/regional unit.[9,15]***
- There is no consensus about the safest mode of delivery in women with type IV EDS. Some have advised an elective Caesarean section[9,15] at 32–34 weeks[4] while others have advised against surgery due to severe intraoperative and postoperative complications.[1,10,16,17,]
- ***A decision to advise a Caesarean section should therefore be individualized.***
- All resuscitative and prophylactic measures should be planned and in place before delivery takes place.
- In the ***mild classic form (type II) EDS, cervical incompetence is often a feature and a prophylactic cervical cerclage suture may need to be considered.***
- The newborn has a 50% chance of inheriting EDS type IV.
- ***Use of FBS, FSE, forceps, or ventouse-assisted vaginal delivery of an infant with known or potential EDS*** should be avoided because of the risk of infant haematomas and skin lacerations.
- Breech presentation, potentially related to hypotonia, is also more common with an affected infant. Other fetal malpositions (face and brow) as well as growth restriction have been reported with hypermobility-type EDS.

Information for patients

Please see Information for patients: Ehlers–Danlos syndrome and pregnancy (p. 531)

References

1. Germain DP. Clinical and genetic features of vascular Ehlers-Danlos syndrome. Int J Vasc Surg 2002;16: 391–397.
2. Dutta I, et al. Pregnancy and delivery in Ehlers-Danlos syndrome (hypermobility type): review of the literature. Obstetrical and Gynecological Int 2011;2011: 306413.
3. Pepin M, et al. Clinical and genetic features of Ehlers-Danlos syndrome type IV, the vascular type. N Engl J Med 2000;342: 673–680.
4. Lurie S, et al. The threat of type IV Ehlers Danlos syndrome on maternal well-being during pregnancy: early delivery may make the difference. J Obstet Gynaecol 1998;18: 245–248.
5. Rudd NL, et al. Pregnancy complications in type IV Ehlers-Danlos syndrome. Lancet 1983;1: 50–53.
6. Brees CK, Gall SA. Rupture of the external iliac artery during pregnancy: a case of type IV Ehlers-Danlos syndrome. J Ky Med Assoc 1995;93: 553–555.
7. Peaceman AM, Cruikshank DP. Ehlers-Danlos syndrome and pregnancy: association of type IV disease with maternal death. Obstet Gynaecol 1987;69: 428–431.
8. Hammond R, Oligbo N. Ehlers Danlos syndrome type IV and pregnancy. Arch Gynecol Obstet 2012;285: 51–54.
9. Erez Y, et al. Ehlers-Danlos type IV in pregnancy. A case report and a literature review. Fetal Diag Ther 2007;23: 7–9.
10. Volkov N, et al. Ehlers-Danlos syndrome: insights on obstetric aspects. Obstet Gynaecol Surv 2006;62: 51–57.
11. Golfier F, et al. Hypermobility type of Ehlers-Danlos syndrome: influence of pregnancies. Clin Genet 2001;60: 240–241.
12. Dill-Russell P, Jones LS. Anaesthesia for caesarean section in a patient with Ehlers-Danlos syndrome and mitral valve prolapse. Int J Obstet Anesth 2001;10: 192–197.
13. De Vos M, et al. Preterm premature rupture of membranes in a patient with the hypermobility type of the Ehlers-Danlos syndrome. A case report. Fetal Diagn Ther. 1999;14: 244–277.
14. Lind J, Wallenburg HCS. Pregnancy and the Ehlers-Danlos syndrome: a retrospective study in a Dutch population. Acta Obstet Gynecol Scand 2002;81: 293–300.
15. Walsh CA, Foley ME. Ehlers-Danlos syndrome in pregnancy. Fetal Diagn Ther 2008;24: 79.
16. Germain DP. Ehlers-Danlos syndrome type IV. Orphanet J Rare Dis 2007;2: 32.
17. Bjorck M, et al. Fatal bleeding following delivery: a manifestation of the vascular type of Ehlers Danlos syndrome. Gynecol Obstet Invest 2007;63: 173–175.

- Clinical manifestations of **Ehlers–Danlos syndrome (EDS)** vary from mild to life-threatening, depending on the type of EDS
- Because of the varying degrees of severity and multiorgan involvement which may signpost a wide range of potential type-specific problems, obstetric, anaesthetic, and haematological plans have to be devised on a case-by-case basis and communicated to all involved in the care of the mother and neonate
- It is essential that these multidisciplinary plans are well documented and in place by mid-pregnancy as the risk of preterm labour is high

Pre-pregnancy assessment and counselling

- Pre-pregnancy multidisciplinary assessment including genetic counselling is crucial for subsequent maternal and neonatal outcomes. Primary care physicians need to instigate such referrals in all women with any type of EDS of reproductive age intending to get pregnant
- Pre-pregnancy counselling is essential in patients with EDS, especially of classic severe type I and type IV who must be fully counselled about the 1 in 3 chances of dying due to a major complication during pregnancy, especially at delivery and postpartum. Pregnancy is not advisable in this group
- Pre-pregnancy confirmation of the type of EDS is essential to guide management plans and to allow discussion of chances of offspring inheriting condition
- Pre-pregnancy biochemical and molecular tests, genetics, and rheumatological assessment will help define the type of EDS, though overlap of features can make this complex
    - ◆ Any patient with **vascular (type IV) EDS** going ahead with pregnancy must receive tertiary centre care during pregnancy and delivery. Immediate referral from a DGH is mandatory in such cases
    - ◆ Delivery of a **classic severe (type I) EDS or type IV EDS patient** is best arranged in a centre with interventional radiology facilities available round the clock for emergency uterine artery embolization
- Multidisciplinary care is mandatory, with prompt and effectively documented communication between all involved in the care of the mother and the newborn
- GP or community midwife refers patient with EDS to maternal medicine clinic within the first trimester

↓

First visit to maternal medicine clinic

- Try to establish type of EDS; ascertain whether patient intends to continue pregnancy, especially women with type IV EDS
- Urgent referral to rheumatology and genetics if not previously initiated through primary care
- Refer to haematologist to exclude platelet dysfunction
- Refer for senior anaesthetic review and detailed plan for labour and delivery
- If vascular (type IV) EDS, immediate referral to tertiary centre for ongoing antenatal and intrapartum care
- Ensure physiotherapist support throughout pregnancy and in puerperium, especially in hypermobility (type III) EDS. Ensure patient has physio contact number
- If any orthostatic tachycardia (especially in type III EDS), refer to cardiologist with ECG and ECHO.
- If hypermobility (type III) EDS, serial cervical length scans at 14,18, and 22 weeks for signs of cervical incompetence. If found, consider cervical cerclage after due counselling
- Arrange serial growth scans with Dopplers from 26 weeks at 3–4 week intervals and maternal medicine clinic review on same day as scans
- Patient to continue routine community midwife antenatal checks according to NICE protocol

↓

Further visits to maternal medicine clinic (26, 30, 34, 37, and 40 weeks)

- Assess progress of pregnancy, symptomatology, fetal growth and activity
- Prophylactic steroids to be considered at about 26–28 weeks
- Formulate joint plans for delivery with anaesthetic and haematology colleagues. Cardiology and rheumatology input as indicated
- Ensure continued physiotherapist support
- If platelet dysfunction reported, seek haematologist's advice
- Decisions and advice regarding mode and timing of delivery in an individualized case-to-case basis. Generally in types II and III, elective Caesarean section only if history of severe recurrent hip subluxation/dislocation or for other obstetric indications. Normal vaginal delivery otherwise feasible in milder cases. Early delivery (<40 weeks) may be indicated if serial scans and Doppler studies indicate IUGR
- Arrange for 4 units crossmatched blood
- ***Document in labour notes—'increased risk of PPH, therefore active management of third stage'***
- **Document in labour notes—'avoid FSE, FBS, ventouse, or forceps'** if baby suspected to have EDS by prior genetic studies
- Neonatologists to be alerted when patient presents in labour or for planned Caesarean section—**document on the 'Baby' page of notes**

14.2 Marfan's Syndrome

FACT FILE

- **Marfan's syndrome** is an **autosomal dominant disorder.** The main areas affected in Marfan's syndrome are the skeleton, eyes, heart, and aorta.
- The diagnosis of Marfan's is based on the **Ghent criteria**[1] and relies on history, physical examination, and a molecular genetics test.
- Marfan's may not have been diagnosed before pregnancy and recognized only after complications develop.
- Because pregnancy-associated complications may be life-threatening,[1,2,3,4,5,6,7,8] physicians caring for women of childbearing age should be aware of the diagnostic criteria and potential problems.
- The syndrome involves multiple organ systems and the diagnosis requires a multidisciplinary approach by specialists in cardiology, ophthalmology, radiology, and clinical genetics.
- **80% of patients with Marfan's syndrome have cardiac involvement**, most commonly:[1,4,6,8,9]
  - mitral valve prolapse
  - mitral regurgitation
  - aortic root dissection.
- **Those with cardiac lesions tend to have offspring with cardiac abnormalities**. The risk of inheritance by the offspring is at least 50%. Also, clinical presentation being variable, though the mother may only have a mild form, the offspring could express a severe form of the disease.[1]
- Other features of Marfan's include:
  - increased height
  - arm span> height
  - joint laxity
  - highly arched palate
  - dislocation of the lens, glaucoma, cataracts, or retinal detachment
  - depressed sternum
  - scoliosis
  - pronounced stretch marks.
- The physiological and hormonal changes of pregnancy can increase cardiovascular strain and produce changes in the collagen of the blood vessel walls.
- In pregnancy, Marfan's carries the risk of aortic dissection and aortic rupture, with an overall expected rate of aortic dissection of approximately 3%. Aortic dissection occurs in 1% in women with aortic diameter of less than 4 cm **but in about 10% in high-risk patients (aortic root diameter >4 cm, rapid dilatation, or previous dissection of the ascending aorta)**.
- Although uncommon, aortic dissections can also occur in women with a normal-size aorta and therefore an event-free pregnancy cannot be guaranteed in women with Marfan's even in the presence of normal aortic diameter.[1]
- Most dissections (80%) are type A, i.e. involving the ascending aorta. **Nearly 90% of these occur antenatally and a quarter of these prove to be fatal**. Type B, involving only the descending aorta, which is not associated with previous aortic root enlargement or aneurysm, accounts for 20%.
- Maternal mortality from vascular dissection and rupture has been reported as 0.74 per 100 000 maternities in the Netherlands[9] and 0.76 per 100 000 in the UK.[10]
- Risk of aortic dissection and rupture during pregnancy[11] is increased when there is:
  - pre-existent or progressive aortic root dilatation (10% risk if aortic root dilatation is >4 cm)
  - a positive family history of dissection or aortic rupture.
- ***Care in pregnancy needs to be multidisciplinary with the involvement of the cardiologist, maternal medicine obstetrician, anaesthetist, radiologist, cardiothoracic and vascular surgeons, and midwives.***
- ***Referral to a tertiary/regional unit with cardiothoracic surgical facilities may need to be considered in any case of Marfan's with heart and/or aortic involvement.***
- ***The development of aortic dissection in the mother carries a substantial risk to the fetus. In addition, Marfan's is associated with a high rate (40%) of obstetric complications such as premature rupture of membranes resulting in premature delivery and increased perinatal mortality in the offspring.***

Pre-pregnancy evaluation and advice

- Pre-pregnancy evaluation and advice from specialist cardiology tertiary/regional centre is essential.
- The management of patients with Marfan's should ideally start before conception.[1,4]
  - The patient should undergo a careful cardiovascular evaluation, with echocardiogram, CT, and/or MRI.
  - Patients should be informed about potential pregnancy-related maternal complications.
  - High risk of the offspring inheriting the syndrome with a possibly more severe expression of the disease.
  - Blood pressure needs close follow-up during pregnancy.
  - Women with a history of aortic valve replacement with a mechanical prosthesis should be informed of the complexity and risk of anticoagulation in pregnancy.
  - The likelihood of morbidity and possibly reduced longevity even after successful pregnancy.
  - ***Pregnancy is to be strongly discouraged if the aortic root dilatation is greater than 4–4.5 cm pre-conception.***[10]
  - ***Patients at high risk, particularly if the aortic root dilatation is greater than 4.5 cm, should be offered corrective surgery before embarking on a pregnancy.***
  - Women with Marfan's must be informed that they have a 1% risk of aortic dissection during pregnancy, even in the presence of a normal sized aorta.[4]
  - Women with other pre-existing risk factors[9] for vascular dissection or rupture such as essential hypertension, obesity, and smoking should have their blood pressure lowered and offered help to lose weight and stop smoking.

Management during pregnancy

- If aortic root dilatation is greater than 4 cm or there is a progression of aortic root enlargement, beta-blockers should be promptly commenced despite the small risk of fetal growth restriction, bradycardia, neonatal hypoglycemia, hyperbilirubinemia, etc. Such side effects should therefore be anticipated by the clinicians.
- Hypertension should be aggressively treated with beta-blockers as such peaks of hypertension can lead to aortic dissection.
- The use of propranolol is not ideal in pregnancy because it may trigger uterine activity. The use of selective β-1 receptor blockers such as **metoprolol may therefore be preferred during pregnancy**. Higher dose of beta-blockers may be needed to achieve adequate heart rate control during pregnancy. When initiated during pregnancy, the dose of beta-blockers should be titrated to reduce the resting maternal heart rate by at least 20%.[1]
- During pregnancy, echocardiography to measure the aortic root diameter is essential.
- For patients with normal-size aorta, antenatal visits should be scheduled every month, and an echocardiogram should be scheduled during each trimester and before the delivery.
- In patients with aortic diameter 4 cm or greater, progressive dilatation, or a history of previous aortic surgery for aortic dilatation or dissection, **an echocardiographic examination should be performed every 4–6 weeks**.

- Patients must be made aware of symptoms such as sudden tearing or 'ripping' kind of chest pain radiating to the back, nausea, sweating, palpitations, and difficulty breathing that accompany type A dissection of the aorta. In contrast, dissection of the descending aorta (type B) may have few symptoms.
- Vaginal delivery is safe in patients with Marfan's-affected women who have no significant cardiovascular involvement and normal aortic diameter (<4 cm).
- To minimize the stress of labour, epidural anaesthetic should be used to reduce pain, and forceps or ventouse may be advisable to shorten the second stage of labour.
- Both systolic and diastolic blood pressures increase markedly during uterine contractions and pain. These changes should be anticipated and prevented with epidural anaesthetic and beta-blockers.
- Delivery in a tertiary/regional unit with immediate and round-the-clock cardiothoracic surgical facilities is highly recommended in any woman with significant aortic root dilatation. Close liaison with the cardiologists at both the local hospital and in the tertiary/regional unit is mandatory during the antenatal care of any patient with Marfan's.
- **Elective Caesarean section under regional block is the safest mode** of delivery for patients with aortic root dilatation. As the risk of aortic dissection continues even after delivery, cardiovascular surgery for aortic repair is performed usually in the postnatal period in the tertiary/regional cardiovascular referral centre.
- Every effort must be made to decrease or minimize haemodynamic changes associated with vaginal delivery.
- **Ergometrine should be avoided** as it can cause a sudden, significant increase in the volume of blood re-entering maternal circulation, thus provoking decompensation of the heart.
- The risk of emergency cardiac surgery for aortic dissection or rupture is high. Therefore, if there is progressive, more than a 10-mm increase of the aortic root diameter within the first 20 weeks of pregnancy, the options should include termination of the pregnancy to allow elective cardiac surgery. These decisions should be made with the patient and at the tertiary/regional referral centre.
- If there is a type A dissection, immediate surgery should ensue. In general, after 28–30 weeks gestation, a Caesarean section under general anaesthetic should be followed by cardiac surgery.
- In those with type B dissection conservative medical treatment may be advised by cardiologists in the absence of signs of rupture or hypotension and hypo-perfusion.[9] However, delivery of the fetus should be considered as the fetal mortality is high in type B dissection.
- In addition to genetic linkage that can be done in early pregnancy, a fetal echocardiography may be performed in the third trimester for the diagnosis of cardiac manifestations of Marfan's in the fetus, such as atrioventricular valve regurgitation, dilatation of the aortic root, etc. Neonatal examination and follow up is recommended.

Information for patients

Please see **Information for patients: Marfan's syndrome and pregnancy** (p. 531)

References

1. Goland S, Elkayam U. Cardiovascular problems in pregnant women with Marfan syndrome. Circulation 2009;119: 619–623.
2. Lachandani S, Wingfield M. Pregnancy in women with Marfan's syndrome. Eur J Obstet Gynecol 2003;110: 125–130.
3. Lipscomb KJ, et al. Outcome of pregnancy in women with Marfan's syndrome. Br J Obstet Gynaecol 1997;104: 201–206.
4. Goland S, et al. Pregnancy in Marfan syndrome: maternal and fetal risk and recommendations for patient assessment and management. Cardiol Rev 2009;17: 253–262.
5. Rahman J, et al. Obstetric and gynecologic complications in women with Marfan syndrome. J Reprod Med 2003;48: 723–728.
6. Tutarel O, et al. Pregnancy in a Marfan patient with pre-existing aortic dissection. Int J Cardiol. 2007;114: E36-L
7. Meijboom LJ, et al. Obstetric complications in Marfan syndrome. Int J Cardiol 2006;110: 53–59.
8. Mulder JM, et al. Pregnancy and Marfan syndrome: an on-going discussion. J Am Coll Cardiol 2012;60: 230–232
9. La Chapelle CF, et al. Maternal mortality attributable to vascular dissection and rupture in the Netherlands: a nationwide confidential enquiry. BJOG 2012;119: 86–93.
10. Lewis G, ed. Saving mother's lives: reviewing maternal deaths to make motherhood safer 2003–2005. The Seventh Report on Confidential Enquiries into Maternal Deaths in the United Kingdom. London: CEMACH, 2007.
11. Adamson DL, et al. Cardiac disease in pregnancy. In: Maternal medicine, ed. Greer I, et al. London: Churchill Livingstone Elsevier, 2007.

Essential pre-pregnancy multidisciplinary assessment and counselling

- Risk stratification for a woman known to have **Marfan's syndrome:** Careful assessment of cardiovascular state with clinical examination, ECHO, CT, MRI
- Discuss risks of complications during pregnancy, especially in those with aortic root dilatation
- Inform patient of 1% risk of **aortic root dissection**, a life-threatening occurrence, even if normal aortic measurements pre-pregnancy. In general, if aortic root diameter is <4 cm, risk of aortic dissection approximately 1%; if ≥4 cm, risk as high as 10%
- In high-risk patients, corrective surgery to be offered before a pregnancy
- Risk of offspring inheriting Marfan's is 50%. Also, even if maternal cardiovascular manifestations are minimal, offspring could inherit a severe form of CVS abnormality
- BP control vital in pregnancy: Use of beta-blockers highly likely with potential of causing IUGR, neonatal bradycardia, hyperbilirubinaemia, hypoglycaemia
- If rapid aortic root dilatation in first half of pregnancy, might even need to consider TOP to save maternal condition from further deterioration
- Contraception: Progesterone implant or LNG-IUS; **not for COCP**

↓

GP or community midwife refers patient as soon as possible in early 1st trimester to maternal medicine antenatal clinic or joint obstetric–cardiology clinic

↓

First visit to maternal medicine or specialist clinic

- Confirm she wants to continue pregnancy, confirm viability and dates
- Urgent ECHO to stratify risk and to plan management
- Multidisciplinary care: Individualized multidisciplinary care pathways must be planned on a case-by-case basis involving tertiary, secondary, and primary care
- Close communication with cardiology

Mild–moderate risk (1% risk of aortic root dissection)

- No aortic root dilatation or aortic root diameter <4 cm
- No rapid dilatation of aortic root
- No previous aortic surgery

↓

- Rigorous monitoring and control of BP. Dose of beta-blockers to be titrated to reduce resting maternal heart rate by 20%
- Patient to be made aware of symptoms suggestive of aortic dissection—severe tearing pain radiating to the back, vomiting, sweating, palpitations, shortness of breath, etc.
- Referral to anaesthetist
- Monthly antenatal checks
- Serial growth and liquor scans from 26 weeks if on beta-blockers
- ECHO assessment in each trimester and before term, as advised by cardiologist

↓

Delivery and postpartum

- Inform neonatologist if mother has been on beta-blockers; also as baby has 50% chance of inheritance
- Vaginal delivery generally safe if no cardiovascular involvement
- Epidural recommended
- Second stage cut short with assisted instrumental delivery with ventouse or forceps
- Ergometrine contraindicated
- Continued cardiovascular vigilance postpartum

High risk (10% risk of aortic root dissection)

- Aortic root diameter ≥4 cm
- Rapid increase of aortic root diameter of >10 mm in the first 20 weeks of pregnancy
- Previous aortic surgery for aortic root dissection

↓

- Beta-blockers to be commenced without delay
- Refer to tertiary centre
- ECHO may be advised at 4–6 week intervals
- Rigorous monitoring and control of BP. Dose of beta-blockers to be titrated to reduce resting maternal heart rate by 20%
- If rapidly progressive dilatation of aorta increased by >10 mm in the first half of pregnancy from early pregnancy dimensions, TOP may need to be considered and urgent aortic surgery undertaken
- Patient to be made aware of symptoms suggestive of aortic dissection—severe tearing pain radiating to the back, vomiting, sweating, palpitations, shortness of breath, etc.
- If type A dissection, urgent aortic surgery indicated
- If type B dissection, conservative treatment but high fetal loss rate
- Refer to anaesthetist
- Serial scans from 26 weeks if on beta-blockers

↓

Delivery and postpartum

- Inform neonatologist if mother has been on beta-blockers; also as baby has 50% chance of inheritance
- Elective Caesarean section under regional block
- Ergometrine contraindicated
- Continued cardiovascular vigilance postpartum

15 Maternal Bowel Disease

15.1 Inflammatory Bowel Disease

FACT FILE

- **Inflammatory bowel diseases (IBD)** include chronic illnesses characterized by inflammation of the intestinal tract, most common of which are **ulcerative colitis** (UC) and **Crohn's disease.**[1]
- Both Crohn's and UC tend to present in young adulthood.
- The natural course of IBD has periods of relapse followed by periods of remission.[2]

Epidemiology and pregnancy outcomes

- Prevalence of UC is about 0.8–1.0 per 1000 in the general population.
- Prevalence of Crohn's disease is about 0.5 per 1000 in the general population.
- UC is more common in women and is more commonly seen in pregnancy.
- UC affects only the colon and presents with diarrhoea, blood, and mucus per rectum and lower abdominal pain.
- Nutritional problems are not uncommon in those with IBD including vitamin B_{12}, iron, folate deficiencies as well as protein and fat malabsorption.
- Crohn's occurs equally in both men and women and can affect **any part** of the gastrointestinal tract.
- A quarter of female patients will conceive after the diagnosis is made.
- Most patients with IBD can expect to have uneventful pregnancies.
- There is no evidence that pregnancy causes disease progression; it may even have a beneficial effect with fewer flares in later years.[3,4]
- The majority (80–90%) of women with IBD have full-term normal deliveries.
- ***Disease activity at the time of conception strongly influences the course of disease during pregnancy.***[1]
- If the disease has been quiescent at time of conception, it will remain so in about two-thirds of patients.
- If the disease is active at the time of conception, two-thirds of patients will have ongoing active disease and the condition deteriorates in up to 60% of patients.[5]
- Disease relapses can, however, can still occur in 20–30% of patients with inactive disease at the time of conception. Even those with excellent disease control have been shown to be at increased risk of pregnancy complications compared with the general population.[6]
- After birth, the risk of a flare is increased if the disease has been active during the last few weeks of pregnancy.
- Pregnant women with inactive IBD have little increased risk of adverse pregnancy outcomes.[7]
- Miscarriage rates can be as 35% in patients with active disease.
- Nutritional malabsorption problems in IBD could also contribute to intrauterine growth restriction (IUGR) and low birth weight.[8]
- Increased risk of IUGR (almost doubled in IBD), preterm delivery, small for gestational age, and adverse perinatal outcomes in Crohn's disease, especially if the disease is active.
- Other associations with IBD that may be relevant to pregnancy are extra-intestinal and include arthritis, gallstones, erythema nodosum, and an increased risk of venous thrombosis.
- Because of the increased risk of adverse outcomes in pregnant women with IBD, the management of pregnancy should be by a multidisciplinary team which includes the obstetric specialist, midwives, gastrointestinal specialist nurse, and the gastroenterologist.

Pre-conception care

- Ideally, issues relating to conception and pregnancy should be discussed with the patient with her GP, the gastroenterologist, and the maternal medicine obstetrician before starting a pregnancy. GPs should facilitate such pre-pregnancy referrals.
- To ensure better outcomes, pregnancy should be planned during a time of disease remission if possible, with disease control achieved before conception.
- Women with IBD should be advised to start high-dose folic acid (5 mg/day), which can be continued throughout the pregnancy, due to their poorer intestinal absorption of folate. Other nutritional supplements such as calcium and vitamin D or other multivitamins may also be required, particularly if extensive small-bowel resection has been performed.
- Smoking worsens the severity of disease in women with Crohn's disease. Smoking has been found to be the primary cause for relapses of IBD during pregnancy, which is in turn linked to low birth weight. Women with Crohn's disease who smoke have a higher risk of IUGR and preterm labour as well as venous thromboembolism. **Pre-conception counselling should include advice to stop smoking to achieve an improvement in disease activity.**[9]
- ***It is vitally important to allay the patient's fears about continuing or initiating IBD medication during pregnancy.***
  - She should be advised that pregnancy outcomes are far worse if the disease flares up during any stage of pregnancy.
  - IBD medications are all generally safe and used extensively during pregnancy. Patient taking drugs such as methotrexate or mycophenolate mofetil should stop these for at least 3 months before conception and take high-dose folic acid.
  - The medical management of IBD during pregnancy, with a few exceptions, should follow the same lines as out of pregnancy.

Management of IBD during pregnancy

- Women with IBD may be inclined to stop taking their drugs during pregnancy because of a perceived risk of causing congenital malformations in the developing fetus.
- ***It is vital, however, that the patient remains in remission during the pregnancy and she must be strongly reassured and discouraged from stopping her medication without consultation with the gastroenterologist.***[10,11]
- Assessment of IBD in pregnancy[1] is based on clinical factors such as abdominal pain, stool frequency, and rectal bleeding. C-reactive protein is also used. Assessment by endoscopic investigation using flexible sigmoidoscopy is safe in pregnancy, although colonoscopy should be avoided.
- Commonly used drugs in IBD[3] include aminosalicylates such as sulfasalazine and mesalazine as well as corticosteroids and thiopurines including azathioprine and 6-mercaptopurine. These are safe and well tolerated in pregnancy. Other drugs such as ciclosporin and tacrolimus may also be used under supervision.
- Thiopurines such as azathioprine and 6-mercaptopurine are the cornerstone of IBD management by reducing relapses, closing fistulas, and allowing steroid reduction and withdrawal.[12,13]
- These drugs do not significantly increase the incidence of stillbirth, low birth weight, or miscarriage.

- Aminosalicylates such as sulfasalazine can interfere with folate absorption. Pre-pregnancy advice should include high-dose folic acid 5 mg from at least 3 months prior to conception and continued throughout pregnancy.
- Aminosalicylates in the form of foam enemas or suppositories as topical agents are also entirely safe for use during pregnancy.
- Methotrexate is contraindicated in pregnancy due to the teratogenic effect. Women on methotrexate must have stopped the drug for at least 6 weeks before conception.
- Metronidazole and ciprofloxacin are the antibiotics most often used in Crohn's. Metronidazole[3] is best avoided in the first trimester, and during breastfeeding. Ciprofloxacin is also contraindicated for breastfeeding but is considered safe during pregnancy.[2,10]
- Infliximab (anti-TNF-alpha)[3] is transferred across the placenta and not enough is known about the effect on the neonate. The advice is that it is best avoided in the last trimester of pregnancy and while breastfeeding, although recent studies have shown it is nor transferred in breast milk.[13,14,15]
- Rarely, surgery for obstruction, haemorrhage, perforation, or toxic megacolon may be required during pregnancy and should not be delayed because of the pregnancy.[16] There is an increased risk of preterm labour and pregnancy loss associated with surgery during pregnancy.[10]

Management of pregnancy with IBD

- Advise continuation of high-dose folate (5 mg/day) supplementation throughout pregnancy. Also note that iron, calcium, vitamin D, and other vitamin deficiencies as well as hypoproteinaemia are more common and relevant supplementation may need to be prescribed.
- Continuation of the medications for the IBD.
- Pregnant patients need access to the gastroenterology specialist nurse.
- Routine anomaly scan.
- Serial growth scans from 26 weeks.
- Any relapses of the disease should be treated aggressively because active disease carries the greatest risk to the fetus. Regular clinical assessments are required during pregnancy.
- If the patient has been on long-term steroids, a glucose tolerance test needs to be performed at about 26–28 weeks pregnancy.
- If the patient has been on steroids for disease control, document the need for bolus doses of hydrocortisone 100 mg IV every 6–8 h during labour and for delivery.
- Those with IBD are at increased risk of venous thromboembolism, and thromboprophylaxis must be considered particularly when there are additional risks such as obesity and Caesarean section.
- The patient should be advised to aim for a vaginal delivery unless there is active perianal disease. **Caesarean section should be reserved for obstetric indications. Caesarean section is not indicated for those with inactive disease and those without perianal disease.**
- Caesarean section should be considered in patients with
  - impaired anal continence
  - those with extensive perineal scarring and loss of skin elasticity (because episiotomy or tears may result in the formation of a fistula)[17]
  - ileal pouch–anal anastomosis.
- A Caesarean section in such patients should be performed by or under the supervision of a senior experienced obstetrician
- **Early induction of labour is not required** unless there are obstetric indications such as IUGR.

Postnatal management

- The risk of a flare during the puerperium is increased if the disease has been active in the last few weeks of pregnancy.
- Advise the patient not to stop medication during the puerperium as this will cause a relapse.
- **Encourage breastfeeding.** There is good evidence that breastfeeding can actually reduce the risk of the infant developing IBD in later life. Patients who wish to breastfeed may decide to stop their IBD medication due to fear of their effect on the baby. Reassure them that the safety of aminosalicylates, azathioprine, 6-mercaptopurine, and prednisolone is well established. Advise the patient to breastfeed just before the day's medication dose.
- ***Drugs contraindicated while breastfeeding: methotrexate, ciprofloxacin, metronidazole and loperamide; also best to avoid infliximab, although it has been found not to be transferred in breast milk.***[15]
- Very occasionally, diarrhoea can occur in breastfed infants when the mother is on aminosalicylates such as sulfasalazine. Although this is very rare the mother must be informed about it.

Information for patients

Please see Information for patients: Inflammatory bowel disease (Crohn's, ulcerative colitis) and pregnancy (p. 532)

References

1. Ferguson CB, et al. Inflammatory bowel disease in pregnancy. BMJ 2008; 337: 170–172.
2. Caprilli R, et al., for the European Crohn's and Colitis Organisation (ECCO European evidence based consensus on the diagnosis and management of Crohn's disease: special situations.) Gut 2006; 55 (Suppl 1): i36–i58.
3. Nwokolo CU, et al. Surgical resections in parous patients with distal ileal and colonic Crohn's disease. Gut 1994; 35: 220–223.
4. Riis L, et al. Does pregnancy change the disease course? A study in a European cohort of patients with inflammatory bowel disease. Am J Gastroenterol 2006; 101: 1539–1545.
5. Norgard B, et al. Disease activity in pregnant women with Crohn's disease and birth outcomes: a regional Danish cohort study. Am J Gastroenterol 2007; 102: 1947–1954.
6. Mahadevan U, et al. Pregnancy outcomes in women with inflammatory bowel disease: a large community-based study from Northern California. Gastroenterology 2007; 133: 1106–1112.
7. Cornish J, et al. A meta-analysis on the influence of inflammatory bowel disease on pregnancy. Gut 2007; 56: 830–837.
8. Moser MA, et al. Crohn's disease, pregnancy, and birth weight. Am J Gastroenterol 2000; 95: 1021–1026.
9. Agret F, et al. Impact of pregnancy on the clinical activity of Crohn's disease. Aliment Pharmacol Ther 2005; 21: 509–513.
10. Smith MA, Sanderson JD. Management of inflammatory bowel disease in pregnancy. Obstet Med 2010; 3: 59–64.
11. Connell W, Miller A. Treating inflammatory bowel disease during pregnancy: risks and safety of drug therapy. Drug Safety 1999; 21: 311–323.
12. Francella A, et al. The safety of 6-mercaptopurine for childbearing patients with inflammatory bowel disease: a retrospective cohort study. Gastroenterology 2003; 124: 9–17.
13. Katz JA, et al. Outcome of pregnancy in women receiving infliximab for the treatment of Crohn's disease and rheumatoid arthritis. Am J Gastroenterol 2004; 99: 2385–2392.
14. Vasiliauskas EA, et al. Case report: evidence for transplacental transfer of maternally administered infliximab to the newborn. Clin Gastroenterol Hepatol 2006; 4: 1255–1258.
15. Stengel JZ, Arnold HL. Is infliximab safe to use while breastfeeding? World J Gastroenterol 2008; 14: 3085–3087.
16. Hill J, et al. Surgical treatment of acute manifestations of Crohn's disease during pregnancy. J R Soc Med 1997; 90: 64–66.
17. Ilnyckyj A, et al. Perianal Crohn's disease and pregnancy: role of the mode of delivery. Am J Gastroenterol 1999; 94: 3274–3278.

CARE PATHWAY

Pre-pregnancy assessment and counselling for a women with inflammatory bowel disease (IBD)

- Disease and medication assessment and optimization
- Pregnancy best planned during a time of disease remission. Good control to be achieved before conception
- Nutritional assessment, optimize nutrition
- High-dose folic acid (5 mg/day) from at least 3 months before conception and continued throughout pregnancy ; also iron, multivitamin especially vitamin D, calcium. May need vitamin B_{12} supplements
- Advise patient to stop smoking
- Advise patient not to stop IBD drugs without consulting gastroenterologist as relapses worsen pregnancy outcomes
- Advise that most IBD drugs are safe during all stages of pregnancy and for breastfeeding. Drugs like methotrexate, mycophenolate mofetil, and ciprofloxacin to be stopped 3 months before conception. If metronidazole required, avoid in 1st trimester
- Reassure her that most women have a full-term normal delivery despite the IBD, provided the disease is in remission before and during pregnancy
- Give patient the gastroenterology specialist nurse helpline contact number

↓

GP or community midwife refers patient with IBD to maternal medicine clinic within first trimester

↓

First visit to maternal medicine or specialist antenatal clinic

- Confirm viability, assess IBD, and review medication
- Continue high-dose folic acid supplementation throughout pregnancy, also of iron, vitamin D, calcium. Vitamin B_{12} if found to be deficient
- Emphasize need to continue IBD medication throughout pregnancy and while breastfeeding to stay in remission. Advise **not to stop medication without prior consultation with the gastroenterologist** as relapse associated with poor pregnancy outcomes
- Arrange routine dating and anomaly scans, serial growth scans at about 28, 32, and 36 weeks(or according to individual unit's serial scan protocol) with antenatal clinic follow-up on same day
- Multidisciplinary care with gastroenterology team—regular assessment of IBD
- Refer to gastroenterologist for urgent assessment if not had one within last 6 months
- Give contact details for gastroenterologist specialist nurses (if not done already)
- Advise to continue routine community midwife antenatal checks according to NICE protocol
- If on long-term steroids, arrange GTT at 26–28 weeks gestation
- Assess risk for thromboembolism—risk of VTE increased in those with IBD

↓

Further visits to maternal medicine or specialist antenatal clinic (28, 32, and 36 weeks)

- Assess pregnancy, ensure consistent growth and liquor on serial scans
- Confirm has had recent gastro follow-up
- If GTT is abnormal, refer to joint obstetric–diabetic antenatal clinic
- Confirm compliance with IBD medication and continuing high-dose folic acid
- Low threshold for thromboprophylaxis as increased risk of VTE with IBD
- Reassure patient that any flares will need vigorous treatment during pregnancy to reduce risks to baby

↓

Labour, delivery, and postpartum

- If patient has been on long-term prednisolone, document need for IV hydrocortisone boluses 100 mg 6–8 hourly for labour, delivery, or just before Caesarean section
- Aim for vaginal delivery unless there is active perianal disease. Vaginal delivery advisable even if the patient has had previous colostomy or ileostomy
- No need for early IOL unless other problems such as IUGR. If all well, book routine post-dates IOL at 40^{+11} (or according to individual unit's post-dates IOL protocol)
- **Caesarean section if active perianal disease, previous ileal pouch, anal anastomoses, extensive perianal scarring**. Otherwise Caesarean section only for obstetric indications
- Book Caesarean section at about 38–39 weeks with senior consultant supervision, **puerperal thromboprophylaxis**
- Ensure follow-up in place with gastro team
- Discuss risks of puerperal flare-ups and advise not to stop medication
- Encourage breastfeeding—most drugs are safe. If on oral prednisolone or azathioprine advise to try to breastfeed just before day's medication dose is taken, thus allowing a 4 h gap before next feed
- Contraception advice before discharge: **Not for COCP**, as IBD associated with risk of VTE

16 Maternal Musculoligamental Conditions

16.1 Symphysis Pubis Dysfunction, Pelvic Girdle Pain

FACT FILE

- **Symphysis pubis dysfunction (SPD), pelvic girdle pain, or pelvic joint pain** are all terms applied to symptoms of pain of varying degrees experienced around the pelvis, especially over the symphysis pubis.
- Though the term 'symphysis pubis dysfunction' was coined recently, it describes pregnancy symptoms that have been around for a long time, 2–3 million years in fact! Ever since humans began to walk on two feet (*Homo erectus*),[1] the female pelvis has had to undergo various essential evolutionary adaptations. These adaptations have not only evolved to bear the weight of an advanced pregnancy but are also designed to undergo the adequate expansion needed to allow the downward passage of a term baby at childbirth.
- In any pregnancy, the pelvic girdle has to bear the pressure and weight of the pregnant uterus and contents, which increase as gestation advances. In addition, the pelvic ligaments become softer and more stretched as a result of hormonal changes from the early weeks of pregnancy.
- This does not mean that the symptoms experienced by the individual woman can be underestimated or ignored as the inevitable consequence of pregnancy. Early recognition and appropriate management with adequate help and support are vital.
- SPD is therefore neither a newly discovered ailment nor is it a 'disease of pregnancy'. It affects every pregnancy although to varying degrees of severity. It can range from being a discomfort to being debilitating enough to affect day-to-day activity and in a few cases keep a woman more or less housebound.
- Appropriate information and education of pregnant women and their partners/families is essential, as is the uniformity of the advice offered by all healthcare professionals including community midwives, GPs, physiotherapists, chiropractors, obstetricians etc. It is important to ensure that the pregnant woman who is already experiencing pain and discomfort due to SPD does not receive mixed messages or conflicting opinions from different healthcare professionals.

What is SPD?

- The pelvis is essentially composed of four jointed bones: the sacrum and coccyx at the back and the two innominate (hip) bones which curve around the sides to meet at the front. These two halves of the pelvis are connected in front by the symphysis pubis. The joint is composed of fibrin and cartilage forming a ligament which is responsive to pregnancy hormones (relaxin and progesterone) produced from the early weeks of pregnancy. The symphysis pubis ligament therefore softens and stretches as a result of weightbearing as well as the hormonal effects of pregnancy. The pubic ligaments need to bear the weight of pregnancy while attempting to maintain the balance and stability essential for mobility.
- After any pregnancy, **irrespective of the mode of delivery**, the pelvic ligaments never resume their pre-pregnancy dimensions, which results in their being left permanently stretched before any subsequent pregnancy.
- SPD refers to symptoms of pain and discomfort[2] particularly with movement or abduction of the legs.

Gestation at presentation

- Softening of the ligaments responsive to the hormonal milieu takes place from early pregnancy. In some women these symptoms start from early in the first trimester, in others only after delivery. This is itself enough reason not to regard either early induction of labour or Caesarean section as 'cures' for SPD.
- Most women notice increasing symptoms of SPD from around the middle of pregnancy.

Symptoms

- Pain over the pelvic joint in the front as well as in the groins and the lower back worsening with change of position and movement are the common symptoms.
- These can be accompanied by a grinding sensation or a 'clicking' feeling in the pubic area, particularly on movement involving change of any position.

Diagnosis

- The symptoms are themselves diagnostic of the condition. Urinary tract infections which can produce pain/discomfort over the pubic area do not vary with change of position or activity but need to be excluded.
- There is actually no agreed objective diagnostic criterion to either estimate the prevalence of SPD or to accurately assess the benefits of any interventions offered.
- The ligaments of the symphysis pubis joint usually appear on imaging as a 'gap' of 4–5 mm during the non-pregnant state with a further stretching by 2–3 mm during pregnancy.
- Tenderness over the symphysis pubis joint exacerbated by abduction of the legs is as diagnostic as any imaging technique such as plain radiography, ultrasound, or MRI.
- Unnecessary ultrasound scans or exposure to fetal irradiation cannot be justified for a condition like SPD where an accurate history of clinical symptoms is just as effective in obtaining the diagnosis.
- ***It is very important to recognize that there is no correlation between the severity of the symptoms to the actual width of the symphyseal gap in SPD.***
- ***The management of SPD is not dependent on measurement of the symphyseal gap but on the severity of symptoms.***
- Some women develop severe symptoms with no more than the normal range of the symphyseal ligament width while others are not affected even when there is a gap of 10 mm—a rare situation called **symphysis pubis diastasis**.
- The use of unnecessary investigations and/or obstetric interventions are therefore unnecessary and can lead to iatrogenically created problems.

Management

- ***SPD is not a disease. It is a pregnancy condition and can therefore only be 'managed' not 'cured'.***[3,4,5,6]
- Usually the pregnant woman reports symptoms of SPD to the community midwife. **The physiotherapist attached to maternity** is the appropriate healthcare professional to whom the community midwife needs to make a direct referral. A direct referral from the community midwife or GP will avoid unnecessary delay in the woman accessing the right assessment, advice, and support.
- Advice regarding posture and position as well as tips to make normal daily activities less painful will be given by the physiotherapists and the community midwives.
- Other strategies such as the use of support pelvic girdles or Tubigrip and pelvic muscle stabilizing exercises are the standard strategies, with supplementary analgesia or alternative therapies such as acupuncture[4] being helpful in some cases. Antenatal exercises especially 'aquanatal' exercises, have also been shown to be beneficial.

- 75–80% of women report an improvement in their symptoms with physiotherapy strategies such as the trochanteric or support belts or pelvic tubular stockinette along with muscle stabilizing exercises.
- Sometimes the symptoms are associated with misalignment of one or more pelvic joints. In such cases it may be possible for the physiotherapist to realign the joints. However, in many cases the misalignment can recur due to the laxity of the ligaments, therefore appropriate management is the key.
- A **pelvic support belt** or **tubular stockinette** worn correctly over the lower abdomen and pelvic area exerts a small amount of force and aids in restoring stability to the pelvic girdle.
- Elbow crutches or walking frames may be occasionally required when stability of movement is compromised.
- In any pregnant patient, should there be prolonged periods of reduced mobility below knee compression stockings are to be recommended.

Analgesia

- For regular analgesia an analgesic such as paracetamol is probably most effective. Codeine-based analgesics within normal dosage limits, used to top up regular doses of paracetamol on occasions, may be required in some cases. These can however cause constipation, which in turn adds to the woman's discomfort.
- Other painkillers such as non-steroidal anti-inflammatory drugs (NSAIDs)—ibuprofen, aspirin, etc.—are contraindicated in pregnancy due to their potential harmful effects on the baby.
- Great care must be taken before opiates are prescribed for SPD. The woman can become habituated to opiates such as oromorph, with resultant side effects.
- Strong reassurance of the pregnant woman emphasizing that the SPD is time limited and not dangerous to the mother or the fetus is crucial to overall management.
- Contact with self-help support groups should be encouraged and provided to women with SPD.
- With appropriate patient education and support and the above advice offered uniformly by all the healthcare professionals involved, expectations can be managed and safe supportive strategies offered.

Interventions to be avoided

- ***SPD is not an indication for unnecessary and potentially risky interventions such as Caesarean sections or early induction of labour.***
- Interventions with their attendant risks such as failed induction necessitating emergency Caesarean section, or risks of haemorrhage, infection, or thromboembolism cannot be justified nor are they effective in the management of SPD.

Management during labour and delivery

- ***There is no reason why a normal vaginal delivery cannot be the aim in any woman with SPD, neither is there any evidence that vaginal delivery makes the condition of SPD any worse.***
- The woman should be encouraged to devise a birth plan taking SPD into account and to inform the midwife at the time of admission to delivery suite in labour about SPD symptoms and the range of movements possible without eliciting pain.
- On admission, the midwife will assess and document the range of pain-free movements possible in the lower spine and hips.
- Mobility should be encouraged with care taken not to position the labouring woman in any position outside her normal comfortable range for a prolonged period.
- Before any internal examination, the woman should be advised to adopt a comfortable position.
- Separation of the legs should be kept to a minimum.
- Excessive forced hip abduction that puts strain on the pubis, such as placing the woman's feet on the attendant's hips, should be avoided.
- Lithotomy position, if required, should be used for as short a time as required and both legs should be moved passively and simultaneously.
- ***Use of epidural analgesia is not contraindicated for women with SPD but care needs to be taken to ensure that the legs are not excessively abducted due to the absence of the sensation of pain.***
- The use of upright or forward-leaning or side-lying positions should be encouraged.
- Use of the birthing pool for both pain relief and delivery may be beneficial if there are no contraindications for a pool birth.

Postpartum

- The symptoms of SPD can resolve within a varying length of time following delivery. Some women notice an immediate improvement, for others it is more gradual over several days or weeks.
- It is beneficial for women with persistent pelvic pain to self-refer to the physiotherapist attached either to the maternity unit or to their GP surgery, for up to 6–8 weeks postpartum.
- Most women (>95%) are fully recovered within 3 months of delivery.

Breastfeeding

- SPD does not hinder breastfeeding, nor do the usual painkillers used for the symptoms of SPD.

Recurrence in subsequent pregnancy

- There is no way of predicting whether SPD will recur in a subsequent pregnancy. After the completion of any pregnancy, irrespective of factors such as mode of delivery, indication for mode of delivery, length of labour, the pelvic ligaments remain permanently more stretched than their pre-pregnancy dimensions.
- A woman can give herself some protection against further pelvic girdle problems by working on exercises to strengthen her core muscles. From 4–6 weeks onwards, postnatal exercise classes, Pilates, core stability exercise, yoga or tai chi are all appropriate. A women's health physiotherapist can give further advice on this.
- The symptoms of SPD may be expected to recur in a subsequent pregnancy in up to 65–85% of women. However, early recognition and appropriate referral to physiotherapy can alter the course of SPD symptoms in a subsequent pregnancy.
- The general advice is for new mothers to try to avoid a subsequent pregnancy until the baby is walking independently, as lifting a child will be especially difficult if SPD symptoms recur in a subsequent pregnancy.

Contact

The Association of Chartered Physiotherapists in Women's Health (ACPWH): <http://www.acpwh.org.uk>

Information for patients

Please see Information for patients: Symphysis pubis dysfunction and pregnancy (p. 533)

References

1. Simpson SW, et al. A female Homo erectus pelvis. Science 2008; 322 (5904): 1089–1092.
2. Jain S, et al. Symphysis pubis dysfunction: a practical approach to management. Obstetrician and Gynaecologist 2006; 8: 153–158.
3. Wainwright M, et al. Symphysis pubis dysfunction: improving the service. Br J Midwifery 2003; 11: 664–667.
4. Elden H, et al. Effects of acupuncture and stabilising exercises as adjunct to standard treatment in pregnant women with pelvic girdle pain: randomised single blind control trial. BMJ 2005; 330: 761.
5. Mason G, Pearson A. Symphysis pubis dysfunction. J Assoc Chartered Physiother Womens Health 2000; 87: 3–4
6. Leadbetter RE, et al. Symphysis pubis dysfunction: a review of the literature. J Matern Fetal and Neonatal Med 2004; 16: 349–354.
7. Wu WH, et al. Pregnancy-related pelvic girdle pain (PPP), I: Terminology, clinical presentation, and prevalence. Eur Spine J 2004; 13: 575–589.
8. Vleeming A, et al. European guidelines for the diagnosis and treatment of pelvic girdle pain. Eur Spine J 2008; 17: 794–819.

CARE PATHWAY

Woman reports symptoms of **symphysis pubis dysfunction (SPD)** to GP or community midwife

↓

Prompt direct referral to maternity physiotherapist, not to an obstetric antenatal clinic

↓

- Advice regarding activities of daily living, pacing, posture, and self-help
- Use of gym balls
- Core stability exercises
- Pelvic support belts or tubular stockinette
- Crutches or walking frames in severe cases

↓

- Graduated compression stockings if severe limitation of mobility

↓

- Aquanatal exercises after 20 weeks
- ? Additional complementary therapies, e.g. acupuncture

↓

GP or community midwife

- Offer support and reassurance
- Analgesia advice/prescription (by GP) if required
- Contact number, websites of support groups
- Routine low-risk antenatal care in community following NICE' guidelines
- From as early as possible after symptoms present, reinforce message that SPD is not an indication for earlier IOL or for a Caesarean section
- Conflicting advice between community and hospital, physiotherapists, or among junior/senior obstetricians should be avoided
- Patient education
- Management of expectations
- Discussion of Birth Plan
- If mobility restricted, ensure graduated compression stockings are being used

↓

Labour and delivery

- Aim for normal vaginal delivery, pool birth possible
- Midwife to assess and document range of pain-free movements on admission
- Appropriate analgesia
- Epidural not contraindicated but care with positioning needed
- Avoid overabduction/prolonged lithotomy

16.2 Fibromyalgia, Chronic Fatigue Syndrome

FACT FILE

- **Fibromyalgia syndrome (FMS) and chronic fatigue syndrome (CFS)** are poorly understood chronic conditions with a considerable overlap of symptomatology, clinical features and response to management modalities. Whether they are the same condition or otherwise is debatable but beyond the remit of this chapter.
- Fibromyalgia syndrome (FMS) literally means muscle pain.
- Fibromyalgia is a condition characterized by chronic widespread pain and fatigue. It is not an uncommon condition, with a 2% incidence in the general population,[1] affecting both men and women.
- Some reports have shown that symptoms of FMS can worsen during pregnancy, although this view has proven inconclusive.
- FMS is not pregnancy-specific, although it is more common in women of childbearing age.
- Likewise there need not be any change in the management of pregnancy labour, delivery, or postpartum due to FMS.
- Most pregnant women will usually have had FMS diagnosed before pregnancy.

Aetiology

- The **causation** of FMS remains unclear. Several aetiologies have been postulated including disordered sleep,[2] circadian rhythm abnormalities,[3] cortisol imbalance,[4] alteration in pain modulatory neuropeptides,[5] genetic abnormalities, psychiatric disorders, environmental stressors,[6] and underlying muscle metabolic disease.[7] No definitive causation has been found to date
- FMS is a common chronic disorder characterized by low-grade widespread musculoskeletal pain, fatigue (CFS),multiple tender soft tissue points throughout the body, and poor sleep patterns.
- The tender spots are usually in precise localized areas in the neck, spine, shoulders, and hips.

Diagnosis

- The **diagnostic criteria** include pain lasting for longer than 3 months on both sides of the body, involving the upper and lower halves of the body, and presence of at least 11 out of 18 specific tender points over the body.[8]
- Other symptoms that can accompany the above in those with FMS include morning stiffness, depression, anxiety, light unrefreshing sleep, lack of concentration, headaches, abdominal discomfort, and paraesthesias.
- Diagnosis of FMS is controversial as there are no laboratory tests and the various symptoms described are non-specific.
- Diagnosis is made more difficult as symptoms tend to be sporadic and there are no clearly defined diagnostic tests.
- With the frequent association of anxiety and depression, there may be a psychosomatic aspect to FMS but this is not clearly defined. Links between FMS and infectious agents, autoimmune conditions, and irritable bowel syndrome have been studied without a definitive connection being established.
- Laboratory tests to exclude hypothyroidism, rheumatoid arthritis, or lupus-like autoimmune conditions are needed before a diagnosis of FMS or CFS is made.
- As FMS is a chronic and long-standing condition, the above tests would usually have been done at some point of time before onset of this pregnancy.

Management

- The management guidelines offered here apply equally to both FMS and CFS.
- **Treatment** poses a challenge as the causation has not been identified. Traditionally, In non-pregnant populations, tricyclic antidepressants, selective serotonin reuptake inhibitors (SSRIs) and serotonin-norepinephrine reuptake inhibitors (SNRIs), anticonvulsants, opioid analgesics, sedatives, hypnotics, and anti-inflammatories have been used with varying degrees of symptom control achieved.
- Pain control in pregnancy is achieved with analgesics such as paracetamol or application of warmth, or topical application of anti-inflammatory gels or patches such as diclofenac. Oral NSAIDs are, however, contraindicated in pregnancy, and opiates such as morphine sulfate solution can lead to habituation and sometimes produce unwanted complications for the mother as well as the neonate. A small dose of amitriptyline after the end of the first trimester is relatively safe.
- ***The best treatment for chronic pain during pregnancy is exercise, massage therapy, rest and relaxation. Suitable exercises may include yoga, aquanatal exercises, Pilates, and stretching, especially back stretching.***

Information for patients

Please see Information for patients: Fibromyalgia, chronic fatigue syndrome, and pregnancy (p. 534)

References

1. Wolfe F, et al. The prevalence and characteristics of fibromyalgia in the general population. Arthritis Rheum 1995; 38: 19–28.
2. Moldofsky H, et al. Musculosketal symptoms and non-REM sleep disturbance in patients with 'fibrositis syndrome' and healthy subjects. Psychosom Med 1975; 37: 341–351.
3. Martinez-Lavin M, et al. Circadian studies of autonomic nervous balance in patients with fibromyalgia: a heart rate variability analysis. Arthritis Rheum 1998; 41: 1966–1971
4. Crofford LJ, et al. Basal circadian and pulsatile ACTH and cortisol secretion in patients with fibromyalgia and/or chronic fatigue syndrome. Brain Behav Immun 2004; 18: 314–325.
5. Russell IJ, et al. Cerebrospinal fluid biogenic amine metabolites in fibromyalgia/ fibrositis syndrome and rheumatoid arthritis. Arthritis Rheum 1992; 35: 550–556.
6. Bradley LA. Pathophysiology of fibromyalgia. Am J Med 2009; 122 (Suppl): S22–30.
7. Abdullah M, et al. Mitochondrial myopathy presenting as fibromyalgia: a case report. J Med Case Reports 2012; 6: 55.
8. Wolfe F, et al. The American College of Rheumatology 1990 Criteria for the Classification of Fibromyalgia. Report of the Multicenter Criteria Committee. Arthritis Rheum 1990; 33: 160–172.

- Most women with **fibromyalgia (FMS) or chronic fatigue syndrome (CFS)** will have reported symptoms of these chronic conditions to their GP before pregnancy
- After exclusion of thyroid disorders or autoimmune conditions as well as neurological or muscular disorders, a diagnosis of FMS or CFS may have been reached based on clinical manifestations
- Management strategies during pregnancy are similar to those outside of pregnancy, **except that some medications are unsuitable or contraindicated in pregnancy**
- Mild aerobic exercises, swimming, walking, etc. are advised to reduce muscle tenderness and improve muscle fitness. Activity must be paced, i.e. it is important that the woman does not do too much on a good day (because she feels she should be doing more) and then be incapable of anything for 2 days afterwards
- Local application of warmth and massage to the points of muscle tenderness will give short-term relief
- Cognitive therapy has also been shown to be very helpful
- Medication: The GP may already have prescribed a short course of a low-dose antidepressant. Newer drugs such as centrally acting analgesics (e.g. tramadol, gabapentin) are best avoided during pregnancy although small doses of amitriptyline after the first trimester are considered relatively safe
- ***Painkillers like aspirin, ibuprofen, and naproxen are not only of little value in treating FMS but are also contraindicated during pregnancy***
- Some women notice a significant improvement in their chronic symptoms during pregnancy, probably due to the effect of progesterone, while others note a worsening, especially of sleep problems
- Medications to aid sleep are not effective in FMS because they do not induce deeper sleep nor eliminate pain or fatigue. Instead, it is advisable for a daily schedule to be developed and adhered to—e.g. exercises during the day, massage, relaxation, avoiding caffeine and other stimulants close to bedtime
- Treatment without medications of any sort has been shown to be as effective for FMS as drug-based strategies
- Responses to medications vary and may diminish over time. They are not usually a long-term treatment strategy

Pregnancy and FMS/CFS

- There is no evidence that FMS/CFS adversely affect pregnancy outcomes, either materno-fetal or neonatal
- ***Management of the pregnancy, labour, and delivery does not differ from that of the routine low-risk antenatal care as defined by the NICE guidelines***
- The care will be almost entirely community based with easier access and help to achieve a holistic approach to the management
- Community-based clinical psychology services may be accessed by the community healthcare professionals if considered necessary
- ***There is no reason to advise unnecessary hospital admission for 'rest' in women with FMS***
- FMS does not cause problems with conceiving, and does not cause miscarriages, preterm births, nor any problems with the fetus/baby
- ***Unnecessary interventions such as early IOL or Caesarean section on demand (if the woman fears her ability to achieve effective 'pushing' in the second stage) are not only to be actively discouraged but also regarded as potentially dangerous interventions, the risks of which far outweigh any perceived benefit. Caesarean sections or early IOL are to be performed for valid obstetric reasons only***
- Support, encouragement, and appropriate patient education and information from community healthcare staff will help manage patients expectations
- **The symptoms of FMS do not impair muscle strength or tone for 'pushing' in the second stage.** There is no increase in the rate of assisted vaginal deliveries (forceps, ventouse) in these groups of women
- FMS does not interfere with breastfeeding ,unless the woman is on certain antidepressants contraindicated for breastfeeding
- An epidural for pain relief is as safe and effective for women with FMS as it is for the general population of labouring women
- The length of hospital stay for the mother or the baby should not be affected by FMS or CFS
- Adequate support at home for the mother and the baby should be ideally arranged during the pregnancy itself. **Vigilance for development of postnatal depression must be maintained.**

Unless there are any other indications warranting a referral to a hospital specialist antenatal clinic, patients with FMS or CFS should receive all their antenatal care in the community according to the NICE low-risk guidelines

17 Maternal Skeletal Disorders

17.1 Achondroplasia

FACT FILE

Epidemiology

- **Achondroplasia** is the most common form of short-limbed dwarfism.[1]
- It is an autosomal dominant condition, with more than 80% being the result of sporadic *de novo* mutations. Most infants with achondroplasia are born to parents of normal stature.
- Incidence ranges from 1:15 000 to 1:33,000 pregnancies.[1]
- Achondroplasia occurs in all ethnic groups and with equal frequency in males and females.
- It is caused by mutations in the gene for fibroblast growth factor receptor 3 (*FGFR3*) on chromosome 4p16-3.[2]
- Abnormal endochondral ossification with resultant short stature and disproportionately shortened limbs with short, thick tubular bones and flat vertebral bodies.[3,4]
- Membranous ossification not affected, so skull and facial bones are normal.
- Achondroplasia can be diagnosed by characteristic clinical and radiographic findings in most affected individuals.[5] Routine gene testing is not necessary except when the clinical diagnosis is in doubt.
- In individuals in whom there is diagnostic uncertainty or atypical findings, molecular genetic testing can be used to detect a mutation in *FGFR3*, the only gene known to be associated with achondroplasia.[2]

Clinical features

- Short stature[3,4]: average male adult height is 131 cm (4 ft 4 in) and for adult females it is 124 cm (4 ft).
- Normal mental and sexual development.
- Delayed milestones in infancy and childhood.[3,4]
- Sleep and breathing problems such as obstructive apnoea; most respiratory problems result from restrictive lung disease due to decreased chest size or upper airway obstruction.
- Other features include disproportionate short stature[3,4], with shortening of the proximal segment of the limbs, a prominent forehead (bossing), a flattened mid- face, and an average-sized trunk. The head usually appears relatively large compared with the body.
- Obesity is a marked feature. Obesity can aggravate the morbidity associated with lumbar stenosis and joint problems as well as contribute to early mortality from cardiovascular complications.[8]
- The most common complication in adulthood is lumbosacral spinal stenosis with compression of the spinal cord or nerve roots leading to back ache, thoracolumbar kyphosis (gibbus)—usually treatable by surgical decompression, if diagnosed at an early stage.[9]
- Lifespan may be normal unless complications with hydrocephalus arise in infancy or childhood, when mean survival could be 10% less than in the general population.[10,11,12]

Genetic counselling

- Recurrence risk in a sibling of a child affected by achondroplasia born to unaffected parents is approximately 1:443 (0.2%).
- Recurrence risk in a sibling of a child affected by achondroplasia born to one affected parent is 50%.
- If the woman has achondroplasia and her spouse is of normal stature, there is a 50% risk in each pregnancy of having a child with achondroplasia.[4,10,11]
- If both partners have achondroplasia, in any one pregancy there is a 25% chance of an unaffected offspring of average stature, a 50% chance of an offspring having heterozygous achondroplasia, and a 25% of an offspring having homozygous achondroplasia (a lethal condition) where it is are stillborn or dies shortly after birth.
- Homozygous achondroplasia can usually be diagnosed prenatally.
  - **Prenatal testing** for pregnancies at increased risk is possible by chorionic villus sampling (CVS) at 9–12 weeks gestation and identification of the mutation in the *FGFR3* gene on chromosome 4.
  - **Prenatal diagnosis** from DNA extracted from fetal cells harvested at CVS can be done in 'high-risk' cases where one or both parents are affected, but only after the mutation has been identified in the affected parent(s).
  - **Prenatal diagnosis** from DNA extracted from fetal cells derived by amniocentesis can also be offered in 'low-risk' pregnancies of normal-statured parents where routine ultrasound scans have unexpectedly revealed short fetal limbs (usually not apparent till the third trimester).
  - **Non-invasive prenatal diagnosis** of fetal achondroplasia using circulating fetal DNA in maternal plasma has been reported.[12]

Pregnancy in an achondroplastic mother

There is limited information regarding obstetric outcomes and complications.[13]

- Prenatal assessment and counselling including genetic counselling should be offered.
- Prenatal assessment should include baseline pulmonary function tests to aid evaluation and advice
- Problems such as pre-eclampsia, polyhydramnios, respiratory compromise, contracted pelvis necessitating lower section Caesarean section, prematurity, and increased intrapartum and neonatal mortality, have been reported.
- Worsening respiratory compromise especially in the third trimester, therefore repeat pulmonary function tests especially in the third trimester and review by respiratory physician at regular intervals during pregnancy.
- Worsening neurological symptoms due to severe lordosis.
- Delivery is invariably by planned Caesarean section.
- Referral to anaesthetic high-risk clinic for review by a senior anaesthetist must be organized as soon as possible.
- Pregnant patients with achondroplasia are at high risk in terms of anaesthesia and obstetric outcomes.
- There are risks involved for both general and regional anaesthetic in achondroplastic patients.[14,15,16] There are several reports,[14,15,16,17] however, on the successful use of both modalities of anaesthetic for Caesarean section in achondroplastic pregnant women.
- Individualized anaesthetic plans for Caesarean section must be made and potential risks discussed with the patient.

Information for patients

Please see Information for patients: Achondroplasia and pregnancy (p. 534)

References

1. Orioli IM, et al. The birth prevalence rates for the skeletal dysplasias. J Med Genet 1986; 23: 328–332.
2. Bellus GA, et al. Achondroplasia is defined by recurrent G380R mutations of FGFR3. Am J Hum Genet 1995; 56: 368–373.
3. Spranger JW, et al. Bone dysplasias: an atlas of genetic disorders of skeletal development, 2nd ed. Oxford: Oxford University Press, 2002, pp. 336–338.

4. Pauli RM. Achondroplasia. In: Cassidy SB, Allanson JE, ed., Management of genetic syndromes 3rd ed. New York: John Wiley & Sons, 2010, pp. 17–37.
5. Krakow D, et al. Use of three-dimensional ultrasound imaging in the diagnosis of prenatal-onset skeletal dysplasias. Ultrasound Obstet Gynecol 2003; 21: 467–472.
6. Wynn J, et al. Mortality in achondroplasia study: A 42-year follow-up. Am J Med Genet A 2007; 143: 2503–2511.
7. Hecht J.T., et al. Mortality in achondroplasia. Am J Hum Genet 1987; 41: 454–464.
8. Hecht JT, et al. Obesity in achondroplasia. Am J Med Genet 1988; 31: 597–602.
9. Laederich MB, Horton WA. Achondroplasia: pathogenesis and implications for future treatment. Curr Opin Pediatr 2010; 22: 516–523.
10. Gooding HC, et al. Issues surrounding prenatal genetic testing for achondroplasia. Prenat Diagn 2002; 22: 933–940.
11. Mettler G, Fraser CF. Recurrence risk for sibs of children with 'sporadic' achondroplasia. Am J Med Genet 2000; 90: 250–251.
12. Lim JH, et al. Non-invasive prenatal detection of achondroplasia using circulating fetal DNA in maternal plasma. . J Assist Reprod Genet 2011; 28: 167–172.
13. Chetty S, et al. Management of pregnancy in women with genetic disorders, part 1: disorders of the connective tissue, muscle, vascular, and skeletal systems. Obstet Gynecol Surv 2011; 66: 699–709.
14. Morrow MJ, Black IH. Epidural anaesthesia for Caesarean section in an achondroplastic dwarf. Br J Anaesth 1998; 81: 619–621.
15. Huang J, Babins N. Anesthesia for cesarean delivery in an achondroplastic dwarf: a case report. AANA J 2008; 76: 435–436.
16. Ravenscroft A, et al. Spinal anesthesia for emergency caesarean section in an achondroplastic dwarf. Anaesthesia 1998; 53: 1236–1237.
17. McGlothlen S. Anesthesia for caesarean section for achondroplastic dwarf: a case report. AANA J 2000; 68: 305–307.

Pre-pregnancy genetic counselling for a women with achondroplasia

- If partner of normal stature, 50% chance of baby having achondroplasia
- If both partners have achondroplasia, 50% risk of affected baby, 25% risk of homozygous achondroplasia (lethal), and 25% chance of unaffected baby
- Antenatal diagnosis available with CVS/amniocentesis, procedure-related risk of miscarriage to be discussed. Type of parental mutation to be established
- ***Pre-pregnancy baseline pulmonary function tests***

↓

GP or community midwife refers woman to specialist antenatal clinic

↓

First visit to specialist antenatal clinic

- Confirm pregnancy, establish dates
- Explore patient and partner's views about invasive testing, explaining procedure-related miscarriage rate
- If they opt for invasive testing, CVS if gestation between 9–12 weeks, amniocentesis if >12 weeks
- Refer to pulmonary physician for continued assessments in each trimester with pulmonary function tests
- Discuss increased vigilance for pregnancy complications such as preterm labour, pre-eclampsia, polyhydramnios, respiratory compromise especially in 3rd trimester
- Referral to senior anaesthetist for review in high-risk anaesthetic clinic
- Consider low-dose aspirin for pre-eclampsia prophylaxis

↓

Further visits to specialist antenatal clinic

- Serial ultrasound scans at regular intervals to monitor fetal growth, measurement of femur length, any development of polyhydramnios or hydrocephaly
- If ultrasound features of fetal achondroplasia seen, discuss with parents and arrange to meet neonatologist/paediatricians
- Increasing evidence of respiratory compromise might warrant early delivery. Give prophylactic corticosteroids to accelerate fetal lung maturity if considering delivery before 35 weeks gestation
- Delivery invariably by elective Caesarean section. Multidisciplinary team meeting with maternal medicine obstetrician, senior anaesthetist, midwife, pulmonary physician neonatologist to discuss time and arrangements for elective Caesarean section
- Detailed plan for type of anaesthetic to be devised by anaesthetic consultant on an individual basis consulting with obstetrician and respiratory physician and discussed with patient
- Plans to include conduct of emergency Caesarean delivery if labour contractions starts or in the event of SROM before date of elective Caesarean section

17.2 Osteogenesis Imperfecta

FACT FILE

Epidemiology

- **Osteogenesis imperfecta (OI)**, also known as **brittle bone disease**, is a group of inherited connective tissue disorders where there is defective synthesis or abnormal structure of type I collagen, the major protein constituent of bone and other connective tissues.
- OI typically involves bones, teeth, ligaments, and eyes and is characterized by fragile bones that break easily. Other features of OI may include hyperhidrosis, hyperthermia, poor dentition, platelet dysfunction, cor pulmonale, and congenital heart disease.[1,2,3,4]
- Overall incidence of all types of OI varies from 1:10 000 to 1:12 000.[5,6,7]
- The clinical phenotype ranges from mild to severe and lethal forms.[8,9,10,11]
- Four types have been described and serve as a clinical framework for diagnosis[5] (see Table 17.1).

Diagnosis

- In all forms of OI, histological and biochemical diagnosis obtained from skin biopsy and examining collagen type I content in fibroblasts for deficiency or defective structure.
- Carrier testing: in families in whom the gene mutation responsible for the disease has been identified; other relatives may be offered tests for the disease itself or for the carrier state.
- In pregnancy, molecular diagnosis is available for families at increased risk of OI by analysis of placental cells drawn at CVS or fetal cells from an amniocentesis sample.[12,13]

Effects of OI on pregnancy

- A high incidence of breech presentation has been reported in infants with OI.[13]
- Very few evidence-based guidelines exist for either the management of pregnancies in women with OI or management of pregnancy when the fetus is found to be affected by OI.
- Some have suggested elective Caesarean section if the fetus is suspected to have a more severe form of OI, based on the hypothesis that a Caesarean section is more controlled and less traumatic than vaginal delivery.[14]
- However, when the fetus is suspected to have a lethal or extremely severe form of OI, delivery by Caesarean section is not actively recommended because of increased maternal morbidity and little evidence of improved outcomes for the neonate.[15]
- When counselling parents of a fetus with suspected OI, one of the most important aspects is to discuss whether a Caesarean section delivery could improve survival and decrease neonatal morbidity.
- Method of delivery must be individualized on a case-by-case basis considering both maternal and fetal risks.
- If a vaginal delivery is chosen, care must be taken to avoid assisted instrumental deliveries if possible, to minimize the risk of intracranial trauma.
- Caesarean delivery does not alter the prognosis of infants with lethal disease forms. Similarly, Caesarean delivery does not necessarily reduce the number of fractures in infants with non-lethal forms of OI.[13] In mild forms of fetal OI where fractures are infrequent, Caesarean section may afford some protection against fractures.

Table 17.1 Types of osteogenesis imperfecta

Type of OI	*Inheritance pattern*	*Incidence per live births*	*Age when symptoms appear*	*Clinical features*	*Progression and outcome*
Type 1	Most common form of OI; about 70% of all OI Autosomal dominant One parent usually has mild or severe form of OI Risk of offspring being affected is 50% in each pregnancy	~1:30 000	Infancy Seldom diagnosed in utero by antenatal scans	Fractures, especially vertebral and long bones, are common but usually heal without much deformity Fewer fractures as adults Biphosphonate treatment in those prone to multiple fractures may help Blue sclera, thin skin, hearing loss, hypermobile joints, scoliosis	Fertility not affected Main pregnancy symptoms -back-ache (13%) and vertebral fractures(4%) Compatible with normal life expectancy
Type 2	Most severe form, 10% of all OI Fresh mutation as all born to healthy parents or one parent has a form of mosaicism Risk of second child affected if previous child had OI type 2 is ~6%	1:60 000	In utero Antenatal scans show multiple fractures, hypomineralization of calvarium (fetal cranium),concertina effect of femur due to multiple fractures and rib fractures, etc.	Multiple fractures in all bones	Most die in early childhood or during process of delivery
Type 3	Severe form, 20% of all OI Usually autosomal dominant, with 50% chance of affected offspring Significant numbers are autosomal recessive, when risk of affected offspring for each pregnancy is ~25%	1:70 000	50% detected antenatally, 50% in infancy	Antenatal scans may show fractures, bones bend and break In childhood, severe deformities, short stature and disability, tooth enamel poor Biphosphonates ineffective in this form of OI	By age of 6 multiple fractures and severe deformities Reduced life expectancy due to complications
Type 4	Autosomal dominant Risk of recurrence similar to type 1	Very rare	Infancy Not usually detected by antenatal scans	Severity between OI types 1 and 3 Fractures of vertebrae and long bones. Fractures mostly before puberty, fewer as adults Sclerae not blue in adults	Compatible with normal life expectancy

Management of pregnancy in women with OI

- There is a 50% chances of the fetus having OI in each pregnancy of an OI mother, due to autosomal dominance.
- Physiological changes of pregnancy when superimposed on the limitations and disabilities of OI, especially in the more severe forms, can be challenging.
- In severe forms of OI, type 3 OI in particular, worsening bone abnormalities with stress fractures due to weightbearing and cardiac and pulmonary compromise can increase maternal morbidity.[1]
- Pregnancy complications that can be anticipated in pregnancy in a patient affected by OI include preterm delivery, preterm premature rupture of membranes, pre-eclampsia, anaemia, calcium deficiency, fetal malpositions, IUGR, and uterine atony with postpartum haemorrhage (PPH).[4,8,14]
- PPH could also result from coexistent platelet dysfunction, capillary fragility, and reduced levels of factor VIII, all being secondary to deficient collagen binding which results in friable tissues and an inadequate vasoconstrictive response to bleeding.
- Multidisciplinary, multispecialty management is essential in pregnancies in women with OI. Referral of severe cases of OI to tertiary centres is recommended.
- Early referral for senior anaesthetic assessment and review is essential, as is referral to the pulmonary physician and cardiologists.
- If platelet abnormalities are noted, haematological opinion must be sought.
- Low-dose aspirin from the first trimester for pre-eclampsia prophylaxis must be considered and vigilance maintained for the development of pre-eclampsia.
- Serial fetal growth scans must be maintained whether the fetus is affected with OI or not.
- Anticipation of PPH, due either to atonicity or to platelet abnormalities, should prompt active management of the third stage with high-dose oxytocin infusion in addition to routine bolus dose of oxytocin or oxytocin with ergometrine.[10] Arrangements for adequate cross-matched blood stores, fresh frozen plasma, etc. must be made antenatally.
- There are particular challenges facing anaesthetic management of women with OI. Respiratory compromise with reduced vital capacity could be present due to restrictive pneumopathy arising from vertebral and rib fractures, pectus excavatum, etc.[4,16] Further anaesthetic problems can arise from immobility of the cervical spine, and hyperthermia provoked by general anaesthetic agents such as succinylcholine and inhalational anaesthetics.[17]
- Pre-existing platelet abnormalities,[18] abnormalities of the spine, and neural compression as a result of multiple fractures and kyphoscoliosis could interfere with neuro-axis block or make the level of the blockade unpredictable.
- Individualized plans for both mode of delivery and type of anaesthetic for either an elective or emergency Caesarean section must be discussed with the patient, shared with all concerned in her care, and clearly documented in the notes.
- Routine thromboprophylaxis guidelines should be followed but with care to ensure appropriate weight-adjusted doses of low molecular weight heparin.

Information for patients

Please see **Information for patients: Osteogenesis imperfecta and pregnancy** (p. 535)

References

1. Glosten B. Osteogenesis imperfecta. In:Gambling DR, Douglas MJ, ed. Obstetric anesthesia and uncommon disorders. Philadelphia: WB Saunders, 1998, pp. 213–218.
2. Rocke DA, Moodley J. Trauma and orthopedic problems. In:Datta S, ed. Anesthetic and obstetric management of high-risk pregnancy 2nd ed. St. Louis: Mosby, 1996, pp. 296–310.
3. Partridge BL. Skin and bone disorders. In:Benumof JL, ed. Anesthesia and uncommon diseases 4th ed. Philadelphia: WB Saunders, 1998, pp. 423–456.
4. Vogel TM, et al. Pregnancy complicated by severe osteogenesis imperfecta: a report of two cases. Anesth Analg 2002; 94: 1315–1317.
5. Sillence DO, et al. Genetic heterogeneity in osteogenesis imperfecta. J Med Genet 1979; 16: 101–116.
6. Orioli IM, et al. The birth prevalence rates for the skeletal dysplasias. J Med Genet 1986; 23: 328–332.
7. Andersen PE Jr, Hauge M. Osteogenesis imperfecta: a genetic, radiological, and epidemiological study. Clin Genet 1989; 36: 250–255.
8. Litos M, et al. Osteogenesis imperfecta and pregnancy. Eur J Obstet Gynecol Reprod Biol 2008; 136: 126–127.
9. Michell C, et al. Osteogenesis imperfecta. Curr Orthop 2007; 21: 236–241.
10. Sharma A, et al. Osteogenesis imperfecta in pregnancy: two cases reports and review literature. Obstet Gynecol Surv 2001; 56: 563–566.
11. Mcallion SJ, Paterson CR. Musculoskeletal problems associated with pregnancy in women with osteogenesis imperfecta. J Obstet Gynaecol 2002; 22: 169–172.
12. Pepin M, et al. Strategies and outcomes of prenatal diagnosis for osteogenesis imperfecta: a review of biochemical and molecular studies completed in 129 pregnancies. Prenat Diagn 1997; 17: 559–570.
13. Cubert R, et al. Osteogenesis imperfecta: mode of delivery and neonatal outcome. Obstet Gynecol 2001; 97: 66–69.
14. Marini JC. Osteogenesis imperfecta: comprehensive management. Adv Pediatr 1988; 35: 391–426.
15. Brons JT, et al. Prenatal ultrasonographic diagnosis of osteogenesis imperfecta. Am J Obstet Gynecol 1988; 159: 176–181.
16. Cho E, et al. Anaesthesia in a parturient with osteogenesis imperfecta. Br J Anaesth 1992; 68: 422–423.
17. Porsborg P, et al. Osteogenesis imperfecta and malignant hyperthermia: Is there a relationship? Anaesthesia 1996; 51: 863–865.
18. Douglas MJ. Platelets, the parturient and regional anesthesia. Int J Obstet Anesth 2001; 10: 113–120.

Pre-pregnancy assessment and genetic counselling

- Usually patient has already had genetic tests and is aware of type of osteogenesis imperfecta (OI)
- Detailed history, including frequency and type of fractures, any pelvic fractures, previous operations, any cardiorespiratory problems, bleeding problems, and previous obstetric history (if multip)
- Genetic counselling: Refer for expert genetic counselling if not already done. Type of OI may have been ascertained by skin biopsy and analysis of fibroblasts. Obtain family history of other individuals with OI—50% chance of offspring being affected in every pregnancy, type of OI usually of the same type as the mother's—occasionally symptoms may be more or less severe
- Baseline pulmonary function tests if restrictive thoracic capacity due to vertebral or rib fractures—referral to pulmonary physician recommended
- Discuss pregnancy management, potential risks and outcomes
- Discuss how physiological changes of pregnancy could add to any already existing cardiopulmonary compromise. Also, increased risk of pregnancy complications (e.g. preterm labour, pre-eclampsia, PPROM, IUGR, fetal malpositions especially breech, PPH) which will require careful surveillance and appropriate multidisciplinary management

↓

Referral from GP or community midwife to specialist antenatal clinic as early as possible in 1st trimester

↓

First visit to specialist antenatal clinic

- Confirm pregnancy, establish viability and dates
- Discuss prenatal diagnosis. If patient opts for it, either CVS or amniocentesis
- Consider low-dose aspirin for pre-eclampsia prophylaxis
- Check FBC, seek haematology opinion if any platelet problems and a previous history of blood clotting problems
- Refer to anaesthetic high-risk clinic for assessment by senior anaesthetist
- Refer to pulmonary physician for baseline measurements of pulmonary function and assessment
- Arrange serial scans for fetal growth, and for any signs of in-utero fractures
- Discuss increased risks of some pregnancy complications (e.g. pre-eclampsia, preterm labour, PPROM) and awareness of symptoms to report
- Continue routine antenatal care with community midwife
- ***Refer to tertiary centre in cases of severe OI***

↓

Further visits to specialist antenatal clinic

At suggested intervals of 4 weeks from about 24 weeks gestation:

- Assess pregnancy progress, fetal serial scans, and any sign of in-utero fractures. Malpositions (especially breech) more common in OI
- Enquire about any respiratory problems
- Confirm patient has been reviewed by senior anaesthetist and at regular intervals during pregnancy by the respiratory physician
- Multidisciplinary team discussion regarding mode of delivery and anaesthetic involved—discuss with patient—delivery invariably by elective Caesarean section.
- ***Documentation of plans for both emergency and elective Caesarean delivery, shared with all involved with patient's care***
- Increasing respiratory compromise might necessitate early delivery
- Mode and timing of delivery and type of anaesthetic to be individualised according to maternal and fetal conditions

17.3 Kyphoscoliosis

FACT FILE

Epidemiology

- **Kyphoscoliosis** (KS) is a bony spinal deformity characterized by excessive posterior curvature (kyphosis) and lateral curvature (scoliosis).
- Aetiology is unknown in most cases (70% of KS is of idiopathic origin). Other rare causes include tuberculosis, severe osteoporosis, neuromuscular disease such as poliomyelitis, connective tissue disorders such as Marfan's, Ehlers–Danlos syndrome, etc.[1]
- Idiopathic KS occurs in infantile, juvenile, and adolescent forms.
- KS can occur at any age but clinical manifestations are seen most commonly at periods of rapid growth.
- Both women and men are affected, but there is a female preponderance of 1:2 to 1:3 for reasons that are so far unknown.
- Prevalence in the general adult population reported to be approximately 8% (data from USA).[2]
- Incidence amongst pregnant women varies between 1 in 1470 to about 1 in 12 000.[3]

Pathophysiology

- Thoracic KS causes a significant reduction in the number of alveoli of the lungs, thus predisposing these patients to impaired gas exchange and pulmonary hypertension.
- Increased risks of respiratory compromise and premature death in severe untreated cases of KS resulting from significant reduction in lung volumes, pulmonary hypertension and cardiorespiratory failure has been reported.[4]
- Compression of the lungs by the malformation of the thoracic cage causing atelectasis can further worsen the respiratory compromise.
- The combined effect of kyphosis and scoliosis is worse than either abnormality on its own.
- Respiratory problems during sleep include hypoxaemia and hypercapnia due to hypoventilation.[5]
- The **Cobb's angle** is a radiological measurement made on an AP view of the spinal radiograph to evaluate the severity of KS. It **correlates well with pulmonary function tests**.

Effect of KS on pregnancy

- Preterm labour and delivery are the most common effects.[6]

Effect of pregnancy on KS

- Those with a stable curvature do not usually worsen in pregnancy whereas those with unstable curvatures show a worsening, especially if the pre-pregnancy curvature was greater than 25 degrees.[7]
- Respiratory complications such as increasing breathlessness are seen in about 17% of women during pregnancy.[8,9]
- In the face of severe restrictive pulmonary compromise, resulting in a vital capacity of less than 1 litre, the patient needs to be advised not to get pregnant.
- ***Maternal mortality and morbidity are directly linked to the degree of such respiratory compromise***. As a general rule, if the lung capacity is 50% or more of the predicted volume, the pregnancy can proceed normally.[8,10]
- The severity of pulmonary impairment correlates with the Cobb's angle, the number of vertebrae involved and a higher site (more cephalad) of the curvature.[11]
- ***Maternal mortality is significantly raised if the vital capacity is less than 1.25 litres.***[1]
- ***Pre-pregnancy assessment by the respiratory physician and subsequent counselling by the specialist obstetrician is thus of paramount importance.***

Management of pregnancy[1]

- Referral to a **senior anaesthetist** for assessment and consultation must be made as soon as possible during pregnancy.[12,13]
- Similarly, referral to the **respiratory physician** for ongoing assessments and input into management plans is essential.
- Ideally, the patient should be assessed routinely in the respiratory medicine unit, at least once in 2 months during pregnancy for measurements of the vital capacity, forced expiratory volume, tidal volume, functional residual capacity, oxygen saturation, and ECG if needed. Arterial blood gas measurements will be required if there is any suspicion of hypoventilation which can result in hypoxaemia and hypercapnia.
- In severe cases, cardiac strain can result secondary to respiratory compromise. Cardiology referral must be made as soon as possible and cardiology input sought in the joint multidisciplinary management.
- Serial growth scans with Doppler flow indices are required.
- If there is worsening maternal respiratory compromise in the third trimester, early delivery, probably by Caesarean section, may be required.
- If the pelvis is misshapen or malpresentations are found, delivery by LSCS is indicated.
- Similarly if evidence of IUGR is confirmed by ultrasound scans and Dopplers, early delivery needs to be considered.
- Cases of KS can pose **serious anaesthetic challenges** during labour and for delivery, either vaginal or Caesarean section.
- It is of vital importance that anaesthetic management plans for both elective and emergency situations are drawn up well ahead of time and disseminated to all involved or likely to be involved in the patient's intrapartum care. Clear documentation in the notes (both the main and patient's hand-held notes) is essential.
- The patient may have had prior surgical correction of the KS with insertion of a metal rod such as the Harrington rod.[13] Spinal fusion with autologous grafting from the iliac bone may have been previously performed.[14] Anaesthetic management plans to provide analgesia for labour and delivery or anaesthetic for a planned or emergency Caesarean section will need to take these factors into account.
- ***It is vital that all pregnant women with KS, with or without previous corrective surgery, be referred as soon as possible in pregnancy to the anaesthetic high-risk antenatal clinic.***[1] ***This will allow the senior anaesthetist an opportunity for a thorough assessment and for management plans to be discussed, drawn up, and disseminated long before the estimated date of delivery.***

Information for patients

Please see Information for patients: Kyphoscoliosis and pregnancy (p. 536)

References

1. Rocke DA, Moodley J. Orthopedic problems: kyphoscoliosis. In: Datta S, ed., Anesthetic and obstetric management of high-risk pregnancy 2nd ed. St. Louis: Mosby, 1996.
2. Carter OD, Haynes SG. Prevalence rates for scoliosis in US adults: Results from the first National Health and Nutrition Examination Survey. Int J Epidemiol 1987; 16: 537–544.
3. Kopenhager T. A review of 50 pregnant patients with kyphoscoliosis. Br J Obstet Gynaecol 1977; 84: 585–587.
4. Pehrsson K, et al. Lung function in adult idiopathic scoliosis: A 20 year follow up. Thorax 1991; 46: 474–478.

5. Midgren B, et al. Nocturnal hypoxaemia in severe scoliosis. Br J Dis Chest 1988; 82: 226–236.
6. Betz RR, et al. Scoliosis and pregnancy. J Bone Joint Surg Am 1987; 69: 90–96.
7. Blount WP, Mellencamp D. The effect of pregnancy on idiopathic scoliosis. J Bone Joint Surg Am 1980; 62: 1083–1087.
8. Sawicka EH, et al. Management of respiratory failure complicating pregnancy in severe kyphoscoliosis: A new use for an old technique? Br J Dis Chest 1986; 80: 191–196.
9. Siegler D, Zorab PA. Pregnancy in thoracic scoliosis. Br J Dis Chest 1981; 75: 367–370.
10. Berman AT, et al. The effects of pregnancy on idiopathic scoliosis: A preliminary report on eight cases and a review of the literature. Spine 1982; 7: 76–77.
11. Veliath DG, et al. Parturient with kyphoscoliosis (operated) for caesarean section. J Anaesthesiol Clin Pharmacol 2012; 28: 124–126.
12. Gupta S, Singariya G. Kyphoscoliosis and pregnancy—a case report. Indian J Anaesth 2004; 48: 215–220.
13. Crosby ET, Halpern SH. Obstetric epidural anaesthesia in patients with Harrington instrumentation Can J Anesth 1989; 36: 693–696.
14. Feldstein G, Ramanathan S. Obstetrical lumbar epidural anesthesia in patients with previous spinal fusion for kyphoscoliosis. Anesth Analg 1985; 64: 83–85.

CARE PATHWAY

Pre-pregnancy assessment and counselling for a women with kyphoscoliosis

- Pre-pregnancy assessment by respiratory physician and subsequent counselling by specialist maternal medicine obstetrician
- Pulmonary function tests: Measurement of vital capacity (VC), forced expiratory volume, tidal volume, functional residual capacity, O_2 saturation, etc. ECG, arterial O_2 especially if hypoventilation
- Radiological measurement of Cobb's angle and of pelvic shape as indicated
- Discussion of multidisciplinary management during a future pregnancy
- Discussion of increased chances and surveillance for preterm delivery, fetal growth restriction, and respiratory complications
- If pelvis is misshapen, increased chances of requiring Caesarean section
- If severely compromised pulmonary function with VC <1 litre, advise against pregnancy due to increased morbidity, even mortality.

↓

GP or community midwife to refer early in 1st trimester to specialist antenatal clinic/maternal medicine clinic

↓

First visit to maternal medicine or specialist antenatal clinic

- Assess pregnancy, note most pulmonary function test findings
- Refer to respiratory physician for ongoing assessment and joint management during pregnancy
- Refer to senior obstetric anaesthetist for assessment and management plans
- In severe cases, urgent referral for cardiological assessment and opinion—may need transfer to a tertiary unit for continued pregnancy care and delivery
- Organize serial fetal growth scans

↓

Further visits to maternal medicine or specialist antenatal clinic

- Ideally, regular pulmonary assessments need to continue every 2 months during pregnancy
- Early discussions regarding mode and timing of delivery
- Clear and timely dissemination of management plans for labour and delivery, including anaesthetic plans, to all those involved in her care
- If pelvis misshapen, delivery by Caesarean section
- ***If worsening respiratory function in 3rd trimester in severe cases, early delivery may be indicated, most likely by Caesarean section. Close liaison with respiratory physician and cardiologist essential in such cases. May need transfer to tertiary unit***
- Preoperative assessment by experienced anaesthetist

18 Maternal Obesity

18.1 Obesity and Pregnancy

FACT FILE

- **Obesity** is a major health risk and these risks increase with the degree of obesity (see Table 18.1).
- Maternal obesity is a major cause of obstetric morbidity and mortality. The prevalence of obesity has reached epidemic proportions and 33% of pregnant women in the UK are now overweight or obese.[1]
- In the Seventh Report of the Confidential Enquiries into Maternal Deaths in the United Kingdom (CEMACE),[2] approximately 35% of all the women who died during pregnancy, labour, and postpartum were obese.
- Also, 30% of mothers who had a stillbirth or neonatal death were obese.[3]
- Obesity in pregnancy is defined as a body mass index (BMI) of 30 kg/m^2 or more at the first antenatal consultation.
- Obesity is a recognized high risk factor for a range of antenatal, intrapartum, and postnatal complications for both mother and baby.[1,2,3,4] It also poses important occupational health and safety issues for staff caring for obese women.
- During any pregnancy, the overall weight gain to be expected is related to the pre-pregnancy weight (see Table 18.2). The figure typically quoted is 12–14 kg, which is the average associated with the best and safest outcome of pregnancy.
- 2–6 kg of this weight gain is an increase in the mother's body fat.
- For each extra kg in addition to the maternal booking weight of the mother (average 61 kg) the birth weight of the baby increases by 9 g.
- The more weight gained during pregnancy (over and above that of the baby and the total weight of the uterus), the greater will be the weight subsequently retained. This is compounded by successive pregnancies where weight is progressively increased.
- The risk of pre-eclampsia, gestational diabetes mellitus (GDM), large-for-gestational-age babies, Caesarean section and stillbirth is linearly related to interpregnancy weight gain.[5]
- A weight loss of at least 4.5 kg before the second pregnancy reduces the risk of developing GDM by up to 40%.[6]
- About half of the body fat gained by the mother during pregnancy is deposited around the abdomen, which itself carries higher health risks.
- Modest weight gain during pregnancy is essential. Women should not therefore actively diet or seriously reduce their intake during pregnancy. Doing so will compromise important micronutrients such as iron, zinc, calcium, and folate, as well as failing to meet the extra energy requirements of pregnancy.
- Active programmes for weight loss should be put into practice before and after a pregnancy, not during. Lifestyle changes such as weight reduction and exercise are firmly in the control of the individual.
- ***The advice therefore is to eat a healthy diet during pregnancy and then to lose weight after childbirth and before the next pregnancy.***

Antenatal and intrapartum risks of obesity

- ***Women with a booking BMI of 30 or more should have an informed discussion antenatally about possible intrapartum complications associated with a high BMI, and management strategies considered. This should be documented in the notes.***[1]
- **Gestational diabetes** (GDM):[4] Overweight and obese women are at much higher risk of developing diabetes brought on by their pregnancy. This in turn, leads to a much higher risk of developing non-insulin-dependent diabetes within 10 years of first developing GDM.
- **Vitamin D deficiency**: Pre-pregnancy BMI is inversely associated with serum vitamin D concentrations among pregnant women. Obese women (BMI ≥30) are at increased risk of vitamin D deficiency compared to women with a healthy weight (BMI <25).[7]
- **Hypertension, pregnancy-induced hypertension, pre-eclampsia**:[8] The risk doubles with each 5–7 kg excess weight gain in pregnancy.
- Increased risk of **preterm labour.**
- **Thromboembolism**: The risk of DVT/PE is increased 2–2.5 times in the obese pregnant patient.[9] Women with a booking BMI of 30 or more requiring pharmacological thromboprophylaxis should be prescribed doses appropriate for maternal weight, in accordance with the RCOG clinical guideline.[10]
- All women with a BMI of 40 or more should be offered postnatal thromboprophylaxis regardless of their mode of delivery.[9,10]
- **Increased risk of congenital anomalies**:[11] Neural tube defects such as spina bifida,[12] omphalocele, heart defects, etc.

Table 18.1 WHO definition of obesity

Classification	*Early pregnancy BMI (kg/m^2)*	*Risk of obstetric/anaesthetic complications*
Normal range	18.5–24.9	No increased obstetric or maternal risk
Overweight	25–29.9	No increased obstetric or maternal risk
Obese I	30–34.9	Mildly increased risks
Obese II	35–39.9	Moderately increased risks
Obese III[a]	≥40	Significant/serious maternal, fetal, and anaesthetic risks

[a] Category Obese III is also known as morbid obesity.

Reproduced with kind permission from the World Health Organization. <http://apps.who.int/bmi/index.jsp?introPage=intro_3.html>

Table 18.2 Recommendations for total weight gain during pregnancy by pre-pregnancy BMI

Pre-pregnancy BMI	Category	*Total weight gain range (singleton pregnancy)*	*Rates of weight gain: 2nd & 3rd trimesters (average range per week)*
18.5–24.9	Normal weight	11–16 kg (25–35 lbs)	0.45 kg (1 lb)
25–29.9	Overweight	7–11 kg (15–25 lbs)	0.27 kg (0.6 lb)
≥30	Obese	5–9 kg (11–20 lbs)	0.22 kg (0.5 lb)

Reprinted with permission from 'Weight gain during pregnancy: Re-examining the Guidelines', Report Brief, 2009, by The Institute of Medicine of the National Academies, Courtesy of the National Academies Press, Washington, D.C.

- **Poorer views on ultrasound scan**: The greater the obesity, the less the accuracy of obtaining good views for both anomaly screening and biometry.
- **Problems with external monitoring of the fetus** in women with category III obesity and above.
- **Abnormal fetal growth**: Macrosomia and IUGR.
- **Increased risk of intrauterine death**: 2–4-fold increase.
- Obese women face a **decreased choice** for home births, water births, etc.
- **Increased risk of failed induction of labour** (up to 40% in obese women), failure of induction, as well as of increased chances of Caesarean section (double the non-obese rate), especially emergency Caesarean section (up to 50%). In the absence of other obstetric or medical indications, obesity alone is not an indication for induction of labour and a normal birth should be encouraged.
- **Failure to progress in labour, poor contractions, dysfunctional labour.**[13]
- **Inadequate analgesia, failed epidurals.**
- **Anaesthetic risks**, including the risk of aspiration of gastric contents under general anaesthesia, difficult endotracheal intubation and postoperative atelectasis.[14]
- ***Technically difficult Caesarean sections with both anaesthetic and surgical risks. Therefore, increased perioperative morbidity, even mortality.***
- **Postpartum haemorrhage.**
- **Shoulder dystocia, meconium aspiration, fetal distress.**
- **Increased perinatal mortality rates** (stillbirths and neonatal deaths).[15,16,17,18]
- **Increased risk of unsuccessful VBACs** (successful VBACs <15–20%).[19]
- **Unsuccessful external cephalic version *(ECV)*.**

Postnatal risks of obesity

- **Wound complications** after operative delivery or perineal trauma.
- **Infections**:[20] wound, endometritis, perineum, UTI, respiratory.
- **Thromboembolic events.**
- **Longer hospital stay.**
- **Failure to establish breastfeeding** due perhaps to an inadequate prolactin response.

Anaesthetic complications and problems

- Elective surgery in the obese is high risk.[1,14]
- Emergency surgery in the obese is extremely high risk
- Problems with positioning of the patient may be encountered.
- **Inadequate or failed regional analgesia**: Though regional anaesthetic for surgery or labour analgesia is favoured over a general anaesthetic, it is more difficult to site, spread of local anaesthetic may be unpredictable, the epidural catheter is more likely to dislodge, and regional analgesia may work unevenly.[21]
- **Oxygenation difficulties** due to abdominal pressure.
- **Airway maintenance problems**: Intubation may be impossible, especially in emergency settings.
- Non-invasive BP cuffs may be less reliable.
- **Care in the high-dependency unit (HDU) or ICU** may be required in some morbidly obese pregnant women.

Pre-pregnancy advice

Pre-pregnancy advice should include:

- Information and advice about the risks of obesity during pregnancy and childbirth must be offered to women of childbearing age with a BMI of 30 or more and they must be supported to lose weight before conception.[1]
- Discussion of the importance of healthy diet and exercise.
- Referral to dietitian.
- Screening for type 2 diabetes, hypertension, hypercholesterolemia, and cardiovascular disease.
- Peri-pregnancy high-dose folic acid (5 mg/day) should be considered.[1,22]
- As this cohort of patients are at high risk of developing pregnancy-induced hypertension and pre-eclampsia, advise **low-dose aspirin** to commence from early in first trimester, continued till end of pregnancy.

Management guidelines in pregnancy

- Medical issues related to the risks and management of obesity in pregnancy (see 'Antenatal and intrapartum risks of obesity') need to be discussed in **an open and non-judgemental manner, handled with dignity and respect**. It is important however, that these issues are not neglected or side-stepped due to reticence of the healthcare staff to engage in such discussions, because such pregnancies are indeed high risk from a purely medical point of view.
- Remember that an obese woman can feel uncomfortable or upset if discussions with professionals are felt to be derogatory or insulting. Professionals likewise often feel embarrassed about broaching the topic of weight in pregnancy. **Sensitive and sympathetic discussions can bridge this gap and the role of the midwife is paramount in this.**
- At booking it is mandatory that the BMI is calculated and recorded in the notes by the community midwife. Weight recording must be in kilograms, not in pounds or stones!
- At booking and at the first visit to the hospital antenatal clinic, the high BMI should be discussed with the patient.
- **It is not uncommon for women in the overweight and obese categories to fail to have identified their own weight category.** Calculation and discussion of the BMI may therefore be the first step.
- According to NICE guidelines,[3] community midwives should refer patients classed as obese category I or above (i.e. BMI >30) to a specialist antenatal clinic for shared antenatal care. There are differences in local prevalence of maternal obesity, and resource implications for local healthcare organizations. By local consensus some maternity units might reset the referral criteria to a hospital-based antenatal clinic as a BMI of 35 or even 38. Initial discussions should include additional risks in pregnancy and need for greater surveillance offered by the hospital.
- Early booking is recommended for all women with a booking BMI greater than 40 to enable management plans to be put in place.
- Ensure that the woman is taking high-dose folic acid 5 mg/day, and advise that this is continued till end of 12 weeks gestation.
- All pregnant women with a BMI of 30 or more must be advised to take 10 micrograms vitamin D supplementation daily during pregnancy and while breastfeeding.
- Prescribe low-dose aspirin 75 mg/day from first trimester to end of pregnancy.
- All those with a booking BMI of 30 will need to have a screening glucose tolerance test (GTT) at about 26–28 weeks gestation according to NICE guidelines.[3]
- If there has been a previous history of gestational diabetes or consecutive episodes of glycosuria in the obese pregnant woman, an early GTT (at 14–16 weeks) is required to detect pre-existing type 2 diabetes. If this early GTT is normal, a standard 26–28-week GTT must be performed to detect gestational diabetes.
- All BP readings for those in category II obesity and above should be taken using the large cuff in the hospital as well as in the community.
- Pregnant women with a booking BMI of 40 or more should have an antenatal consultation with an obstetric anaesthetist, so that potential difficulties with venous access, regional or general anaesthesia can be identified. **An anaesthetic management plan for labour and delivery should be discussed and documented in the medical records.**[1,21]
- Overweight women at booking must be given a target for weight gain in pregnancy according to their category (see Table 18.2). Giving overweight/obese women the same targets for weight gain during pregnancy as women of normal weight might contribute to excess weight gain.[23,24]
- Once the risks associated with obesity and excessive weight gain have been discussed, referral to the dietitian is recommended. A diet and activity plan and a target range for weight gain during

pregnancy should be agreed with the woman. This should be documented in the hand-held notes and referred to by the community midwife and by the hospital antenatal team in subsequent visits.

- The limitations of ultrasonography and symphysiofundal measurements in obese women must be recognized.
- Wide BP cuffs must be consistently used consistently both in the community and in hospital, with documentation in the notes made at the booking or the first hospital antenatal clinic visit.
- Specific plans for labour and delivery must be discussed and documented in the notes.[1] These include:
  - Women with a BMI of 40 or more should have venous access established early in labour.
  - All women with a BMI of 30 or more should be recommended to have active management of the third stage of labour.
  - Women with a BMI of 30 or more having a Caesarean section have an increased risk of wound infection, and should receive prophylactic antibiotics at the time of surgery.
  - Women undergoing Caesarean section who have more than 2 cm subcutaneous fat should have suturing of the subcutaneous space in order to reduce the risk of wound infection and wound separation.[25]
  - Postnatal thromboprophylaxis with weight -dependent doses of LMWH.
- **Obese women who have had a previous Caesarean section have a lower successful VBAC rate,**[19] which needs to be taken into account when options for mode of delivery are discussed.
- As a Caesarean section is itself a more risky procedure in an obese woman, the decision to attempt a trial of labour has to be individualized after various risks have been fully explored with the patient and documented.
- Advice regarding care of abdominal or perineal wound must be given.
- All women who have been diagnosed with gestational diabetes should have a postnatal GTT at 6 weeks, should be advised to have annual screening for cardiometabolic risk factors, and should be offered lifestyle and weight management advice.

Information for patients

Please see Information for patients: Obesity and pregnancy (p. 536)

References

1. CMACE/RCOG Joint Guideline Management of Women with Obesity in Pregnancy. London: Centre for Maternal and Child Enquiries and the Royal College of Obstetricians and Gynaecologists, 2010
2. Lewis G, ed. Saving mothers' lives: reviewing maternal deaths to make motherhood safer 2003-2005. The Seventh Report of the Confidential Enquiries into Maternal Deaths in the United Kingdom. London: CEMACH, 2007.
3. NICE. Obesity: guidance on the prevention, identification, assessment and management of overweight and obesity in adults and children. GC43. London: National Institute for Health and Care Excellence, 2006.
4. Chu SY, et al. Maternity obesity and risk of gestational diabetes mellitus. Diabetes Care 2007; 30: 2070–2076.
5. Villamor E, Cnattingius S. Interpregnancy weight change and risk of adverse pregnancy outcomes: a population-based study. Lancet 2006; 368 (9542): 1164–1170.
6. Glazer NL, et al. Weight change and the risk of gestational diabetes in obese women. Epidemiology 2004; 15: 733–737.
7. Bodnar LM, et al. Prepregnancy obesity predicts poor vitamin D status in mothers and their neonates. J Nutr 2007; 137: 2437–2442.
8. O'Brien TE, et al. Maternal body mass index and the risk of preeclampsia: a systematic overview. Epidemiology 2003; 14: 368–374.
9. James AH, et al. Venous thromboembolism during pregnancy and the post-partum period: incidence, risk factors, and mortality. Am J Obstet Gynecol 2006; 194: 1311–1315.
10. RCOG Green-top Guideline No. 37. Reducing the risk of thrombosis and embolism during pregnancy and puerperium. London: Royal College of Obstetricians and Gynaecologists, 2009.
11. Waller DK, et al. Prepregnancy obesity as a risk factor for structural birth defects. National Birth Defects Prevention Study. Arch Pediatr Adolesc Med 2007; 161: 745–750.
12. Rasmussen SA, et al. Maternity obesity and the risk of neural tubal defects: a meta-analysis. Am J Obstet Gynecol 2008; 198: 611–619
13. Ehrenberg HM, et al. Maternal obesity, uterine activity, and the risk of spontaneous preterm birth. Obstet Gynecol 2009; 113: 48–52.
14. Saravanakumar K, et al. The challenges of obesity and obstetric anaesthesia. Curr Opin Obstet Gynecol 2006; 18: 631–635.
15. Chu SY, et al. Maternal obesity and risk of cesarean delivery: a meta-analysis. Obes Rev 2007; 8: 385–394.
16. Kristensen J, et al. Pre-pregnancy weight and the risk of stillbirth and neonatal death. BJOG 2005; 112: 403–408.
17. Sebire NJ, et al. Maternal obesity and pregnancy outcome: a study of 287,213 pregnancies in London. Int J Obes Relat Metab Disord 2001; 25: 1175–82.
18. Lu GC, et al. The effect of the increasing prevalence of maternal obesity on perinatal morbidity. Am J Obstet Gynecol 2001; 185: 845–849.
19. Goodall PT, et al. Obesity as a risk factor for failed trial of labor in patients with previous Cesarean delivery. Am J Obstet Gynecol 2005; 192: 1423–1426.
20. Myles TD, et al. Obesity as an independent risk factor for infectious morbidity in patients who undergo Cesarean delivery. Obstet Gynecol 2002; 100: 959–964.
21. Hood DD, Dewan DM.Anesthetic and obstetric outcome in morbidly obese parturients. Anesthesiology 1993; 79: 1210–1218.
22. Mojtabai R. Body mass index and serum folate in childbearing age women. Eur J Epidemiol 2004; 19: 1029.
23. Stotland NE. Obesity and pregnancy. BMJ 2009; 338: 107–110.
24. Stotland NE, et al. Body mass index, provider advice, and target gestational weight gain. Obstet Gynecol 2005; 105: 633–638.
25. National Institute for Health and Clinical Excellence. Caesarean section. London: Royal College of Obstetricians and Gynaecologists, 2004.

CARE PATHWAY

Community midwife or GP at booking

- Calculate and document BMI (recording weight in kilograms, not in pounds or stones)
- Share BMI chart with **obese patient**, explaining the particular BMI category she fits into
- Possible associated risks during pregnancy and delivery, hence the referral to the hospital specialist clinic
- Discuss importance of healthy diet and exercise, give information booklet about healthy eating in pregnancy
- For any woman with a booking BMI ≥35 or an arm diameter of >35 cm, BP recorded with large cuff
- If BMI >40 (morbid obesity) refer woman to anaesthetic high- risk clinic irrespective of proposed mode of delivery
- Refer woman for shared antenatal care to hospital specialist antenatal clinic
- Arrange GTT at 28 weeks. **(Note: Some regional/local guidelines may vary from NICE guidelines due to resource constraints, offering GTT only to those with BMI >35. NICE guidelines recommend GTT screening for all with BMI >30.)**
- If previous history of gestational diabetes, arrange GTT for 16 weeks. If this is normal, arrange repeat GTT at 28 weeks pregnancy
- High-dose folic acid (5 mg/day) from before pregnancy till end of 12 weeks gestation
- If raised BP at booking or previous history of PIH/pre-eclampsia, advise low-dose aspirin

↓

First visit to specialist antenatal clinic

- Non-judgemental, sensitive, but open discussion regarding additional risks of obesity during pregnancy, delivery, and postpartum
- Discussion of the woman's BMI category and level of obstetric, anaesthetic, and fetal risks (see Table 18.1)
- Discuss increased risks of congenital abnormalities, PIH, pre-eclampsia, gestational diabetes, thromboembolism, fetal growth problems, poorer views on scan, less accurate clinical measurement, etc.
- High-dose folic acid (5 mg/day) till end of 12 weeks gestation
- Low-dose aspirin to continue till end of pregnancy
- All BP measurements with large cuff
- Advise smoking cessation, offer help and support with this
- Discuss optimum level of pregnancy weight gain according to individual booking BMI category (see Table 18.2)
- Refer to dietitian for review of diet, to agree plan of healthy eating, expected weight gain, and exercise regime during pregnancy
- Arrange detailed scan with specific notation in request form about increased BMI of mother—longer ultrasound appointment time might be required
- GTT at 16 weeks if previous history of gestational diabetes—if normal, arrange repeat GTT at 28 weeks
- For those without previous gestational diabetes, arrange GTT at about 26–28 weeks
- Arrange growth scans at locally agreed frequencies, e.g. one scan as minimum at about 34 weeks gestation or two scans at 30 and 35 weeks gestation with same-day review after scan in hospital antenatal clinic
- If booking BMI ≥50, inform delivery suite and wards as special equipment may need to be kept ready and accessible
- Thromboembolism prophylaxis according to RCOG guidelines—mandatory
- Refer to anaesthetic clinic if BMI ≥40 (according to locally agreed guidelines)
- Further antenatal visits to hospital clinic to be individualized according to any comorbidities (see relevant Comorbidity pathways)
- Antenatal visits to community midwife to continue

↓

Comorbidity pathways

- ***Gestational diabetes***
  - Transfer care to combined obstetric–diabetes clinic
  - Gestational diabetes care pathway to be followed (Chapter 9.1, pp 201–202)
- ***PIH/pre-eclampsia:***
  - See PIH/pre-eclampsia pathway (Chapter 5, pp. 152–157)
  - Refer to hypertension/pre-eclampsia guidelines
- ***Suspected IUGR***—see IUGR pathway (Chapter 26.1, p. 421)
- ***Suspected macrosomia***—see macrosomia pathway (Chapter 26.2, pp 424–425)
- ***Previous Caesarean Section***—see previous Caesarean section pathway (Chapter 22.1, p. 350) **Discuss lower rates of successful VBAC in obesity as well as increased surgical and anaesthetic risks with Caesarean section**

↓

Further visits to specialist antenatal clinic

- Presentation check with scan at each hospital visit, especially in women who are morbidly obese
- Discuss mode of delivery
- Discuss with patient that unless previous history of significant shoulder dystocia with a macrosomic baby, routine early IOL before 40 weeks has not been shown to be of benefit and increases risks of failed IOL and therefore a potentially complicated Caesarean section
- Offer P/V for a 'stretch and sweep' at about 39–40 weeks, **document modified Bishop's score**
- **Clear documentation in notes regarding thromboprophylaxis** following either Caesarean section or vaginal delivery according to RCOG risk-category based guidelines
- Encourage breastfeeding
- Discuss future contraception: **Not for COCP**
- **Encourage active weight loss after postpartum and before starting next pregnancy**

18.2 Pregnancy after Bariatric Surgery

FACT FILE

- With the epidemic of obesity in the population, there is a very significant increase of obesity in women of childbearing age. As the overall prevalence of obesity has increased in the general population, so it has among pregnant women.
- More than 1 in 3 pregnant women in the UK is obese.[1] The UK prevalence of women with a known BMI of 35 or more (class II and class III obesity) at any point in pregnancy, who give birth $\geq 24^{+0}$ weeks gestation, is 5%.[2]
- There are considerable risks of maternal and perinatal morbidity and mortality in obese pregnant women. Obesity in pregnancy is associated with an increased risk serious adverse outcomes, including miscarriage, congenital anomaly, thromboembolism, gestational diabetes, pre-eclampsia, dysfunctional labour, higher Caesarean section rate, postpartum haemorrhage, wound infections, lower breastfeeding rates, stillbirth, and neonatal death.[3,4,5]
- The Confidential Enquiry into Maternal and Child Health's report on maternal deaths in the 2003–2005 triennium[3] showed that 28% of mothers who died were obese, whereas the prevalence of obesity in the general maternity population within the same time period was 16–19%.[1]
- A similar disproportionate mortality trend had also been seen in the previous triennial period:[4] of all women who died during pregnancy, childbirth, or postpartum in 2000–2002 in the UK, 35% were obese. Of those who had a stillbirth or neonatal death, 30% were obese.
- Non-surgical weight loss programmes include behavioural changes, diet, exercise, and pharmacological agents.
- ***Bariatric surgery, however, has been shown to be the most effective therapy available for morbid obesity in the longer term (up to 10 years after surgery).***[6,7,8]
- The two most common bariatric surgery procedures are:
  - **laparoscopic adjustable gastric band (LAGB)**, which acts by restricting gastric capacity
  - **Roux-en-Y gastric bypass (RYGB)**, which works by a combination of food restriction with a certain degree of malabsorption by shortening the length of the intestinal tract.
- In LAGB, an inflatable silicon gastric band is placed horizontally at the proximal part of the stomach (fundus). The band can be inflated or deflated with fluid through a subcutaneous port to create a smaller or larger pouch capacity. Restricting the pouch capacity leads to an earlier feeling of satiety and therefore reduced calorie intake.[9]
- Both types of bariatric surgery procedures have a complication rate of about 5%.
- Increasing numbers of women are now getting pregnant having had bariatric surgery. They present a relatively new high-risk pregnancy group with specific challenges that need to be taken into account during their antenatal, intrapartum, and postnatal care.
- ***The care of these women should ideally start from pre-pregnancy with targeted assessment and counselling.***
- There is increasing evidence that weight loss after bariatric surgery may improve both maternal and fetal outcomes. Lower rates of obesity-linked pregnancy complications such as gestational diabetes and hypertensive disorders of pregnancy including pre-eclampsia and fetal macrosomia have been reported.[9,10,11]
- However, not all studies show a reduced incidence of macrosomia after bariatric surgery or a reduction in miscarriage and preterm delivery rates.[10]
- Some significant complications in pregnancies after previous bariatric surgery include maternal intestinal obstruction, gastrointestinal perforation, and haemorrhage as well as nutritional deficiencies which may have a fetal impact.
- IUGR rates have been reported to be higher in pregnancies after bariatric surgery.
- There are reports of an increase in Caesarean rates after bariatric surgery, mainly attributed to previous Caesarean sections (pre-bariatric surgery) in this obese population.
- After bariatric surgery, many patients still remain obese (30–80%).[10,11]

Pre-pregnancy

- Contraception and pre-pregnancy counselling should be mandatory in any woman of reproductive age undergoing bariatric surgery.[10]
- The weight loss following bariatric surgery can restart ovulation, leading to unplanned pregnancies. Also, there is an increased risk of oral contraception failure after bariatric surgery due to malabsorption. Therefore, the non-oral route of contraception in the form of progesterone implant or the intrauterine levonorgestrel-loaded Mirena® may need to be advised.
- The patient should be advised to wait for 12–24 months after bariatric surgery before getting pregnant as this is the time of most rapid weight loss and the micronutrient depletion may not be conducive to the developing fetus.[9,10,11]
- The most common nutritional deficiencies afterbariatric surgery are of protein, iron, folic acid, calcium, and vitamins B_{12}, B_1, D, and K.
- A broad pre-pregnancy evaluation of the levels of these nutrients and vitamins will allow supplementation of those in deficit, starting even before a pregnancy is established. Referral to a dietitian is also advisable.
- Supplements can start in oral form; sometimes the parenteral route may be necessary if there is severe malabsorption.
- It is not clear whether high-dose folic acid (5 mg/day) is required to try to prevent neural tube defects, especially in those who have had the RYGB which results in malabsorption. Care must be taken to ensure there is no concomitant vitamin B_{12} deficiency present before prescribing high-dose folic acid to prevent subacute degeneration of the cord.
- As a minimum, the routine dose of folic acid 400 micrograms must be advised.
- Oral ferrous sulfate (or fumarate which is sometimes better tolerated), and multivitamin supplements are advisable.
- If vitamin B_{12} deficiency is detected, 3-monthly IM injections of vitamin B_{12} may need to be continued throughout pregnancy.

Antenatal care

- ***Proper management during pregnancy is essential to optimize maternal and neonatal outcomes in this group of high-risk pregnancies. Antenatal care must be commenced as soon as possible in the first trimester to treat any nutritional deficiencies.***
- ***Multidisciplinary collaborative care with the bariatric surgeons, dietitian, obstetric specialist in high-risk pregnancies, and midwife is required.***
- ***Advise folic acid 5 mg/day till end of the first trimester.***
- The type of gastric procedure needs to be first established and details obtained from the bariatric surgeon/centre where it was performed.
- Referral to the dietitian for advice regarding a healthy and varied diet.
- Nutritional supplements must be tailored to the individual patient and the type of bariatric surgery she has had.
- If the patient is still obese, low-dose aspirin to reduce risk of pre-eclampsia.
- 'Active band management' where fluid is released or reduced through the subcutaneous port may be required to allow less gastric constriction to relieve nausea and vomiting during the first trimester. The band can be reinflated, if necessary, after the hyperemesis settles.

- Gastrointestinal symptoms such as nausea, vomiting, and abdominal pain, which are otherwise common in pregnancy, should be investigated with care in a woman who has had previous bariatric surgery. Diagnosis of complications related to bariatric surgery, such as bowel obstruction, internal hernias, or anastomotic leaks could otherwise be delayed or missed.
- Intestinal obstruction occurs mainly due to adhesions from previous surgery. It can occur when the expanding uterus puts pressure on the intestine, or when the baby's head descends into the pelvis. Intestinal obstruction may also be encountered postpartum when there is rapid uterine involution.
- Intestinal herniation and obstruction are serious complications that need urgent recognition and intervention.
- ***A considerable proportion of patients (30–80%) remain obese after bariatric surgery and therefore continue to have obesity-related risks.***
- Detailed study of the fetal spine is required as there may have been insufficient folic acid absorption.
- As there is an increased incidence of IUGR, serial growth scans may need to be considered from about 28 weeks onwards at monthly intervals.
- ***Screening for gestational diabetes is required in all such cases but the standard GTT may not be tolerated in those who have developed post-bariatric surgery dumping syndrome.***
- **Dumping syndrome** can occur after gastric bypass procedures if the patient consumes refined sugars or high-glycaemic carbohydrates which cause the stomach to empty rapidly into the small intestine. This can result in abdominal cramps, bloating, nausea, vomiting, and diarrhoea.
- Patients with dumping syndrome cannot tolerate the standard sugary drink of 75 g glucose employed in the GTT. These patients may require **alternative measures to screen for gestational diabetes** such as measuring fasting and then postprandial 2-h blood sugars for about a week between 26–28 weeks. This needs to be discussed with the diabetologist.
- ***After gastric bypass surgery, the absorptive surface of the small intestine is decreased, with less time for absorption. Therefore any drug preparation that is in a slow-release form is not recommended in these patients.***[7] Oral solutions or rapid release preparations should be used instead.
- Prescribe oral water-soluble vitamin K 10 mg/day from about 37 weeks onwards.
- **Previous bariatric surgery should not alter the course of labour and delivery.**[9,10] It must be borne in mind that many of these patients remain obese and the baby might be macrosomic.
- ***Bariatric surgery itself is not an indication for Caesarean section.***[9,10,12]
- Breastfeeding must be encouraged. Sometimes if there is poor maternal fat absorption and low vitamin B_{12} levels this can reduce the energy content of breast milk and affect postnatal growth of the baby.[10,11,12]

Information for patients

Please see Information for patients: Pregnancy after gastric band or gastric bypass procedure (p. 538)

References

1. Heslehurst N, et al. Trends in maternal obesity incidence rates, demographic predictors, and health inequalities in 36,821 women over a 15-year period. BJOG 2007; 114: 187–194.
2. Centre for Maternal and Child Enquiries (CEMACE). Maternal obesity in the UK: findings from a national project. London: CEMACE, 2010 <http://www.cmace.org.uk>.
3. Lewis G, ed. Confidential Enquiry into Maternal and Child Health. Saving mothers' lives: reviewing maternal deaths to make motherhood safer 2003-2005. The Seventh Report of the Confidential Enquiries into Maternal Deaths in the United Kingdom. London: CEMACH, 2007.
4. Confidential Enquiry into Maternal and Child Health (CEMACH). Why mothers die 2000-2002: The Sixth Report of the Confidential Enquiries into Maternal Deaths in the United Kingdom. London: Royal College of Obstetricians and Gynaecologists, 2004.
5. CMACE/RCOG Joint Guideline. Management of women with obesity in pregnancy. London: Centre for Maternal and Child Enquiries and the Royal College of Obstetricians and Gynaecologists, 2010.
6. Maggard MA, et al. Pregnancy and fertility following bariatric surgery: a systematic review. JAMA 2008; 300: 2286–2296.
7. Buchwald H, et al. Bariatric surgery: a systematic review and meta-analysis. JAMA 2004; 292: 1724–1737 (erratum in JAMA 2005; 293: 1728).
8. Colquitt JL, et al. Surgery for morbid obesity. Cochrane Database Syst Rev 2005; 4: CD003641.
9. ACOG Practice Bulletin. Bariatric Surgery and Pregnancy 2009; 105: 1–9.
10. Hezelgrave NL, Oteng-Ntim E. Pregnancy after bariatric surgery: a review. J Obes 2011; 501939.
11. Guelinckx I, et al. Reproductive outcomes after bariatric surgery: a critical review. Hum Reprod Update 2009; 15: 189–201.
12. Abodeely A, et al. Pregnancy outcomes after bariatric surgery: maternal, fetal, and infant implications. Surg Obes Relat Dis 2008; 4: 464–471.

CARE PATHWAY

Pre-pregnancy counselling

Ideally, pre-pregnancy counselling includes discussions about:

- Advice to defer pregnancy for 12–24 months after bariatric surgery
- Effective contraception to avoid an unplanned pregnancy—oral contraception less effective, so advise alternative contraception, e.g. progesterone implant or LNG-IUS (Mirena®)
- Pre-pregnancy evaluation of any nutritional deficiencies
- Supplements to be prescribed according to type of **bariatric surgery** and of the deficient nutrient/vitamins
- If no vitamin B_{12} deficiency found, pre-pregnancy high-dose folic acid (5 mg/day) can be prescribed with advice to continue till end of 12 weeks of pregnancy
- If high-dose folic acid is not prescribed, advise usual 400 micrograms folic acid
- Vitamin B_{12} deficiency to be treated with 3-monthly IM injections
- Oral ferrous sulfate (or fumarate) with multivitamins can be advised
- Refer to dietian to assess and advise a healthy and varied diet

↓

Referred by GP or community midwife to specialist antenatal clinic

↓

First visit to specialist antenatal clinic

- Check viability and dates, detailed history
- Confirm type of bariatric surgery and details requested for any follow-up due with bariatric unit
- Check early pregnancy levels of serum iron, ferritin, folic acid, vitamin B_{12}, calcium, vitamin D
- Refer to dietitian to assess patient's diet and results of above tests to detect any nutritional deficiencies that need correction
- Advise 1st-trimester high-dose folic acid (5 mg/day) if no vitamin B_{12} deficiency, otherwise routine 400 micrograms. Prescribe 10 micrograms vitamin D od throughout pregnancy and lactation
- If still obese, low-dose aspirin prophylaxis as in obesity care pathway (p. 310)
- Assess severity of hyperemesis gravidarum. If severe, gastric band may need temporary deflation till symptoms settle
- Warn patient to be aware that signs of complications of bariatric surgery could initially mimic normal pregnancy symptoms—she should report these to midwife, GP, or specialist obstetrician
- Routine anomaly scan as well as serial growth scans monthly from 28 weeks with same-day reviews in specialist antenatal clinic
- Due to possible dumping syndrome if patient has had gastric by-pass, arrange alternative method of gestational diabetes screening at 26–28 weeks: refer to endocrinologist
- If on any slow-release medications, change these to oral solution or rapid-release forms
- Advise continued routine antenatal care with community midwife meanwhile

↓

Further visits to specialist antenatal clinic (at about 28, 32, and 36 weeks)

- Frequency of subsequent visits depends on any comorbidities that might develop in course of pregnancy
- Check progress of pregnancy, fetal growth
- Repeat serum iron, ferritin, folic acid, vitamin D, and calcium levels at about 28 and 34–36 weeks gestation
- Refer to bariatric surgeon or general surgeon if any bariatric surgery linked problems for joint input
- Gastric band may require deflation via subdermal port in the 3rd trimester
- Prescribe oral water-soluble vitamin K 10 mg from about 37 weeks gestation

↓

Labour, delivery, and postpartum

- ***No change in management of labour and delivery just on basis of previous bariatric surgery, no indication for Caesarean section or early IOL unless for other obstetric indications***
- Encourage breastfeeding

Pre-pregnancy counselling

First visit to specialist antenatal clinic

Labour, delivery, and postpartum

19 Maternal Malignancy

19.1 Malignancy and Pregnancy

FACT FILE

Epidemiology

- Although cancer is the second most common cause of death during reproductive years, it is relatively rare, occurring in only 1 in 1000 pregnancies.
- The most common malignancies with relevance to pregnancy, either a previous history of, or those occurring during a pregnancy or within 1 year postpartum are of the breast, cervix, leukaemia, lymphoma, melanoma, thyroid, ovary, and colon.
- Approximately 11 000 patients between 15–40 years of age, male and female, are diagnosed with cancer each year.
- With improved cancer survival rates greater than 75% in general, more survivors can now consider pregnancy, particularly with greater access to fertility treatments.
- Patients need full information at the time of diagnosis of cancer and prior to potentially gonadotoxic treatment or surgical procedures about possible effects on future fertility.[1]
- Greater awareness of treatment modalities and their effects on future fertility, especially the potential impact on sperm, ovaries, uterus, and cervical function have led to new management techniques for anticipated gonadal damage.[2,3,4,5]
- In the overall female population, half of all cancers are those affecting the breast, cervix, and thyroid.
- Also, 1 in 1000 pregnancies is complicated by gestational trophoblastic neoplasia.
- ***Cancers complicating pregnancy and lactation are those that occur during gestation or within 1 year postpartum.***[1]
- The presence of pregnancy may have a direct (e.g. hormonal) or an indirect effect on the course and management of disease.
- If malignancy is diagnosed for the first time during a pregnancy, it is not unusual for there to have been a delay in diagnostic workup and treatment.

Malignancy diagnosed during pregnancy

- When diagnosed during pregnancy,[1] patients have to deal with the impact of having cancer, the immediate consequences of disease and treatment, worries about how these might affect the fetus, longer term impact on survival, and future fertility issues.[2,3,4,5]
- Maternal wishes are extremely important in making any decision regarding choice of treatment.
- The management of any pregnant patient with current cancer or one who has been successfully treated previously for cancer, needs to be by a **specialist multidisciplinary team consisting of the patient herself, the medical oncologist, maternal medicine consultant obstetrician, midwife, clinical geneticist, haematologist, anaesthetist, and neonatologist.**
- A clear plan of action must be documented with the proviso that it might need to be altered with changes in the cancer growth, changes due to advancing pregnancy or the state of health of the patient. Updated plans must be widely circulated to all key members of the multidisciplinary team as well as to the patient and her partner/family.
- ***In general, malignant conditions during pregnancy are not associated with poor perinatal outcomes.***
- When a diagnosis of cancer is made during pregnancy, this is bound to be a great shock to the pregnant woman and her immediate family. Especially if the decision to terminate the pregnancy has been made to enable appropriate cancer therapy to be started, she will need additional emotional support from trained bereavement counsellors or through Macmillan cancer nurses.

Chemotherapy during pregnancy

- Almost all cytotoxic drugs cross the placenta and can theoretically be teratogenic by affecting the mechanism of cell division in the first trimester.
- The fetus is most susceptible between 5 and 10 weeks gestation.
- If the fetus is exposed to a single cytotoxic drug at this time, the estimated risk of major malformation is about 10%.[6]
- If it is exposed to several chemotherapeutic agents, the risk increases to 25% (compared with 1–3% in the general population). Fetal demise may also occur with increased risk of miscarriage.[6]
- Exposure to anticancer drugs **after** the first trimester does not seem to be associated with increased teratogenicity.
- After the first trimester, any effect is likely to be IUGR or pancytopenia at birth; 30% of babies who have had in-utero exposure to chemotherapy will display pancytopenia at birth.
- As fetal brain development continues throughout pregnancy, exposure to antineoplastic drugs later in pregnancy may theoretically affect neurodevelopment; however, there is little supporting literature.
- The impact of fetal exposure to chemotherapy on the future rate of malignancy in childhood or adolescence or on subsequent fertility of the offspring remains poorly defined.

Radiotherapy and pregnancy

- Radiation is used both for diagnostic and therapeutic purposes. Exposure to less than 0.05 Gy does not increase the teratogenic risks.[6]
- The cumulative exposure due to diagnostic imaging and radiation treatment may increase the risk to the fetus, causing central nervous system (CNS) abnormalities such as microcephaly and developmental delays.
- Ionizing radiation is a known CNS teratogen and may be a greater risk to the fetus than the cancer itself.

Obstetric outcomes in cancer survivors (pregnancies post-cancer treatment)

- **Post-chemotherapy effects** on female reproductive organs: Chemotherapy effects the ovaries, but has no direct effect on the cervix or on the uterine capacity.
- **Post-radiotherapy impact** on female reproductive system:
  - ovarian damage of both germ cell and endocrine components
  - partial or whole uterine irradiation can lead to amenorrhoea,
  - decreased uterine capacity and endometrial thickness, reduced vascular supply
  - cranial irradiation: amenorrhoea due to damage to the hypothalamic–pituitary axis.
- ***In general, however, good pregnancy outcomes can be expected.***
- No excess risk of death in survivors during subsequent pregnancy.
- No increase in fetal malformation rates if treatment completed at least 1–2 years before pregnancy.
- No significant increase in perinatal mortality in subsequent pregnancy.
- Some studies[7,8,9,10] have indicated an increased incidence of IUGR, Caesarean section, and preterm delivery in pregnancies of

cancer survivors. Oestrogen deficiency produced by chemo- or radiotherapy, vascular insufficiency, fibrosis, or decreased uterine capacity have been postulated as reasons.

- **Data from Scottish Registry (2002):**[8] Increased risk of postpartum haemorrhage (56%); higher incidence of Caesarean sections and assisted instrumental vaginal deliveries (33%); higher rates of preterm delivery (33%); no increase in perinatal mortality.
- **Childhood Cancer Survivor Study (2002):**[9] Increased risk of IUGR and low birth weight babies in women who have received pelvic irradiation in the past; increased risk of preterm labour.
- **Norwegian Cancer and Birth Registries Study (2005):**[10] Infants an average 130 g lighter at birth; delivered on average 6 days earlier; Caesarean delivery more likely.

Specific obstetric and anaesthetic issues associated with previous anthracycline chemotherapy

- Anthracyclines (e.g. daunorubicin, doxorubicin) are cytotoxic antibiotics.
- Previous treatment with the anthracyclines can, in some instances, lead to cardiomyopathy and nephrotoxicity.
- If given in childhood, anthracyclines can cause a dose-dependent myocyte damage, impaired cardiac growth, permanent cardiac dysfunction, poorly compliant myocardium, and a poor response to pre- and afterload.
- A pre-pregnancy cardiac ± renal assessment with relevant specialists and maternal medicine obstetric advice is recommended.
- Management of pregnancy with previous anthracycline-derived sequelae will need to be multidisciplinary including assessment by a senior anaesthetist.
- Continued close surveillance is essential.
- ***Prior renal damage could mask signs of gestational diabetes, pre-eclampsia.***
- Clear plans for care in pregnancy, labour, and delivery are required incorporating anaesthetic/analgesia plans for labour and delivery.
- During labour and delivery, expert care for fluid management, regional block is recommended.
- If cardiomyopathy or cardiac dysfunction has been identified, ergometrine/oxytocin with ergometrine are contraindicated as uterotonics for third-stage labour management. Also, care is needed with oxytocin bolus doses as hypotension may occur due to decreased cardiac reserve.

Recommended interval between end of cancer treatment and starting a pregnancy

- **Breast cancer:**[2]
  - Advise contraception for 2–3 years with non-hormonal contraception, longer if high-grade tumours. The risk of late recurrence is 2–3 % up to 10 years, 1–2% up to 15 years.
  - If on tamoxifen, treatment is needed for at least 5 years, and then stopped for a minimum of 3 months before pregnancy.
  - Pregnancy if on tamoxifen may be associated with craniofacial abnormalities, such as Pierre Robin sequence, Goldenhar syndrome, and abnormal development of genitalia.[10]
- **Thyroid cancer:**[6]
  - Avoid pregnancy for at least 12 months after radio-iodine isotope treatment.
- **Gestational trophoblastic neoplasia including placental site trophoblastic tumours** (PSTT):
  - Avoid pregnancy for 1 year, avoid oral contraceptives.
- **Melanoma:**[1]
  - Advise delaying pregnancy for 2–5 years, depending on the thickness of the melanoma.

Some individual malignancies

See Chapter 19.2 for fact file and care pathway for **breast cancer**.

Leukaemia

- Pregnancy and leukaemia are rarely associated due to decreased fertility.[1]
- The course of either acute or chronic leukaemia is **not** altered by pregnancy, based on the limited data available.[1,6,7,8,9]
- The earlier the diagnosis is made during pregnancy, the higher the perinatal mortality—this may be due to maternal anaemia, thrombosis, etc.
- Acute leukaemia is highly malignant but potentially curable. Without treatment, maternal death can occur within 2 months. Therefore, the most effective chemotherapeutic regimen is recommended, irrespective of gestation, associated risks of fetal demise, or teratogenicity.

Thyroid cancer[6]

- Papillary adenocarcinoma is the commonest thyroid malignancy.
- Peak incidence is at 30–35 years of age.
- Pregnancy has negligible effect on the thyroid cancer.
- Prognosis is generally favourable with appropriate treatment although diagnosis is likely to be delayed, masked by pregnancy symptoms.
- In early disease, treatment can be deferred to the postpartum period.
- Surgery can be undertaken any time after the first trimester.
- In more advanced disease, surgical excision followed by postpartum radio-iodine is indicated.
- Treatment usually consists of tumour ablation with radio-iodine, but this is contraindicated in pregnancy. Radioactive iodine therapy is deferred to after delivery.
- Contact with the infant should be avoided for several days post-radioiodine.
- Pregnancy is best deferred to 12 months after radio-iodine exposure. Patients should be advised to use effective contraception for at least 12 months after radio-iodine therapy has been completed.

Melanoma

- One-third of women diagnosed with malignant melanoma are of reproductive age.
- No difference in survival rates between melanomas diagnosed out of pregnancy to those diagnosed during a pregnancy, when controlled for tumour thickness.[1,6,7,8,11]
- Symptoms and prognosis are the same as in women who are not pregnant.
- Localized melanoma: Wide local excision around the site with wide margins performed irrespective of pregnancy status. Sentinel lymph node biopsy should be performed if the melanoma is greater than 2 mm thickness.
- More advanced cases (>4 mm thickness) should be considered for adjuvant therapy with high-dose interferon, though this is contraindicated in pregnancy.
- In those who have received previous treatment for melanoma, pregnancy itself does not alter prognosis.[1]
- Recurrences can occur in lymph nodes or internal organs, with a small potential risk of spread to the fetus.
- ***Melanoma is the most common malignancy to metastasize to placenta. Careful examination of the placenta is mandatory.***
- In women with advanced (stage III and IV) melanoma, the placenta should be examined to exclude metastatic melanomas. **If these are present, there is a 20% risk of the baby dying due to transplacental spread of melanoma.**
- Poor neonatal outcome in primary fetal melanomas.
- ***Usual advice is to defer pregnancy for at least 3–5 years after a diagnosis has been made because of the high risk of recurrence during this time frame.***

Lymphomas

- Lymphoma is the fourth most frequent malignancy diagnosed during pregnancy.[12]
- Coincident lymphoma and pregnancy is rare, variously reported as occurring in 1 in 1000[13] to 1 in 6000 deliveries.[12]
- With the trend for pregnancies to be deferred to later age there is an increased incidence of lymphoma in the mother.
- Additionally, the incidence of AIDS-related non-Hodgkin's lymphoma (NHL) during pregnancies in developing countries is high, despite highly active antiretroviral therapy.[14,15]

- Staging of lymphomas diagnosed during pregnancy requires imaging techniques such as radiography, ultrasonography, or MRI.
- Chest and abdominal CT scan are to be avoided in pregnancy.
- Biopsy of a lymph node is required for a secure diagnosis of lymphoma.
- Hodgkin's lymphoma (HL) is the most common type of lymphoma during pregnancy.

Non-Hodgkin's lymphoma

- Mean age at diagnosis of NHL is about 42 years[12] therefore with the recent trend to defer pregnancies into the fourth decade, it is likely to be diagnosed more often.
- Risk factors include being white, or having an inherited immune disorder/autoimmune disease or when immunosuppressed due to HIV/AIDS, post-organ transplant or having had previous treatment for HL.
- NHL often has unusual manifestations and their diagnosis is frequently delayed. These patients usually have aggressive, advanced-stage disease and a poor outcome.[12,13]
- Investigations during pregnancy do not differ from the non-pregnant in order to establish a diagnosis.
- NHL during pregnancy appears to have a more aggressive histology with the most common being large B-cell or peripheral T-cell lymphomas.
- In NHL during pregnancy, serum levels of the enzyme lactate dehydrogenase (LDH) are assessed to help determine prognosis. Elevated LDH levels denote aggressive disease and carry a poorer prognosis.
- **Prognosis** depends on:
  - the type and stage of the cancer
  - the level of LDH in the blood.
- Most NHL that occur during pregnancy are of the aggressive variety rather than of a low-grade, slow-growing indolent type, therefore delaying treatment of aggressive lymphoma until after the birth of the baby may lessen the mother's chances of survival. Immediate treatment is often recommended, even during pregnancy.
- NHL during pregnancy is also staged according to the rate of growth of the tumour as well as location of the affected lymph nodes.
- MRI, ultrasound scan, bone marrow biopsy, and lumbar puncture are used safely during pregnancy to stage the NHL.
- The treatment options are dependent on:
  - the type and stage of the cancer
  - the wishes of the patient
  - the patient's age and general health
  - which trimester of pregnancy the diagnosis has been made in.
- Different types of treatment options that need to be individualized
  - radiation therapy
  - chemotherapy
  - watchful waiting.
- ***Example A: Aggressive NHL diagnosed in first trimester of pregnancy*.**
  - Medical oncologist may advise termination of pregnancy (TOP) so that treatment with high-dose combination chemotherapy with or without radiation can be commenced.
- ***Example B: Aggressive NHL diagnosed in second or third trimester of pregnancy*.**
  - When possible, treatment is postponed until after an early delivery is achieved before chemotherapy or radiotherapy are started.
  - However, sometimes urgent treatment is required to increase the mother's chance of survival.
- ***Example C: Indolent (low-grade, slow-growing) NHL during pregnancy*.**
  - Treatment can be delayed until after pregnancy with a 'watch and wait' approach.

Hodgkin's lymphoma

- HL primarily affects young adults.
- A significant number of patients can look forward to prolonged survival.
- The median age at diagnosis is 30 years.
- Approximately 70% will be cured as a result of first or second-line treatment.
- Pregnancy is itself not a risk factor for HL.
- Most studies suggest that the disease probably has little or no effect on the pregnancy and vice versa.[13]

Hodgkin's lymphoma first diagnosed in pregnancy

- Presentation, clinical behaviour, prognosis, and histological subtypes of HL during pregnancy do not differ from those of the non-pregnant women of similar age. However, **treatment options are different in pregnancy**.
- Presenting symptoms: Painless, swollen lymph nodes in neck, underarm or groin, fever of non-specific origin, drenching night sweats, weight loss, itchy skin, and feeling very tired.
- MRI is the preferred tool for staging evaluation.
- Prognosis depends on stage of cancer and treatment options. Most pregnant patients with newly diagnosed Hodgkin's HL can be cured.
- The 20-year survival of those women where HL was diagnosed during pregnancy and appropriately treated is no different from matched non-pregnant women.[13]

Treatment

- Treatment choice must be individualized depending on:
  - patient's wishes
  - severity and pace of the cancer
  - length of remaining gestation.
- If HL is diagnosed in the first trimester of pregnancy, this is not an absolute indication for TOP.
- If the tumour presents in an early stage above the diaphragm and is of a slow-growing variety, patients can be followed carefully with plans to deliver early and then proceed with definitive therapy.
- Alternatively, supradiaphragmatic radiation while shielding the uterus.
- Chemotherapy administered in the first trimester can be associated with congenital abnormalities in up to 33% of cases and is therefore not usually recommended.
- Beyond the first trimester, the management options for women with Hodgkin's disease include:[10]
  - observation until disease progression or delivery
  - single-agent vinblastine
  - modified or standard combination chemotherapy, and radiation therapy (with appropriate shielding)
  - in the second half of pregnancy, most patients can be followed carefully, and definitive surgery postponed until delivery is arranged from 32–36 weeks.
- If chemotherapy is unavoidable, e.g. in symptomatic advanced-stage disease, vinblastine alone can be given intravenously, every 2 weeks until delivery.
- Alternatively, a short course of radiation with suitable shielding could be used prior to delivery in cases of respiratory compromise due to a rapidly enlarging mediastinal mass.
- Combination chemotherapy appears safe in the second half of pregnancy.
- Steroid therapy is also employed for the autoimmune effect as well as for hastening fetal pulmonary maturity, especially important if early delivery is planned.

Pregnancy following previous treatment for HL and NHL

- Especially in younger women, following a temporary phase of subfertility, recovery of fertility can occur especially when non-gonadotoxic chemotherapy or ovary-shielding radiotherapy has been used.
- A future pregnancy after previous treatment for HL does not increase the chances of relapse.
- There is little evidence that previous treatment leads to increased risks of perinatal loss or congenital malformations.
- Patients should be advised to use effective contraception for at least 2 years following completion of treatment.[5] This is to differentiate those who might have recurrence during this period

which would require very aggressive therapy, the latter being incompatible with pregnancy.

- After previous treatment (either radiotherapy or chemotherapy) for cancer, the average age of menopause takes place some 10 years earlier than normal. The patient, therefore, should be advised not to unduly delay pregnancy after 1–2 years after treatment completion.[5]

Information for patients

Please see Information for patients: Cancer and pregnancy (p. 538)

References

1. Pavlidis NA. Coexistence of pregnancy and malignancy. Oncologist 2002;7: 279–287.
2. RCP. Effects of cancer treatment on reproductive functions. Report of a Working Party. London: Royal College of Physicians, 2008.
3. RCOG Green-top Guideline No. 12. Pregnancy and Breast Cancer. London: Royal College of Obstetricians and Gynaecologists, 2011.
4. Gelb AB, et al. Pregnancy-associated lymphomas. Cancer 1996;78: 304–310.
5. RCP, RCR, RCOG, Cancerbackup. The effects of cancer treatment on reproductive functions: guidance on management. Report of a Working Party. London: Royal College of Physicians, 2007.
6. Shafi MI, Karim SA. Malignant disease in pregnancy. In: Greer IA, et al., ed., Maternal medicine. Edinburgh: Churchill Livingstone Elsevier, 2007.
7. Clark H, et al. Obstetric outcomes in cancer survivors. Obstet Gynecol 2007;110: 849–854.
8. Green DM, et al. Pregnancy outcome of female survivors of childhood cancer: a report from the Childhood Cancer Survivor Study. Am J Obstet Gynecol 2002;187: 1070–1080.
9. Fosså SD, et al. Parenthood in survivors after adulthood cancer and perinatal health in their offspring: a preliminary report. J Natl Cancer Inst Monogr 2005;34: 77–82.
10. Berger JC, Clericuzio CL. Pierre Robin sequence associated with first trimester fetal tamoxifen exposure. Am J Med Genet 2008;146A; 2141–2144.
11. Koren G, et al. The Motherisk guide to cancer in pregnancy and lactation, 2nd ed. Toronto: Motherisk Program, 2005.
12. Pereg D, et al. The treatment of Hodgkin's and non-Hodgkin's lymphoma in pregnancy. Haematologica 2007;92: 1230–1237
13. Pohlman B, Macklis RM. Lymphoma and pregnancy. Semin Oncol 2000;27: 657–666.
14. Diamond C, et al. Changes in acquired immunodeficiency syndrome-related non-Hodgkin lymphoma in the era of highly active antiretroviral therapy: incidence, presentation, treatment, and survival. Cancer 2006;106: 128–135.
15. Cheung MC, et al. AIDS-related malignancies: emerging challenges in the era of highly active antiretroviral therapy. Oncologist 2005;10: 412–426.

CARE PATHWAY

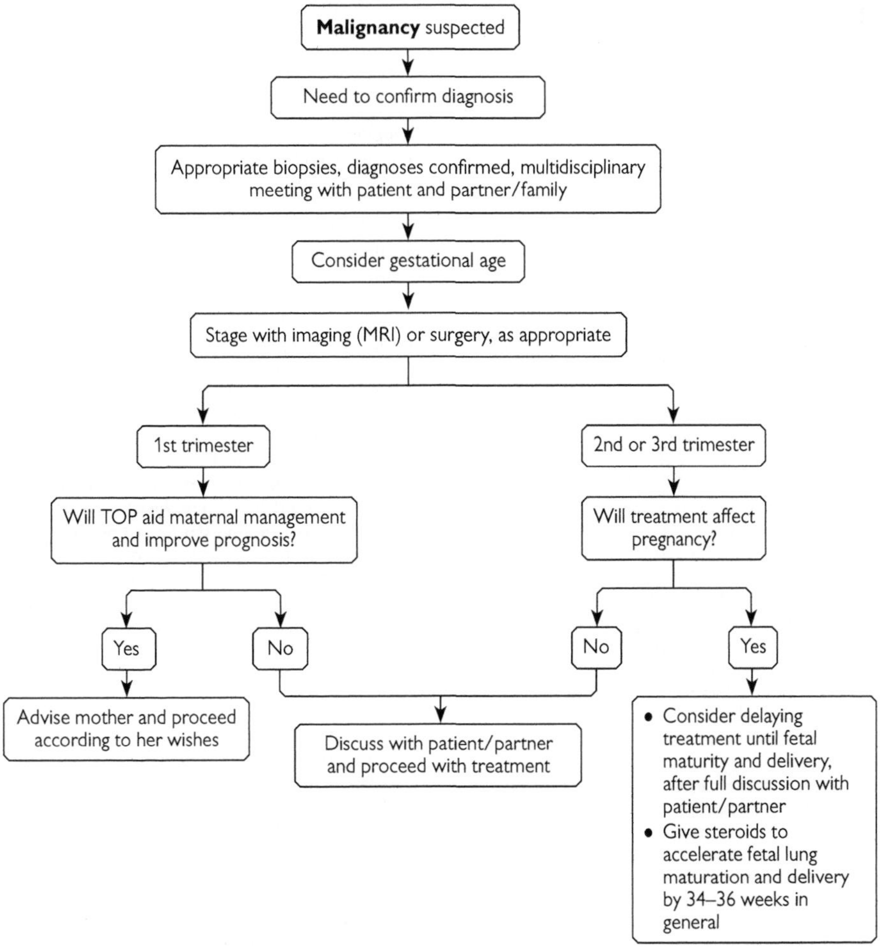

19.2 Breast Cancer

FACT FILE

Epidemiology

- **Breast cancer** is the most common malignancy in women, with a lifetime risk of about 11% in the UK (1 in 9).[1] About 3% of all breast cancers are diagnosed either during pregnancy or during lactation.[2]
- Over 90% of women with disease localized to the breast and who have received appropriate treatment have a high probability of long-term survival.
- Over 70% of women presenting with early breast cancer can now expect to be alive without evidence of disease at 10 years.
- The 5-year survival rate is around 80% for the under 50s age group.[1]
- Women with metastatic disease have a median survival of 2 years.
- Adjuvant chemotherapy in the treatment of breast cancer reduces the annual risk of recurrence and death by 40% and 30% respectively.
- Nulliparity is a well-recognized risk factor, as are early menarche and later age at first pregnancy. With the present trend towards deferring pregnancies into the late third or fourth decade, an increase in breast cancer rates may be expected.
- A few studies have indicated that there may be a transient short-term increased risk of developing breast cancer in the first 3–4 years after a full-term delivery.[3] This transient risk appears to be reduced if the pregnancy ended preterm or as a miscarriage, suggesting an effect linked to pregnancy duration.[4]
- Breastfeeding, especially if carried on for longer, has a weakly protective benefit in reducing the risk of breast cancer.[5]
- In premenopausal women, chemotherapy may induce a premature menopause especially if an alkylating agent (e.g. cyclophosphamide) has been used, as the ovary is chemosensitive. However, chemotherapy-induced ovarian suppression may only be temporary in younger women.
- Pregnancy increases risk of breast cancer in carriers of the *BRCA1* and *BRCA2* mutations. In this instance, parous carriers of the mutations are at increased risk of breast cancer by the age of 40, compared with nulliparous carriers of the same mutations.[6] Each pregnancy in these women seems to increase the risk.
- Women who have completed adjuvant treatment for early breast cancer may wish to start a family or have more children. 7% of women who are fertile after treatment for breast cancer will subsequently have children.[2]

Pregnancy-associated breast cancer

- Breast cancer is the most common solid tumour to be diagnosed during pregnancy and occurs in 1 in 3000 pregnancies.[7]
- **Pregnancy-associated breast cancer is defined as breast cancer diagnosed during pregnancy, within the first postpartum year, or any time during lactation.**[8] The prognosis in this group, especially in women less than 30 years of age, is worse than in those diagnosed at other times, usually because the disease is at a more advanced stage.[9]
- A pregnant woman has a 2.5-fold higher risk of presenting with advanced breast cancer than a non-pregnant woman.[7]
- A delay in establishing a diagnosis due to the difficulty in distinguishing between physiological breast changes in pregnancy and lactation and the sinister changes of cancer, as well as a resultant delay in initiating treatment, contribute to the greater incidence of late-stage disease in this group.
- Reports quote 5-year survival rates of 40–73% in pregnancy-associated breast cancer.[10]
- **Presentation in pregnancy** is usually as a painless mass. Any lump persisting for more than 2–4 weeks needs urgent investigation, although 80% are benign.
- Less common presentations:
  - A bloody discharge from the nipple.
  - Indurated erythematous breast (with or without the classic peau d'orange sign).
  - The 'milk rejection' sign where the baby rejects the breast which has a hitherto undiagnosed cancer.

Imaging

- Imaging modalities during pregnancy need to take into account the effect of radiation exposure to the fetus as well as the high false-positive and false-negative rates caused by physiological changes in the breast tissue during pregnancy and lactation.
- **Ultrasonography** is a safe first imaging modality to assess a discrete lump. Ultrasound can distinguish a solid from a cystic lesion of the breast, but not between malignant from benign appearances. Also used to detect liver metastasis.
- **Mammography**, though within the safety threshold of fetal radiation exposure, is not a first-line imaging modality as it is less sensitive due to the physiological changes, especially the increased density of the parenchyma seen in pregnancy· Mammography (with fetal shielding) is used to assess the extent of the disease and to assess the contralateral breast.[1]
- ***CT and isotope-bone scans are contraindicated during pregnancy but can be employed after delivery.***
- **MRI: There are few studies to ascertain usefulness in pregnancy.** Non-contrast MRI of thoracolumbar spine can be employed to detect bone metastasis.
- **Chest radiograph** with adequate shielding of the abdomen is safe as the fetal radiation exposure is 0.01 mGy, well below the threshold dose of no more than 100 mGy.[11] Chest radiography is used for further staging of the cancer.

Diagnosis

- Any woman presenting with a breast lump during pregnancy should be referred to the specialist breast team. Imaging and treatment planning should be multidisciplinary with good communication between the specialist breast team, the consultant obstetrician, midwife, and GP. The key coordinator is usually the breast care nurse.[1]
- Histological diagnosis is established from a ultrasound guided core needle or excisional biopsy.
- **The pathologist must be informed that sample is from a pregnant or lactating woman.**
- A fine needle aspiration for cytology is less useful during pregnancy and lactation as it has a high false-positive rate[12] due to the hyperproliferative cellularity of breast tissue during pregnancy and lactation.

Staging

- As in non-pregnant women the TNM staging system of the American Joint Committee on Cancer is used.
- Common sites of metastasis are the bones, liver and lungs.
- Staging for metastases is indicated only when there is increased clinical suspicion.[1]

Pathology

- Breast cancers during pregnancy tend to be high-grade infiltrating ductal carcinomas[13] with larger tumour size and greater node involvement.
- The grade, receptor status, and human epidermal growth factor receptor-2 (HER2) need to be defined to assist further treatment planning.[1]

Treatment

- To a large extent the choice and timing of treatment modalities depend on the gestational age of pregnancy and the wishes of the pregnant woman. Multispecialty and multiprofessional (oncology and obstetric/midwifery) team approach to both discussions with the pregnant woman and her partner/family, and management is recommended.

- A decision to continue the pregnancy or not needs to be made by the patient and her partner after careful discussion of the prognosis, treatment, and future fertility with the multidisciplinary team. It is essential that the multidisciplinary team (MDT) review outcomes are forwarded to the consultant obstetrician and the GP.[1]
- Pregnancy termination does not improve prognosis but may have to be considered by the woman or the couple when a stage IV breast cancer is detected in the first trimester, to allow immediate treatment with chemotherapy. It may also need to be discussed in cases of late-stage aggressive high-grade disease where survival is expected to be shorter than the time to achieve fetal viability.
- If the decision is to continue with the pregnancy, the options then lie between early delivery, if the fetus is viable followed by definitive treatment, versus initiation of treatment while the pregnancy continues.
- Immediate treatment is associated with better results in breast cancer (see Table 19.1) while poor outcomes due to disease progression are seen if treatment is delayed or declined.[14] The patient and her family need to be made aware of this during multidisciplinary discussions

Surgery

- Breast surgery can be safely performed in any trimester of pregnancy.
- Surgery is usually the first-line treatment with a modified radical mastectomy or lumpectomy with axillary clearance as the definitive procedure of choice for stages I–III disease.[15] The safety and efficacy of sentinel lymph node biopsy during pregnancy is not proven and it is not to be used in these cases.
- In general, breast-conserving surgery is not recommended in pregnancy[21] except in the third trimester close to delivery when it can be combined with axillary clearance.[16,17] In this situation, radiotherapy could be delayed till after delivery to a maximum of 12 weeks.[14,18]
- There is a high rate of nodal involvement in pregnancy-associated breast cancer and axillary lymph node clearance is to be performed in all cases of invasive disease.[15] Postoperative chemotherapy is indicated due to the high risk of axillary node involvement.
- In women in whom wide local excision has been performed, adjuvant radiotherapy is required to prevent local recurrence. Further surgery may be required if the excision margins are not clear of the malignancy.

Radiotherapy

- This is not recommended during the first trimester due to adverse effects that can cause miscarriage, teratogenicity, IUGR, microcephaly, neurodevelopmental defects, etc., as well as a possible role in childhood malignancies.
- Later in pregnancy, radiotherapy has been used in selected cases, with adequate lead shielding.[19]

Chemotherapy

- Chemotherapy is required to treat the high-grade invasive disease that is usually associated with pregnancy-related breast cancer.
- Chemotherapy is contraindicated in first trimester due to embryotoxic and teratogenic effects.
- It is safe in the second and third trimesters although may be associated with IUGR, low birth weight, preterm labour, transient neonatal tachypnoea, and transient maternal and neonatal leucopenia especially if administered less than 3 weeks before delivery.

Table 19.1 Nettleton's model of delayed systemic treatment and increased risk (in percentage) of axillary node involvement in pregnancy-associated early-stage primary breast cancer

Delay in treatment	*Less aggressive tumour (doubling time of 130 days)*	*Aggressive tumour (doubling time of 65 days)*
1 month	0.9%	1.8%
3 months	2.6%	5.2%
6 months	5.1%	10.2%

Data from Nettleton J et al., Breast cancer—during pregnancy: quantifying the risk of treatment delay, *Obstetrics and Gynecology*, 1996, 87, 3, pp. 414–418.

- Serial ultrasound scans to monitor fetal growth are recommended if chemotherapy is used.
- The timing of delivery in relation to chemotherapy must be considered with care. It is advisable therefore to plan delivery and stop chemotherapy 2–3 weeks before this.
- Systemic chemotherapy is the treatment of choice after the first trimester in those with stage IV disease.
- If the diagnosis of advanced disease is made in the first trimester, TOP needs to be discussed to allow initiation of systemic chemotherapy.
- Drug regimes are similar to those used in non-pregnant women.
- Early commencement of chemotherapy following surgery has better outcomes than when it is delayed for more than 3 weeks post-surgery.[20]
- Supportive measures to control nausea and vomiting associated with pregnancy include odansetron, steroids, and $5HT_3$-serotonin antagonists.
- Cyclophosphamide, doxorubicin and fluorouracil have a good safety record in pregnancy.[21]
- Anthracyclines are among the most effective drugs in breast cancer and doxorubicin is most widely used in pregnancy.
- Methotrexate, idarubicin, epirubicin, and trastuzumab are contraindicated at any stage of pregnancy.[22]

Hormone therapy

- Tamoxifen exposure in the first trimester has been associated with miscarriages, congenital abnormalities[23,24] including craniofacial abnormalities such as the Goldenhaar (oculoauriculovertebral dysplasia) or Pierre Robin syndrome, as well as ambiguous genitalia. Little information is available about this non-steroidal oestrogen in pregnancy but it is advisable to discontinue use during pregnancy. The half-life of tamoxifen is about 6 weeks, therefore ideally the drug should have been stopped at least 8 weeks before conception.
- Tamoxifen exposure at any stage of pregnancy is not, however, usually regarded as medical grounds for TOP.[25]

Multidisciplinary management

- If the woman is undergoing chemotherapy, serial growth scans may be considered.
- If delivery is planned before 36 weeks, steroids can be used to accelerate fetal lung maturity.
- Ideally, a 2–3 week chemo-free period is advisable before a planned delivery to reduce risks of maternal and fetal leucopenia at delivery and after.
- Caesarean section is only for standard obstetric indications.
- Lactation is contraindicated during chemotherapy and radiotherapy. All chemotherapeutic drugs are transferred through breast milk and may cause neonatal leukopenia and provoke infection. An interval of at least 14 days is required between the last chemotherapy session and to the start of breastfeeding to allow drug clearance from breast milk.[1]

Contraception

- Oral hormonal contraceptives (both combined and progesterone-only) are contraindicated in women with current or recent breast cancer whether the tumour is hormone-receptor positive or negative.[26]
- Although there is a case for oral contraception after 5 years free of recurrence, there is still insufficient evidence to recommend this.[1]
- The levonorgestrel intrauterine system (LNG-IUS, Mirena®) may reduce the risk or tamoxifen-related endometrial abnormalities, but further evidence of its safety in breast cancer survivors is recommended.[1]
- Inert intrauterine devices or barrier method of contraception may be used.

Pregnancy in survivors of breast cancer

Pre-pregnancy counselling

- It is recommended that pregnancy should be delayed for at least 2 years in order to ensure that any potential risks to the fetus from chemotherapy exposure have been minimized,[27] although this interval has been challenged in recent times with advances in adjuvant chemotherapy.[27]

- Delay also allows the peak incidence of breast cancer recurrence to pass. This timescale also helps differentiate those with a better chance of long-term survival from those with more aggressive disease.
- No adverse effects of subsequent pregnancies on long-term survival of treated breast cancer women have been reported.
- If on tamoxifen, this should be stopped for at least 8–12 weeks before a pregnancy is established.
- Any routine imaging is best done before a pregnancy is established.
- **5-year survival rates:**[28]
    - for women who start a pregnancy less than 6 months after cancer treatment: 54%
    - for women who start a pregnancy between 6 months and 2 years after cancer treatment: 78%
    - for women who start a pregnancy more than 5 years after cancer treatment: 100%.
- In women with **stage IV disease** (5-year survival <15%), it is advisable **not** to consider a pregnancy.
- Women with **stage III disease** are advised to consider deferring a pregnancy for at least 5 years after treatment.
- Similarly, those with **recurrent Stage I or II tumours** are advised not to contemplate conception because of the intensity of the treatment required and the poor prognosis.[7]

Optimal management of pregnancy following treated early-stage breast cancer

- Joint management: oncologist, obstetrician, midwife, anaesthetist, and breast surgeon.
- If previous adjuvant chemotherapy included anthracyclines there is a risk of anthracycline-related cardiomyopathy or pulmonary fibrosis in rare cases. Echocardiography must therefore be performed during pregnancy in such women to detect signs of cardiomyopathy with referral to cardiology and pulmonary medicine.
- During pregnancy, imaging by ultrasound is best, though detection of metastases is more difficult.
- Reassure the woman that successful breastfeeding with the unaffected breast is entirely feasible and that breastfeeding does not increase risk of recurrence.
- Previous chemotherapy does not affect the safety of breastfeeding.
- Previous radiotherapy may cause fibrosis, thereby impairing lactation.
- Suppression of lactation does not affect long-term prognosis.

Treatment for recurrence or metastases of breast cancer during pregnancy

- Multidisciplinary decisions, with mother's wishes being of paramount importance.
- Initial surgical excision may be planned, with chemotherapy postponed to after delivery, though chemotherapy may become necessary after the first trimester.
- Cyclophosphamide during second and third trimesters can be associated with IUGR, preterm labour, even intrauterine death, though rare.
- Most infants exposed to combination chemotherapy after the first trimester have no long-term major problems.
- **TOP: no benefit seen on outcome of breast cancer**
- Radiotherapy though not absolutely contraindicated with adequate shielding, is best deferred to after delivery.

General treatment principles for disease recurrence during pregnancy

Chemotherapy

- Almost all cytotoxic drugs cross the placenta and affect cell division.
- Used in first trimester, they can cause fetal death, miscarriage, or teratogenicity.
- The period of maximal fetal susceptibility is 5–10 weeks gestation.
- Exposure to single-agent chemotherapy at this stage has been associated with a 10% major malformation rate, whereas with combination chemotherapeutic drugs this risk is up to 25%.
- Antineoplastic drugs after the first trimester are not associated with teratogenicity as organogenesis is complete. Brain development continues throughout pregnancy, however, and the impact of maternal chemotherapy on long-term fetal neurodevelopment is currently unclear.

Radiation

- Radiation exposure of less than 0.05 Gy is not associated with an increased teratogenic risk.
- Imaging for malignancy requires much higher exposure and therefore there are risks, especially to the CNS with increased rate of fetal microcephaly and developmental delay. Damage caused is related to dose, time, and gestational age.

Information for patients

Please see **Information for patients: Breast cancer and pregnancy** (p. 539)

References

1. RCOG Green-top Guideline No. 12. Pregnancy and breast cancer. London: Royal College of Obstetricians and Gynaecologists, 2011.
2. Ring AE, et al. Breast cancer and pregnancy. Ann Oncol 2005;16: 1855–1860.
3. Lambe M, et al. Maternal risk of breast cancer following multiple births: a nation-wide study in Sweden. Cancer Causes Control 1996;7: 533–538.
4. Hsieh CC, et al. Delivery of premature newborns and maternal breast-cancer risk. Lancet 1999;353: 1239.
5. Breast cancer and breastfeeding: collaborative reanalysis of individual data from 47 epidemiological studies in 30 countries, including 50302 women with breast cancer and 96973 women without the disease. Collaborative Group on Hormonal Factors in Breast Cancer. Lancet. 2002;360 (9328): 187–195.
6. Jernstrom H, et al. Pregnancy and risk of early breast cancer in carriers of BRCA1 and BRCA2. Lancet 1999;354: 1846–1850.
7. Johannsson O, et al. Pregnancy-associated breast cancer in BRCA1 and BRCA2 germ-line mutation carriers. Lancet 1998;352: 1359–1360.
8. Saunders CM, Baum M. Breast cancer and pregnancy: a review. J R Soc Med 1993;86: 162–165.
9. Kroman N, et al. Breast Cancer Cooperative Group. Pregnancy after treatment of breast cancer - a population-based study on behalf of Danish Breast Cancer Cooperative Group. Acta Oncol 2008;47: 545–549.
10. Ives AD, et al. The Western Australian gestational breast cancer project: a population-based study of the incidence, management and outcomes. Breast 2005;14: 276–282.
11. 20th International Commission on Radiological Protection. The 2007 Recommendations of the International Commission on Radiological Protection. Ann ICRP 2007;37: 1–332.
12. Brenner R, et al. Stereotactic core-needle breast biopsy: a multi-institutional prospective trial. Radiology 2001;218: 866–872.
13. Middleton LP, et al. Breast carcinoma in pregnant women: assessment of clinicopathologic and immunohistochemical features. Cancer 2003;98: 1055–1060.
14. Nettleton J, et al. Breast cancer during pregnancy: quantifying the risk of treatment delay. Obstet Gynecol 1996;87: 414–418.
15. SIGN Guideline No. 84. Management of breast cancer in women. Edinburgh: Scottish Intercollegiate Guidelines Network, 2005.
16. Annane K, et al. Infiltrative breast cancer during pregnancy and conservative surgery. Fetal Diagn Ther 2005;20: 442–444.
17. Kuerer HM, et al. Conservative surgery and chemotherapy for breast carcinoma during pregnancy. Surgery 2002;131: 108–110.
18. Whelan TJ, et al. Group BCDS. Breast irradiation in women in early stage invasive breast cancer following breast conserving surgery. Cancer Prev Control 2002;1: 228–240.
19. Fenig E, et al. Pregnancy and radiation. Cancer Treat Rev 2001;27: 1–7.
20. Colleoni M, et al. Early start of adjuvant chemotherapy may improve treatment outcome for premenopausal breast cancer patients with tumors not expressing estrogen receptors. The International Breast Cancer Study Group. J Clin Oncol 2000;18: 584–590.
21. Karin M, et al. Treatment of pregnant breast cancer patients and outcomes of children exposed to chemotherapy in utero. Cancer 2006;107: 1219–1226.

22. Watson WJ. Herceptin (transtuzumab) therapy during pregnancy: association with reversible anhydramnios. Obstet Gynecol 2005;105: 642–643.
23. Issacs R, et al. Tamoxifen for systemic treatment of advanced breast cancer during pregnancy: case report and literature review. Gynecol Oncol 2001;80: 405–408.
24. Braems G, et al. Use of tamoxifen before and during pregnancy. Oncologist 2011;16: 1547–1551.
25. UKTIS. Use of tamoxifen in pregnancy. UK Teratology Information Service, 2009. <http://www.uktis.org/docs/tamoxifen.pdf>
26. Gaffield ME, Culwell KR. New recommendations on the safety of contraceptive methods for women with medical conditions: World Health Organization's medical eligibility criteria for contraceptive use, 4th ed. IPPF Medical Bulletin 2010; 44 (1)
27. Gwyn K, Theriault R. Breast cancer during pregnancy. Oncology 2001;15: 39–51.
28. Averette HE, et al. Pregnancy after breast carcinoma: the ultimate medical challenge. Cancer 1999;85: 2301–2304.

CARE PATHWAY

Pregnancy-Associated Breast Cancer: Early Stage Disease (I or II)

- Multidisciplinary approach involving the oncology, breast surgery, obstetric and midwifery teams working with the pregnant woman and her partner/ family
- Any woman discovered to have a lump in the breast that has persisted for more than 2 weeks must be referred to the breast specialist team without delay
- Any imaging modality involving X-ray irradiation to be use adequate thickness lead shielding
- Multidisciplinary team review outcome shared with obstetric consultant and GP

Breast cancer diagnosed during pregnancy

- Stage of disease and gestational age to inform discussions with patient
- If decision is for pregnancy continuation, the choice is between
  - early delivery, if the fetus is viable, followed by definitive treatment, or
  - initiation of treatment while the pregnancy continues

Early stage disease (stage I or II)

1st trimester / 2nd trimester

Modified radical mastectomy and chemotherapy after 14 weeks gestation

- Serial fetal growth scans
- Discuss chemotherapy as contraindication for breastfeeding
- Timing of delivery to 2–3 weeks after last chemo session to avoid maternal and neonatal leukopenia—inform paediatrics, vigilance for infections and active treatment
- Steroids, if delivery <36 weeks
- Caesarean only for standard obstetric indications
- Contraceptive advice—not for hormonal contraception; advice to defer pregnancy for about 2 years, but individualized advice

3rd trimester

28–32 weeks during ongoing pregnancy

Either modified radical mastectomy + chemotherapy

Or breast-conserving surgery with axillary clearance

- Deliver at ≈34 weeks after prophylactic steroids
- After delivery, chemotherapy ± radiotherapy ± hormone therapy
- Advise not to breastfeed
- Non-hormonal contraception

>32 weeks Plan delivery by ≈34 weeks

- Steroid prophylaxis
- Discuss delivery
- Discuss chemotherapy being a contraindication for breast feeding
- Breast surgery followed by chemotherapy ± radiotherapy ± hormone therapy
- Discuss contraception: No hormonal methods

Adapted from Padmagirison R et al., Management of breast cancer during pregnancy, *The Obstetrician and Gynaecologist*, 12, pp. 186–192, Wiley. © 2010 Royal College of Obstetricians and Gynaecologists, with permission.

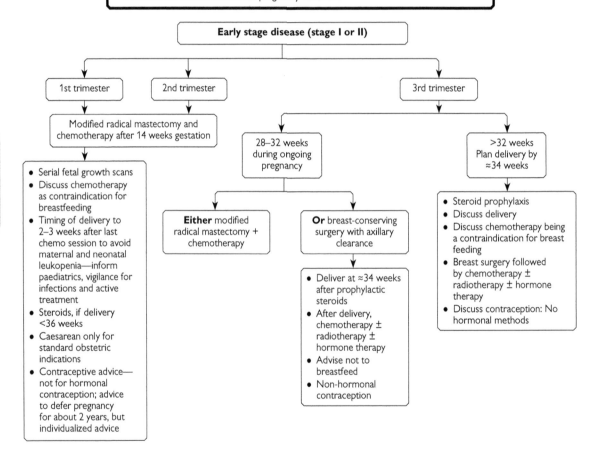

Pregnancy-associated breast cancer: late stage disease (III or IV)

- Multidisciplinary approach involving the oncology, breast surgery, obstetric, and midwifery teams working with the pregnant woman and her partner/family.
- Any woman discovered to have a lump in the breast that has persisted for more than 2 weeks must be referred to the breast specialist team without delay
- Any imaging modality involving X-ray irradiation to use adequate thickness lead shielding.
- Multidisciplinary team review outcome shared with obstetric consultant and GP

Breast cancer diagnosed during pregnancy

- Stage of disease and gestational age to inform discussions with patient
- If decision is for pregnancy continuation, the choice is between
  - early delivery, if the fetus is viable, followed by definitive treatment, or
  - initiation of treatment while the pregnancy continues

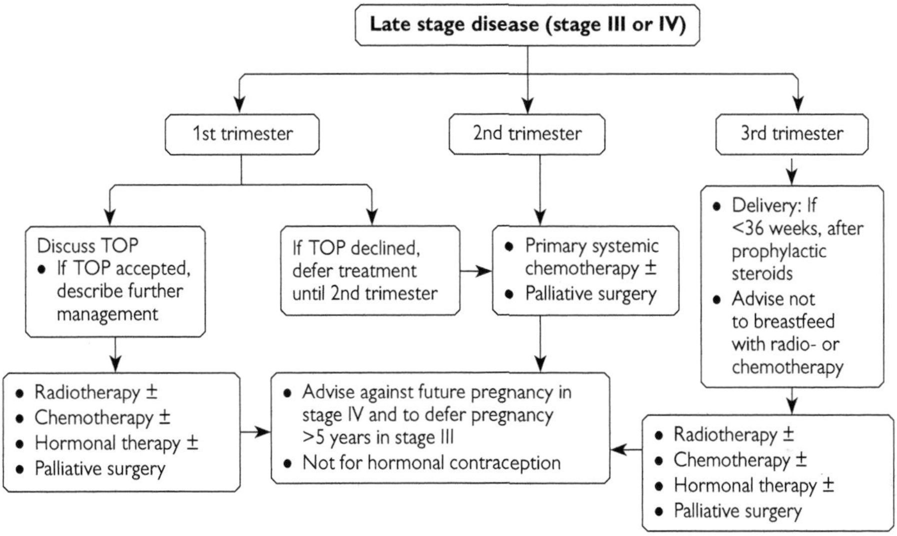

Adapted from Padmagirison R et al., Management of breast cancer during pregnancy, *The Obstetrician and Gynaecologist*, 12, pp. 186–192, Wiley. © 2010 Royal College of Obstetricians and Gynaecologists, with permission.

20 Pregnancy in the Mother Post Organ Transplant

20.1 Kidney Transplant

FACT FILE

Post-transplant and pre-pregnancy assessment and counselling

- While fertility is impaired in those with chronic kidney disease (CKD), end-stage kidney failure, or those on dialysis, it is restored within 1–12 months of a successful renal transplant.[1,2]
- Pregnancy after renal transplantation is not uncommon and occurs in 5–12% of women who have undergone kidney transplantation and are of childbearing age. Only 50% of these pregnancies is planned.[2]
- Pregnancy is ideally **deferred to 12–18 months after transplantation**, as this is the time when maximum use of potentially embyrotoxic and teratogenic drugs as well as optimal immunosuppression is being aimed at.
- **Optimal contraception** should be initiated before transplantation because of the rapid return of fertility post transplantation. A low-dose combined pill or the progesterone-only pill, progesterone depot injections, or subdermal implant may be used. Intrauterine devices (IUDs) were not regarded as suitable as they require an intact immune system for maximal efficacy. However, given the special requirements in post-transplant patients a levonorgestrel-loaded IUD (Mirena®) is probably the best option as it is long lasting, has a very low failure rate, and is reversible, allowing the patient to get pregnant without delay on removal. Interactions with other medications are highly unlikely.[2]
- Successful pregnancy outcome rates of 95–97% or more are reported in post-transplant patients when the pregnancy progresses beyond the first trimester.
- Current recommendation is that the post-renal transplant woman can proceed to get pregnant when the graft is functioning well,[1,3] i.e.
  - serum creatinine less than 125 micromol/litre
  - total protein excretion in 24-h urine is less than 500 mg
  - no fetotoxic or teratogenic medications are being used
  - Immunosuppressant drugs are at a stable dose at maintenance levels.
- Immunosuppressant drugs such as mycophenolate mofetil or sirolimus are contraindicated in pregnancy and will need to be changed, at least 6 weeks pre-conception, to regimes including prednisolone, azathioprine, ciclosporin, or tacrolimus.
- Women must be reassured about the safety of these drugs, which have been widely used in pregnancy with a good safety record. Reduction of the dose or stopping these immunosuppressive drugs can cause graft rejection. The drug levels of these medications should be monitored during pregnancy and maintained at pre-pregnancy levels.
- Pregnancy outcomes and effects on the allograft depend on pre-pregnancy baseline serum creatinine levels, presence or absence of hypertension, extent of proteinuria, and/or diabetes. The better the graft function at conception, the lower the pregnancy complications or adverse effects on the allograft function.
- If serum creatinine levels are less than 100 micromol/litre at time of conception there is no adverse effect on long-term graft survival. If this level is in excess of 125 micromol/litre, the graft survival is reduced to 65% three years later.[3]
- The incidence of pregnancy complications in post-transplant women is nearly 50% including hypertension, pre-eclampsia, IUGR, preterm delivery, graft rejection, and recurrent UTIs.

Pre-pregnancy evaluation

- Rubella immunization, a live vaccine, **cannot be administered after transplantation**, therefore must be administered ***before*** transplantation and antibody status confirmed.
- Rhesus compatibility of patient and transplant donor: check Rh (D) antibody at booking.
- Hepatitis B and C, cytomegalovirus (CMV), HIV, toxoplasmosis, rubella: counsel before pregnancy, offer rubella and Hep B vaccination.
- Check lupus anticoagulant, cardiolipin antibodies.
- Advise to stop smoking.
- Peri-pregnancy folic acid.
- Consider low-dose aspirin.
- Review all medications.
- Refer for genetic issues if polycystic kidney disease or vesicoureteric reflux that has led to chronic renal disease due to inheritance patterns.

Principles of antenatal management

Due to the rate of complications, these pregnancies are high risk and need close multidisciplinary input from the transplant nephrologist, specialist high-risk pregnancy obstetrician, transplant surgeon, urologist, and midwife. *This usually takes place in a tertiary setting.*

- Careful monitoring and tight BP control at below 140/90 mmHg are vital. The patient can be trained to monitor BP daily.
- Optimal choice of antihypertensives depend on level of hypertension. Methyldopa, labetalol, nifedipine ± thiazide diuretics are first-line agents. For more urgent control hydralazine, labetalol, or nifedipine can be employed. ACE inhibitors and angiotensin receptor blockers are contraindicated in pregnancy.
- Low-dose aspirin 75 mg oral to be continued throughout pregnancy
- As a model schedule for antenatal checks, the American Society of Nephrologists has suggested these antenatal visits could be once in 2–3 weeks till 20 weeks gestation, then every fortnight till 28 weeks and weekly thereafter.[1]
- In the UK, with input from primary care GPs and midwives as well as care shared with the local hospital, this schedule could be adapted to be make it less tedious for patients attending tertiary hospital clinics each time.
- UTIs occur in about 40% of post-transplant pregnancies, though pyelonephritis is rare. MSU must be sent at each antenatal visit to the hospital or community clinic, with prompt treatment of any infection. Some may require long-term suppressive antibiotics.
- FBC and serum calcium checks every month with treatment of anaemia, maintenance of normal calcium levels by adjustment of calcium and vitamin D supplements, as required, to prevent either hypo- or hypercalcaemia.
- Regular assessments of renal function, serum levels of immunosuppressants.
- Liver function tests every 6–8 weeks.
- Vigilance for superadded pre-eclampsia is required as this occurs in 15–25% of post-transplant pregnancies.
- If increasing and dense proteinuria, increase risk for thromboembolism, prophylaxis must be instituted.
- High risk for preterm delivery (about 50–64% are born <37 weeks)[1] mainly due to maternal or fetal complications rather than spontaneous preterm labour. Prophylactic steroids (beta- or

dexamethasone) for accelerated fetal lung maturity if more than 23 weeks and up until 35 weeks gestation.

- Fetal growth restriction is found in more than 30–50% of pregnancies. Serial growth liquor and Doppler monitoring from 24–26 weeks gestation at frequencies as per individual unit's protocols for growth scans and Doppler studies.
- ***CMV titres at the start of pregnancy and repeated in each trimester if the woman is CMV negative, as this is the most serious viral infection in post-transplant pregnancies.***
- Glucose tolerance test (GTT) at 26–28 weeks as many are on steroids (prednisolone) and tacrolimus.
- Proteinuria itself, without deteriorating renal function or hypertension, is not an indication for delivery.[3]
- If graft rejection is suspected, this can only be diagnosed by renal biopsy.
- The presence of the allograft kidney does not obstruct a vaginal delivery. Although a Caesarean section is required only for obstetric indications, the rate of lower segment Caesarean section (LSCS) in this group is high.
- Clear instructions must be documented regarding:
  - Care to avoid fluid overload, especially water retention secondary to oxytocin.
  - Prophylactic antibiotics for all interventions including episiotomy.
  - Steroid bolus with 100 mg hydrocortisone IM/IV every 6–8 h during labour to cover delivery, and the immediate postpartum period.
  - ACE inhibitors can be used for BP control after delivery.
- Breastfeeding, though traditionally contraindicated in patients on immunosuppressive drugs, is probably safe in those not on ciclosporin. The recent consensus is that breastfeeding need not be strictly contraindicated.[4]
- Inform paediatricians if parental history of polycystic kidneys or vesicoureteric reflux to initiate further paediatric follow-up.
- Continue low molecular weight heparin prophylaxis for up to 6 weeks after delivery in those with dense proteinuria.[5]
- Confirm ongoing nephrology follow-up appointments are in place before postnatal discharge.

Information for patients

Please see Information for patients: Pregnancy after kidney transplant (p. 540)

References

1. McKay DB, Josephson MA. Pregnancy after kidney transplantation. Clin J Am Soc Nephrol 2008;3: S117–S125
2. Ramhendar T, Byrne P. Use of the levonorgestrel-releasing intrauterine system in renal transplant recipients: a retrospective case review. Contraception 2012;86: 288–289.
3. Nelson-Piercy C. Renal disease. In: Handbook of maternal medicine, 4th ed. London: Informa Health Care, 2010.
4. McKay D, Josephson M. Reproduction and transplantation: Report on the AST consensus conference on reproductive issues and transplantation. Am J Transplant 2005;5: 1–8.
5. Carr S. Pregnancy and the renal transplant recipient. In: Davison JM, et al, ed., Renal disease in pregnancy. London: RCOG Press 2008.

Post renal transplant and pre-pregnancy

- Advise patient to defer pregnancy by 12–24 months after transplant; advise reliable, effective, and safe contraception
- Discuss parameters for ideal time to conceive—when the graft is functioning well, there is only minimal hypertension or proteinuria, immunosuppression is stable with drugs without fetotoxic/teratogenic potential
- Confirm rubella immune (**vaccination pre-transplant**), Hep B, C and HIV status
- Check blood group and any antibodies especially Rh(D)
- Advise smoking cessation
- Check for lupus and antiphospholipid syndrome, diabetes if not previously done
- Advise peri-pregnancy folic acid till end of 12 weeks
- ***Assess medications:***
  - If on ACE inhibitors or ARBs, change at least 6 weeks pre-pregnancy to methyldopa or labetalol ± nifedipine
  - Mycophenolate mofetil or sirolimus must be stopped and immunosuppression achieved with agents such as prednisolone, azathioprine, tacrolimus, or ciclosporin
  - Stop statins, biphosphonates
- Warn patient not to reduce or stop prescribed immunosuppressants due to any teratogenic concerns as risk of graft rejection otherwise high. Reassure regarding safety record of prescribed medications
- Consider low-dose aspirin prophylaxis
- Genetic referral if previous history of renal failure due to polycystic kidney disease or reflux nephropathy
- Advise prevention of UTIs. Some may need low-dose long-term antibiotic prophylaxis
- Pregnancy care should to be multidisciplinary, mainly in a tertiary centre with transplant nephrologist, urologist, specialist obstetrician, etc.
- Some aspects of antenatal care can be shared between local DGH and primary care to reduce inconvenience of patient's weekly trips to tertiary unit. Good communication is vital
- Reassure patient that pregnancies conceived at the optimal time and those that proceed beyond the 1st trimester have a 95–97% good outcome rate
- Instruct patient regarding home monitoring of BP

↓

Prompt referral, usually to tertiary unit from primary care, once pregnancy established. Subsequent antenatal care can be shared between local DGH and tertiary unit as well as with community midwife for routine antenatal checks

↓

First visit to maternal medicine or joint obstetric–renal clinic

- Confirm dates, viability, routine booking bloods plus renal and liver function tests, serum calcium, ferritin, folate, etc.
- Review medications: If on ACE inhibitors or ARBs, change to methyldopa or labetalol
- Biphosphanates and statins to be stopped if not done already
- High-dose folic acid (5 mg/day) till end of 12 weeks gestation, continue till end of pregnancy if on azathioprine, tacrolimus
- Low-dose aspirin (75 mg/day), to continue throughout pregnancy
- Advise patient not to reduce or stop taking immunosuppressant drugs as graft rejection can occur otherwise
- Regular BP monitoring—patient can check daily with home monitor
- BP levels to be maintained <140/90, ideally with antihypertensives suitable in pregnancy. Arrange regular BP series in day assessment unit once a fortnight till 28 weeks, then weekly
- Baseline renal function tests, LFTs, serum calcium, ferritin, folate
- Check CMV IgM titres, if negative, repeat titres in each trimester
- Arrange genetic counselling if maternal history of renal failure due to polycystic kidney disease or reflux nephropathy
- MSU to be sent at each visit—vigilance for UTIs
- Further appointments co-ordinated between tertiary unit and DGH
- Routine anomaly scan at about 20 weeks, arrange further scans at about 26 weeks, then at 3–4 week intervals
- Arrange GTT at 26–28 weeks if patient on prednisolone or tacrolimus

↓

Further visits to maternal medicine or joint obstetric–renal clinic (at individualized intervals)

- Renal function tests including serum creatinine, electrolytes, uric acid, and 24 h urine for total protein—at frequencies as directed by nephrologist
- Monthly FBC, Hb, platelets in particular—haematinics to be prescribed if anaemic. Monthly serum calcium levels to exclude either hypo- or hypercalcaemia
- Serum measurement of immunosuppressant levels as directed by transplant nephrologist
- MSU for C&S at each visit both in hospital and community, immediate antibiotic treatment, low-dose prophylaxis/maintenance antibiotics in certain cases
- GTT at 26–28 weeks if on tacrolimus, prednisolone. Commence diabetes management if abnormal GTT (see diabetes care pathway, pp. 201–202)
- LFTs at 6–8 weekly intervals
- CMV IgM titres in each trimester if CMV −ve at start of pregnancy
- Detailed anomaly scan at 20 weeks
- Ensure is continuing prescribed medications
- Serial scans for growth and liquor ± UA Doppler from 24–26 weeks at 3–4 weekly intervals, more frequently if indicated
- Vigilance for pre-eclampsia
- If increasing or dense proteinuria, thromboprophylaxis with LMWH and below-knee compression stockings, to be continued for up to 6 weeks postpartum
- Reassure patient that the transplanted kidney does not cause obstruction during vaginal delivery

↓

Delivery and postpartum

- Caesarean section for obstetric indications such as severe pre-eclampsia, IUGR, etc.
- Antenatal referral to paediatricians if fetal polycystic kidneys or vesicoureteric obstruction suspected
- Discuss breastfeeding, as not entirely contraindicated according to recent reports

↓

Clear documentation in notes (on intrapartum, neonatal, and postnatal pages)

- Care to avoid fluid overload, especially water retention secondary to syntocinon
- Prophylactic antibiotics for any procedure including episiotomy or repair of tear
- If patient has been on prednisolone, bolus doses of 100 mg IM/IV hydrocortisone at 6–8 hourly intervals during labour as well as to cover delivery
- Alert neonatologists if suspected fetal polycystic kidneys or vesicoureteric obstruction for neonatal scans
- ACE inhibitors can be reintroduced if necessary, after delivery
- Ensure continued nephrology follow-up appointments are in place before discharge
- If dense proteinuria, to continue thromboprophylaxis for about 6 weeks postpartum with below-knee compression stockings
- Advise contraception—Avoid COCP. Mirena® (LNG-IUS) or progesterone intradermal implant ideal

20.2 Other Organ Transplants

FACT FILE

- Following improved success of transplantation surgery and immunosuppressant therapies, more women can survive and have children.
- Information obtained from large transplant pregnancy registries[1,2,3] is used to study data about pregnancy outcomes, maternal complications and graft function and any long-term infancy/childhood risks.
- Kidney transplant is the most common solid organ transplant.
- Pregnancies are most commonly reported after kidney transplants.
- More pregnancies are being reported after liver, pancreas, heart, bowel, pancreas–kidney, heart–lung, liver–kidney transplants.[1,4,5,6]
- Survival rates, graft loss, and rejection rates associated with pregnancy vary according to the organ involved, underlying pathology, and comorbidities such as hypertension or diabetes.[1]

Kidney transplant

- Long-term graft survival does not seem to be affected by pregnancy, even several pregnancies.
- In those with a previously stable graft, pregnancy does not affect renal function.[7,8]
- In those with pre-existing renal graft **dysfunction** and/or hypertension needing antihypertensives, there is further elevation of the serum creatinine during pregnancy which does not return to pre-pregnancy levels. Subsequent renal function may be adversely affected in such cases.[1,2]

Liver transplant

- Fewer adverse events reported in pregnancy than in other solid organ transplants.
- Liver enzymes may remain elevated in pregnancy but without jaundice, usually settle to normal values with a dose increase of immunosuppressants or a bolus course of steroids[9]

Heart transplant

- The normal haemodynamic changes of pregnancy and post-delivery do not seem to increase the risk of heart failure in those who have had a heart transplant.[2,6]
- No increase has been reported either with pregnancy complications or adverse outcomes or with graft rejection, whether it be one or more pregnancies.

Lung or heart–lung transplant

- Lung transplants are most commonly performed for cystic fibrosis.
- They are associated with increased incidence of pregnancy complications such as preterm birth, IUGR, and infection.
- Greater graft rejection rates and higher graft loss rates 2 years after delivery with increased long-term morbidity and mortality have been reported with pregnancy.[1,10]
- Genetic counselling is important before pregnancy to discuss cystic fibrosis inheritance by offspring.

Pancreas–kidney transplant

- Recipients who have had long-standing diabetes may have underlying vascular disease. Good metabolic control is otherwise seen in pregnancy.
- Worsening glucose control may be an indication of graft rejection warranting investigation.[4,11]
- Pregnancy complications such as fetal loss are seen in nearly one-third of pregnancies. Preterm delivery (77%), pre-eclampsia (34%), pyelonephritis (42%), low birth weight (62%), and hypertension (66%) are more frequent with simultaneous kidney–pancreas transplantations.[10]

Immunosuppresants

- Most pregnant women are on maintenance doses of a combination of corticosteroids, calcineurin inhibitors, macrolides, and/or antimetabolites. Such combination therapy helps decrease the risk of toxicity from high doses of single immunosuppressive drugs, while not reducing efficacy.[1,12]
- Certain immunosuppressant medications, especially in high doses, may have an impact on the pregnant woman and the fetus/neonate (see Table 20.1) while others are entirely contraindicated due to their embryotoxicity and/or teratogenicity.

Pre-conception assessment and counselling

- Pre-pregnancy planning involving transplant team and specialist obstetrician is highly recommended.
- Ethical issues regarding life expectancy, long-term child care, etc. should be discussed with sensitivity.
- Discussion regarding the cause of original disease for which transplantation was required and any continuing sequelae need identification.
- Women with post-transplant organ dysfunction should be advised to defer any pregnancy till evaluation for severity of organ damage or progression of disease.
- Reassure the patient that the majority of women will have no allograft dysfunction during pregnancy if the graft has been stable and there are minimal comorbidities.
- Renal transplant patients with elevated serum creatinine levels in excess of 1.4 mg/dL should be counselled to reconsider plans for a pregnancy as they have poor pregnancy prognosis and an increased

Table 20.1 Immunosuppressants: possible effects on mother and baby

Immunosuppressant drug (category)	*Mode of action*	*Maternal effects with high doses*	*Possible pregnancy complication*
Prednisolone (corticosteroid)	Leukocyte inhibition	Cushingoid facies, hypertension, gestational diabetes, osteopenia, peptic ulceration, psychiatric disturbances, poor wound healing	Preterm rupture of membranes
Azathioprine (antimetabolite)	Inhibition of clonal-T cell proliferation	Anaemia, leukopenia	No specific effect reported
Ciclosporin (calcineurin inhibitor)	Block cytokine production needed for T cell activation and proliferation	Hypertension, nephrotoxicity, hirsutism	No specific effect reported
Tacrolimus[a] (macrolide antibiotic, also a calcineurin inhibitor)	Calcineurin inhibitor, powerful inhibitor of helper T cell function	Nephrotoxicity,(therefore must not be given with ciclosporin), hypertension, diabetes, neurotoxicity	Neonatal hyperkalaemia, cardiomyopathy
Mycophenolate mofetil	Inhibitor of purine synthesis	**Contraindicated in pregnancy**: embryotoxic, teratogenic	**Contraindicated in pregnancy**

[a] Monthly blood concentration measurement and dosage adjustment.

risk of graft dysfunction with progression to end-stage renal failure within 2 years after delivery.[10]

- Pregnancy is optimally timed at least 1 year after transplantation to allow time for graft stabilization and to reduce dosages of immunosuppressant drugs to maintenance levels.[3,10]
- Possible complications, such as hypertension, diabetes, repeated infections, or smoking, that could affect graft function as well as have an adverse impact on pregnancy outcomes must be discussed.
- Underlying hypertension not only affects graft function but also can also lead to pregnancy complications. ACE inhibitors and angiotensin receptor blockers should be discontinued before pregnancy and methyldopa or labetalol substituted.
- Those who have had pre-existing diabetes before transplantation, or develop diabetes after immunosuppressant therapy, must be encouraged to achieve optimal glucose control before embarking on a pregnancy.
- Transplant patients have a greater chance of developing osteopenia, osteoporosis and fractures. Calcium supplementation 1000 mg/day and vitamin D 0.25 micrograms/day should be initiated before pregnancy.[1]
- Folic acid should be commenced before pregnancy and continued till 13 completed weeks of gestation.
- Pre-pregnancy immune status for rubella, varicella, toxoplasmosis, CMV, parvovirus, herpes simplex and hepatitis should be checked.
- Live virus vaccines for rubella and varicella should have been given, if indicated by the immune status, before transplantation, as these are contraindicated when immunosuppressants are used.
- Similarly hepatitis, influenza, and pneumococcal vaccines are best given and immune seroconversion checked before transplantation.

Management of pregnancy

- ***Multidisciplinary team management is essential***.
- Apart from the routine pregnancy bloods at the initial booking, liver function tests and serum creatinine levels as well as a 24-h urine collection (for total protein, creatinine clearance) is recommended.
- Hyperemesis in early pregnancy may cause inadequate immunosuppressant drug levels, and thereby inadequate immunosuppression, risking graft rejection. Medication dosages may need to be adjusted as guided by serum drug levels and frequent clinical and biochemical tests to monitor the function of the transplanted organ are required.
- Vigilance must be maintained throughout pregnancy for the development of complications such as pregnancy-induced hypertension, worsening of pre-existing hypertension, gestational diabetes, pre-eclampsia, preterm labour, fetal growth restriction, and maternal UTIs, pyelonephritis, etc.
- Continue calcium and vitamin D supplementation throughout pregnancy
- As these patients are at high risk of developing pre-eclampsia, low-dose aspirin prophylaxis from 13 weeks gestation onwards must be considered.
- Routine monthly midstream urine cultures are advisable.
- ***It is important that the location of the transplanted organ is clearly documented in the notes to prevent inadvertent surgical damage should an emergency Caesarean section becomes necessary***.
- An early GTT (at about 16 weeks gestation) is recommended for those on tacrolimus and/or steroids. If normal, this should be repeated at about 26–28 weeks gestation to exclude gestational diabetes. Liver transplant patients have a high likelihood of developing diabetes (37%) of which half are gestational diabetes.[13]
- Hypertension should be treated aggressively in order to prevent graft organ damage and pregnancy complications. Antihypertensives that are appropriate for pregnancy need to be used, sometimes in combination.
- **Signs of pre-eclampsia** such as elevated liver enzymes, thrombocytopenia, hypertension, significant proteinuria, or hyperuricaemia can mimic acute organ rejection, drug toxicity, or disease progression.
- If advised by renal physicians and the transplant team, the patient may even need an organ biopsy to achieve diagnostic differentiation. Delay in diagnosis with the assumed diagnosis of pre-eclampsia may jeopardize graft function and long-term survival of the patient.
- If anaemia is detected, serum iron and ferritin levels, folate, vitamin B_{12}, and reticulocyte count need to be evaluated and necessary supplements advised.
- Gastric irritation in those on long-term steroids should be managed with H_2 receptor blockers or proton pump inhibitors.
- Detailed anomaly scan at about 20 weeks should be followed by serial fetal growth ultrasound scans at monthly intervals from about 26 weeks onwards.
- Tests for fetal well-being with biophysical profile studies, umbilical artery Dopplers, ± cardiotocography may be considered from 32–34 weeks onwards, if indicated.[1,14]
- Early involvement of senior obstetric anaesthetist to plan analgesia/anaesthesia for labour and delivery or for a Caesarean section is mandatory, especially with heart–lung transplants.

Delivery and postpartum

- In the absence of obstetric complications such as pre-eclampsia or IUGR, delivery at term can be anticipated.
- Caesarean sections are more common in transplant patients mainly due to associated obstetric problems; in the absence of such complications, a vaginal delivery is entirely feasible.
- At Caesarean section extra care must be taken to identify and stay clear of the intra-abdominal/pelvic graft. With renal transplants great care must be taken to avoid ureteric injury as the ureter may be superior to the uterine artery, thus entering the bladder over the lower uterine segment.
- Epidural analgesia is recommended for labour.[15]
- Immunosuppressant medication must be continued during labour and postpartum.[2]
- Safety of **breastfeeding** in women on immunosuppressants remains controversial.[1]
- Combined oral **contraceptives** are contraindicated with most immunosuppressants. The progesterone-only pill, implant, or the levonorgestrel-loaded IUD (Mirena®) are acceptable contraceptive choices.

Information for patients

Please see Information for patients: Pregnancy after a transplant operation (p. 540)

References

1. Mastrobattista JM, Gomez-Lobo V Pregnancy after solid organ transplantation. Obstet Gynecol 2008;112: 919–932.
2. Sibanda N, et al. Pregnancy after organ transplantation: a report from the U.K. Transplant Pregnancy Registry. Transplantation 2007; 83: 1301–1307.
3. McKay DB, et al. Reproduction and transplantation: report on the AST Consensus Conference on Reproductive Issues and Transplantation. Am J Transplant 2005;5: 1592–1599.
4. Bramham K, et al. Pregnancy in pancreas-kidney transplant recipients: report of three cases and review of the literature. Obstet Med 2010;3: 73–77.
5. Källén B, et al. Pregnancy outcome after maternal organ transplantation in Sweden. BJOG 2005;112: 904–909.
6. Troché V, et al. Pregnancy after heart or heart-lung transplantation: a series of 10 pregnancies. BJOG 1998;105: 454–458.
7. Naqvi R, et al. Outcome of pregnancy in renal allograft recipients: SIUT experience. Transplant Proc 2006;38: 2001–2002.
8. Armenti VT, et al. Report from the National Transplantation Pregnancy Registry (NTPR): outcomes of pregnancy after transplantation. Clin Transpl 2005: 69–83.
9. Jain AB, et al. Pregnancy after liver transplantation with Tacrolimus immunosuppression: a single center's experience update at 13 years. Transplantation 2003;76: 827–832.
10. Armenti VT, et al. Report from the National Transplantation Pregnancy Registry: outcomes of pregnancy after transplantation. Clin Transpl 2006: 57–70.

11. Barrou BM, et al. Pregnancy after pancreas transplantation in the cyclosporine era: report from the International Pancreas Transplant Registry. Transplantation 1998;65: 524–527.
12. Ekberg H Reduced exposure to calcineurin inhibitors in renal transplantation. N Engl J Med 2007;357: 2762–2775.
13. Nagy S, et al. Pregnancy outcome in liver transplant recipients. Obstet Gynecol 2003;102: 121–128.
14. Stratta P, et al. Pregnancy in kidney transplantation: satisfactory outcomes and harsh realities. J Nephrol 2003; 16: 792–806.
15. Wu D, et al. Pregnancy after thoracic organ transplantation. Semin Perinatol 2007;31: 354–362.

CARE PATHWAY

Pre-pregnancy advice after organ transplantation

- Advise pregnancy is deferred for at least 1 year post-transplant and advise effective contraception meanwhile. COCP contraindicated. Progesterone-only pill, implant, or Mirena ideal
- Assess graft function
- Discuss any ethical issues with sensitivity
- Check immune status for Hep B and C, CMV, toxoplasmosis, herpes simplex, rubella, etc.
- Assess immunosuppression therapy, mycophenolate mofetil, sirolimus contraindicated for pregnancy
- Assess comorbidities (e.g. hypertension, diabetes): optimize control, change ACE inhibitors or ARBs to pregnancy-appropriate antihypertensives (e.g. methyldopa, labetalol)
- Baseline kidney and liver function tests
- Vaccinations if needed (e.g. for hepatitis, tetanus, pneumococcus, HPV, influenza)
- Pre-pregnancy folic acid, vitamin D, and calcium supplementation
- Explore cause of original disease and any persistent sequelae (e.g. hypertension, vasculitis)
- Genetic referral if lung transplant done for cystic fibrosis
- Discuss effect of pregnancy on allograft function
- Discuss possible complications of the original condition, the transplant and subsequent immunosuppressant therapy on pregnancy (e.g. miscarriages, premature birth, pre-eclampsia, IUGR, hypertension, gestational diabetes, etc.)
- Discuss effect of pregnancy on allograft function
- Reassure patient that most women will have no allograft dysfunction during pregnancy, especially if graft is stable and any comorbidities are well controlled

↓

Antenatal management

In specialist maternal medicine antenatal clinic, or joint obstetric antenatal clinics with transplant team

- Accurate dating and confirmation of viability
- Folic acid till 13 weeks gestation
- Continuation of calcium and vitamin D supplementation throughout pregnancy
- Clinical and laboratory monitoring of graft function status of transplanted organ and levels of immunosuppressant drugs, as appropriate
- Clear documentation of location of transplanted organ in abdomen/pelvis to avoid inadvertent injury if emergency LSCS required
- Regular antenatal assessments—suggested frequency: every 4 weeks until about 32 weeks, every 2 weeks till 36 weeks, and weekly thereafter
- In those on steroids/tacrolimus, early GTT at 16 weeks, if normal, repeat at 26–28 weeks
- Optimal management of gestational diabetes
- Monthly MSU, aggressive management of any UTI
- Surveillance for bacterial and viral infections
- Aggressive management of hypertension with pregnancy appropriate drugs
- Vigilance for signs of graft rejection
- Early referral to senior anaesthetist for assessment and plans for analgesia, anaesthetic for labour, delivery or for Caesarean section (emergency and elective)
- Fetal surveillance: 1st-trimester scan, targeted and detailed fetal anomaly scan at about 20 weeks, serial growth scans monthly from about 26 weeks
- BPP/Dopplers ± CTG after about 32 weeks—may be optional in individual cases
- Close surveillance for pre-eclampsia, nephropathy, hypertension: remember signs could be similar to drug toxicity, acute graft rejection or progressive disease. Organ biopsy may be recommended by renal physicians, transplant team

↓

Postpartum

- Breastfeeding may be appropriate with some immunosuppressants
- Contraception advice—Not for COCP. Progesterone implant or Mirena® can be recommended

Data from: Mastrobattista JM and Gomez-Lobo V, Pregnancy after solid organ transplantation, *Obstetrics and Gynecology*, 2008, 112, 4, pp. 919–932; and Armenti VT et al., Report from the National Transplantation Pregnancy Registry (NTPR): outcomes of pregnancy after transplantation, *Clinical Transplant*, 2005, pp. 69–83.

21 Maternal Enzymatic Abnormalities

21.1 C_1 Inhibitor Deficiency

FACT FILE

- **C_1 inhibitor deficiency (C_1INHD)**[1,2] is characterized by intermittent episodes of soft tissue swelling and angio-oedema.
- **C_1INHD or hereditary angio-oedema** is an autosomal dominant disorder with a prevalence of 1 in 50 000.
- This is an autosomal dominant condition with a 50% chance of the offspring inheriting the condition.
- Hereditary angio-oedema is a potentially life-threatening condition which can complicate pregnancy.
- In 20% of patients there is no family history, the condition being caused by a new mutation.
- These attacks are not histamine-mediated and do not respond to antihistamines or corticosteroids.

Sites and complications of angio-oedema

- The face and limbs are most commonly affected although any part of the body may be involved.
- Greatest risks are when the mouth, tongue, upper respiratory tract, and bowels are involved.
- The soft tissue swelling may progress for 24–48 h and depending on the site and severity, may be painless and without accompanying itching, urticaria, or local heat.
- **Laryngeal oedema** may present with hoarseness and/or change in the quality or loss of voice as well as difficulty in breathing. **This is a life-threatening emergency requiring urgent treatment** due to the potential for asphyxiation.
- Angio-oedema of the bowel walls leading to severe intractable abdominal pain and vomiting, symptoms may mimic acute appendicitis, or intestinal obstruction.

Triggers for development of angio-oedema

- In 50% of episodes, the patient herself can identify a trigger.
- Triggers include trauma (often mild) or a surgical procedure.
- Trauma to the mouth and pharynx (intubation or any dental procedure) are particularly likely to induce laryngeal oedema.
- There are some reports of pregnancy worsening the disease[3] and even contributing to premature labour and stillbirth.[4,5]
- Other triggers are prolonged pressure on any site, infection, emotional stress, early pregnancy, and the postnatal period.
- ACE inhibitors, which are anyway contraindicated in pregnancy, may also trigger angio-oedema.

Management during pregnancy [1,2,6]

- Patients should be managed individually with input from the wider multidisciplinary team.
- Severe attacks during pregnancy should be treated with concentrate as in the non-pregnant patient. Severe cases may require regular C_1INH replacement therapy.[1]
- Close liaison with the medical and anaesthetic teams is very important.
- Although attacks of angio-oedema are more common during early pregnancy, symptoms are reported to be reduced during pregnancy. There are reports of increased attacks in the postnatal period.[1]
- Drugs such as stanozolol danazol or tranexemic acid, which are generally used outside of pregnancy for prophylaxis against angio-oedema, are however contraindicated in pregnancy.
- Referral to the anaesthetic high-risk clinic is essential in pregnancy.
- Clear peripartum management plans along with an anaesthetic plan need to be drawn up and clearly documented in the hospital records and hand-held notes as well as widely dispersed to all concerned in the care of the patient.
- Early communication with the pharmacist, with the clinical lead in the emergency department and midwifery lead in delivery suite is recommended.
- It is likely that the patient has already been reviewed by a clinical geneticist to identify whether she has the hereditary form of angio-oedema. Referral to genetics, if not done so already, should be instigated as the hereditary form is autosomal dominant with a 50% chance of the baby inheriting it.
- Effective communication between the team involved in the individual patient's care and dissemination of information to health professionals as well as to the patient and partner or relatives are crucial.[1]
- **Home possession of C_1INH concentrate**[1]**:** C_1INH deficiency patients will have been offered the opportunity to keep a therapeutic dose of C_1INH concentrate at home, sufficient to treat a laryngeal emergency, as 50–75% have a life-threatening attack at some time.[4] **Ensure that the patient has this at home**.

Short-term prophylaxis for labour, delivery, or surgery (including Caesarean section)

- There is little evidence that complications from C_1INH deficiency are any more common in vaginal delivery.
- Human C_1INH concentrate should be administered immediately upon the onset of labour or for elective Caesarean section. As it is effective for 24 h, a second dose is required only if the patient is undelivered by this time.
- ***Note: Multiple doses of the human C_1INH concentrate must be kept available at all times during the patient's hospital stay.***
- ***The safest obstetric approach appears to be to administer a pre-delivery infusion of 500–1000 U C_1INH concentrate.***
- In a low-risk pregnancy without pretreatment with C_1INH concentrate, it is recommended that C_1INH should be available in the delivery suite.
- There may be local swelling of the vulva and infusion sites, but this does not usually require treatment unless urethral obstruction is a problem.[7]
- If an operative delivery is undertaken, regional analgesia is preferable to endotracheal intubation in order to avoid laryngeal trauma.
- In all situations, the clinician should be aware that the postpartum period is one when there is a high risk of acute attacks.

Treatment of acute severe attack involving the upper airways or gut

- **General supportive measures** including clearing and maintenance of the airways, rehydration, and analgesia for abdominal pain.
- **Human C_1INH concentrate** must be kept readily available in the emergency department as well as in the delivery suite whenever a patient with C_1INH deficiency is booked for delivery at the hospital. This is to be ordered from the pharmacy on a named-patient basis.

- This concentrate is the treatment of choice for swelling within the mouth, of the tongue and throat as well as for severe abdominal pain. **The usual dose is 500–1500 plasma units by slow IV injection. A second dose should be available without delay if so required.**
- ***Note: Human C_1INH concentrate is a non-licensed drug and a blood product. As such, the patient must be made aware of these facts and the discussion documented in both the hand-held maternity notes as well as the main hospital notes during the first visit to the specialist antenatal clinic.***
- Trust guidelines regarding the use of blood products must be followed, including a record of the batch number in the main notes at the time of administration.
- Fresh frozen plasma (FFP) is an acceptable alternative when C_1INH concentrate is not available, but can cause a temporary worsening of swelling.[8]
- Antihistamines are ineffective in C_1INH deficiency.

Contraception

- **Oestrogens should be avoided.** The use of combined oral contraceptives can exacerbate symptoms.[9] A recent study reported that over 60% of hereditary angio-odema patients have more frequent attacks when on oestrogens.[9]
- In general, progesterone-only pills such as levonorgestrel are preferred. Progesterone may have a mildly protective effect. No published data are available about any contraindications for intrauterine devices.
- ***Remind the patient to always wear a MedicAlert bracelet.***

Information for patients

Please see Information for patients: C_1 inhibitor deficiency and pregnancy (p. 540)

References

1. Gompels MM. C1 inhibitor deficiency: consensus document. Clin Exp Immunol 2005; 139: 379–394.
2. Bork K, et al. Clinical studies of sudden upper airway obstruction in patients with hereditary angioedema due to C1 esterase inhibitor deficiency Arch Intern Med 2003; 163: 1229–1235.
3. Logan RA, Greaves MW. Hereditary angio-oedema:treatment with C1 esterase inhibitor concentrate. J R Soc Med 1984; 77: 1046–1048.
4. Raychaudhuri K, et al. Termination of pregnancy in a patient with hereditary angioedema. Br J Hosp Med 1997; 58: 287–288.
5. Nielsen EW, et al. Hereditary angio-oedema: new clinical observations and autoimmune screening, complement and kallikrein-kinin analyses. J Intern Med 1996; 239: 119–130.
6. Bouittet L, et al. Angioedema and oral contraception. Dermatology 2003; 206: 106–109.
7. Chappatte O, de Swiet M. Hereditary angioneurotic oedema and pregnancy. Case reports and review of the literature. Br J Obstet Gynaecol 1988; 95: 938–942.
8. Galan HL, et al. Fresh frozen plasma prophylaxis for hereditary angioedema during pregnancy. A case report. J Reprod Med 1996; 41: 541–544.
9. Bork K, et al. Recurrent episodes of skin angioedema and severe attacks of abdominal pain induced by oral contraceptives or hormone replacement therapy. Am J Med 2003; 114: 294–298.

For urgent advice on **C_1 inhibitor deficiency** contact senior pharmacist on call or haematologist

GP or community midwife refers patient to maternal medicine or specialist antenatal clinic as early as possible in the 1st trimester

↓

First visit to maternal medicine or specialist antenatal clinic

- Note history of any recent attacks
- Check whether patient has dose of C_1 esterase concentrate at home and that both partners have been trained to administer it. If not, organize without delay
- Remind patient to wear MedicAlert at all times
- Discuss triggers for angio-oedema
- Advise to report early to emergency department or delivery suite if symptoms develop, especially breathing problems, swelling of mouth, tongue, or throat
- ***Refer to high-risk anaesthetic clinic as a priority***
- Refer to genetics team, if patient has not been reviewed already
- If already confirmed to have hereditary angio-oedema, 50% chance of offspring inheriting the same—discuss with patient. Inform paediatricians antenatally
- Inform patient and document that C_1 inhibitor concentrate is a non-licensed blood product, but a life- saving drug
- Inform chief pharmacist, emergency department, and delivery suite leads to ensure that multiple doses of C_1 inhibitor concentrate, on a named patient basis, are readily available at both sites. **Document this in both hand-held and main notes**
- ***Ensure that an 'Alert' (electronic and/or paper) is placed on the patient records***
- Clear documentation in both hand-held and main notes regarding prophylactic dose of C_1 inhibitor concentrate as a slow IV infusion of 500–1500 plasma units (as advised by senior pharmacist) to be given at start of labour or before LSCS
- Inform patient that **her condition in itself is not an indication for early IOL or LSCS**
- Routine antenatal checks with community midwife to continue, according to NICE low-risk schedule

↓

Further visits to maternal medicine or specialist antenatal clinic (at about 34 and 40 weeks)

- Assess pregnancy, any recent angio-oedema flares? What steps were taken?
- Ensure patient has had an anaesthetic review
- Ensure the availability of C_1 inhibitor concentrate in emergency department as well as in delivery suite and that all medical and midwifery staff are aware of its location
- Exclude any precipitating triggers for attacks of angio-oedema, if possible (e.g. prompt treatment of any infection)
- Reiterate that **early IOL or LSCS are required only for obstetric indications**, not C_1 inhibitor deficiency per se

↓

Delivery and postpartum

- Date for routine post-date IOL (avoiding weekends) at about 40^{+10-11} or according to individual unit's post-dates IOL policy
- At the time of postnatal discharge, advise and document discussion regarding contraception—COCP contraindicated

21.2 Mastocytosis

FACT FILE

Aetiology and pathogenesis

- **Mastocytosis**, also called **systemic mast cell disease**, is a rare heterogeneous disorder, where due to an excessive accumulation of mast cells, an immediate hypersensitivity reaction is triggered which, in severe cases, can result in hypotension, shock and death.
- Mast cells are found in the perivascular spaces of most tissues of a normal person. They have an active role in the mediation of the body's immune system by the release of proinflammatory and vasoactive mediators including histamines, triggered by exposure to stimuli such as allergens.
- Mast cells have both oestrogen and progesterone receptors and are present in the myometrium and the placenta.[1] In any normal pregnancy, mast cells are known to increase in the myometrium with progress of pregnancy, but the effect of this is unclear.[2]
- Mastocytosis is characterized by an increase in mast cells in the skin, lymph nodes, liver, spleen, and bone marrow.
- The aetiology is unknown, most likely multifactorial. A genetic component may be involved, though this is not entirely clear.
- The mechanism thought to be involved in most patients is a genetic change in a protein called KIT on the mast cell which results in too many of these cells accumulating in various parts of the body. These cases result from a genetic mutation which causes the overactivation of the receptor (c-KIT) that controls mast cell growth and proliferation. This mutation is believed to cause the abnormal accumulation of mast cells in certain tissues.
- These mutations in the c-KIT proto-oncogene are passed down through families in an autosomal dominant fashion.
- There are some familial cases of mastocytosis and related mast cell disorders. More commonly, within a family, members may have different disorders which are all linked by irregular mast cell activity.

Clinical manifestations

- Two forms of mastocytosis exist: **cutaneous** and **systemic. Although an individual may have one or the other form, in some people the cutaneous and systemic forms of mastocytosis may coexist.**
- **Cutaneous mastocytosis** is the most common form of mastocytosis and usually affects only children (in 75% of cases aged 1–4 years) of age and appears as skin lesions without a systemic component. This variety of mastocytosis usually resolves spontaneously by the time puberty is reached.
- There are three main types of **systemic mastocytosis:**[3] (1) indolent mastocytosis, (2) mastocytosis with an associated haematological disorder, and (3) aggressive mastocytosis. The incidence of systemic mastocytosis is approximately 1 in 150 000.
- Most common is the **indolent variety** (90% of cases) where symptoms are usually mild to moderate, characterized by **urticaria pigmentosa**, with small reddish-brown skin macules or papules. Pruritus, skin flushing,[4] episodes of anaphylaxis, dyspepsia, gastrointestinal symptoms including abdominal pain, vomiting and diarrhoea, vascular instability, osteoporosis, mood changes, headaches, peripheral neuropathy tiredness, etc. may be variously present.
- Hepatosplenomegaly and lymphadenopathy may be present as well as anaemia or cytopenias if there is bone marrow involvement.
- Those with urticaria pigmentosa display skin lesions which when stroked or rubbed become red, swollen, and itchy (the classic Darier's sign) due to mast cell degranulation induced by the physical stimuli.

Triggers for attacks

- These include:
  - physical stimuli, e.g. heat, cold, friction, sunlight, perfumes
  - stress
  - certain foods, e.g. shellfish, cheese, preservatives, flavourings
  - alcohol
  - insect bites
  - certain infections which may be bacterial, viral, or fungal.
- ***Attacks can also be triggered in different patients with mastocytosis by certain medications such as aspirin, other NSAIDs, certain anaesthetic agents, opioids, atracurium, hyoscine, procaine, tubocurarine, dextran, certain radiographic dyes, and even some antibiotics.***[4]

Diagnostic tests

- These include skin biopsy, elevated serum tryptase levels (>20 ng/ml),[1,5] elevated urine histamine levels, and molecular testing.
- Other investigations: full blood count, renal function tests, liver function tests, and clotting studies.
- In systemic mastocytosis, depending on the symptomatology, other tests such as ultrasound of abdominal organs, or chest radiograph (for presence of lymphadenopathy) may be required. Investigations such as skeletal radiographs, bone marrow biopsy, endoscopy, or bone density scan are invariably avoided during pregnancy.

Management

- Management is mainly symptomatic and by avoidance of known allergens.
- Patients are encouraged to wear a MedicAlert bracelet and carry an emergency treatment protocol card from their specialist.
- Those with frequent anaphylactic episodes are advised to carry injectable adrenaline (epinephrine) in the form of a pen for emergencies.
- Despite the variety of symptoms, treatment with H_1 and H_2 antagonists such as chlorphenamine and cimetidine is most effective in the majority.
- In mastocytosis that coexists with haematological disorders, treatment of the latter allows remission of mastocytosis.[1] Mast cell stabilizers such as sodium cromoglicate, nedocromil, and ketotifen are also used, but the safety of nedocromil and ketotifen in pregnancy is yet to be established.
- Alpha- and beta-blockers and cholinergic antagonists are contraindicated in those with systemic forms of mastocytosis.
- Any drug known to trigger an anaphylactic reaction must be scrupulously avoided and great care taken with those that the patient has not been hitherto exposed to.
- Vaccinations can be given unless there has been an allergic reaction previously. Usually most reactions are mild, with low-grade pyrexia that responds to paracetamol. It is also advisable for patients to take an antihistamine on the day and to continue this for a few days after the vaccination in order to dampen symptoms such as urticaria or flushing due to mast cell mediator release.

Pregnancy management in women with an established diagnosis of mastocytosis

- ***This follows the same principles as listed in the previous section.***
- Vitamin D and calcium supplements need to be considered in pregnancy.
- Some women (20%) may experience worsening of urticaria pigmentosa and other mast cell-related symptoms in pregnancy and in the puerperium while 33% notice an improvement and the rest have no change in their symptoms.[5,6]
- Oral prednisolone may be required to control mastocytosis-related symptoms. If so, bolus IV hydrocortisone 100 mg every 6–8 h must be given during labour and to cover delivery, in order to prevent Addisonian crisis. Similar hydrocortisone cover would be required before a Caesarean section.

- Conservative intrapartum management includes continuation of adequate prophylactic H_1 and H_2 antihistamine therapy with immediate treatment with IV adrenaline (epinephrine) (1:10 000 dilution) if needed.
- Local anaesthetics such as lidocaine can be used safely.
- Referral to the high-risk anaesthetic clinic for review is required during pregnancy.
- Agents used for regional analgesia and oxytocics are usually well tolerated but senior anaesthetic advice should be sought if general anaesthetic is to be used.
- In those with mastocytosis-related dyspepsia, an improvement seems to be noticed during the weeks or months of breastfeeding.[1]
- There is little information about the optimal contraceptive for affected women. Unless there is a specific reaction to any type of hormonal contraception or if is triggered by barrier methods in a particular patient, general options for contraception can be offered.

Information for patients

Please see **Information for patients: Mastocytosis and pregnancy** (p. 541)

References

1. Worobec AS, et al. Mastocytosis complicating pregnancy. Obstet Gynecol 2000; 95: 391–395.
2. Rudolph MI, et al. Distribution of mast cells and the effect of their mediators on contractility in human myometrium. Br J Obstet Gynaecol 1993; 100: 1125–1130.
3. Metcalfe DD. Classification and diagnosis of mastocytosis: current status. J Invest Dermatol 1991; 96: 2S–4S.
4. Gupta S, et al. Intrapartum management of a patient with urticaria pigmentosa. Int J Obstet Anesth 1998; 7: 261–262.
5. Watson KD, et al. Systemic mastocytosis complicating pregnancy. Obstet Gynecol 2012; 112: 486–489.
6. Donahue JG, et al. Cutaneous mastocytosis complicating pregnancy. Obstet Gynecol 1995; 85: 813–815.

Mastocytosis: Management principles in general

- Advise avoidance of allergens, including any drug that could trigger anaphylaxis
- Symptomatic treatment
- Advise patients to wear MedicAlert bracelets and carry emergency treatment protocol card
- For those prone to frequent attacks, advise carrying an adrenaline self-injecting pen
- H1 and H2 antagonists—mainstay of treatment
- Alpha- and beta-blockers are contraindicated in those with systemic mastocytosis
- Necessary vaccinations with antihistamine cover

↓

Management during pregnancy

- Includes all the above principles
- Advise women that symptoms including urticaria pigmentosa may worsen in 20% either during pregnancy or in the puerperium
- Vitamin D and calcium supplements advisable throughout pregnancy
- Oral prednisolone may be required for symptom control
- If oral prednisolone has been required during pregnancy, remember to document need for hydrocortisone bolus cover during labour /delivery or for Caesarean section
- ***Refer to senior anaesthetist***
- Document instructions for intrapartum and postnatal care management:
  - Continuation of adequate prophylaxis with H1 and H2 antagonists
  - Local anaesthetics (e.g. lidocaine) and regional anaesthetics are well tolerated but senior anaesthetist advice to be sought if general anaesthetic needed
  - Oxytocics well tolerated
  - No contraindication for breastfeeding
  - Any form of contraception can be used unless previous adverse reaction to oral contraceptive pill (combined or progesterone only).

21.3 Phenylketonuria

FACT FILE

Epidemiology and inheritance

- **Phenylketonuria (PKU)** is the most common inborn error of protein metabolism. Phenylalanine is an essential amino acid necessary for normal growth and development.
- Incidence of 1 in 10 000 to 1 in 15 000 live births (1 in 4500 in N. Ireland).[1,2,3]
- ***PKU is an autosomal recessive disorder characterized by deficiency of the enzyme phenylalanine hydroxylase (PAH) that catalyses the conversion of phenylalanine (Phe) to tyrosine.***
- This leads to elevated levels of phenylalanine and its metabolites and low plasma tyrosine levels.
- In PKU, levels of phenylalanine are usually more than 1.2 mmol/litre with little or no PAH.
- The PAH locus of the *PKU* gene is located on chromosome 12.
- In the general population of the UK, 1 in 60 are carriers of the gene.
- If the mother has PKU and the father is a carrier, 50% of the offspring will have PKU.

Maternal PKU

- **Maternal PKU** is where maternal levels of phenylalanine are elevated and can cause damage to a developing fetus.
- In maternal PKU, due to the 1:1.5 gradient of phenylalanine across the placenta, the fetus is exposed to higher concentrations of phenylalanine than found in maternal serum. Serum phenylalanine levels that are safe in adults prove harmful to the fetus due to this concentrating action by the placenta.
- There is a distinct difference in outcomes between the offspring of maternal PKU and of a child born with PKU (e.g. the offspring of two carriers or father with PKU). While the child born with PKU can be managed well right from birth with dietary modifications, a child exposed in utero to high maternal levels of phenylalanine can suffer irreversible damage.
- In the less severe form, hyperphenylalaninaemia, there are lower maternal serum levels of phenylalanine, but the fetus is still at risk.
- Control of serum phenylalanine must be **strictly within the range 60–240 μmol/litre, both preconceptually and throughout pregnancy**.

Adverse outcomes of untreated maternal PKU

- **Untreated maternal PKU** can lead to significant adverse outcomes for the offspring during pregnancy as well as neonate, infant, and child due to the irreversible brain damage suffered in utero.[1,2,3,4,5,6]

During pregnancy

The higher the maternal serum phenylalanine levels the greater the degree of fetal damage especially during the period of embryogenesis and organogenesis, resulting in:

- Spontaneous miscarriages (24%)
- Fetal microcephaly (73%)
- Fetal growth restriction (40%)
- Congenital cardiac defects (10%)
- Craniofacial dysmorphia
- Major bowel anomalies (1–2%).

In the neonate

- Abnormal neurological findings
- Postnatal growth restriction

In the child

- Severe psychomotor problems
- Mental impairment
- Poor cognition
- Behavioural difficulties
- Eczema, rashes

Pre-pregnancy assessment and counselling

- In women of reproductive age, the features of PKU are the same as those of other PKU-affected individuals in the general population, depending to a large extent on severity of the condition and dietary control since childhood.[7]
- Compliance with dietary control needs to be lifelong but in reality many young women stop adherence to dietary restrictions or use of special dietetic formulations by the time they reach adolescence. Many are lost to follow-up.[5,7]
- They may have lower IQs than population averages[8] and exhibit behavioural aberrations. They may also be prone to greater levels of anxiety and depression. These factors must be taken into consideration when advising dietary compliance before and during pregnancy. Additional support must be available to these women in order to reduce the adverse impact on the next generation.
- Ideally, pre-conceptual education, counselling, and advice should be commenced in adolescence by paediatricians or paediatric nurse specialists and reinforced by GPs who are most likely to see the young woman seeking contraception.
- Information regarding the importance of compliance to dietary advice in order to maintain levels of serum phenylalanine to not more than 240 μmol/litre before conception and throughout pregnancy must be reiterated.[7]
- Women with PKU will find these levels are tighter than what they have been used to in childhood and adolescence. The reasons for such strict control before and during pregnancy must be explained and, in addition, written information and website links must be provided.
- The serious adverse effects of poorly controlled maternal PKU on the fetus, newborn, and child must be emphasized. The direct relationship between higher maternal phenyalanine levels, especially around the critical weeks of embryogenesis and organogenesis, with the frequency of fetal abnormalities, poor fetal outcomes, and intellectual impairment must be explained.
- Dietary compliance should start before pregnancy and contraception advised till maternal phenyalanine levels have consistently been between 60 and 240 μmol/litre for a minimum of 4 consecutive weeks.[1,7]
- A dietician with experience in PKU and metabolic disease will be required to instruct the patient about dietary protein restriction, provide practical advice on diet preparation and use of food lists (see Table 21.1), especially if the mother has not recently had a protein-restricted diet.
- Dietary supplements of phenyalanine-free protein, additional supplements of mineral and vitamins (especially vitamin B_{12} and folic acid) are essential in the pre-pregnancy and pregnancy dietary regime.
- Before and during pregnancy, weekly blood tests need be arranged to monitor maternal phenyalanine levels and food intake adjusted accordingly.
- During pregnancy, ultrasound scans and fetal ECHO will be employed to try to detect abnormalities and to assess progressive fetal growth.
- The patient should expect multidisciplinary team management involving the specialist dietician, maternal medicine obstetrician, metabolic disease physician, midwife, clinical nurse specialist, neonatologist, and metabolic biochemistry monitoring service.[1,2]
- Care during pregnancy will be coordinated with specialist teams based in tertiary/regional centres working closely with local community and hospital healthcare professionals.[1]

Table 21.1 Food items that can be included or need to be avoided in women with PKU before and during pregnancy

Foods to avoid	*Foods to include*
Meat	Most fruit
Eggs	Some vegetables
Chicken	Sugar
Fish	Butter
Milk	Boiled sweets
Cheese	Low-protein flour
Other dairy products	Low-protein bread
Nuts	Low-protein pasta
Biscuits	Low-protein biscuits
Bread	Low-protein energy bar
Cakes	Egg substitute
Pasta	
Aspartame (Nutra-Sweet)	

Data from: National Society for Phenylketonuria, Management of PKU. A consensus document for the diagnosis and management of children, adolescents and adults with phenylketonuria, Feb 2004; and Recommendations on the dietary management of phenylketonuria. Report of Medical Research Council Working Party on Phenylketonuria, *Archives of Disease in Childhood*, 1993, 68, pp. 426–427.

Antenatal management

- Multidisciplinary team management with liaison with community staff.
- Support and encouragement to maintain compliance with diet.
- Weekly blood phenyalanine measurements coordinated with specialist teams at tertiary/regional centres. Diet adjustments to be monitored by specialist dietician to maintain phenyalanine levels at 60–240 μmol/litre.
- Peri-pregnancy folic acid.
- Increase phenyalanine-free protein supplements to maintain total daily protein intake of approximately 70 g.[1,7]
- Hyperemesis in early pregnancy may make compliance with the special diet particularly difficult.
- Energy supplements may be required as well as other vital minerals and vitamins such as iron, calcium, zinc, vitamin B_{12}, vitamin D, and folic acid.
- Normal pregnancy weight gain is to be aimed for.[9] Rates of microcephaly and congenital cardiac disease may be reduced by ensuring essential maternal nutrient intake while controlling phenyalanine levels.

Fetal surveillance

- Apart from routine viability and dating scan in the first trimester, a detailed anomaly scan at about 20 weeks should be followed up with fetal echocardiography. Referral to a tertiary/regional fetal medicine centre may be required.
- Severe cardiac abnormality, if found, could prompt parents to request termination of pregnancy. Prenatal diagnosis of fetal cardiac anomaly may influence delivery being arranged in a centre with paediatric cardiac facility.
- Serial scans to measure head circumference to attempt to detect microcephaly. Referral to a fetal medicine centre may be required. Microcephaly could become evident only in late second or in the third trimester.[9]

Delivery and after birth

- Decisions regarding mode of delivery must be made on the basis of obstetric indications, not on the basis of the mother's PKU status.
- Breastfeeding is to be encouraged.
- Advice regarding effective contraception is vital before postnatal discharge.
- The baby should undergo routine PKU screening at 6–14 days. Initial neonatal examination must be by a senior neonatologist.[1,2,7]
- Long-term follow-up of the infant must be maintained. The birth and follow-up must be registered with the PKU Register.

Information for patients

Please see **Information for patients: Phenylketonuria and pregnancy** (p. 542)

References

1. National Society for Phenylketonuria. Management of PKU. A consensus document for the diagnosis and management of children, adolescents and adults with phenylketonuria, 2014 <http://www.nspku.org/publications/publication/management-pku>.
2. Krishnamoorthy U, Dickson M. Maternal phenylketonuria in pregnancy. Obstetrician and Gynaecologist 2005; 7: 28–33.
3. Smith I, et al. Review of neonatal screening programme for phenylketonuria. BMJ 1991; 303: 333–335.
4. Rouse B, et al. Maternal phenylketonuria pregnancy outcome: a preliminary report of facial dysmorphology and major malformations. J Inherit Metab Dis 1990; 13: 289–291.
5. Koch R, et al. Outcome implications of the International Maternal Phenylketonuria Collaborative Study (MPKUCS). Eur J Pediatr 1994; 155Suppl 1: 5162–5164.
6. Lenke RR, Levy HL. Maternal PKU and hyperphenylalaninemia. An international survey of the outcome of untreated and treated pregnancies N Engl J Med 1980; 303: 1202–1208.
7. Recommendations on the dietary management of phenylketonuria. Report of Medical Research Council Working Party on Phenylketonuria Arch Dis Child 1993; 68: 426–427.
8. Costello PM, et al. Intelligence in mild phenylketonuria. Eur J Pediatr 1994; 153: 260–263.
9. Joe TR, Clarke MD. The Maternal Phenylketonuria Project: a summary of progress and challenges for the future. Pediatrics 2003; 112; 1584–1586.

CARE PATHWAY

Pre-pregnancy counselling for a woman with phenylketonuria (PKU)

- Discuss frequent serum phenylalanine (Phe) level monitoring every week, sometimes more frequently : discuss compliance with special diet
- Confirm patient is in close contact with specialist dietitian and nurse from regional PKU centre
- Discuss how dietary control with special diet to keep blood levels of Phe with critical range of 60–240 µmol/litre needs to start from before conception and continued throughout pregnancy
- Explain that worse the control, the higher the Phe levels. Fetal abnormalities, mental impairment, etc. directly proportional to levels of maternal PKU
- Fetal development starts as early as 5 weeks gestation when pregnancy might not have been suspected by woman. Therefore, tight control to achieve safe Phe range needs to start pre-pregnancy
- Describe increased risks of miscarriage, fetal developmental abnormalities of heart, brain, later mental impairment, etc., could be reduced by tight dietary compliance started from before conception
- Specialist dietician to assess and advise on dietary adjustments, supplementation
- Emphasize need for deferring pregnancy using effective contraception till at least 4 consecutive weekly serum Phe levels are within the safe range of 60–240 µmol/litre
- Prescribe oral supplements of folic acid, also of vitamin D, B_{12}, calcium, iron, as required
- Folic acid to be continued till end of first trimester
- Discuss plan of care during future pregnancy, once or twice weekly blood samples for Phe levels to continue, the specialist team at regional PKU centre working closely with patient, community, and local hospital healthcare professionals
- Patient's visits to the regional PKU clinic usually every 1–2 months during pregnancy
- Ultrasound scans at regular intervals to assess fetal structures and organs, sequential growth, head measurements, as well as fetal ECHO for detection of any cardiac abnormalities will be done either in the local unit or in fetal medicine tertiary centre if any problems are suspected
- Discuss chances of inheritance by offspring—approximately 1:100 if father of baby is a carrier. Partner's carrier state may be difficult and unnecessary to identify as >400 different mutations of PKU
- Management of the pregnancy, labour, and delivery no different from that of women without PKU except for tighter serum Phe levels
- Give written information and website links to the National Society for Phenylketonuria (<http://www.nspku.org>)

Close liaison with and multidisciplinary input from regional PKU specialist team, local specialist dietitian, maternal medicine specialist, neonatologist, metabolic biochemistry, clinical nurse specialist, etc.

GP or community midwife refers patient with PKU asap in 1st trimester to maternal medicine or specialist antenatal clinic

↓

First visit to maternal medicine or specialist antenatal clinic

- Confirm viability and dates
- Ensure frequent Phe serum sample monitoring is in place; assess most recent results and advise accordingly
- Reiterate optimal range to be maintained throughout pregnancy
- Admission may be required for dietary stabilization—specialist dietitian supervision
- Confirm she is on folic acid, to continue at least till end of first trimester
- Other supplements (e.g. Phe-free protein supplements, vitamin B_{12}, vitamin D, calcium, iron, etc.)
- Further scans, fetal ECHO either in local unit or tertiary fetal medicine referral centre
- Frequency of further appointments to be individualized
- Routine antenatal care in community to continue

↓

Further visits to maternal medicine or specialist antenatal clinic

- Continued frequent blood samples for Phe level monitoring with specialist dietitian overseeing dietary adjustments to maintain safe range of maternal Phe
- Fetal anomaly scan at about 20 weeks
- Fetal ECHO in either local unit or at tertiary fetal medicine centre
- Serial growth scan to try to identify fetal microcephaly, IUGR
- If severe congenital heart abnormality identified and confirmed, patients might consider TOP
- In other less severe abnormalities, place of delivery to decided according to availability of paediatric cardiac surgical facility
- Inform neonatologists regarding maternal PKU status
- Admission for dietary surveillance and stabilization occasionally required
- Routine pregnancy blood tests with continued community midwife antenatal checks
- Aim for normal pregnancy weight gain, dietician to advise.
- Mode and time of delivery should depend on obstetric factors, not maternal Phe levels

↓

Postpartum

- Neonatal screening according to routine at 6–10 days of life
- Long-term follow-up of baby
- Contraception advice before discharge
- Encourage pre-pregnancy assessment and counselling before next pregnancy
- Vigilance by community team for postnatal depression

21.4 Alpha-1 Antitrypsin Deficiency

FACT FILE

- **Alpha-1 antitrypsin (AAT) deficiency** is an inherited disorder that can cause lung disease in adults and liver disease in adults and children.
- AAT is a protease inhibitor, synthesized in the liver, which protects lung alveolar tissues from destruction by neutrophil elastase.

Epidemiology

- AAT deficiency is a common autosomal recessive condition with an incidence of 1:1600 to 1:1800.
- Almost all those affected by AAT deficiency are white and of northern European descent.
- AAT deficiency is genetic condition due to inheriting two deficient PI alleles from the *AAT* gene locus on chromosome 14.[1] The most common deficiency allele is *PiZ*.
- For a couple with one affected child, the risk is 25% in every subsequent pregnancy.
- When only one parent carries the *Z* allele (or *S* allele), there is no risk that any of their offspring will have the disease.

Clinical manifestations of AAT deficiency and prognosis

- Clinical manifestations and therefore morbidity and mortality show considerable variation.[1,2,3,4,5]
- Emphysema in the young adult is the most obvious pulmonary manifestation and most deaths are due to progressive emphysema.
- Liver disease, especially neonatal cholestasis, can also be a feature and can progress to cirrhosis or even carcinoma in later life.
- Lung disease attributable to AAT deficiency does not occur in childhood, but is **closely linked to smoking** in adults. Membranoproliferative glomerulonephritis, panniculitis, and necrotizing vasculitis are associations with AAT in adult life.[6,7]
- Tobacco smoking is associated with rapid progression of pulmonary disease.
- After the age of 30–35 years there is an accelerated decline in forced expiratory volume in one second (FEV_1) which is considerably worsened by cigarette smoking. In a non-smoker, symptoms are generally seen at around 50 years of age, while smokers will be symptomatic by 30–40 years.[8]
- Although life expectancy is more difficult to estimate with accuracy, a combination of three studies gives a mean age of death of 50 years in smokers, compared with 66 years in non-smokers.

Pregnancy and AAT

- **Pregnancy can result in life-threatening decrease of pulmonary function in severely affected women**. A fall of nearly 50% in FEV_1 has been reported.[1,2]
- In other cases where there has been only mild airflow limitation, pregnancy has been relatively well tolerated.
- Although in normal pregnancies breathlessness is a common feature in the third trimester, this does not alter normal vital capacity.
- In those with respiratory compromise, pregnancy can cause increasing maternal hypoxaemia and resulting IUGR of the fetus.[1]
- In extreme cases, cor pulmonale could also result in pulmonary hypertension with high maternal mortality.

Pre-pregnancy assessment and counselling

- Pre-pregnancy assessment and counselling are vital.
- This should include discussion about ideal contraception which would be progesterone implant or levonorgestrel intrauterine system (Mirena®). Because of associated liver damage, combined oral contraceptive with oestrogen is strictly contraindicated.
- ***As part of pre-pregnancy counselling the patient must be encouraged to have yearly flu immunization (including H1N1) as well as the one-off immunization against pneumococcus.***
- During pre-pregnancy counselling, **the patient must receive unequivocal advice regarding smoking cessation and abstinence from alcohol** to improve both maternal and fetal outcomes.
- Strategies for smoking cessation (see Chapter 24.5) must be offered.

Antenatal care

- The care of any pregnant woman with AAT deficiency must necessarily be multidisciplinary with close involvement of tertiary/regional centres. The pulmonary physician, maternal medicine obstetrician along with the midwife, gastrointestinal or hepatology specialist, anaesthetist, intensive care physician, and respiratory nurse should be actively involved in the antenatal and postnatal care.
- Frequent and close respiratory function monitoring should be conducted monthly throughout pregnancy, sometimes more frequently. Close communication must be maintained amongst the different clinicians involved.
- If emphysema is a feature, treatment follows similar lines as in the non-pregnant with bronchodilators, inhaled steroids, or short courses of oral prednisolone. Antibiotics are required in chest infections to prevent development of worsening pulmonary sequelae.
- **IV AAT replacement**: A pooled, purified, human plasma protein concentrate replacement for the missing enzyme has been shown in some studies to be beneficial, but no randomized controlled studies are available to unequivocally prove that IV augmentation therapy improves survival or slows the rate of emphysema progression.[9]
- If longer-term steroids are required in pregnancy, a glucose tolerance test needs to be performed at about 26–28 weeks.
- Frequent maternal arterial blood gas measurements may be required throughout pregnancy.
- In those with a hepatic element to the AAT deficiency, close monitoring of liver function tests are required.
- **Serial monthly fetal growth scans** need to start from about 26 weeks gestation.

Planning for labour and delivery

- The timing, mode, and place of delivery need careful consideration.[1,2,3,4]
- If the patient has been on steroids for a few weeks, prophylactic bolus doses of IV hydrocortisone 100 mg every 6–8 h for labour and to cover delivery are required. Similarly, a bolus dose is to be given just before a Caesarean section is commenced.
- During labour and delivery, some commonly used **medications should be avoided** because of their tendency to cause bronchoconstriction. These include:
  - prostaglandin F2-alpha
  - ergotamine
  - morphine
  - diclofenac.
- Other medications pose no significant threat and some have a bronchodilating effect. **Safe drugs for use in labour and delivery** include:
  - oxytocin
  - prostaglandin E2 (dinoprostone)
  - fentanyl
  - epidural anaesthesia
  - magnesium sulfate.

- Clear documentation regarding drugs to avoid in labour and after delivery must be recorded in both the main notes as well as in the hand-held notes.
- In cases of deteriorating respiratory function and capacity, an elective Caesarean section under regional block needs to be discussed and clear documentation of these plans shared with the patient and all concerned in her care.
- Careful monitoring of postoperative lung function and interventions to prevent pulmonary oedema or infection should be rigorously followed.
- Vaginal delivery is not precluded especially in multiparous women with a mild form of the disease but may require a shortened second stage with assisted instrumental delivery.
- Pneumothorax and pneumomediastinum could occur in the second stage due to straining against a closed glottis.[3] Assisted vaginal delivery with an epidural is a safer option to reduce the expulsive effort required by the patient.
- Routine measurement of the baby's cord gases (pH and actual base-excess) is recommended especially if there has been chronic maternal hypoxaemia.
- Before discharge, confirm that support with childcare is available.
- Effective and safe contraception must be emphasized.
- Arrangements for subsequent follow-up with the pulmonary physician ± hepatologist must be organized and communicated to the patient.

Information for patients

Please see **Information for patients: Alpha-1 antitrypsin (AAT) deficiency and pregnancy** (p. 542)

References

1. Dempsey OJ, et al. Severe α-1 antitrypsin deficiency and pregnancy. Eur Respir J 1999; 13: 1492–1494.
2. Giesler CF, et al. Alpha-1 antitrypsin deficiency. Severe obstructive lung disease and pregnancy. Obstet Gynaecol 1977; 49: 31–34.
3. Atkinson AR. Pregnancy and alpha-1 antitrypsin deficiency. Postgrad Med J 1987; 63: 817–820.
4. Kuller JA, et al. Alpha-1 antitrypsin deficiency and pregnancy. Am J Perinatol 1995; 12: 303–305.
5. Silverman EK, Sandhaus RA. Alpha-1 antitrypsin deficiency. N Engl J Med 2009; 360: 2749–2757.
6. Elzouki AN, et al. Severe alpha1-antitrypsin deficiency (PiZ homozygosity) with membranoproliferative glomerulonephritis and nephrotic syndrome, reversible after orthotopic liver transplantation. J Hepatol 1997; 26: 1403–1407.
7. O'Riordan K, et al. Alpha 1-antitrypsin deficiency associated panniculitis: resolution with intravenous alpha 1-antitrypsin administration and liver transplantation. Transplantation 1997; 63: 480–482.
8. Primhak RA, Tanner MS. Alpha-1 antitrypsin deficiency. Arch Dis Child 2001; 85: 2–5.
9. Stoller JK, Aboussouan LS. α1-Antitrypsin deficiency 5: Intravenous augmentation therapy: current understanding. Thorax 2004; 59: 708–712.

CARE PATHWAY

AAT: Pre-pregnancy assessment and counselling is ideal. Immunization against pneumococcus and yearly flu immunization (including swine flu) must be advised

GP or community midwife refers patient to maternal medicine clinic or a specialist antenatal clinic in the 1st trimester

↓

First visit to maternal medicine or specialist antenatal clinic

- Confirm dates and viability. Detailed history to establish pulmonary ± hepatic manifestations, medications, etc.
- Check whether seen recently by respiratory physician and extent of pre-pregnancy pulmonary function and capacity
- If liver disease, check last review of LFTs by hepatologist
- Advise **smoking cessation**, offer help and support with this
- Advise to take folic acid till end of 1st trimester
- Arrange fetal growth scans once a month from 26 weeks
- If on oral steroids, GTT at 26–28 weeks
- Liaise with respiratory specialist and hepatologist with regular reviews throughout pregnancy
- Discuss autosomal recessive inheritance, referral to genetics if patient has not previously had this
- Refer to anaesthetic high-risk clinic
- Maternal medicine/specialist antenatal clinic reviews approximately once 6 weeks till 24–26 weeks, then once a month with serial growth scans on the same day
- Community midwife antenatal checks as per routine NICE schedule
- Referral to or advice from tertiary centre as directed by DGH respiratory physician in severe cases

↓

Further visits to maternal medicine or specialist antenatal clinic

- Assess pregnancy, maternal symptoms, symptoms and signs of any respiratory impairment
- Assess fetal growth, movements
- Check results of recent lung and liver function tests
- Close collaboration with respiratory physician and hepatologist
- Ensure has had anaesthetic review
- In-patient admission may be required if signs of worsening lung function

↓

Delivery and postpartum

- Collaborative decision regarding place, timing, and mode of delivery to be made on a case-by-case basis
- ***If severe pulmonary impairment delivery by elective Caesarean section under regional block may be indicated***
- Detailed plan shared with patient and all concerned in her care
- Inform neonatologist regarding maternal α-1 AT deficiency—baby will need thorough examination
- **Clear documentation in notes** regarding labour and delivery:
  - Avoid ergometrine, prostaglandin $F_2\alpha$, morphine, or diclofenac
  - If vaginal delivery planned, clear instruction in notes to cut short second stage with assisted instrumental delivery
  - If on long-term oral steroids, bolus doses of IV hydrocortisone 100 mg every 6–8 h for labour and delivery or just before a Caesarean section
  - Cord gases to be checked
  - Careful post-op lung function assessments, avoid pulmonary oedema/infection
  - Before discharge, discuss safest forms of **contraception**. COCP contraindicated, advise progesterone implant or LNG-IUS (Mirena)
  - Ensure mother has adequate help at home
  - Subsequent pulmonary/hepatic follow-up arrangements in place
  - No contraindications for breastfeeding if mother is not too exhausted.

22 Previous Pregnancy Problems

22.1 Previous Caesarean Section

FACT FILE

- The rate of Caesarean sections in England was nearly 25% (24.8%) in 2010.[1]
- Nine percent of women giving birth in England and Wales have had a previous Caesarean section.[2] In those who have had at least one previous Caesarean section, the repeat Caesarean section rate in England and Wales was found to be 67% in the 2001 Sentinel audit. The same study identified a successful (vaginal birth after Caesarean section) VBAC rate of 33% in those who had had one previous Caesarean section.[2]
- Each maternity unit in the UK has its own structure of antenatal clinics where women with previous Caesarean section(s) are seen in a subsequent pregnancy. These may involve 1–2 visits to a general obstetric clinic in the hospital with most of the care delivered in the community, or in a designated previous Caesarean section clinic led by an obstetrician and/or clinic midwife. In the latter instance, the routine community-based care will also continue and the obstetrician will need to be involved when the final decision regarding mode of delivery is agreed with the patient, ideally at about 36 weeks gestation.
- In some units, women with one previous uncomplicated Caesarean section will be directed to a senior midwife-led antenatal clinic with the obstetrician involved only at the final decision-making stage at 36 weeks gestation.
- Women who have had a complicated previous Caesarean section or more than one previous Caesarean section will be seen by the obstetric team on a shared care basis.
- Those women who have had one previous uncomplicated Caesarean section, but have developed problems or complications during the current pregnancy, will have their antenatal care directed to the appropriate obstetrician-led antenatal clinic.
- In some units, if an elective repeat caesarean section (ERCS) has been finalized after discussions at the 36-week visit, it is common practice for the patient's informed signed consent to be obtained at the time by the obstetrician.[3] In other units, the relevant information (printed version) is given to the patient and her signed informed consent obtained on the day of the ERCS by the surgeon or assistant doctor.[3]
- Similarly, arrangements regarding mandatory MRSA swabs and anaesthetic review a few days before the planned date for the ERCS, etc. are individualized to each maternity unit, depending on local resources and structure.
- A clear plan for delivery should be discussed and documented in the notes in the event of labour commencing before the planned date for an ERCS, as about 10% of those scheduled for ERCS will go into labour before 39 weeks gestation[4] (see Figure 22.1).
- In the UK, in general, antenatal counselling and care of women after previous Caesarean section are based on the RCOG Green-top guideline,[5] NICE Clinical Guideline,[6] and NCCWCH clinical guideline.[7]
- Incidences of placenta praevia[8,9,10,11] and placenta accreta[12,13,14] are increased in women who have had previous Caesarean section, with the risk increasing with the number of Caesarean sections a woman has had. It is therefore imperative that the placenta should be carefully localized. If the placenta is found to be low-lying and anterior, further imaging to gain more information about possible morbid adherence should be arranged (see Chapter 29.1 on placenta praevia and morbid adherence of placenta).

Fetal risks

- The risk of antepartum stillbirth after 34 weeks and especially after 39 weeks gestation is doubled in women who have had a previous Caesarean section compared to those who have not (4 per 1000 compared to 2 per 1000).[15]
- There is an increased risk of perinatal mortality which is largely due to the increased risk of antepartum stillbirth after 40–41 weeks gestation in planned VBAC when the patient has not started spontaneous labour. This is no higher than if the woman were labouring for the first time but higher compared to an ERCS (0.1%) at 39 weeks gestation.
- Fetal acidosis and hypoxic encephalopathy are more common with VBAC in general (both successful and failed VBAC), although the risks are small.
- Compared with infants delivered by women by vaginal delivery, those delivered by elective Caesarean section had an increased risk of respiratory morbidity at any gestational age before 40 weeks, particularly if undertaken before the onset of labour. A nearly fourfold increased risk was found at 37 weeks gestation and a threefold increase in risk at 38 weeks gestation, whereas the risk was doubled in infants delivered at 39 weeks gestation.[16,17,18]
- The fundamental question raised by the ASTECS (Antenatal Steroids for Term Elective Caesarean Section) trial study is 'Do antenatal corticosteroids administered before elective Caesarean section at term alter the subsequent development of asthma and are there possible adverse consequences?'.[17] In this study, 48 h before the elective Caesarean section, women in the case group received two intramuscular doses of 12 mg of betamethasone, separated by 24 h.
- Antenatal betamethasone decreases the number of admissions with respiratory distress, especially transient tachypnoea of the newborn, by 50% and may be of benefit in reducing the long-term risk of developing asthma.
- These findings imply that antenatal steroids can aid the clearing of lung fluid after delivery when an elective Caesarean section is performed before 39 weeks gestation.
- The likely benefits of antenatal betamethasone should be compared with those of delaying Caesarean section until 39 weeks when possible.

Counselling

- Women who have had one previous uncomplicated lower segment Caesarean section (LSCS) and have no complications in their present pregnancy should be offered the option of planned VBAC or the alternative of ERCS[5] (see Figure 22.1).
- VBAC in **multiple pregnancy** has to be approached with caution and offered only in well-selected cases. There is a 3–5-fold increased risk of scar dehiscence seen in VBAC with twins, although 70% will deliver vaginally.[18]
- **In general, women who have had one previous uncomplicated Caesarean section should be informed that they have a 72–76% success rate for a planned VBAC.**[5,19,20]
- When counselling women who have had one previous uncomplicated LSCS, their intentions for further pregnancies must be taken into consideration. ERCS appears to be associated with a lower peripartum hysterectomy rate when there is only one further pregnancy. However, if more children are planned, VBAC carries a lower risk of subsequent peripartum hysterectomy.[13]
- A final decision for preferred mode of delivery should be agreed between the woman and her obstetrician before the expected or planned date for delivery, ideally at about 36–37 weeks gestation, after fetal presentation is confirmed.

- **VBAC may be considered even in those who had had 2 previous uncomplicated Caesarean sections, but carries an increased risk of scar rupture.**

A guide to estimating chances of success for attempted VBAC

- If the patient has had a previous successful vaginal delivery as well as a previous Caesarean section, she has a 80–90% chance of another successful VBAC.[4,15]
- If the previous vaginal delivery was a previous VBAC, the chances of a successful VBAC are increased for this pregnancy. However, close maternal and fetal surveillance should not be relaxed during labour.
- After one previous uncomplicated Caesarean section, e.g. for fetal distress in early labour or for breech, and provided the indication for Caesarean section was not dystocia (CPD), there is a 70–80% chance of a successful VBAC.
- If increased BMI and the previous Caesarean section was for failure to progress (presumed dystocia), chances for a successful VBAC are less than 40%.
- If the patient has had a previous unsuccessful trial of instrumental delivery, proceeding to Caesarean section, her chances of a successful VBAC are perhaps only 50%.

Contraindications for VBAC

- Previous classical, Delee, inverted T, or inverted J uterine incision
- Previous uterine rupture
- Three or more Caesarean sections
- Placenta praevia
- Breech or malpresentations
- Myomectomy when the uterine cavity has been breached
- HIV women not on any retroviral therapy or where viral load is in excess of 400 copies/ml despite retroviral therapy
- Other relative contraindications include multiple pregnancy and suspected IUGR.

Unsuccessful VBAC

The following factors are more likely to result in a failed VBAC[5,21,22,23,24,25,26] and need to be discussed with the patient during counselling to enable her to make the best informed choice (see Figure 22.1).

- Labour is induced, even without PGE_2
- No previous vaginal birth
- BMI >30
- Two previous Caesarean sections instead of only one
- Previous Caesarean section for dystocia
- VBAC attempted at or after 41 weeks
- Baby's birth weight estimated at over 4 kg
- Previous preterm Caesarean section
- Short interval between previous Caesarean section and present conception (<18 months); this is associated with a greater risk of scar rupture as well
- Cervical dilatation at admission less than 4 cm
- Short maternal stature, big baby
- No epidural.

Figure 22.1 Previous Caesarean section: model checklist to aid mode of delivery discussion in subsequent pregnancy. This checklist, based on the current UK guidelines,[5,6,7] can be used by either the obstetrician or the lead midwife for the mandatory documentation[5] required regarding the antenatal counselling and discussions with the woman, usually carried out before 20 weeks gestation. This documentation can also be shared with the patient, depending on local arrangements, to accompany the RCOG patient information leaflet.[21]

For Obstetricians and Midwives

Date:..................

Signature and name (in capitals) of Obstetrician or lead Midwife: ....

....

Designation...

Patient Details (addressograph)

EDD (by first trimester scan dates).....................................
Gestational age at this consultation (in weeks).............................

Antenatal counselling discussions have included the following:
(Please tick as appropriate):

- ☐ Present pregnancy assessed
- ☐ No contraindication for vaginal birth
- ☐ Previous pregnancy – details of labour, delivery, operative details, including type of uterine incision, any extension of scar especially into upper segment or into cervix, post- operative complications reviewed if notes available. If previous delivery has been elsewhere, details to be requested from the other hospital if feasible
- ☐ Risk factors for unsuccessful VBAC discussed with patient
- ☐ Success rate for attempted VBAC discussed with patient

The following specific risks and benefits of VBAC have been discussed (Please tick as appropriate):

- ☐ A planned VBAC carries a risk of uterine rupture of about 0.5% versus practically no risk of uterine rupture if undergoing a planned repeat elective Caesarean section
- ☐ Uterine rupture of the previous scar is a rare outcome, but is associated with significant maternal and perinatal morbidity and mortality

- ☐ A failed VBAC carries higher risks of maternal complications than ERCS, especially uterine rupture, fetal acidosis, hypoxic ischaemic encephalopathy, sepsis, need for blood transfusion, PPH, hysterectomy etc.
- ☐ Fetal acidosis and hypoxic encephalopathy are more common with VBAC in general (both successful and failed VBACs), although the risks are small.
- ☐ A planned VBAC carries a small 2-3/10,000 additional risk of perinatal death.
- ☐ Attempting a VBAC probably reduces the risk of respiratory problems of baby after birth compared to ERCS.
- ☐ There is an increased risk of admission of the baby to SCBU with respiratory distress even when an elective caesarean section is performed at term (from 37 weeks).
- ☐ Continuous intrapartum electronic fetal monitoring is necessary during labour if VBAC is planned.
- ☐ Intrapartum care would need to be in a unit where there is immediate access to C/S and on-site blood transfusion services.
- ☐ For an attempted VBAC, discussion regarding the risk of uterine rupture should detail:-
  - ◆ There is a 2-3 fold increased risk of uterine rupture and around 1.5 fold increased risk of Caesarean section if labour has been induced or augmented in an attempted VBAC, compared to spontaneous start of labour.
  - ◆ There is a 16-fold higher risk of uterine rupture seen if labour is induced with prostaglandin compared to ERCS.
  - ◆ Higher risk of uterine rupture for women whose labours were induced even without prostaglandin (80 per 10,000).
  - ◆ Augmentation with oxytocin, if required, would be undertaken cautiously, with a low threshold for C/S particularly if dystocia is suspected
  - ◆ VBAC may be considered even when the woman has had 2 previous C/S but there is an increased risk of scar rupture.
- ☐ **Risk of anaesthetic complications** is very low whether VBAC or ERCS under regional block.
- ☐ **Risks and benefits of ERCS** including:
  - ◆ Increasing number of repeat Caesarean sections deliveries increases the risks of placenta praevia (30-60% rise), placenta accreta/percreta as well as of antepartum stillbirth.
  - ◆ *The risk of IUD in those with previous Caesarean section increases after 39-40 weeks, and the more the number of previous Caesarean sections, the greater this risk.*
  - ◆ Therefore, for a planned ERCS, the ideal time to perform this would be at close to 39 weeks gestation. For a planned VBAC, if labour has not started spontaneously by 40 weeks and an ARM is not feasible, then an elective Caesarean section is advisable and conducted at or before 41 weeks.
  - ◆ Increased risk of injuries to bladder, bowels, uterus, hysterectomy, ICU admissions, blood transfusions, length of hospital stay with repeated Caesarean sections.
  - ◆ Risk of hysterectomy increases linearly with an increase in number of Caesarean sections.
- ☐ *A clear management plan for delivery, should labour commence before the date of the planned ERCS, has been discussed and documented.*

Data from: RCOG Green-top Guideline No. 45, *Birth after previous Caesarean birth*, 2007, Royal College of Obstetricians and Gynaecologists; NICE clinical guideline 132, *Caesarean section*, 2011, National Institute for Health and Clinical Excellence, www.nice.org.uk/cg132; and National Collaborating Centre for Women's and Children's Health, *Caesarean section*, 2004 [www.rcog.org.uk/index.asp?PageID=694].

Information for patients

Please see Information for patients: Pregnancy after previous Caesarean section (p. 543)

References

1. Hospital Episode Statistics. Maternity data 2009–10. <http://www.hesonline.nhs.uk/Ease/servlet/ContentServer?siteID=1937&category ID=1475>.
2. Thomas J, Paranjothy S. The National Sentinel Caesarean Section Audit Report. London: RCOG Press, 2001.
3. GMC. Consent guidance: patients and doctors making decisions together. <http://www.gmc-uk.org>
4. Landon MB, et al. Maternal and perinatal outcomes associated with a trial of labor after prior cesarean delivery. N Engl J Med 2004; 351: 2581–2589.
5. RCOG Green-top Guideline No. 45. Birth after previous Caesarean birth. London: Royal College of Obstetricians and Gynaecologists, 2007.
6. NICE Clinical Guideline. Caesarean section. CG132. London: National Institute for Health and Clinical Excellence, 2011 <http://www.nice.org.uk/cg132>.
7. National Collaborating Centre for Women's and Children's Health. Caesarean section. London: RCOG Press; 2004 <http://www.rcog.org.uk/index.asp?PageID=694>.
8. Rasmussen S, et al. Obstetric history and the risk of placenta previa. Acta Obstet Gynecol Scand 2000; 79: 502–507.
9. Ugyur D, et al. Multiple repeat caesarean section:is it safe? Eur J Obstet Gynecol Reprod Biol 2005; 119: 171–175.
10. Gilliam M, et al. The likelihood of placenta previa with greater number of cesarean deliveries and higher parity. Obstet Gynecol 2002; 99: 976–980.
11. Lydon-Rochelle M, et al. First-birth cesarean and placental abruption or previa at second birth. Obstet Gynecol 2001; 97: 765–769.
12. Miller DA, et al. Clinical risk factors for placenta previa-placenta accreta. Am J Obstet Gynecol 1997; 177: 210–214.
13. Pare E, et al. Vaginal birth after caesarean section versus elective repeat caesarean section: assessment of maternal downstream health outcomes. BJOG 2006: 113: 75–85.
14. Clark SL, et al. Placenta previa/accreta and prior cesarean section. Obstet Gynecol 1985; 66: 89–92.
15. Smith GCS, et al. Caesarean section and risk of unexplained stillbirth in subsequent pregnancy. Lancet 2003; 362: 1779–1784.
16. Hansen AK, et al. Risk of respiratory morbidity in term infants delivered by elective caesarean section: cohort study. BMJ 2008; 336: 85.
17. Stutchfield P, et al. Antenatal betamethasone and incidence of neonatal respiratory distress after elective caesarean section: pragmatic randomised trial. BMJ 2005; 331 (7518): 662–664.
18. Sansregret A, et al. Twin delivery after a previous Caesarean: a twelve-year experience. J Obstet Gynaecol Can 2003; 25: 294–298.
19. Guise JM, et al. Safety of vaginal birth after cesarean: a systematic review. Obstet Gynecol 2004; 103: 420–429.
20. Chauhan SP, et al. Maternal and perinatal complications with uterine rupture in142,075 patients who attempted vaginal birth after cesarean delivery: a review of the literature. Am J Obstet Gynecol 2003; 189: 408–417.
21. RCOG Patient Information. Birth after previous caesarean—information for you. London: RCOG, 2008 <http://www.rcog.org.uk>.
22. Ball E, Hinshaw K. The current management of vaginal birth after previous caesarean delivery. Obstetrician and Gynaecologist 2007; 9: 77–82.
23. Lydon-Rochelle M, et al. Risk of uterine rupture during labor among women with a prior cesarean delivery. N Engl J Med 2001; 345: 3–8.
24. Scott JR. Avoiding labor problems during vaginal birth after cesarean delivery. Clin Obstet Gynaecol 1997; 40: 533–541.
25. Lin c, Raynor BD. Risk of uterine rupture in labor induction of patients with prior cesarean section: an inner city hospital experience. Am J Obstet Gynecol 2004; 190: 1476–1478.
26. Gyamfi C, et al. Increased success of trial of labor after previous vaginal birth after cesarean. Obstet Gynecol 2004; 104: 715–719.

CARE PATHWAY

Two or more previous Caesarean sections

16 weeks

- Routine examination.
- Ascertain patient's future pregnancy plans
- Discuss birth options—risks and benefits of **elective repeat Caesarean section (ERCS)**, or **vaginal birth after Caesarean section (VBAC)**
- Discuss tubal ligation if appropriate **
- Discuss increased risk of scar rupture/hysterectomy
- Increased risk of placenta praevia/accreta
- Discuss increased risk of stillbirth after 40 weeks in those with previous Caesarean section, especially multiple sections
- Explain why an elective Caesarean section is advisable at 39 weeks
- Discuss and give checklist/fact file
- Complete checklist for doctors and midwives
- Community midwife to continue routine antenatal care meanwhile, if otherwise uncomplicated

If patient insists on VBAC after two previous Caesarean sections, refer her to consultant antenatal clinic at about 20–24 weeks gestation

36 weeks*

- Routine examination and check placental site
- Further imaging studies if suspicion of placenta accreta. Re-discuss plans
- Obtain informed consent if opts for repeat Caesarean section
- If elective Caesarean section is decided on, give date for 39 weeks, may need to be earlier if previous multiple Caesarean sections
- Discuss information sheet previously given
- Arrange anaesthetic pre-op appointment
- If tubal ligation** as well, **document discussion** re: irreversibility, failure rate, Mirena®, etc.
- Advise to come in immediately to the delivery suite if labour, SROM, or 'show'
- Advise patient to see community midwife weekly till date for Caesarean section
- Advise patient to be vigilant about fetal movements

***** *Note: If the patient wishes to discuss any issue from her checklist, the community midwife can arrange for her to have an extra appointment in an obstetric antenatal clinic***

***** A request for tubal ligation and the required counselling should have been conducted during the pregnancy and agreed to at least 1 week prior to the Caesarean section (NICE guidelines). Documentation of discussions regarding irreversibility, failure rate (3–4 per 1000), increased risk of menorrhagia and of ectopic, alternatives such as LNG-IUS (Mirena®), and vasectomy should be complete and clear in the case notes***

One previous LSCS

16 weeks

- Routine examination
- Confirm no contraindications for vaginal delivery
- Establish patient's preference
- Ascertain her plans for future pregnancies
- Check details of previous labour, partogram, operative details, type of uterine incision, post-op complications
- *Inform patient what her chances of successful VBAC are likely to be, based on above details
- Discuss maternal risks and benefits of both VBAC and **elective repeat Caesarean section (ERCS)**
- **If decision is for ERCS, explain why it is done at 39 weeks
- **Clearly document plans if labour starts before date of ERCS**
- Complete and sign checklist, arrange further appointment for 36 weeks in antenatal clinic
- Give information sheets about both VBAC and ERCS and checklist
- Community midwifery care meanwhile for routine antenatal care if pregnancy remains uncomplicated

36 weeks if ERCS chosen

36 weeks if VBAC attempt chosen*

- Assess pregnancy to date, check placental site
- Check presentation. If non-cephalic, advise ERCS at 39 weeks
- If cephalic, ascertain patient's choice once again
- Briefly re-discuss risks and benefits of VBAC vs ERCS
- Explain why IOL with PGE2 (dinoprostone) is not generally recommended.
- Explain why delivery is best achieved not later than 40–41 weeks due to increased risk of IUD
- Explain why there is an increased risk of scar rupture in induced labour compared to spontaneous onset of labour
- Arrange for either artificial rupture of membranes (ARM) or elective Caesarean section at 40–41 weeks—prepare as for elective Caesarean section
- Obtain informed consent for LSCS if ARM not feasible on the day of Caesarean section
- Give patient both VBAC and Caesarean section leaflets
- If patient chooses VBAC but has high BMI (>38) arrange an anaesthetic appointment as if for elective Caesarean section
- Patient to see community midwife weekly meanwhile
- Advise patient to be vigilant of fetal movements
- Advise patient to report without delay if any 'show', SROM, or contractions commence
- Inform patient of need for close maternal and electronic fetal heart rate monitoring when in active labour
- Advise epidural in labour

22.2 Previous Obstetric Anal Sphincter Injuries

FACT FILE

- Previous **obstetric anal sphincteric injuries (OASIS)** including third- and fourth-degree perineal tears, can lead to subsequent physical and psychological complications affecting the quality of life due to perineal pain, dyspareunia, sphincteric weakness, or faecal incontinence.[1,2]
- **Third-degree tears** involve disruption of the vaginal epithelium, perineal skin, perineal body, and anal sphincter muscles. This should be further subdivided into:
  - **IIIa:** partial tear of the external sphincter involving less than 50% thickness
  - **IIIb:** more than 50% of thickness involved or complete tear of the external sphincter
  - **IIIc:** internal sphincter also torn.
- **Fourth-degree tear:** A third-degree tear **plus** disruption of the anal ± rectal epithelium.
- Reported incidence of third- and fourth-degree OASIS is 1–10% of all vaginal deliveries.[3,4,5,6,7]
- Many risk factors for OASIS have been identified including primiparity, instrumental vaginal delivery, larger babies, and previous female genital mutilation.[6,7,8,9]. Other risk factors such as older mothers,[10,11] or induction of labour,[12,13] prolonged second stage of labour,[14,15], or inherent predisposition (e.g. a short perineal body),[14] have also been identified in some studies, but not in others.[16,17,18]
- Some studies indicate a fourfold increased risk of recurrence of OASIS in a second pregnancy and if OASIS had been incurred in two previous deliveries, a tenfold increased risk for the third delivery.[9,16,19]
- The risk of recurrence of OASIS in the course of a subsequent delivery seems to be particularly associated with forceps delivery or a baby weighing more than 3.5 kg.[9,16,19] Subsequent delivery by ventouse does not seem to be associated with such an increased recurrence risk of OASIS.[16]
- Others have not found an increased risk of OASIS in women with previous OASIS.[9,19]
- An increased elective Caesarean rate in a second pregnancy has been seen in women with one previous OASIS compared to those without such a history.(6% vs 1.5% respectively)[16] and after OASIS has occurred in both a first and a second delivery, the planned Caesarean rate tends to be 13-fold higher than when no previous OASIS has occurred.
- The desire to have another pregnancy and the subsequent delivery rate are not generally affected by the previous history of OASIS, albeit with more women choosing to have an elective Caesarean section in the next pregnancy.[16]

Post-OASIS management and pre-pregnancy advice

- When a delivery has resulted in OASIS, physiotherapy referral must be offered before discharge and advice regarding pelvic floor exercises must be given.[20]
- In the event of the patient continuing to experience poor anal sphincteric tone or faecal incontinence, a gynaecology referral must be arranged.
- For patients who continue to have problems with faecal urgency or incontinence or pain, referral must be considered to a specialist gynaecology clinic or to a colorectal surgeon for endoanal ultrasonography and anorectal manometry to be considered.
- A small number of women may require referral to a colorectal surgeon for consideration of secondary sphincter repair.
- Women should be advised that 60–80% will be asymptomatic at 12 months and the prognosis following standard repair technique is good.

If seen for pre-pregnancy advice[20]

- Discuss injury sustained during childbirth, preferably with the benefit of the case notes.
- If continued sphincter problems are reported, assess sphincter tone.
- Advice concerning mode of delivery in a subsequent pregnancy should include:
  - The risk of worsening symptoms with a subsequent vaginal delivery if there has been continued faecal incontinence following the previous delivery with OASIS.
  - That there is little evidence to support the role of prophylactic episiotomy in subsequent pregnancies.
  - Those women who have sustained extensive obstetric and sphincter injury and are left symptomatic and/or have abnormal endoanal ultrasonography/manometry should have the option of elective Caesarean section in a future pregnancy. This must be clearly documented in the notes.[20]

Information for patients

Please see **Information for patients: Previous third- and fourth-degree tears** (p. 543)

References

1. Samarasekara DN, et al. Long-term anal continence and quality of life following postpartum anal sphincter injury. Colorectal Dis 2008; 10: 793–799.
2. Haadem K, et al. Long-term ailments due to anal sphincter rupture caused by delivery—a hidden problem. Eur J Obstet Gynecol Reprod Biol 1988; 27: 27–32.
3. Groom KM, Paterson-Brown S. Can we improve on the diagnosis of third degree tears? Eur J Obstet Gynecol Reprod Biol 2002; 101: 19–21.
4. Laine K, et al. Changing incidence of anal sphincter tears in four Nordic countries through the last decades. Eur J Obstet Gynecol Reprod Biol 2009; 146: 71–75.
5. Baghestan E, et al. Trends in risk factors for obstetric anal sphincter injuries in Norway. Obstet Gynecol 2010; 116: 25–34.
6. Christianson LM, et al. Risk factors for perineal injury during delivery. Am J Obstet Gynecol 2003; 189: 255–260.
7. Räisänen S, et al. The increased incidence of obstetric anal sphincter rupture—an emerging trend in Finland. Prev Med 2009; 49: 535–540.
8. Kudish B, et al. Trends in major modifiable risk factors for severe perineal trauma, 1996-2006. Int J Gynaecol Obstet 2008; 102: 165–170.
9. Edwards H, et al. Is severe perineal damage increased in women with prior anal sphincter injury? J Matern Fetal Neonatal Med 2006; 19: 723–727.
10. Hornemann A, et al. Advanced age is a risk factor for higher grade perineal lacerations during delivery in nulliparous women. Arch Gynecol Obstet 2010; 281: 59–64.
11. Angioli R, et al. Severe perineal lacerations during vaginal delivery: The University of Miami experience. Am J Obstet Gynecol 2001; 182: 1083–1085.
12. Nakai A, et al. Incidence and risk factors for severe perineal laceration after vaginal delivery in Japanese patients. Arch Gynecol Obstet 2006; 274: 222–226.
13. Hirayama F, et al. Prevalence and risk factors for third-and fourth-degree perineal lacerations during vaginal delivery: a multi-country study. BJOG 2012; 119: 340–347.
14. Power D, et al. Obstetric anal sphincter injury: how to avoid, how to repair a literature review. 2006 J Fam Pract; 55: 193–200.
15. Utz-Billing I, Kentenich H. Female genital mutilation: an injury, physical and mental harm. J Psychosom Obstet Gynaecol 2008; 29: 225–229.
16. Baghestan E, et al. Risk of recurrence and subsequent delivery after obstetric anal sphincter injury. BJOG 2012; 119: 62–69.
17. Landy HJ, et al. Characteristics associated with severe perineal and cervical lacerations during vaginal delivery. Obstet Gynecol 2011; 117: 627–635.
18. Eskander O, Shet D. Risk factors for 3rd and 4th degree perineal tear. J Obstet Gynecol 2009; 29: 119–122.
19. Dandolu V, et al. Risk of recurrence of anal sphincter lacerations. Obstet Gynecol 2005; 105: 831–835.
20. RCOG Green-top Guideline No. 29. The management of third- and fourth-degree perineal tears. London: Royal College of Obstetricians and Gynaecologists, 2007.

22.3 Previous Postpartum Haemorrhage

FACT FILE

- Primary **postpartum haemorrhage (PPH)** occurs in 4–6% of all pregnancies,[1,2] with uterine atonicity accounting for 75–90% of primary PPH.[2]
- Secondary PPH occurs in 1–3% of all deliveries, the most common aetiology being retained placental tissue.[3]
- The incidence of retained placenta is 1–6%.[4]
- Both PPH and manual removal of placenta (MROP) have a high incidence of recurrence.[5]
- Risk of recurrence is 8–28% for **primary PPH**[1,3] and 19% for **secondary PPH**.[3]
- Risk of recurrence for **retained placenta** is 16–30%.[6,7]
- **One of the most important risk factors for PPH is a history of previous PPH.**[1,2,3,4,8]
- In those who have had PPH in a first pregnancy, about 15% will have recurrent PPH in their second pregnancy, representing a greater than threefold increased risk of recurrent PPH compared to those who did not have a PPH in the first pregnancy.[5]
- The recurrence risk is nearly 22% for women who have had two prior PPHs, a fivefold increase compared to women who have not had PPH in either of the two previous pregnancies.[5]
- With a history of previous PPH in a first pregnancy, even if a second pregnancy had a normal third stage of labour without PPH, the risk of PPH continues to be as high as 20% in a third pregnancy.
- Any pregnant woman with a past history of PPH or MROP must be referred for at least one consultation from the community to a specialist antenatal clinic.
- A **careful analysis of the previous notes** (if the PPH in a prior pregnancy occurred in the same hospital) is essential to determine the aetiology. If the episode occurred elsewhere an effort must be made to obtain the details of the event.

Risk factors

Certain risk factors in the current pregnancy in a woman who already has had PPH in a previous pregnancy, increases her overall risk several fold:

- Overdistension of uterus (multiple pregnancies, macrosomia, polyhydramnios)
- Induction of labour
- Antepartum haemorrhage
- Coagulation disorders
- Previous Caesarean section
- Grand multiparity
- Fibroid uterus
- Placenta praevia.

Contributory factors for the past PPH which could be identified from previous records include:

- Tone:
  - multiparity
  - polyhydramnios, multiple gestation
  - prolonged labour ± augmentation
  - uterine atony
  - antepartum haemorrhage
  - uterine inversion
  - operative delivery
- Tissue:
  - fibroid uterus
  - retained placenta or blood clots
  - abnormal placentation (praevia, placenta accreta, percreta)
  - connective tissue disorders such as Marfan's or Ehler–Danlos syndrome
- Trauma:
  - lower genital tract lacerations
  - uterine rupture
- Coagulation disorders:
  - if on anticoagulants
  - inherited coagulation disorders, e.g. von Willebrandt disease (vWD)
  - HELLP
  - DIC
- ***A history of previous PPH is the strongest predictor for recurrent PPH.***[1,2,3,4,5,6]
- ***A history of previous retained placenta needing MROP increases the recurrence risk of the same in 16–30% of cases, thereby increasing the risk of PPH as well.***[4]
- Correction of anaemia before delivery is essential.
- Any woman with a **known coagulation disorder** has an ongoing recurrence risk of PPH.
- vWD is the most common inherited bleeding disorder, with the risks or primary PPH quoted as 16–29% and of secondary PPH quoted as 20–28%.
- Any history of abnormal bleeding especially with respect to menorrhagia and excessive bleeding at the time of any injury or surgical/dental procedures warrants further investigations to exclude any inherited bleeding disorder.
- Carriers of haemophilia A (factor VIII deficiency) or of B (factor IX deficiency) have a high rate of PPH, both primary and secondary (21% and 10% respectively).
- Patients with immune thrombocytopenia (ITP) have an increased risk of PPH in up to 25% of cases.
- Connective tissue disorders, such as Ehlers–Danlos or Marfan's, increase the risk of PPH due to uterine atony.

Interventions to reduce recurrence of PPH

- Predicting the risk of PPH is an essential part of antenatal screening and preventive management as well as preparation for recurrence of PPH which continues to be an important cause of maternal mortality worldwide.
- It is essential that the third stage of labour in women with a previous PPH history should be managed with vigilance, anticipating potential haemorrhage.[9,10]
- The patient should be appropriately counselled about the potential for recurrence and recommended preventive measures.
- Anaemia must be optimally corrected.
- Risk factors, including bleeding history, should be identified.
- As preparation for recurrence of PPH, document the following in notes (both hand-held and hospital):
  - IV access in labour.
  - Group and save when admitted in labour.
  - Blood products (if known bleeding disorder) to be kept available.
  - Active management of third stage with routine 5 iu oxytocin bolus IM as well as additional oxytocin infusion 40 iu in 500 ml normal saline run for 4–6 h following either a vaginal or Caesarean section delivery.
  - Carbetocin, especially in the context of Caesarean section.
- Allow spontaneous separation of the placenta before removal by controlled cord traction at Caesarean section.[9]

Information for patients

Please see Information for patients: Previous postpartum haemorrhage and/or retained placenta (p. 543)

References

1. Combs CA, et al. Factors associated with postpartum haemorrhage with vaginal birth. Obstet Gynecol 1991; 77: 69–76.

2. RCOG Green-top Guideline No. 52. Postpartum haemorrhage, prevention and management. London: Royal College of Obstetricians and Gynaecologists, 2009 and 2011.
3. Hoveyda F, MacKenzie IZ. Secondary post-partum haemorrhage: incidence, morbidity and current management. BJOG 2002; 108: 927–930.
4. Kominiarek MA, Kilpatrick SJ. Postpartum hemorrhage: a recurring pregnancy complication. Semin Perinatol 2007; 31: 159–166.
5. Ford JB, et al. Postpartum haemorrhage occurrence and recurrence: a population-based study. Med J Aust 2007; 187: 391–393.
6. Tandberg A, et al. Manual removal of the placenta: incidence and clinical significance. Acta Obstet Gynecol Scand 1999; 78: 33–36.
7. Titiz H, et al. Manual removal of the placenta: a case control study. Aust N Z J Obstet Gynaecol 2001; 41: 41–44.
8. Hall MH, et al. Concomitant and repeated happenings of complications of the third stage of labour. BJOG 1985; 92: 732–738.
9. McCurdy C, et al. The effect of placental management at cesarean delivery on operative blood loss. Am J Obstet Gynecol 1992; 167: 1363.
10. de Bernis L, et al. Managing complications in pregnancy and childbirth: a guide for midwives and doctors. Geneva: World Health Organization, 2003.

Community midwife refers patient with **previous PPH** to a specialist antenatal clinic for at least one consultation

↓

First visit to specialist antenatal clinic

- Detailed history including that of any bleeding disorders in family or personally
- Analyses of previous pregnancy records (if available) to identify aetiology of previous PPH—? atonic ? traumatic? retained placenta/products ? coagulation disorder
- Discuss recurrence risks with patient and recommended preventive measures
- Identify any additional risk factors in this pregnancy*.
- Identify placental site in this pregnancy
- Correction of anaemia during pregnancy is essential.
- Document instructions for care during labour, e.g.
  - IV access, group and save
  - blood products to be available (if any known bleeding disorders)
  - active management of 3rd stage with oxytocin bolus IM or IV as well as syntocinon infusion to run for 4–6 h following delivery, either vaginal or Caesarean section
  - Consider carbetocin, especially in the context of Caesarean section
- Refer back to midwifery-led care for rest of care during pregnancy

↓

Routine community midwife-led antenatal care (according to NICE guidelines) continues as long as no additional risk factors* for PPH develop during pregnancy

↓

Prompt referral back to specialist hospital antenatal clinic if any additional risk factors* develop during pregnancy

↓

Management according to Care pathways for individual risk factors

***Additional risk factors for PPH that may develop during current pregnancy**

- Antepartum haemorrhage
- Low-lying placenta/praevia
- Overdistension of uterus due to polyhydramnios, macrosomia, multiple pregnancy
- Anaemia
- Fibroid uterus
- Thrombocytopenia (newly diagnosed)
- Short interpregnancy interval from previous Caesarean section with placenta anterior and praevia in current pregnancy.
- HELLP, DIC, etc.

22.4 Previous Pre-Eclampsia

FACT FILE

See also Chapter 5, Hypertension in pregnancy

- Hypertensive disorders during pregnancy remain one of the leading causes of maternal death in the UK.[1]
- Women with a previous pregnancy complicated by pre-eclampsia have an increased risk for recurrence in subsequent pregnancies.[2,3,4]
- **Pre-eclampsia** complicates approximately 5–10% of nulliparous pregnancies[5] and 2–4% of all pregnancies.
- Pre-eclampsia is twice as common in primigravidae as in multiparas.
- Recurrence risk is as high as 50% for those who have had severe pre-eclampsia in an initial pregnancy.
- Although pre-eclampsia tends to be mainly a disease of first pregnancies, many risk factors for pre-eclampsia will persist in subsequent pregnancies,[6] such as:
  - chronic hypertension
  - diabetes
  - gestational diabetes
  - vascular and connective tissue disease
  - nephropathies
  - lupus and antiphospholipid syndrome
  - thrombophilias
  - obesity
  - Afro-Caribbean ethnicity
  - maternal age >35 years
  - family history of pre-eclampsia.
- The rate of recurrence of pre-eclampsia seems to be influenced by the severity and gestation at onset of pre-eclampsia in the previous pregnancy.[3,7,8,9,10,11] The highest rates of recurrence are found when the pre-eclampsia in the previous pregnancy was early, severe or complicated by eclampsia, HELLP syndrome, or fetal growth restriction.
- In women who have had previous severe pre-eclampsia in the second trimester, the risk of recurrence is significant (75%). Of these, nearly 33% developed recurrent pre-eclampsia at less than 28 weeks, another 33% at 28–36 weeks, and a the remainder at 37–40 weeks.[12]
- Women with pre-existing chronic hypertension have a higher rate of pre-eclampsia in a subsequent pregnancy as well as of preterm birth, IUGR, placental abruption and perinatal death.[8]
- ***All these pregnancy complications seem to have a common link with abnormal or impaired placentation.***

Screening tools for pre-eclampsia in those at risk of recurrence

- ***Research models[13,14,15,16] have been designed for the early screening for pre-eclampsia using combinations of maternal characteristics and history as well as Doppler studies of uterine artery pulsatility indices, maternal mean arterial pressure, and biochemical parameters, which can give clues to impaired placental function such as serum pregnancy associated plasma-protein A (PAPP-A) and placental growth factor (PlGF).***
- Failure of physiological transformation of the spiral arteries in placental bed biopsies has been associated with high impedance to blood flow in the uterine arteries and decreased perfusion of the placenta, which has been considered to play a role in the pathophysiology of pre-eclampsia. An abnormal uterine artery Doppler flow typically characterized by a persistence of the postsystolic notch and high resistance indices has been associated with a higher risk of developing early-onset than late-onset pre-eclampsia.[16]
- ***An imbalance between circulating angiogenic factors such as vascular endothelial growth factor (VEGF) and placental growth factor (PlGF), and antiangiogenic factors such as soluble vascular endothelial growth factor receptor-1 (sVEGFR-1), also referred to as soluble fms-like tyrosine kinase-1 (sFlt1), and the soluble form of endoglin (sEng) appears to be key to the pathophysiology of pre-eclampsia.***[15,16]
- ***Changes in the maternal plasma concentrations of angiogenic factors (such as PlGF and VEGF) and antiangiogenic factors (such as sEng and sVEGFR-1) precede the clinical presentation of pre-eclampsia.***[15,16]

Strategies to help reduce or prevent risk of recurrent pre-eclampsia

- **Pre-pregnancy counselling** including in-depth history, review of previous pregnancy details and results of investigations including placental pathology if available, arranging additional investigations as necessary, and planning for a next pregnancy, is vital.[3]
- A careful history including:
  - Gestational age at which pre-eclampsia was detected in a previous pregnancy: **early onset** before 34 weeks gestation; **intermediate onset** 34–37 weeks gestation; **late onset** after >37 weeks gestation
  - Pre-existent chronic diseases, comorbidities
  - History of pre-eclampsia in close family members—mother, sister.
- Women at particularly high risk of recurrence of pre-eclampsia including those who have had previous early-onset, severe pre-eclampsia, HELLP syndrome, eclampsia, fetal growth restriction, abruption of the placenta, oligohydramnios, perinatal death, a strong family history, or autoimmune conditions such as systemic lupus erythematosus (SLE) or antiphospholipid syndrome (APS) should receive targeted attention to try to reduce or prevent risk of pre-eclampsia recurrence.
- If the pathology report of the placenta from the previous pregnancy is available, evidence of reduced volume of intervillous spaces, massive intervillous fibrin deposition, reduced surface areas of terminal villi, infarcts or thrombi especially when accompanying fetal growth restriction may trigger further investigations such as screening for SLE or thrombophilias (acquired and inherited).
- Advise regarding loss of weight if obesity is an issue.
- Ensure optimal diabetic control if there is pre-pregnancy diabetes.
- If any underlying renal pathology is suspected, pre-pregnancy serum creatinine, 24-h urine for total protein, full blood count, uric acid, urinalysis, etc.
- At present, there is sufficient evidence only for prophylaxis with antiplatelet therapy i.e. low-dose aspirin started from early pregnancy (12 weeks gestation onwards and continued till the end of pregnancy) which has been shown to reduce the risk of recurrence of pre-eclampsia by up to 19%.[17,18]
  - As the transformation of the spiral arteries with increased interstitial trophoblast penetration occurs from 9–16 weeks gestation, some have suggested that low-dose aspirin needs to be commenced much earlier in gestation, from 8 weeks, and continued to the end of pregnancy.[19]
  - Effective counselling must be provided to the patient about the safety of low-dose aspirin and that only low-dose (75 mg) aspirin prophylaxis must be used. If the distinction between low-dose (75 mg/day) aspirin and high-dose or adult strength aspirin (150–300 mg/day) is not explained, non-compliance resulting from fear that aspirin would harm the fetus or the pregnant woman is not uncommon.
  - A meta-analysis of 11 randomized controlled trials of low-dose aspirin prophylaxis in pregnancy did not find an association between aspirin and either abruption of the placenta or perinatal mortality or morbidity.[20]
  - **High-dose aspirin** consumption close to delivery can result in maternal and fetal clotting abnormalities such as increased maternal bleeding and neonatal intracranial haemorrhage.[21,22]

- ◆ Maternal effects were seen with doses of 1500–2500 mg/day, and neonatal effects with doses of 325–1500 mg/day.[23,24]
- There is insufficient evidence to support of calcium, vitamins C and E, or fish oil supplements or progesterone as being effective prophylactic strategies.

Information for patients

Please see **Information for patients: Previous pre-eclampsia** (p. 544)

References

1. The Confidential Enquiry into Maternal and Child Health (CEMACH). Saving mothers' lives: reviewing maternal deaths to make motherhood safer 2003-2005. The Seventh Report of the Confidential Enquiries into Maternal Deaths in the UK. London: CEMACH, 2007.
2. Mostello D, et al. Recurrence of pre-eclampsia: effects of gestational age at delivery of the first pregnancy, body mass index, paternity, and interval between births. Am J Obstet Gynecol 2008; 199: 55–57.
3. Dildy GA III, et al. Preeclampsia recurrence and prevention. Semin Perinatol 2007; 31: 135–141.
4. McDonald SD, et al. The recurrence risk of severe de novo pre-eclampsia in singleton pregnancies: a population -based cohort. BJOG 2009; 116: 1578–1584.
5. Sibai BM, et al. The Calcium for Pre-eclampsia Prevention (CPEP) Study Group Risk Factors associated with preeclampsia in healthy nulliparous women. Am J Obstet Gynecol 1997; 177: 1003–1010.
6. ACOG Practice Bulletin No. 33. Diagnosis and management of pre-eclampsia and eclampsia. Obstet Gynecol 2002; 99: 159–167.
7. van Rijn BB, et al. Outcomes of subsequent pregnancy after first pregnancy with early-onset preeclampsia. Am J Obst Gynecol 2006; 195: 723–728.
8. Sibai BM, et al. Pregnancies complicated by HELLP syndrome (hemolysis, elevated liver enzymes, and low platelets): subsequent pregnancy outcome and long-term prognosis. Am J Obstet Gynecol 1995; 172: 125–129.
9. Chames MC, et al. Subsequent pregnancy outcome in women with a history of HELLP syndrome at 28 weeks of gestation. Am J Obstet Gynecol 2003; 188: 1504–1507.
10. Hnat MD, et al. Perinatal outcome in women with recurrent preeclampsia compared with women who develop preeclampsia as nulliparas. Am J Obstet Gynecol 2002; 186: 422–426.
11. Trogstad L, et al. Recurrence risk of preeclampsia in twin and singleton pregnancies. Am J Med Genet 2004; 126: 41–45
12. Sibai BM, et al. Severe preeclampsia in the second trimester: recurrence risk and long-term prognosis. Am J Obstet Gynecol 1991; 165: 1408–1412.
13. Poon LCY, et al. Hypertensive disorders in pregnancy: screening by systolic diastolic and mean arterial pressure at 11-13weeks. Hypertension in Pregnancy 2011; 30 (1): 93–107
14. Poon LCY, et al. Hypertensive disorders in pregnancy: screening by uterine artery Doppler at 11-13weeks. Ultrasound Obstet Gynecol 2009; 34: 142–148.
15. Kusanovic JP, et al. A prospective cohort study of the value of maternal plasma concentrations of angiogenic and anti-angiogenic factors in early pregnancy and midtrimester in the identification of patients destined to develop preeclampsia. J Matern Fetal Neonatal Med 2009; 22: 1021–1038.
16. Mikat B. Early detection of maternal risk for preeclampsia. ISRN Obstet Gynecol 2012; 2012: 172808.
17. Duley L, et al. Antiplatelet agents for preventing pre-eclampsia and its complications. Cochrane Database Syst Rev 2004; CD004659.
18. Coomarasamy A, et al. Aspirin for prevention of preeclampsia in women with historical risk factors: a systematic review. Obstet Gynecol 2003; 101: 1319–1332.
19. Carbillon L, Uzan S. Early treatment with low-dose aspirin is effective for the prevention of preeclampsia and related complications in high-risk patients selected by the analysis of their historic risk factors. Blood 2005; 105: 902–903.
20. Hauth JC, et al. Low-dose aspirin: lack of association with an increase in abruptio placentae or perinatal mortality. Obstet Gynecol 1995; 85: 1055–1058.
21. Schiff E, Mashiach S. The use of low dose aspirin in pregnancy. Am J Reprod Immunol 1992; 28: 153–156.
22. Stuart MJ, et al. Effects of acetylsalicylic acid ingestion on maternal and neonatal hemostasis. N Engl J Med 1982; 307: 909–912.
23. Valcamonico A, et al. Low dose aspirin in pregnancy: a clinical and biochemical study of effects on the newborn. J Perinat Med 1993; 21: 235–240.
24. Sibai BM, et al. Low dose aspirin in pregnancy. Obstet Gynecol 1989; 74: 551–556.

CARE PATHWAY

Assessment, investigations, and counselling

(ideally following the pregnancy with severe **pre-eclampsia** or before a next planned pregnancy)

- Discuss pathophysiology of pre-eclampsia, degrees of severity, association with other pregnancy complications such as IUGR, preterm birth, abruption, etc.
- Discuss recurrence rates and increased incidence in older mothers, those with strong family history of pre-eclampsia, Afro-Caribbean origin
- From history and notes, establish gestation at time of onset of pre-eclampsia, severity, and management
- Identify any comorbidities and their control—e.g. diabetes, pre-existent chronic hypertension, nephropathies, autoimmune conditions (lupus, APS), known thrombophilia, obesity, vascular and connective tissue disorders, etc.
- If not investigated already, screening for lupus, APS, etc.
- Review previous placental pathology if available
- Advise weight loss if obese.
- Optimization of control in diabetes, chronic hypertension, renal disease—multidisciplinary care (see individual care pathways)
- If pre-existent renal impairment, arrange pre-pregnancy baseline renal function tests (see care pathway for renal disease, p. 162)
- If APS confirmed, discuss role of low-dose aspirin with prophylactic LMWH. If lupus alone, aspirin prophylaxis from early first trimester
- Recommend low-dose aspirin is commenced from 1st trimester and continued during course of pregnancy
- Discuss and communicate plan of care in future pregnancy to GP, community midwife, and patient, including increased vigilance for pre-eclampsia
- In women with chronic hypertension, ensure antihypertensives such as ACE inhibitors, ARBs, and statins are switched to labetalol or methyldopa before pregnancy or immediately after pregnancy test is positive—include in communication to GP and patient

↓

Early referral in 1st trimester from community to specialist antenatal clinic, care shared with community

↓

First visit to specialist antenatal clinic

- If patient is on antihypertensives, ensure she is on pregnancy-compatible drugs
- Low-dose aspirin from 12 weeks gestation
- If severe pre-eclampsia in a previous pregnancy, according to local unit policy and availability, consider early screening predictors for recurrence risk—e.g. uterine artery pulsatility index, maternal mean arterial pressure, serum PAPP-A, placental growth factor
- If APS +ve, prophylactic LMWH added to low-dose aspirin from early first trimester. Also TED precautions

↓

Continued surveillance for signs and symptoms of pre-eclampsia

- Describe symptoms that patient needs to take note of and report promptly
- Self-monitoring of BP and urine
- Community midwife checks and day assessment unit monitoring of BP, proteinuria at regular intervals especially from 24–26 weeks gestation onwards
- Serial growth scans according to local unit policy
- Further follow-up antenatal clinic visits on a case-by-case basis
- Ensure the patient is on low-dose aspirin
- ***If recurrence of pre-eclampsia, continue management according to Care pathway 5.1***

↓

Further visits to specialist antenatal clinic

- Continued surveillance for maternal and fetal well-being and fetal biometry as previously planned
- If comorbidities present, multidisciplinary input to optimize control (see relevant care pathways, eg diabetes, chronic hypertension, renal disease, acquired thrombophilias, etc.)
- Timing and mode of delivery individualized on a case-to case-basis

22.5 Previous Shoulder Dystocia

FACT FILE

- **Shoulder dystocia** is a largely unpredictable and an unpreventable event. Incidence of shoulder dystocia is rising due to increasing maternity obesity and rising birth weight.
- Shoulder dystocia is defined as any vaginal cephalic delivery where additional obstetric manoeuvres are required to release the baby's shoulders after delivery of the head and when gentle downward traction has failed.[1,2]
- Though rare (incidence 0.6%),the condition carries a high perinatal morbidity and mortality, even when appropriately managed.[3,4]
- Maternal morbidity, especially PPH (11%) and fourth-degree perineal tears, are sequelae of delivery when shoulder dystocia occurs.[1,3,4]
- Risk factor assessments are not sufficiently predictive to allow prevention of shoulder dystocia in the large majority of cases.
- In the vast majority of cases, shoulder dystocia occurs when no risk factors are identifiable.
- Brachial plexus injury complicates 4–16% of such deliveries.[4,5] Fewer than 10% of these results in permanent brachial plexus damage.[6]
- Up to 27% of shoulder dystocia will be complicated by some maternal and/or fetal injury with 10% left with permanent sequelae.
- Not all injuries are due to excessive traction. There is good evidence not only that maternal propulsive forces can contribute to such injuries but that brachial plexus injuries can also occur without shoulder dystocia being encountered at vaginal delivery and even at uncomplicated Caesarean sections (4–16%).[7,8]

Fetal size and shoulder dystocia

- The large majority of infants with a birth weight of 4.5 kg or more do not develop shoulder dystocia.[9]
- 48% of incidences of shoulder dystocia occur in infants with a birth weight less than 4 kg.[10]
- Clinical risk estimation is unreliable and even third-trimester ultrasound scans have a 10–20% margin for error for actual birth weight. The larger the baby, the greater is this margin of error.
- High maternal BMI (>30 kg/m^2) is a well-recognized risk factor, and with increasing levels of maternal obesity the estimation of birth weight by any means is unreliable.
- Clinicians must always be alert to the possibility of shoulder dystocia with any delivery.
- ***There is no evidence to support induction of labour in women without diabetes at term where the fetus is thought to be macrosomic.***[1]
- ***Elective Caesarean section is not recommended for suspected fetal macrosomia (estimated fetal weight >4.5 kg) without diabetes.***
- However, the American College of Obstetricians and Gynaecologists (ACOG) has recommended that an estimated fetal weight of over 5 kg should prompt consideration of delivery by Caesarean section, despite the limitations of fetal size assessment.[11] The larger the infant, the more likely is the brachial plexus injury to be permanent rather than transient.[12]

Risk of recurrence of shoulder dystocia in a subsequent pregnancy

- A history of shoulder dystocia in a prior delivery carries a risk of recurrence of 10–16%.[13,14] A prior history of shoulder dystocia is indeed the single greatest risk factor for shoulder dystocia with odds ratio of 7–10 times that of the general population.[4]
- Either elective Caesarean section or vaginal delivery can be appropriate after previous shoulder dystocia.[1] Given the unpredictable nature of shoulder dystocia and the 10–16% risk of recurrence, the patient's choice of mode of delivery is an important factor to consider.
- When offering recommendations for the next delivery, factors to be considered are the details of the previous delivery proforma completed for shoulder dystocia (standardized shoulder dystocia proforma), the severity of any previous neonatal or maternal injury, fetal size, maternal BMI, and maternal choice.
- Apart from a history of shoulder dystocia in a prior pregnancy, other risk factors include maternal obesity and a disproportionate ultrasound measurement of enlarged abdominal circumference (AC) compared to head circumference (HC).
- ***The most common way to assess accelerated truncal growth is the HC:AC ratio. If this is below 0.9 near term, the risk for shoulder dystocia may be increased, even when the overall estimated fetal weight has not surpassed the 90th percentile.***[13]
- Pelvimetry (radiographic or CT) has no proven value in predicting shoulder dystocia or cephalopelvic disproportion.
- Many women may opt for a vaginal delivery in a subsequent pregnancy after a previous mild–moderate shoulder dystocia in a preceding pregnancy. In such cases, an epidural is recommended from early labour. A senior obstetrician must be alerted when maternal 'pushing down' efforts are commenced. These plans should be documented in the labour page of the notes.

Information for patients

Please see Information for patients: Previous birth complicated by shoulder dystocia (p. 544)

References

1. RCOG Green-top Guideline No. 42. Shoulder dystocia. 2nd ed, London: Royal College of Obstetricians and Gynaecologists, 2012
2. Draycott TJ, et al. Improving neonatal outcome through practical shoulder dystocia training. Obstet Gynecol 2008; 112: 14–20.
3. Al Hadi M, et al. Shoulder dystocia: risk factors and maternal and perinatal outcome. J Obstet Gynaecol 2001; 21: 352–354.
4. Gherman RBC et al. Obstetric manoeuvres for shoulder dystocia and associated fetal morbidity. Am J Obstet Gynecol 1998; 178; 1126–1113.
5. Acker D, et al. Risk factors for shoulder dystocia. Obstet Gynecol 1985; 66: 476–480.
6. Gherman RB, et al. Spontaneous vaginal delivery: a risk factor for Erb's palsy? Am J Obstet Gynecol 1998; 178: 423–427.
7. Sandmire HF, Demott RK. Erb's palsy without shoulder dystocia. Int J Gynaecol Obstet 2002; 78: 253–256.
8. Gherman RB, et al. Brachial plexus palsy associated with cesarean section: an in-utero injury? Am J Obstet Gynecol 1997; 177: 1162–1164
9. Naef RW III, Martin JN Jr. Emergent management of shoulder dystocia. Obstet Gynecol Clin North Am 1995; 22: 247–259.
10. Baskett TF, Allen AC. Perinatal implications of shoulder dystocia. Obstet Gynecol 1995; 86: 14–17.
11. Sokol RJ, Blackwell SC. Shoulder dystocia. Int J Gynaecol Obstet 2003; 80: 87–92.
12. Gherman RB, et al. Comparison of shoulder dystocia -associated transient and permanent brachial plexus palsies. Obstet Gynecol 2003; 102: 544–548.
13. Gurewitsch ED, et al. After shoulder dystocia: managing the subsequent pregnancy and delivery. Semin Perinatol 2007; 31: 185–195.
14. Lewis DF, et al. Recurrence rate of shoulder dystocia. Am J Obstet Gynaecol 1995; 172: 1369–1371.

CARE PATHWAY

Details of previous pregnancy, labour, and delivery

- Elicit details of previous pregnancy, results of GTT if performed, trajectory of fetal growth if serial scans had been performed
- Review details from notes of the previous labour and delivery, whether labour was induced or spontaneous, type of analgesia in labour, length of second stage, whether delivery was assisted instrumental or spontaneous vaginal delivery, manoeuvres that were employed to deliver shoulders with reference to previous partogram, delivery notes, and shoulder dystocia proforma if one was completed. Note birthweight of baby
- If delivery was in a different hospital, request pregnancy and intrapartum details
- Enquire about degree of brachial plexus injury of previous child, any residual weakness

↓

Assessing patient-specific recurrence risk of shoulder dystocia

- Note booking BMI
- Note whether patient has had any previous vaginal delivery without shoulder dystocia
- If previous macrosomic baby, arrange for a GTT at 26–28 weeks
- Serial scans to assess trajectory of fetal growth, especially any evidence of asymmetric growth
- Ponderal indices to assess accelerated truncal growth. If HC:AC ratio near term is below 0.9, increased risk of shoulder dystocia, even if overall estimated fetal weight has not exceeded the 90th centile

↓

Discussion and documentation

- With information obtained, discuss options
- Discuss risk of recurrence of shoulder dystocia (10–16%), mode and timing of delivery: explain no evidence that early IOL is of benefit, greater risk of failed IOL and emergency Caesarean section
- Elicit patient's views on mode of delivery
- Advise epidural in good time once in active labour
- Elective Caesarean section can be offered if estimated fetal weight is >5000 g in non-diabetics and >4500 g in diabetic gravidae.
- **Document** need for experienced obstetrician and midwife to be present/available at delivery
- **Document** discussions and plans for delivery in patient's notes

22.6 Previous Second-Trimester Pregnancy Loss or Very Pre-Term Birth < 26 Weeks Gestation

FACT FILE

- **Preterm birth** is the biggest single cause of neonatal mortality and morbidity.[1]
- Incidence: 7–10% of all births.[1]
- More than 50% of preterm births arise in pregnancies without obvious risk factors.
- 35% of all neonatal deaths in singleton pregnancies and 55% of neonatal deaths in multiple pregnancies are due to pulmonary effects of prematurity.
- ***Risk assessment is a key feature of antenatal care and in particular of the first antenatal visit.***

Aetiological factors

Aetiological factors are often multiple and can include:

- **A history of a previous second-trimester pregnancy loss or preterm birth is perhaps the strongest predictor of risk of recurrence.**[1,2,3] Increased risk of recurrence in subsequent pregnancy after one previous preterm birth is approximately 15%. After two previous preterm births, risks of recurrence is up to 42%. The gestational age of the previous preterm birth closely approximates the gestational age of subsequent delivery ± 2 weeks.
- **A short interpregnancy interval**[4] is an independent risk factor for preterm delivery.
- **Smoking** is related to a 40% increase in risk of preterm birth: advise the woman to stop, and offer necessary help and support.
- ***Fetal anomalies:***
  - structural.
  - chromosomal.
- **Multiple pregnancies:** fetal death rate 18.5 vs 6.2/1000 in singletons.
- ***Placental/umbilical cord risk factors:***
  - abruption
  - cord accident
  - uteroplacental insufficiency
- ***Maternal risk factors:***
  - vascular disease (see Chapter 1)
  - diabetes (see Chapter 9)
  - obesity (see Chapter 18)
  - SLE, APS (see Chapter 13)
  - uterine abnormalities, e.g. bicornuate/septate uterus, large intramural fibroids
  - periodontal disease: if dental health is poor, encourage early dental assessment and care during pregnancy.
- **Thrombophilias** (see Chapter 1.2): 15% of white European populations have some form of thrombophilia. This is responsible for around 50% of all maternal thromboembolic events in pregnancy and also linked to an increased risk of fetal demise in some studies. Many adverse pregnancy outcomes are associated with characteristic placental lesions involving thrombosis. Inherited conditions include:
  - factor V Leiden mutation
  - prothrombin *G20210A* gene mutation (heterozygous)
  - antithrombin III deficiency
  - protein S deficiency
  - protein C deficiency.
- **Cervical insufficiency** (see Chapter 11): This is defined as inability of the uterine cervix to retain a pregnancy in the absence of contractions or labour and associated with painless cervical dilation. Cervical shortening, funnelling, and history of previous preterm delivery are independent contributors for preterm delivery.
- **Infection** is an important factor in up to 40% of cases, although aetiology is often multifactorial. Infections can be vaginal, urinary tract, or periodontal.
  - There is a significant association between abnormal genital flora **such as bacterial vaginosis (BV) and related organisms**[5] and adverse outcome of pregnancy whether late miscarriage, preterm pre-labour rupture of the membranes, or preterm birth.
  - The earlier in pregnancy abnormal genital flora occurs, the greater the risk of preterm birth.
  - A positive screening test for BV at 26–32 weeks is associated with a 1.5–2-fold increased risk of preterm birth but would miss cases of late miscarriages and very early preterm birth. In contrast, a positive screen in the second trimester is associated with a 3–7-fold increased risk of late miscarriage or preterm birth.
  - If BV +ve at 16 weeks then 50% continue to have BV at 33 weeks.
  - If BV −ve at 16 weeks then <2% continue to have BV at >33 weeks.
  - BV is usually a marker for mycoplasma.
  - BV is not always isolated in a high vaginal swab (HVS).
  - BV alone increases risk of preterm birth by threefold. With mycoplasma in addition, the risk increased by 30%.
  - Therefore the recommendation is for **prophylactic clindamycin cream for vaginal application at 16 weeks gestation (once in 24 h for 7 days) repeated at 22 weeks gestation.**[1,5]
  - There is no standard HVS screening programme for BV in the UK. Some studies have shown a 60% decrease in the incidence of preterm birth with the use of clindamycin vaginal cream in low-risk women.[5,6,7,8]
  - Once treated at 16 weeks gestation, the recurrence rate of BV is 6.3% at 22 weeks and 1.3% at 28–34 weeks.
- There is increasing evidence for the use of **progesterone** in the management of a pregnancy with a history of previous preterm labour or second-trimester pregnancy loss,[9,10,11,12,13] although the Royal College of Obstetricians and Gynaecologists endorses current recommendations that, in women at high risk of preterm delivery, progesterone administration should be restricted to clinical trials. Progesterone pessaries are is the preparation used (400 mg/day PR or PV) till the risk of early premature delivery has passed.
- ***Each day between 24–26 weeks gestation improves survival outcome by 3% in neonates.***

Information for patients

Please see Information for patients: Previous premature birth or late miscarriage (p. 544)

References

1. 46th RCOG Study Group: Preterm birth. London Royal College of Obstetricians and Gynaecologists, 2004.
2. Romero R, et al. The preterm parturition syndrome. BJOG 2006; 113 Suppl 3: 17–42.
3. McManemy J, et al. Recurrence risk for preterm delivery. Am J Obstet Gynecol 2007; 196: 571–576.
4. Smith GCS, et al. Interpregnancy interval and risk of preterm birth and neonatal death. BMJ 2003; 327 (7410): 313.
5. Nelson DB, Macones G. Bacterial vaginosis in pregnancy: current findings and future directions. Epidemiol Rev 2002; 24: 102–108.
6. Hauth JC, et al. Reduced incidence of preterm delivery with metronidazole and erythromycin in women with bacterial vaginosis. N Engl J Med 1995; 333: 1732–1736.

7. Lamont RF, et al. Intravaginal clindamycin to reduce preterm birth in women with abnormal genital tract. Obstet Gynecol 2003; 101: 516–522.
8. Ugwumadu A, et al. Effect of early oral clindamycin on late miscarriage and preterm delivery in asymptomatic women with abnormal vaginal flora and bacterial vaginosis: a randomised controlled trial. Lancet 2003; 361 (9362): 983–988.
9. Kiss H, et al. Prospective randomised controlled trial of an infection screening programme to reduce the rate of preterm delivery. BMJ 2004; 329: 371.
10. Fonseca EB, et al. Progesterone and the risk of preterm birth among women with a short cervix, for the Fetal Medicine Foundation Second Trimester Screening Group. N Engl J Med 2007; 357: 462–469.
11. SOGC Technical Update No. 202. The use of progesterone for prevention of preterm birth. Ottawa: Society of Obstetricians and Gynaecologists of Canada, 2008.
12. ACOG Committee Opinion No. 419. Use of progesterone to reduce preterm birth. American College of Obstetricians and Gynecologists. Obstet Gynecol 2008; 112: 963–965.
13. Dodd JM, Crowther CA. The role of progesterone in prevention of preterm birth. Int J Womens Health 2009; 1: 73–84.

CARE PATHWAY

Community midwife refers pregnant woman with **previous one or more 2nd-trimester pregnancy loss or preterm delivery** to a specialist antenatal clinic

↓

First visit to specialist antenatal clinic (before 12 weeks)

- ***Refer to letter/notes from post-pregnancy loss/preterm delivery counselling that patient might have already had which might include detailed plans for future pregnancy management***
- If not seen for post-pregnancy loss counselling after the previous pregnancy, obtain detailed history of previous pregnancy, events leading up to miscarriage/preterm delivery to help find any cause—IUD? cervical insufficiency? preterm labour? infection? multiple pregnancy? fetal abnormality? uterine abnormality? autoimmune conditions? thrombophilia?, etc.
- Discuss recurrence risk depending on details obtained from the past history and investigations that might have identified a cause for the pregnancy loss
- If applicable, advise stop smoking and/or use of illicit drugs
- If not done previously, APS, SLE screening; Thrombophilia screening if relevant to history
- Prescribe prophylactic clindamycin cream PV at 16 weeks, repeat at 22 weeks (a week's course each time)
- Low-dose aspirin till end of pregnancy if lupus +ve. If APS +ve, add dalteparin—see lupus, APS pathways (pp. 272, 273)
- Consider progesterone 400 mg pessary OD either PR or PV from 12 weeks till approximately 34 weeks gestation

↓

If previous history of one or more mid- trimester pregnancy loss(es) and history suggestive of cervical insufficiency, arrange scans at about 14,18, 22 weeks to confirm viability and assess cervical length ± funnelling

↓

- If cervix is ≤25 mm before 24 weeks of gestation. consider cervical cerclage (ultrasound-indicated cerclage)
- Before suture insertion, screening for aneuploidy and attempt to exclude lethal/major fetal abnormality recommended
- Explain procedure, risks. Give info leaflet
- Arrange cervical cerclage under spinal anaesthetic in maternity theatre

↓

Perioperative antibiotics and progesterone (Cyclogest 400 mg PR or PV OD) till approximately 34 weeks gestation may be recommended

↓

- Subsequent visits to antenatal clinic 2 weeks after cerclage
- No further routine cervical scans required
- Serial fetal growth scans 28, 32, 36 weeks with same-day specialist antenatal clinic visits (or according to individual unit's serial growth scans)
- Arrange for suture removal at 37 weeks
- Rest of pregnancy as normal. IOL at 40+ weeks

If no pathological cervical changes on TVS →

No specific cause identified for previous early preterm delivery or late 2nd-trimester pregnancy loss—history not suggestive of cervical insufficiency

↓

- Prophylactic clindamycin PV at 16 and 22 weeks, each a 7-day course
- Continue daily progesterone pessaries till about 34 weeks
- Further specialist antenatal clinic at 24 weeks
- Serial growth scans at about 28, 32, 36 weeks with same-day antenatal clinic follow-up (or according to individual unit's serial scan protocol)
- Routine community midwifery visits to continue according to NICE protocol
- If no SLE/APS, and no growth problems in serial scans, IOL at 40+ weeks according to individual unit's protocol
- Earlier IOL if APS/SLE +ve or IUGR on scans (see relevant care pathways)

↓

Routine community midwifery visits according to standard NICE protocol to continue

22.7 Previous Perinatal Loss

FACT FILE

Incidence and aetiology

- **Stillbirth** unfortunately remains relatively common and occurs in 1 in 200 of all births, with an overall adjusted stillbirth rate of 3.9 per 1000.[1]
- One-third of stillbirths are of small for gestational age babies[2,3] and up to 50% are classified as unexplained.[4]
- The stillbirth rate has remained at about the same rate from 2000, probably attributable to the rising levels of obesity[5] and pregnancies in older women.[6,7,8]
- Adverse events in a previous pregnancy could be due to a wide range of conditions.
- A previous history of intrauterine fetal death (IUFD) or stillbirth or peripartum death defines the current pregnancy as 'high risk',[9,10,11,12,] mainly because of the increased risk of obstetric and perinatal complications including pre-eclampsia, abruption, fetal growth restriction and low birth weight, preterm delivery, and increased intervention rates. Consultant-led care based mainly, though not exclusively, in the hospital is advisable.
- The serious emotional and psychological effects of **IUFD** and **stillbirth**, quite apart from the physical effects, must not be underestimated. The mother's level of anxiety in a subsequent pregnancy are likely to be profound.

Post-pregnancy loss counselling

- Such patients should, ideally have received thorough post-pregnancy loss counselling after the previous pregnancy loss, and have also have had all relevant investigations completed.
- The cause of the stillbirth or IUFD, if found, should have been discussed with the parents as well as any recurrence risk and any preventive measures. It must be noted, however, that 12–50% of stillbirths may remain unexplained even after investigations.[6,9]
- Plans for a future pregnancy management will ideally have been discussed with a consultant obstetrician before the start of the next pregnancy.
- General advice such as smoking cessation, weight loss if overweight, routine peri-pregnancy folic acid, rubella vaccination, etc. should be offered pre-pregnancy.
- A short interpregnancy interval (<6 months) after a previous stillbirth has been associated with a higher rate of adverse pregnancy outcomes in a subsequent pregnancy.[13,14,15] This is an important aspect to be emphasized during post-pregnancy counselling after a previous stillbirth or perinatal mortality.
- Several studies have shown that women with a past history of stillbirth have a 12-fold increased risk of **intrapartum stillbirth as well as an increased risk of placental abruption and pre-eclampsia.**[9,16,17,18] The increased risk of stillbirth after a previous infant mortality was particularly marked (a twofold increase) in the black population in one study.[15]
- An increased incidence of **ischaemic placental disease, fetal distress, extreme preterm delivery**, early intrauterine death between 20–28 weeks and **early neonatal mortality have also been found in subsequent pregnancies.**[16,19]
- This increased risk is independent of fetal congenital anomalies or underlying maternal conditions.[12]
- In women with a previous history of unexplained stillbirth, a four times greater than expected rate of gestational diabetes was found in one study.[10]
- Women with thrombophilic defects including deficiency of antithrombin, protein C, or protein S may have a higher risk of fetal loss due to placental insufficiency,[20] which is itself caused by maternal/placental vessels being more prone to thrombosis.[21,22] Thromboprophylaxis during pregnancy in women with deficiency of antithrombin, protein C, or protein S has been shown to significantly reduce the risk of late fetal loss.[21,23]
- Screening for such thrombophilias is recommended as an integral part of follow-up investigations after an unexplained stillbirth, especially if the woman has a strong family history or a personal history of thromboembolic conditions or if the stillbirth fetus was growth restricted[24] or the IUFD was associated with abruption of the placenta.
- A significantly higher rate of factor V Leiden and prothrombin *G20210A* mutations are found in placentas with thrombotic events compared with normal placentas.[25]
- Even if permission for a post-mortem is withheld, the placenta must be sent for histological analysis and if relevant, samples also sent for virological and microbiological investigations. Placental disease,[25,26] which accounts for a significant proportion of stillbirths, cannot be detected otherwise and may hinder information shared with the parents at the post-pregnancy loss counselling or for management plans to be put in place for a subsequent pregnancy.
- Care providers must be aware of the increased risk of postnatal depression in women who have had a previous IUFD, found particularly in those where there is a short interval (<12 months) between the previous IUFD and a new conception.[27]
- Reassurance, support, and good communication backed up with relevant investigations, close monitoring as indicated, and any necessary and timely intervention/s are vital.

Principles of management of a subsequent pregnancy

The underlying principles of management of any subsequent pregnancy after a previous adverse obstetric history resulting in the loss of a baby are:

- To get as much information as possible about the previous pregnancy/delivery with results of investigations correspondence, etc. in order to analyse any risk of recurrence and quantify this risk, if possible.
  - If the woman has had the previous pregnancy loss in the same hospital, detailed analysis of the notes of that pregnancy, results of investigations (including post-mortem findings, if performed) and relevant correspondence is necessary.
  - If the previous pregnancy loss had occurred in another hospital, all efforts must be made to obtain details from that hospital as soon as possible, after booking has been completed in this pregnancy.
- Apart from medical management of the subsequent pregnancy, the emotional and psychological element involved should be recognized and due care and support provided.
- An individualized plan of care should be designed for this pregnancy, involving the patient/partner from the onset.
- Any necessary investigations or monitoring should be organized as required.
- Although there is little evidence for the benefits of serial ultrasonography in a subsequent pregnancy after a previous stillbirth, serial ultrasound can provide much valued reassurance for parents and must be considered, although the timing and frequency are not established for certain.[28]
- Good communication with community healthcare providers should be maintained throughout the pregnancy.
- Referral to a tertiary centre may be indicated, especially if rare genetic or inherited metabolic disease was involved in the loss of the previous baby.
- Timely intervention based on the above factors is essential.
- Although there is limited evidence to support early planned delivery in a subsequent pregnancy, the emotional and psychological stress of the parents and the awareness of increased risk of recurrence of pregnancy loss often prompts obstetricians worldwide to consider delivery by about 38–39 weeks, even if no other risk factors or complications have been identified.

- Higher rates for induction of labour and instrumental or Caesarean section delivery in subsequent pregnancies [9,10] are mainly due to obstetric intervention.[10,29]
- Reassurance and emotional support must underpin good medical care at both primary care and hospital level.
- ***Note: In the event of any ongoing medico-legal issues associated with a previous pregnancy which resulted in an adverse outcome, it is advisable not to comment on causation or quality of care, as these are probably being dealt with at a different level. Duty and remit of care lies with the current pregnancy.***

Previous information to aid antenatal care in present pregnancy

Although it is impossible to design a 'one size fits all' guideline to embrace all conditions that might have caused a previous pregnancy loss, the following points provide a general guide.

Previous second-trimester miscarriages

See individual guidelines for the following:

- Suspected cervical incompetence
- Associated maternal conditions, e.g. obesity, diabetes, smoking, SLE, APS, thrombophilias, renal disease, infections.

Intrauterine fetal death/stillbirth

- Previous chromosomal abnormalities or congenital malformations: check results of any post-mortem, karyotyping, or genetic counselling.
- Multiple pregnancy: The previous pregnancy, if a multiple pregnancy, would have had significantly increased risks compared to a subsequent singleton pregnancy, although underlying maternal risk factors should not be discounted without adequate investigations.
- Associated maternal conditions: Refer to individual guidelines in other chapter.
- Previous placental insufficiency: See IUGR guidelines for care in this pregnancy.
- Previous placental abruption: Seek any associated risk factors such as smoking, hypertension, SLE, APS, or thrombophilias, referring to individual guidelines for care in this pregnancy.
- Previous blood group incompatibilities, haemolytic anaemia, stillbirth, or neonatal death: see individual guidelines.
- Previous unexplained stillbirth: A disappointingly large number of stillbirths (12–50%) occur without any risk factors or causation being identified.
- However, 10–15% of unexplained stillbirths have been found to be due to silent fetomaternal haemorrhage and it is worth checking the result of the previous Kleihauer test, which is recommended as part of IUFD investigations at the time.
- If the previous pregnancy was an IVF pregnancy, there is a slightly higher risk of sudden IUFD compared to a subsequent spontaneously conceived pregnancy, especially after 40 weeks gestation.

Intrapartum or early neonatal death

Reasons may be multifactorial. Check the previous notes for the following:

- Preterm or post-mature (>42 weeks)
- Preterm premature rupture of membranes
- Meconium aspiration
- Chorioamnionitis, ascending infection, septicaemia
- Birth weight
- Oligo- or polyhydramnios
- Post-mortem reports/histology, microbiology of the placenta, karyotype results if available
- Associations with abruption, pre-eclampsia, hypertension, IUGR, etc.
- Multiple pregnancy
- Any documentation of a complicated labour and delivery, e.g. multiple attempts to deliver, significant shoulder dystocia, any subsequent birth trauma
- Documentation of cord pH and base excess of both umbilical artery (UA) and umbilical vein (UV) to indicate or exclude possible birth asphyxia
- Summary of neonatal period from SCBU.

Planned antenatal care

Planned antenatal care should be individualized in every woman, guided by the events of the previous pregnancy loss. In general:

- If the patient is a smoker and/or an user of illicit drugs, advise immediate cessation and refer to the anti-smoking coordinator or to the substance abuse midwife respectively, with the patient's consent.
- Ensure patient is on peri-pregnancy folic acid (higher dose of 5 mg indicated if previous history of neural tube defect, if patient is on antiepileptic medication or drugs for inflammatory bowel disease, or is diabetic).
- Early dating and viability scan.
- CVS/amniocentesis if indicated by previous history.
- Low-dose aspirin from early in first trimester if SLE positive and low molecular weight heparin (LMWH) added to low-dose aspirin from first missed period if APS is positive.
- LMWH in the presence of previously identified coexistent thrombophilia.
- If not performed previously, screening for SLE, APS, and thrombophilias.
- Robust BP control with antihypertension medication suitable for pregnancy as well as prophylactic low dose aspirin in those who have associated hypertension. Regular BP monitoring to continue both in the day assessment unit and in the community.
- Routine anomaly scan at about 20 weeks gestation to detect any congenital anomaly, especially those with an increased risk of recurrence.
- Multidisciplinary referral and joint management as required if coexistent maternal conditions/diseases exist.
- If history of preterm delivery, PPROM may have been due to possible bacterial vaginosis—clindamycin vaginal cream prophylaxis for 5–7 days at 16 weeks, repeated at 22 weeks.
- If tests for SLE or APS are positive, uterine artery Doppler at 20–22 weeks may be considered. This is not, however, a mandatory part of antenatal care in most clinical settings and the results should not deflect attention from continued close surveillance for pre-eclampsia.
- In cases of previous macrosomia/polyhydramnios, glucose tolerance test (GTT) at 28 weeks or an earlier GTT at 16 weeks if there is a history of previous gestational diabetes.
- Referral to regional centre for red cell incompatibility if indicated by rising titres.
- Continued vigilance for pre-eclampsia, abruption, recurrence of obstetric cholestasis.
- Fetal monitoring from approximately 26–28 weeks to include:
  - Serial growth scans ± Doppler
  - BPP and CTG as indicated
  - Patient to be informed about maintaining vigilance for daily fetal movements, with the aid of a fetal movement chart if necessary.
- Decisions regarding induction of labour before 40 weeks or delivery by elective LSCS must be made on a case-to-case basis by a senior clinician, and clear documentation to this effect is mandatory.
- Any special instructions for intrapartum care or care of the neonate should be clearly documented.
- Referral to a neonatologist during the pregnancy, and/or to a tertiary centre if indicated, should be promptly organized and followed through as relevant.
- Patient education starting from early pregnancy should include advice about recognizing and prompt reporting of symptoms such as decreased fetal movements, abdominal pain, vaginal bleeding, symptoms suggestive of pre-eclampsia, etc.
- ***While there is no guarantee for a successful outcome for any pregnancy, careful planning, monitoring, and management***

with patient involvement at each stage will hopefully result in a happier outcome than that of her previous pregnancy.

Information for patients

Please see Information for patients: Stillbirth (p. 545)

References

1. Confidential Enquiry into Maternal and Child Health (CEMACH). Perinatal mortality 2007: United Kingdom. CEMACH: London, 2009.
2. Vergani P, et al. Identifying the causes of stillbirth: a comparison of four classification systems. Am J Obstet Gynecol 2008; 199: 319.e1–4.
3. Gardosi J, et al. Classification of stillbirth by relevant condition at death (ReCoDe): population based cohort study. BMJ 2005; 331: 1113–1117.
4. Confidential Enquiry into Maternal and Child Health (CEMACH). Perinatal mortality 2006: England, Wales and Northern Ireland. CEMACH: London, 2008.
5. Stephansson O, et al. Maternal weight, pregnancy weight gain, and the risk of antepartum stillbirth. Am J Obstet Gynecol 2001; 184: 463–469.
6. Fretts RC. Etiology and prevention of stillbirth. Am J Obstet Gynecol 2005; 193: 1923–1935.
7. Cnattingius S, et al. Delayed childbearing and risk of adverse perinatal outcome. A population-based study. JAMA 1992; 268: 886–890.
8. Raymond EG, et al. Effects of maternal age, parity, and smoking on the risk of stillbirth. Br J Obstet Gynaecol 1994; 101: 301–306.
9. Black M, et al. Obstetric outcomes subsequent to intrauterine death in the first pregnancy. BJOG 2008; 115: 269–274.
10. Robson S, et al. Subsequent birth outcomes after an unexplained stillbirth: preliminary population-based retrospective cohort study. Aust N Z J Obstet Gynaecol 2001; 41: 29–35.
11. Robson S, et al. Obstetric management of the next pregnancy after an unexplained stillbirth: an anonymous postal survey of Australian obstetricians. Aus N Z J Obstet Gynaecol 2006; 46: 278–281.
12. Heinonen S, Kirkinen P. Pregnancy outcome after previous stillbirth resulting from causes other than maternal conditions and fetal abnormalities. Birth 2000; 27: 33–37.
13. Moore T, et al. Interconception care for couples after perinatal loss: comprehensive review of the literature. J Perinat Neonatal Nurs 2011; 25: 44–51.
14. Conde-Agudelo A, et al. Birth spacing and risk of adverse perinatal outcomes: a meta-analysis. JAMA 2006; 19;295: 1809–1823.
15. August EM, et al. Infant mortality and subsequent risk of stillbirth: a retrospective cohort study. BJOG 2011; 118: 1636–1645.
16. Sharma PP, et al. Stillbirth recurrence in a population of relatively low-risk mothers Paediatr Perinat Epidemiol 2007; 21: 24–30.
17. El-Bastawissi AY, et al. History of fetal loss and other adverse pregnancy outcomes in relation to subsequent risk of preterm delivery. Matern Child Health J 2003; 7: 53–58.
18. Reddy UM. Prediction and prevention of recurrent stillbirth. Obstet Gynecol 2007; 110: 1151–1164.
19. Getahun D, et al. The association between stillbirth in the first pregnancy and subsequent adverse perinatal outcomes. Am J Obstet Gynecol 2009; 201: 378.e1–6.
20. Alonso A, et al. Acquired and inherited thrombophilia in women with unexplained fetal losses. Am J Obstet Gynecol 2002; 187: 1337–1342.
21. Korteweg FJ, et al. Fetal loss in women with hereditary thrombophilic defects and concomitance of other thrombophilic defects: a retrospective family study. BJOG 2012; 119: 422–430.
22. Sarig G, et al. Thrombophilia is common in women with idiopathic pregnancy loss and is associated with late pregnancy wastage. Fertil Steril 2002; 77: 342–347.
23. Folkeringa N, et al. Reduction of high fetal loss rate by anticoagulant treatment during pregnancy in antithrombin, protein C or protein S deficient women. Br J Haematol 2007; 136: 656–661.
24. Weiner Z, et al. Thrombophilia and stillbirth: possible connection by intrauterine growth restriction. BJOG 2004; 111: 780–783.
25. Mousa HA, Alfirevici Z. Do placental lesions reflect thrombophilia state in women with adverse pregnancy outcome? Hum Reprod 2000; 15: 1830–1833.
26. Stallmach T, Hebisch G. Placental pathology: its impact on explaining prenatal and perinatal death. Virchows Arch 2004; 445: 9–16.
27. Hughes PM, et al. Stillbirth as risk factor for depression and anxiety in the subsequent pregnancy: cohort study. BMJ 1999; 318: 1721–1724.
28. RCOG Green-top Guidelines No. 55. Late intrauterine fetal death and stillbirth. London: Royal College of Obstetricians and Gynaecologists, 2010.
29. Gold KJ, et al. How physicians cope with stillbirth or neonatal death: a national survey of obstetricians. Obstet Gynecol 2008; 112: 29–34.

23 Fertility-Related Issues

23.1 Singleton IVF Pregnancy

FACT FILE

Singleton pregnancies resulting from assisted reproductive techniques are dealt with in this chapter although multiple pregnancies share the same problems with further increased risks. For multiple pregnancies, see 'Multiple pregnancy' under the subheading 'Fetal conditions'

- Subfertility affects one in seven couples in the UK.[1]
- It is estimated that about 2–4% of all babies born nowadays in developed countries are conceived by assisted reproductive techniques (ART).[2]
- In-vitro fertilization (IVF) and associated laboratory techniques such as intracytoplasmic sperm injection (ICSI) blastocyst culture can have an effect not only on the course of the pregnancy but also on neonatal health compared to spontaneously conceived pregnancies.
- The absolute risks of poor pregnancy outcomes appear small and the majority of births after ART are uncomplicated.
- Multiple pregnancies are associated with significant maternal and perinatal risks, and with IVF there is a significant increase in multiple gestations compared with spontaneous conception. Multiple pregnancies remain the most common risk associated with IVF and related techniques.
- However, even **singleton pregnancies conceived after IVF** or related ART[1,2,3,4,5,6,7] or those singletons spontaneously conceived following a long period of subfertility are at increased risks of adverse perinatal outcomes.[8,9]
- Underlying maternal factors rather than ART methods themselves may play a significant role in causing such outcomes.
- Clinicians need to be aware of and remain vigilant about increased risk of pregnancy complications.
- Although most such pregnancies progress without complications and result in good maternal and perinatal outcomes, couples attempting ART need to be given accurate information about the risks of adverse reproductive outcomes.

Pre-ART assessment and counselling

- The importance of pre-ART assessment and counselling cannot be overemphasized.
  - A thorough history should be obtained to recognize any pre-existing medical conditions or fetal abnormalities in the family in order to facilitate referral to appropriate maternal medicine or medical team or for genetic counselling.
  - Optimal control of chronic medical conditions such as diabetes, renal disease, anaemia, epilepsy, and hypertension should be achieved.
  - Retinopathy and nephropathy screening and, if required, treatment should be completed before conception to reduce risk of deterioration.
  - Drug therapy for epileptic patients should be reviewed aiming for good control with monotherapy. Similarly antihypertensive drugs such ACE inhibitors, ARBs, or beta-blockers (excepting labetalol) must be preferably changed to labetalol or methyldopa leading up to and during pregnancy.
  - Couples considering IVF–ICSI for male factor infertility must be made aware and if need be, referred for genetic counselling, as there is an increased risk of chromosomal abnormalities. They should be informed that prenatal diagnosis by chorionic villus sampling (CVS) or amniocentesis is available once they conceive.
  - Strategies aimed to optimize maternal health must be discussed. This includes advice regarding healthy diet and lifestyle modifications especially regarding smoking, alcohol, or substance misuse. Weight management is essential.
  - Peri-pregnancy folic acid must be advised to reduce the risk of neural tube defects in the fetus by up to 75%. A higher dose of 5 mg/day may be necessary in women with history of neural tube defects in the past, obesity, diabetes, anticonvulsant therapy, alcohol abuse, inflammatory bowel disease, and malabsorption syndromes.
  - Vitamin D supplementation (10 micrograms/day) should be offered for all women during pregnancy and while breastfeeding, especially in women with darker skin such those as of South Asian, African, Caribbean, or Middle Eastern descent as well as obese women or those who have limited direct skin exposure to sunlight.
  - Rubella status should be checked; vaccination should be offered to women who are non-immune.
- Obstetricians caring for these pregnancies need to formulate an individualized care pathway from peri-conception to the puerperium, with the aim of preventing or reducing the risks for maternal and perinatal morbidity[2] (see Care Pathway)

Maternal morbidity

- **Increasing maternal age** is a well-recognized risk factor for pregnancy complications. Women having IVF or those who have conceived after a prolonged period of subfertility are more likely to be older.
- Studies which have compared age-matched controls have shown an increased risk of pregnancy complications in those who have conceived by ART such as IVF or spontaneously after a long period of infertility.[10,11,12,13]
- Pregnancy complications include a higher incidence of ectopic pregnancies and spontaneous miscarriage (17–32%),[2] pre-eclampsia, essential or pregnancy-induced hypertension, diabetes or gestational diabetes, placenta praevia (3–6-fold increase), obstetric haemorrhage, and increased Caesarean section rates.
- Pre-existing comorbidities can cause further complications in such pregnancies, highlighting how crucial the role of pre-IVF counselling is.
- Vigilance for the development of some of these comorbidities and appropriate screening is advisable.
- Low-dose aspirin from the first trimester and continued till the end of pregnancy needs consideration in those at higher risk of pre-eclampsia.
- **Women with donated egg IVF pregnancies have a sevenfold increased risk of pregnancy-induced hypertension compared with pregnant women who have IVF with their own eggs.**[1,10] This is a group where prophylactic low-dose aspirin should be considered.

Perinatal risks associated with IVF

- Increased risk of **congenital malformations** is seen in infants born as a result of IVF compared with spontaneous conception, even correcting for multiple pregnancies. Congenital anomalies are slightly increased (by 15–40%) compared with spontaneously conceived children after adjustments for relevant confounders.[1,2,3,4,5] While this reflects a significant relative risk, as these abnormalities are relatively rare the absolute risk remains low. Such anomalies include gastrointestinal, cardiovascular, and septal heart defects and trachea-oesophageal or anorectal atresia.[13,14]

- **Genetic risks** including chromosomal anomalies, microdeletion of the long arm of the Y chromosome as well as genomic imprinting errors, the latter resulting in conditions such as Beckwith–Widemann syndrome, Prader–Willi Syndrome, or Angelman syndrome, have been reported as occurring more frequently with IVF and related laboratory procedures. This could be due to transmission of genetic factors or as a result of the procedure itself.[1,2,3,4]
- **Low birth weight** (<2.5 kg) and **very low birth weight** (<1.5 kg) have been shown to be significantly more frequent with IVF than in spontaneously conceived babies, even correcting for maternal age.[1,2,5,6,7] The risk of low birth weight is nearly doubled and there is a nearly threefold increased risk of very low birth weight babies following IVF compared with spontaneous conceptions. This could be associated to some extent with the increased rates of prematurity.
- **Preterm delivery:** Increased risks of [1,2,5,6,7] in those with subfertility who have conceived singleton pregnancies by IVF and related techniques compared with spontaneously conceived singletons: a twofold increased risk of birth before 37 weeks gestation and a threefold increased risk of birth before 32 weeks.
- **Small for gestational age:** A 40–60% increased risk of SGA in IVF singletons compared with spontaneous singletons.[2,5,7] **Serial growth scans** are therefore indicated.
- **Perinatal mortality:** A threefold increased risk of perinatal death is seen in singleton pregnancies conceived spontaneously but after a long period of infertility, compared with singletons spontaneously conceived without any delay in conception.[5,6,7]
- **Perinatal deaths:** Some studies[6,7,9,15] quote a higher rate (**a four-fold increase**) in singletons conceived by IVF compared with spontaneous conceptions where there has been no undue delay in conception. This might be, to some extent, due to a shortened mean gestational age seen with IVF versus spontaneously conceived singletons. In practice, **IOL at about 40 weeks would seem a logical and reasonable intervention in IVF pregnancies**.

Long-term outcomes

- ***ART itself, after adjustment for confounding factors such as low birth weight and prematurity, does not seem to be related to any increased risk of cerebral palsy***.
- Similarly, current evidence remains either insufficient or inconclusive about any association of ART with childhood malignancies or cardiovascular and metabolic problems in future life.[2]
- ***These issues must be discussed at the time of the first visit to the hospital antenatal clinic if pre-ART information regarding such issues is missing or inadequate***.

Information for patients

Please see Information for patients: Pregnancy conceived by IVF or related techniques (p. 545)

References

1. RCOG Perinatal risks associated with IVF. Scientific Impact Paper No. 8. London: Royal College of Obstetrics and Gynaecology, 2012.
2. Talaulikar VS, Arulkumaran S Maternal, perinatal and long-term outcomes after assisted reproductive techniques (ART): implications for clinical practice. Eur J Obstet Gynecol Reprod Biol 2013;170: 13–19.
3. Rimm AA, et al. A meta-analysis of controlled studies comparing major malformation rates in IVF and ICSI infants with naturally conceived children. J Assist Reprod Genet 2004;21: 437–443.
4. Hansen M, et al. Assisted reproductive technologies and the risk of birth defects: a systematic review. Hum Reprod 2005;20: 328–338.
5. McDonald SD, et al. Perinatal outcomes of singleton pregnancies achieved by in vitro fertilisation: a systematic review and meta-analysis. J Obstet Gynaecol Can 2005;27: 449–459.
6. Helmerhorst FM, et al. Perinatal outcomes of singletons and twins after assisted conception: a systematic review of controlled studies. BMJ 2004;328: 261–265.
7. Jackson RA, et al. Perinatal outcomes in singletons following in vitro fertilisation: a meta-analysis. Obstet Gynecol 2004;103: 551–563.
8. Jaques AM, et al. Adverse obstetric and perinatal outcomes in subfertile women conceiving without assisted reproductive technologies. Fertil Steril 2010;94: 2674–2679.
9. Draper ES, et al. Assessment of separate contributions to perinatal mortality of infertility history and treatment: a case-control analysis. Lancet 1999;353: 1746–1749.
10. Wiggins DA, Main E Outcomes of pregnancies achieved by donor egg in vitro fertilization—a comparison with standard in vitro fertilization pregnancies. Am J Obstet Gynecol 2005;192: 2002–2006.
11. Reddy UM, et al. Infertility, assisted reproductive technology, and adverse pregnancy outcomes: executive summary of a National Institute of Child Health and Human Development workshop. Obstet Gynecol 2007;109: 967–977.
12. Healy DL, et al. Prevalence and risk factors for obstetric haemorrhage in 6730 singleton births after assisted reproductive technology in Victoria Australia. Hum Reprod 2010;25: 265–274.
13. Reefhuis J, et al. Assisted reproductive technology and major structural birth defects in the United States. Hum Reprod 2009;24: 360–366.
14. El-Chaar D, et al. Risk of birth defects increased in pregnancies conceived by assisted human reproduction. Fertil Steril 2009;92: 1557–1561.
15. Wisborg K, et al. IVF and stillbirth: a prospective follow-up study. Hum Reprod 2010;25: 1312–1316.

Pre-pregnancy assessment and counselling

- Detailed history, appropriate referral and optimal control of chronic conditions (e.g. diabetes, hypertension, renal disease, epilepsy, anaemia, etc.); genetic referral if male factor infertility
- Review of drugs (e.g. anticonvulsants, antihypertensives)
- Advice regarding lifestyle factors—healthy diet, cessation of smoking, alcohol, substance abuse cessation, weight management
- Folic acid, vitamin D supplementation
- Rubella status check, vaccination if not immune

↓

GP or community midwife refers woman with **ART-achieved singleton pregnancy** to a specialist antenatal clinic

↓

First visit to specialist antenatal clinic

- Obtain history of any pre-existent hypertension, renal disease, epilepsy, diabetes, other chronic conditions
- Review current medication; changes to be made as necessary, especially antihypertensives
- Ensure patient is on appropriate doses of folic acid and vitamin D, prescribe low-dose aspirin to continue throughout pregnancy
- Scan for viability, dates
- Thromboembolism risk assessment
- Review medications that might have been advised by the IVF unit (e.g. progesterone, LMWH, aspirin 75 mg, etc.)
- Explain **and document** that most pregnancies progress without problems and with good maternal and neonatal outcomes, but a small risk of adverse outcomes such as
  - chromosomal abnormalities
  - congenital malformations
  - premature labour
  - IUGR, therefore serial growth scans indicated.
  - placental dysfunction, and therefore delivery advisable by 40 weeks
  - pre-eclampsia, pregnancy induced hypertension
- Prescribe low-dose aspirin and advise to continue till end of pregnancy, especially if essential hypertension or IVF with egg donation
- GTT at 26–28 weeks if additional risk category (e.g. ethnic origin, obesity, previous polycystic ovarian syndrome)
- Confirm whether patient chooses/declines trisomy screening
- Consider serial scans for about 28, 32, and 36 weeks or according to individual unit's serial scan protocol
- Arrange for specialist antenatal clinic hospital follow-up on same day as scans at 32 and 36 weeks
- Continued community midwife antenatal checks as normal routine avoiding overlap

↓

Further visits to specialist antenatal clinic (at about 32 and 36 weeks, with scan)

- Specify in 20 week anomaly scan request form that it is an IVF pregnancy—careful assessment for congenital anomalies and placental localization. If low-lying placenta, rescan at 34 weeks to establish placental site to guide decision about timing and mode of delivery
- Serial scans for growth, liquor volume—see IUGR care pathway (p. 421) if IUGR suspected
- Assess progress of pregnancy
- Discuss reasons for advising delivery by 40 weeks and with patient's consent, book date for IOL at about 40 weeks, earlier if any fetal growth concerns, pre-eclampsia

↓

Delivery and postpartum

- Recommend intrapartum electronic fetal heart rate monitoring in labour for early detection of potential hypoxia
- Caesarean section for obstetric reasons; decision regarding mode of delivery after thorough discussion of risks and benefits, especially in relation to future pregnancies
- Encourage breastfeeding

23.2 Surrogacy

FACT FILE

- In cases where female infertility is due to uterine factors such as having had a hysterectomy or radical trachelectomy of the cervix, congenital absence of the uterus, or severe abnormalities of the Müllerian duct, or when the health of the woman could be seriously jeopardized by pregnancy and delivery, surrogacy may be an option that couples would like to consider. Increasingly surrogacy has been sought by single-sex couples (e.g. male partners in a civil partnership or marriage).
- **Surrogacy** involves implanting an embryo into the uterus of another woman who will then carry the pregnancy and give birth as a 'surrogate mother'.[1]
- A **surrogate mother** as defined in the British Medical Association report[2] is a woman who carries a fetus and bears the baby on behalf of another person or persons, having agreed to surrender that baby to this or these persons at birth or shortly thereafter. The couple who are intending to parent a child resulting from a surrogate pregnancy are known as the **commissioning parents**.[3,4]
- In the UK, payment for surrogacy is not allowed and is illegal: only the 'reasonable expenses' of the surrogate mother can be compensated. Only altruistic surrogacy is recognized by the law in the UK: that is, where the surrogate mother agrees to carry a baby for reasons other than financial gain.[5]

Types of surrogacy

There are two forms of surrogacy.

Partial (also called 'traditional' surrogacy)

- In **artificial partial surrogacy** the surrogate mother undergoes artificial insemination by the sperm from the commissioning male partner/husband of the infertile woman. The oocyte is supplied by the surrogate mother herself. In such a case the baby is biologically related to the surrogate mother and the commissioning father. In this type of surrogacy, the artificial insemination can be performed in a fertility clinic or at home.
- In **natural partial surrogacy**[3,4] the commissioning father has intercourse with another woman, i.e. the surrogate mother, who thereby donates her oocyte, carries the pregnancy, and gives birth to a child that is genetically and biologically hers.
- In either of the above forms of traditional/partial surrogacy (whether by artificial or natural means), the commissioning woman is a **social mother** till the parental order has been obtained, after which, she is known as the **legal mother**. The commissioning father, though the genetic father of the child, can become the legal father only after the parental order has been completed.

Gestational surrogacy (also known as complete, full, host, or IVF surrogacy

- This form of surrogacy is possible only with the use of assisted conception techniques such as IVF, where embryo/embryos formed in vitro from the egg and sperm of the commissioning couple are transferred into the surrogate mother who is genetically unrelated to the offspring. Gestational surrogacy allows women with clearly defined medical problems to have their own genetic children.

Legal and ethical aspects of surrogacy

- In the UK, surrogacy is a private social arrangement carried out by the commissioning parents and the surrogate mother and, in the case of traditional surrogacy, does not need to be either recorded for data collection or regulated. An estimation of the number of surrogate pregnancies per year can only be derived in the case of gestational surrogacies involving fertility clinics licensed by the Human Fertilization and Embryology Authority (HFEA), as well as the number of couples obtaining the legally required **parental order**. Data about pregnancy from privately arranged traditional surrogacy agreements that do not involve health services (NHS or private sector) or social services are therefore unavailable.
- The UK is one of the few European countries where surrogacy is legal, permitting altruistic but not commercial surrogacy.[3] Gestational surrogacy is fully regulated in the UK.
- There are widely differing laws regarding surrogacy in different countries. There are also considerable variations in the religious and cultural attitudes to surrogacy, as might be expected.
- Before embarking on surrogacy both parties need to be thoroughly counselled about the medical and psychological risks, and legal issues that may be involved. Gestational surrogacy undertaken in a HFEA-licensed fertility unit will be able to benefit from such in-depth counselling.[3]
- As **surrogacy arrangements are not legally binding**, both parties need to draw up a contract involving solicitors; even so, implementation may give rise to a number of legal and ethical challenges, such as:
  - The surrogate mother may decline to give up the baby, especially in partial surrogacy where she is the genetic mother as well.
  - The commissioning couple may decline to take the baby, if he/she is born with physical or mental defects.
  - To what extent can the commissioning couple coerce the surrogate mother to undergo screening or invasive diagnostic procedures such as amniocentesis and then undergo a termination of pregnancy if an abnormality is diagnosed?
  - Can the surrogate mother change her mind and seek pregnancy termination?
  - To what extent can the commissioning couple control the lifestyle of the surrogate mother including smoking, substance and alcohol abuse, etc.?
  - Who makes the decisions during pregnancy, labour, and delivery? If it generally agreed that the surrogate mother has this right in any decision concerning her own health,[2] while the commissioning couple can make those decisions pertaining to the baby exclusively. In reality, there are few occasions where decisions pertain only to the baby and not the pregnant woman.
  - How legally binding can any pre-pregnancy surrogacy agreement be, even one drawn up with the advice and involvement of solicitors? Could they not be challenged on other legal grounds?
- Given the serious ethical and psychological challenges that surrogacy involves, it is surprising to find that only 4% of surrogacy arrangements fail due to the surrogate mother declining to give up the baby.[6,7] Other studies have also found that the emotional bond and affection of the commissioning mother for the baby is the same whether surrogacy was achieved by traditional (partial) or gestational (IVF) methods.[8,9]
- Postpartum depression rates are not increased above average in surrogate mothers.[6,10]
- ***Interestingly, the majority of legal or ethical problems seem to be associated with traditional (partial) surrogacy compared with gestational or host surrogacy.***[3]

The legal standpoint

- ***The surrogate mother is always the legal mother.***[5]
- If the surrogate mother has a partner, he is the legal father unless he can 'show that he did not consent to his wife/ common-law wife being inseminated with the sperms of the biological father', in this case the commissioning male.[5]
- If the insemination treatment took place in a licensed fertility clinic and the surrogate mother does not have a partner, the child is legally fatherless at birth.
- The commissioning couple become legal parents only when they apply for a parental order or apply to adopt the child, even if both are the genetic parents of the baby (in full or gestational surrogacy).

- This would mean that if the commissioning couple changed their minds during a surrogate pregnancy (e.g. due to split-up of their relationship), the surrogate mother and her partner, if she has one, will of necessity be the ones legally responsible and liable for the child.
- A parental order, which is issued only 6 weeks after the baby's birth, has the same legal status as an adoption, only it can be achieved quicker in a case of surrogacy and is obtained by application to the courts. In the interim, the surrogate mother and the commissioning father could sign a **parental responsibility agreement** allowing them equal rights over decisions made for the welfare of baby after birth.
- An application for a parental order must be made within 6 months of the baby's birth. One or both of the commissioning parents must live within the UK and the baby must reside with them.

Medical aspects in a surrogate pregnancy

- ***Clinical pregnancy rates of about 40% per transfer are achieved with gestational surrogacy and 60% of surrogate mothers achieve live birth in IVF surrogacy.***[3]
- There is a risk of transmission of infections such as HIV, Heb B, Hep C, especially with unregulated self-insemination.
- Testing for genetically transmissible conditions is recommended.
- Ideally the surrogate mother should be in a good physical and mental state with no risk factors such as smoking, substance and alcohol abuse, or obesity.
- It is preferable that a potential surrogate mother is not older than 35 years of age and has already had at least one previous delivery, as the risk of complications are far higher in a primigravida.
- Risks involved with a IVF surrogate pregnancy seem to be similar to those of any IVF-derived pregnancy or insemination with the same number of fetuses.[3,4,10,11,12]

Medico-legal aspects of surrogacy

- All those involved in the care of a surrogate pregnancy should be aware of the legal issues surrounding surrogacy as well as the ethical issues that can arise if there are conflicts of interest.[5,13,14]
- The guidelines of the Royal College of Midwives[13] dealing with care of surrogate mothers during pregnancy and birth are equally applicable to obstetricians. Strict confidentiality has to be maintained regarding the individual's surrogacy arrangements, recognizing that her care needs to be the same as that of any pregnant woman, offered with respect and without prejudice.[13,14]
- If any conflict of interest arises between the parties concerned, the legal duty of care for the midwives and doctors should be with the surrogate mother and the baby and not the commissioning parents.[13,14]
- The healthcare professionals should, however, endeavour to build a supportive alliance between the surrogate mother and the commissioning parents, thus ameliorating those situations where a conflict of interests may arise.
- Medico-legal challenges can centre around the issue of consent. A surrogate mother has the legal right to accept or decline any investigation or treatment, as has any other pregnant woman.
- Care must be taken to ensure that the surrogate mother is not being coerced or compelled to give her consent by the commissioning parents. This is specially so when the surrogate mother is a friend or a relative of the commissioning couple.
- The surrogate mother alone has the right to determine what information about the pregnancy could be shared with the commissioning couple and healthcare professionals are duty bound to comply with this. The commissioning couple may have access to the surrogate mother's medical information regarding this pregnancy only with the pregnant woman's explicit consent.[14]
- The surrogate mother, with the advice of healthcare professionals, has the sole right to decide about pain relief in labour, mode of delivery, etc.
- If problems are anticipated with the baby, the paediatricians must be informed in advance, so that they are also aware of the legal aspects. This may help prevent potential risk of breach of confidentiality as well as establishing who has the legal right to participate in decisions that might be required for the neonate's care soon after delivery.
- Legal advice should be sought without delay in rare instances of the surrogate mother wishing to exercise her rights by withholding consent for medically advised interventions during labour, which could result in potential intrapartum or neonatal death or morbidity for the infant.
- In the postnatal period, the question arises about who needs to be consulted about decisions that might be required in the neonate's care especially if the baby is preterm or born in poor condition. If a parental responsibility agreement has not been signed, it is the surrogate mother who has the right to enter into such a decision-making until the baby is 6 weeks old and a parental order has been obtained by the commissioning parents.
- The question of breastfeeding or artificial feeding is preferably resolved by both parties before embarking on the surrogacy arrangement. Healthcare professionals should endeavour to support this previous arrangement, if it is in the best interests of the baby.
- If the surrogate mother does not wish to breastfeed, antilactogenic agents can be offered.
- ***The care of a surrogacy during pregnancy, labour, delivery, and after, presents formidable challenges such that every surrogate pregnancy must be regarded as high-risk.***

References

1. Schenker JG, Frenckel DA. Medico-legal aspects of in-vitro fertilization and embryo transfer practice. Obstet Gynecol Surv 1987;41: 405–413.
2. British Medical Association. Surrogacy: ethical considerations. Report of the Working Party on Human Infertility Services. London: BMA Publications, 1990.
3. Brinsden PR. Gestational surrogacy. Hum Reprod Update 2003;9: 483–491.
4. Schenker JG, Eisenberg VH. Surrogate pregnancies:ethical, social and legal aspects. Prenat Neonat Med 1996;1: 29–37.
5. Bhatia K, et al. Surrogate pregnancy: an essential guide for clinicians. Obstetrician and Gynaecologist 2009;11, 49–54.
6. Jadva, V, et al. Surrogate mothers: motivations, experiences and beyond. Hum Reprod 2003;18: 2196–2204.
7. Fischer S, Gillman, I. Surrogate motherhood: attachment, attitudes and social support. Psychiatry 1991;54: 13–20.
8. Golombok S, et al. Families created through a surrogacy arrangement: parent-child relationships in the first year of life. Dev Psychol 2004;40: 400–411.
9. Ber R. Ethical issues in gestational surrogacy. Theor Med Bioeth 2000;21: 153–169.
10. Söderström-Anttila V, et al. Experience of in-vitro fertilization surrogacy in Finland Acta Obstet Gynecol Scand 2002;81: 747–752.
11. Corson SL, et al. Gestational carrier pregnancy. Fertil Steril 1998;69: 670–674.
12. Parkinson J, et al. Perinatal outcome after in-vitro fertilization-surrogacy. Hum Reprod 1999;14: 671–676.
13. RCM. Surrogacy: Defining motherhood. London: Royal College of Midwives, 1997.
14. ACOG Committee Opinion No 397. Surrogate motherhood. American College of Obstetricians and Gynecologists. Obstet Gynecol 2008;111: 465–470.

23.3 Contraception with Medical Conditions

FACT FILE

- ***Contraceptive advice for those with underlying medical conditions has to be considered with care, taking several factors into account:***
- The underlying medical condition and comorbidities that may be present.
- Potential impact of the specific contraceptive on the underlying medical condition and any comorbidities, if present.
- Medications that are required for certain chronic medical conditions may alter the effectiveness of the contraceptive and vice versa.
- Different dosages and methods of delivery of certain hormonal contraceptives may have different actions and associated risks for an underlying medical disease.
- Efficacy of the contraceptive method is dependent on how consistent the user is with the correct use of the method. For example, the percentage of unplanned pregnancies within the first year of use of combined oral contraceptives (COC), if used 'perfectly' by women is quoted to be 0.3%; however, in reality, with 'typical' use, the failure rate is up to 8%.
- Maternal mortality is known to be significantly higher in women with coexistent medical conditions than in healthy women without such problems. In a few medical conditions, pregnancy is strongly discouraged as the mortality rates approach 50%. It is therefore, of extreme importance that the most effective and reliable contraception is advised as a next unintended pregnancy could result in maternal mortality or severe morbidity.

Increased risk as a result of unintended pregnancy

- Conditions that expose a woman to increased risk are[2]
  - breast cancer
  - complicated valvular heart disease
  - diabetes: insulin-dependent; with nephropathy/retinopathy/neuropathy or other vascular disease; or of more than 20 years duration
  - endometrial or ovarian cancer
  - epilepsy
  - high blood pressure (systolic >160 mmHg or diastolic >100 mmHg)
  - HIV/AIDS
  - ischaemic heart disease
  - malignant gestational trophoblastic disease
  - malignant liver tumours (hepatoma) and hepatocellular carcinoma of the liver
  - schistosomiasis with fibrosis of the liver
  - severe (decompensated) cirrhosis
  - sickle cell disease
  - STI
  - stroke
  - systemic lupus erythematosus (SLE)
  - thrombogenic mutations
  - tuberculosis.

(Reproduced with kind permission from World Health Organization, *Medical Eligibility Criteria for Contraceptive Use*, Fourth Edition, 2009, © 2010 World Health Organization. <http://apps.who.int/iris/handle/10665/44433>.)

- Before deciding on the best contraceptive when there is an underlying medical disease, the following must be considered:[2]
  - efficacy
  - thrombotic risk
  - arterial risk
  - infective risk
  - bleeding risk(for those on anticoagulants)
  - drug interactions
  - ease of use
  - necessity for anaesthetic for application/insertion of the contraceptive or for tubal ligation or occlusion.
- **WHO classifies contraceptive agents into four categories, depending on their suitability for use in coexistent medical disease**[1] (see Table 23.1).

Table 23.1 Medical conditions and choice of contraceptive agents (WHO classes 1–4)

Condition	*COC*	*CIC*	*P/R*	*POP*	*LNG/ETG*	*Cu-IUCD*	*LNG-IUD*
Multiple risk factors for arterial cardiovascular disease (older women, smoking, diabetes, hypertension)	3/4	3/4	3/4	2	2	1	1–2
Hypertension							
(a) BP not regularly evaluated	3	3	3	2	2	1	2
(b) Adequately controlled hypertension with regular BP evaluation	3	3	3	1	1	1	1
(c) Elevated BP levels (properly taken at regular intervals):							
• BP 140–159/90–99	3	3	3	1	1	1	1
• BP ≥160/ ≥100 mmHg	4	4	4	2	2	1	2
(d) Vascular disease	4	4	4	2	2	1	2
History of high BP during pregnancy (current BP is measured and is normal)	2	2	2	1	1	1	1
Known thrombophilias (factor V Leiden, prothromin mutation, protein C, S, and antithrombin deficiencies)	4	4	4	2	2	1	1–2
Current and previous history of ischaemic heart disease	4	4	4	2-3	2–3	1	2–3
Stroke, history of cerebrovascular accident	4	4	4	2–3	2–3	1	2
Valvular heart disease							
(a) Uncomplicated	2	2	2	1	1	1	1
(b) Complicated (pulmonary hypertension, risk of atrial fibrillation)	4	4	4	1	1	2	2

Table 23.1 Medical conditions and choice of contraceptive agents (WHO classes 1–4) (*continued*)

Condition	*COC*	*CIC*	*P/R*	*POP*	*LNG/ETG*	*Cu-IUCD*	*LNG-IUD*
Systemic lupus erythematosus							
(a) With positive APS antibodies	4	4	4	3	3	1–1	3
(b) Severe thrombocytopenia	2	2	2	2	2	3–2	2
(c) Immunosuppressive treatment	2	2	2	2	2	2–1	2
(d) None of the above	2	2	2	2	2	1–1	2
Epilepsy							
Not on any treatment	1	1	1	1	1	1	1
On anticonvulsants:							
(a) Phenytoin, carbamazepine, topiramate, primidone, barbiturates	3	2	3	3	2	1	1
(b) Lamotrigine	3	3	3	1	1	1	1
History of cholestasis							
(a) Pregnancy related	2	2	2	1	1	1	1
(b) Past COC related	3	2	3	2	2	1	2
Diabetes							
(a) History of gestational disease	1	1	1	1	1	1	1
(b) Non-vascular disease	2	2	2	2	2	1	2
(c) Nephropathy/ retinopathy/neuropathy	3–4	3–4	3–4	2	2	1	2
(d) Other vascular disease or disease of >20 years duration	3–4	3–4	3-4	2	2	1	2
Thyroid disorders							
(a) Simple goitre	1	1	1	1	1	1	1
(b) Hyperthyroid	1	1	1	1	1	1	1
(c) Hypothyroid	1	1	1	1	1	1	1
Uterine fibroids							
(a) That distort the uterine cavity	1	1	1	1	1	4	4
(b) That do not distort the uterine cavity	1	1	1	1	1	1	1
Haemoglobinopathy							
(a) Thalassaemia	1	1	1	1	1	2	1
(b) Sickle cell disease	2	2	2	1	1	2	1

COC, combined oral contraceptive; CIC, combined injectable contraceptive; P/R, combined contraceptive patch/combined contraceptive vaginal ring; POP, progesterone-only pill; LNG/ETG, levonorgestrel and etonogestrel implant; Cu-IUCD, copper intrauterine contraceptive device; LNG-IUD, levonorgestrel-releasing intrauterine contraceptive device.

Adapted with kind permission from World Health Organization, *Medical Eligibility Criteria for Contraceptive Use*, Fourth Edition, 2009, © 2010 World Health Organization. <http://apps.who.int/iris/handle/10665/44433>. Data from Dhanjal MK, Contraception in women with medical problems, *Obstetric Medicine*, 2008, 1, pp. 78–87.

- **Class 1:** A condition for which there is no restriction for the use of the contraceptive method.
- **Class 2:** A condition where the advantages of using the method generally outweigh the theoretical or proven risks.
- **Class 3:** A condition where the theoretical or proven risks usually outweigh the advantages of using the method.
- **Class 4:** A condition which represents an unacceptable health risk if the contraceptive method is used.

(Reproduced with kind permission from World Health Organization, *Medical Eligibility Criteria for Contraceptive Use*, Fourth Edition, 2009, © 2010 World Health Organization. <http://apps.who.int/iris/handle/10665/44433>.)

References

1. WHO. Improving access to quality care in family planning. Medical eligibility criteria for contraceptive use, 4th ed. Geneva: World Health Organization, 2009.
2. Dhanjal MK. Contraception in women with medical problems. Obstet Med 2008;1: 78–87.

24 Other Maternal Conditions

24.1 Unbooked Pregnancies or Poor Attenders

FACT FILE

- About 1% of women who deliver in the UK do so without having had any antenatal care.[1,2]
- All maternity care, including the antenatal, intrapartum, and postnatal period, is free to all who have a legal right to free NHS services. This includes not only the pregnancy and postnatal care but also free prescriptions and dental care during pregnancy and for 1 year after childbirth.
- This is in stark contrast to several countries in the world where the costs of paying for medical care during pregnancy and childbirth from one's own pocket, or through medical insurance, are prohibitive. In other countries the long travel and distances involved that make medical services less accessible are factors that deter women from seeking antenatal care.
- A small minority of women do not access the high-standard pregnancy services that are free in countries such as UK and Finland, where travel distances and available modes of transport do not generally pose any serious problems. Reasons for those who either book late or not at all or are serial non-attenders at antenatal clinics are very varied.[1,2,3]

Patient profile

- In the group of women who are unbooked, book late in pregnancy, or miss several antenatal appointments, there is an over-representation of those who are young (teenagers), of low socio-economic status, low levels of education, unemployed, single unsupported status, high parity, alcohol and substance abusers, and immigrant women from ethnic non-English-speaking backgrounds.[2,4,5,6,7,8,9]
- The incidence of domestic violence in this vulnerable group of women must also be considered as a contributory factor.[10,11]

Outcomes

- What these varied groups have in common, however, is the fact that they share the risk of adverse pregnancy outcomes, both maternal and perinatal.
- *Saving Mothers' Lives* (2007)[4] highlighted the fact that vulnerable women are at higher risk of death during or after pregnancy than other women. The vulnerable women with socially complex lives who died were far less likely to seek antenatal care early in pregnancy or to stay in regular contact with maternity services. Overall, 17% of the women who died from direct or indirect causes had booked for maternity care after 22 weeks of gestational age or had missed more than four routine antenatal visits, compared with 2% of the general population.
- **Pregnancy complications** in these women include increased rates of preterm births, low birth weight, stillbirths, chorioamnionitis, abruption, and neonatal deaths as well as maternal mortality due to severe pre-eclampsia/eclampsia, overwhelming sepsis, uterine rupture, major placental abruption, PPH, pulmonary embolism, or arterial thrombosis.[1,4,12]
- Recent NICE guidelines (2010)[13] address the complex and multiagency involvement and planning needed to help improve accessibility of maternity services to these socially disadvantaged groups.

References

1. Raatikainen K, et al. Under-attending free antenatal care is associated with adverse pregnancy outcomes. BMC Public Health. 2007;7: 268.
2. Tucker A, et al. The unbooked mother: a cohort study of maternal and fetal outcomes in a North London Hospital. Arch Gynecol Obstet 2010;281: 613–616.
3. Macfarlane A. Birth counts: statistics of pregnancy and childbirth, Volume I. London: The Stationery Office, 2000.
4. CEMACH. Saving mothers' lives: reviewing maternal deaths to make motherhood safer—2003–2005. The Seventh Report of the Confidential Enquiries into Maternal Deaths in the United Kingdom. London: CEMACH, 2007.
5. Kupek E, et al. Clinical, provider and socio-demographic predictors of late initiation of antenatal care in England and Wales. BJOG 2002;109: 265–273.
6. McCaw-Binns A, et al. Under-users of antenatal care: a comparison of non-attenders and late attenders for antenatal care, with early attenders. Soc Sci Med 1995;40: 1003–1012.
7. Delvaux T, et al. Barriers to prenatal care in Europe. Am J Prev Med 2001;21: 52–59.
8. Murray L, et al. Self-exclusion from health care in women at high risk for postpartum depression. J Public Health Med 2003;25: 131–137.
9. Herbst MA, et al. Relationship of prenatal care and perinatal morbidity in low-birth-weight infants. Am J Obstet Gynecol 2003;189: 930–933.
10. Berenson AB. Perinatal morbidity associated with violence experienced by pregnant women. Am J Obstet Gynecol 1994;170: 1760–1766.
11. Yost NP, et al. A prospective observational study of domestic violence during pregnancy. Obstet Gynecol 2005;106: 61–65.
12. Treacy A, et al. Perinatal outcome in unbooked women at the Rotunda Hospital. Ir Med J 2000;95: 44–47.
13. NICE guideline. Pregnancy and complex social factors: a model for service provision for pregnant women with complex social factors. CG110. London: National Collaborating Centre for Women's and Children's Health, 2010.

24.2 Teenage Pregnancies

FACT FILE

This fact file addresses only the obstetric and perinatal aspects of **early teenage pregnancies (<15 years of age)** as the other aspects, though crucial, are beyond the remit of this volume.

- The UK has the highest teenage pregnancy rate in western Europe.
- Teenage pregnancies represent very complex challenges involving socio-economic, educational, political, and social factors as well as medical and mental health issues.
- Pregnancies in young teenagers are well recognized to be associated with increased risks of pregnancy complications such as preterm labour, IUGR, pre-eclampsia, anaemia, chorioamnionitis, neonatal morbidity and mortality, and continuing health and social problems facing the offspring.[1,2,3,4,5,6,7,8]
- The risk of maternal mortality in teenage pregnancies was highlighted in the Confidential Enquiry into Maternal Death Report of 2001[9] where there were 14 deaths of teenage mothers less than 18 years, of which 5 were in girls under 15 years of age. High rates of domestic violence, poor attendance at antenatal clinics or late booking of pregnancy, and homelessness were noted.
- Smoking rates are particularly high in teenage girls and in pregnant teenage girls compared with pregnant older mothers.[10,11] Smoking is recognized to have a dose-related impact on placental abruption and fetal and neonatal problems including decreased birth weight and preterm birth.[12]
- While a marked fall has been observed in fetal growth after 36 weeks gestation in pregnant adolescents who smoke, at least 10% of adolescent smokers have pregnancies affected by severe and early growth restriction even before 32 weeks gestation.[13]
- Multifactorial influences, such as gynaecological immaturity, associated smoking, alcohol and substance abuse, poor nutrition, and inadequate usage of antenatal services,[1,14,15] all contribute to the poor outcomes seen in teenage pregnancy.[16] It is difficult to separate biological factors, lifestyles, and socio-economic conditions in this context.[14,17]
- Correcting for smoking and for poor use of antenatal services as confounding factors, two studies showed that, after multiple logistic regression analyses, no significantly increased risk of poor perinatal outcomes was found in teenage pregnancies.[16,18] This has been refuted by other studies which found that the increased risk of adverse perinatal outcomes remains independent of confounding factors such as smoking, poor nutrition, or non-attendance for antenatal care.[19,20]
- Pregnancy at the stage of incomplete gynaecological maturity can impose a competition for essential nutritional supply between the teenage mother's own growth requirements and that of the developing fetus.[19,21,22]
- Such a competitive biological environment compounded by smoking and poor nutrition, invariably seen in this group of pregnant mothers, can have an adverse effect on the feto-placental unit.
- Some teenagers may have poor eating habits, neglect to take any supplements such as folic acid or iron, and are less likely to gain an adequate amount of weight during pregnancy.[22]
- Other risks faced by teenage mothers include that of sexually transmitted diseases, especially gonorrhoea, herpes, and chlamydia.[23,24]
- Teenagers, especially those in the older teen group (17–19 years of age), have been found, in several studies, to have lower Caesarean section and vaginal operative deliveries compared with adults.[7,10]
- Postnatal depression, problems with breastfeeding, and repeated pregnancies in the teenage years are also more likely in this group.[25]
- Every effort must be made to offer effective contraceptive advice to teenage mothers both in the hospital and in primary care, addressing not only contraceptive requirements but also prevention of sexually transmitted diseases.

Targeted antenatal care

- Active encouragement from primary health care professionals to attend antenatal clinics. These, if possible and resources permitting, may be midwifery led, located in the community after school hours, and meant for young pregnant teenagers who would otherwise might be reluctant to attend hospital-based antenatal clinics. Once their trust and confidence has improved, they may show greater willingness to attend hospital clinics, should any problems be identified in the community.[21]
- Gestational age must be confirmed by scan as soon as possible. Unfortunately as many of these young mothers are late bookers or poor attenders, the opportunities for first-trimester scan and folic acid supplementation during the first trimester are often lost.
- At the first visit, improved nutrition and issues concerned with smoking, alcohol, or substance abuse must be explored and advice regarding support for cessation offered. Family set-up and support available must be explored.
- Though not usually feasible during the first antenatal check, enquiry must be made into any domestic violence or housing issues.
- Early referral to social services is important and is usually initiated in primary care. Confirmation by midwifery and/or medical staff in the hospital that such a referral has been made (especially in those <15 years of age) is advisable.
- Information regarding pregnancy care and labour and delivery must be presented in a format that appeals to and can be understood by young teenagers.
- All interaction must be devoid of judgemental or patronizing overtones.
- Vigilance must be maintained for the development of pre-eclampsia, fetal growth restriction, preterm labour, etc.
- The young mother should be instructed to report symptoms that may be suggestive of pre-eclampsia, abruption, preterm labour, preterm rupture of membranes, etc.
- If IUGR is suspected on clinical examination, further management should follow the same guidelines as in the adult pregnant woman.
- If there are signs of obvious maternal undernutrition ± smoking, serial growth scans may be required.
- The care of teenage pregnancy and after must be essentially multidisciplinary with good mutual communication.

References

1. Fraser AM, et al. Association of young maternal age with adverse reproductive outcomes. N Engl J Med 1995;332: 1113.
2. Scholl TO, et al. Prenatal care and maternal health during adolescent pregnancy: a review and meta-analysis. J Adolesc Health 1994;15: 444–456.
3. Miller HS, et al. Adolescence and very low birthweight infants: a disproportionate association. Obstet Gynecol 1996;87: 83–88.
4. Olausson PO, et al. Teenage pregnancies and risk of late fetal death and infant mortality. Br J Obstet Gynaecol 1999;106: 116–121.
5. Knoje JC, et al. Early teenage pregnancy in Hull. Br J Obstet Gynaecol 1992;99: 969–973.
6. Nebot M, et. Adolescent motherhood and socio-economic factors. An ecological approach. Eur J Public Health 1997;7: 144–148.
7. Jolly MC, et al. Obstetric risks of pregnancy in women less than 18 years old. Obstet Gynecol 2000;96: 962–966.
8. van der Klis KA, et al. Teenage pregnancy:trends, characteristics and outcomes in South Australia and Australia. Aust N Z J Public Health 2002;26: 125–131.
9. CEMACH. Why mothers die 1997–1999. The Confidential Enquiries into Maternal Deaths in the United Kingdom. London: RCOG Press, 2001.
10. Lao TT, Ho LF. Obstetric outcome of teenage pregnancies. Hum Reprod 1998;13: 3228–3232.
11. Lee KS, et al. Maternal age and incidence of low birth weight at term a population study Am J Obstet Gynecol 1998;158: 84–89.

12. Kyrklund-Blomberg NB, Cnattingius S. Preterm birth and maternal smoking: risks related to gestational age and onset of delivery. Am J Obstet Gynecol 1998;179: 1051–1055.
13. Delpisheh A, et a. Adolescent smoking in pregnancy and birth outcomes. Eur J Public Health 2006;16: 168–172.
14. Amini SB, et al. Births to teenagers: trends and obstetric outcomes. Obstet Gynecol 1996;87: 668–674.
15. Ukil D, Esen UI. Early teenage pregnancy outcome: a comparison between a standard and a dedicated teenage antenatal clinic. J Obstet Gynaecol 2002;22: 270–272.
16. Smith GC, Pell JP. Teenage pregnancy and risk of adverse perinatal outcomes associated with first and second births: population based retrospective cohort study. BMJ 2001;323: 476.
17. Chandra PC, et al. Pregnancy outcomes in urban teenagers. Int J Gynaecol Obstet 2002;79: 117–122.
18. Raatikainen K, et al. Good outcome of teenage pregnancies in high-quality maternity care Eur J Public Health 2006;16: 157–161.
19. Chen X-K., et al. Teenage pregnancy and adverse birth outcomes: a large population based retrospective cohort study. Int. J. Epidemiol 2007;36: 368–373.
20. Horgan RP, Kenny LC. Management of teenage pregnancy. Obstetrician and Gynaecologist 2007;9: 153–158.
21. Baker P, et al. Teenage pregnancy and reproductive health. RCOG Summary Review. London: RCOG Press, 2007.
22. Kircgengast S, Hartmann B. Impact of maternal age and maternal somatic characteristics on newborn size. Am J Hum Biol 2003;15: 220–228.
23. Martin IMC, Ison CA . Rise in gonorrhoea in London, UK. Lancet 2000;355: 623.
24. Wiesenfeld HC, et al. Self-collection of vaginal swabs for the detection of Chlamydia, gonorrhea, and trichomoniasis: opportunity to encourage sexually transmitted disease testing among adolescents. Sex Transm Dis 2001;28: 321–325.
25. Motil KJ, et al. Lactational performance of adolescent mothers shows preliminary differences from that of adult women. J Adolesc Health 1997;20: 442–449.

24.3 Women Declining Blood or Blood Products, Jehovah's Witnesses

FACT FILE

This fact file deals mainly with the multidisciplinary planning and preparation for labour, delivery, and postpartum required in **the antenatal period** for women who **decline blood or blood transfusion products**. The ethical and legal aspects as well as actual intrapartum techniques are mentioned only briefly as they are not the primary focus of this fact file.

- Women who decline blood and blood products may do so on religious grounds (Jehovah's Witnesses) or because they fear the risk of blood-transmitted infections.
- Among these groups, variation may exist in what is acceptable to some women but not to others. The degree of risk that a woman may be willing to accept under varying circumstances can also differ and it is crucial that various scenarios are discussed and the woman's opinion and wishes documented accordingly.
- Some women may not be aware that immunoglobulin products such as anti-D are derived from human blood products, as are clotting factors.
- While autologous blood transfusion may be acceptable to those who decline blood or blood products because of fear of infection, this may not be so for some Jehovah's Witnesses.
- By UK law, a woman who is competent may voluntarily and autonomously decline any treatment even if it leads to her death.[1] Also, no one can refuse treatment on behalf of another competent individual (e.g. a relative cannot make decisions regarding refusal or acceptance of blood as long as the woman is deemed competent).
- Advance directives to decline blood/blood products are legally valid and to breach them would amount to assault/battery.[2]
- Although the woman may have expressed her wish and/or has drawn up an **advance directive** to decline blood or blood products during antenatal discussions, she might autonomously change her mind during an emergency situation without any coercion from relatives or from the professionals caring for her. Provided she is deemed capable of giving consent and coercion can be excluded, her willingness to accept blood/blood products under these circumstances must be documented and will supersede her opinion expressed in the antenatal period.
- It must be recognized that even among Jehovah's Witnesses, individuals may vary in their beliefs and willingness to accept different degrees of risk. It is important that these parameters are discussed on an individual case-by-case basis rather than just assuming that the Watch Tower Society's blood policy is acceptable to all members of the Jehovah's Witness denomination.[3]

Antenatal management

- Antenatal counselling should involve frank and open discussions. Exploring the woman's beliefs and preferences under various scenarios and meticulous documentation of her choices is mandatory.
- Multidisciplinary planning by involving senior obstetrician, anaesthetist, and haematologist as well as the Patient Advisory Liaison Service (and the NHS Trust's legal team, if necessary), is essential.

Pre-pregnancy

- Ideally, women who have been identified in primary care as those likely to decline blood/blood products, and are planning to get pregnant should have their haemoglobin checked and all efforts made to optimize the levels before commencing a pregnancy.
- Insight provided from primary care colleagues as to the extent the woman's preferences are influenced by those of her partner/family or other members of the Jehovah's Witnesses would be invaluable in subsequent discussions during pregnancy.
- ***If the woman is on anticoagulants or has an inherited coagulation disorder, she should ideally be referred for formal pre-pregnancy counselling.***
- Likewise, women with other risk factors for postpartum haemorrhage such as those who have had previous PPH, grand multiparity, fibroid uterus, previous pregnancy where morbid adherence of the placenta had been identified, previous multiple Caesarean sections, previous classical uterine incision, etc. should preferably be identified in the community and referred for pre-pregnancy counselling.

At the booking visit

- It is essential that all women are asked at their booking visit whether they have any views regarding receiving blood/blood products in an emergency situation. If the woman declines, enquiry should be made (and documented) into her grounds for declining blood/blood products.
- Such a pregnancy comes into the high-risk category and she must be referred to a specialist clinic to see the consultant obstetrician.[2]
- Those who are Rhesus negative must receive information that anti-D immunoglobulin is derived from human blood products and the implications of not receiving it during pregnancy/postpartum.
- Similarly when routine 'booking bloods' are taken, the significance of 'group and save' must be clearly discussed. If the woman wishes to avoid this, her informed decision must be respected.[2]

Specialist antenatal clinic consultations

- It is essential to establish the relationship of any person accompanying the pregnant woman by polite enquiry. The woman's preferences might be less than autonomous and heavily influenced by her 'companion' in some cases. Additional insight may be provided by primary care professionals.
- Discussion should encompass detailing those situations during childbirth or postpartum which may normally warrant blood transfusions. The extent to which the individual is prepared to take the risk, including that of mortality, under varying circumstances, must be ascertained and documented.
- In Rhesus-negative patients, it is essential they understand the implications for a subsequent pregnancy of declining anti-D immunoglobulin, a blood-derived product
- The implications of declining blood must be discussed. A 6% rate of postpartum haemorrhage has been established in studies of obstetric outcomes in Jehovah's Witnesses.[4,5] Various large reports including the Confidential Enquiries into Maternal Mortality have shown a 44-fold to 100-fold increased risk of death in women declining blood compared with the general population.[4,5,6]
- The grounds for her declining blood or blood products must be explored. If it is fear of infection, explain that since 2006 donated blood undergoes **leucodepletion** to reduce the risk of infection, and anyone who has received a blood transfusion since 1980 is excluded from the pool of donors to further minimize the chances of CJD.[2]
- Every attempt must be made to improve iron stores to avoid anaemia. Oral iron (e.g. ferrous sulfate) is sufficient in most cases, but where anaemia is discovered late in pregnancy or if the woman is resistant to or unable to tolerate oral iron, IV iron–sucrose complex may be required to produce a more rapid rise of haemoglobin.[7]
- Joint multidisciplinary plans [8] must be discussed with the patient and her partner and input obtained from the anaesthetist, haematologist and blood bank, interventional radiologist, and intensivist as well as the patient's GP and community midwife.
- The woman must be referred to the anaesthetic high-risk clinic and close communication maintained with the anaesthetists.[9] A clear management plan can then be devised and shared with the patient and all those involved in her care.[10]
- Ultrasound identification of the placental site is essential to exclude placenta praevia in such cases. If there is a suspicion that an anterior placenta praevia may be morbidly adherent to

a previous uterine scar, MRI may help to clarify this.[11] If placenta praevia or accreta are detected, further discussion with the woman at this point is advisable. The woman may review her objections to accepting blood/blood products when presented with this information.

- Similarly, other risk factors, such as heritable clotting disorders, or if the woman is on anticoagulants or has a multiple pregnancy, or has fibroids (especially if intramural or submucous in location), must be identified and the patient counselled accordingly.
- If, on the other hand, there is no change to her declining blood transfusion, it may be safer to recommend that delivery is organized at a tertiary referral centre with access to interventional radiology, recombinant factor VII, and level 3 intensive care facilities as well as cell salvage if the patient is willing to accept this.
- Antenatal discussion regarding her stance on blood conservation techniques such as intraoperative cell salvage and infusion of the salvaged blood[12,13] should take place and be clearly documented in the case notes.[14,15]
- Women who decline blood/blood products must be encouraged to complete an advance directive, which is a legally binding document.[2]
- Instructions regarding proactive intrapartum/postpartum measures such as insertion of a wide-bore Venflon and blood sent for urgent FBC check once labour is established, active management of third stage,[16] prompt suturing of any perineal trauma, early recourse to surgical techniques such as balloon tamponade (e.g. the Rusch intrauterine balloon or the Bakri SOS balloon for multiple complex vaginal tears) or the B-Lynch suture, access to interventional radiology,[17,18] etc. must be clearly documented in both the patient's hand-held and hospital notes.
- A longer-acting oxytocin derivative, **carbetocin**, is licensed in the UK and Ireland and several European countries specifically for the prevention of PPH in the context of Caesarean section or women at risk of PPH.[19,20,21,22,23]
- Carbetocin is a long-acting synthetic analogue of oxytocin with a half-life of 30 min (vs 1.5 min for syntocinon).
- ***For PPH prophylaxis, a single injection of 100 micrograms carbetocin given as a slow IM injection over 1 min after delivery of the placenta has been shown to be twice as effective as 8 h of syntocinon infusion.***[24]
- Carbetocin has been shown to provide more sustained uterine contractions after delivery of the placenta, and also increases the amplitude of contractions.[24]
- Carbetocin has been shown to reduce the need for repeat syntocinon bolus injections as well as of blood transfusion.[24,25]
- ***Carbetocin may therefore be the ideal prophylactic uterotonic agent in Jehovah's Witnesses.***
- Communication with senior midwifery colleagues to ensure availability of carbetocin and of tamponade balloons in delivery suite is essential.
- If interventional radiology facilities are locally available, the radiologist must be kept informed during pregnancy and labour.
- It is recommended that the woman is seen by both a consultant obstetrician and a consultant anaesthetist at the onset of labour in order to decide on a final plan with the patient.[8]

References

1. ReT (Adult: Refusal of Medical Treatment) All Eng Law Rep 1992;4: 649–670.
2. Currie J, et al. Management of women who decline blood and blood products in pregnancy. Obstetrician and Gynaecologist 2010;12: 13–20.
3. Elder L. Why some Jehovah's Witnesses accept blood and conscientiously reject official Watchtower Society blood policy. J Med Ethics 2000;26: 375–380.
4. Singla A, et al. Are women who are Jehovah's witnesses at risk of maternal death? Am J Obstet Gynecol 2001;185: 893–895.
5. Massiah N, et al. Obstetric care of Jehovah's Witnesses: a 14-year observational study. Arch Gynecol Obstet 2007;276: 339–343.
6. Hibbard BM, et al., ed. Report on Confidential Enquiries into Maternal Deaths in the United Kingdom 1991–1993. London: HMSO, 1996, pp. 32–44.
7. Al-Momen A, et al. Intravenous iron sucrose complex in the treatment of iron deficiency anaemia during pregnancy. Eur J Obstet Gynecol Reprod Biol 1996;69: 121–124.
8. Lewis G, ed. Saving mothers' lives: reviewing maternal deaths to make motherhood safer, 2003-2000. The Seventh Report of the Confidential Enquiries into Maternal Deaths in the United Kingdom. London: CEMACH, 2007.
9. OAA/AAGBI. Guidelines of obstetric anaesthetic services, revised ed. London: Obstetric Anaesthetists' Association/Association of Anaesthetists of Great Britain and Ireland, 2005, p. 25
10. AAGB. The management of anaesthesia for Jehovah's Witnesses, 2nd ed. London: Association of Anaesthetists of GB and Ireland, 2005.
11. Warshak CR, et al. Accuracy of ultrasonography and magnetic resonance imaging in the diagnosis of placenta accrete. Obstet Gynecol 2006;108: 573–581.
12. NICE Interventional. Procedure Guidance 144 Intraoperative blood salvage in obstetrics. London: National Institute of Health and Clinical Excellence, 2005.
13. British Committee for Standards in Haematology Blood Transfusion Task Force. Guidelines for the clinical use of red cell transfusion. Br J Haematol 2001;113: 24–31.
14. Hall M. Guidelines for management and treatment of obstetric haemorrhage in women who decline blood transfusion. In: Lewis G, Drife J, ed. Why mothers die 2000–2002. The Sixth Report of the Confidential Enquiries into Maternal Deaths in the United Kingdom. London: RCOG Press 2004, pp. 94–95.
15. RCOG Green-top Guideline No. 47. Blood transfusion in obstetrics. London: Royal College of Obstetricians and Gynaecologists, 2008.
16. Prendiville WJ, et al. Active versus expectant management in the third stage of labour. Cochrane Database Syst Rev 2009; 3.
17. RCOG Good Practice Series 6. The role of emergency and elective interventional radiology in postpartum haemorrhage. London: Royal College of Obstetricians and Gynaecologists, 2007.
18. Yoong W, et al. Balloon tamponade for postpartum vaginal lacerations in a woman refusing blood transfusion. Int J Gynecol Obstet 2009;106: 261.
19. Dansereau J, et al. Double-blind comparison of carbetocin versus oxytocin in prevention of uterine atony after cesarean section. Am J Obstet Gynecol 1999;180 (3 Pt 1): 670–676.
20. Boucher M, et al. Comparison of carbetocin and oxytocin for the prevention of postpartum hemorrhage following vaginal delivery: a double-blind randomized trial. J Obstet Gynaecol Can 2004;26: 481–488.
21. Attilakos G., et al. Carbetocin versus oxytocin for the prevention of postpartum haemorrhage following caesarean section: the results of a double-blind randomised trial. BJOG 2010;117: 929–936.
22. Leung SW, et al. A randomized trial of carbetocin versus Syntometrine in the management of the third stage of labour. BJOG 2006;113: 1459–1464.
23. Su LL, et al. Oxytocin agonists for preventing postpartum hemorrhage. Cochrane Database Syst Rev 2007;3: CD005457.
24. Farine D. Prevention of postpartum haemorrhage. Oral presentation and abstract at the 17th World Congress on Obstetrics, Gynecology and Infertility (COGI), Lisbon, 2012.
25. Leduc D, et al. SOGC Clinical Practice Guideline No. 235. Active management of the third stage of labour: prevention and treatment of postpartum hemorrhage. Ottawa: Society of Obstetricians and Gynaecologists of Canada, 2009.

CARE PATHWAY

Pre-pregnancy

- Optimization of haemoglobin in primary care prior to pregnancy
- Referral to specialists for pre-pregnancy counselling if additional risk factors—e.g. anticoagulants, inherited clotting disorders, grand multiparity, previous PPH, previous multiple Caesarean sections, previous morbid adherence of placenta, fibroid uterus, etc.

↓

Booking visit

- **Establish and document reasons for declining blood**—religious grounds or fear of blood-transmitted infections?
- Attempt to ascertain how much of the decision is autonomous or influenced by others
- Before taking routine booking bloods, explain purpose of sample sent for group and save. If patients declines G&S, document and highlight in notes
- If known to be Rh(D) −ve, enquire whether or not she has received anti-D immunoglobulin in previous pregnancy and postpartum, as this is a blood-derived product. **Document in notes**
- Refer to see consultant obstetrician in a specialist antenatal clinic

↓

In specialist antenatal clinic

- Enquire politely about relationship of accompanying person to patient. Also note any information provided by primary care
- Explore whether she is declining blood due to religious grounds or fear of acquiring infection. If the latter, explain that since 2006, leucodepletion carried out in processing donated blood, thus significantly reducing infection risks
- Discuss scenarios during and after childbirth that may arise when rapid blood transfusion could be lifesaving to the mother and the baby. Explanation to include the fact that women who decline blood have a 44-fold to 100-fold increased risk of death compared to general population
- Explore limits of what is acceptable or not to patient, e.g. cell salvage, autologous transfusion, etc. **Document in notes**
- Encourage her to complete an advance directive
- If she is Rh (D) −ve, and declines anti-D, explain implications of alloimmunization in this or a future pregnancy. **Document discussion**
- Organize multidisciplinary input from consultant anaesthetist, haematologist, interventional radiology, senior midwifery staff
- Ascertain location of placenta and if previous Caesarean sections and anterior low-lying placenta, MRI for possible placenta accreta
- If other high risk factors are present (e.g. multiple pregnancy, placenta praevia, possible morbid adherence of placenta, if patient has a blood clotting disorder, or is on anticoagulant therapy), discuss even greater risk of massive PPH and mortality if patient declines blood transfusion. Consider arranging delivery in a tertiary unit with access to interventional radiology, cell salvage, etc.
- **Optimize iron stores**. If intolerance or resistance to oral iron, consider iron–sucrose IV infusion
- Ensure Rusch and/or Bakri balloons are available in delivery suite for tamponade in case of PPH
- **Documentation in notes** to include instructions for labour and delivery:
  - Active management of third stage. **Consider carbetocin 100 micrograms as a slow IM injection over 1 min** after delivery of placenta, rather than o bolus. If carbetocin unavailable, after oxytocin or oxytocin with ergometrine bolus in third stage, high-dose oxytocin infusion to follow for several hours
  - Patient not to be left unattended for at least 1 hour after delivery, frequent checks of uterine tone, excess lochia, vital signs mandatory
  - Prompt institution of medical uterotonics, B-Lynch suture or Rusch intrauterine tamponade balloon insertion if atonic uterus or Bakri balloon if multiple complex vaginal tears
  - Consultant obstetrician, anaesthetist, senior midwifery staff to be closely involved and kept updated throughout
  - **Interventional radiologist availability and contact to be documented** if service available locally
- Inform the patient that despite her advance directive prepared during pregnancy, should she, in the case of an emergency at childbirth or after delivery, change her mind regarding blood transfusion and if she is conscious and competent to give consent without coercion, this would override the advance directive and she would then be given the necessary blood/blood products

24.4 Antidepressants, Anxiolytics, and Antipsychotics During Pregnancy and Lactation

FACT FILE

- This fact file aims to address the common clinical situation of women who are already on antidepressants, anxiolytics, or antipsychotic medication and have concerns about the safety of these medications during pregnancy and breastfeeding. General principles and advice regarding some commonly used drugs are addressed but the list is not exhaustive.
- The multidisciplinary management of antenatal and postnatal mental health problems is of great importance but outside the remit of this book. The reader is referred to the NICE guidelines[1] for comprehensive information, including individualized treatment for different mental health diseases.

Antidepressants

General principles

- Depression in pregnancy and during breastfeeding is a common problem.
- Treatment mainly involves pharmacotherapy and/or psychotherapy.
- Antidepressants including selective serotonin reuptake inhibitors (SSRIs) and serotonin norepinephrine reuptake inhibitors (SNRIs) are the most commonly used drugs.
- Most antidepressants can take 3 weeks to 3 months before the full benefit is perceived.
- Many pregnant or recently delivered women may be reluctant to take antidepressant medication for fear of any harm being caused to the developing fetus or the breastfed baby.
- Clinicians may be uncertain about the safety of some antidepressants during pregnancy or breastfeeding and therefore reluctant to prescribe them.
- ***Exposure to any class of antidepressants is not on its own, grounds for termination of pregnancy.***[2]
- Women usually stop their antidepressant medication abruptly as soon as they realize they are pregnant. In this group, up to 75% may develop a recurrence of depression before delivery.[3,4] Careful assessment of the relative risks may be required to reassure women that continuing with the medication may be appropriate.
- Relapse rates are high if the medication is abruptly discontinued.[5]
- Anxiety and depression, if unrecognized and untreated, can have significant impact on the well-being of the mother as well as in her bonding with the baby.
- Very careful assessments should include the risk of self-harm or suicide.
- The risks of not treating or discontinuing antidepressant treatment must be balanced against the fetal risks on an individual case-by-case basis.[6,7]
- All SSRIs and SNRIs can be transmitted through the placenta in varying degrees.
- Sertraline and its metabolite as well as paroxetine (which has no active metabolite) are transmitted at lower rate than fluoxetine and its metabolite norfluoxetine.[6]
- The present recommendation is to continue whichever antidepressant medication that has been found to be most suitable and effective to the individual woman throughout pregnancy.[1]
- It is further recommended that an antidepressant the woman has responded to favourably before pregnancy is not routinely changed during pregnancy.[1]
- Treatment with a single antidepressant is preferable to the use of multiple drugs.
- Some studies[8,9] have found a link between maternal antenatal depression and shorter gestational length and lower birth weight, although there is no consensus about this.

Recommendations from NICE guidelines

NICE recommendations regarding prescribing antidepressants pre-pregnancy, during pregnancy, and during lactation include the following:[1]

- In women with mild–moderate depression, non-pharmacological approaches such as cognitive behavioural therapy and self-help strategies such as computerized cognitive therapy are to be considered.
- If the signs of depression appear to have receded before a pregnancy is established, a trial of gradual tapering and cessation of the medication may be successful, but vigilance must be maintained for signs of relapse.[3]
- Discussions with patient, sometimes including her partner/family as appropriate with her consent, before starting treatment should address the following:
  - There is some uncertainty about all the risks, especially possible long-term risks to the child, associated with certain antidepressant medications.
  - The background risk of fetal malformations (minor to major) in any unselected population is about 2–4%, irrespective of antidepressants or otherwise.
  - The pros and cons of treatment and of not treating the mental health disorder.
- Clear documentation of the discussions held (in some settings, even an audiotaped record) is essential for medico-legal reasons.
- Providing written information about any risks of a particular drug, as well as care during pregnancy, and extra vigilance for early detection of any possible problems during pregnancy, is good practice.
- Choose a medication with the lowest risk profile for the mother and fetus/infant.
- Start at the lowest dose and slowly increase if required.
- If preterm delivery is a possible risk with the selected antidepressant, inform patient of signs of preterm labour and action that is required in this context.
- If fetal growth restriction is a reported risk, arrange for serial growth scans, maintaining clinical surveillance for possible IUGR.
- Neonatal staff must be informed about the particular antidepressant the mother is taking.
- Similarly, decisions to stop antidepressants in a woman with a mental disorder who is planning a pregnancy, is pregnant, or is lactating should take the following into consideration:
  - NICE guidance (Section 6) on the particular mental health disorder[1]
  - possible risks to the mother and fetus/infant of not treating the disorder
  - any possible effects on fetus/neonate during the drug withdrawal phase.

Some common antidepressants

- If the woman conceives on paroxetine, or is on the drug before pregnancy and is planning to get pregnant, paroxetine must be promptly stopped because of its teratogenic potential, especially of causing heart defects. An alternative antidepressant needs to be prescribed without delay.
- Tricyclic antidepressants such as amitriptyline, imipramine, and nortriptyline have fewer recognized side effects during pregnancy than SSRIs, but a higher fatality index in case of an overdose.
- SSRIs in the first trimester have been reported to be associated with increased risk of miscarriages, cardiac and other malformations.[10,11,12,13,14]
- SSRIs after 20 weeks gestation can rarely be associated with fetal persistent pulmonary hypertension. The neonatologists must be duly informed regarding maternal SSRIs.

- SSRIs may be associated with a small but significant risk of preterm delivery and lower birth weight, therefore serial growth scans are required.[8]
- SSRIs continued in the third trimester may also cause mild respiratory distress, irritability, constant crying, and feeding problems in the neonate which are usually self-limiting and settle within 2–4 weeks.[4,15,16] Rarely intraventricular haemorrhage may result.[15,16,17]
- Among the SSRIs, fluoxetine has a long half-life active metabolite and the fewest known risks during pregnancy.
- Venlafaxine a SNRI antidepressant, may cause hypertension and potentiate drugs which increase the risk of bleeding. It has a higher fetal toxicity profile than SSRIs and some tricyclic antidepressants with overdose. It is transmitted in significant amounts in breast milk and is to be avoided during breastfeeding. Venlafaxine is also more difficult to withdraw and ideally a change to a safer drug is best managed several months before conception.[18]

During breastfeeding

- Although all antidepressants carry a risk of withdrawal/toxicity in the infant, this is usually self-limiting and mild. The neonate, especially if premature or small for dates, must be monitored for adverse effects such as drowsiness, jitteriness, hyperexcitability, or feeding problems. Other problems such as cardiac dysrhythmias, intestinal motility disorders, and urinary retention are rare.[2]
- If clinically appropriate, the dose of antidepressants should be tapered 3–4 weeks before the expected date of delivery to minimize neonatal withdrawal symptoms.
- During breastfeeding, while nortriptyline (imipramine, and sertraline (Lustral, Zoloft) are present in relatively low concentrations in breast milk, citalopram), escitalopram, and fluoxetine are present in relatively high levels.
- SSRIs are, in general, highly protein-bound, therefore only small amounts are transmitted in breast milk. The effects on the infant are not completely understood.

Benzodiazepine anxiolytics

- These include diazepam, lorazepam, oxazepam, and chlordiazepoxide.
- Although effective, they can produce dependence.
- **Benzodiazepines should not be routinely prescribed or continued during pregnancy** to treat anxiety, panic attacks, etc.
- Gradual withdrawal is advisable during pregnancy.
- Benzodiazepines have a teratogenic potential and can cause cleft palate.
- They can also cause the floppy baby syndrome in the neonate, neonatal hypothermia, and respiratory depression.[2,9]

Antipsychotics

- Certain drugs such as amisulpride, risperidone, and sulpiride can result in high prolactin levels which may actually interfere with fertility in those trying for a pregnancy.
- Clozapine should not be prescribed during either pregnancy or breastfeeding as it can result in agranulocytosis in the fetus and breastfed neonate.
- Problems such as gestational hypertension and excess weight gain can result from the use of olanzapine in pregnant women, especially in some ethnic groups and in women who are already obese.
- Depot antipsychotics are to be avoided during pregnancy as they can cause extrapyramidal symptoms in the baby even after several months.
- Quetiapine, used in depression in bipolar disorder, can cause extrapyramidal and withdrawal syndrome in the neonate if used in the third trimester.

Valproate

- If valproate is being used in the treatment of bipolar disorder, and the woman is planning a pregnancy, valproate is preferably stopped and an alternative (usually one of the antipsychotics) prescribed.
- If there is no suitable alternative to valproate, due to the significantly increased risks of neural tubal defects, high-dose (5 mg/day) folic acid should be prescribed in any woman aiming to get pregnant and the dose of valproate should preferably not exceed 1 g/day in divided slow-release form.[1,2]

Lithium (Camcolit, Liskonum, Priadel)

- Lithium is used in the prophylaxis and treatment of mania or depression associated with bipolar disorders or to augment other antidepressants in treatment-resistant depression.
- Its use is associated with a significant increase in fetal cardiac abnormalities and it should not be prescribed during pregnancy.
- If a woman on lithium is planning a pregnancy or unexpectedly conceives while on the medication and if she is stable with a **low risk of relapse**, she should be advised to gradually discontinue lithium over 4 weeks although cardiac malformation may have already occurred.
- If the woman is unstable or is at **high risk of relapse**, options are to gradually change to an alternative antipsychotic, or stop lithium in the first trimester and restart in the second trimester, provided the woman does not intend to breastfeed.
- If lithium is continued during pregnancy, fetal cardiac scan and serial growth scans are recommended.
- Serum lithium levels need to be checked every 4 weeks till 36 weeks, then weekly till delivery and within 24 h after delivery.
- Continuous fetal monitoring with adequate hydration to avoid lithium toxicity is essential during labour.
- Newborns of mothers on lithium can show toxicity or withdrawal symptoms including irritability, floppiness or increased tone, feeding or sleeping difficulties, tremors, and rarely seizures.
- High concentrations are found in breast milk, therefore lithium is not recommended during breastfeeding.[19]

References

1. NICE Clinical Guideline. Antenatal and postnatal mental health. CG 45. London: National Institute for Health and Clinical Excellence, 2007 <http://nice.org.uk/guidance/CG45>.
2. National Teratology Information Service <www.UKTIS.org> (For NHS health professionals only: Tel. 0844 892 0909, 9.00–17.00 Monday to Friday; outside of these hours, urgent enquiries only).
3. Williams AS. Antidepressants in pregnancy and breastfeeding. Aust Prescr 2007;30: 125–127.
4. Austin MP. To treat or not to treat: maternal depression, SSRI use in pregnancy and adverse neonatal effects. Psychol Med 2006;36: 1663–1670.
5. Einarson A, et al. Discontinuing antidepressants and benzodiazepines upon becoming pregnant. Beware of the risks of abrupt discontinuation. Can Fam Physician 2001;47: 489–490.
6. Misri S, et al. The use of antidepressants in pregnancy and lactation. BC Med J 2005;47: 139–142.
7. Martins C, Gaffin EA. Effects of early maternal depression on patterns of infant-mother attachment: A meta-analytic investigation. J Child Psychol Psychiatry 2000;41: 737–746.
8. Oberlander TF, et al. Neonatal outcomes after prenatal exposure to selective serotonin reuptake inhibitor antidepressants and maternal depression using population-based linked health data. Arch Gen Psychiatry 2006;63: 898–906.
9. van den Bergh BR, et al. Antenatal maternal anxiety and stress and the neuro behavioural development of the fetus and child: links and possible mechanisms. A review. Neurosci Biobehav Rev 2005;29: 237–258.
10. Kulin NA, et al. Pregnancy outcome following maternal use of the new selective serotonin reuptake inhibitors: a prospective controlled multicentre study. JAMA 1998;279: 609–610.
11. Alwan S, et al. National Birth Defects Prevention Study. Use of selective serotonin-reuptake inhibitors in pregnancy and the risk of birth defects. N Engl J Med 2007;356: 2684–2692.
12. Louik C, et al. First-trimester use of selective serotonin-reuptake inhibitors and the risk of birth defects. N Engl J Med 2007;356: 2675–2683.
13. Wogelius P, et al. Maternal use of selective serotonin reuptake inhibitors and risk of congenital malformations. Epidemiology 2006;17: 701–704.

14. Berard A, et al. First trimester exposure to paroxetine and risk of cardiac malformations in infants: the importance of dosage. Birth Defects Res B Dev Reprod Toxicol 2007;80: 18–27.
15. Nordeng H, Spigset O. Treatment with selective serotonin reuptake inhibitors in the third trimester of pregnancy: effects on the infant. Drug Saf 2005;28: 565–581.
16. Chambers CD, et al. Selective serotonin-reuptake inhibitors and risk of persistent pulmonary hypertension of the newborn. N Engl J Med 2006;354: 579–587.
17. Lattimore KA, et al. Selective serotonin reuptake inhibitor (SSRI) use during pregnancy and effects on the fetus and newborn: a meta-analysis. J Perinatol 2005;25: 595–604.
18. Ilett KF, et al. Distribution of venlafaxine and its O-desmethyl metabolite in human milk and their effects in breastfed infants. Br J Clin Pharmacol 2002;53: 17–22.
19. Viguera AC, et al. Lithium in breast milk and nursing infants: clinical implications. Am J Psychiatry 2007;164: 342–345.

24.5 Smoking in Pregnancy

FACT FILE

- The risks of **smoking** in pregnancy for both the mother and the baby are well recognized.
- The adverse effects of smoking are seen throughout pregnancy and the sequelae last beyond the birth.
- Smoking is the one modifiable cause of several adverse pregnancy outcomes and its cessation is entirely under the control of the individual woman.
- It is estimated that about 20% of women smoke during pregnancy.[1,2,3]
- In the first trimester, smoking increases the risk of miscarriage by 20–80% compared with women who do not smoke.[4]
- In the second and third trimesters, the risk of abruption is increased, postulated to be due to the hypoxia induced by increased carbon dioxide levels.
- The reduced levels of oxygenation may also cause enlargement of the placental surface area and therefore the increased incidence of placenta praevia found among smokers.[3]
- Preterm delivery and intrauterine growth restriction (IUGR) are also increased, linked to the relatively poor placental function compared with non-smokers.[5,6]
- Increased incidence of neonatal death, sudden infant death syndrome, childhood asthma, atopy, etc.
- Smoking also decreases breast milk production. There is insufficient evidence regarding the effects of neonatal ingestion of breast milk containing higher levels of nicotine.
- The effect of smoking on neurodevelopment is not clear but it may be associated with cognitive and learning defects.

Smoking cessation

- All pregnant women who smoke must receive advice and support to stop.[6,7] Cessation interventions should be offered throughout pregnancy, not just at the beginning. A Cochrane meta- analysis showed that women who received smoking cessation intervention had a 70% improvement in cessation rates.[8]
- **Brief interventions** consist of one-to-one counselling sessions and the supply of self -help material.
- A Swedish study showed that 29% of women manage to give up smoking completely during pregnancy. The majority of women, about 1 in 5, who quit smoking do so prior to or just after their first prenatal consultation.[9] Those who continue to smoke after the initial intervention are more likely to do so throughout pregnancy.
- Cognitive behavioural therapy (CBT), education, and motivational strategies including feedback, though effective, are expensive and cannot be provided to all pregnant smokers.
- **Nicotine replacement therapy** (NRT: patches, gum, spray, lozenge) is presently the most common pharmacotherapy intervention. There have been reports of increased incidence of congenital abnormalities, pre-eclampsia, preterm birth, etc.[9] Therefore only the lowest doses of NRT, used intermittently and preferably **after organogenesis is complete at 12 weeks** are recommended.
- Newer pharmacotherapeutic agents under research include the antidepressant bupropion and varenicline.
- Other strategies such as acupuncture, acupressure, and hypnotherapy are also tried, but have not been proven to be effective.[10]

Information for patients

Please see Information for patients: Stopping smoking in pregnancy (p. 546)

References

1. Statistics on women's smoking status at time of delivery: England, October to December, 2011 (Q3—quarterly report). Health and Social Care Information Centre <http://www.hscic.uk>.
2. Bittoun R, Femia G Smoking cessation in pregnancy Obstet Med 2010;3: 90–93.
3. Cnattingius S. The epidemiology of smoking during pregnancy: smoking prevalence, maternal characteristics, and pregnancy outcomes. Nicotine Tob Res 2004;6: S125–140.
4. Castles A, et al. Effects of smoking during pregnancy: five meta-analyses. Am J Prev Med 1999;16: 208–215.
5. Jauniaux E, Burton GJ. Morphological and biological effects of maternal exposure to tobacco smoke on the fetoplacental unit. Early Hum Dev 2007;3: 699–706.
6. NICE Guideline. Quitting smoking in pregnancy and following childbirth. PH26. London: National Institute for Health and Clinical Excellence, 2010.
7. NICE Pathway. Smoking cessation in maternity services. London: National Institute for Health and Clinical Excellence, 2012.
8. Lumley J., et al. Interventions for promoting smoking cessation during pregnancy. Cochrane Database Syst Rev 2009;3; 1–163.
9. Pollak KI, et al. Nicotine replacement and behavioral therapy for smoking cessation in pregnancy. Am J Prev Med 2007;33; 297–305.
10. White AR, et al. Acupuncture and related interventions for smoking cessation. Cochrane Database Syst Rev 2006;1: CD000009.

Booking visit

- All midwives and staff working with **pregnant smokers** need to advise and provide women with information about the risks of smoking to her and the unborn child, including smoking by partners/ family members
- Enquire about smoking status. Does she smoke? Anyone in the household?
- Use CO breath test
- Record smoking status and CO level in the hand-held notes
- Refer any of the following to NHS Stop Smoking Services:
  - women who say they smoke
  - women with a CO reading around 7 ppm
  - women who say that they have stopped smoking in the last 2 weeks
- ***Give NHS Pregnancy Smoking Helpline number (0800 1699 169) and local number and record this in in hand-held notes***

At next appointment

Check if referral was taken up

No

- Ask if she is interested if stopping smoking
- Offer another referral to NHS Smoking Services
- Record in hand-held notes

Yes

- Provide positive feedback and record in hand-held notes

Referral accepted

- Refer to NHS Stop Smoking Services
- Give NHS Pregnancy Smoking Helpline number(0800 1699 169) and local number.
- Record this in hand-held notes

Referral declined

- Accept answer non-judgementally
- Leave offer of help open
- Record in hand-held notes
- Review at a later appointment

- Review at subsequent appointments as appropriate, offer appropriate feedback
- Record in hand-held notes

National Institute for Health and Clinical Excellence (2010) Adapted from *PH26 Quitting smoking in pregnancy and following childbirth*. London: NICE. Available from www.nice.org.uk/PH26. This information was accurate at the time of press. For any further updates to this information, please visit the NICE website.

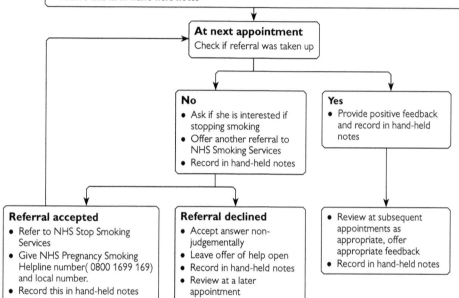

24.6 Alcohol in Pregnancy

FACT FILE

- Several drugs and chemicals have teratogenic effects especially around the time of organogenesis. **Alcohol (ethanol)** is one of them and has a dose-dependent effect on pregnancy.
- Offspring of mothers who have consumed ethanol during pregnancy have been known to suffer malformations, pre- and postnatal growth deficits, craniofacial dysmorphism, mental retardation, and behavioural abnormalities.[1]
- **Fetal alcohol syndrome (FAS):** If a pregnant woman drinks ethanol heavily and repeatedly, there is a 6–10% chance of the fetus developing FAS.[1] The principal features of FAS are prenatal and postnatal growth deficiency, short stature, neurodevelopmental defects and delay, microcephaly, characteristic facial dysmorphism, and fine motor dysfunction.
- Neural tube defects, cleft palate, cardiac anomalies, and altered palmar creases are seen in FAS. One-third of children with alcohol embryopathy will have congenital cardiac problems.
- Drinking that is less heavy but still habitual can cause a range of alcohol-induced neurobehavioural defects, collectively known as **fetal alcohol spectrum disorder**,[2] manifested as hyperactivity, attention deficits, motor coordination abnormalities, and neuropsychological impairment.
- **Binge drinking** is particularly harmful in pregnancy as the developing fetus is exposed to greater peaks of blood ethanol concentrations which can cause orofacial clefts, renal malformations, and intrauterine fetal death.[3,4,5]
- The amount of alcohol consumed, the length of time of alcohol exposure, and the developmental stage of the fetus at exposure determine effects on fetal development and later sequelae.
- Alcohol drinking, even in moderate amounts, is associated with an increased risk of first-trimester spontaneous miscarriages.
- Alcohol-induced fetal damage may manifest immediately after birth, in infancy, or even later in life, especially if the central nervous system (CNS) is involved.
- ***Although organogenesis is complete in all other areas by the end of the first trimester, the CNS, especially the cerebral cortex, continues to develop throughout pregnancy and early postnatal life. The cerebellar cortex develops during the second and third trimesters. The effect of psychotropic agents such as ethanol can therefore affect CNS development throughout pregnancy, leading to changes in intellectual capacity, learning ability, attention span, and behaviour.***[1]
- Alcohol misuse in pregnancy often coexists with poor nutrition, other substance abuse, and smoking, which can further increase risks of brain damage to the fetus.
- **Advice to women in the UK** regarding the safety of alcohol and the quantity that is considered harmful was revised by the Department of Health[6] and the RCOG statement[7] in 2006.
- ***The revised advice states that pregnant women or women trying to conceive should avoid drinking alcohol.***
- ***However, if they choose to drink, healthcare professionals should advise that in order to minimize risks to the baby, they should not consume more than 1–2 units, once or at most twice a week, and should avoid binge drinking altogether.***
- ***This is at variance with recommendations from other countries (USA, France, Denmark, Spain, Norway, Netherlands, Germany, Canada, Australia, New Zealand etc) where the unequivocal message is that women should avoid alcohol entirely while pregnant or trying to conceive because damage can occur in the earliest weeks of pregnancy, even before a woman knows that she is pregnant.***
- Pregnancy seemed to affect a positive change in the drinking pattern of the most women in a large Swedish study.[8] Of heavy (hazardous) drinkers, 60% consumed no alcohol once pregnancy was confirmed, and the rest reported a decreased frequency of alcohol consumption per month.

Management of alcohol misuse in pregnancy

Screening tools

- Tools such as the **T-ACE test** need to be used for appropriate screening for the use of alcohol and illicit drugs by all healthcare professionals from primary care to hospital antenatal clinics.[2,9]
- The **T-ACE test** is a validated screening four-question test to identify risky drinking in pregnant women. It asks the following questions:
  1. Does it take (**T**) more than three drinks to make you feel high?
  2. Have you ever been annoyed (**A**) by people's criticism of your drinking?
  3. Are you trying to cut down (**C**) on drinking?
  4. Have you ever used alcohol as an eye opener (**E**) in the morning?
- ***A positive response to question 1 scores 2 points and positive responses to any of the other questions score 1 point each. A positive response to two of these four questions is considered to indicate possible alcohol abuse or dependence, as does a total score of 2 or more points.***

(Data from Sokol RJ, Finding the Risk Drinker in Your Clinical Practice. In: Robinson G and Armstrong R (eds.), *Alcohol and Child*/ Family Health: Proceedings of a Conference with Particular Reference to the Prevention of Alcohol-Related Birth Defects, Vancouver, BC, 1988.)

Brief interventions for harmful drinking

- **Brief intervention** is a technique to motivate harmful drinkers to change their drinking behaviour.
- It consists of a short one-to-one counselling session, lasting for about 10–15 min, by a healthcare professionals such as a GP, practice nurse, or and midwife in an antenatal clinic.[10]
- Large studies in antenatal settings have shown that such brief interventions achieved significant decrease in or even abstinence from drinking in those with highest levels of drinking.[11,12]

Pregnancy management

This includes:

- Assessment of nutritional state, enquiry into other substance misuse, smoking, social circumstances, family support, etc.
- Initial booking bloods to include Hep C, Hep B screening after full explanation and patient's consent. Booking bloods must include baseline liver function tests (LFTs).
- Ultrasound scans at 12 weeks, 16 weeks (to exclude neural tube defects, orofacial clefts), detailed anomaly scan at 20 weeks followed by serial growth scans.
- The paediatricians must be informed to be aware of the possibility of FAS and long-term sequelae.
- LFTs can be repeated at about 34–36 weeks gestation.
- Breast milk contains the same level of alcohol as maternal serum, hence in heavy drinkers the fetus could display signs of drowsiness, weakness, deep sleep, decreased milk ejection reflex, etc.[1]
- Discussion regarding contraception before discharge from hospital.

Treatment of severe alcohol misuse or alcohol dependence

- This needs multidisciplinary management in pregnancy.
- Such women should be referred to specialist services for treatment. Antenatal clinics run by specialist midwives acting as liaison between the alcohol and substance addiction and social services teams, the hospital obstetrician, and the GP.[2]
- Detoxification programmes need to be undertaken in an inpatient setting with monitoring of maternal and fetal well-being.

Information for patients

Please see Information for patients: Alcohol and pregnancy (p. 546)

References

1. Ornoy A, Ergaz Z. Alcohol abuse in pregnant women: effects on the fetus and newborn, mode of action and maternal treatment. Int J Environ Res Public Health 2010;7: 364–379.
2. Guerrini I, et al. Pregnancy and alcohol misuse. BMJ 2009;338: 829–832.
3. Strandberg-Larsen K, et al. Binge drinking in pregnancy and risk of fetal death. Obstet Gynecol 2008;111: 602–609.
4. Aliyu MH, et al. Alcohol consumption during pregnancy and the risk of early stillbirth among singletons. Alcohol 2008;42: 369–374.
5. Slickers JE, et al. Maternal body mass index and lifestyle exposures and the risk of bilateral renal agenesis or hypoplasia: the National Birth Defects Prevention Study. Am J Epidemiol 2008;168: 1259–1267.
6. DH. Updated alcohol advice for pregnant women. London: Department of Health, 2007.
7. RCOG Statement No. 5. Alcohol consumption and the outcome of pregnancy. London: Royal College of Obstetricians and Gynaecologists, 2006.
8. Goransson M, et al. Fetus at risk: prevalence of alcohol consumption during pregnancy estimated with a simple screening method in Swedish antenatal clinics. Addiction 2003:98: 1513–1520.
9. WHO. Brief intervention for hazardous and harmful drinking. Geneva: World Health Organization, 2001 <http://whqlibdoc.who.int/HQ/2001/WHO_MSD_MSB_01.6b.pdf>.
10. NICE Evidence briefing. Prevention and reduction of alcohol misuse, 2nd ed. London: National Institute for Health and Clinical Excellence, 2005 <http://www.nice.nhs.uk/nicemedia/documents/alcoholeb2ndedition_summary.pdf>.
11. Chang G, et al. Brief intervention for prenatal alcohol use. Obstet Gynaecol 2005;105: 991–998.
12. DH. Drug misuse and dependence: UK guidelines on clinical management. London: Department of Health, 2007.

CARE PATHWAYS

Antenatal management of alcohol misuse in pregnancy

Individual care pathways must be designed on a case-to-case basis

In primary care

- GPs, practice nurses, and/or midwives need to assess the amount of alcohol consumption in women intending to conceive and women with newly confirmed pregnancy to advise abstinence
- A screening test such as the T-ACE test needs to be used to screen for high or hazardous alcohol misuse
- Pre-pregnancy advice to include smoking cessation as well as stopping any illicit substance use
- Primary care is best placed to assess social circumstances and liaise with specialist services such as local substance and alcohol misuse teams, social services, etc.
- Brief intervention to be undertaken by primary care healthcare professional (e.g. GP, community midwife)
- Fetal risks to be clearly explained and reiterated at each visit. Set limits of no more than 1–2 UK units once or twice a week if abstinence cannot be achieved
- Refer to hospital specialist antenatal clinic with liaison midwife coordinating multidisciplinary team involvement in patient's care
- After explanation and with patient's consent, in addition to routine booking bloods, consider baseline LFTs, screening for Hep C, Hep B

↓

In hospital specialist antenatal clinic

- At the first specialist antenatal clinic visit, assess pregnancy, check viability and dates, assess patient's general health including exclusion of any hepatomegaly, signs of portal hypertension
- Explain that fetal risks are directly proportional to amount of alcohol consumed, reiterate total abstinence is safest. DH and NICE guideline-based limits of no more than 1–2 UK units once or twice a week if abstinence cannot be achieved
- Check LFTs if not already done. Refer to physicians (hepatologist) for postpartum follow-up if chronic alcoholism and liver problems
- Specify maternal alcohol usage in all scan request forms. Viability and dating scan at 12 weeks to be followed by scan at 16 weeks to exclude neural tube defects, any orofacial clefts, etc. Anomaly scans at about 20 weeks and 24 weeks for detailed assessment of fetal brain, heart and kidneys, facial anatomy, etc.
- Subsequent serial scans for fetal growth from about 26 weeks onwards. If IUGR suspected, follow care pathway for IUGR (p. 421)
- Neonatologists/paediatricians to be informed of maternal alcohol misuse in order to check newborn for signs of fetal alcohol syndrome and for subsequent follow-up of infant and child
- Antenatal and postnatal care arrangements coordinated by liaison midwife for continuing support from social services and specialist team for alcohol and substance abuse and for continued support along with community midwife, health visitor, and GP postpartum
- Contraception advice before discharge

Alcohol cessation pathway

Booking appointment
- Ask all women about alcohol use
- Record in notes

Ask
- Do you drink?
- If so, how many units?
- Discuss health benefits of stopping

No alcohol
- Congratulate non-drinkers and those who have stopped once pregnancy was recognized
- Reinforce health benefits

Explain T-ACE questionnaire
- If patient is interested, assess degree of alcohol consumption using T-ACE questionnaire

Hazardous levels
- Specialist referral to drug and alcohol team
- Inform GP and obstetrician
- Ensure close liaison and follow-up

Assist by
- Providing information and advice on health benefits during a one-to-one brief intervention
- Requesting patient to complete a diary of alcohol intake, reminding her that home measures are often larger than pub measures

Follow-up
- Discuss diary and follow-up progress
- Remind her of health benefits of ceasing to drink alcohol and risks of continued drinking for her and her baby's health
- Re-assess using the T-ACE questions.

Reduced use, but not stopped completely
- Identify problems that are impeding patient's attempts to stop alcohol
- Reinforce health benefits of stopping alcohol for herself and the developing fetus

Stopped alcohol
- ***Congratulate her on her success***
- Review during routine antenatal care

Adapted with kind permission from 'Women, Pregnancy & Substance Misuse Protocol - The Highland Good Practice Guide'. <http://www.forhighlandschildren.org/4-icspublication/index_76_2618347006.pdf>.

24.7 Substance Abuse in Pregnancy

FACT FILE

- **Use of illicit drugs** is not uncommon in women of childbearing age and during pregnancy.
- This is associated with significant risks to the mother and the baby (fetus and neonate).[1,2,3,4,5,6,7] Illicit substances are detectable in the placenta by 12 weeks gestation and are associated with congenital and developmental abnormalities.
- It is difficult to precisely determine the effect of any single illicit drug on pregnancy outcomes due to high rates of multiple-substance abuse, also concurrent use of alcohol and smoking.
- Medical comorbidities are often present, such as anaemia, poor nutrition, cellulitis, abscesses, thromboembolic blood-borne infections such as Hep C, HIV, and other STIs as well as psychiatric morbidity.
- Adverse social circumstances, poor nutrition, low levels of family support, domestic violence, and delayed or poor utilization of antenatal services further confound illicit substance use during pregnancy.
- Many drug users have additional financial and housing problems; some have other children removed into care.
- In keeping with their chaotic lifestyle, it is not uncommon for these patients to miss numerous clinic appointments both in primary and hospital-based care.
- However, there is evidence that when there is well directed and comprehensive support from health and social care services, improved pregnancy outcomes can be expected. It is essential that a coordinated multiagency network that is readily accessible is in place.[2]
- The recognition that this group of pregnant women have differing needs, particular difficulties, and complications, and that their care requires multispecialty input starting from pre-pregnancy and continuing after childbirth, is of paramount importance.
- Pregnancy presents a good opportunity to undertake screening, and offer education and interventions to try to decrease the risky lifestyle choices of women using illicit substances.
- There is increased maternal motivation and a greater awareness of possible adverse effects on their babies during pregnancy.[1] Studies have shown a decrease in the use of illicit substances in pregnant compared with non-pregnant women.[2]
- This decrease may, however, be due to low rates of self-reporting by pregnant women to try to avoid stigmatization, fear of facing judgemental attitudes, legal implications, or the threat of the baby being removed into care.
- Recommencement of substance abuse is common within 3 months of childbirth.[1]

Substances commonly used in pregnancy

Marijuana

- ***Hallucinogen: Main psychoactive ingredient Δ-tetrahydrocannabinol (THC).***
- Also known as 'hashish', 'joint', 'cannabis', 'draw', 'blow', 'hash', 'grass', 'dope'.
- Most widely used substance during pregnancy.
- Effects on pregnancy and fetus still unclear as there is often multisubstance abuse in addition.
- Freely crosses placenta, with vasoconstrictive effect on placental microcirculation.
- IUGR because of chronic fetal hypoxia as marijuana produces carbon monoxide levels five times higher than cigarette smoking.
- Conflicting reports of links to preterm delivery, neural tube defects, and neurobehaviour in infancy and childhood.

Opioids

- ***Heroin, morphine, fentanyl, dihydrocodeine, and methadone. Oral, SC, IM, or IV route.***
- Heroin also known as 'skag,' 'brown', 'gear'.
- Maternal complications include infectious complications such as abscesses, cellulitis, thrombophlebitis, or blood-borne viruses (e.g. Hep C, Hep B and HIV), risk of overdose, and acute withdrawal.[1]
- Risks to the baby include IUGR, preterm delivery, increased need for NICU admission and **neonatal abstinence syndrome (NAS)**. Symptoms of NAS appear within 24–72 h of birth and include tremors, sweating, fever, respiratory distress, hyperactivity, hypertonicity, convulsions, and high-pitched cry.
- All pregnant women who are opioid dependent must be offered methadone replacement therapy. Methadone is a legal alternative.
- Methadone replacement prevents acute withdrawal risks, improves maternal health status, and reduces fetal and neonatal morbidity and incidence of NAS.
- Methadone has a longer half-life and allows for greater stability, and reduces the risk of infection from injecting opioids.
- Women should, however, be informed that methadone treatment can lead to more severe and longer-lasting withdrawals in the neonate.

Cocaine

- ***In powder form, usually sniffed, injected or smoked, applied intranasally or transmucosally. Crack ('freebase', 'rocks') is a smokable form of cocaine.***
- The teratogenicity of cocaine is not completely defined. Cardiac, CNS, genitourinary, gastroschisis, and limb malformations have been reported.
- Can cause miscarriages, premature rupture of membranes, preterm delivery, small for dates, IUGR.
- Cocaine causes vasoconstriction resulting in reduced oxygen supply to the fetus, leading to IUGR which involves the brain growth as well.
- Neurobehavioural defects persist after birth.
- Maternal morbidity related to cocaine can include hypertension and/or seizures resembling pre-eclampsia/eclampsia, myocardial infarction, pulmonary oedema.
- Maternal blood pressure and uterine vascular resistance are both increased, while uterine blood flow is decreased by cocaine.
- Incidence of arterial thrombosis is also increased.
- **Abruption** of the placenta is thus more common in those on cocaine.

Amphetamine/methamphetamine

- ***CNS stimulant; taken by snorting, orally, or injected. Also known as 'whizz', 'speed', 'billie', etc.***
- Maternal cardiovascular complications include hypertension, hyperthermia, tachycardia, cardiac arrhythmias, stroke, and myocardial infarction.
- Pregnancy complications include premature rupture of membranes, placental abruption, IUGR, preterm delivery, intrauterine infections, and stillbirth.

Ecstasy

- ***3,4-methylenedioxymethamphetamine (MDMA). Derived from amphetamines, so similar profile,***
- Causes a small (0.6 °C) rise in core body temperature, which may contributes to association with congenital abnormalities.

Benzodiazepines

- ***Diazepam, temazepam, chlorodiazepoxide: Tranquillizers, CNS depressants. Common street drugs. Temazepam now classified as Schedule 3 drug.***
- May be associated with cleft palate.
- Newborns may display withdrawal symptoms such as hypotonia, hypothermia, hyperbilirubinaemia, poor feeding, or respiratory difficulties.

Volatile substance/solvents

- ***Glue, paint, petrol.***
- Sniffing solvents during pregnancy is associated with IUGR, increased NICU admissions, stillbirth.
- Maternal risks are of cardiac arrest, asphyxia, inhalation of vomit, etc.

Hallucinogens

- ***LSD ('acid'), psilocybin ('magic mushroom').***
- Alter perception, cause illusions and visual hallucinations, profound psychological effects, flashbacks which can persist for years; repeated use can cause prolonged psychosis.
- Effects on pregnancy as yet undefined.

Pre-conception care and interventions in substance abusers

- Pre-pregnancy contact with addiction services affords an opportunity to engage with the woman of reproductive age who may or may not want to get pregnant.
- Discussions regarding contraception, dietary assessment and advice, avoidance of high-risk activities and prescribing peri-pregnancy folic acid should be conducted in a sensitive, non-judgemental manner.
- Those wishing to conceive may be anxious about blood-borne viral diseases (HIV, Hep C) as well as other STIs. Screening before pregnancy can be offered to them.
- Immunization for Hep B and rubella can be arranged.
- Pre-pregnancy baseline urine test for opioid concentration before conversion to the methadone replacement and repeated urine tests to ensure that there are no opioids being used during the methadone programme.
- Adequate information including printed versions of information sheets should be given regarding the misuse of substances and their potential impact on pregnancy outcomes, risks to the developing baby or the mother herself.
- Worsening of these risks with concomitant use of alcohol and smoking should be highlighted and patient referred to support services and addiction services for help to give up these high-risk lifestyle choices.
- Women should be informed of the care they can expect to receive during pregnancy, multidisciplinary support, use of drugs or replacement programme, and how the specialist liaison midwife would coordinate her care.
- If there are psychotic manifestations or psychiatric issues, pre-pregnancy referral to and assessment by the mental health team is mandatory.
- If the woman agrees, early referral to the local alcohol and substance abuse community services is recommended if she has not self-referred already.
- A nominated key worker should be identified to coordinate her care, interfacing both hospital and primary care services and acting as liaison with all the other professionals involved.
- If assistance with social services, housing and probation officers, welfare rights advisor is required, the designated key worker/coordinator should undertake to do so.

Antenatal management: general principles

- The patient requires care that is individualized and multidisciplinary team-based.
- The multidisciplinary team will usually consist of the community midwife and substance and alcohol service counsellor, the GP, social worker and mental health professional as well as hospital specialist midwife serving as the key link, obstetrician, neonatologist, and anaesthetist.
- Care must be individualized to address the specific issues concerning each pregnant substance abuser. All care must be delivered in a non-judgemental manner at every point of contact.

Booking visit

- Once the patient presents to the GP or to addiction services or Druglink stating that she is pregnant, an appointment must be made as soon as possible for the community midwife to arrange the booking visit.
- This needs to be in a venue that is acceptable to the patient in order to reduce non-attendance for future appointments.
- Early morning appointments in the are unlikely to be attended. Also, waiting for a long time to be seen in clinic can be distressing especially if the patient is suffering withdrawals.
- During this first visit, a detailed history needs to be obtained as it will form the basis of further care planning and coordinating services. [9] The details of all the drugs used, pattern, route and frequency, concomitant smoking, and alcohol misuse must be established. Enquire if partner is using drugs as well.
- If she is using IV drugs, enquire about needle techniques and safe practice, and provide information about safe needle exchanges.
- The community midwife will establish the approximate gestational age and explore the patient's views on proceeding with the pregnancy if she is in the early stages and has not yet decided. She should be offered appropriate information and directed for counselling.
- Dietary assessment and advice regarding folic acid if still within the first trimester must be offered.
- Booking bloods may need to be taken at another date if there has been recent IV drug use. Some women prefer to draw the blood samples themselves.
- Screening tests including Hep B, Hep C, HIV must be fully explained and taken with the patient's consent.
- Referral to the substance misuse coordinating midwife should be organized and the patient informed about who is to be her key contact during pregnancy.
- The pregnant woman must be encouraged to accept referral to specialist services such as local Druglink or addiction team so that early liaison can be established to maximize support.
- The patient and her partner should receive information about the risks of substance abuse to the developing fetus.
- If appropriate, referral to the social worker at an early stage will help assessment of the patient's needs.
- The high-risk circumstances must be clearly explained and shared care encouraged. The patient must be reassured that hospital appointments will be kept to the minimum required by her clinical needs.

Subsequent appointments in hospital antenatal clinic

- Clear documentation of management plans and good communication are of vital importance.
- The same senior obstetrician should ideally see all women who misuse substances at this initial hospital visit and ongoing follow-up and assessment. This builds up the confidence of the patient and a reduced tendency for non-attendance.
- Such pregnancies are high-risk because of the associated medical and social problems.
- Arranging antenatal clinic visits on the same day as an ultrasound scan helps improve attendance. Ideally, these could be planned for 20, 28, 32, and 36 weeks following a scan on each of those occasions. Additional visits may need to be arranged if any complications develop.
- The majority of antenatal care can continue meanwhile in the community: for example, at 16, 24, 34, 38 weeks gestation and weekly thereafter till delivery.
- Vigilance must be maintained for hypertension, IUGR, abruption, preterm labour. Likely symptoms must be explained to the patient and contact details about who and where to report to without delay.
- Referral to the anaesthetic high-risk clinic is necessary to discuss plans for analgesia, assess venous access, etc. Those who are opioid dependent will often require higher dose of analgesics and develop cross-tolerance to CNS depressants including anaesthetic agents, especially opiate analgesics and benzodiazepine.
- The coordinator/specialist liaison midwife, working with the addiction services team, will ensure the patient is fully informed of the risks, has access to counselling and social services help, and oversee her supportive care or the methadone replacement programme.

- At about 28–30 weeks a planning meeting for pre-birth discussions needs to be held, to which the patient is invited as well as all professionals involved with her including the assigned social worker.
- Child protection agencies must be informed through mandatory reporting channels if specific child protection issues are recognized or suspected.
- ***Unless there is a danger of heightened harm towards the unborn baby, the patient must be informed of statutory obligations. It must be made clear to the mother that substance abuse is, on its own, not a reason for child protection concerns. Concerns regarding parenting that warrant child protection are not inevitable consequences of substance abuse.***
- Unless specific obstetric indications such as IUGR, pre-eclampsia, or abruption arise, there is no need to change routine obstetric care or for interventions such as early IOL or Caesarean section.
- The neonatologists must be informed about maternal substance misuse so that the baby can be monitored for withdrawal symptoms and treated accordingly.
- Increased risks of infection, thrombophlebitis, etc. must be recognized.
- Breastfeeding is not contraindicated if the patient is on less than 50 mg methadone. Breastfeeding is particularly helpful in preventing or reducing the severity of neonatal withdrawal symptoms. Weaning should likewise be gradual.
- Before discharge from the hospital, clear plans for continued multidisciplinary support from outreach teams must be organized and contraceptive advice offered. Long-acting progesterone implants or a levonorgestrel intrauterine system (Mirena®) are the most effective options.
- Confidentiality must be maintained and the patient's drug use not disclosed to anyone unless they are directly involved in her or her baby's care. The patient may choose what is written in her hand-held notes and if information is recorded and made accessible to others without the patient's knowledge, this might represent a breach of trust.

Information for patients

Please see **Information for patients: Substance misuse and pregnancy** (p. 546)

References

1. Scott K, Lust K. Illicit substance use in pregnancy—a review. Obstet Med 2010;3: 94–100.
2. NICE Guideline. Pregnancy and complex social factors: a model for service provision for pregnant women with complex social factors. CG110. London: National Collaborating Centre for Women's and Children's Health/National Institute for Health and Care Excellence, 2010.
3. Hoare J. Drug misuse declared: findings from the 2008/09 British Crime Survey England and Wales. London: Home Office Statistical Bulletin, 2009.
4. Buehler BA, et al. Teratogenic potential of cocaine. Semin Perinatol 1996;20: 93–98.
5. Elliot L, et al. Case-control study of a gastroschisis cluster in Nevada. Arch Pediatr Adolesc Med 2009;163: 1000–1006.
6. Fried PA. Marijuana use during pregnancy: consequences for the offspring. Semin Perinatol 1991;15: 280–287.
7. Schempf A. Illicit drug use and neonatal outcomes: a critical review. Obstet Gynecol Surv 2007;62: 749–757.

CARE PATHWAY

Pre-conception care
- Advice on reproductive and sexual health and **substance misuse (smoking, alcohol, drugs)**
- Advice on care during pregnancy, folic acid

↓

Confirmation of pregnancy
- Woman attends GP/midwife or addiction service
- Pregnancy test positive, refer for booking appointment

↓

8–12 weeks: booking appointment
- Detailed history, ongoing assessment of substance misuse—smoking and alcohol (ACE questionnaire), use of other drugs
- Commence ongoing pregnancy risk assessment
- Refer to substance/alcohol specialist liaison midwife
- Give information, obtain consent for blood-borne virus testing
- Give hand-held notes
- Discuss other screening tests
- Discuss information sharing, confidentiality reassurance, seek formal consent for multiagency working including social services, if appropriate
- Clarify professional responsibility and identify key link(s) for patient to contact
- Non-attendance to be followed up by community midwife ± GP

↓

1st-trimester ultrasound scan
- Specify maternal substance use in scan requests, to allow focus on anomaly, growth, etc. in subsequent scans
- Dating scan ± nuchal fold thickness scan

↓

15–17 weeks gestation: hospital specialist antenatal clinic
With both consultant obstetrician and liaison midwife:
- Discuss and agree care plans for pregnancy as well as management of substance misuse. Document the plans and share with patient and those involved with her care and that of the yet-to-be-born baby; discuss risks of substance misuse for patient and her baby
- Ensure continuous liaison with appropriate multiagencies
- Further hospital antenatal visit to follow after scans on the same day, preferably afternoon appointments at 20, 24, 28, 32, 36 weeks
- Non-attendance to be followed up by community midwife ± GP
- Give information re risks of IUGR, abruption, hypertension
- Refer to anaesthetic high-risk clinic

↓

Approx. 20 weeks gestation: anomaly scan
- Review by Liaison midwife
- Assessment of pregnancy, of mother and of any continued drug use

↓

Approx. 22–26 weeks gestation
Community midwife/liaison midwife and addiction services specialist ± social worker follow-up keeping appointments to minimum and avoiding duplication:
- Monitor substance misuse/compliance
- If on methadone programme, urine/blood checks to detect any continued illicit substance misuse
- Monitor progress of pregnancy
- Inform neonatologists and special care baby unit (SCBU) about maternal substance use, especially in the event of preterm delivery.

↓

28 weeks: planning meeting for pre-birth discussion

With patient and key multiagency care providers:

- Discuss social circumstances, risk re-assessment
- Discuss Neonatal Abstinence Scoring (NAS) system
- Review of growth scan results, follow-up scans at 32 and 36 weeks
- Discuss infant feeding
- Routine blood tests

32 weeks antenatal appointment

- ***Child protection case conference, if needed, not routinely just on basis of maternal substance misuse***
- Review scan for fetal growth.
- Confirm has had anaesthetic review
- Discuss labour and delivery plans
- Reiterate NAS
- If on methadone programme, urine/blood checks to detect any continued illicit substance misuse

36 weeks: antenatal check

- Assess pregnancy progress
- Assess fetal growth scan results
- Monitor drug/ alcohol use, routine blood tests
- Discuss breastfeeding, future contraception

38 and 40 weeks antenatal checks

- Monitor drug/alcohol use
- Assess pregnancy, fetal movements
- Offer routine 'stretch and sweep' at 40 weeks
- After discussions with patient, book IOL according to unit policy at 40^{+10-11}, if no obstetric indications for early IOL or Caesarean

Delivery and postpartum hospital stay

- Liaison re pregnancy outcome
- NAS assessment and care in SCBU if identified
- Discharge arrangements including prescription and contraception plans
- Follow postnatal care plan/inform GP, health visitor
- Discharge information
- Breastfeeding support if required (not to breastfeed if HIV +ve)

10 days: postnatal care

- Continue multidisciplinary support
- Continue NAS assessment and care as indicated
- Monitor drug/alcohol use
- Relapse prevention support
- Reiterate contraception
- Review care plan

Adapted with kind permission from Whittaker A (2011) *The essential guide to problem substance use during pregnancy: a resource book for professionals, London,* DrugScope. ISBN 978-1904319535 http://www.nhslothian.scot.nhs.uk/MediaCentre/Publications/ForProfessionals/Documents/SubstanceMisusePregnancy.pdf

24.8 Hyperemesis Gravidarum

FACT FILE

- Although 80–90% of pregnant women experience nausea and vomiting, only 0.5–3% experience the severe form known as **hyperemesis gravidarum (HG)**.[1,2]
- HG is generally defined as severe nausea and intractable vomiting before 22 weeks gestation, leading to fluid, electrolyte and acid imbalance, nutrition deficiency, ketonuria, more than 3 kg or 5% weight loss, requiring hospital admission.
- The incidence of HG varies between different ethnic groups.
- HG usually occurs between week 5 and week 10 of gestation, the peak incidence of onset being week 9. Resolution of HG is usually by 20–22 weeks gestation; however, in 10% symptoms will persist throughout pregnancy.[1]
- HG is most prevalent during, but not limited to, the first trimester of pregnancy when both the corpus luteum and the placenta are producing hormones and the body is adapting to the pregnant state.
- HG, though self-limiting, can be life-threatening and treatment must be commenced immediately. Before the introduction of IV fluid therapy, the mortality from HG was 159 maternal deaths per million births in Great Britain.[3]
- Severe nausea and vomiting remain as one of the leading causes for hospitalization during pregnancy.[4] It is estimated that 206 h are lost from paid work for each woman who has nausea and vomiting in early pregnancy.[5]
- Multifactorial factors including hormonal (hCG, progesterone, oestrogen, thyroid, leptin, adrenal hormones), immunological, and *H. pylori* infection, as well as psychosomatic influences, have all been implicated in HG.

Risk factors

- Risk factors include obesity, multiple pregnancy, trophoblastic disorders, HG in previous pregnancy, nulliparity, metabolic causes (e.g. hyperthyroidism, hyperparathyroidism, hepatic dysfunction, impaired lipid metabolism), and eating disorders such as bulimia or anorexia[6] as well as women of Asian descent in the UK.[7]
- Other conditions should be excluded especially if severe nausea and vomiting is present before 8–9 weeks or after 20–22 weeks gestation, such as any underlying disorders or related symptoms suggesting other pathology may be involved (see Figure 24.1).
- Clinical symptoms are usually non-specific; unusual causes of nausea and vomiting should be excluded.

Maternal and fetal outcomes

- HG can cause severe distress in affected women due to loss of time from work, a reduced quality of life, and the psychological burden of not feeling well for several weeks or months, which in turn may result in family problems such as care of the other children.
- The psychosomatic aspects of hyperemesis can be considerable and can present in the form of secondary depression, which affects up to 7% of patients with HG.[8]
- In severe cases, HG can even result in rupture of oesophageal varices, Mallory–Weiss syndrome, pneumothorax, peripheral neuropathy, or Wernicke's encephalopathy due to lack of thiamine.
- HG occurring in the second trimester has been shown to double the risk of developing early onset pre-eclampsia, a threefold increased risk of placental abruption, and a 39% increased risk of a SGA baby.[9] Such placental dysfunction disorders have not been observed in women presenting with HG in the first trimester.

Investigations required

- Laboratory investigations should include:
  - Haematocrit, electrolytes, urea, thyroid function tests, LFTs especially transaminases and bilirubin; magnesium levels need to be checked if hyperemesis is severe or if potassium is less than 3.0 mmol/litre.
  - Urinalysis for ketones, nitrites, leucocytes, casts and culture and sensitivity of a midstream sample of urine. If glycosuria in addition to ketonuria is found, diabetes to be excluded.

Figure 24.1 Conditions associated with nausea and vomiting in pregnancy.

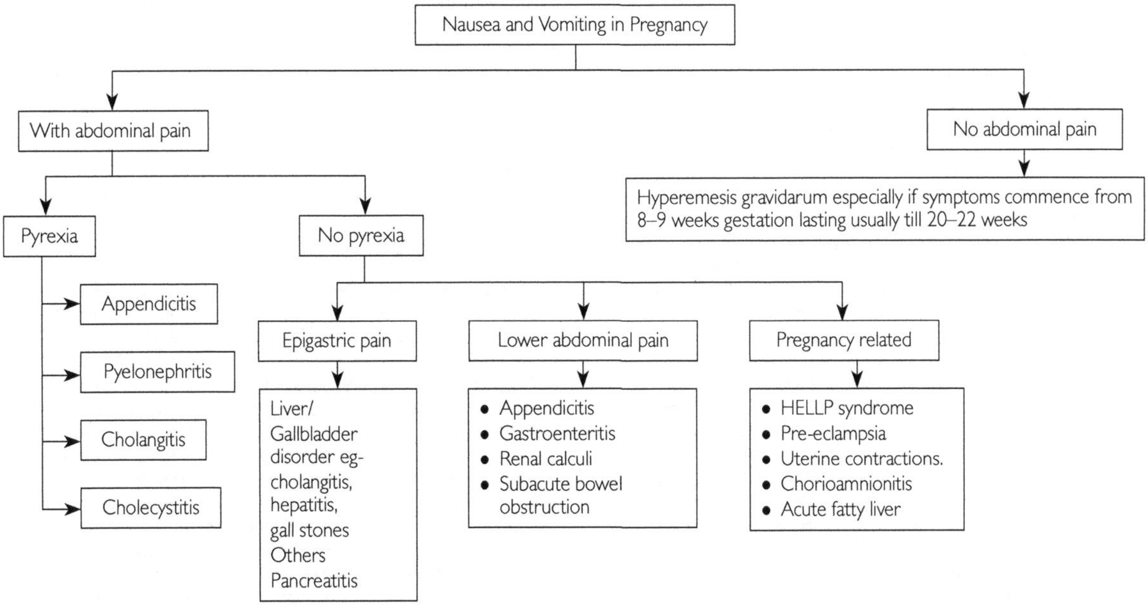

- Other investigations such as serum amylase need to be performed as necessary according to any associated symptoms.
- Ultrasound scan if not previously performed to exclude multiple pregnancy, hydatidiform mole as well as gallstones, renal calculi, etc.
- HG is characterized by dehydration, acidosis due to lack of nutrition, alkalosis due to loss of hydrochloride, and hypokalaemia. The metabolic imbalance that accompanies HG is not present in the normal nausea and vomiting seen in 80–90% of all pregnant women.[6]
- Liver function abnormalities have been reported in up to 67% of HG patients, with elevations of either aspartate aminotransferase or alanine aminotransferase being observed in 50%. Liver enzyme abnormalities were found to be associated with a later onset of HG, more severe ketonuria, and hyperthyroidism.[10]
- Liver enzymes return to normal soon after the vomiting resolves and adequate nutrition is resumed. The liver enzyme abnormalities are a result rather than the cause of HG and are probably due to the combined effect of hypovolaemia, malnutrition, and lactic acidosis in HG.
- Transient gestational thyrotoxicosis is found in up to two-thirds of women suffering from HG. This condition may be partly caused by the high levels of HCG that are often seen in patients with HG since HCG and thyroid stimulating hormone (TSH) have a very similar protein structure. This enables HCG to act like thyrotrophin receptor hormone (TRH) and hyperstimulate the thyroid.[11]
- In transient gestational thyrotoxicosis associated with HG, free T3 and free T4 are usually in the normal range, with reduced levels of TSH.
- For a diagnosis of transient gestational thyrotoxicosis of HG to be made, apart from the above thyroid function findings, there would have to be no previous history of thyrotoxicosis before the pregnancy, no clinical signs of hyperthyroidism, and no thyroid antibodies present.[6]
- Transient gestational thyrotoxicosis may last up to the 18th week of gestation and does not require treatment.

Treatment

- Since the causation of HG involves multifarious factors, treatment of this condition should be multimodal, ranging from dietary and lifestyle advice, to psychosomatic counselling. IV fluid replacement is necessary as well as administration of antiemetics.
- Management of HG depends on the severity.

Management in primary care

- Most cases of HG are dealt with almost exclusively by GPs.[12]
- Most cases are self-limiting and settle without complications as the pregnancy progresses.
- Nausea and vomiting in pregnancy are usually associated with favourable pregnancy outcomes.
- In cases of severe vomiting, multiple pregnancy and hydatidiform mole must be considered in early pregnancy while nausea and vomiting could be part of the symptomatology of pre-eclampsia in later pregnancy.
- Iron supplements may sometimes trigger nausea and vomiting and are worth stopping till HG settles.
- Admit to hospital if symptoms are severe despite 24 h of medication (e.g. inability to tolerate liquids without vomiting), or there is evidence of dehydration or suspicion of complications or if significantly abnormal urea and electrolytes (sodium <120 mmol/litre) are found.
- Seek specialist advice from an obstetrician if the woman has elevated urine ketone levels despite drug treatment or in the event of haematemesis.
- Have a lower threshold for admitting to hospital or seeking specialist advice if the woman has a coexisting condition (e.g. diabetes) which may be adversely affected by nausea and vomiting.
- Reassure the woman that nausea and vomiting are a normal part of pregnancy and that pregnancy outcomes are generally better for women who have nausea and vomiting in early pregnancy.
- Advise rest and drinking little and often rather than in large amounts, as this may help to prevent vomiting.
- The following advice may also be tried:
  - Eating small, frequent meals high in carbohydrate and low in fat (cold meals may be more easily tolerated if nausea is smell-related).
  - Eating plain biscuits about 20 min before getting up.
  - Ginger.
  - Avoiding cold, tart, or sweet beverages.
  - Acupressure.
- The cornerstone of **non-pharmacological therapy of HG** is avoidance of environmental triggers such as stuffy rooms, odours (e.g. perfume, food, smoke), heat, humidity, noise, and visual or physical motion (e.g. flickering lights, driving).
- Electrolyte replacement drinks and oral nutritional supplements are advisable for ensuring maintenance of electrolyte balance and an adequate intake of calories.
- All women with nausea and vomiting in pregnancy should be advised to seek urgent medical advice if they experience:
  - very dark urine, or no urination for more than 8 h
  - abdominal pain or fever
  - severe weakness or feeling faint
  - vomiting blood.
  - repeated, unstoppable vomiting.
  - inability to keep down food or fluids for 24 h.
- Consider **drug treatment** only if initial treatments (e.g. dietary advice, rest) have failed and the woman has persistent, severe symptoms that prevent daily activities, or increased urine ketone levels.
- ***All antiemetics are unlicensed for treatment of nausea and vomiting in pregnancy!***
- If an antiemetic is required in pregnancy, prescribe oral promethazine (25 mg at bedtime) or alternatively oral cyclizine (50 mg tds), and reassess after 24–48 h (checking for dehydration).
- If the response after 24–48 h is good, continue promethazine/cyclizine.
- If the response is inadequate, the woman is not dehydrated, and there is no ketonuria, switch medication to oral metoclopramide 10 mg tds or oral prochlorperazine 10 mg tds or buccal 3–6 mg bd for another 24–48 h and reassess. Seek specialist advice from an obstetrician if there is an inadequate response to antiemetics and/or the woman is dehydrated or has ketonuria.

Management in hospital

- Admission to hospital is indicated when persistent vomiting continues after rehydration and outpatient management has not worked, especially after three or more previous attendances for day case rehydration.
- Assessment for clinical dehydration, general condition, weight measurement, investigations as specified above (see 'Investigation required').
- Other causes for vomiting to be excluded.
- The treatment goals in patients with nausea and vomiting of pregnancy are to:
  - reduce symptoms through changes in diet/environment and by medication.
  - correct complications of nausea and vomiting (e.g. fluid depletion, hypokalaemia, and metabolic alkalosis).
- In patients with severe dehydration or ketonuria, inpatient admission is required. Sometimes hospitalization alone, even if not for overnight stay, is sufficient to improve symptoms.
- The primary therapeutic step is total food withdrawal.
- The treatment of dehydration is of paramount importance. Maintaining hydration or, in the case of severe dehydration achieving rapid and sufficient rehydration, is the most important intervention. Rehydration is most easily and quickly accomplished intravenously and this reduces adverse symptoms very effectively.
- Volume and electrolyte replacement (at least 3 litres/day), correction of potential electrolyte imbalance, administration of vitamins.
- Initial IV fluid should be normal saline with 20 mmol potassium. Glucose-containing (carbohydrate-rich) IV fluids must be avoided to start with, as they may precipitate Wernicke's encephalopathy.

- Initial rehydration with lactate administration using Hartman's is not optimal and also contraindicated before thiamine replacement.
- **First -line antiemetic therapy** includes one or a combination of the following:
  - dopamine antagonist phenothiazines, e.g. prochlorperazine
  - metoclopramide
  - antihistamines (e.g. cyclizine).
- **Second- line therapy:** In addition to a first-line drug, if needed, ondansetron or promethazine can also be used in severe cases of HG.
- ***Third- line therapy:***
  - Steroids: Hydrocortisone
  - Pyridoxine (vitamin B_6) improves mild to moderate nausea, but does not significantly reduce vomiting. The mechanism for the therapeutic effect of pyridoxine in women with nausea is unknown. The initial dose of pyridoxine is 25 mg orally every 6–8 h; the maximum dose suggested for pregnant women is 200 mg/day, but cumulative doses up to 500 mg/day appear to be safe.
- Acid-reducing medications can be used as adjunctive therapy. In women with heartburn/acid reflux and nausea/vomiting of pregnancy, acid-reducing therapy (e.g. antacids, H_2 blockers, proton pump inhibitors) combined with antiemetic medication has been found to result in significant improvement in symptoms within 3–4 days after beginning therapy.[13]
- Pharmacological acid-suppressive therapy with H_2 receptor antagonists, ranitidine and cimetidine, or proton pump inhibitors such as omeprazole appears to be safe during pregnancy.
- In order to determine whether an underlying *H. pylori* infection is (partially) causative, *H. pylori* testing may be performed. In the event of a positive result, H_2 blockers (e.g. cimetidine) or proton pump inhibitors (e.g. omeprazole) can be added to infusions.
- If HG is refractory to treatment, corticoids (e.g. hydrocortisone) may also be used.[14] IV administration may be preferable to oral administration, particularly in refractory cases, as the effect is greater and more rapid.
- The transplacental passage of prednisolone is limited to around 10%.[15] Corticosteroids are considered to be safe and have no known adverse effects for the fetus, especially when used in the second trimester.
- Steroids may have an impact on causing a small increased risk of facial cleft palate and/or cleft lip, especially when used in the first trimester.
- Use ranitidine orally or IV if heartburn is present.
- If steroids have been used for more than 2 weeks during the pregnancy, IV hydrocortisone cover must be offered during labour and delivery.
- Similarly in cases of longer term steroid use, a GTT at about 28 weeks is needed to exclude steroid-induced gestational diabetes.
- The use of total parenteral nutrition (TPN) is controversial and it should only be used as a last resort when all other treatments have failed, as it can be associated with severe complications such as thrombosis, metabolic disturbances, and septicaemia.[2,16] A nasogastric tube is uncomfortable and is also associated with hazards.[17] Both modalities require hospitalization and being attached to intrusive tubes and are inferior to steroid therapy in restoring well-being.
- Treatment should be continued until vomiting ceases or occurs less than three times a day. Subsequent food reintroduction should be carried out gradually.
- VTE assessment must be performed on admission and antiembolic stockings and LMWH prescribed to all clinically dehydrated patients.
- Termination of pregnancy in extreme cases of HG when all measures have not succeeded has been reported in about 2% of pregnancies complicated by HG.[14,18]

Information for patients

Please see **Information for patients: Hyperemesis gravidarum** (p. 546)

References

1. Gadsby R, et al. A prospective study of nausea and vomiting during pregnancy. Br J Gen Pract 1993;43: 245–248.
2. Jueckstock JK, et al. Managing hyperemesis gravidarum: a multimodal challenge. BMC Med 2010;8: 46–54.
3. Michelini GA. Hyperemesis gravidarum. Emedicine 2002, July 12, Section 2.
4. Miller F. Nausea and vomiting in pregnancy: the problem of perception—is it really a disease? Am J Obstet Gynecol 2002; 186 Suppl: S182–S183.
5. Mazzotta P, et al. Attitudes, management and consequences of nausea and vomiting of pregnancy in the United States and Canada. Int J Gynaecol Obstet 2000;70: 359–365.
6. Mylonas I, et al. Nausea and vomiting in pregnancy. Dtsch Arztebl 2007;104: A1821–1826.
7. Price A, et al. Asian women are at increased risk of gestational thyrotoxicosis. J Clin Endocrinol Metab 1996;81: 1160–1163.
8. Poursharif B, et al. The psychosocial burden of hyperemesis gravidarum. J Perinatol 2008;28: 176–181.
9. Bolin M, et al. Hyperemesis gravidarum and risks of placental dysfunction disorders: a population-based cohort study. BJOG 2013;120: 541–547.
10. Verberg MFG, et al. Hyperemesis gravidarum, a literature review. Hum Reprod Update 2005;11: 527–539.
11. Rodien P, et al. Abnormal stimulation of the thyrotrophin receptor during gestation. Hum Reprod Update 2004;10: 95–105.
12. Clinical Knowledge Summaries: Nausea and vomiting in pregnancy. <http://www.cks.nhs.uk/nausea_vomiting_in_pregnancy>
13. Gill SK, et al. The effect of acid-reducing pharmacotherapy on the severity of nausea and vomiting of pregnancy. Obstet Gynecol Int 2009;2009: 1–4.
14. Al-Ozairi E, et al. Termination is not the treatment of choice for severe hyperemesis gravidarum: Successful management using prednisolone. Obstet Med 2009;2: 34–37.
15. Beitins IZ, et al. Transplacental passage of prednisolone and prednisolone in pregnancy near term. J Pediatr 1972;81: 936–945.
16. Holmgren C, et al. Hyperemesis in pregnancy: an evaluation of treatment strategies with maternal and neonatal outcomes. Am J Obstet Gynecol 2008;198: e1–4.
17. Hutchinson R, et al. A case of intramural oesophageal dissection secondary to nasogastric tube insertion. Ann R Coll Surg Engl 2008;90: W4–7.
18. Mazzotta P, et al. Factors associated with elective termination of pregnancy among Canadian and American women with nausea and vomiting of pregnancy. J Psychosom Obstet Gynaecol 2001;22: 7–12.

Guide for in-patient admission

- Severe symptoms **of HG** despite 24 h of medication (inability to tolerate liquids without vomiting); persistent large ketones on urinalysis even after day case rehydration
- Evidence of dehydration or suspicion of complications or if significantly abnormal urea and electrolytes (sodium <120 mmol/litre) are found
- If there is a coexisting condition (e.g. diabetes)
- If rehydration and outpatient management has not worked, especially after 3 or more previous attendances for day-case rehydration
- Haematemesis
- Severe abdominal pain or symptoms suggesting a different pathology

↓

Initial assessment; investigations to exclude other aetiology and to confirm HG

- **History** of any abdominal pain, pyrexia, colour of urine, pre-existing medical problems such as diabetes, thyroiditis or hyperthyroidism, hyperparathyroidism; recently commenced oral iron supplements or antibiotics, weight loss, bowel movements, etc
- **Signs** of clinical dehydration, weight, pulse, temperature, BP
- **Blood tests:** Haematocrit, electrolytes, urea, thyroid function tests, liver function tests especially transaminases and bilirubin; magnesium levels if potassium <3.0 mmol/litre. Other investigations as indicated by any additional symptoms
- **Urine analysis:** Ketones, nitrites, leucocytes, casts; culture and sensitivity of a mid-stream sample of urine. If glycosuria present as well as ketonuria, consider diabetes
- **Ultrasound scan:** Exclude multiple pregnancy, molar pregnancy, and if symptoms of abdominal/flank pain scan to exclude renal or gall bladder stones

↓

Management

- Even while investigations are in progress, institute IV fluids, antiemetics. Nil by mouth
- Oral nutrition to be stopped
- Fluid and electrolyte replacement: Initial IV fluid should be normal saline with 20 mmol potassium, 2 litres over 4–6 h. After thiamine supplementation, Hartman's solution can be used. Avoid glucose-containing solutions
- Thiamine—oral supplementation 50 mg three times a day. If patient unable to tolerate oral thiamine discuss IV thiamine administration with pharmacist
- Further fluid and electrolyte management according to U&E results and presence of ketonuria
- Withhold oral iron, advise patient to avoid any identified triggers for nausea and vomiting
- First dose of antiemetic IV or IM on admission; continue regular antiemetics by IV or IM route till patient able to tolerate food without vomiting
- Regular doses of antiemetics to continue—do not stop antiemetics after initial temporary abatement of symptoms, as HG will recur otherwise
- Antiemetics in a stepped-up regime (see below)
- **Nutrition:** Once dehydration (no ketonuria) and electrolyte imbalance corrected, start with small oral sips of clear fluids, advancing gradually to solids as tolerated. Dietitian must be involved. As a last resort, TPN to be considered
- Antiembolic stockings and prophylactic LMWH (weight adjusted)
- Accurate fluid balance chart, weekly weighing if still in-patient, urinanalysis on each specimen
- Emotional and psychological support and encouragement
- Discharge with oral thiamine, folic acid (if <13 weeks gestation)and oral or PR antiemetics

Stepped-up antiemetic regime

- **First-line therapy:** one or a combination of two of the following:
  - Proclorperazine 12.5 mg deep IM injections or 25 mg PR suppositories followed by oral or rectal maintenance doses of 5–10 mg twice or three times daily
  - Cyclizine as IM or IV injection 50 mg/ml 3 times daily
  - Metoclopramide IM injection 5–10 mg over 1–2 min 3 times daily or oral 5–10 mg 3 times daily
- **Second-line therapy:** Ondansetron first as IV injection 4–8 mg 12 hourly for 2 doses then 8 mg oral twice daily or 16 mg PR once daily. This is in addition to a first-line drug
- **Third-line therapy:** Steroids—IM hydrocortisone 100 mg twice daily initially, then oral prednisolone 20 mg for 7 days, tapering doses thereafter

24.9 Domestic Violence

FACT FILE

Incidence and forms of domestic violence in the UK

- Violence may take the form of physical, sexual, or psychological abuse where the perpetrator seeks control over their victim.
- Domestic violence in pregnancy is, in the vast majority, mostly inflicted by the present sexual partner, an ex-partner, or another member of the extended family in certain cultural groups, which may result in isolation from the outside world.
- This may cause alienation of the victim from the outside world. The health service may be their only point of contact and chance to disclose.
- 1 in 4 women are said to be victims of domestic violence during their lifetime,[1,2] although this is bound to be an underestimate.
- On average, it takes an average of 35 episodes of violence before help is sought and most women will only volunteer information if asked directly.

Effect of domestic violence during pregnancy and puerperium

- In as many as 30% of cases, domestic violence seems to either start or to escalate during pregnancy and after delivery.[3] The risk of moderate to severe violence appears to be greatest in the postpartum period. In the CEMACH report of 2005,[4] 11 new mothers were murdered by their partners within 6 weeks of delivery.
- 12% of the 378 women whose deaths were included in the 1997–99 Confidential Enquiry on Maternal Deaths had voluntarily reported domestic violence to a healthcare professional during their pregnancy.[5]
- The pattern of assault may alter, with pregnant women being 13 times more likely to be struck on the abdomen and breasts.
- Violence may be aimed directly at the unborn child. Physical injuries to live fetuses include broken bones, stab wounds, and fetal death.[3]
- Pregnancy may be a consequence of rape.
- The psychological and social consequences of domestic violence include alcohol and drug dependence, suicide attempts, depression, and post-traumatic stress disorder.
- The effects of domestic violence on women include:
  - 15 times more likely to use alcohol
  - 9 times more likely to use drugs
  - 3 times more likely to have mental ill health
  - 5 times more likely to attempt suicide.
- Domestic violence can also cause miscarriage,[5,6,7] premature delivery,[8] low birth weight,[9] abruption,[10] stillbirth,[11] and maternal death, in-utero brain damage, or impaired neurobiological brain development leading to mental and physical disability of the child.
- Domestic violence affects all social classes and ethnic groups.
- Between 5% and 11% of women who present acutely to a hospital emergency department do so as a result of domestic violence.
- They are more likely to be pregnant, present with multiple injuries including fractures, abdominal injuries, injuries to the arm and face, have delayed presentation, or lost consciousness. They may initially state that their injury was due to a fall down the stairs.[12]
- Pregnant women who have suffered a history of domestic violence within the last 12 months may present with late booking, spurious labour, significant backaches, headaches, hyperemesis.[13] Vague unresolved admissions to the antenatal ward can be associated with domestic violence in the current pregnancy.
- Another study examined the incidence of preterm labour and found this to be 4.1 times greater (incidence 17%) in those who experienced severe violence as compared with those who experienced no maternal abuse during pregnancy.[10]

Indicators of domestic abuse relevant to maternity care[13]

- Late booking and/or poor attendance or non-attendance at antenatal clinics.
- Repeat attendances at antenatal clinics, the GP surgery or emergency departments for minor injuries or trivial or non-existent complaints or unexplained admissions.
- Non-compliance with treatment regimens/early self- discharge from hospital.
- Repeat presentation with depression, anxiety, self-harm, and psychosomatic symptoms.
- Injuries that are untended and of several different ages, especially to the neck, head, breasts, abdomen, and genitals.
- Minimalization of signs of abuse on the body.
- Sexually transmitted diseases and frequent vaginal or urinary tract infections and pelvic pain.
- Poor obstetric history: for example, repeated miscarriage or terminations of pregnancy) stillbirth or preterm birth, intrauterine growth restriction/low birth weight, unwanted or unplanned pregnancy.
- The constant presence of the woman's partner at examinations, who may be domineering, answer all the questions for her, and be unwilling to leave the room.
- The woman appears evasive or reluctant to speak or disagree in front of her partner or a member of the partner's family.

Interaction between healthcare professionals and victims of domestic violence

- Victims of domestic violence are often reluctant to seek professional help or are unaware of the possibility of accessing such help.[14] They may be overwhelmed by the involvement of multiple agencies. Others, especially recent arrivals into the country, may not be familiar with antenatal care services and may find it hard to communicate with healthcare staff. They may fear backlash from the perpetrator of violence if their effort to seek help is discovered.
- Victims might fear both the perpetrator and professionals. Perpetrators may have used professional response to domestic violence that the victim fears as a threat (you are an unfit mother; the children will be taken into care, etc.).
- Women may have gone to great lengths to disguise domestic violence for a number of reasons (guilt, fear of perpetrator, fear of losing the children).
- Questions about domestic violence must be asked in a sympathetic way.[15,16]
- Domestic violence is a challenging and difficult area for any healthcare professional to explore, especially in the relatively short interaction involved during the span of a pregnancy. Despite this, it is incumbent upon all staff to be able to raise the subject with all pregnant women, irrespective of class or ethnic origin.
- The community midwife is in a privileged position, due to the nature of her role and the encounters with the pregnant woman, sometimes in her home setting, to enquire about and receive disclosures about the domestic situation.
- There is clear evidence that routine enquiry in a confidential setting, ensuring that the pregnant woman understands that adequate support, appropriate referral, and follow-up mechanisms are available, would see a sixfold increase in the identification of domestic violence.[15]
- The mechanism and structure as well as the requisite training for health care professionals has been defined by the NICE Clinical Guideline[14] and the guidelines of the Department of Health for responding to domestic abuse.[16]

Information for patients

Please see **Information for patients: Domestic violence during pregnancy** (p. 547)

References

1. Knox E. Perinatal review: domestic violence. Birmingham: Perinatal Institute, 2001 <http://www.perinatal.nhs.uk/reviews/dv/dv_intro.htm>.
2. Home Office. Domestic violence: findings from a new British Crime Survey self-completion questionnaire. London: Home Office, 1999.
3. Mezey GC, Bewley S. Domestic violence and pregnancy: risk is greatest after delivery BMJ 1997;314: 1295.
4. Lewis G, et al. Why mothers die: report from the Confidential Enquiries into Maternal Deaths in the United Kingdom 2000–2002. CEMACH. London: RCOG Press, 2005.
5. CEMACH. Why mothers die 1997–1999. Confidential Enquiries into Maternal Deaths. London: RCOG Press, 2001.
6. Mezey GC. Domestic violence in pregnancy. In: Bewley S, ed., Violence against women. London: RCOG Press, 1997.
7. Mezey GC, Bewley S. Domestic violence: prevalence in pregnant women and associations with physical and psychological health. Euro J Obstet Gynecol Reprod Biol 2004;113: 6–11.
8. Webster J, et al. Pregnancy outcomes and healthcare use: effects of abuse. Am J Obstet Gynecol 1996;174: 760–767.
9. Shah PS, Shah J. Maternal exposure to domestic violence and pregnancy and birth outcomes: a systematic review and meta-analyses. J Womens Health 2010;19: 2017–2029.
10. Shumway J, et al. Preterm labor, placental abruption, and premature rupture of membranes in relation to maternal violence or verbal abuse. J Matern Fetal Med 1999;8: 76–80.
11. Mezey G, et al. An exploration of the prevalence, nature and effect of domestic violence in pregnancy. ESRC study, 2000.
12. Spedding RL, et al. Markers for domestic violence in women. J Accid Emerg Med 1999;16: 400–402.
13. Centre for Maternal and Child Enquiries (CMACE). Saving mothers' lives: reviewing maternal deaths to make motherhood safer: 2006–08. The Eighth Report on Confidential Enquiries into Maternal Deaths in the United Kingdom. BJOG 2011;118Suppl. 1: 1–203.
14. NICE Clinical Guideline. Pregnancy and complex social factors. CG110. London: National Institute for Health and Clinical Excellence, 2010.
15. Price S, et al. Does routine antenatal enquiry lead to an increased rate of disclosure of domestic abuse? Evidence Based Midwifery 2007;5; 100–106.
16. DH. Responding to domestic abuse. A handbook for healthcare professionals. London: Department of Health, 2005.

24.10 Periodontal Disease and Pregnancy Outcomes

FACT FILE

- Increasing evidence is emerging to suggest that maternal periodontitis and gingivitis may be risk factors for pregnancy complications such as miscarriages, preterm birth, intrauterine growth restriction (IUGR), or pre-eclampsia, but further studies are needed to establish an irrefutable causal link.[1,2,3,4,5,6,7,8,9]
- Periodontal disease includes **gingivitis** (an inflammatory condition of the soft tissues surrounding a tooth or the gingiva) and **periodontitis** (which involves destruction of the supporting structures such as periodontal ligament, bone, dental cement, or soft tissues).
- Periodontal disease is caused by overgrowth of certain bacterial species, mainly Gram-negative, anaerobic bacteria that flourish in subgingival sites.
- Prevalence in adults has been reported varying between 10 and 60% depending on diagnostic criteria used in different studies.[10,11,12]
- Periodontal disease is an infectious disease found in nearly 25% of women.[13]
- Periodontitis is usually chronic and insidious with pain usually developing late in the disease process when bone and tooth loss occur.

Pathogenesis and perinatal effects

- ***Periodontal disease may pose a greater risk for preterm labour and lowbirth weight than even alcohol consumption or smoking.***
- Obstetricians, midwives, and GPs must therefore be aware of the possible link between poor dental health and adverse pregnancy outcomes.
- Periodontal disease is both preventable and curable, therefore improving periodontal health both before and during pregnancy may help prevent or reduce the occurrence of adverse pregnancy outcomes.
- It is well recognized that genitourinary infections are implicated in a significant proportion of preterm deliveries and in preterm premature rupture of membranes. Such infections induce the release of inflammatory mediators such as interleukin 1 (IL-1), tumour necrosis factor alpha(TNF-α), and prostaglandin E_2(PGE_2) which trigger preterm labour and PPROM.
- Other generalized systemic infections such as viral infections may also lead to preterm deliveries.
- Chronic periodontal disease can also produce local and systemic host responses leading to transient bacteraemia. Lipopolysaccharide (LPS) endotoxins that enter gingival tissue produce high levels of proinflammatory cytokines (e.g. tumour necrosis factor).[14]
- About 40% of all pregnancies are associated with fetal IgM antibody response that can be identified in the placenta mounted against organisms of maternal oral origin.
- If there is poor or inadequate oral hygiene, periodontal bacteria can accumulate in gingival crevices forming an organized structure called a **bacterial film**.
- Such bacterial microfilms can lead to direct destruction of periodontal structures but also cause maternal sepsis, thus disseminating throughout the body to trigger a systemic inflammatory response.[14]
- Periodontitis can act as a source of **Gram-negative anaerobic bacteria** growing in the subgingival sites as well as of inflammatory mediators that can affect the feto-placental unit through the circulating blood and lead to pregnancy complications.
- Some case-control and cohort studies have shown a strong association (risk increased by up to 7.5–20%) between periodontal disease and pregnancy complications,[1,2,3,4,12,15] whereas others have failed to demonstrate such a causal link.[7,16]
- The main differences between these studies are most likely to be accounted for by definitions of periodontal disease and differences in populations in terms of periodontal health and poor pregnancy outcomes, as well as confounding factors such as poor socio-economic class, smoking, diabetes, hypertension, etc.[7]
- In those studies that showed such a positive association, periodontal disease preceded the pregnancy complications and not vice versa.[1,2,3,4,12,15]
- The risk of preterm delivery, especially the very preterm, appears to be particularly associated with **progressive** periodontal disease.[13]
- Interventional studies treating periodontal disease in one group and not in the other, have shown a reduction of adverse pregnancy outcomes in the treated group.[17,18]
- The dental interventions in these studies consisted of **plaque control instructions, scaling, and root planing with or without the use of chlorhexidine mouth rinse or metronidazole**. Such periodontal treatments employed in these studies have suggested a reduction in the incidence of preterm labour and lowbirth weight.
- More studies are needed, however, to establish a firm link that periodontal treatment of the mother will improve pregnancy and neonatal outcomes.

References

1. Offenbacher SJ, et al. Periodontal infection as a possible risk factor for preterm low birth weight. Periodontology 1996;67:1103–1113.
2. Goepfert AR, et al. Periodontal disease and upper genital tract inflammation in early spontaneous preterm birth. Obstet Gynecol 2004;104:777–783.
3. Radnai M, et al. A possible association between preterm birth and early periodontitis: a pilot study. J Clin Periodontol 2004;31:736–741.
4. Jarjoura K, et al. Markers of periodontal infection and preterm birth. Am J Obstet Gynecol 2005;192:513–519.
5. Sembene M, et al. Periodontal infectionin pregnant women and low birth weight babies. Odontostomatol Trop 2000;23:19–22.
6. Louro PM, et al. Periodontal disease in pregnancy and low birth weight. J Pediatr (Rio J) 2001;77:23–28.
7. Davenport ES, et al. Maternal periodontal disease and preterm low birthweight: case-control study. J Dent Res 2002;81:313–318.
8. Jeffcoat MK, et al. Periodontal disease and preterm birth: results of a pilot intervention study. J Periodontol 2003;74:1214–1218.
9. Xiong X, et al. Periodontal disease and adverse pregnancy outcomes: a systematic review. BJOG 2006;113:135–143.
10. Papapanou PN. Periodontal diseases: epidemiology. Ann Periodontol 1996;1:1–36.
11. Albandar JM, Rams TE. Global epidemiology of periodontal diseases: an overview. Periodontology 20002002;29:7–10.
12. Offenbacher S, et al. Maternal periodontitis and prematurity. Part I: Obstetric outcome of prematurity and growth restriction. Ann Periodontol 2001;6:164–174.
13. Bobetsis YA, et al. Exploring the relationship between periodontal disease and pregnancy complications. JADA 2006; 137:7s–11 S
14. Garcia RI, et al. Relationship between periodontal disease and systemic health. Periodontol 20002001;25:21–36.
15. Boggess KA, et al. Maternal periodontal disease is associated with an increased risk for preeclampsia. Obstet Gynecol 2003;101:227–31
16. Moore S, et al. A prospective study to investigate the relationship between periodontal disease and adverse pregnancy outcome. Br Dent J 2004;197:251–258.
17. Mitchell-Lewis D, et al. Periodontal infections and pre-term birth: early findings from a cohort of young minority women in New York. Eur J Oral Sci 2001;109:34–39.
18. Lopez NJ, et al. Periodontal therapy may reduce the risk of preterm low birth weight in women with periodontal disease: a randomized controlled trial. J Periodontol 2002;73:911–924.

24.11 Ophthalmologic Considerations in Pregnancy and Puerperium

FACT FILE

Physiological ocular changes in pregnancy.

Several areas and functional aspects of the eyes undergo some change during a normal pregnancy.[1]

Cornea

- Slight increase in corneal thickness, especially in third trimester, probably due to oedema, reverts to normal in postpartum.[1]
- Increase in corneal curvature seen in pregnancy, which may continue for several months postpartum. Reversal after cessation of breastfeeding.
- Reversible decrease in lens accommodation sometimes seen in pregnancy.
- Due to increase in corneal curvature, thickness, and changes in the tear film, contact lenses may be less well tolerated during pregnancy.
- Women are therefore advised to wait for several weeks postpartum, until refraction is stabilized, before obtaining a new prescription for lenses.[2]

Intraocular pressure

- Decreases in pregnancy, persisting for several months postpartum.
- In pregnant women with pre-existing glaucoma, an improvement is often seen.[3]

Visual field

- Asymptomatic visual field changes may occur in pregnant women possibly due to the normal and slight increase in the size of the pituitary gland if it affects the optic chiasm.[4] These asymptomatic changes could include a degree of bitemporal loss, concentric constriction and enlarged blind spots. These are entirely reversible changes with spontaneous correction postpartum.
- Any symptomatic visual field changes during pregnancy or the puerperium, must, however, be rigorously investigated.[1]

External changes

- External changes such as drooping of the eyelids (ptosis) due to fluid retention and chloasmic pigmentation of the eye area are sometimes seen in normal pregnancy.[1] They are reversible changes that warrant no treatment other than reassurance.

Ocular changes associated with certain high-risk pregnancies

Pre-eclampsia and eclampsia

- Ocular sequelae are reported in up to a third of these cases (25% in pre-eclampsia, 50% in eclampsia),[5,6,7] including blurred vision, diplopia, scotomas.
- **Retinopathy, optic neuropathy, serous detachments, and occipital cortical changes** are the ocular manifestations that can be seen in association with fulminant pre-eclampsia or eclampsia.
- **Retinopathy** associated with pre-eclampsia is similar to hypertensive retinopathy with narrowing of the retinal arteriole, which can be focal or diffuse. Retinal haemorrhages, oedema, exudates ('cotton wool'exudates), and nerve infarcts can also be seen. Most, though not all, of these changes are reversible once pre-eclampsia resolves.
- The worse the pre-eclampsia, the greater the degree of retinopathy.
- In those with additional comorbidities such as diabetes, chronic hypertension, lupus, antiphospholipid syndrome, or renal disease, the retinopathy associated with pre-eclampsia is usually more severe.
- ***Optic nerve changes seen in pre-eclampsia / eclampsia include papilloedema, acute ischaemic optic neuropathy, even optical atrophy.***
- **Serous exudative retinal detachments** are usually bilateral more often seen in cases of impending eclampsia or eclampsia. Most resolve after a few weeks postpartum.
- **Loss of vision due to cortical blindness** as a result of cerebral oedema is likewise reported in severe pre-eclampsia/eclampsia.[8] Resolution of the cerebral oedema can lead to visual recovery in such patients.
- Visual changes in the postpartum period could rarely be the only sign of impending seizures in a woman with minimal signs of pre-eclampsia during pregnancy, labour, and delivery.[9]

Occlusive vascular disorders

- Both retinal arterial and venous occlusions have been reported in about 10% of certain coagulopathies seen in pregnancy such as **disseminated intravascular coagulopathy (DIC), thrombotic thrombocytopenic purpura (TTP), amniotic embolism, or antiphospholipid syndrome (APS).** Retinal vein occlusions are less common than arterial occlusions.
- In DIC, the choroid is a common ocular site to be involved. Visual loss can result from choroidal infarction or haemorrhage. Serous retinal detachment can resolve along with the DIC, but retinal pigmentary changes are usually left behind as a permanent feature.
- TTP is a rare disorder characterized by small vessel thrombosis, thrombocytopenia, microangiopathic haemolytic anaemia, renal dysfunction, and fever. Visual symptoms may occur due to serous retinal, detachment optic nerve oedema, retinal haemorrhage, etc.
- In APS, vascular thrombosis can be seen in the retina, choroid, optic nerve, visual pathway, and ocular motor nerves.[10,11,12]

Effect of pregnancy on pre-existing ophthalmologic disorders

Diabetic retinopathy

- Pregnancy can cause **worsening of pre-existing diabetic retinopathy**,[13] especially if the retinopathy was severe at the time of conception, if the glycaemic control is poor during pregnancy, or if the diabetes has been long-standing as well as if there is coexistent hypertension.
- Even among those who have had **no diabetic retinopathy at the time of conception**, approximately 10% can show some background changes, although very few (<0.2%) progress to a stage of proliferative retinopathy.
- Among those patients with **non-proliferative nephropathy**, 50% may show a worsening of this during pregnancy with about 10% also demonstrating proliferative changes. **An ophthalmologic examination is required at least once each trimester in such patients**.
- Diabetic women who commence pregnancy with **proliferative retinopathy**[14] need to have **monthly ophthalmologic examinations as a worsening is seen in about 45%**. In those who have had laser treatment before pregnancy, the risk of progressive proliferative retinopathy is reduced by 50%.
- Laser photocoagulation, is therefore recommended before pregnancy in those with severe non-proliferative or proliferative retinopathy.
- In diabetic women with superadded pre-eclampsia, **macular oedema** is a common finding, although this resolves spontaneously postpartum.

Intracerebral tumours[7]

- **Pituitary tumours:**
  - Enlargement during pregnancy of previously asymptomatic pituitary adenomas or microadenomas could be heralded by ophthalmologic symptoms such as visual field changes and/or visual acuity loss.
  - Of the symptomatic pituitary adenomas during pregnancy, a small number will require multispecialty involvement of ophthalmologists, endocrinologist, maternal medicine

obstetrician and the neurosurgeon to decide the most appropriate treatment—medical, surgical, or radiation.
    - An acute increase of the pituitary size due to infarction or haemorrhage can present as sudden onset of headache or visual field loss, or even visual loss.[4,6] This warrants prompt neurosurgical assessment with a view to surgical decompression. Pituitary apoplexy as a result of infarction can result in total pituitary failure (Sheehan's syndrome).
- **Meningiomas**:
    - Benign, slow-growing tumours but can enlarge rapidly in pregnancy causing severe symptoms such as decreased visual acuity, visual field loss, disc oedema, or oculomotor palsy.[8]
    - Conservative management in asymptomatic or minimally symptomatic pregnant women, but if symptomatic, neurosurgery usually required as these tumours are not sensitive to radiation or chemotherapy.

Connective tissue disorders (sarcoidosis, ankylosing spondylitis, rheumatoid arthritis, Sjögren's, dermatomyositis, polymyositis, etc.)

- There is usually an improvement in the ocular symptoms, mainly of uveitis, of these conditions during pregnancy.[7,8] This reflects systemic improvement, mainly because of the natural immunosuppression and higher circulating steroid levels seen in pregnancy. Relapses are, however, likely in the puerperium.

Ocular toxoplasmosis

- If the pregnant woman is known to have **congenital toxoplasmosis** acquired when she herself was a fetus, reactivation of ocular toxoplasmosis during pregnancy can occur with the presence of active toxoplasmic retinochoroiditis or scarring.[15] These are not signs of a fresh infection.
- In such recurrent disease the mother has already developed antibodies that protect the fetus and any risk of the fetus acquiring congenital toxoplasmosis is negligible.
- In cases where the pregnant woman has contracted active toxoplasmosis during the current pregnancy, ophthalmological examination is recommended every 3 months for the mother as well as close neonatal investigations and follow-up.

Idiopathic intracranial hypertension

Formerly called benign intracranial hypertension or pseudotumourcerebrii.

- Pregnancy does not increase the risk of developing idiopathic intracranial hypertension (IIH). Those who have pre-existing IIH have similar outcomes as in the non-pregnant. Ocular problems including papilloedema or transient visual disturbances are not uncommon.
- Acetazolamide has been shown to have a teratogenic potential in animal studies and is therefore best avoided in the first trimester, though can be used after embryogenesis is complete at the end of 12 weeks gestation.
- Diuretics might cause electrolyte and placental blood flow changes and are therefore used with care in pregnancy.
- Visual acuity and fields should be carefully monitored every 2 months during pregnancy. Any impairment of visual acuity or visual fields should be treated promptly with corticosteroids.
- Glucocorticoids, acetazolamide, diuretics and even serial lumbar puncture[16,17] are used to lower intracranial pressure in severe IIH to prevent permanent visual loss.
- Except in severe or untreated cases of IIH, labour and normal vaginal delivery are to be aimed for with Caesarean section reserved for obstetric indications. The obstetric management should remain unchanged if there are no signs of progressively worsening papilloedema and/or visual loss.

Glaucoma

- Pre-existing glaucoma may improve during pregnancy.
- Early referral to the ophthalmologist is recommended during pregnancy.
- Treatment options need to be modified during pregnancy.[18,19,20,21]
- Beta-blockers such as timolol are either avoided during pregnancy or the minimal dose is used.
- Systemic carbonic anhydrase blockers such as acetazolamide have potential teratogenic effects, though only in animal studies. They can be used with safety after the first trimester. The use of topical acetazolamide appears to be safe in pregnancy, especially when the patient is instructed to occlude the nasolacrimal duct and the punctum to reduce the amount absorbed by the nasal mucosa.
- Miotics such as pilocarpine appear to be safe in pregnancy, with the exception of demecarium.

High myopia, previously treated retinal detachment

- Until recently, obstetric concerns about possible retinal re-detachment or tears in those with high myopia or a previous history of treated retinal detachment (an opinion not shared by retinal detachment surgeons), resulted in advice supporting early induction of labour, avoiding vaginal delivery involving maternal bearing-down efforts, even advocating elective Caesarean section. This has led to unnecessary interventions being recommended.
- A recent retrospective study from Poland[22] has shown that in over 2% of Caesarean sections in that country were purely for ocular indications including myopia, glaucoma, or previous retinal detachment, though fully treated.
- More recent studies and expert ophthalmologic opinion have shown no deleterious effects on the retina, even with normal bearing-down efforts.[23,24,25] With a better understanding of the pathophysiology of 'rhegmatogenous' retinal detachment (RRD) there is **no evidence of increase in intra-ocular pressure with the Valsalva-like manoeuvres and increased intra-abdominal pressure associated with bearing-down efforts in the second stage of labour**.[24,25,26,27] Intraocular pressure can only be increased by blockage of the aqueous drainage in the anterior chamber of the eye, such as in glaucoma.
- Also, increased intraocular pressure is not a risk factor for RRD.[24,27]
- Patients with either high myopia or previously treated retinal detachment must therefore be strongly reassured about the safety of normal delivery, without any requirement to have elective Caesarean section, or early induction, or even second stage curtailed by forceps or ventouse.[22,24,25]

Retinoblastoma

- Retinoblastoma is a tumour arising from the retina of the eye that usually develops in children but can also occur in adults.[28] It is an autosomal dominant condition and all such individuals have a 1 in 2 chance of passing the defective gene on to their children, who then develop the eye tumour. As the condition is increasingly diagnosed early and treated successfully, most patients survive into adulthood.
- Both the woman and her partner, if either is a survivor of retinoblastoma, need to be counselled regarding the possibility of prenatal diagnosis. If genetic testing has already identified the tumour-predisposing mutation, fetal DNA obtained by chorionic villus sampling or amniocentesis can be analysed to confirm or exclude the diagnosis.[29] In cases where the causative mutation is unknown, ultrasound of the fetal eyes may successfully identify a fetal retinoblastoma.[30]

References

1. Sunness JS. The pregnant woman's eye. Surv Ophthalmol 1988;32:219–238.
2. Imafidon CO, Imafidon JE. Contact lenses in pregnancy. BJOG 1992;99:865–867.
3. Razeghinejad MR, et al. Pregnancy and glaucoma. Surv Ophthalmol 2011;56:324–335.
4. Elster AD, et al. Size and shape of the pituitary gland during pregnancy and postpartum: measurement with MR imaging. Radiology 1991;181:531–535.
5. Folk JC, Weingeist TA. Fundus changes in toxaemia. Ophthalmology 1981;88:1173–1174.
6. Park AJ, et al. Visual loss in pregnancy. Surv Ophthalmol 2000;45: 223–230.
7. Schultz KL, et al. Ocular disease in pregnancy. Curr Opin Ophthalmol 2005;16:308–314.
8. Thorsrud A, Kerty E. Combined retinal and cerebral changes in a pre-eclamptic woman. Acta Ophthalmol 2009;87: 925–926.
9. Watson DL, et al. Late postpartum eclampsia: an update. South Med J 1983;76:1487–1489.

10. Gass JD. Central serous chorioretinopathy and white subretinal exudation during pregnancy. Arch Ophthalmol 1991;109:677–681.
11. Chang M, Herbert WN. Retinal arteriolar occlusions following amniotic fluid embolism.. Ophthalmology 1984;91:1634–1637.
12. Durrani OM, et al. Primary anti-phospholipid antibody syndrome (APS): current concepts. Surv Ophthalmol 2002;47:215–238.
13. Sheth BP. Does pregnancy accelerate the rate of progression of diabetic retinopathy?: an update. Curr Diab Rep 2008.;8(4):270–273.
14. Reece EA, et al. Retinal and pregnancy outcomes in the presence of diabetic proliferative retinopathy. Reprod Med 1994;39:799–804.
15. Garweg JG. Reactivation of ocular toxoplasmosis during pregnancy. BJOG 2005;112:241–242.
16. Huna-Baron R, Kupersmith, MJ. Idiopathic intracranial hypertension in pregnancy. J Neurol 2002;249:1078–1081.
17. Badve M, McConnell MJ. Idiopathic intracranial hypertension in pregnancy treated with serial lumbar punctures. Int J Clin Med 2011;2:9–12.
18. Johnson SM, et al. Management of glaucoma in pregnancy and lactation. Surv Ophthalmol 2001;45:449–454.
19. Vaideanu D, Fraser S. Glaucoma management in pregnancy: a questionnaire survey. Eye (Lond) 2007;21:341–343.
20. Chung CY, et al. Use of ophthalmic medications during pregnancy. Hong Kong Med J 2004;10:191–195.
21. Sharma S, et al. Pregnancy and the eye. Obstetrician and Gynaecologist 2006;8:141–146.
22. Socha MW, et al. Retrospective analysis of ocular disorders and frequency of caesarean sections for ocular indications in 2000–2008—our own experience. Ginekol Pol 2010;81:188–191.
23. Feghali M, et al. Association of vaginal delivery efforts with retinal disease in women with type I diabetes. J Matern Fetal Neonatal Med 2012;25:27–31.
24. Papamichael E, et al. Obstetric opinions regarding the method of delivery in women that have had surgery for retinal detachment. JRSM Short Rep 2011;2:24.
25. Inglesby DV, et al. Surgery for detachment of the retina should not affect a normal delivery. BMJ 1990;300:980.
26. Neri A, et al. The management of labor in high myopic patients. Eur J Obstet Gynecol Reprod Biol 1985;23:277–279.
27. Landau D, et al. The effect of normal childbirth on eyes with abnormalities predisposing to rhegmatogenous retinal detachment. Graefs Arch Clin Exp Ophthalmol 1995;233:598–600.
28. Patni S, Gandhi A. Pregnancy and the eye. Obstetrician and Gynaecologist 2007;9:136a–137.
29. Pierro L, et al. Prenatal detection and early diagnosis of hereditary retinoblastoma in a family. Ophthalmologica 1993;207:106–111.
30. Salim A, et al. Fetal retinoblastoma. J Ultrasound Med 1998;17:717–720.

25 Multiple Pregnancies

25.1 Multiple Pregnancies: General Points

FACT FILE

- The incidence of **multiple births** has risen in the last 30 years.[1] Multiple births currently account for 3% of live births.
- This rising multiple birth rate is due mainly to the increased use of assisted reproduction techniques (ART), including in-vitro fertilization (IVF). Up to 24% of 'successful' IVF procedures result in multiple pregnancies.[2]
- **Fertility tourism,** a more recent phenomenon, has also contributed to higher-order multiple pregnancies resulting from IVF performed in countries that have fewer regulations governing numbers of embryos transferred.
- Other changes in population dynamics, including increasing maternal age at conception and immigration from regions where spontaneous multiple pregnancies are more common, have also contributed to the rise.
- Multiple pregnancies, whether conceived spontaneously or as a result of ART, are undoubtedly more complex compared with singleton pregnancies, with higher risks for the mother and babies.[1,3,4] The higher the order of multiple fetuses, the greater these risks.
- Due to the higher risk of complications, women with multiple pregnancies need closer and more frequent surveillance during pregnancy. This, as well as the pressure on neonatal services, represents a significant impact on NHS resources, even without accounting for the long-term care costs of chronic disability of some of the babies.
- In addition, due to the increased risks and need for frequent surveillance, psychological stress and concerns about the economic impact may add to the anxieties of the woman and her family.

Risks of multiple pregnancies

- **Maternal mortality associated with multiple births is 2.5 times that for singleton births.**[1,3,4]
- In general, an increased risk of **miscarriage, hyperemesis gravidarum, anaemia** (both microcytic and megaloblastic due to folic acid deficiency), **hypertensive disorders** including pre-eclampsia which could be of early onset and severe, **placental abruption, gestational diabetes, obstetric cholestasis**, increased need for **operative delivery, postpartum haemorrhage** and its sequelae as well as **puerperal problems** including **psychological problems** are more common with multiple gestations.
- The risk of **pre-eclampsia** in twin pregnancies is almost three times that for singleton pregnancies, and the risk is increased nine-fold in triplet pregnancies.
- All the minor ailments and discomforts of pregnancy are more marked in multiple gestation.
- The risk of **preterm birth** is significantly higher in multiple pregnancies than in singleton, with 50% of twins being born preterm (before 38 weeks). About 10% of all twins are born before 32 weeks gestation. The duration of pregnancy decreases with the increasing number of fetuses.
- The higher incidence of preterm birth in multiple pregnancies is inevitably associated with increased **neonatal mortality and long-term morbidity** including cerebral palsy, global developmental delay, and chronic lung disease.
- Prematurity accounts for 65% of neonatal deaths among multiple births, compared with 43% in singleton births.[5]
- The **stillbirth rate** in multiple pregnancies is higher than in singleton pregnancies: in 2009 the stillbirth rate was 12.3 per 1000 twin births and 31.1 per 1000 triplet and higher-order multiple births, compared with 5 per 1000 singleton births.
- Risks and outcomes are also influenced by the chorionicity and amnionicity of the multiple pregnancy. The phenomenon of **twin-to-twin transfusion syndrome (TTTS)** seen in 10–15% of monochorionic twin pregnancies, can also occur in monochorionic and dichorionic triplet pregnancies, hence the collective terminology **feto-fetal transfusion syndrome (FFTS)**.
- About 20% of all stillbirths in multiple pregnancies are due to FFTS. It is also associated with a significantly increased risk of neurodevelopmental morbidity.
- Monochorionic, monoamniotic **(MCMA)** pregnancies although rare (only 1–2% of MC pregnancies are MA) they face additional risks and poor outcomes such as **cord entanglement**.
- Increased rates of **intrauterine growth restriction (IUGR)** and **congenital abnormalities** are found with multiple pregnancies, independently contributing to the perinatal mortality and morbidity.
- Major congenital abnormalities are 4.9% more common in multiple pregnancies than in singleton pregnancies.

Management principles

- ***A definitive antenatal diagnosis of chorionicity is necessary at the earliest opportunity so that the pregnancy can be identified as the relatively less complicated dichorionic (DC) variety or the higher-risk MC type.***[1,3]

Pre-pregnancy

- Risk of multiple pregnancy is increases to 20–40% in women undergoing treatment cycles with ovulation induction agents; an increase of 5–10% is seen with clomifene citrate.
- The pregnancy risks with ART are also dependent on the number of embryos, zygotes, or oocytes returned.
- The best method of reducing the number of all multiple pregnancies achieved by ART is to reduce the number of embryos, zygotes, or oocytes transferred after full discussion of risks and benefits with the couple.

Models of antenatal care

- **Modified shared care** with both hospital-based and primary care is ideal, both for the psychological benefit of the pregnant mother and to reduce the inconvenience of her having to travel for numerous hospital visits if all her antenatal care were to be provided only in the hospital. Similarly, efforts to combine ultrasound scan appointments, fetal surveillance sessions, or blood pressure series, if indicated, with the antenatal clinic visit will reduce the number of visits to the hospital she would otherwise have to make.
- More care which is delivered closer to home, working on locally agreed algorithms **based on NICE and RCOG guidelines, needs to be planned and shared with the patient**.
- **Dating ultrasound scan in the first trimester:** If a multiple pregnancy is diagnosed, viability, the number of fetuses, chorionicity, and amnionicity should be established with visualization of either a lambda or 'T' sign.
- Aneuploidy screening needs to be discussed and offered if the patient chooses. Discordant nuchal translucency (NT) measurements in the first trimester may indicate fetal aneuploidy, trisomy, or triploidy if DC or early TTTS in MC multiple pregnancies.

- Other signs such as discordant bladder or crown–rump length (CRL) measurements may indicate early TTTS in MC pregnancy, though there are still some questions about their significance and sensitivity.
- Frequent antenatal visits shared with primary care allow extra vigilance for the early detection of PIH/pre-eclampsia.
- Iron and folate supplementation may be indicated from the second trimester to the end of pregnancy due to the high incidence of maternal anaemia.
- Anomaly scan at about 20 weeks, due to the increased risk of congenital anomalies in multiple pregnancies, especially cardiac defects.
- Schedule for scanning varies according to chorionicity and must be planned accordingly.
- There is no evidence that prophylactic cervical cerclage, tocolytics, or bed rest help prevent preterm labour/delivery in multiple pregnancies.[1]
- NICE[1] recommends that women with twin and triplet pregnancies are informed of their increased risk of preterm birth and about the benefits of targeted corticosteroids when there was an immediate risk of preterm birth.
- There is less evidence for the benefits of the role of untargeted (routine) single course of corticosteroids in multiple pregnancy based on current literature, although NICE acknowledges the urgent need for better research into this.
- ***Targeted prophylactic steroids are recommended as a single course (two split doses).***
- ***Documented discussion regarding the overall risks of multiple pregnancies, particularly of the type the patient is carrying, recognition of symptoms which might indicate complications and how to seek immediate advice and help, and continued structure of antenatal care needs to take place at the first clinic visit in the hospital. The patient can be offered an information leaflet regarding her particular type of multiple pregnancy.***

Ultrasound determination of chorionicity

- **Ultrasound examination at 6–9 weeks gestation:** Thick septum between chorionic sacs indicates DC twins. Non-identification of the Lambda sign at 10–14 weeks scan is definite proof of MC pregnancy.[4]
- Sonographic examination of the base of the inter-twin membrane at its attachment to the placenta at 10–13+ weeks for the presence or absence of the lambda sign (twin peak sign) or the 'T' sign to distinguish DC from MC pregnancies.
- There is regression of the lambda sign with advancing gestation. By 20 weeks gestation, only 85% of DC pregnancies demonstrate the lambda sign. Absence of the lambda sign after 20 weeks does not, therefore, exclude dichorionicity.
- If the first ultrasound examination is delayed until 16–18 weeks, chorionic status is more difficult to determine and an opportunity to plan successful management of TTTS may already have been missed.
- Chorionicity, rather than zygosity is the main factor determining pregnancy outcomes (see Table 25.1).

Risk of complications

Miscarriage and late second-trimester pregnancy loss

- In a singleton pregnancy if a scan at 13 weeks shows a live fetus, rate of subsequent miscarriage or fetal death before 24 weeks gestation is only about 1%.
- In DC twins the risk is 2–4% and in MC twins up to 10%. The latter is due to the effect of severe early-onset TTTS.

Perinatal mortality

- PNMR for twins is 5–7 times higher than in singletons, mainly due to prematurity related complications. This is worse with MC than DC twin pregnancies.
- In MC twins, TTTS is an added complication to that of prematurity.

Early preterm delivery

- Risk of spontaneous delivery at 24–32 weeks in singletons is about 1%.
- In DC twins, this is up to 5–10%; in MC twins 10–15%.
- Almost all babies born before 23 weeks die and almost all babies born after 32 weeks survive.
- In those born between 24 and 32 weeks, there is a higher risk of neonatal death and cerebral palsy (CP) in the survivors.

IUGR

- In singletons, prevalence of babies with birth weight below the fifth centile is 5%.
- In DC twins it is approximately 20 % for each twin.
- In MC twins it is approximately 30% for each twin.
- In MC twins, detection of early IUGR before 24 weeks gestation carries a poor prognosis for one or both babies.
- Also, chance of IUGR for both twins is 2% in DC and 8% in MC pregnancies.

Pre-eclampsia

- Prevalence is four times greater in twins than singletons with little difference between MC and DC twins.

Table 25.1 Chorionicity and pregnancy complications

	Singleton	*Dichorionic*	*Monochorionic*
Miscarriage after 1st trimester and late 2nd trimester fetal loss	1%	2–4%	10%
PNMR		5–7 times higher than for singletons	Worse with MC twins due to additional problems of TTTS
Early preterm delivery (24–32 weeks)	1%	5–10%	10–15%
IUGR (<5th centile) IUGR in both twins	5%	20% 2%	30% 8%
Pre-eclampsia	7–10% of all primips	4 times greater in twins (slightly more in MC twins than DC)	
IUD of one twin		Increased risk of preterm labour. 5–10% risk of PNMR or CP in survivor	30% risk of PNMR or CP in survivor
Structural defects		Same as in singleton	2–3 times higher than in singleton

CP, cerebral palsy; DC, dichorionic; IUD, intrauterine death; IUGR, intrauterine growth retardation; MC, monochorionic; PNMR, perinatal morality rate; TTTS, twin-to-twin transfusion syndrome.

Data from: *Multiple pregnancy: the management of twin and triplet pregnancies in the antenatal period*, National Collaborating Centre for Women's and Children's Health, commissioned by the National Institute for Health and Clinical Excellence, 2011, RCOG Press; Braude P, *One child at a time: reducing multiple births after IVF*. Report of the Expert Group on Multiple Births after IVF, 2006, <http://www.hfea.gov.uk/docs/MBSET_report.pdf>; and RCOG Green-top Guideline No. 51, *Management of monochorionic twin pregnancy*, 2008, Royal College of Obstetricians and Gynaecologists.

Death of one fetus

- In DC pregnancy there is increased risk of preterm delivery.
- In DC twins there is a 5–10% risk of death or CP in surviving twin.
- In MC twins there is at least a 30% risk of death or neurological handicap of the surviving co-twin.
- Spontaneous reduction in fetal number and an embryo may disappear; the **'vanishing twin'** syndrome. An association between first-trimester vanishing twin syndrome and aetiology of spastic CP in the survivor has been mooted but further research is awaited.

Structural defects

- In dizygotic twins the prevalence of structural defects per fetus is the same as in singletons, whereas in monozygotic twins it is 2–3 times higher than in singletons.
- If the abnormality in one twin is non-lethal, but may well result in serious handicap, the parents need to decide whether the potential burden of the affected child is enough to risk the loss of the normal twin from feticide-linked complications.
- When the abnormality is lethal, it is best to avoid such a risk to the normal fetus, unless the abnormality in the affected twin itself threatens the survival of the normal twin.
- In the case of DC pregnancies, feticide can be carried out by intracardiac injection of KCl, whereas in MC pregnancies, feticide will necessitate occlusion of the umbilical cord vessels.

TTTS

- In MC twin pregnancies, placental vascular anastomoses allowing communication of the two fetoplacental circulations maybe of various types:
    - arterio-arterial (a-a)
    - veno-venous (v-v)
    - **arterio-venous (a-v):** deep in placenta with superficial feeder vessels.
- In 30% of MC twin pregnancies, an imbalance in the net flow of blood from one fetus (the donor) to the other (the recipient), results in TTTS. In about half of these, the condition is severe and carries a very poor outcome.
- Severe TTTS becomes apparent at 16–24 weeks pregnancy. In advanced cases, the classic features of a **'stuck twin'** are seen clearly on scan.

Early prediction of TTTS

- Ultrasound of MC pregnancies at 11–14 weeks gestation may show increased NT in one or both of the fetuses. The increased nuchal fold thickness in at least one twin in a MC twin pregnancy indicates that 30% will subsequently develop TTTS compared with 10% in those who do not develop TTTS.
- Other early ultrasound markers of severe TTTS may be abnormal Doppler flow velocity waveform in the ductus of the recipient twin.
- Inter-twin membrane folding is another sign of TTTS seen in 30% of all MC twins at 15–17 weeks gestation.

Pathophysiology and antenatal treatment options

- Superficial connections between vessels of like type (i.e. a-a or v-v) are visualized with colour-flow Dopplers. A-a connections are not the basis for TTTS; in fact, they are protective against development of TTTS. V-v connections are rare, and commonly associated with poor outcomes.
- **A-v anastomoses are found deep in the parenchyma of the placenta:** This zone of placental parenchyma is supplied with umbilical arterial blood from one twin (donor) but from which venous blood is inappropriately returned to the other twin (recipient) instead of back to the donor twin. Solitary a-v anastomoses are rare, but make TTTS inevitable. Usually, an a-a anastomoses also coexists that protects the twins from the harmful effects of an a-v connections that otherwise can prove disastrous.
- In TTTS, the donor is growth-retarded from the earliest stage. Arterial hypoperfusion of the viscera, especially of the kidneys, leads to oligohydramnios. The recipient becomes hypervolaemic and compensates with polyuria, producing polyhydramnios, cardiac failure, hydrops fetalis, and ultimately fetal death.
- The development of polyhydramnios is often abrupt and quite dramatic with maternal abdominal discomfort and respiratory distress, premature ROM and/or preterm labour. At this stage, any intervention for fetal salvage is virtually impossible.
- In contrast, presymptomatic oligo/polyhydramnios is anticipated by early and frequent ultrasound studies of MC twin pregnancies. Any intervention to increase fetal survival must be carried out before death of the first twin, as delayed intervention will not prevent multiorgan damage to the survivor.
- Repeated therapeutic amnioreduction: Survival potential for treated fetuses is approximately 50%. Even if untreated, 20% may also survive.
- Fetoscopic laser occlusion of chorionic plate vessels (a-v anastomoses) or septal puncture of the dividing membrane are interventions still within the remit of research centres.

Twin reversed arterial perfusion sequence or TRAP sequence

- 1% of monozygotic twin pregnancies is an **acardiac twinning**, the most extreme form of TTTS. The underlying mechanism is probably disruption of normal vascular perfusion leading to maldevelopment in the recipient twin

Chromosomal defects in multiple pregnancies

- Prenatal diagnosis is complicated as it could lead to higher rates of miscarriage.
- Selective feticide can result in miscarriage or severe preterm delivery several weeks later.
- Selective feticide after 16 weeks is associated with a threefold increase in risk compared with fetal reduction before 16 weeks.
- Amniocentesis in twins is effective in providing a reliable karyotype for both fetuses and has a procedure-related loss rate of approximately 2–3%.

Cerebral palsy in multiple pregnancies

- The risk of cerebral palsy (CP) is higher in premature births and in low birth weight (LBW) infants.[7] As both preterm birth and LBW are more common in multiple pregnancy, the risk of CP is considerably increased.[8]
- Rates of CP[9,10,11] are about 2 per 1000 in liveborn **singletons**, 7.4 per 1000 in liveborn **twins**, and 28 per 1000 in liveborn **triplets**. The higher the number of fetuses, the higher the risk of CP—an increase that is exponential.
- 30 of 1000 VLBW singletons (<1.5 kg birth weight) have CP; 100 of 1000 VLBW twins have CP.
- Although LBW and preterm births are the most significant risk factors for CP, in multiple pregnancies, the prevalence of CP is increased compared with singletons even when the birth weight is more than 2.5 kg or gestational age more than 37 weeks.[9,12,13] This suggests that 'term' occurs earlier in multiple gestations, a fact borne out by increased mortality[14] and morbidity[15] rates of twins when pregnancy lasts beyond 38 weeks gestation, supporting the practice of delivering hitherto uncomplicated twins no later than 37–38 weeks gestation.
- Multifetal pregnancies conceived by ART or iatrogenic multiple pregnancies have high rates of CP compared with spontaneously conceived multiple pregnancies. The risk is greater when three embryos are transferred compared with two, or after a reduction of triplets to twins.[16]
- Brain damage in the survivor following fetal death of one twin is almost exclusively seen in MC (2/3 of monozygotic twins), in which intertwined placental connections are always found. TTTS of varying degrees is seen in 10–15% of MC twins. In such cases there is a 20% risk of cerebral impairment in the survivor,[17,18] due to either embolic or ischaemic phenomena. **If one twin dies in utero, the rate of CP increases by 100 times in the liveborn co-twin compared with a liveborn singleton. If one twin dies in utero, there is a 1 in 12 chance that the survivor has CP.**
- MC placentation is one of highest risk factors for CP and severe disability in preterm babies of multiple pregnancies.[19]
- Long-term neurodevelopmental morbidity is also seen in MC pregnancies with TTTS when both twins have survived.[20]

Consensus view

(from RCOG 50th study group on multiple pregnancy, 2007[3])

- All women with a multiple pregnancy should be offered an ultrasound examination at 10–13 weeks gestation to assess:
  - viability
  - chorionicity
  - risk assessment for risk of trisomies
  - risk assessment (in MC twins) for TTTS
  - major congenital malformation.
- All MC twins should have a detailed ultrasound assessment including extended views of the fetal heart at about 20 weeks, repeated if necessary at 22–24 weeks.
- MC twins require increased ultrasound surveillance at 2-week intervals from 16 weeks gestation onwards to detect TTTS and growth discordance.
- NT-based screening for aneuploidy is the preferred choice in multiple pregnancy.
- Twin pregnancy where a fetal anomaly is detected should be referred to a regional fetal medicine unit as soon as possible.
- Organization of antenatal multiple pregnancy clinics should be facilitated by care pathways and allow easy referral to fetal medicine centres when appropriate.
- Multidisciplinary multiple pregnancy clinics with lead clinicians with experience in management of multiple pregnancies and scanning should be organized in each unit. This should include the vital role of midwives.
- The survivor after a co-twin demise in MC twins should have follow-up ultrasound and, if normal, an MRI examination of the fetal brain 2–3 weeks after death of the co-twin. Referral to a regional fetal medicine unit is required in this situation. Counselling should include the possible long-term neurological morbidity in the survivor.
- In view of the increased risk of stillbirth in twins, delivery is recommended between 37 and 38 weeks in DCDA twins and between 36 and 37 weeks in MCDA twins if there are no other indications for an earlier delivery.
- Specific information, including documentation regarding analgesia, delivery, postnatal care, and breastfeeding should be shared with the patient. Information leaflets to be given and additional support from TAMBA and the Multiple Birth Foundation as well as the locally run twins antenatal classes should be encouraged.
- Watch for early signs of perinatal psychiatric disturbances which are increased after multiple births.

Indications for referral to a regional fetal medicine centre[1]

- MCMA triplet pregnancies
- MCDA triplet pregnancies
- DCDA triplet pregnancies
- Pregnancies complicated by any of the following:
  - discordant fetal growth
  - fetal anomaly
  - discordant fetal death
  - FFTS.

Information for patients

Please see **Information for patients: Multiple pregnancies** (p. 547)

References

1. National Collaborating Centre for Women's and Children's Health. Multiple pregnancy: the management of twin and triplet pregnancies in the antenatal period. Commissioned by the National Institute for Health and Clinical Excellence. London: RCOG Press, 2011.
2. <http://www.hfea.gov.uk/docs/MBSET_report.pdf>
3. RCOG Green-top Guideline No. 51. Management of monochorionic twin pregnancy. London, Royal College of Obstetricians and Gynaecologists, 2008.
4. Consensus views arising from the 50th Study Group: Multiple pregnancy. In:Kilby M, et al., ed., Multiple pregnancy. London: RCOG Press, 2006, pp. 283–286.
5. <http://cemach.interface-test.com/getattachment/4cc984be-9460-4cc7-91f1-532c9424f76e/Perinatal-Mortality-2006.aspx>
6. Blickstein I. Cerebral palsy in multifoetal pregnancies. Dev Med Child Neurol 2002; 44: 352–355.
7. Luke B, Keith LG. The contribution of singletons, twins, and triplets to low birthweight, infant mortality, and handicap in the United States. J Reprod Med 1992; 37: 661–666.
8. Javier Laplaza F et al. Cerebral palsy in twins. Dev Med Child Neurol 1992; 34: 1053–1063.
9. Williams K, et al. Cerebral palsy: effects of twinning, birthweight, and gestational age. Arch Disease in Child Fetal Neonatal Ed 1996; 75: F178–182.
10. Liu J, et al. Cerebral palsy and multiple births in China. Int J Epidemiol 2000; 29: 292–299.
11. Grether J K, et al. Twinning and cerebral palsy: experience in four northern California counties' births, 1983 through 1985. Pediatrics 1993; 92: 854–858.
12. Pharoah POD, Cooke T. Cerebral palsy and multiple births. Arch Dis Child Fetal Neonat Ed 1996; 75: F174–177.
13. Minakami H, Sato I. Reestimating date of delivery in multifoetal pregnancies. JAMA;1996; 275: 1432–1434.
14. Luke B, et al. The cost of prematurity: a case-control study of twins vs singletons. Am J Public Health 1996; 86: 809–814.
15. Blickstein I, Weissman A. Estimating the risk of cerebral palsy following assisted conceptions. N Engl J Med 1999; 341: 1313–1314.
16. Kiely JL, et al. Contribution of the rise in multiple births to a potential increase in cerebral palsy. Pediatr Res 2000; 47: 314A (abstract)
17. Pharoah PO, Adi Y. Consequences of in-utero death in a twin pregnancy. Lancet 2000; 355: 1597–1602.
18. Pharoah PO. Cerebral palsy in the surviving twin associated with infant death of the co-twin. Arch Dis Child Fetal Neonatal Ed 2001; 84: F111–116.
19. Burguet A, et al. Some risk factors for cerebral palsy in very premature infants: importance of premature rupture of membranes and monochorionic twin placentation. Biol Neonate 1999; 75: 177–186.
20. Cincotta RB, et al. Long term outcome of twin-twin transfusion syndrome. Arch Dis Child Fetal Neonatal Ed 2000; 83: F171–176.

CARE PATHWAY Pertaining to Twin Pregnancies

1st trimester: routine booking in community

↓

Routine 1st-trimester scan detects multiple pregnancy: number of fetuses, dates, viability, chorionicity, any major congenital malformation, NT scan if patient opts for aneuploidy screening

↓

Immediate referral to Multiple pregnancy clinic and inform screening midwife

Dichorionic twins

First visit to antenatal clinic (at 16 weeks)

- Routine antenatal checks
- **Discuss and document increased risks of multiple pregnancy, need for delivery by $37–37^{+6}$ weeks**, symptoms patient should to be aware of, when and how to seek advice
- Consider iron and folic acid supplementation to prevent maternal anaemia.
- Consider low-dose aspirin
- Discuss role of targeted steroids
- Outline plan of care, give info leaflets
- Encourage contact with TAMBA, local multiple pregnancy support groups
- Advise continued care shared with community midwife in between but not overlapping hospital appointments.

- ***20 weeks:***
  - Detailed anomaly scan with appointment with antenatal clinic or community midwife if NAD on scan
  - Check Hb result, consider iron, folic acid supplementation

- ***If 20 week scan shows discordant size or anomaly:***
  - Counsel in multiple pregnancy clinic
  - Urgent referral to tertiary fetal medicine unit

- **24, 28, 32 weeks:** Antenatal clinic and scans to screen for IUGR each time, BP, urine
- **28 weeks:** Routine bloods
- **32 weeks:** Discuss del at about 37 weeks, intrapartum and postnatal care

22, 26, 30, 34 weeks (approx.): ***To see community midwife***—vigilance for pre-eclampsia, discuss breastfeeding, home support, postnatal care, management of late pregnancy discomforts

- **36 weeks:**
  - Scan, screen for IUGR, presentation of first twin, placental edge localization if previously low
  - Clinic appointment: BP, urine; discuss mode and timing of delivery. If hitherto uncomplicated pregnancy, offer elective birth at about $37–37^{+5}$ weeks; arrange this, discuss intrapartum care, breastfeeding; check routine bloods
- ***If elective delivery at 37 weeks declined, reiterate increased risk of fetal death after 38 weeks, offer weekly scans and Dopplers as well as appointment with specialist obstetrician***

Monochorionic twins

Scan: any NT, bladder, CRL discrepancy may indicate early TTTS or growth discordance

Prompt tertiary fetal medicine referral if:

- MCMA twins or MCDA with TTTS
- Discordant growth
- Anomaly or fetal death of one twin **at any gestational age**

If MCDA, **at 16 weeks:**

- Scan for TTTS, arrange scans every 2 weeks thereafter
- Routine pregnancy assessments
- **Discuss and document** increased risks of MCDA twins, symptoms to be aware of, how and when to seek help, role of targeted steroids
- Consider folic acid and iron supplementation to prevent maternal anaemia
- Consider low-dose aspirin
- Outline plan of care, give info leaflets
- Encourage contact with TAMBA, local twins groups
- Care with community midwife without overlapping hospital appointments

Community visits to continue at individualized intervals to continue vigilance for pre-eclampsia, discuss breastfeeding, home support, postnatal care, late pregnancy discomforts

Further visits to antenatal clinic

- ***18 weeks:***
  - Scan for TTTS
  - Multiple pregnancy clinic **(MPC)** for routine checks
- ***20, 22, and 24 weeks:***
  - Detailed anomaly scans including fetal ECHO/cardiac scans with Doppler at 20–22 weeks
  - TTTS screening at each scan
  - MPC follow-up appointments: BP, urine,
  - Check Hb result at 20 wks, consider folic acid, iron supplements
- ***26 weeks onwards at 2–3 weekly intervals:***
  - Scans for IUGR with MPC follow-up appointments
  - Vigilance for pre-eclampsia, anaemia
  - Routine bloods at 28 weeks
  - Individualize prophylactic steroids (targeted)
- ***32 and 34 weeks:***
  - Scans for IUGR, presentation of first twin, placental edge localization if previously low
  - MPC appointment for routine checks
  - Discuss timing elective delivery at $36–36^{+5}$ weeks if pregnancy uncomplicated till then
  - Discuss mode of delivery, intrapartum care, breastfeeding
- ***If elective delivery at 36 weeks declined, reiterate increased risk of fetal death after 37 weeks, offer weekly scans and BPP as well as appointment with specialist obstetrician***

25.2 Dichorionic Twins

FACT FILE

- **Twin clinic/multiple pregnancy clinic**: Lead clinician with multidisciplinary team
- Ultrasound at 10–13 weeks:
  - viability
  - chorionicity
  - nuchal fold thickness for aneuploidy if patient wishes.
- Ultrasound scan at about 20 weeks for anomalies
- Ultrasound serial scans for growth 28, 32, 36 weeks.

Booking visit in hospital antenatal clinic

- **Discuss and document risks of multiple pregnancy** including preterm labour and delivery, pre-eclampsia, IUGR of one or both twins, malpresentations, gestational diabetes, abruption, obstetric cholestasis, increased risk of operative delivery, PPH, reasons why delivery is advised between 37 and 38 weeks gestation.
- Explain **symptoms that might indicate complications** and contact numbers for the mother to report these to obtain advice and help.
- Consider **low-dose aspirin** from 12 weeks gestation to reduce the risk of pre-eclampsia in later pregnancy in this group at higher risk, especially if primigravida, older age group, obese or with pre-existent hypertension or diabetes or pre-eclampsia in a previous pregnancy.
- Discuss **targeted corticosteroids**.
- **Discuss plans for monitoring and care** for rest of pregnancy.[1,2]
  - Arrange subsequent visits to the hospital antenatal clinic for 24, 28, 32, 36 weeks, combining serial growth scans at 28, 32 and 36 weeks.
  - Advise visits to community midwife/GP, ideally at 16, 22, 26, 30, 34, and 37 weeks, to alternate with the hospital antenatal clinic visits.
- Explain that all discomforts of pregnancy from hyperemesis to pelvic girdle pain are likely to be magnified in a twin pregnancy and that the woman may need to seek to take maternity leave earlier than in a singleton pregnancy.
- Vigilance for pre-eclampsia, IUGR, and anaemia which might require iron and folic acid supplementation. Check presentation of leading twin at 36 weeks.
- If complications that require referral to a tertiary fetal medicine unit[1] occur, prompt referral after due explanation to the woman and partner/family is required.
- In uncomplicated DCDA pregnancies, arrange delivery between 37 and 38 weeks if the woman is still undelivered.
  - Elective lower-segment Caesarean section (LSCS) at about 38 weeks if leading twin is in a non-cephalic presentation.
  - Consider elective LSCS at about 37–38 weeks if previous Caesarean section. Document placental site in notes.
  - Induction of labour at about 38 weeks if the leading twin is in cephalic presentation.
  - Advise an epidural for analgesia in labour as in 30% of DCDA twins the second twin may need internal manipulation for delivery which would be aided by having a working epidural on board.
  - Document the increased risk of PPH and the prophylactic measures to be adopted.
  - Delivery needs to be in the hospital within an unit with all facilities for continuous electronic fetal monitoring, immediate access to Caesarean section, and neonatal care facilities

References

1. National Collaborating Centre for Women's and Children's Health. Multiple pregnancy: the management of twin and triplet pregnancies in the antenatal period. Commissioned by the National Institute for Health and Clinical Excellence. London: RCOG Press, 2011.
2. Consensus views arising from the 50th Study Group: Multiple Pregnancy. In: Kilby M, et al., ed. Multiple pregnancy. London: RCOG Press, 2006, pp. 283–286.

25.3 Monochorionic Twins

FACT FILE

- **MC twin** pregnancy is one in which both babies share a single placenta.
- About 30% of all twin pregnancies are MC.
- Of all twin pregnancies, 1% are MCMA.
- In 3% of MC placenta, due to very early separation, two placental masses may be seen on scan mimicking dichorionic pregnancy.[1]
- Chorionicity is best determined before 14 weeks of pregnancy by ultrasound scan and it is recommended that a photographic record is maintained of the membrane attachment to the placenta.[2] If there is any ambiguity, a second opinion, particularly from a specialist, should be obtained without delay as chorionicity becomes harder to determine after 14 weeks gestation.
- Ultrasound determination of chorionicity has been shown to be about 96% accurate in a retrospective study[3] where the presence of a lamba or 'twin peak' sign in DCDA twins and a 'T' sign in MCDA twins is seen at the junction of the membrane–placenta insertion.
- Outcomes in MC twins are worse than in DC twins with a higher fetal loss rate especially due to second-trimester loss (e.g. perinatal mortality in MC twins of 11.6% compared with 5% in DC twins[4]) though the risk persists even into the third trimester (e.g. perinatal loss of MC twins after 24 weeks of 4.9% vs 2.8% for DC twins[5]).
- In MC twin pregnancies, if one twin dies there is an increased risk of death (12%) or neurological impairment (18%) in the other, considerably higher than in DC twin pregnancies. Such cases must be referred to a regional fetal medicine centre for assessment and management, which is likely to be complex, including fetal brain imaging in the survivor with MRI. Conservative management is usually advised unless there are acute changes in the CTG or evidence of fetal anaemia (abnormal peak systolic velocity in the middle cerebral artery Doppler).
- When one twin has been found to have a severe fetal anomaly, referral must be made to a regional fetal medicine centre as soon as possible. Intracardiac feticide is not an option in MC pregnancies due to shared vessels. Cord coagulation by bipolar diathermy or intrafetal laser ablation may be required.[6]
- As in any multiple pregnancy, **an ultrasound scan at 10 – 14 weeks is aimed at establishing:**
  - number of fetuses
  - viability
  - chorionicity
  - NT in those women who wish to have aneuploidy screening
  - signs of TTTS in MC twins.

Uncomplicated MCDA twin pregnancies

Recommended ultrasound schedule

- An ultrasound assessment at 2–3-week intervals from 16 weeks gestation is recommended throughout the pregnancy.[2,7] Between 16 and 24 weeks gestation, the aim is to detect any signs of TTTS. After 24 weeks, in addition, the primary aim is to detect concordant or discordant fetal growth restriction.
- If complications develop, more frequent ultrasound assessments are indicated.
- After 24 weeks, in addition to fetal biometry and amniotic fluid measurements (deepest pool in each sac in MCDA twins), umbilical artery Dopplers in each cord may be indicated.

Mode and timing of delivery

- Delivery at 36–37 weeks is recommended unless there are specific indications for earlier delivery.[2] Discussions regarding timing and mode of delivery need to take place at 32–34 weeks, if the MCDA pregnancy has been uncomplicated till then.
- Aiming for a vaginal delivery in the absence of complications such as TTTS, growth restriction, or specific situations such as first twin presenting as breech or a previous Caesarean section, is an acceptable option.
- Close electronic CTG monitoring is essential in labour due to the risk of intrapartum TTTS.

TTTS in MCDA twin pregnancies

- ***TTTS is a particular problem with MC twins, occurring in about 10–15%, arising due to vascular anastomoses between umbilical circulations of both twins. There is also a higher incidence of unequal placental sharing and velamentous cord insertions seen in MC pregnancies affected with TTTS.***[2,7]
- In TTTS, unidirectional a-v connections are more likely than the protective bidirectional a-a anastomosis. V-v anastomoses are also more common in TTTS.
- Though TTTS can occur with both MCDA and MCMA twins, it is more common with MCDA pregnancies.
- It is relatively less common for TTTS to develop for the first time after 24 weeks, although the risk of late-onset TTTS (>26 weeks) can continue[2] even into the intrapartum period.
- Another problem recognized in MC twin pregnancies, even in the absence of TTTS, is discordance in growth,[7,8] which can be of early onset. In MCDA affected by non-TTTS growth discrepancy, there is no polyhydramnios in one sac; instead oligohydramnios is often detected in the smaller twin with normal amniotic fluid in the other sac.

Ultrasound diagnosis of TTTS

Ultrasound diagnosis of TTTS is based on finding:[2]

- A single placental mass.
- Concordant gender.
- Oligohydramnios with a maximum vertical pocket depth of less than 2 cm in one sac and polyhydramnios in the other sac (≥8 cm at <20 weeks and ≥10 cm at >20 weeks gestation).
- Discordant bladder appearances, indicating severe TTTS.
- Signs of haemodynamic and cardiac compromise including hydrops, pericardial and pleural effusions, or ascites, seen in severe cases of TTTS. In such cases fetal echographic studies may be indicated.
- Discrepancy in NT and crown–rump length (CRL) measurements may predict TTTS, although this is still debated. Some studies suggest that a difference of 10% in CRL[9] or of 20% in NT between 11 and 13^{+6} weeks[9] as predictors of TTTS developing before 20 weeks gestation.

The Quintero classification system

- **Grading or staging of TTTS** is generally according to the Quintero system of classification (Table 25.2), although the course of TTTS can be unpredictable, involving rapid change from one grade to the other.
- There is still some controversy regarding the Quintero classification, with suggestions that fetal echocardiographic structural and functional assessments of MC twins with or at the risk of TTTS should be an additional criterion to the Quintero classification.[11]

Management of TTTS

- Any TTTS in a MC twin pregnancy is best managed in conjunction with a regional fetal medicine unit for multidisciplinary specialist input.[2]
- In early (<24–26 weeks) TTTS, laser ablation of shared vessels may be considered instead of amnioreduction or septostomy.[12]
- In cases of severe TTTs, especially when there is recurrence after laser ablation (as seen in about 14%[13]) in specialist centres, termination of pregnancy or selective feticide may be a viable option for some couples.[13]
- It is unclear what the frequency and modality of fetal surveillance should be after laser ablation or amnioreduction. Weekly biometry,

Table 25.2 The Quintero classification system

Stage	*Classification*
I	There is a discrepancy in amniotic fluid volume with oligohydramnios of a MVP ≤2 cm in one sac and polyhydramnios in other sac (MVP ≥8 cm). The bladder of the donor twin is visible and Doppler studies are normal
II	The bladder of the donor twin is not visible (during period of examination, usually around 1 h) but Doppler studies are not critically abnormal
III	Doppler studies are critically abnormal in either twin and are characterized as abnormal or reversed end-diastolic velocities in the umbilical artery, reverse flow in the ductus venosus, or pulsatile umbilical venous flow
IV	Ascites, pericardial or pleural effusion, scalp oedema, or overt hydrops present
V	One or both babies are dead

MVP, maximum vertical pocket.

Data from Quintero RA et al., Staging of twin-twin transfusion syndrome, *Journal of Perinatology*, 1999, 19, pp. 550–555.

Doppler assessments, and brain imaging has been suggested by some, with delivery (invariably by LSCS at this gestation) following steroid adminstration.[15,16]

MCMA pregnancies

- MCMA pregnancies have the worst outcomes among all varieties of twins and a survival rate of about 60% can be expected.[17] Most have signs of cord entanglement. Elective delivery is usually recommended by Caesarean section at 32 weeks.

Conjoint twins

- Conjoint twins occurs in 1 in 90 000 to 1 in 100 000 pregnancies.
- They are usually diagnosed by scan from the mid-first trimester and additional colour Doppler and 3D scan studies are required to determine prognosis and enable plans for management.
- One study reported a 20% termination of pregnancy requested by parents and an overall individual survival rate at discharge of about 25%.[18]

Management of MCDA twin pregnancy in a district general hospital

Booking visit in hospital antenatal clinic

- **Discuss and document:** Risks of multiple pregnancy particularly MC twins including preterm labour and delivery, TTTS, pre-eclampsia, IUGR, abruption, malpresentations, increased risk of operative delivery, risk of IUD, need for delivery at 36– 37 weeks gestation, PPH.[7]
- Discuss plans for monitoring and pattern of care for rest of pregnancy,
- Advice about iron, folic acid, and vitamin D supplements.
- Advise women to take 75 mg of aspirin daily from 12 weeks until the birth of the babies, especially if they have one or more of the following risk factors for hypertension:[7]
  - first pregnancy
  - age 40 years or older
  - pregnancy interval of more than 10 years
  - BMI of 35 or more at first visit
  - family history of pre-eclampsia.
- Arrange subsequent ultrasound scans visits at 2–3-week intervals from 16 weeks gestation, attempting to combine clinic visits during the same session to reduce inconvenience for patients of several visits to the hospital.
- Community midwife visits should continue but not overlap in the same week as hospital clinic appointments.
- Discussion about aneuploidy screening as well as scan detection of discordant malformations and the possible management dilemma that might arise needs to be mentioned at this visit.
- Information regarding symptoms that might suggest development of complications such as sudden abdominal distension causing considerable maternal discomfort, difficulty breathing, or shortness of breath might indicate acute TTTS. Similarly, advise about immediately reporting vaginal bleeding, rupture of membranes, preterm contractions, etc.
- In addition, a printed information leaflet about MC pregnancies including a standard care schedule can be shared with the patient and her family/partner.

Subsequent antenatal visits

- Vigilance maintained for TTTS, IUGR, pre-eclampsia; consider prophylactic steroids if early delivery is considered a possibility.
- Continued ultrasound surveillance. If TTTS, early discordant growth, or IUD of one twin is detected, referral to the regional fetal medicine centre must be organized without delay.
- Consider folic acid and/or iron supplements to avoid or treat maternal anaemia.
- In hitherto uncomplicated MCDA pregnancies, determine the presentation of leading twin as well as site of the placenta at about 34 weeks gestation.
- **At 32–34 weeks**: Discuss plans for delivery. A vaginal delivery can be aimed for if there are no contraindications such as breech presentation in twin 1 or previous Caesarean section, and if the pregnancy progresses without fresh problems till 36–37 weeks.
- Discuss continuous monitoring of twins in labour (risk of TTTS persists even during labour) and early recourse to Caesarean section if any problems develop.
- Elective LSCS at 36–37 completed weeks if leading twin is in a non-cephalic presentation.
- Elective LSCS at about 36 completed weeks if previous Caesarean section.
- IOL at 36–37 weeks if leading twin is cephalic in presentation and pregnancy uncomplicated so far.
- **Document instructions in notes about vigilance needed** for the high risk of PPH, whether vaginal or abdominal route of delivery, and due prophylactic measures that need to be employed.

References

1. Lopriore E. Twin pregnancies with two separate placental masses can still be monochorionic and have vascular anastomoses. Am J Obstet Gynecol 2006; 194: 804–808.
2. RCOG Green-top Guideline No.51. Management of monochorionic twin pregnancy. London, Royal College of Obstetricians and Gynaecologists, 2008.
3. Lee YM, et al Antenatal sonographic prediction of twin chorionicity. Am J Obstet Gynecol 2006; 195: 863–867.
4. Hack KE, et al. Increased perinatal mortality and morbidity in monochorionic versus dichorionic twin pregnancies: clinical implications of a large Dutch cohort study. BJOG 2008; 115: 58–67.
5. Sebire NJ, et al. The hidden mortality of monochorionic twin pregnancies. Br J Obstet Gynaecol 1997; 104: 1203–1207.
6. Lewi L, et al. Pregnancy and infant outcome of 80 consecutive cord coagulations in complicated monochorionic multiple pregnancies. Am J Obstet Gynecol 2006; 194: 782–789.
7. National Collaborating Centre for Women's and Children's Health. Multiple pregnancy: the management of twin and triplet pregnancies in the antenatal period NICE guidelines. Commissioned by the National Institute for Health and Clinical Excellence. London: RCOG Press, 2011.
8. Sebire NJ, et al. Intertwin disparity in fetal size in monochorionic and dichorionic pregnancies. Obstet Gynecol 1998; 91: 82–85
9. El Kateb A, et al. First-trimester discordance in crown-rump length predicts timing of development of twin-twin transfusion syndrome:OP05. 02. Prenat Diagn 2007; 27: 922–925.
10. Kagan KO, et al. Discordance in nuchal translucency thickness in the prediction of severe twin-to-twin transfusion syndrome. Ultrasound Obstet Gynecol 2007; 29: 527–532.
11. Quintero R A, et al. Staging of twin-twin transfusion syndrome. J Perinatol 1999; 19: 550–555.
12. Roberts D, et al. Interventions for the treatment of twin-twin transfusion syndrome. Cochrane Database Syst Rev 2008; CD002073.
13. Robyr R.Prevalence and management of late fetal complications following successful selective laser coagulation of chorionic plate anastomoses in twin-to-twin transfusion syndrome. Am J Obstet Gynecol 2006; 194: 796–803.

14. Taylor MJ, et al. Ultrasound-guided umbilical cord occlusion using bipolar diathermy for Stage III/IV twin-twin transfusion syndrome. Prenat Diagn 2002; 22: 70–76.
15. Consensus views arising from the 50th Study Group: Multiple Pregnancy. In:Kilby M, et al., ed. Multiple pregnancy. London: RCOG Press, 2006, pp. 283–286.
16. Blickstein I, et al. The Istanbul international consensus statement on the perinatal care of multiple pregnancy. J Perinat Med 2007; 35: 465–467.
17. Ezra Y, et al. Intensive management and early delivery reduce antenatal mortality in monoamniotic twin pregnancies. Acta Obstet Gynecol Scand 2005; 84: 432–435.
18. Agarwal U, et al. Vaginal birth of conjoined thoracopagus: a rare event. Arch Gynecol Obstet 2003; 269: 66–67.

26 Fetal Growth Issues

26.1 Intrauterine Growth Restriction (Previous or Current Pregnancy)

FACT FILE

Definitions

- The term growth restriction (**IUGR**) is used interchangeably with fetal growth restriction (**FGR**).
- IUGR is not synonymous with small for gestational age (**SGA**). SGA refers to a **birth weight that is below the 10th percentile for gestational age**. Not all fetuses with IUGR are classified as SGA, and vice versa.[1,2]
- The SGA category includes pathologically growth-restricted fetuses and fetuses that are just constitutionally small.
- An SGA fetus can thus result due to IUGR or be constitutionally small without any IUGR. For example, as many as 70% of fetuses who, at birth, weigh below the 10th percentile for gestational age are small simply because of constitutional factors such as female sex or maternal ethnicity, parity, or body mass index (BMI); they are not at high risk of perinatal mortality or morbidity.[1,3]
- IUGR refers to a pattern of restricted intrauterine fetal growth that deviates from expected norms, whereas SGA is a category assigned on the basis of birth weight.
- IUGR refers to a condition in which the fetus has failed to achieve its genetically determined growth potential. This is a functional definition which is aimed at identifying the cohort of fetuses at greater risk of perinatal problems.[1,2]
- Factors such as **racial differences** (e.g. babies of Indo-Asian ethnicity are generally smaller), **short maternal and /or paternal stature**, as well as the **reassurance of sustained fetal growth with absence of other signs of uteroplacental insufficiency** (e.g. oligohydramnios, abnormal Doppler findings) are most likely to indicate a **constitutionally small but healthy baby**.
- Similarly, not all fetuses with IUGR need to be SGA, i.e. less than the 10th centile for abdominal circumference or estimated weight for the gestational age.[4]
- Because the diagnosis can be confirmed with certainty only after the birth of the baby, a significant number of fetuses that are SGA but healthy will be subjected to intensive monitoring protocols and iatrogenic preterm delivery.
- IUGR can be **symmetrical** or **asymmetrical**.
- **Symmetrical IUGR** may represent a global insult that occurs early in pregnancy due to causes such as chromosomal abnormalities, viral infections, or fetal alcohol syndrome.
- **Asymmetrical IUGR** is more likely due to reduced nutrients and diminished gas exchange. In asymmetrical growth restriction, the brain-sparing effect may result in differential fetal growth patterns with a greater reduction in abdominal circumference than in head circumference.
- In asymmetrical IUGR, the brain-sparing effect results in redistribution of blood flow patterns with relatively increased blood flow to the brain, heart, adrenals, and placenta, and diminished flow to the bone marrow, muscles, lungs, GI tract, and kidneys.
- IUGR fetuses are at greater risk of complications[5,6,7] such as stillbirth, birth hypoxia, meconium aspiration, hypoxic ischaemic encephalopathy, impaired neurodevelopment, neonatal death, and possibly type 2 (non-insulin-dependent) diabetes and hypertension in adult life.
- ***The most common pathophysiological findings in IUGR due to uteroplacental causes is inadequate invasion of maternal spiral arteries by the trophoblast as well as increased blood viscosity.***

Common factors for constitutionally small SGA fetuses

- Ethnicity (Generally, babies of Indo-Asian origin tend to be smaller.)
- Maternal size
- Female infant
- First pregnancy.

Common risk factors for IUGR

Several factors, sometimes acting together, can lead to IUGR.[8]

- Smoking: vigilance is to be maintained to detect IUGR of late onset[8]
- Alcohol, illicit drugs
- Poor maternal nutrition, social disadvantage
- Chronic hypertension especially if associated with atherosclerosis
- Pregnancy-induced hypertension
- Maternal diseases such as renal, cardiac, severe asthma, hyperthyroidism, haemoglobinopathies
- Autoimmune conditions, e.g. lupus, antiphospholipid syndrome, IgA nephropathy
- Connective tissue disorders, e.g. rheumatoid arthritis, Sjögren's, sclerosing dermatomyositis, scleroderma
- Maternal medication, e.g. antiepileptics, immunosuppressants, some antidepressants
- Maternal diabetes with diabetic vasculopathy—indicated by nephropathy, retinopathy, and hypertension
- Chromosomal abnormalities of fetus (usually causes symmetric IUGR with normal liquor volume and normal Dopplers). Up to 20% of IUGR babies may have chromosomal abnormalities ± structural abnormalities.
- Uterine malformations, large submucosal fibroids, or uterine septum
- Fetal infection in utero
- Decreased uteroplacental blood flow
- Repeated abruption of the placenta, bleeding during pregnancy
- Thrombophilias
- Placental factors—thrombosis, infarction, and vasculitis—usually associated with maternal hypertension, diabetes, or autoimmune conditions.
- Multiple pregnancies, especially twin-to-twin transfusion syndrome (TTTS) in monochorionic twins.

Perinatal implications

IUGR can cause a variety of perinatal complications,[9] including:

- Fetal morbidity and mortality, iatrogenic prematurity with need for induction of labour or Caesarean delivery, fetal compromise in labour.
- Neonatal problems such as increased rates of necrotizing enterocolitis, neonatal mortality, thrombocytopenia, temperature instability, renal failure.

Clinical assessment of IUGR

- ***No single biometric or Doppler measurement on its own can be predictive of IUGR, but screening is important to identify at-risk fetuses.***
- Women who have a major risk factor should be referred for serial ultrasound measurement of fetal size and assessment of well-being with umbilical artery (UA) Doppler from 26–28 weeks of pregnancy.

- Composite abnormal results such as a small fetus with reduced biometric measurements, reduced liquor, or abnormal uterine artery Doppler may indicate an at-risk fetus.[1]
- If the patient has an underlying maternal disease known to be associated with increased risk of IUGR, serial ultrasonography should be planned during the pregnancy.
- In such cases, after the anomaly scan at about 20 weeks gestation, repeat scans are usually scheduled at 28, 32, and 36 weeks to assess fetal growth, evidence of asymmetry, and liquor volume.
- Screening in the general population relies on symphysio-fundal height (SFH) measurements, as part of routine antenatal care from 20 weeks gestation until term. **Abdominal palpation has, however, limited accuracy for the prediction of a SGA neonate.**

Clinical symphysio-fundal height

- Clinical SFH measurements have poor sensitivity (27%) and specificity (88%) in the third trimester with less than 30% SGA detected.[10] Serial SFH measurements plotted on a chart, preferably a customized chart, and especially if performed by the same examiner, may improve detection rates.[11]
- The accuracy of fundal height measurements is limited (particularly in obese patients, large fibroids, or hydramnios) but a discrepancy of greater than 2–3 cm between observed and expected measurements should prompt further should be referred for serial ultrasound assessments of fetal size.
- Women with a single SFH measurement which plots below the 10th centile or serial measurements which demonstrate slow or static growth by crossing centiles should be referred for ultrasound measurement of fetal size.
- If IUGR is suspected, clinical examination must be supplemented with ultrasound serial biometric tests.[1]
- **Customized fundal height charts** adjusted for physiological variables such as maternal height, weight, ethnic group, and parity have been shown to improve the accuracy of predicting a SGA baby.[11,12,13,14]

Laboratory tests

- Biochemical markers performed as part of the routine trisomy screening offered at 12–13 weeks gestation include alpha-fetoprotein and PAPP-A. A low level (<0.415 MoM) of the first-trimester marker PAPP-A is a strong indicator of subsequent IUGR and delivery of a SGA neonate.[1]
- Second-trimester Down's syndrome markers have limited predictive accuracy for delivery of a SGA neonate.[1]

Ultrasound investigations

(apart from the routine dating and anomaly scans)

Fetal biometry

- The **Shepard** and **Aoki** formulae[15,16] are recommended for estimating fetal weight, and have been validated for birth weights of 2.08–4.43 kg.
- The **Hadlock** formula[17] may be more appropriate when the fetus is expected to be very small.
- Serial measurements of abdominal and head circumference and estimated fetal weight are performed with measurement of the amniotic fluid volume.
- Serial measurements of abdominal circumference (AC) and estimated fetal weight (EFW) below the 10th centile, representing growth velocities, are better than single estimates of AC or EFW in predicting IUGR.[12]
- In women having serial assessment of fetal size, use of a customized fetal weight reference may improve the prediction of normal perinatal outcome.
- Use of a customized fetal weight reference may improve prediction of a SGA neonate and adverse perinatal outcome.
- Where the fetal AC or EFW is below the 10th centile or there is evidence of reduced growth velocity, women should be offered serial assessment of fetal size and UA Doppler.[1]
- Biometric tests, if performed serially, indicate the velocity of fetal growth.
- Up to 19% of fetuses with AC and EFW below the 5th centile may have chromosomal defects.
- Structural and/or karyotypic abnormalities may result in symmetrical IUGR with normal liquor volume and normal uterine or UA Dopplers. Karyotyping, even late amniocentesis if necessary, must therefore be considered.

Liquor volume

- Amniotic fluid index (AFI) and measurement of the deepest pool may have a similar implications, but interpretation of amniotic fluid volume should be based on single deepest vertical pocket.[1]
- Reduction in liquor volume (LV) may be associated with increased perinatal morbidity and mortality.
- Decreased LV is associated with an increased risk of Caesarean section for fetal distress and Apgar score of less than 7 at 5 min. Reduced LV has been associated with increased perinatal mortality compared with those with normal LV.[1]
- Severe oligohydramnios without an obvious cause is a sinister sign, associated with a high mortality rate.
- Ultrasound assessment of amniotic fluid volume should not be used as the only form of surveillance in SGA fetuses.[1]

Doppler studies

Uterine artery Dopplers

- In high-risk populations, uterine artery Doppler at 20–24 weeks gestation has a moderate predictive value for a severely SGA neonate.[1]
- Only women who have three or more minor risk factors may be referred for **uterine artery Doppler** at 20–24 weeks. It has limited or no benefit to mother or baby in a low-risk population.
- Repeating uterine artery Doppler is of limited value. Women with an abnormal uterine artery Doppler at 20–24 weeks (defined as a pulsatility index (PI) >95th centile) and/or notching should be referred for serial ultrasound measurement of fetal size and assessment of well-being with UA Doppler commencing at 26–28 weeks.
- Women with a normal uterine artery Doppler do not require serial biometry or assessments of well-being with UA Doppler unless they develop specific pregnancy complications, such as antepartum haemorrhage or hypertension. However, they should be offered a scan for fetal size and umbilical artery Doppler during the third trimester.

Umbilical artery Doppler

- In normal pregnancies, UA resistance shows a steady decline as gestation advances; this may **not** occur in fetuses faced with uteroplacental insufficiency and **abnormal UA Doppler waveforms may be found in association with IUGR**.
- The most commonly used measures of gestational age-specific UA resistance are the pulsatility and resistance indices. As the insufficiency progresses, **end-diastolic velocity is absent and is finally reversed**.
- A significant difference in mean birth weight and perinatal mortality has been demonstrated for **absent** end-diastolic velocity (20%) and for **reversed** end-diastolic velocity (68%).[18]
- The abnormal status of UA blood flow may strengthen a diagnosis of IUGR providing early evidence of circulatory abnormalities in the fetus. This allows the clinician to identify the fetus at risk and to prompt fetal surveillance and further management of the pregnancy.
- Monitoring high-risk fetuses with UA Doppler has been shown to reduce perinatal mortality and morbidity. UA Doppler surveillance also reduces the rates of antenatal admissions and induction of labour and does not lead to an increased interventions rate.[1]
- ***Doppler must be used as the primary surveillance tool in suspected IUGR.***[19]
- When UA Doppler flow indices are normal it is reasonable to repeat surveillance every 14 days.
- More frequent Doppler surveillance may be appropriate in severe SGA.

- ***When UA Doppler flow indices are abnormal (pulsatility or resistance index more than 2 SDs above mean for gestational age) and delivery is not indicated, repeat surveillance twice weekly in fetuses with end-diastolic velocities present and daily in fetuses with absent/reversed end-diastolic frequencies.***
- Fetuses with an elevated UA systolic-to-diastolic ratio have been shown to have a 10-fold increase in the rate of admission to and the duration of stay in the neonatal intensive care unit (NICU) as well as in the frequency and severity of respiratory distress syndrome.[20]
- Equally, no fetus with normal Doppler measurements was delivered with documented metabolic acidaemia.[20]
- The **resistance index (RI) has been shown to be best for predicting poor outcomes** such as SGA, poor Apgar scores, pathological CTG, low umbilical cord pH, and NICU admission.[21]
- If increased resistance is found (high RI) a repeat assessment in 1 week is recommended.
- The SGA baby is likely to be a 'normal but small ' if the anomaly scan (± karyotyping) and UA Dopplers have shown no abnormalities.[1]
- In such cases, outpatient management of the mother and monitoring at fortnightly intervals appear to be generally sufficient.[1]
- Absent end-diastolic flow in the UA Doppler may have a long latency interval before fetal compromise becomes sufficient to justify delivery before 32 weeks. Specialized fetal assessments (such as ductus venosus Doppler) should therefore take place before planning delivery based on UA Doppler alone before 32 weeks gestation.

Middle cerebral artery

- ***In the preterm SGA fetus, middle cerebral artery (MCA) Doppler has limited accuracy to predict acidaemia and adverse outcome and should not be used to time delivery.***[1]
- MCA PI and MCA peak systolic velocity (PSV) in term growth-restricted fetuses are further refinements in the detection of a fetus at risk.
- While an abnormal PI precedes an abnormal PSV, the PI demonstrates an inconsistent pattern. MCA-PSV, however, shows a consistent increase in blood velocity and a decrease immediately prior to fetal demise.[22]
- In the term SGA fetus with normal UA Doppler, an abnormal MCA Doppler (PI <5th centile) has moderate predictive value for acidosis at birth and should be used to time delivery.[1]

Ductus venosus Doppler

- Venous Doppler flow patterns measured at the ductus venosus (DV), umbilical vein (UV), inferior vena cava (IVC), and other sites, provide information about fetal cardiovascular and respiratory responses in relation to the intrauterine environment.
- DV Doppler has moderate predictive value for acidaemia and adverse outcome.
- DV Doppler should be used for surveillance in the preterm SGA fetus with abnormal **UA Doppler, and used to time delivery**.
- These measurements, especially of the DV, have been shown to become typically abnormal when a fetus is severely compromised,[23] predicting poor perinatal outcomes within 0–7 days.
- Near term, venous Doppler abnormalities may **not** in fact be observed before severe fetal compromise or even death occurs.
- This may provide additional information for the timing of delivery, especially in very preterm pregnancies (<32 weeks gestation).

Biophysical profile

- ***Biophysical profile (BPP) should not be used for fetal surveillance in preterm SGA fetuses.***
- The BPP is not designed to predict the size of the fetus, unlike serial biometric measurements. **It is designed to predict fetal well-being, i.e. decreased likelihood of fetal acidaemia.**
- ***A BPP score ≤ 4 is considered abnormal.***[1]
- In a high-risk pregnancies the BPP has a good negative predictive value, i.e. fetal death is rare with a normal BPP.
- ***When primary surveillance with UA Doppler is abnormal, a BPP is likely to be useful given its good negative predictive value in high-risk populations.***

Strategies for IUGR

- Various strategies have been tried to promote intrauterine growth and thus decrease perinatal morbidity and mortality, but with limited success.
- The most important strategy is smoking cessation.
- Improved and balanced nutrition in undernourished women is also important.
- Smoking cessation and avoiding use of illicit drugs, as well as good nutrition, should begin pre-pregnancy and be continued throughout.
- Bed rest as a way to promote fetal growth has shown no effect.[1]
- Low-dose aspirin versus placebo **after** a diagnosis of IUGR based on abnormal UA Doppler findings has not been shown to make a difference.[1]
- Low-dose aspirin commenced from 13 weeks gestation has been found to counteract inadequate invasion of maternal spiral arteries by the trophoblast as well as reduce blood viscosity in up to 19% of women with a previous history of pre-eclampsia.[24,25] A similar pathology is postulated for IUGR due to uteroplacental insufficiency. In women who have had a previous SGA baby with IUGR, prophylactic low-dose aspirin from the end of the first trimester must therefore be considered.
- Similarly, there is insufficient evidence at present for strategies including maternal hyperoxygenation or specific nutritional supplements.[26]
- Prophylactic administration of steroids when delivery is anticipated in preterm gestation (<36 weeks) is essential, as it is in appropriately grown fetuses of similar gestation.

Antenatal management

- ***All women should be assessed at booking for risk factors for a SGA fetus/neonate to identify those who require increased surveillance***[1] ***(see Table 26.1).***

If previous history of IUGR

- ***The recurrence risk was found in one study to be 29% if the first pregnancy was affected, and 44% if two pregnancies have been affected.***[27]
- At the first visit (≤13 weeks):
  - Detailed history to exclude risk factors.
  - Appropriate advice regarding stopping illicit drugs, smoking, etc.
  - Lupus and antiphospholipid (APS) screening in cases of previous severe IUGR, especially of early onset (<32 weeks gestation and baby weighed <10th centile).
  - Consider low-dose aspirin 75 mg daily from 12 weeks till the end of pregnancy. The role of aspirin is to decrease blood viscosity in the uteroplacental microcirculation, thereby improving blood flow.[28,29]
  - If a woman has had one previous IUGR baby followed by subsequent normally grown baby/babies, a single extra scan at 34 weeks is generally sufficient if all clinical findings are satisfactory.
  - If the IUGR in previous pregnancy resulted in a baby's birth weight less than 20% of expected birth weight for that gestation, serial scans are recommended at 28 and 32 weeks gestation.
  - If the previous IUGR baby's birth weight was less than 10% of the expected birth weight for that gestation, serial scans are recommended at 28, 32, and 36 weeks.
  - If there are no growth concerns for the fetus in this pregnancy, interventions such as early induction of labour or Caesarean section should not be based purely on the previous obstetric history of IUGR.

If IUGR suspected during this pregnancy

Early-onset growth restriction

- If severe SGA is identified at around 20 weeks, referral for a detailed fetal anatomical survey and UA Doppler by a fetal medicine specialist is indicated.
- Karyotyping should be offered in severely SGA fetuses with structural anomalies and in those detected before 23 weeks of gestation, especially if UA Doppler is normal.

- Serological screening for congenital cytomegalovirus (CMV) and toxoplasmosis infection should be offered in severely SGA fetuses.
- Testing for syphilis and malaria should be considered in high-risk populations.

If severe and of early onset (<32 weeks gestation)

- Once IUGR has been detected, the management of the pregnancy should depend on a surveillance plan that reduces the risks of neonatal morbidity and mortality while maximizing gestational age.
- The goal of management is to deliver the most mature fetus in the best physiological condition possible, before acidaemia and chronic hypoxia set in.
- Thrombophilia screen (lupus, APS).
- Chromosomal or any congenital abnormality to be excluded especially in symmetrical IUGR with normal liquor and Doppler.
- Maternal serology for CMV, toxoplasmosis, syphilis (if not previously performed), if hydramnios or polyhydramnios occurs with IUGR.
- Scan and Doppler studies.
- One in 5 severely growth-restricted fetuses will show episodes of unprovoked bradycardia. CTG monitoring at frequencies should be decided on a case-by- case basis, but CTG should not be used as the only form of surveillance in IUGR fetuses.[1]
- Corticosteroids in anticipation of early delivery, if indicated at 36 weeks gestation or earlier.
- After discussions with patient, a management plan is to be developed, including mode of delivery.
- The timing of delivery must be individualized and will depend on the aetiology, severity, and gestational age.

Severe IUGR detected after 32 weeks gestation

- If absent or reversed diastolic flow is found, admission, close surveillance with BPP, MCA PI, and repeated CTGs is called for. Reversed end-diastolic flow indicates need for delivery within days as it is associated with increased perinatal morbidity and mortality.
- CTG should not be used as the only form of surveillance in SGA fetuses.
- Prophylactic steroids if gestation is less than 36 weeks.
- Consider delivery if gestation is more than 34 weeks in the presence of absent or reversed end-diastolic flow. Admit, give steroids and plan delivery within 48 h.
- IUGR with oligohydramnios—consider delivery at 36–37 weeks.

Moderate IUGR

- Consider induction of labour (IOL) if cephalic presentation and if the cervix is favourable at about 37–38 weeks gestation.[30]
- The presence of end-diastolic flow is insensitive at a gestation of 37 weeks. An increased UA PI or an abnormal cerebroplacental ratio even in the presence of positive end-diastolic velocities may suggest that the fetus is at increased risk of perinatal death, and delivery at or by 37 weeks needs to be considered.
- If absent or reversed end-diastolic flow is detected, admit, give steroids if less than 36 weeks gestation and plan to deliver.

Optimum gestation to deliver the IUGR fetus

- In the preterm IUGR fetus with absent or reversed end-diastolic velocity in the UA detected prior to 32 weeks of gestation, delivery is recommended when DV Doppler becomes abnormal or UV pulsations appear, provided the fetus is considered viable and after completion of steroids.[1]
- Even when venous Doppler is normal, delivery is recommended by 32 weeks of gestation and should be considered between 30 and 32 weeks.
- If MCA Doppler is abnormal, delivery should be recommended no later than 37 weeks.
- In the IUGR fetus detected after 32 weeks of gestation with an abnormal UA Doppler, delivery no later than 37 weeks is recommended.
- In the IUGR fetus detected after 32 weeks with normal UA Doppler, a senior obstetrician should be involved in determining the timing and mode of birth of these pregnancies.
- Delivery should be offered at 37 weeks.

Mode of delivery

- Current data **does not justify a policy of elective Caesarean section for all IUGR babies.**
- In the IUGR fetus with normal UA Doppler or with abnormal UA PI but where the end-diastolic velocity is present, IOL can be offered. Rates of emergency Caesarean section are, however, increased.
- Continuous fetal heart rate monitoring is recommended from the onset of uterine contractions.
- In the IUGR fetus where absent or reversed end-diastolic velocity is seen in the UA Doppler, delivery by Caesarean section is recommended.
- IUGR associated with absent or reversed end-diastolic flow requires delivery by lower-segment Caesarean section (LSCS).
- If severe IUGR + oligohydramnios and an unfavourable cervix, elective Caesarean section is often indicated.
- Acute pathological features of the antenatal CTG with unprovoked decelerations or sustained lack of variability and absent accelerations are indications for an emergency Caesarean section.

Placental pathology

- Sending the placenta for examination (histology, microbiology, virology) in cases of severe growth restriction or IUGR with polyhydramnios when an infective cause is suspected is highly recommended.
- Histopathological studies of the placenta in IUGR[31] may indicate abnormalities of the maternal spiral arterioles, dysregulated villous vasculogenesis, abundant fibrin deposition. etc. Chronic histiocytic intervillositis of unknown aetiology is a rare placental inflammatory disease, associated with severe obstetric complications including IUGR.

Information for patients

Please see Information for patients: The small baby (p. 549)

Table 26.1 Risk factors for an **SGA neonate**. High risks are emphasized in bold

Risk category	*Definition of risk*	*Risk estimate*
Maternal risk factors		
Age	≥35 years	
	>40 years	**High risk (OR = 3.2)**
Parity	Nulliparity	
BMI	<20 or >30	
Maternal substance abuse	Smoker 1–10 cigarettes/day	
	Smoker ≥11 cigarettes/day	**High risk (OR = 2.21)**
	Cocaine	**High risk (OR = 3.23)**
IVF	Singleton	
Previous pregnancy history		
Previous SGA baby		**High risk (OR = 3.9)**
Previous stillbirth		**Highest risk (OR = 6.4)**
Pre-eclampsia		
Pregnancy interval <6 months		
Pregnancy interval >60 months		
Maternal medicine history		
Maternal SGA (if info. available)		**High risk (OR = 2.64)**

Table 26.1 *(Continued)*

Risk category	*Definition of risk*	*Risk estimate*
Chronic hypertension		High risk (OR = 2.5)
Diabetes and vascular disease		Highest risk (OR = 6)
Renal impairment		Highest risk (AOR = 5.3)
Antiphospholipid syndrome		Highest risk (RR = 5.5)
Paternal SGA (if info. available)		High risk (OR = 3.47)
Current pregnancy—contributory factors		
Threatened miscarriage (heavy bleeding like a period)		High risk (AOR = 2.6)
Echogenic bowel seen on scan		High risk (AOR = 2.1)
Pre-eclampsia		High risk (AOR = 2.26)
Severe pregnancy-induced hypertension		High risk (RR = 2.5)
Placental abruption		High risk (OR = 1.3–4.1)
Unexplained APH		High risk (OR = 5.6)
Low PAPP-A (0.4 MoM)		High risk (OR = 2.6)
Low maternal weight gain in pregnancy		High risk (OR = 4.9)

AOR, adjusted odds ratio; BMI, body mass index; IVF, in vitro fertilization; OR, odds ratio; RR, relative risk; SGA, small for gestational age.

Reproduced from: Royal College of Obstetricians and Gynaecologists. Bacterial sepsis in pregnancy. Green-top Guideline No. 64a. London: RCOG; 2012, with the permission of the Royal College of Obstetricians and Gynaecologists

References

1. RCOG Green-top Guideline No. 31. The investigation and management of the small-for-gestational-age fetus, 2nd ed. London: Royal College of Obstetricians and Gynaecologists, 2013.
2. McIntire DD, et al. Birthweight in relation to morbidity and mortality among newborn infants. N Engl J Med 1999;340: 1234–1238.
3. Gardosi J. New definition of small for gestational age based on fetal growth potential. Horm Res 2006;65: 15–18.
4. Chard T, et al. Evidence of growth retardation in neonates of apparently normal weight. Eur J Obstet Gynecol Reprod Biol 1992;45: 59–62.
5. Kaijser M, et al. Perinatal risk factors for ischemic heart disease: disentangling the roles of birth weight and preterm birth. Circulation 2008;117: 405–410.
6. Hallan S, et al. Effect of intrauterine growth restriction on kidney function at young adult age: the Nord Trøndelag Health (HUNT 2) Study. Am J Kidney Dis 2008;51: 10–20.
7. Tideman E, et al. Cognitive function in young adults following intrauterine growth restriction with abnormal fetal aortic blood flow. Ultrasound Obstet Gynecol 2007;29: 614–618.
8. Severi FM, et al. Intrauterine growth retardation and fetal cardiac function. Fetal Diagn Ther 2000;15: 8–19.
9. Bernstein IM, et al. Morbidity and mortality among very-low-birth-weight neonates with intrauterine growth restriction. Am J Obstet Gynecol 2000;182 (1 Pt 1): 198–206.
10. Jelks A, et al. Clinician bias in fundal height measurement. Obstet Gynecol 2007;110: 892–899.
11. Gardosi J, Francis A. Controlled trial of fundal height measurement plotted on customised antenatal growth charts. Br J Obstet Gynaecol 1999;106: 309–317.
12. De Jong CL, et al. Customized fetal weight limits for antenatal detection of fetal growth restriction. Ultrasound Obstet Gynecol 2000;15: 36–40.
13. Gardosi J, et al. Customised antenatal growth charts. Lancet 1992;339: 283–287.
14. Clausson B, et al. Perinatal outcome in SGA births defined by customised versus population-based birthweight standards. BJOG 2001;108: 830–834.
15. Shepard MJ, et al. An evaluation of two equations for predicting fetal weight by ultrasound. Am J Obstet Gynecol 1982;142: 47–54.
16. Aoki M. Fetal weight calculation; Osaka University method. In: Yoshihide C, ed., Ultrasound in obstetrics and gynaecology 2nd ed. Kyoto: Kinpodo, 1990.
17. Hadlock FP, et al. Estimation of fetal weight with the use of head, body, and femur measurements—a prospective study. Am J Obstet Gynecol 1985;151: 333–337.
18. Chien PF, et al. How useful is uterine artery Doppler flow velocimetry in the prediction of pre-eclampsia, intrauterine growth retardation and perinatal death? An overview. BJOG 2000;107: 196–208.
19. Alfirevic Z., Neilson JP. Doppler ultrasonography in high-risk pregnancies: systematic review with meta-analysis. Am J Obstet Gynecol 1995;172: 1379–1387.
20. Baschat AA, Weiner CP. Umbilical artery Doppler screening for detection of the small fetus in need of antepartum surveillance. Am J Obstet Gynecol 2000;182 (1 Pt 1): 154–158.
21. Maulik D, et al. Comparative efficacy of umbilical arterial Doppler indices for predicting adverse perinatal outcome. Am J Obstet Gynecol 1991;164: 1434–1439.
22. Mari G, et al. Middle cerebral artery peak systolic velocity: a new Doppler parameter in the assessment of growth-restricted fetuses. Ultrasound Obstet Gynecol 2007;29: 310–316.
23. Bilardo CM, et al. Relationship between monitoring parameters and perinatal outcome in severe, early intrauterine growth restriction. Ultrasound Obstet Gynecol 2004;23: 119–125.
24. CLASP: a randomised trial of low-dose aspirin for the prevention and treatment of pre-eclampsia among 9364 pregnant women. CLASP (Collaborative Low-dose Aspirin Study in Pregnancy) Collaborative Group. Lancet 1994;343 (8898): 619–629.
25. Say L, et al. Maternal nutrient supplementation for suspected impaired fetal growth. Cochrane Database Syst Rev 2003; CD000148.
26. Say L, et al. Maternal oxygen administration for suspected impaired fetal growth. Cochrane Database Syst Rev 2003; CD000137.
27. Abuzzahab MJ, et al. IGF-I receptor mutations resulting in intrauterine and postnatal growth retardation. N Engl J Med 2003; 349: 2211–2222.
28. Harrington K, et al. A prospective management study of slow-release aspirin in the palliation of uteroplacental insufficiency predicted by uterine artery Doppler at 20 weeks. Ultrasound Obstet Gynecol 2000;15: 13–18.
29. Boers KE, et al. Induction versus expectant monitoring for intrauterine growth restriction at term: randomised equivalence trial (DIGITAT). BMJ 2010;341: c7087.
30. Baschat AA, Hecher K. Fetal growth restriction due to placental disease. Semin Perinatol 2004;28: 67–80.
31. Scifres CM, Nelson DM. Intrauterine growth restriction, human placental development and trophoblast cell death. J Physiol 2009;587: 3453–3458.

CARE PATHWAY

Screening pathway for the small-for-gestational-age neonate

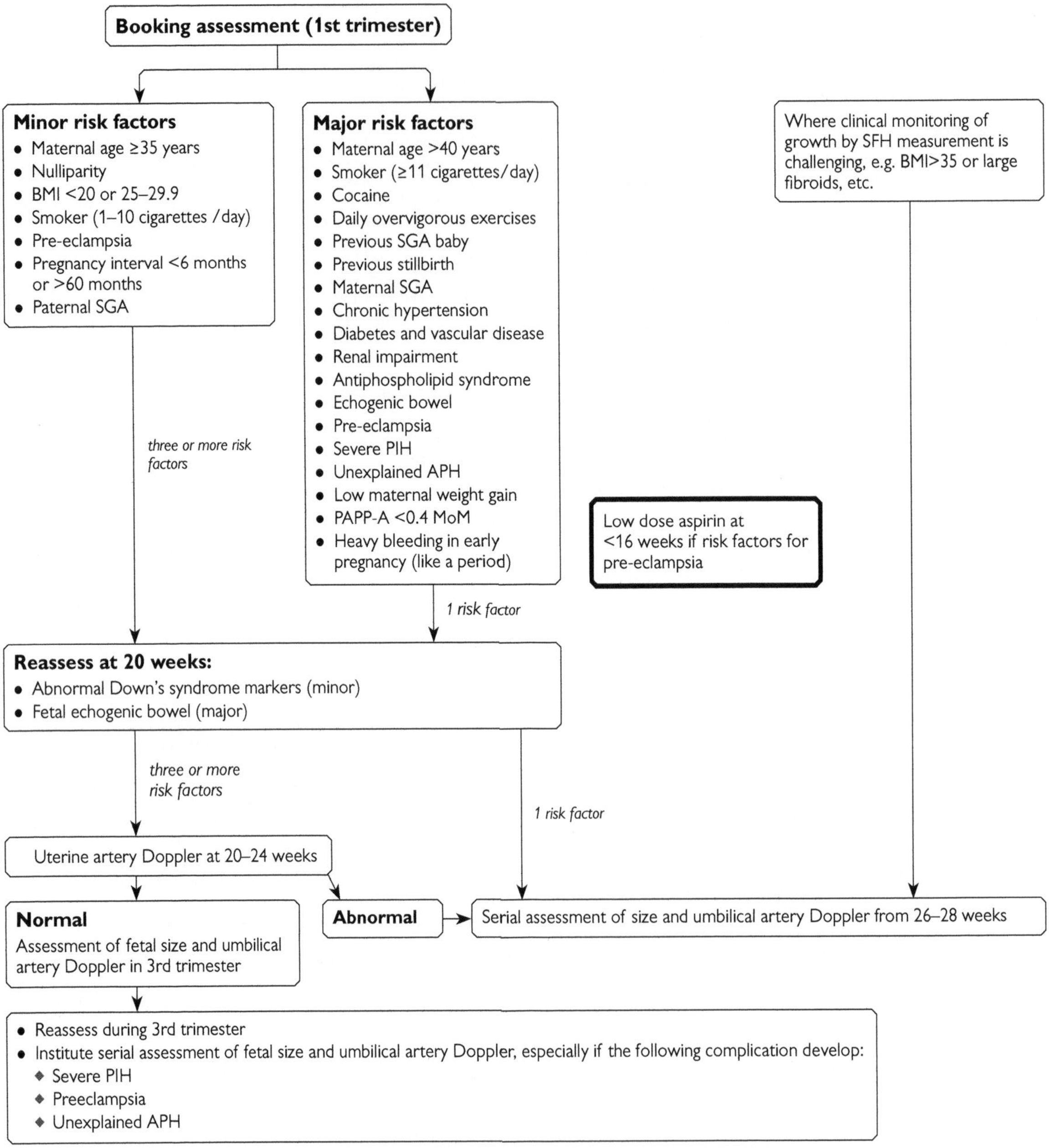

Reproduced from: Royal College of Obstetricians and Gynaecologists. Investigation and management of small for gestational age fetus. Green-top Guideline No. 31. London: RCOG; 2013, with the permission of the Royal College of Obstetricians and Gynaecologists

Management if IUGR suspected in present pregnancy

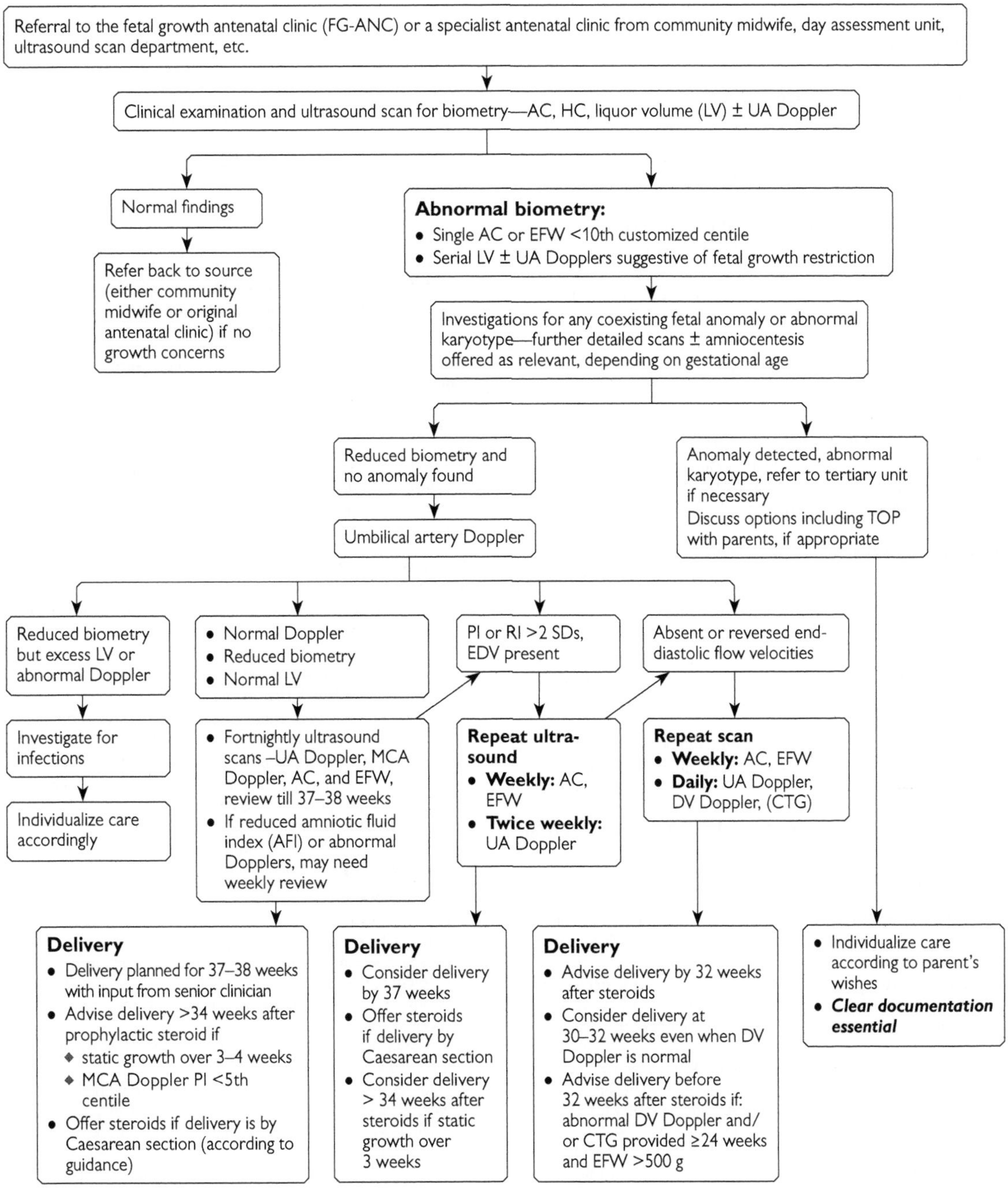
Referral to the fetal growth antenatal clinic (FG-ANC) or a specialist antenatal clinic from community midwife, day assessment unit, ultrasound scan department, etc.
Clinical examination and ultrasound scan for biometry—AC, HC, liquor volume (LV) ± UA Doppler
Normal findings
Refer back to source (either community midwife or original antenatal clinic) if no growth concerns
Abnormal biometry:
• Single AC or EFW <10th customized centile
• Serial LV ± UA Dopplers suggestive of fetal growth restriction
Investigations for any coexisting fetal anomaly or abnormal karyotype—further detailed scans ± amniocentesis offered as relevant, depending on gestational age
Reduced biometry and no anomaly found
Anomaly detected, abnormal karyotype, refer to tertiary unit if necessary
Discuss options including TOP with parents, if appropriate
Umbilical artery Doppler
Reduced biometry but excess LV or abnormal Doppler
• Normal Doppler
• Reduced biometry
• Normal LV
PI or RI >2 SDs, EDV present
Absent or reversed end-diastolic flow velocities
Investigate for infections
Individualize care accordingly
• Fortnightly ultrasound scans –UA Doppler, MCA Doppler, AC, and EFW, review till 37–38 weeks
• If reduced amniotic fluid index (AFI) or abnormal Dopplers, may need weekly review
Repeat ultra-sound
• Weekly: AC, EFW
• Twice weekly: UA Doppler
Repeat scan
• Weekly: AC, EFW
• Daily: UA Doppler, DV Doppler, (CTG)
Delivery
• Delivery planned for 37–38 weeks with input from senior clinician
• Advise delivery >34 weeks after prophylactic steroid if
◆ static growth over 3–4 weeks
◆ MCA Doppler PI <5th centile
• Offer steroids if delivery is by Caesarean section (according to guidance)
Delivery
• Consider delivery by 37 weeks
• Offer steroids if delivery by Caesarean section
• Consider delivery > 34 weeks after steroids if static growth over 3 weeks
Delivery
• Advise delivery by 32 weeks after steroids
• Consider delivery at 30–32 weeks even when DV Doppler is normal
• Advise delivery before 32 weeks after steroids if: abnormal DV Doppler and/ or CTG provided ≥24 weeks and EFW >500 g
• Individualize care according to parent's wishes
• Clear documentation essential

Reproduced from: Royal College of Obstetricians and Gynaecologists. Investigation and management of small for gestational age fetus. Green-top Guideline No. 31. London: RCOG; 2013, with the permission of the Royal College of Obstetricians and Gynaecologists

26.2 Large for Gestational Age in Non-Diabetic Mothers

FACT FILE

- **Large for gestational age:** Defined as estimated fetal weight (EFW) greater than the 90th centile for the given gestational age.
- **Macrosomia** is variously defined[1,2,3] as the newborn's birth weight being in excess of 4 kg or 4.5 kg, regardless of gestational age. The diagnosis of macrosomia can therefore be only be made after birth.

What is known about LGA and macrosomia

- An increase of 15–25% in the last 2–3 decades in many countries of women delivering large babies.
- Prevalence of babies born with a birth weight of more than 4 kg is about 10% and this is rising.[4,5,6].
- Increased maternal, fetal, and neonatal morbidity associated with fetal macrosomia.
- **Maternal risks** associated with fetal macrosomia include injury to the birth canal (third- and fourth-degree perineal tears, cervical, vaginal lacerations), obstructed labour, chorioamnionitis, increased chances of Caesarean section, postpartum haemorrhage.
- **Fetal risks** include birth trauma (3–7%), including shoulder dystocia, brachial plexus injury, and intrapartum mortality.
- Risk of shoulder dystocia rises from 1.4% of all vaginal births to 9–24% in macrosomia.[6]
- **Neonatal risks** include hypoglycaemia and electrolyte imbalances (in 50%), early neonatal death due to asphyxia, increase in postneonatal deaths with a doubling of rate of sudden infant death syndromes compared with average-size babies.[4]
- Long-term risks include childhood obesity and type 2 diabetes.
- Factors that influence birth weight, apart from genetic and racial variations, are male sex, post-dates, maternal gestational diabetes or pre-existent diabetes, maternal obesity, and excessive weight gain during pregnancy.
- Although maternal gestational diabetes and pregestational diabetes are risk factors for fetal macrosomia, the great **majority of macrosomic infants are born to non-diabetic mothers.**[7]

What is less well known about LGA and macrosomia

Accurate prediction

- Most macrosomic babies may not have identifiable risk factors. Even with identified risk factors, there is no combination of these to be able to accurately predict macrosomia. Both clinical estimation and ultrasound measurements show significant variations and inaccuracies.
- Serial measurements of SFH, preferably by the same person, may lessen the variation, especially if customized with maternal variables such as age, BMI, parity, and birth weight of previous babies (if multiparous).
- Ultrasound measurements of AC and EFW also have a low sensitivity, low positive predictive value, and high negative predictive value. A combination of AFI and biometry for EFW may improve the positive predictive value if performed in mid-third trimester.[4] However, NICE guidelines on antenatal care for low-risk pregnancies[8] do not support ultrasound estimation of fetal size for suspected LGA in a low-risk population.
- The larger the fetus, the more inaccurate the ultrasonographic prediction of EFW.
- ***There does not appear to be any difference between ultrasound estimation of EFW and clinical estimation by an experienced assessor.***

Antenatal management

- **Consensus** regarding the management of LGA/suspected fetal macrosomia **is lacking.**
- ***IOL at 38–40 weeks gestation for suspected fetal macrosomia has shown no improvement in perinatal outcomes while increasing emergency Caesarean section rate.***[4,7]
- **Elective Caesarean section** has been employed to prevent maternal perineal trauma or brachial plexus injuries in suspected macrosomia. It is estimated that as many as 3700 elective Caesarean sections need to be performed in order to prevent one case of permanent nerve injury.[9] This has to be considered in addition to the surgical and anaesthetic risks associated with any Caesarean section, especially in the presence of maternal obesity.
  - ***Elective Caesarean section cannot therefore be justified if suspected macrosomia is the only indication.***
  - ***Elective Caesarean appears be beneficial only if the fetus is suspected to be more than 5 kg in a non-diabetic mother.***[4]

Fetal macrosomia suspected in a woman who has had a previous Caesarean section

- This offers another management dilemma. The chances of a successful vaginal birth after Caesarean section (VBAC) are diminished if there are additional risk factors such as maternal obesity, the indication for the previous Caesarean section being failure to progress especially in the second stage or a failed trial of instrumental delivery, a previous macrosomic baby, or when the woman has not had any previous vaginal delivery.

Previous shoulder dystocia

- Shoulder dystocia has a recurrence rate of 2–16%.
- If there has been shoulder dystocia **with permanent nerve injury**, an elective Caesarean delivery is a reasonable option (also see Chapter 22.5 on previous shoulder dystocia).
- ***To help make management decisions the following points need to be discussed with the mother:***
  - That not all cases of shoulder dystocia result in permanent nerve damage; most present as transient weakness.
  - 50% of cases of shoulder dystocia are in babies of less than 4 kg.
  - 33% of cases of permanent nerve damage occur even when there has not been any shoulder dystocia at birth and can occur even after an apparently uncomplicated Caesarean delivery.
  - A significant number of shoulder dystocia cases actually occur **antenatally** for ill-defined reasons.

Labour and delivery

- Expectant management of spontaneous onset of labour is entirely reasonable, once a detailed discussion has been had with the pregnant woman to explain the uncertainties involved in EFW prediction, risks and benefits of both expectant management and of any interventions, as well as the intrapartum care she would receive.
- In a large study, 88% of women who laboured with an LGA baby achieved a vaginal delivery.[10]
- Epidural analgesia for labour and delivery should be considered, when shoulder dystocia is anticipated in cases of suspected fetal macrosomia, in order to assist in the manipulations required to deliver the baby.
- Clear documentation for senior obstetric and midwifery staff should be readily available, in cases where shoulder dystocia is a possibility. The use of a shoulder dystocia proforma is strongly recommended.
- All staff must have regular updated drills for shoulder dystocia management.

Information for patients

Please see Information for patients: The large baby (p. 550)

References

1. Berkus MD, et al. The large fetus. Clinical Obstet Gynecol 1999;42: 766–784.

2. Boulet SL, et al. Macrosomic births in the United States: determinants, outcomes and proposed grades of risk. Am J Obstet Gynecol 2003;188: 1372–1378.
3. Martin JA, et al. Births: final data for 2004. Natl Vital Statist Rep 2006;55: 1–101.
4. Aye SS, et al. Management of large-for-gestational-age pregnancy in non-diabetic women. Obstetrician and Gynaecologist 2010;12: 250–256.
5. Kramer MS, et al. Why are babies getting bigger? Temporal trends in fetal growth and its determinants. J Pediatr 2002;141: 538–542.
6. Pundir J, Sinha P. Non-diabetic macrosomia: an obstetric dilemma. J Obstet Gynaecol 2009;29: 200–205.
7. Ben-Haroush A, et al. Induction of labor in pregnancies with suspected large-for-gestational- age foetuses and unfavourable cervix. Eur J Obstet Gynaecol Reprod Biol 2004;116: 182–185.
8. NICE Clinical Guideline: Antenatal Care. CG62. London: National Institute for Clinical Excellence, 2008, updated 2010 <www.nice.org.uk/CG062>.
9. Rouse DJ, et al. The effectiveness and costs of elective cesarean delivery for fetal macrosomia diagnosed by ultrasound. JAMA 1996;276: 1480–1486.
10. Walsh CA, et al. Recurrence of fetal macrosomia in non-diabetic pregnancies. J Obstet Gynaecol 2007;27: 374–378.

CARE PATHWAY

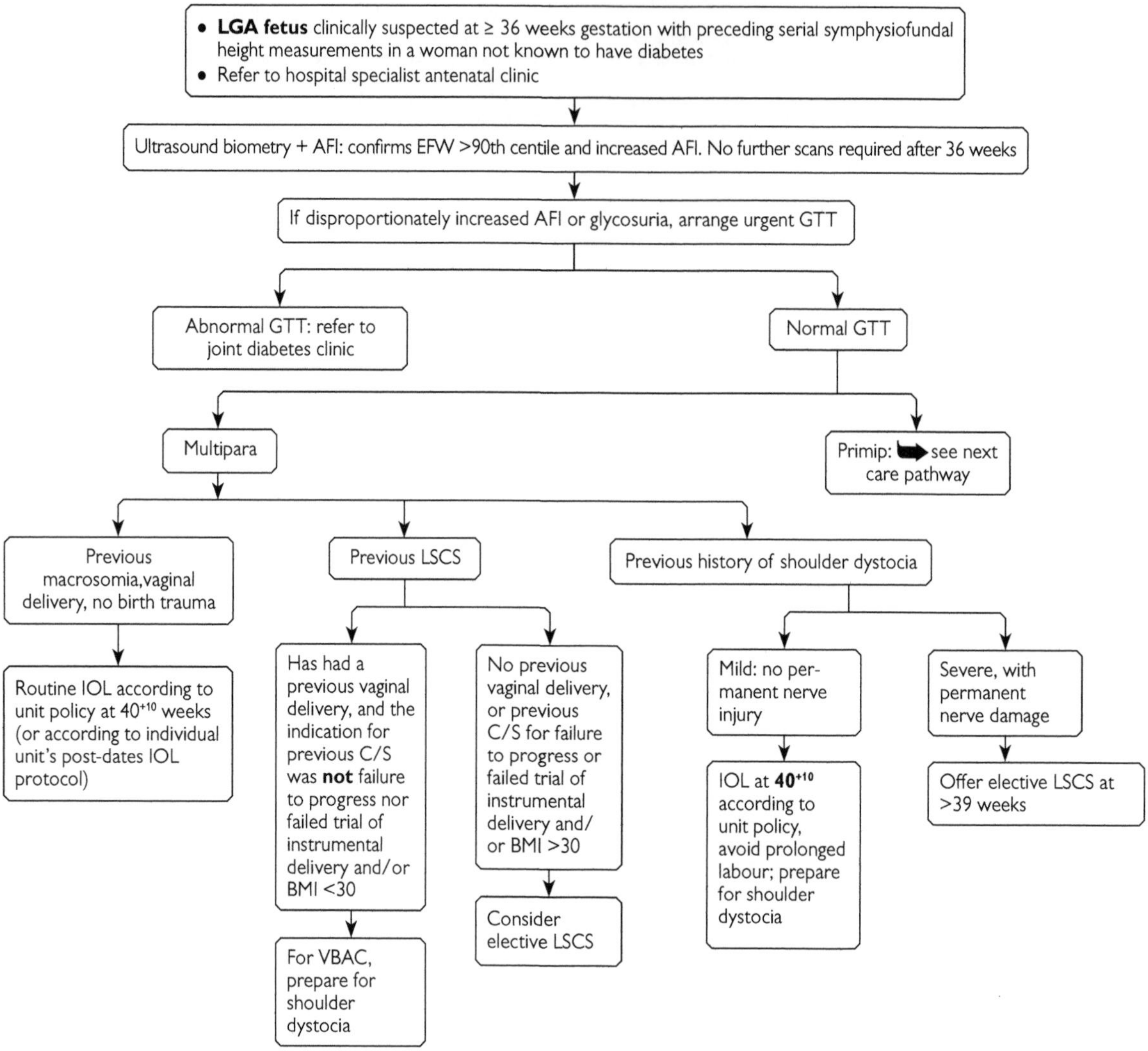

• LGA fetus clinically suspected at ≥ 36 weeks gestation with preceding serial symphysiofundal height measurements in a woman not known to have diabetes
• Refer to hospital specialist antenatal clinic
Ultrasound biometry + AFI: confirms EFW >90th centile and increased AFI. No further scans required after 36 weeks
If disproportionately increased AFI or glycosuria, arrange urgent GTT
Abnormal GTT: refer to joint diabetes clinic
Normal GTT
Multipara
Primip: see next care pathway
Previous macrosomia, vaginal delivery, no birth trauma
Previous LSCS
Previous history of shoulder dystocia
Routine IOL according to unit policy at 40^{+10} weeks (or according to individual unit's post-dates IOL protocol)
Has had a previous vaginal delivery, and the indication for previous C/S was not failure to progress nor failed trial of instrumental delivery and/or BMI <30
No previous vaginal delivery, or previous C/S for failure to progress or failed trial of instrumental delivery and/or BMI >30
Mild: no permanent nerve injury
Severe, with permanent nerve damage
For VBAC, prepare for shoulder dystocia
Consider elective LSCS
IOL at 40^{+10} according to unit policy, avoid prolonged labour; prepare for shoulder dystocia
Offer elective LSCS at >39 weeks

Adapted from Aye SS et al., Management of large for gestational age pregnancy in non-diabetic women, The Obstetrician and Gynaecologist, 12, 4, pp. 250–256, Wiley. © 2010 Royal College of Obstetricians and Gynaecologists, with permission.

Management of LGA in primips

Clinical suspicion of LGA, patient referred to hospital antenatal clinic from primary care

↓

Scan confirms growth at 36 weeks >90th centile and ↑ AFI, no further scans needed after 36 weeks

↓ (two branches)

- GTT if glycosuria/disproportionately ↑AFI
- Abnormal GTT: refer to joint diabetes clinic

GTT if glycosuria/disproportionately ↑AFI ↓

Normal GTT

↓

- Assess maternal BMI, parental habitus. Discuss options, pros and cons of expectant management vs interventions and invite mother's views
- Cervical assessment with 'stretch and sweep' of cervix and membranes at 40–41 weeks if possible
- Assess Bishop's score

↓ (two branches)

Favourable cervix

↓

- Induction of labour at 40^{+10} weeks gestation(according to individual unit's post-date IOL policy)
- Advise epidural
- Prepare for shoulder dystocia management, PPH prophylaxis

Unfavourable cervix, low Bishop's score and, if in addition, maternal obesity

↓

Discuss options, pros and cons of expectant management vs interventions and long-term risks

↓ (two branches)

- If decides on vaginal delivery, await spontaneous onset of labour, otherwise IOL with PGE2 around 41 weeks; advise epidural; preparation for shoulder dystocia; PPH and VTE prophylaxis
- **Document 'Early recourse to LSCS'** if no descent of head

- If opts for elective LSCS, arrange for about 40 weeks gestation under regional block
- If maternal morbid obesity, ensure anaesthetic assessment has already taken place, otherwise arrange urgently. PPH & VTE prophylaxis

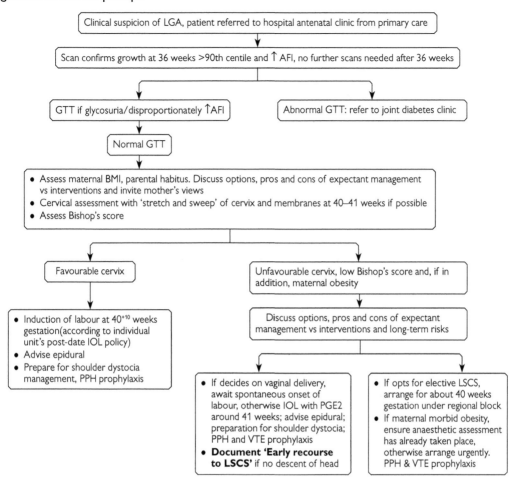

27 Fetal Abnormalities

27.1 Fetal Hydronephrosis

FACT FILE

Epidemiology and pathogenesis

- **Fetal hydronephrosis** is the commonest anomaly detected on antenatal mid-trimester ultrasound scanning, accounting for up to 50% of all detectable fetal anomalies.
- The estimated prevalence is quoted as approximately 2–5.5% of all pregnancies.[1,2,3,4]
- Hydronephrosis is the term used to describe dilatation of the renal collecting system.
- Hydronephrosis may have several causes.
- **It is very important to recognize that hydronephrosis is not synonymous with obstruction in all cases. In most cases, in fact, hydronephrosis is diagnosed without any overt urinary tract obstruction**, when the antero-posterior diameter (APD) of the renal pelvis exceeds the range for that gestational age.
- Antenatal hydronephrosis can be the result either due to **non-obstructive processes** such as vesicoureteric reflux or prune belly syndrome, or **obstructive lesions** such as pelviureteric obstruction (PUO).
- A significant number of fetal hydronephrosis cases are physiological renal pelvic dilatation, where spontaneous resolution is common either antenatally or after birth, with 50% of neonates showing no hydronephrosis on the postnatal ultrasound.
- Of the remaining 50% of neonates in whom hydronephrosis was diagnosed antenatally, a range of uropathies are diagnosed, most commonly PUO seen in 64% and vesicoureteral reflux, megaureter. or posterior urethral valves accounting for the rest.
- The incidence of significant renal impairment associated with antenatal hydronephrosis is about 0.2–0.9%.[5]
- About 5% of babies with mid-trimester fetal hydronephrosis is detected (1 in 1000 total births) require postnatal surgical intervention.[6]
- Ultrasonography can identify the fetal bladder and kidneys by 15 weeks gestation, a central echo (renal sinus) by about 18–20 weeks gestation,[5] and internal renal architecture and anomalies can be assessed by 20 weeks gestation.
- The benefit of prenatal fetal surgery for hydronephrosis, such as bilateral ureterostomies, open vesicostomies, or fetal cystoscopic ablation of posterior urethral valves, remains controversial due to lack of data regarding success as well as the high complication rates.[7,8]
- Interventions such as repeated amnio-infusions to try to reduce the risk of pulmonary hypoplasia[9] as well as to assist in placement of percutaneous shunts may be offered in tertiary centres in selected cases.

Embryology

- The ureteric bud develops from the mesonephric (Wolffian) duct in the fifth week of gestation, starting as a solid cord that lengthens and canalizes to allow uninterrupted flow of urine. Meanwhile, the renal parenchyma develops with most nephrons present by mid-second trimester. The bladder and urethra develop from the urogenital sinus at 10 and 12 weeks gestation respectively.
- Fetal kidneys begin to produce hypotonic urine at 5–9 weeks gestation. In the presence of progressive renal damage, the urine becomes isotonic, with raised levels of sodium, calcium, and chloride as well as osmolality which may indicate potentially irreversible renal dysplasia.[10]

Imaging

- The rate of prenatal abnormalities detected by screening ultrasound varies with the timing of fetal imaging. Detection rates increase when ultrasound is performed at mid-trimester compared with earlier scanning.[2] If ultrasound assessment at the time of the 'routine' anomaly scan at about 20 weeks shows mild dilation of the renal pelvis as an isolated finding, evaluation later in gestation is used to guide postnatal management.
- Further scans will help delineate renal architecture, size, parenchymal echogenicity, amniotic fluid volume, bladder dimensions, and filling.[11]
- Increased echogenicity may indicate renal dysplasia.
- Calyceal dilatation or the 'eggshell sign' indicates increased intrarenal pressure due to an obstructive process.[12]
- A thorough search for associated structural abnormalities or markers suggestive of chromosomal anomalies during the ultrasound assessment is essential.
- Chromosomal analysis should be offered in such cases.
- Fetal hydronephrosis can be classified as **mild, moderate, or severe** using a system based on measurement of renal pelvic APD.[1,4,13]

Prognosis

- A diagnosis of fetal hydronephrosis during pregnancy can provoke considerable anxiety for parents. Most fetuses with mild hydronephrosis have an excellent neonatal prognosis and parents need to be made aware of this (see Table 27.1).
- All cases of mild–severe hydronephrosis detected antenatally must be referred for multispeciality evaluation and assessment to a regional fetal medicine centre.
- Prenatal interventions such as may be considered in tertiary centres.
- In those with features indicating very poor prognosis, after sharing in-depth information with the parents, the option of termination must be discussed.
- It is crucial that several factors are taken into account during discussions regarding possible outcomes and prognosis.

Table 27.1 Degree of fetal hydronephrosis and postnatal prognosis

Fetal hydronephrosis classification	*Renal pelvic APD (mm)*		*Postnatal prognosis*
	Second trimester	Third trimester	
Mild	>4 to <7	>7 to ≤9	Excellent
Moderate	7–10 ± presence of calyceal dilatation	9–15 ± presence of calyceal dilatation	Thorough urological assessment and long-term follow-up required
Severe	≥10 ± presence of calyceal dilatation	≥15 ± presence of calyceal dilatation	Thorough urological assessment and long-term follow-up required Higher rates of renal impairment and need for postnatal surgery if calyceal dilatation present as well

Factors that must be considered

- **The underlying aetiology:** Obstructive lesions, particularly if bilateral, can cause greater damage to the developing kidneys compared to non-obstructive causes for hydronephrosis. This differentiation is therefore of paramount importance. Sometimes, however, such differentiation may be possible only after birth of the baby.
- The degree of hydronephrosis and the stage of pregnancy it develops in, whether it is unilateral or bilateral, resultant oligohydramnios and timing of its occurrence, as well as the presence or absence of other coexistent malformations or chromosomal anomalies, must be considered.
- Unilateral as well as non-obstructive lesions have a significantly better prognosis than bilateral and obstructive ones. For example, unilateral renal obstruction has a survival rate of nearly 100% with less than one-quarter of these children requiring surgery at 4 years follow-up.[14,15]
- In bilateral renal obstruction, oligohydramnios indicates an adverse outcome, especially when detected in the second trimester.[16,17] With oligohydramnios, pulmonary hypoplasia can be expected as well as compression deformities of the skeletal system. Anhydramnios with bilateral renal obstruction (Potter's syndrome) is incompatible with survival.
- The earlier the lesion develops, the greater the impact on the fetal kidneys and lungs and overall outcome.
- When the lesion is detected only in the third trimester, the mortality rate is about 13%.[18] Lesions detected in the second trimester with oligo- or anhydramnios have a high fatality rate of nearly 83–100%.[19]
- Normally the fetal bladder should be visualized with functional emptying once in 30–60 min. A bladder that is distended and does not empty in this manner can suggest posterior urethral valves or prune belly syndrome.
- When massive dilatation of the bladder and sometimes of the ureters is seen (megacystis, megaureters), it indicates obstructive urethral atresia which is almost always fatal. Megacystis is defined by a simple formula, with the fetal bladder sagittal length being greater than the gestational age plus 12.[20]
- In a significant number with fetal bilateral hydronephrosis and oligohydramnios, up to 55%,[21,22] associated structural (usually cardiac, brain, spine) or chromosomal anomalies are also found, which, if present pose a worse prognosis.

Neonatal management

- **Postnatal ultrasound assessment** is mandatory. If persisting hydronephrosis is confirmed, urgent paediatric urology evaluation is essential for all babies where antenatal hydronephrosis has been detected.
- Serially repeated ultrasonographic assessments are recommended starting after about 2 days of birth in order to avoid underestimation of any hydronephrosis when the neonate is relatively dehydrated.[23]
- Most babies with mild hydronephrosis or simple unilateral hydronephrosis persisting in the postnatal period have good outcomes[6] and are usually discharged home by paediatricians with prophylactic antibiotics to prevent UTIs, depending on the underlying cause of renal dilatation. Plans for further follow-up imaging and outpatient reviews will be arranged by the paediatric team.
- **When there is a high risk of demise in the antenatal or postnatal period or severe pulmonary complications**, such as with bilateral hydronephrosis (moderate or severe) with distended bladder, oligohydramnios, **referral to a tertiary fetal medicine centre is highly recommended**.
- Depending on the individual case, these babies may need delivery in a tertiary unit as they require level 3 cardiopulmonary support and may also require early intervention by paediatric urology.

Information for patients

Please see **Information for patients: Antenatal fetal hydronephrosis** (p. 551)

References

1. Pates JA, et al. Prenatal diagnosis and management of hydronephrosis. Early Hum Dev 2006;82: 3–8.
2. Fefer S, Ellsworth P. Prenatal hydronephrosis. Pediatr Clin N Am 2006;53: 429–447.
3. Gunn TR, et al. Antenatal diagnosis of urinary tract abnormalities by ultrasonography after 28 weeks' gestation: incidence and outcome. Am J Obstet Gynecol 1995;172: 479–486.
4. Lee RS, et al. Antenatal hydronephrosis as a predictor of postnatal outcome: a meta-analysis. Pediatrics 2006;118: 586–593.
5. Yiee J, Wilcox D. Management of fetal hydronephrosis. Pediatr Nephrol 2008;23: 347–353.
6. Sairam S, et al. Natural history of fetal hydronephrosis diagnosed on mid-trimester ultrasound. Ultrasound Obstet Gynecol 2001;17: 191–196.
7. Harrison MR, et al. Fetal surgery for congenital hydronephrosis. N Engl J Med 1982;306: 591–593.
8. Quintero RA., et al. Percutaneous fetal cystoscopy and endoscopic fulguration of posterior urethral valves. Am J Obstet Gynecol 1995;172: 206–209.
9. Vergani P, et al. Amnioinfusion for prevention of pulmonary hypoplasia in second-trimester rupture of membranes. Am J Perinatol 1997;14: 325–329.
10. Burghard R, et al. Protein analysis in amniotic fluid and fetal urine for the assessment of fetal renal function and dysfunction. Fetal Ther 1987;2: 188–196.
11. Coplen DE. Prenatal management of hydronephrosis. AUA Update Series Vol. 19. Linthicum, MD: American Urological Association, 2000.
12. Dewan PA, et al. Presence of the eggshell sign in obstructive uropathy. Urology 2002;59: 287–289.
13. Estrada CR Jr. Prenatal hydronephrosis: early evaluation. Curr Opinion Urol 2008;18: 401–403.
14. Lee R, et al. Antenatal hydronephrosis as a predictor of postnatal outcome: a meta-analysis. Pediatrics 2006;118: 586–593.
15. Aksu N, et al. Postnatal management of infants with antenatally detected hydronephrosis. Pediatr Nephrol 2005;20: 1253–1259.
16. Reznik VM, et al. Follow-up of infants with obstructive uropathy detected in utero and treated surgically postnatally. J Pediatr Surg 1989;24: 1289–1292.
17. Shokeir AA, Nijman RJM. Antenatal hydronephrosis: changing concepts in diagnosis and subsequent management. BJU Int 2000;85: 987–994.
18. Bastide A, et al. Ultrasound evaluation of amniotic fluid: outcome of pregnancies with severe oligohydramnios. Am J Obstet Gynecol 1986;154: 895–900.
19. Wigglesworth JS, Desai R. Is fetal respiratory function a major determinant of perinatal survival? Lancet 1982;i(8266): 264–267.
20. Maizels M, et al. Fetal bladder sagittal length: a simple monitor to assess normal and enlarged fetal bladder size, and forecast clinical outcome. J Urol 2004;172: 1995–1999.
21. Reuss A, et al. Non-invasive management of fetal obstructive uropathy. Lancet 1988;ii(8617): 949–951.
22. Ott WJ, Taysi K. Obstetric ultrasonographic findings and fetal chromosomal abnormalities: refining the association. Am J Obstet Gynecol 2001;184: 1414–1420.
23. Wiener JS, O'Hara SM. Optimal timing of initial postnatal ultrasonography in newborns with prenatal hydronephrosis. J Urol 2002;168: 1826–1829.

CARE PATHWAY

2nd- or 3rd-trimester ultrasound scan shows fetal hydronephrosis

- Assess renal pelvic antero-posterior diameter (APD), uni- or bilateral hydronephrosis, amniotic fluid, renal parenchymal texture, renal architecture, any calyceal dilatation, fetal sex, any renal cortical cysts, bladder: any distension, filling, any other structural abnormalities, ultrasound markers of aneuploidies
- Discuss additional tests including karyotyping, scans
- Referral to a tertiary centre may be required for further evaluation

→

- No other abnormalities seen
- Karyotyping normal or declined

→

- **Mild hydronephrosis:** APD <7 mm, unilateral, no oligohydramnios, non-obstructive lesions, no calyceal dilatation or cortical cysts, normal bladder size and function
- Excellent prognosis—reassure parents, only 15–20% of unilateral renal obstruction need surgery in childhood

→

- Serial scans at monthly intervals for APD, liquor, growth
- No change in obstetric management needed for labour and delivery, if no IUGR
- Inform paediatrics for postnatal scanning (>2nd day after birth) and further follow-up if hydronephrosis seen to persist after birth

→

- **Moderate–severe hydronephrosis:** APD 7–15 mm or >15 mm, bilateral, oligohydramnios, echogenic parenchyma, calyceal dilatation, cortical cysts, increased mortality, pulmonary morbidity
- Referral to tertiary centre for multispecialty input, evaluation and discussion with parents

→

No bladder distension

→

- Serial scans once in about 2 weeks, monitor for bladder distension, oligohydramnios, growth
- Amnioinfusions ± stenting may be considered
- No change in obstetric management needed for labour and delivery if no IUGR
- Vigilance for antenatal or intrapartum signs of fetal distress if oligohydramnios ± IUGR present
- Inform paediatrics for postnatal scanning (>2nd day after birth) and paediatric urology follow-up

→

Bladder distension

→

- Generally poor prognosis as suggestive of obstructive process
- In-utero interventions may be considered in tertiary centres in selected cases
- If megacystis/megaureter present, almost always fatal
- Discuss options with parents and tertiary centre
- Options including TOP or a non-interventional, conservative approach
- Proceed according to parents' choice
- If TOP opted for, discuss post-mortem
- If parents wish to continue pregnancy, referral to meet paediatrician/neonatologist

→

Other structural abnormalities seen on scan and/or chromosomal abnormality confirmed with amniocentesis

→

Prognosis can be expected to be poor. Discuss management options including TOP

→

- If parents choose TOP, proceed accordingly
- If karyotyping not previously performed, discuss post-mortem

→

- If parents choose non-interventional approach, discuss expected poor prognosis and conservative management
- Referral to meet paediatrician/neonatologist during pregnancy

27.2 Cervical Teratoma, Fetal Sacrococcygeal Teratoma, Cystic Hygroma

FACT FILE

- Apart from congenital cystic adenomatoid malformation (CCAM) (see chapter 27.5), other fetal tumours such as **sacrococcygeal teratomas, cervical teratomas, or cystic hygromas** can also be diagnosed antenatally on scan.
- Germ cell tumours contain a variety of tissues derived from all three embryonic germ cell layers: ectoderm, mesoderm, and endoderm.
- These are usually benign although the teratomas have a malignant potential.
- These tumours can grow to a large size and are highly vascular. This causes stress on the fetal heart leading to signs of in-utero heart failure and development of non-immune hydrops.
- Polyhydramnios could be seen with teratomas and oligohydramnios with cystic hygromas.
- Non-immune hydrops fetalis, cardiomegaly, placentomegaly, large tumour size, and rapid growth rate carry poor prognosis and fetal mortality is high.

Cervical teratoma

- Cervical teratomas occur as a tumour located in the fetal neck. They appear partly solid and partly cystic and may contain calcifications.[1,2] They are composed of several different types of embryonic tissue. Cervical teratomas often surround vital structures (e.g. oesophagus, trachea, or thyroid), which may cause airway obstruction and neonatal death.[3,4]
- A cervical teratoma is very rare and accounts for about 3–5% of all teratomas.[3,4] It affects both sexes and all ethnicities.
- Serial ultrasound scans are required to monitor the size and vascularity of the tumour, fetal growth, and the amount of amniotic fluid present. Polyhydramnios is often found with large tumours.[3]
- A fetal MRI as well as three-dimensional ultrasonography may be used to get better definition of the airway anatomy as well as of tumour extension.[4,5]
- In the case of highly vascular tumours, a fetal echocardiogram is also recommended.
- Alpha-fetoprotein (AFP) levels in maternal serum are often found elevated in cases of fetal cystic hygromas as AFP is produced by immature fetal cells.
- Preterm labour is common due to significant polyhydramnios,[4] itself caused by oesophageal compression interfering with the baby's ability to swallow amniotic fluid.
- Delivery is best planned at a tertiary referral centre, with the availability of neonatal and paediatric surgery. Airway management at birth is critical, with giant neck masses seen in cervical teratomas. Airway obstruction is life-threatening and associated with a high mortality.
- **EXIT** (ex-intrapartum treatment)[1,2] is a procedure where an airway is surgically established while the baby is still attached to and sustained by the placenta during a Caesarean section, with the mother under general anaesthetic.
- The tumour is surgically removed after the neonate is stabilized. Although a cervical teratoma is usually benign, there is a small possibility of malignancy. If there is complete surgical excision, chemotherapy is not indicated. However, in rare cases of recurrence in immature or malignant tumours, chemotherapy is very effective.
- A cervical teratoma may involve the thyroid and parathyroid glands; these infants may be at risk for hypoparathyroidism, and hypothyroidism. Paediatric endocrinologist input is required after birth and subsequently.
- AFP levels should fall after tumour removal and subsequent AFP levels are used as a screening tool for recurrence.
- Serial physical examination and imaging of the neck area is recommended until 3 years of age.
- The risk of cervical teratoma in a future pregnancy is extremely low.

Sacrococcygeal teratoma

- Sacrococcygeal teratomas (SCT) are the most common variety of teratomas and the most common solid neoplasm in neonates.
- They can be diagnosed prenatally by fetal ultrasound and 50–70% are found during the first few days of life.
- They occur at the base of the spine as a solid or solid-cystic mass and may be highly vascular. Most commonly, teratomas appear as a complex mass with roughly equal amounts of solid heterogeneous and cystic areas with or without septations. Other abnormalities may also be present.[1]
- Sacrococcygeal teratomas are particularly associated with poorly controlled maternal diabetes.
- SCT is very rare with an estimated occurrence between 1 in 35 000 and 1 in 40 000 live births.[2] It is more common in females than males (ratio 4:1).
- The vast majority of these tumours are benign but a few may be malignant.
- SCTs may be classified as **benign (mature)** and **malignant or immature** (composed of embryonic elements).[3] Mature teratomas are most common in neonates (68%) and older children (73%). Immature teratomas are cystic, whereas malignant tumours are solid. Over 50% of SCTs have calcification and ossification.
- The size of a SCT (average 8 cm, range 1–30 cm) does not predict its biological behaviour.[3] SCTs are described according to their size (small, 2–5 cm diameter; moderate, 5–10 cm diameter; large, > 10 cm diameter).[4]
- Serial ultrasounds are required for sequential assessment of the growth of the SCT and the systemic impact on the fetus.
- **Maternal serum AFP levels are elevated in cases of fetal SCT.**
- Polyhydramnios is a common feature and may result in preterm delivery.
- Doppler studies are required to assess the degree of vascularity. Some highly vascular tumours create an arteriovenous shunt resulting in fetal cardiac failure evidenced by hydrops.[5]
- The perinatal mortality rate is high with solid SCTs (46%)[6] compared to more cystic lesions.
- A fetal echocardiogram is recommended to assess the baby's heart function. In some cases, a fetal MRI is helpful in determining tumour size, type and extension.[7,8]
- Advanced hydrops may be associated with placentomegaly and **maternal 'mirror syndrome'**.[9,10]
- Open fetal surgery, is rarely available in the UK. In the US, it has been reserved for babies with highly vascular SCTs who develop hydrops before 30 weeks gestation.[11] Minimally invasive fetal surgical techniques including percutaneous laser therapy are being developed, but have met with limited success thus far and in the UK they are still under trial.[12]
- Delivery should be planned at a tertiary centre equipped with paediatric surgical services.
- Caesarean section is recommended for large tumours to prevent dystocia, tumour rupture, or bleeding.
- After initial stabilization of the baby, the tumour is surgically removed. Solid teratomas may be very vascular and can be associated with significant intraoperative haemorrhage.[13]
- The long-term outlook for babies with SCT is usually very good.[14]
- Regular follow-up of these infants and children up to at least the age of 3 years is required as even benign tumours may recur.

- During follow-up, serum AFP is used as a screening tool to identify tumour recurrence.
- SCTs located mostly in the pelvis may affect the muscles and nerves in the pelvis, altering bowel and bladder function.
- There have been a few reported familial cases of SCT. Type IV SCTs may occur as a familial form inherited as an autosomal dominant condition. In this entity, a presacral mass (teratoma, anterior meningocele, dermoid cyst, lipoma, neurofibroma, enteric cysts, or hamartoma) is associated with anal stenosis and typical scimitar defect of the sacrum. This is often referred to as **Currarino triad**.[4,15]

Cystic hygroma

- Cystic hygroma (CH) refers to a lymphangioma located in the region of the fetal neck. It is a developmental abnormality of the lymphatic system and appears as a mass with multiple cysts which can cause displacement of the normal structures of the neck.[1,2,3]
- CH may be macrocystic, microcystic,or of mixed lesions.
- CH occurs approximately in 1 in every 6000 live births.[2,3]
- CH is often associated with other malformations and chromosomal abnormalities, such as Turner's syndrome, [4] but a CH located in the anterior portion of the neck is usually not associated with a chromosomal abnormality.
- Serial ultrasound scans are required to monitor the size of the mass, to detect non-immune hydrops, ascites, pleural effusions and other defects, andto assess the amount of amniotic fluid volume and fetal growth.[1,3]
- Amniocentesis may be recommended because of the association with chromosomal abnormalities such as Turner's syndrome.[4]
- Fetal prognosis is usually poor, especially with associated chromosomal abnormalities or in the presence of non-immune hydrops fetalis and/or bilateral pleural effusions.[4,5,6,7]
- Compression of the oesophagus by large CH mass can lead to polyhydramnios which, in turn, can precipitate preterm labour.
- Airway obstruction is the main complication of CH in the neck. Airway management at birth is critical with giant neck masses.[4,5,6].
- In the presence of large CH, delivery must be planned in a tertiary centre well equipped with neonatal and paediatric surgery facilities.
- If there is concern about establishing an airway, an ex-uterine intrapartum (**EXIT**) Procedure may be considered, though this is still a rare procedure in the UK.[7] If an endotracheal tube cannot be inserted, a fetal tracheostomy is performed. Occasionally, partial resection of the mass while the baby is still on continued placental support, having been delivered only partially from the uterus, is required to place a tracheostomy.
- Those babies with CH secondary to a chromosomal abnormality will have additional health issues dependent on the underlying diagnosis.
- CH is often an isolated event, with little risk of recurrence. Genetic counselling is advisable if CH was secondary to a chromosomal abnormality.

Management options

All management options for fetal tumours are to be discussed with parents and should involve advice from the fetal unit in the tertiary centre. Options include:

- Termination of pregnancy (TOP) in the presence of signs of increasing fetal compromise and poor fetal prognosis.
- Continuation of pregnancy without intervention to allow nature to take its course
- Elective early Caesarean delivery of the fetus **in the tertiary centre** if signs of increasing fetal problems develop. The parents need to be advised that the prognosis may be poor even if the gestation is approaching term in such cases and clear documentation to this effect made in the notes.
- Fetuses with large neck masses (cervical teratomas or CH) and upper airway obstruction require immediate assessment at birth with emergency tracheotomy performed during an **EXIT procedure Caesarean section**. This involves an airway being surgically established with only the upper part of the fetus delivered at Caesarean section while the fetus is still attached to and sustained by the placenta. The rest of the fetus is delivered as usual after the surgical airway is established.
- Novel techniques involving interventions such as percutaneous laser therapy for fetal tumours are at present undergoing trials for safety and efficacy.
- After birth, the extent of the tumour is assessed and surgery is the mainstay of treatment with the aim of removing the tumour completely to prevent local recurrence.
- CHs are treated with surgery or sclerotherapy.[8,9] Macrocystic lesions may be treated with sclerotherapy whereas microcystic lesions usually require surgical excision.
- CHs are benign lesions; therefore if vital structures are closely involved with the mass, complete removal is neither necessary nor feasible.
- The risk of recurrence is low after therapy.
- The prognosis for neonates who undergo successful surgery is generally good. Additional surgery may be needed and long-term follow-up is required.

Information for patients

Please see Information for patients: Sacrococcygeal teratoma (p. 552); Cystic hygroma (p. 552)

References

Cervical teratomas

1. NICE Interventional Procedures Guidance. Interventional procedure overview of percutaneous laser therapy for fetal tumours. IPG180. London, National Institute for Health and Clinical Excellence, 2006.
2. Liechty KW, et al. Severe pulmonary hypoplasia associated with giant cervical teratomas. J Pediatr Surg 2006;41: 230–233.
3. Hasiotou M, et al. Congenital cervical teratomas. Int J Pediatr Otorhinolaryngol 2004;68: 1133–1139.
4. Herman TE, Siegel MJ. Cervical teratoma. J Perinatol 2008;28: 649–651.
5. Araujo Júnior E, et al. Prenatal diagnosis of a large fetal cervical teratoma by three-dimensional ultrasonography: a case report. Arch Gynecol Obstet 2007;275: 141–144.

Sacrococcygeal teratomas

1. Wells RG, Sty JR. Imaging of sacrococcygeal germ cell tumors. Radiographics 1990;10: 701–713.
2. Winderl LM, Silverman RK. Prenatal identification of a completely cystic internal sacrococcygeal teratoma (type IV). Ultrasound Obstet Gynecol 1997;9: 425–428.
3. Keslar PJ, et al. Germ cell tumors of the sacrococcygeal region: radiologic-pathologic correlation. Radiographics 1994;14: 607–622.
4. Altman RP, et al. Sacrococcygeal teratoma. American Academy of Pediatrics Surgical Section survey. J Pediatr Surg 1973;9: 389–398.
5. Flake AW. Fetal sacrococcygeal teratoma. Semin Pediatr Surg 1993;2: 113–120.
6. Hedrick HL, et al. Sacrococcygeal teratoma: prenatal assessment, fetal intervention, and outcome. J Pediatr Surg 2004;39: 430–438.
7. Kubick-Huch RA. Prenatal diagnosis of fetal malformations by ultrafast magnetic resonance imaging. .Prenat Diagn 1998;18: 1205–1208.
8. Danzer E, et al. Diagnosis and characterization of fetal sacrococcygeal teratoma with prenatal MRI. AJR 2006;187: 350–356.
9. Van Selm M, et al. Maternal hydrops syndrome: a review. Obstet Gynecol Surv 1991;46: 785–788.
10. Heyborne KD, Chism DM. Reversal of Ballantyne syndrome by selective second trimester fetal termination: a case report. J Reprod Med 2000;45: 360–362.
11. Adzick NS. Management of fetal lung lesions. Clin Perinatol 2003;30: 481–492.
12. NICE InterventionalProceduresGuidance. Interventional procedure overview of percutaneous laser therapy for fetal tumours. IPG180. London, National Institute for Health and Clinical Excellence, 2006.
13. Chisholm CA, et al. Prenatal diagnosis and perinatal management of fetal sacrococcygeal teratoma. Am J Perinatol 1999;16: 47–50.
14. Tuladhar R, et al. Review: sacrococcygeal teratoma in the perinatal period. Postgrad Med J 2000;76: 754–759.
15. Samuel M, et al. Currarino triad—diagnostic dilemma and a combined surgical approach. J Pediatr Surg 2000;35: 1970–1974.

Cystic hygroma

1. Benacerraf BR, Frigoletto FD Jr. Prenatal sonographic diagnosis of isolated congenital cystic hygroma, unassociated with lymphedema or other morphologic abnormality. J Ultrasound Med 1987;6: 63–66.
2. Langer JC, et al. Cervical cystic hygroma in the fetus: clinical spectrum and outcome. J Pediatr Surg 1990;25: 58–62.
3. Gallagher PG, et al. Cystic hygroma in the fetus and newborn. Semin Perinatol 1999;23: 341–356.
4. Abramowicz JS, et al. Congenital cystic hygroma of the neck diagnosed prenatally: outcome with normal and abnormal karyotype. Prenat Diagn 1989;9: 321–327.
5. Bernstein HS, et al. Prognosis of fetuses with a cystic hygroma. Prenat Diagn 1991;11: 349–355.
6. Tanriverdi HA. Hygroma colli cysticum: prenatal diagnosis and prognosis. Am J Perinatol 2001;18: 415–420.
7. Ganapathy R, et al. Natural history and outcome of prenatally diagnosed cystic hygroma Prenat Diagn 2004;24: 965–968.
8. Niramis R, et al. Treatment of cystic hygroma by intralesional bleomycin injection: experience in 70 patients. Eur J Pediatr Surg 2010;20: 178–182.
9. Ogita S, et al. Intracystic injection of OK-432: a new sclerosing therapy for cystic hygroma in children. Br J Surg 1987;74: 690–691.

CARE PATHWAY

- Care needs to be individualized on a case-to-case basis with joint interdisciplinary management with the tertiary referral centre
- Tumour usually detected on ultrasound scan in either 1st or 2nd trimester

Fetal teratoma on scan

Hydrops, ascites, pleural, pericardial effusions, cardiomegaly, large tumour size, placentomegaly

↓

Options to be discussed with parents: TOP, conservative expectant management or in-utero fetal surgery in specialist centres

↓

- If parents decide pregnancy is to continue with fetal salvage, continue serial scans
- Vigilance for maternal 'mirror syndrome'
- Fetal surgery by percutaneous techniques only in some specialist centres and as part of trials

↓

- Elective Caesarean section in tertiary centre with neonatal surgical expertise
- ? EXIT procedure to be considered if airway obstruction expected
- Post-delivery surgery after stabilization

→ (to regular follow-up, below)

No hydrops or other features suggestive of poor prognosis

↓

Serial ultrasound scans, MRI or 3D Doppler

↓

- Absence of poor prognostic signs
- Multidisciplinary discussions regarding place, time, and mode of delivery
- If airway obstruction expected, delivery in tertiary centre with neonatal surgical expertise

↓

- Regular follow-up of infants and children for at least 3 years in fetal teratomas
- Outlook generally good

Cystic hygroma detected on scan

↓

- Discuss possible association with chromosomal abnormalities (e.g. Turner's syndrome)
- Discuss amniocentesis

↓

If amniocentesis performed:

If amniocentesis confirms a chromosomal abnormality or further scans show progressive non-immune hydrops/ bilateral pleural effusions:

- Discuss poor prognosis
- Discuss options with parents: TOP or conservative expectant management
- If significant fetal non-immune hydrops is found, vigilance for maternal 'mirror syndrome'

No chromosomal abnormality present, no hydrops or pleural effusions, no other abnormality detected

- Continued serial scans for signs of polyhydramnios, tumour size, fetal growth
- Fetal surgery by percutaneous techniques only in some specialist centres as part of trials
- Delivery plans in tertiary centre
- Large tumour—in general, delivery by Caesarean section; if a small tumour, vaginal delivery possible
- ? EXIT procedure at Caesarean section, if airway obstruction expected
- After delivery, further assessment for treatment(e.g. surgery or sclerotherapy) to be considered
- Long-term follow-up in early childhood necessary
- Low risk of recurrence following treatment

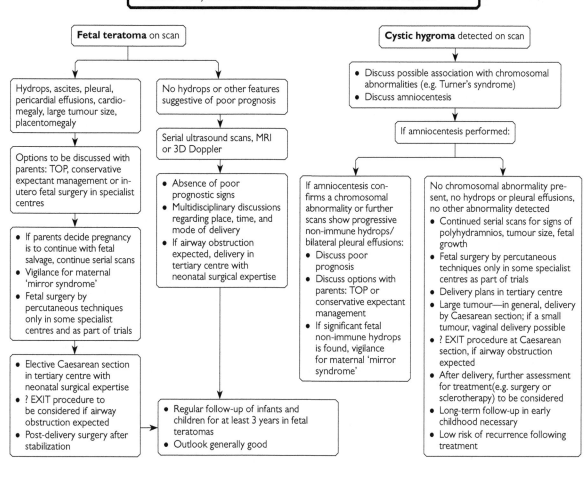

27.3 Fetal Exomphalos, Gastroschisis

FACT FILE

Both **exomphalos and gastroschisis** are defects of the fetal anterior abdominal wall but each has a different aetiology, chromosomal links, associated anomalies, and outcomes (see Table 27.2). Antenatal distinction between the two conditions is therefore crucial for parental counselling, decisions regarding invasive testing, and further management of the pregnancy.

Table 27.2 Comparison between exomphalos and gastroschisis

Feature	*Exomphalos (or omphalocele)*	*Gastroschisis*
Type of defect	• Midline defect where some abdominal contents herniate through the base of the umbilicus and are found outside the abdomen within a thin, translucent avascular sac to which the umbilical cord is attached. The surrounding sac is composed of the baby's parietal peritoneum, intervening layer of mesenchyme (Wharton's jelly), and the amnion • A large exomphalos can contain the stomach, bowel, bladder a portion of the liver, sometimes the spleen and even the ovaries • A small exomphalos may contain just the Meckel's diverticulum	• Malformation of the abdominal wall that presents as protrusion of the viscera through a paraumbilical defect, most often on the right side of a normally sited and intact umbilicus • The defect involves all layers of the abdominal wall, therefore the small bowel eviscerates and floats free in the amniotic fluid, without any membranous covering • Lack of a membranous covering allows the intestinal walls to develop an inflammatory coating and the mesentery to become thickened • The gut is malrotated • In early pregnancy, the bowel loops are found to float freely in the amniotic fluid, and the bowel wall thickness and lumen diameter ($\leq$11 mm) are normal • Later in the pregnancy, significant bowel dilatation (lumen $\geq$17 mm) due to bowel obstruction or perforation can occur • Less commonly, the liver, testes, ovaries are involved
Incidence	• Occurs in 1 in 3000 births[1] • Increases with rising maternal age	• Reported rates vary from 0.1 to 6 per 10 000 total births, with a fourfold increase from 2002–2004 in the UK[2] • Incidence increasing steadily worldwide in last 30 years, especially with young maternal age (<20 years), low social class, poor nutrition, smoking, and substance abuse[3,4] • North–south divide in the UK with more cases reported in northern registers in this time[2] • Up to 40% of babies with gastroschisis born to mothers <20 years old, compared to only 9–10% of overall births[2]
Pathogenesis	• During the 6th week of embryogenesis, the intestines develop rapidly and migrate through the umbilical ring into the umbilical cord. In normal development, the intestines should return into the abdominal cavity within the next 4 weeks with a normal 270° anticlockwise rotation • Exomphalos develops when the intestines do not return to the abdominal cavity, probably due to delayed closure of the lateral folds of the anterior abdominal wall. This is associated with non-rotation or malrotation of the gut	• Gastroschisis results from a vascular compromise of either the right umbilical vein or the omphalomesenteric artery. This might lead to disruption of the umbilical ring, therefore herniation of the abdominal contents • ***Gastroschisis does not usually have a genetic component.*** Only a few familial cases of gastroschisis have been reported[5]
Associated anomalies	• *Chromosomal abnormalities are found in 50–67%*[1] *of exomphalos*, mainly trisomies 13, 14,15, and 18, and triploidies which have a high rate of intrauterine lethality. Trisomy 21, Turner's and Klinefelter's syndromes are also found. Amniocentesis for fetal karyotyping should therefore be offered as this might influence further decisions about management of the pregnancy. • Other severe anomalies accompany exomphalos in about 50–70% of cases, including cardiac defects (VSD, tetralogy of Fallot), neural tube defects, diaphragmatic hernia, arteriovenous malformations • Exomphalos may also occur as a component of Beckwith–Wiedemann syndrome (macroglossia, macrosomia, enlarged kidneys and liver) as well as the pentalogy of Cantrell (ectopia cardis, VSD, sternal and/or diaphragmatic malformations)[6]	• Approximately 80% of gastroschisis occur as isolated defects, while 10–20% may have associated malformations, mainly of the intestinal tract including atresia, stenosis, obstruction may occur. • Other congenital defects such as cardiac defects, hydrocephalus, Meckel's diverticulum, genitourinary tract abnormalities are less frequently seen
Ultrasound findings	• Antenatal ultrasound can detect an exomphalos as a mass that appears solid, is spherical and echogenic, sited close to the abdominal wall. Central herniation within a sac or membrane is seen, into which the umbilical cord is inserted • Following the detection of exomphalos, close scrutiny for other congenital abnormalities as well as **fetal ECHO** is recommended • **Amniocentesis** is advisable after detail explanation of exomphalos and increased chances of fetal karyotypic abnormalities	• Antenatal ultrasound scan can detect multiple free-floating bowel loops close to the anterior abdominal wall. No membranous sac is seen • Either polyhydramnios or oligohydramnios may be seen • Genetic amniocentesis not usually recommended as the vast majority of cases are not associated with chromosomal abnormalities • In some cases associated anomalies can be found
Abnormal biochemical tests	• Maternal l serum AFP is abnormally elevated	• Maternal serum AFP is abnormally elevated in 75–98% of cases, as is amniotic fluid AFP (If amniocentesis has been performed for any other reason or if the antenatal scan cannot exclude a ruptured exomphalos, where the ultrasound images may resemble those of gastroschisis.)

Table 27.2 *(Continued)*

Feature	*Exomphalos (or omphalocele)*	*Gastroschisis*
Management options		
Counselling of parents	• Has to be done with sensitivity and taking into account finding of any karyotypic and/or other congenital anomalies. Referral to fetal medicine unit in tertiary centre is highly recommended to allow the parents to discuss issues with the perinatal and surgical team • If exomphalos is associated with chromosomal anomalies or other structural defects, increased risk of intrauterine death • Neonatal death usually due to presence of other anomalies present in addition to exomphalos (80–nearly 90% of neonatal morbidity due to other coexistent defects) • Approximately 50% of fetuses diagnosed with exomphalos may not survive mainly because of the presence of other abnormalities. • Discussions must include the option of termination, depending on the individual case, and carried out if parents choose this route • If exomphalos is found to be an isolated anomaly, and without chromosomal abnormalities, the outcome for the baby is good after surgical repair • Surgical repair is usually performed, at least as a first-stage procedure, in the early neonatal period (usually within 24–48 h after birth.) • Depending on the size of the defect, staged repair may be required	• Detection of additional abnormalities (found in 10–20% of gastroschisis) may affect the prognosis • In cases of isolated gastroschisis, the overall prognosis is excellent with a survival rate >90% after surgical repair[6] • Referral to a tertiary centre to discuss issues with the fetal medicine and neonatal surgical team, should be offered to parents • Overall prognosis in isolated gastroschisis after surgical repair is excellent (>90% survival rate) • In cases where there is associated severe bowel atresia, the outcomes are not as good and survival can be expected in only about 40% • Surgical repair is usually performed within 24 h of birth • In at least 80% of cases, only a single stage operation is required to close the defect • If the defect is extensive, and /or the abdomen is small in a baby with IUGR, an initial silastic pouch is usually fashioned and delayed closure is performed after gradual reduction over 3–10 days.
Further management in pregnancy	• Serial growth scans including assessment of liquor volume • Prophylactic steroids if signs of preterm labour • Delivery is usually arranged at a tertiary centre with access to neonatal surgery, paediatric cardiology • Unless there are signs of IUGR, delivery at term is reasonable • Most studies have shown no added benefit of Caesarean section with regards to fetal mortality or morbidity compared to vaginal delivery • Many obstetricians would however, advise delivery by Caesarean section in cases of large exomphalos containing a portion of the liver, especially in the absence of chromosomal or other defects	• Serial growth scans with assessment of amniotic fluid volume should be maintained as IUGR is found in about 50% of cases • Polyhydramnios could precipitate premature labour and prophylactic steroids must be considered • Ultrasound signs of fetal bowel obstruction or atresia need monitoring • Delivery is best arranged at a tertiary centre with access to advanced perinatal and neonatal surgical services • Timing of delivery will depend on the presence or absence of IUGR, Doppler. and amniotic volume findings. Some would advise delivery by 37–38 weeks to reduce bowel damage from exposure to amniotic fluid • Although most studies have not shown an added benefit of Caesarean section delivery, in those with large defects especially containing a portion of the liver, many would advise delivery by elective Caesarean section

1. Snijders RJM, et al. Fetal exomphalos and chromosomal defects: relationship to maternal age and gestation. Ultrasound Obstet Gynecol 1995;6: 250–255.
2. Gastroschisis: a growing concern. In: Annual report of the Chief Medical Officer. London, Department of Health, 2004, pp. 41–47.
3. Srivatsava V, et al. Rising incidence of gastroschisis and exomphalos in New Zealand. J Paed Surg 2009;44: 551–555.
4. David AL, et al. Gastroschisis: sonographic diagnosis, associations, management and outcome. Prenat Diag 2008;28: 633–644.
5. Torfs CP, Curry CJR. Familial cases of gastroschisis in a population-based registry. Am J Med Genet 1993;45: 465–467.
6. Poddar R, Hartley L. Exomphalos and gastroschisis. Contin Educ Anaesth Crit Care Pain 2009;9: 48–51.

Information for patients

Please see **Information for patients: Exomphalos and gastroschisis** (p. 553)

CARE PATHWAY

Exomphalos

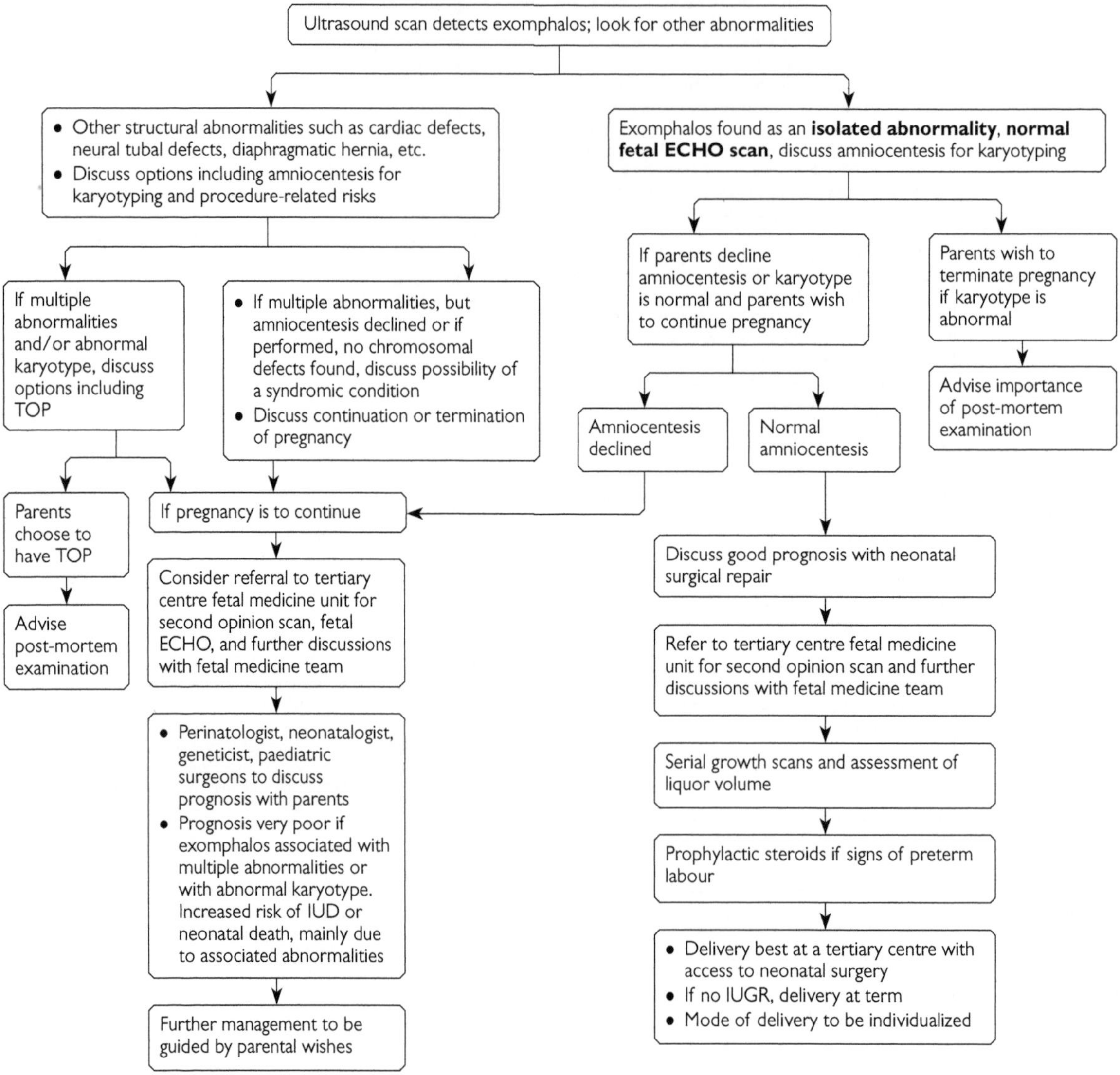

Gastroschisis

Ultrasound scan detects malformation of the abdominal wall, protrusion of the viscera through a paraumbilical defect, most often on the right side of a normally sited and intact umbilicus, and free-floating bowel loops suggestive of gastroschisis

↓

Careful ultrasound scrutiny for other abnormalities, which occur in 10–20% of cases—especially of the intestinal tract including atresia, stenosis, obstruction, cardiac defects, hydrocephalus, rarely genitourinary defects

↓

Reassure parents:

- that gastroschisis is not associated with karyotypic abnormalities in vast majority of cases; therefore **karyotyping not indicated** in **isolated gastroschisis**
- that surgical repair after birth carries excellent prognosis of >90%, but of about 40% if severe bowel atresia develops

↓

Refer to tertiary centre fetal medicine unit

↓

Serial growth scans and liquor assessment

↓

If polyhydramnios and signs of preterm labour, or ultrasound scan shows signs of bowel obstruction or atresia, consider prophylactic steroids

↓

- Delivery in tertiary centre with access to neonatal surgical facilities as best results from surgical repair within 24 h of birth
- Timing of delivery depending on the presence or absence of IUGR as well as Doppler and amniotic volume findings. Some advise delivery by 37–38 weeks to reduce bowel damage from exposure to amniotic fluid
- Although no absolute benefit of Caesarean section demonstrated, in those with large defects—especially containing a portion of the liver—elective Caesarean section usually resorted to.

27.4 Fetal Congenital Diaphragmatic Hernia

FACT FILE

Epidemiology

- **Congenital diaphragmatic hernia (CDH)** arises from the failure of proper fusion of the two halves of the diaphragm, allowing abdominal organs in the developing fetus to migrate into the chest cavity. The diaphragm is fully formed by 9 weeks gestation.
- The most common site for CDH is the left side, through which the stomach, liver, bowels, and spleen can herniate.
- CDH is associated with a high degree of morbidity and mortality, mainly due to pulmonary hypoplasia.
- Incidence is about 1 in 3700 live births,[1] but taking miscarriages, TOPs, and stillbirths into account the incidence is closer to 1 in 2200 pregnancies.
- CDH accounts for 8% of all major congenital defects.
- In about 33% of CDH, additional abnormalities are detected on ultrasound.[2]
- Chromosomal abnormalities are found in approximately 10–30% of cases of CDH.
- Overall prenatal detection rate by scan is about 50–60%.[3]
- Male fetuses are more commonly affected than female (3:2).
- Most are idiopathic.
- Familial CDH occurs in less than 2% of cases[4]. Very rarely, in a small number of families, CDH is part of a genetic syndrome with a risk of recurrence as high as 25%.
- Certain drugs such as thalidomide, quinine, and some antiepileptics have been postulated as causing CDH, although the associations are weak.
- ***For isolated CDH, risk of recurrence in a future pregnancy is approximately 1–2%.***

Classification of CDH

- Classification of CDH is usually according to the location of the defect. Most are left-sided (approximately 90%), while 10% are right-sided and 2% are bilateral. Defects that are posterolateral, known as **Bochdalek hernia**, are most common. A defect in the anterior part of the diaphragm, known as **Morgagni hernia**, is rare.
- CDH may be an isolated finding or it may be part of other structural abnormalities (in up to 40%) involving cardiovascular, genitourinary, and gastrointestinal malformations. The associated abnormalities are usually congenital heart defects (patent ductus arteriosus, ventricular septal defects, tetralogy of Fallot, or cardiac hypoplasia) followed by renal (23%), central nervous system (10%), and gastrointestinal (14%) anomalies.

Differential diagnosis

- The differential diagnosis includes extralobular sequestration, CCAM, congenital lobar emphysema, diffuse pulmonary cysts, and rarely pulmonary agenesis.

Chromosomal abnormalities and syndromes

- Karyotype abnormalities found in 10–30% of antenatally diagnosed fetusus may include various anomalies including **trisomy 13, 18, 21 and Turner's syndrome**.
- The **Plaister–Killian syndrome** (tetrasomy12p mosaicism) may also be associated with CDH.
- Lethal anomalies are present in up to 16% of infants and most of these involve central nervous system anomalies in addition to CDH.
- Other syndromes associated with CDH include **Fryn's**, **Beckwith–Wiedemann**, **VACTERL**, **Klippel–Feil**, and **Cornelia de Lange**.

Prognosis

- Outcomes are better when the CDH is an isolated defect without other malformations or chromosomal abnormalities and delivery takes place in a tertiary hospital with access to expert neonatal and paediatric surgical facilities, Survival rate in these circumstances is more than 50–70%.[3,5]
- Left-sided defects carry better prognosis than right-sided or bilateral defects.
- Ultrasound features indicative of **poor prognosis** are:
  - early diagnosis
  - abdominal organs, especially the liver, sited in the thorax
  - cpolyhydramnios (found in up to 75% of CDH)
  - hydrops fetalis (carries close to a 100% mortality)
  - right-sided and bilateral defects (mortality rate of 80% to 100% respectively)[5]
  - f. significant mediastinal shift
  - large defects seen earlier in gestation (22–25 weeks) allowing a greater volume of abdominal viscera into the thoracic cavity; this, in turn, results in a greater degree of pulmonary hypoplasia and a worse outcome
  - similarly a 'sliding' hernia in which abdominal viscera can move in and out of the thoracic cavity has a better prognosis than one with a fixed large volume of herniated abdominal viscera
  - presence of the stomach in the thoracic cavity has a poor prognosis; fetuses with the stomach below the diaphragm have better survival rates.
- **The lung-to-head ratio (LHR)** as measured by serial ultrasound has been used to predict postnatal outcomes in CDH. As ultrasound scan cannot visualize the actual lung structure, the lung area contralateral to the CDH is obtained by taking the product of the longest two perpendicular linear measurements of the lung (length 1 and length 2) measured at the level of the four-chamber view of the heart on a transverse scan of the fetal thorax. The product is divided by the head circumference (HC) to obtain the LHR[6].
  - lung area = length 1 × length 2
  - LHR = lung area/HC
  - Alternatively, using the manual tracing method[7] the lung area contralateral to the CDH can be obtained by tracing of the limits of the lung.
  - ***If the LHR measures less than 1, a near 100% perinatal mortality can be expected compared to an almost 100% survival if the LHR remains consistently more than 1.4.***

Referral to tertiary centre for antenatal assessments and delivery

- Parents should be referred to a tertiary centre for paediatric surgery consultation as soon as possible after prenatal diagnosis.
- This consulatation includes the initial assessments, serial scans for lung/head ratio and other features indicating prognosis, as well as consideration of in-utero fetal surgery for well-selected cases.[8,9,10,11]
- If the parents opt to continue the pregnancy, the local unit's paediatricians must be informed during pregnancy in the event of the patient presenting to the district general hospital in advanced preterm labour, before the date of the planned delivery in the tertiary centre, thus making in-utero transfer difficult.

Information for patients

Please see Information for patients: Congenital diaphragmatic hernia (p. 553)

References

1. Wenstrom KD, et al. A five-year state wide experience with congenital diaphragmatic hernia. Am J Obstet Gynecol 1991;165: 838–842.
2. Enns GM, et al. Congenital diaphragmatic defects and associated syndromes, malformations, and chromosome anomalies: a retrospective study of 60 patients and literature review. Am J Med Genet 1998;79: 215–225.

3. Graham G, Devine PC. Antenatal diagnosis of congenital diaphragmatic hernia. Semin Perinatol 2005;29: 69–76.
4. Narayan H, et al. Familial congenital diaphragmatic hernia: prenatal diagnosis, management, and outcome. Prenat Diagn.1993;13: 893–901.
5. Adzick NS, et al. Diaphragmatic hernia in the fetus (prenatal diagnosis and outcome in 94 cases). J Pediatr Surg 1985;20: 357–361.
6. Alfaraj MA, et al. Congenital diaphragmatic hernia: lung-to-head ratio and lung volume for prediction of outcome. Am J Obstet Gynecol 2011;205: 43.e 1–8.
7. Peralta CF, et al. Left and right lung volumes in fetuses with diaphragmatic hernia. Ultrasound Obstet Gynecol 2006;27: 551–554.
8. Harrison MR, et al. The fetus with diaphragmatic hernia: pathology, natural history and surgical management. In: The unborn patient: prenatal diagnosis and treatment, 2nd ed. Philadelphia, PA: WB Saunders, 1990, p. 295–312.
9. Harrison MR, et al. Correction of diaphragmatic hernia. J Paediatr Surg 1993;28: 1411–1418.
10. Doyle NM, Lally KP. The CDH Study Group and advances in the clinical care of the patient with CDH. Semin Perinatol 2004;28: 174–184.
11. Doné E, et al. Prenatal diagnosis, prediction of outcome and in utero therapy of isolated congenital diaphragmatic hernia. Prenat Diagn 2008;28: 581–591.

CARE PATHWAY

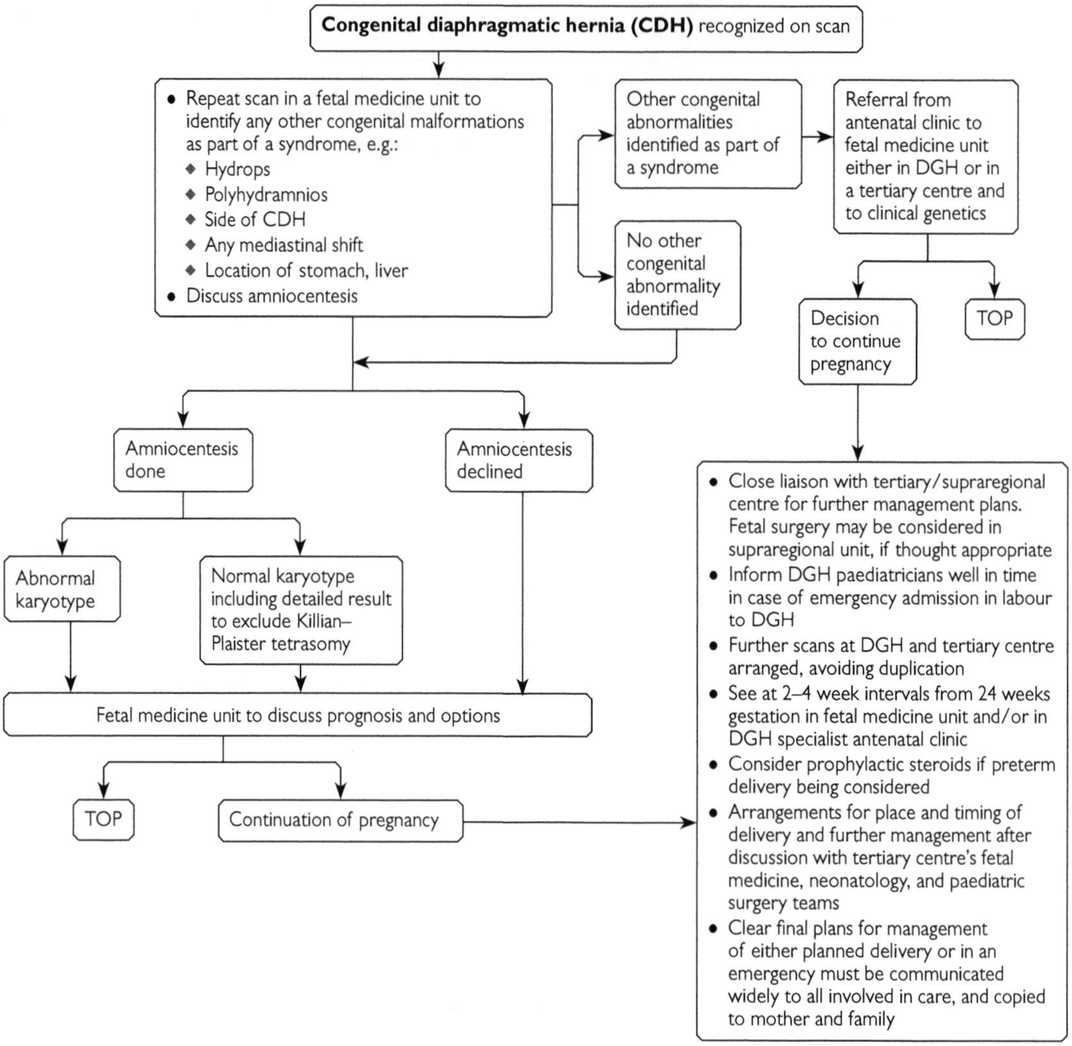

Congenital diaphragmatic hernia (CDH) recognized on scan
• Repeat scan in a fetal medicine unit to identify any other congenital malformations as part of a syndrome, e.g.:
◆ Hydrops
◆ Polyhydramnios
◆ Side of CDH
◆ Any mediastinal shift
◆ Location of stomach, liver
• Discuss amniocentesis
Other congenital abnormalities identified as part of a syndrome
Referral from antenatal clinic to fetal medicine unit either in DGH or in a tertiary centre and to clinical genetics
No other congenital abnormality identified
Decision to continue pregnancy
TOP
Amniocentesis done
Amniocentesis declined
Abnormal karyotype
Normal karyotype including detailed result to exclude Killian–Plaister tetrasomy
Fetal medicine unit to discuss prognosis and options
TOP
Continuation of pregnancy
• Close liaison with tertiary/supraregional centre for further management plans. Fetal surgery may be considered in supraregional unit, if thought appropriate
• Inform DGH paediatricians well in time in case of emergency admission in labour to DGH
• Further scans at DGH and tertiary centre arranged, avoiding duplication
• See at 2–4 week intervals from 24 weeks gestation in fetal medicine unit and/or in DGH specialist antenatal clinic
• Consider prophylactic steroids if preterm delivery being considered
• Arrangements for place and timing of delivery and further management after discussion with tertiary centre's fetal medicine, neonatology, and paediatric surgery teams
• Clear final plans for management of either planned delivery or in an emergency must be communicated widely to all involved in care, and copied to mother and family

27.5 Fetal Congenital Cystic Adenomatoid Malformation or Congenital Pulmonary Airway Malformation

FACT FILE

Epidemiology

- **Congenital cystic adenomatoid malformation or CCAM** (also more recently termed **congenital pulmonary airway malformation, CPAM**) is a rare unilateral congenital abnormality of lung development with proliferation of bronchial structures leading to a solid/cystic mass within the lung.[1,2,3]
- Incidence of antenatally diagnosed CCAM is about 1 in 11 000 to 1 in 35 000.[4,5]
- Most cases are identified by routine ultrasound scans during pregnancy.
- About 85% of CCAM lesions are unilateral.[1,6,7,8]
- There is no known association with chromosomal abnormalities in CCAM,[8]
- Five pathological types are described:
  - **Type 0:** Rare and usually lethal, arises from the trachea or bronchus. Cysts are small.
  - **Type I:** This is the most common type (50–70% of cases). With a small number of large echolucent cysts 2–10 cm in size, it arises from the distal bronchus or proximal bronchiole. Due to the large size of cysts, hydrops is often seen.
  - **Type II:** Accounts for 15–30% of cases and arises from terminal bronchioles, with smaller cysts (0.5–1 cm). This type of CCAM has the highest incidence (up to 60%) of associated anomalies, and prognosis depends on these findings, which include most organ systems.
  - **Type III:** Accounts for 5–10% of cases and probably arises from acinar-like tissue. The cysts are so small (microcysts) that the mass appears to be solid and highly echogenic on ultrasound. The large mass may distort the thoracic contents and affect survival.
  - **Type IV:** Accounts for 5–15% of cases, alveolar in origin. The cysts are as large as 10 cm and have been associated with malignancy.
- CCAMs are usually isolated and sporadic, although they have been associated with other anomalies (mostly cardiac and renal) in 15–20% of cases.[10]

Prognosis

- Overall perinatal mortality rate when an antenatal diagnosis of CCAM has been made is approximately 12% in recent reports,[1,9,10] although higher rates of up to 49% have been reported in older series.[11]
- Preterm delivery and dystocia at birth may also occur with large lesions.[12]
- Large lesions are particularly associated with non-immune hydrops fetalis, mediastinal shift of the heart, and pulmonary hypoplasia.[13]
- Spontaneous antenatal resolution has been reported in 15–76% of CCAM.[1,4,8,10,11,14]
- Peak CCAM growth is noted in at about 28 weeks and in 20% of cases regression begins from 29 weeks.[15]
- Resolution of CCAM on antenatal ultrasound scans or normal chest radiographs after birth is not diagnostic of tumour regression as in the majority of these infants, CCAM is found to persist when CT imaging is undertaken. Due to the false negative rate of neonatal chest radiographs, postnatal CT imaging is mandatory.[16]

Poor prognostic signs in CCAM

Poor prognostic signs in CCAM include:

- Non-immune hydrops (seen in about 18–40%).
- A **CCAM volume ratio (CVR)** is obtained by dividing the CCAM volume by HC to correct for fetal size. A CVR greater than 1.6 is predictive of non-immune hydrops developing in 80% of cases.[14]
- Significant mediastinal shift (seen in about 80%).
- Large size of tumour.
- **Polyhydramnios** (which arises due to oesophageal compression and inability to swallow).
- If tumour is of the microcytic rather the macrocytic variety: survival rates in type I about 69% but 0% in types II and III.
- **Non-immune hydrops** is due to compression of the inferior vena cava and thus restriction of venous return. This, in turn, results in decreased cardiac output and development of effusions.
- **Pulmonary hypoplasia** can also occur due to the presence of the CCAM and this may lead to postnatal respiratory distress.
- Survival rates when non-immune hydrops is present in CCAM is about 50% with expectant management in more recent studies.[1]

Predictable perinatal outcomes

- **CCAM without hydrops:** 95% survival with expectant management only, also 50% could show spontaneous antenatal resolution. In fetuses that do not develop hydrops, postnatal survival has been reported as nearly 100%.[17]
- **CCAM with hydrops:** 95% will die at or shortly after birth with only conservative management. In fetuses with hydrops who undergo prenatal intervention, survival has been reported at a mean of 80%, with rates of up to 100% in those treated by thoracocentesis.[17]
- Premature delivery to salvage a fetus with CCAM and hydrops may still lead to fetal neonatal demise due to severe lung hypoplasia.
- **Type 0 CCAM is considered lethal**. Resection of type I CCAM is considered curative and outcomes are excellent.[10] Outcomes for Type II CCAM depend largely on the presence of associated anomalies. The risk of pulmonary hypoplasia is highest with type III CCAM, given its tendency for growth and mass effect.

Postnatal problems

- Postnatal problems can involve severe respiratory distress, spontaneous pneumothorax, dyspnoea, recurrent infections, and pleural effusions secondary to hydrops.
- Despite the antenatal resolution of CCAM seen on ultrasound, postnatal follow-up is required because of the long-term complications of this malformations including recurrent chest infections and neoplastic change.[1] Malignancies consist mainly of pulmonary blastoma and rhabdomyosarcoma in infants and young children, and bronchio-alveolar carcinoma in older children and adults.
- Not all CCAMs present in the antenatal period. Some cases present only after birth or in childhood with respiratory distress, recurrent chest infections, chest pain, haemoptysis, and failure to thrive.

Antenatal management options

CCAM without hydrops

- In these cases conservative management with regular scans to assess the change in size of the tumour is called for. A significant proportion of these lesions decrease in size and regress spontaneously.
- All these cases must be referred to a tertiary fetal medicine unit at least for initial assessments.
- In-utero percutaneous laser therapy for CCAM is a novel procedure as yet of uncertain safety and efficacy, currently undergoing trials.[12,18] Percutaneous laser therapy is reserved for fetuses that develop signs of cardiac failure (non-immune hydrops). Other percutaneous procedures may include radiofrequency ablation or thermocoagulation with monopolar diathermy.
- Prenatal thoracoamniotic shunts have also been reported to improve outcomes in some cases.
- In-utero fetal surgery in some cases has also been shown to improve survival rates although the morbidity to mother and fetus is significant.[11]

- Multispeciality decisions involving the district general hospital, the tertiary centre, and the parents regarding the place, timing, and mode of delivery must be made on an individualized case-to-case basis.
- All babies diagnosed antenatally require postnatal CT imaging irrespective of signs of antenatal resolution of the CCAM.
- After birth, asymptomatic infants need close follow-up and elective surgery usually within the first year of life. Repeat surgery may also be required in some cases.

CCAM with hydrops

- In the presence of poor prognostic features (such as increasing signs of fetal cardiac failure such as progressive hydrops, effusions, polyhydramnios, large tumour size, or tumour of a microcytic variety), TOP is an option to be discussed.
- Some parents will prefer to continue the pregnancy without intervention in order to let nature take its course. They need appropriate support.
- If the parents have opted for neonatal salvage, early elective Caesarean section in a tertiary centre is appropriate in case significant problems develop, recognizing that the chances of survival are no more than 20–50%.
- Following birth, the extent of the tumour is assessed and surgery is the mainstay of treatment with the aim of removing the tumour completely to avoid local recurrences. Repeat surgery may also be required subsequently.
- The potential for malignant transformation is recognized in all cases of CCAM.
- During pregnancy, referral to a paediatric consultant in the local unit is recommended before 28 weeks gestation, although the patient might already be booked under a tertiary centre multidisciplinary team. In the case of unexpected spontaneous early onset of labour or if any obstetric emergency develops and in-utero transfer is not possible, the paediatricians in the local unit should already have had the opportunity to meet the parents and discuss neonatal outcomes.
- Antenatal management of CCAM should take place with close input from the tertiary fetal centre and delivery needs to be arranged in the tertiary centre.

Information for patients

Please see **Information for patients: Congenital cystic adenomatoid malformation** (p. 554)

References

1. Ierullo AM, et al. Neonatal outcome of antenatally diagnosed congenital cystic adenomatoid malformations. Ultrasound Obstet Gynecol 2005;26: 150–153.
2. Langston C. New concepts in the pathology of congenital lung malformations. Semin Pediatr Surg 2003;12: 17–37.
3. Laberge JM, et al. Asymptomatic congenital lung malformations. Semin Pediatr Surg 2005;14: 16–33.
4. Laberge JM, et al. Outcome of the prenatally diagnosed congenital cystic adenomatoid lung malformation: a Canadian experience. Fetal Diagn Ther 2001;16: 178–186.
5. Gornall AS, et al. Congenital cystic adenomatoid malformation: accuracy of prenatal diagnosis, prevalence and outcome in a general population. Prenat Diagn 2003;23: 997–1002.
6. Wilson RD, et al. Cystic adenomatoid malformation of the lung: review of genetics, prenatal diagnosis, and in utero treatment. Am J Med Genet 2006;140: 151–155.
7. Tran H, et al. Congenital cystic adenomatoid malformation: monitoring the antenatal and short-term neonatal outcome. Aust N Z J Obstet Gynecol 2008;48: 462–466.
8. Azizkhan RG, Crombleholme TM. Congenital cystic lung disease: contemporary antenatal and postnatal management. Pediatr Surg Int 2008;24: 643–657.
9. Sfakianaki AK, Copel JA. Congenital cystic lesions of the lung: congenital cystic adenomatoid malformation and bronchopulmonary sequestration. Rev Obstet Gynecol 2012;5: 85–93.
10. Laje P, Liechty KW. Postnatal management and outcome of prenatally diagnosed lung lesions. Prenat Diagn 2008;28: 612–618.
11. Adzick NS, et al. Fetal lung lesions: management and outcome. Am J Obstet Gynecol 1998;179: 884–889.
12. NICE InterventionalProceduresGuidance. Interventional procedure overview of percutaneous laser therapy for fetal tumours. IPG180. London: National Institute for Health and Clinical Excellence, 2006.
13. Orpen N, et al. Intralobar pulmonary sequestration with congenital cystic adematous malformation and rhabdomyomatous dysplasia. Pediatr Surg Int 2003;19: 610–611.
14. Cass DL, et al. Prenatal diagnosis and outcome of fetal lung masses. J Pediatr Surg 2011;46: 292–298.
15. Duncombe GJ, et al. Prenatal diagnosis and management of congenital cystic adenomatoid malformation of the lung. Am J Obstet Gynecol 2002;187: 950–954.
16. Blau H, et al. Postnatal management of resolving fetal lung lesions. Pediatrics 2002;109: 105–108.
17. Witlox RS, et al. Neonatal outcome after prenatal interventions for congenital lung lesions. Early Hum Dev 2011;87: 611–618.
18. Davenport M, et al. Current outcome of antenatally diagnosed cystic lung disease. J Pediatr Surg 2004;4: 549–556.

CARE PATHWAY

Congenital cystic adenomatoid malformation (CCAM) diagnosed in pregnancy—detected by ultrasound as an isolated abnormality

↓

- Seen in hospital specialist antenatal clinic straightaway
- Nature of lung lesion discussed with parents
- Parents to be reassured that CCAM is not a genetic condition, therefore referral to genetics unnecessary
- Urgent referral to tertiary centre fetal medicine unit for scan and review by fetal medicine specialists, paediatricians and paediatric surgical team
- Follow-up scans arranged at about 2-weekly intervals, alternating with tertiary unit, to detect development of non-immune hydrops, polyhydramnios, mediastinal shift of heart, nature of cysts , size of tumour noting any increase or regression in cysts

↓

CCAM without non-immune hydrops or other poor prognostic factors

↓

- Prognostic factors to be discussed—good prognosis
- Discussions in tertiary unit with paediatric surgeons, paediatricians, and fetal medicine specialists to develop plan of care (both antenatal and postnatal)
- Serial scans alternating with tertiary centre
- Frequency of visits to specialist antenatal clinic in DGH and tertiary centre to be individualized
- Neonatologists at DGH to maintain continued input
- Plans for timing, place, and mode of delivery to be discussed with tertiary centre
- Routine community antenatal checks to continue avoiding overlap with hospital appointments.
- Postnatal CT imaging is essential

CCAM with hydrops ± other poor prognostic signs

↓

- Poor prognosis discussed with parents by fetal medicine specialists, paediatric surgeons, etc. in tertiary centre
- Options for management discussed including:
    - TOP
    - Conservative management without intervention to let nature take its course
    - Elective early Caesarean delivery if significant problems develop, although poor prognosis even if approaching term
- Clear documentation in notes of options discussed and agreed plan
- If pregnancy is to continue, serial scans alternating with tertiary unit
- Continued involvement of local DGH paediatricians
- Frequency of visits to specialist antenatal clinics in tertiary centre/DGH to be individualized
- Place, timing and mode of delivery after discussions with tertiary centre
- In between the essential hospital antenatal appointments, community antenatal checks can be continued

27.6 Fetal Autosomal Recessive (Infantile) Polycystic Kidney Disease

FACT FILE

- ***The terms adult or infantile polycystic kidney disease (PKD) are no longer used because they are inaccurate descriptions: both can involve the presence of renal cysts at any time during an affected person's life, from the prenatal period to adolescence or older.***
- The 'infantile' type is **autosomal recessive** (**ARPKD**) with a recurrence risk of 25%. It is the most common genetic cystic renal disease of infancy and childhood.
- ARPKD is different from the **autosomal dominant** variety ('adult' PKD) in its genetic basis, presentation, treatment and prognosis.

Epidemiology and pathogenesis

- ARPKD is less common than the autosomal dominant ('adult') variety and occurs in 1 in 10 000 to 1 in 40 000 babies, with a carrier frequency of between 1 in 50 and 1 in 70.[1,2]
- The ARPKD gene (*PKDHD1*) is localized to the short arm of chromosome 6.[1]
- If only one parent carries the abnormal gene, the baby cannot get the disease. If both parents carry the gene there is a 1 in 4 chance that the baby will be affected by the disease.
- Both sexes are equally affected. There is no racial predilection.
- ARPKD is characterized by non-obstructive, bilateral, symmetrical dilatation and elongation of 10–90% of the renal collecting ducts As the number of ducts involved increases, the kidneys enlarge. However, the reniform shape of the kidneys is maintained, because the abnormality is in the collecting ducts and the cysts are usually minute (<3 mm).
- Kidneys are bilaterally enlarged and contain large number of cysts throughout. At birth, the interstitium and the rest of the tubules are normal but they may later develop interstitial fibrosis and tubular atrophy that can cause renal failure.
- Liver involvement is seen in the majority of cases of autosomal recessive polycystic kidney disease. Congenital hepatic fibrosis (CHF) may have a more severe clinical manifestation than the renal disease.[5] There may be hepatic involvement with bile duct ectasia (Caroli's disease).
- The renal and hepatic disease tend to show opposite degrees of severity. Generally, the later the manifestation of the renal disease, the more marked is the liver disease.
- Severe cases of liver disease may even progress to cirrhosis with portal hypertension and oesophageal varices in addition to renal involvement.

Prognosis by category of ARPKD

- Prognosis in ARPKD varies, ranging from perinatal death to survival with a milder progressive form which may not be diagnosed until adolescence.
- Babies with less severe renal manifestations who survive the neonatal period may still develop chronic kidney disease, which occurs at varying ages depending on the degree of renal involvement.
- ARPKD has a poor overall prognosis. In severe cases, depending on pulmonary status, early neonatal death occurs due to bilateral pulmonary hypoplasia. In those who survive the neonatal period, renal prognosis has improved over time because of renal transplantation.
- The most common classification of ARPKD, categories 1–4, is based on age at presentation which is in turn related to disease severity:[6,7]

Category 1: Perinatal presentation (Potter's syndrome)

- The baby is born with a very large abdomen due to massive renal enlargement which may complicate delivery. About 90% of the collecting ducts are dilated but the liver is hardly ever involved.
- Severe renal impairment in utero produces oligohydramnios and subsequent pulmonary hypoplasia. Other clinical findings resulting from oligohydramnios include Potter's facies (flattened nose, micrognathia, and large, floppy, low-set ears) and talipes.[1]
- In approximately 75% neonatal death occurs within a week of birth.

Category 2: Neonatal presentation

- Kidneys palpable at birth.
- About 60% of the kidney is affected and there is mild liver disease.
- Though renal impairment less severe in utero with less risk of pulmonary hypoplasia, progressive renal failure results in neonatal death within a few months.

Category 3: Presents in infancy

- Presents when the baby is a few months old.
- Approximately 25% of renal collecting ducts are dilated, with moderate hepatic fibrosis.
- Enlarged kidneys and hepatosplenomegaly on examination.
- Affected babies and children often develop chronic renal failure with or without portal and systemic hypertension.
- The principle cause of mortality is endstage renal failure, usually in adolescence.

Category 4: Presents in childhood

- There is marked liver disease.
- Less than 10% develop renal failure.
- Usually presents between 6 months and 5 years.
- Variable renal enlargement and hepatosplenomegaly.
- Significant liver involvement with portal hypertension.
- Morbidity and mortality are usually due to portal hypertension, including variceal bleeding and thrombocytopenia or anaemia from hypersplenism.
- Mortality is the lowest of the four categories, around 80% surviving beyond the age of 15 years.

Diagnosis

- Antenatal diagnosis of categories 1 and 2 ARPKD may be made by **ultrasound scan** appearances[7,8] of smooth kidney outline with tiny echogenic cysts. Both kidneys are equally affected and with severe bilateral renal disease with oligo/anhydramnios. This results in pulmonary hypoplasia. Large kidneys may appear 'bright' from about 13 weeks and between 20–30 weeks oligohydramnios is detectable. Early ultrasound is not very reliable at detecting the condition. Severe cases of this disease are detected with sonography in utero, with most cases detected in the second or third trimester of gestation. Most of these infants die from pulmonary complications after birth.
- Parents usually ask why the condition was not diagnosed during earlier scans, especially in the first trimester. Large kidneys may appear 'bright' from about 13 weeks but significant oligohydramnios is detectable only on later scans. When there is severe bilateral renal disease, oligo - or anhydramnios are usual accompaniments as well as the bladder not being visualized on the scan. With better definition of the tiny cysts that replace normal renal structure a progressive increase in the size of the kidneys is then established. **Early ultrasound is therefore not very reliable at detecting the condition.**
- ***Prenatal diagnosis is unlikely before the second half of pregnancy unless there are strong reasons to suspect the condition, such as an affected older child.***
- Clinical detection of oligohydramnios or noting a large abdomen on routine late scan later in pregnancy may lead to suspicion of condition. MRI is an useful adjunct, particularly to define lung hypoplasia.

- Genetic testing in ARPKD by linkage analysis is possible where the patient's family has at least one diagnosed index case.

Differential diagnosis

- The differential diagnosis includes Meckel's syndrome, congenital nephrotic syndrome, autosomal dominant polycystic kidneys, glomerulocystic disease, and diffuse cystic dysplasia.

Management once a diagnosis is made

- Just as in any potentially lethal fetal abnormality found at scan, this information needs to be imparted with due sensitivity to the parents.
- When counselling parents, it is important to stress that early diagnostic tests are unreliable in this highly variable condition.[1] TOP may need to be discussed when Potter's syndrome is suspected.
- **Referral to the genetics** service is recommended. The genetic basis of the baby having been so affected must be clearly explained. Both parents must carry the defective gene for 1 in 4 of their offspring to develop the condition (autosomal recessive inheritance). If only one parent is a carrier, none of their offspring can be affected.
- Both parents are carriers, not disease sufferers.
- Finding ARPKD in the baby does not have any bearing on the mother's health either during pregnancy or long term.
- **Care pathways** must be individualized for every pregnancy with an affected fetus on a case-by-case basis because of the varying severity of the condition and its presentation.
- The following general principles should be borne in mind and employed while **counselling parents** who have received such a diagnosis:
  - The condition has a very variable course, ranging from perinatal death to survival with a milder progressive form, which may not be diagnosed until adolescence.
  - Symptoms of ARPKD can start in utero with the scan appearance of oligohydramnios. This often results in pulmonary hypoplasia and neonatal death. Even those babies that survive the neonatal period can develop progressive renal and liver failure resulting in death in the first few months of life, in childhood or in adolescence, depending on the category of ARPKD. Dialysis or kidney transplant are the only modalities employed to treat the kidney failure.
  - Children who survive the first few months/years can have hypertension, frequent UTIs, liver and spleen enlargement, cirrhosis, and progressive liver failure.
  - Newborns with category 1 ARPKD display a typical 'Potter's facies' and in 75%, neonatal death usually occurs in the first week. Parents must be warned, with sensitivity, to expect this.
  - TOP may need to be discussed, especially in categories 1 and 2 ARPKD, and the parents' choice must be respected at all times. Ongoing support and genetics review must be offered and the issue of post-mortem broached with the greatest sensitivity.
  - If the parents decide to continue with the pregnancy, referral to a fetal medicine unit at a tertiary centre is required. Multidisciplinary input is essential involving specialist obstetrician, neonatologist, geneticist, and midwife.
  - Antenatal referral to meet the paediatricians is very useful to discuss prognosis in the immediate postnatal period as well as in the medium to longer term.
- Clear documentation must be made in the main and hand-held notes about the frequency of further antenatal visits and scans as well as the degree of intervention that parents expect to be undertaken at the time of labour/delivery of the affected baby.
- Investigations of the parents will be useful for counselling them regarding chances of recurrence in a subsequent pregnancy.

Information for patients

Please see Information for patients: Autosomal recessive polycystic kidney disease (p. 555)

References

1. Traubici J, Daneman A. High-resolution renal sonography in children with autosomal recessive polycystic kidney disease. AJR Am J Roentgenol 2005;184: 1630–1633.
2. Martinez-Frias ML, et al. Epidemiological aspects of Mendelian syndromes in a Spanish population sample: II. Autosomal recessive malformation syndromes. Am J Med Genet 1991;15;38: 626–629.
3. Zerres K, et al. Mapping of the gene for autosomal recessive polycystic kidney disease (ARPKD) to chromosome 6p21-cen. Nat Genet 1994;7: 429–432.
4. O'Brien K, et al. Congenital hepatic fibrosis and portal hypertension in autosomal dominant polycystic kidney disease. J Pediatr Gastroenterol Nutr 2012;54: 83–89.
5. Halvorson CR, et al. Polycystic kidney disease: inheritance, pathophysiology, prognosis, and treatment. Int J Nephrol Renovasc Dis 2010;3: 69–83.
6. Gunay-Aygun M, et al. Autosomal recessive polycystic kidney disease and congenital hepatic fibrosis: summary statement of a first National Institutes of Health/Office of Rare Diseases conference. J Pediatr 2006;149: 159–164.
7. Tahvanainen E, et al. Polycystic liver and kidney diseases. Ann Med 2005;37: 546–555.
8. Lonergan GL, et al. Autosomal recessive polycystic kidney disease: radiologic-pathologic correlation. RadioGraphics 2000;20: 837–885.

CARE PATHWAY

Scan diagnosis of **autosomal recessive polycystic kidney disease (ARPKD)** usually made at the 20 week anomaly scan or later

↓

Sensitive explanation to parents

- Prognosis*, perinatal mortality mainly due to lung hypoplasia caused by oligo/anhydramnios and constricted space due to pressure exerted of enlarged kidneys
- Also, hepatic fibrosis, which if severe, causes neonatal portal hypertension
- Explanation of autosomal recessive nature of inheritance—both parents must be carriers, referral to genetics for counselling
- Discuss options, including that of termination, conservative expectant management, or management aimed at fetal salvage
- Antenatal management—multidisciplinary input from specialist obstetrician, neonatologist, geneticist, midwives

↓

- Parents choose TOP, especially in types I and II of ARPKD
- Sensitive discussion regarding post-mortem
- Arrange follow-up genetics referral if parents wish

- Parents chose not to have any intervention, and to let nature takes its course
- If IUD, arrange IOL as per local/RCOG protocol. Sensitive discussion regarding post-mortem

---

Parents decide to continue with pregnancy aiming for fetal salvage

↓

- Referral to neonatologists for antenatal consultation to discuss neonatal condition and care at birth and neonatal, infancy, and childhood. Further postnatal problems, hypertension, UTIs, hepatosplenomegaly, cirrhosis and progressive heart failure
- In Potter's syndrome neonatal death can be expected in the first week of birth and parents should be duly warned
- Subsequent serial scans organized at individualized frequency to measure liquor volume and size of kidneys, and identify presence or absence of breathing movements,
- Ascertain what degree of intervention parents expect to be undertaken at time of labour, delivery, and postnatally
- Mode of delivery may depend on parental choice, also size of infant's abdomen. If gross enlargement of fetal kidneys—elective Caesarean section may be indicated

---

*Discussion of prognosis depending on severity, size of fetal kidneys, liver involvement, lung hypoplasia, etc.

- In less severe cases (types III and IV), affected babies and children develop chronic renal failure with or without portal and systemic hypertension
- The principal cause of mortality is end-stage renal failure, usually in adolescence
- Morbidity and mortality are usually due to portal hypertension, including variceal bleeding and thrombocytopenia or anaemia from hypersplenism
- Mortality is the lowest in type IV, around 80% surviving beyond the age of 15 years

27.7 Fetal Cardiac Rhabdomyoma, Tuberous Sclerosis

FACT FILE

- **Cardiac rhabdomyoma**, though rare, is the most common primary fetal and neonatal cardiac tumour accounting for 60–86% of primary fetal cardiac tumours.[1,2]

Pathogenesis and pathology

- Rhabdomyoma is considered to be a hamartoma of immature developing cardiac myocytes.[3,4]
- It is a benign cardiac tumour with no capacity for metastasis or invasion.
- The natural history of rhabdomyomas is regression, usually after 32 weeks gestation.
- Cardiac rhabdomyomas most frequently arise in the right or left ventricular myocardium, but they may also be situated in the atria, the interventricular septum, the epicardial surface, or the cavoatrial junction.
- The position, size and number of intracardiac rhabdomyomas may influence the fetal/neonatal outcomes.
- Large tumour size and fetal hydrops are associated with poor neonatal outcome.[5]
- Reported survival rates of rhabdomyomas range from 81% to 92%.[2]

Diagnosis

- Most rhabdomyomas are discovered in pregnancy as incidental findings detected during a routine anomaly ultrasound scan at about 20 weeks gestation.
- Echocardiography and MRI are the main diagnostic tools for cardiac rhabdomyomas. MRI is also useful in the detection of any cerebral, kidney, or liver lesions of tuberous sclerosis.
- Cardiac rhabdomyomas can appear as well circumscribed, round, hyperechoic echogenic tumours.
- Multiple small rhabdomyomas can appear on ultrasonography and MRI as widespread small military nodules (<1 mm diameter) in a thickened myometrium and are associated with an increased chance of tuberous sclerosis.[2]
- With advanced sonographic, MRI and molecular technologies, fetal diagnosis of rhabdomyomas is crucial.
- Rhabdomyomas are not associated with calcification, which is typically seen in cardiac fibromas.
- Rhabdomyomas can vary from 1 mm to as large as 10 cm in their greatest diameter

Outcomes of rhabdomyoma

- Intrauterine death (IUD) could occur as a result of a large tumour size obstructing inflow or ventricular outflow causing decreased cardiac output or due to arrhythmias, both atrial and ventricular, causing hydrops fetalis. Fetal death could also be a result of atrial and caval hypertension or loss of myometrial function due to extensive tumour involvement.
- Cardiac complications such as arrhythmias, intracardiac obstruction, and cardiac failure are strong predictors of poor neonatal outcomes.[5]
- Regression of the tumour is associated with resolution of arrhythmias. Because most rhabdomyomas regress in size during the third trimester, in the absence of outflow obstruction or arrhythmias, conservative management with close neonatal and infant monitoring is all that is required in the majority of antenatally diagnosed rhabdomyoma. Surgical intervention is only rarely required.[8]

Tuberous sclerosis

- The finding of fetal cardiac rhabdomyoma, especially if multiple, is strongly suggestive of **tuberous sclerosis (TS)**[6] or **Bournville's disease**, which is found in nearly 40–80% of **fetuses** and up to 80% of **neonates** with rhabdomyomas.[2,7,8,9]
- TS is associated with 30% of cases where a solitary rhabdomyoma is found, compared to over 80% of cases where two or more rhabdomyomas are detected antenatally.[9]
- TS is characterized by the triad of **intellectual disability of varying degrees** (53–71%), **epilepsy** (78%), and **facial angiofibromas** (27%).[7,9]
- Epilepsy mostly presents within the first year of life, mainly as infantile spasms.
- More than 50% of the children with TS will have some kind of behavioural problems.
- Other features of TS can include renal involvement such as renal cysts, renal carcinoma, renal angiolipomas, polycystic kidney disease, and pulmonary involvement, which if severe, has a poor prognosis.
- TS is also characterized by hamartomas seen in the brain, heart, kidneys, skin, etc.
- TS can be familial when it is inherited as an autosomal dominant disorder or occur as a sporadic mutation as found in 50% of cases.[10]
- The incidence of TS is about 1 in 6000 to 1 in 10 000 live births, although this incidence is greater if termination of affected pregnancies is included.[11]
- The finding of multiple rhabdomyomas often precedes the development of neurological, renal, and cutaneous manifestations of TS.[9]
- Neonatal seizures are a common feature of TS. MRI may reveal cortical or subependymal tubers. Renal angiomyolipomas usually manifest later.

Antenatal management

- Once fetal cardiac rhabdomyoma or TS is diagnosed, antenatal management should include multidisciplinary input.
- A detailed family history and genetic counselling (three pedigree) should therefore be offered if fetal cardiac rhabdomyoma is detected.
- Antenatal search for extracardiac anomalies and karyotypic abnormalities is recommended.
- Serial growth scans are advisable.
- Antenatal management should include discussions regarding options including TOP in potentially lethal cases.
- In cases of IUD or TOP, the value of post-mortem examination must be discussed in a sympathetic manner.
- In continuing pregnancies, arrangements for labour and delivery should be planned with the tertiary centre to ensure appropriate obstetric and neonatal facilities are readily available. Psychological support for the parents must not be overlooked.
- Long-term prognosis of rhabdomyomas detected antenatally is influenced by the neurological manifestations of TS. Prenatal diagnosis of cerebral lesions is vital for counselling of parents as the presence of non-solitary rhabdomyomas strongly suggests TS and may predict future neurodevelopmental complications,[11,12,13,14] though not in all cases.[5]

Prognosis

- Perinatal mortality rates varying from 0 to 100% for TS have been reported.[1,2]
- Prognosis in TS has been quoted as 30% mortality by the age of 5 and 75% mortality by the age of 20. **These facts are essential when undertaking antenatal counselling of parents, if TS is a strong association with rhabdomyoma.**
- Absence of cerebral involvement on MRI does not exclude subsequent development of TS and the infants need neurological follow-up including MRI for at least 1 year after birth.[6] Although third-trimester cerebral MRI can detect TS-associated cerebral lesions, future neurological outcome is difficult to predict as cerebral lesions can develop progressively after birth.[15]

- **A normal prenatal cerebral MRI is, therefore, not predictive** of subsequent normal neurodevelopmental outcome.[15] Antenatal counselling of parents should highlight this.

Genetic counselling

- Genetic analysis has identified two disease genes, *TSC1* and *TSC2*, located on chromosomes 9 and 16 respectively.
- TS may also be associated with trisomy 21[16] and basal cell naevus syndrome. Karyotyping may be considered.
- Postnatally, stabilization of the neonate, confirmation of the diagnosis, and planning of further management are essential.

Prenatal counselling

- **Pre-pregnancy counselling** should include counselling women at risk, and chromosomal genetic studies.

Mother with TS

- The pregnant woman may herself have TS, in which case increased risks of respiratory failure, spontaneous pneumothorax, severe pre-eclampsia, IUGR, deterioration of renal function, hydrops fetalis, and intrauterine fetal death have been reported.[17,18]

Information for patients

Please see Information for patients: Tuberous sclerosis (p. 555)

References

1. Allan L. Fetal cardiac tumors. In:Allan L,C et al. Textbook of fetal cardiology. London: Greenwich Medical Media, 2000, pp. 358–365.
2. Isaacs H Jr. Fetal and neonatal cardiac tumors. Pediatr Cardiol 2004;25: 252–273.
3. Becker AE. Primary heart tumors in the pediatric age group: a review of salient pathologic features relevant for clinicians. Pediatr Cardiol 2000;21: 317–323.
4. Elderkin RA, Radford DJ. Primary cardiac tumours in a paediatric population. J Paediatr Child Health 2002;38: 173–177.
5. Chao AS, et al. Outcome of antenatally diagnosed cardiac rhabdomyoma: case series and a meta-analysis. Ultrasound Obstet Gynecol 2008;31: 289–295.
6. Vaughan CJ, et al. Tumors and the heart: molecular genetic advances. Curr Opin Cardiol 2001;16: 195–200.
7. Bader RS, et al. Fetal rhabdomyoma: prenatal diagnosis, clinical outcome, and incidence of associated tuberous sclerosis complex. J Pediatr 2003;143: 620–624.
8. Fesslova V, et al. Natural history and long-term outcome of cardiac rhabdomyomas detected prenatally. Prenat Diagn 2004;24: 241–248.
9. Gamzu R, et al. Evaluating the risk of tuberous sclerosis in cases with prenatal diagnosis of cardiac rhabdomyoma. Prenat Diagn 2002;22: 1044–1047.
10. D'Addario V, et al. Prenatal diagnosis and postnatal outcome of cardiac rhabdomyomas. J Perinat Med 2002;30: 170–175.
11. O'Callaghan FJ, et al. The relation of infantile spasms, tubers, and intelligence in tuberous sclerosis complex. Arch Dis Child 2004;89: 530–533.
12. Goodman M, et al. Cortical tuber count: a biomarker indicating neurologic severity of tuberous sclerosis complex. J Child Neurol 1997;12: 85–90.
13. Shepherd CW, et al. MR findings in tuberous sclerosis complex and correlation with seizure development and mental impairment. AJNR Am J Neuroradiol 1995;16: 149–155.
14. Jansen FE, et al. Cognitive impairment in tuberous sclerosis complex is a multifactorial condition. Neurology 2008;70: 916–923.
15. Saada J, et al. Prenatal diagnosis of cardiac rhabdomyomas: incidence of associated cerebral lesions of tuberous sclerosis complex. Ultrasound Obstet Gynecol 2009;34: 155–159.
16. Krapp M, et al. Tuberous sclerosis with intracardiac rhabdomyoma in a fetus with trisomy 21: case report and review of literature. Prenat Diagn 1999;19: 610–613.
17. King JA, Stamilio DM. Maternal and fetal tuberous sclerosis complicating pregnancy: a case report and overview of the literature. Am J Perinatol 2005;22: 103–108.
18. Gupta N, et al. Fetal cardiac rhabdomyoma with maternal tuberous sclerosis complicating pregnancy. Arch Gynecol Obstet 2008;278: 169–170.

CARE PATHWAY

Intracardiac rhabdomyoma diagnosed at a routine anomaly scan at about 20 weeks gestation

↓

Establish position, number, size of intracardiac rhabdomyoma; presence of any other anomalies or of non- immune hydrops

↓

Referral to fetal medicine unit at tertiary centre after due explanation to the pregnant woman

↓

- Multidisciplinary input from specialist team
- Ultrasound scan repeated, also fetal ECHO and MRI—main diagnostic tools, also for detection of other anomalies of cerebrum, kidneys or liver found in **tuberous sclerosis (TS)**
- Discussion of benign nature of rhabdomyoma, natural history usually of regression after 32 weeks, good prognosis if single lesion and absence of arrhythmias or outflow obstruction
- Poor prognosis if multiple tumours and other anomalies suggestive of association with TS
- Presence of multiple rhabdomyomas, other anomalies of lungs, kidneys or cerebral lesion is strongly suggestive of TS, hence poor long-term prognosis—30% mortality by age of 5 years; 75% mortality by age of 20
- Explain to parents that even in absence of cerebral lesion, subsequent neurodevelopmental normality cannot be predicted
- Discuss characteristics of TS even in absence of cerebral lesions: mental disability of varying degrees, epilepsy, and facial angiofibromas

↓

Discuss options including TOP

↓ (two branches)

If parents opt for TOP or in case of IUD, sympathetic discussion to encourage post-mortem

→ Offer genetic counselling and pre-pregnancy counselling before next pregnancy

If parents choose to continue pregnancy
- Multidisciplinary involvement in antenatal and neonatal management
- Serial growth scans
- Continue search for extracardiac anomalies
- Plan for labour and delivery
- Detailed family history and genetic counselling
- Karyotyping to be considered if high possibility of TS

↓

- Delivery ideally in a tertiary centre with appropriate obstetric, neonatal, and neonatal cardiology facilities
- Mode and timing of delivery to be individualized
- Postnatal: Stabilization of neonate, continued close neonatal and infant monitoring, confirm diagnosis, postnatal MRI
- Neonatal seizures common in TS

↓

Offer genetic counselling and pre-pregnancy counselling before next pregnancy

27.8 Fetal Arthrogryposis Multiplex Congenita

FACT FILE

Epidemiology

- **Arthrogryposis multiplex congenita (AMC) or arthrogryposis** for short, is a rare and sporadic fetal abnormality which refers to a **non-progressive** condition characterized by multiple joint contractures found throughout the body and present at birth.
- The main cause of AMC appears to be severely reduced or absent fetal movements as seen in fetal akinesia,[1,2] which leads to congenital joint contractures
- Incidence of AMC is approximately 1 in 2000 to 1 in 12 000 live births,[3] with an equal sex ratio.
- The earlier in gestation that fetal akinesia develops, the more severe the congenital contractures of joints.
- The condition is non-progressive.
- In one-third of cases, a genetic cause may be identified.[1]

Aetiology

Aetiological factors may be intrinsic or extrinsic.

Extrinsic causes

- Fetal movements commence from approximately 7 weeks gestation.[4] **Any curtailment of movements in utero can result in joint contractions** as the connecting tendons are not stretched to their full extent.[5,6]
- Such limitation of fetal movements could result from space constraints such those due to **severe oligohydramnios**, **large fibroids**, or **uterine malformations**.
- Certain maternal conditions[7,8] such as diabetes, myasthenia, infection, or drugs may also be associated with AMC of the fetus.

Intrinsic causes

- Various neurological conditions such as holoprosencephaly, anterior horn cell disease, cerebral hypoplasia, defects in neural migration, or spinal muscular atrophy are the most common causes of AMC, accounting for 70–80%.[9,10,11,12]
- Connective tissue or muscle abnormalities.
- Fetal vascular compromise.
- Chromosomal abnormalities (trisomy 21,18) with dysgenesis of the nervous system.[13]
- Dysplasias of the brainstem nuclei and of the spinal cord such as part of Pierre–Robin syndrome, Zellweger syndrome, etc.

Ultrasound diagnosis

- Diagnosis is usually made in the second trimester either at the time of the routine 20-week anomaly scan or by a scan prompted by the mother complaining of little or no fetal movements.[5,14,15,16]
- Features on the scan may include no fetal movements seen with the baby in a fixed abnormal position with static flexion deformities. Other features such as micrognathia, altered fluid volume, cerebral ventriculomegaly, holoprosencephaly, IUGR, or dysmorphic features may also be detected early in the second trimester. The joints most often affected are the shoulders, elbows, wrists, or distal legs with talipes. In severe cases, almost all joints are affected.[17,18]
- Imaging is focused on flexion, extension of proximal and distal joints, and movements of the jaws and spine.
- AMC may also present with an increased nuchal fold thickness seen at 10–14 weeks gestation,[13] or associated with cystic hygroma,[16] polyhydramnios, multiple diaphyseal fractures,[18] or fetal seizures sometimes visualized in real time during the scan.[19]
- The diagnosis can be arrived at about a week earlier with a 4D scan than a 2D scan (i.e. by about 12–13 weeks gestation.)
- Further confirmation can be obtained by MRI which may also reveal the multiplicity of involved joints, distal muscle atrophy, and pulmonary hypoplasia.

Clinical features

Clinical features include:[20,21]

- Joint contractures causing the involved extremities to be fusiform or cylindrical with thin subcutaneous tissue
- Symmetrical deformities with severity increasing distally; hands and feet are the most malformed
- Muscle atrophy; sometimes whole groups of muscles may be absent
- Lung hypoplasia
- Small chest
- Mid-facial haemangioma
- Small for gestational age
- Abnormalities of the face, jaw, and back
- Limited jaw movement and opening
- Tracheo-oesophageal fistulae
- Cardiac anomalies
- Structural abnormalities of kidneys, ureters, bladder
- Abdominal hernias abnormal genitalia such as cryptorchidism or absent labia majora
- Associated skin, scalp, and nail defects.

Prognosis

- Prognosis can vary.
- In intrinsically derived AMC the prognosis is generally worse due to central nervous system (CNS) involvement compared to AMC due to extrinsic factors such as space limitation.
- Significant morbidity and mortality can result as an effect of lung hypoplasia, respiratory compromise caused by scoliosis as well as CNS dysfunction.
- Problems during delivery arise due to fixed and abnormal fetal positions and fixed inflexible joints
- Fracture of limbs during delivery occurs in 5–10% of cases.[18]
- Antenatal findings indicative of pulmonary insufficiency are absent fetal movements, micrognathia, oligohydramnios, small and thin ribs.
- Ventilator dependence in neonates is associated with poor prognosis.
- In severe cases many will remain partially or totally dependent on others for life whereas in milder cases, a near-normal independent life with a normal lifespan is possible.
- Prognosis depends on the natural history of AMC and its variations as well as response to therapy;[20] for example, contractures may improve or worsen, likewise CNS damage may be lethal, remain stable, or improve.

Pregnancy management when AMC has been diagnosed

- The diagnosis is bound to be shocking for parents and contact details of national or local support groups must be offered.[22]
- Early diagnosis indicates increased severity of the condition.
- Multidisciplinary input is essential,[5] involving specialist obstetrician, neonatologist, geneticist, and midwife. Referral to a fetal medicine unit at a tertiary centre may be required.
- After detailed investigations (scans, MRI, amniocentesis for trisomies) and multidisciplinary input in management plans, the parents must be provided with accurate and appropriate information to enable them to make an informed choice which might include TOP, based on the predicted severity of AMC.
- If the decision for termination is arrived at after 21 completed weeks of gestation, feticide with intracardiac KCl will be required before proceeding with medical induction of labour.
- Sensitive discussions with the parents regarding post-mortem should be undertaken by a senior obstetrician as autopsy can

provide valuable information regarding aetiology and other organs involved, and help provide a recurrence risk.

- If the parents decide to continue with the pregnancy, serial scans to monitor fetal growth, detect polyhydramnios, and confirm fetal position are indicated.
- Early referral to enable parents to meet the paediatrician/neonatologists must be made. The increased chances of perinatal mortality if severe lung hypoplasia is suspected must be explained to parents, as well as the additional long-term care that the child may require.
- Therapies[23] for the child including correction of talipes by appropriate plaster casting, and surgery involving properly sequenced corrective procedures followed by physiotherapy, etc., can be discussed by the consultant neonatologist.
- If the baby lies in a persistent breech or transverse/oblique lie, especially in the presence of polyhydramnios, the patient needs to be advised about the risk of pre-labour rupture of membranes and possible cord prolapse. Advice regarding immediate measures must be offered and emergency contact numbers provided.
- A decision regarding the timing, method, and place of delivery needs to be discussed on an individual case-by-case basis.
- Delivery by Caesarean section may be indicated because of an abnormal position and lie of the baby, the lack of joint flexibility, and the risk of fractures during vaginal delivery.
- Prophylactic steroids must be offered if delivery is planned at less than 36 weeks gestation.
- Referral to clinical genetics after a few weeks following delivery is essential to establish and discuss the mode of inheritance and recurrence risks in a future pregnancy.

Recurrence risk

- Recurrence risk depends on causative factors and mode of inheritance as well as persistence of certain maternal factors.
- Extrinsic factors, such as maternal conditions including diabetes, myasthenia gravis, and uterine malformations, can be expected to persist. Large fibroids or a near-complete uterine septum hindering fetal movements need to be dealt with before commencing a next pregnancy.
- As a genetic cause can be identified in a third of cases,[1,15] the risk of recurrence varies with the type of genetic disorder.[7]

Mode of inheritance and recurrence risk of AMC

- **Autosomal dominant:** As in distal arthrogryposis, where the risk of recurrence is 50%.
- **Autosomal recessive:** Both parents being obligate carriers, the risk of recurrence is 25%.
- **X-linked recessive:** All daughters of affected males are carriers. Fifty per cent of all sons of the carrier female will be affected by AMC and 50% of daughters of female carriers will themselves be carriers of the condition.
- **Mitochondrial mutations:**[11,24] A small proportion of AMC, especially the distal type IIB AMC, are due to mitochondrial mutations inherited exclusively from the mother.
- **Sporadic:** When no specific genetic link is established through the family in the unaffected parents of an offspring with AMC, an empiric 3–5% recurrence risk of recurrence is given for a sibling or the offspring of the affected individual.

Information for patients

Please see Information for patients: Arthrogryposis (p. 556)

References

1. Bamshad M, et al. Arthrogryposis: a review and update. J Bone Joint Surg 2009A;91 suppl 4: 40–46.
2. Porter HJ. Lethal arthrogryposis multiplex congenital (fetal akinesia deformation sequence, FADS). Pediatr Pathol Lab Med 1995;15: 617–637.
3. Hoff JM, et al. Arthrogryposis multiplexa congenita: an epidemiologic study of nearly 9 million births in 24 EUROCAT registers. Eur J Obstet Gynecol Reprod Biol 2011;159: 347–350.
4. de Vries JIP, et al. The emergence of fetal behaviour: qualitative aspects. Early Hum Dev 1982;7: 301–322.
5. Navti OB, et al. Review of perinatal management of arthrogryposis at a large UK teaching hospital serving a multiethnic population. Prenat Diagn 2010;30: 49–56.
6. Witters I, et al. Fetal akinesia deformation sequence: a study of 30 consecutive in utero diagnoses. Am J Med Genet 2002;113: 23–28.
7. Hall JG. Arthrogryposis multiplex congenita: etiology, genetics, classification, diagnostic approach, and general aspects. J Pediatr Orthop B 1997;6: 159–166.
8. Polizzi A, et al. Teratogen update: maternal myasthenia gravis as a cause of congenital arthrogryposis. Teratology 2000;62: 332–341.
9. Laugel V, et al. Cerebro-oculo-facio-skeletal syndrome: three additional cases with CSB mutations, new diagnostic criteria and an approach to investigation. J Med Genet 2008;45: 564–571.
10. Hoff JM, et al. Artrogryposis multiplex congenita—a rare fetal condition caused by maternal myasthenia gravis. Acta Neurol Scand 2006;113 Suppl 183: 26–27.
11. McPherson E, Zabel C. Mitochondrial mutation in a child with distal arthrogryposis. Am J Med Genet 2006;140: 184–185.
12. Bonilla-Musoles F, et al. Multiple congenital contractures (congenital multiple arthrogryposis) J Perinat Med 2002;30: 99–104.
13. Madazli R, et al. Prenatal diagnosis of arthrogryposis multiplex congenita with increased nuchal translucency but without any underlying fetal neurogenic or myogenic pathology. Fetal Diagn Ther 2002;17: 29–33.
14. Kalampokas E, et al. Diagnosing arthrogryposis multiplex congenita: a review. ISRN Obstet Gynecol 2012; 2012: 264918.
15. Rink BD. Arthrogryposis: a review and approach to prenatal diagnosis. Obstet Gynecol Survey 2011;66: 369–377.
16. Scott H, et al. Non-lethal arthrogryposis multiplex congenita presenting with cystic hygroma at 13 weeks gestational age. Prenat Diagn 1999;19: 966–971.
17. Bevan WP, et al. Arthrogryposis multiplex congenita (amyoplasia): an orthopaedic perspective. J Pediatr Orthop 2007;27: 594–600.
18. Chen H, et al. Fetal akinesia and multiple perinatal fractures. Am J Med Genet 1995;55: 472–477.
19. Sheizaf B, et al. Early sonographic prenatal diagnosis of seizures. Ultrasound Obstet Gynecol 2007;30: 1007–1009.
20. Darin N, et al. Multiple congenital contractures: birth prevalence, etiology, and outcome. J Pediatr 2002;140: 61–67.
21. Mennen U, et al. Arthrogryposis multiplex congenita. J Hand Surg [Br] 2005;30: 468–474.
22. McGillivray K, Watson AJ. Congenital arthrogryposis in pregnancy. J Obstet Gynaecol 2002;22: 218–219.
23. Hall JG. Arthrogryposes (multiple congenital contractures). In:Rimoin DL, et al., ed., Principles and practice of medical genetics. London: Churchill Livingstone, 1990;vol. 2, pp. 989–1035.
24. Jiang M, et al. Molecular prenatal diagnosis for hereditary distal arthrogryposis type 2B. Prenat Diagn 2007;27: 468–470.

CARE PATHWAY

Ultrasound features of multiple joint contractures and other features suggestive of **arthrogryposis multiplex congenita (AMC)**—incidental findings at routine anomaly scan at 20 weeks gestation
or
Targeted early 2nd-trimester scan due to family history or past obstetric history of AMC baby

Pregnant woman complains of very little fetal movement or none at all after 18–20 weeks gestation

↓

Ultrasound features of multiple joint contractures and other features suggestive of AMC

↓

Urgent review in specialist antenatal clinic to be seen by fetomaternal obstetrician

↓

First visit to specialist antenatal clinic

- Elicit history:
  - Detailed family history: Whether relative was affected with AMC or any other bone/muscle deformities
  - Detailed past obstetric history: Miscarriages or stillbirths or any such abnormalities?
  - Any history of consanguinity
  - Maternal conditions: Diabetes, myotonic dystrophy, myasthenia gravis, exposure to teratogenic drugs, alcohol, street drugs, medications such as phenytoin that may decrease fetal mobility
  - Any evidence of space-limiting uterine abnormalities such as submucosal or large intramural fibroids, septate or bicornuate uterus
  - Any history of prolonged rupture of membranes leading to oligo- or anhydramnios
  - Maternal infections such as rubella, coxsackie virus, enteroviruses, etc.
  - Bleeding or attempted TOP earlier in pregnancy
- **Clinical examination and repeat ultrasound scan/MRI**: Any evidence of oligo- or polyhydramnios, persistently abnormal lie, bilateral talipes, bilateral joint contractures especially elbows, wrists, ankles. Cylindrical tapering extremities, small thin ribs, restricted chest cavity, any evidence of hydrops, any cardiac or urogenital abnormalities, markers suggestive of aneuploidies, brain or spinal malformations etc. Exclude large fibroids, uterine septum etc. if feasible
- **Discuss suspected diagnosis** of AMC, implications, association with other CNS, connective tissue, muscle abnormalities, fetal akinesia resulting in subsequent complications including pulmonary hypoplasia
- Offer referral to tertiary centre fetal medicine unit and clinical genetics; arrange as indicated
- *Discuss amniocentesis* to exclude associated aneuploidies which might aid informed choice for parents
- Multidisciplinary input and expert opinion from fetal medicine unit at tertiary referral centre
- Discuss rapid karyotype results (FISH), if amniocentesis done
- Sensitive discussion of short, medium, and long-term prognosis to enable informed decision-making by parents
- Discuss options including TOP. Subsequent management depends on parent's wish for TOP or to continue pregnancy

↓

Parents opt for pregnancy termination

- If gestation is >21^{+6} weeks, feticide before medical TOP. Discuss with parents, arrange accordingly
- Consultant or senior obstetrician undertakes sensitive discussions with parents regarding post-mortem
- Autopsy would yield vital information about possible aetiology, any affected internal organs, CNS, CVS, urogenital abnormalities, karyotyping if amniocentesis had been declined, as well as help define recurrence risk for the future
- Referral to genetics post-pregnancy, if appropriate

↓

Post-pregnancy

- Referral to genetics for detailed evaluation including parental investigations and to discuss chances of recurrence in a subsequent pregnancy
- If fetal akinesia was due to space limitation and patient found to have uterine abnormalities such as large fibroids or septum, arrange postnatal review to discuss appropriate management before another pregnancy

Parents opt to continue with the pregnancy

- Antenatal referral to neonatologist to discuss management of neonate and longer-term therapy including sequential surgical corrective procedures, physiotherapy, appropriate casts for talipes
- Serial scans at regular intervals to assess fetal growth, liquor volume, etc.
- If persistent abnormal lie especially in the presence of polyhydramnios, warn patient of the risk of pre-labour rupture of membranes and cord prolapse as well as immediate measures to adopt
- Joint decision with multidisciplinary input regarding timing, site, and mode of delivery
- If delivery is planned for <36 weeks gestation, prophylactic steroids
- High chance of Caesarean section if abnormal lie of baby and to reduce risk of perinatal fractures during vaginal delivery. Attempt to deliver the baby en-caul and with a generous lower segment incision to reduce trauma at delivery

(→ Post-pregnancy)

27.9 Fetal Dandy–Walker Syndrome

FACT FILE

Epidemiology and pathogenesis

- **Dandy–Walker syndrome (DWS) or Dandy–Walker malformation** (DWM) is a rare congenital malformation of the CNS with a reported incidence of 1 in 25 000 to 1 in 35 000 live births[1] and a slight female predominance.
- The original definition of **DWS**[2] included three features: (1) hydrocephalus, (2) partial or complete absence of the cerebellar vermis, and (3) posterior fossa cyst contiguous with the fourth ventricle.
- Classically, posterior fossa cystic malformations have been divided into DWM, Dandy–Walker variant, mega cisterna magna, and posterior fossa arachnoid cyst. Precise differentiation of the malformations may not be possible using imaging studies. DWM, variant, and mega cisterna magna are currently believed to represent a continuum of developmental anomalies of a spectrum that has been termed the Dandy–Walker complex (DWC).[2]
- Approximately 70–90% of patients have hydrocephalus, which often develops postnatally. **DWM** may also be associated with atresia of the foramen of Magendie and, sometimes, the foramen of Luschka. DWM accounts for 1–4% of cases of antenatally detected hydrocephalus.
- Once fetal DWM is suspected, a multidisciplinary approach involving radiologists, obstetric, and genetic specialists as well as midwives and neonatologist is vital.
- Determining the full extent of other abnormalities and results of karyotyping (if performed) will help provide the parents with complete information. The multidisciplinary team can support them in making an informed decision about continuation or termination of the pregnancy.
- Preparing the parents about what to expect of the condition of the neonate and the neonatal care that they can expect and counselling them for future pregnancies is best done by the specialist team involved.

Aetiology and associations

- DWM is frequently associated with brain malformations and disorders of other areas of the CNS including holoprosencephaly, meningoceles, and absence of the corpus callosum. Systemic malformations including cardiac, neural tube, cleft lip/palate, gastrointestinal, urogenital and facial anomalies, and malformations of the face, limbs, fingers, and toes may coexist in DWM.
- DWM may be associated with Mendelian disorders such as Warburg or Meckel syndromes. It may also form part of the PHACES syndrome (**P**osterior fossa anomalies as DWM; **H**aemangioma; **A**rterial lesions of the head and neck; **C**ardiac abnormalities as aortic coarctation; **E**ye abnormalities; and **S**ternal defect).[3]
- DWS may also result from **chromosomal** anomalies or **environmental** factors. There are various types of chromosomal abnormalities associated with DWS, chromosomes 3, 9, 13, and 18 being the most common.[4]
- Environmental factors that may be involved in the causation of DWS include first-trimester exposure to rubella, cytomegalovirus, and toxoplasmosis, and drugs such as isotretinoin, warfarin, and alcohol.
- Marked variation has been shown in the genetics and aetiology of DWM, which is an aetiologically heterogeneous condition.

Recurrence risk

- Parents of children with DWS must be offered genetic counselling if they intend to have more children.
- Recurrence risk for siblings may be high when there is an association with a single-gene disorder.
- If DWM has been shown to be non-syndromic without being associated with Mendelian or chromosomal disorders, there is a low recurrence risk (1–5%).

Diagnosis

- Ultrasound is reliable and accurate for making the diagnosis. In utero, fetal MRI can be used to confirm the diagnosis and also to identify any associated abnormalities. Additional fetal anomalies have been reported in all cases of DWM.[5,6] A careful cardiac evaluation is needed in all infants with DWM for early recognition of potentially serious associated cardiac malformations.[7]
- Comprehensive fetal ultrasound and karyotyping should be offered in any pregnancy where the fetus has DWM. Postnatal imaging should be performed on all fetal DWM.
- Radiologically, patients show elevated imprint of the transverse sinuses with thinning and bulging of the bones of the posterior fossa.

Prognosis and presentation

- The presence of karyotype and associated fetal anomalies can help predict immediate neonatal survival. Overall mortality rates of 12–50% have been reported; associated congenital abnormalities contribute to 83% of postnatal deaths and subnormal intelligence is reported in 40–70% of cases.[8] The isolated Dandy–Walker variant abnormality has the highest incidence of survival, and there are reported cases of people who have had Dandy–Walker variant their entire lives without any symptoms.[9,10].
- In the postnatal period, paediatricians should look for postnatal hydrocephalus even if the ventricular size is normal or slightly dilated on prenatal imaging.[11]
- DWS can appear dramatically or develop gradually. Almost 80% of newborns with DWM may have normal ventricular dimensions, yet by the age of 1 year, 80% will have developed ventriculomegaly.
- Symptoms often occur in early infancy and include developmental delay with slow motor development and abnormally rapid increase in HC with bulging at the back of the skull.
- Affected children present early in life with hydrocephalus associated with a bulging occiput. Posterior fossa signs such as cranial nerve palsies, nystagmus, and truncal ataxia are common. Motor deficits such as with balance, delayed motor development, hypotonic, and ataxia are frequently seen and about half have mental and psychiatric problems.
- Despite early treatment of hydrocephalus, children with DWS may never achieve normal intellectual development with 40–70% showing subnormal intelligence.
- In older children, there may be signs of increased intracranial pressure, such as irritability, vomiting, and convulsions (seizures occur in 15–30%).[1] There may also be signs of cerebellar dysfunction, such as unsteadiness, lack of muscle coordination, or jerky movements of the eyes (nystagmus), and psychiatric problems such as mania.
- There may also be jerky movements of the face and neck and abnormal breathing patterns.
- Prognosis otherwise depends on the severity of the syndrome and associated malformations. The presence of multiple congenital defects may shorten lifespan.
- An impaired respiratory control centre in the brainstem may lead to respiratory failure.

Treatment modalities

- This involves managing the associated problems, e.g. seizure management.
- Shunts to treat associated hydrocephalus can be inserted. These may be to shunt the cyst (cystoperitoneal) or the ventricles (ventriculoperitoneal), or both.

Post-mortem

- A large proportion of DWM pregnancies will be terminated, especially with the identification of associated abnormalities and karyotypic defects.
- In cases of TOP, autopsy is valuable in order to confirm the diagnosis and to provide additional information to help in counselling the parents regarding future pregnancies. Autopsy is considered the gold standard for accurate diagnosis of the fetal abnormality.[1]

Information for patients

Please see **Information for patients: Dandy–Walker syndrome** (p. 557)

References

1. Lavanya T, et al. A case of a Dandy-Walker variant: the importance of a multidisciplinary team approach using complementary techniques to obtain accurate diagnostic information. Br J Radiol 2008;81 (970): e242–245.
2. Altman NR, et al. Posterior fossa malformations. Am J Neuroradiol 1992;13: 691–724.
3. Lopez-Gutierrez JC. PHACES syndrome and ectopia cordis. Interact Cardiovasc Thorac Surg 2011;12: 642–644.
4. Imataka G, et al. Dandy-Walker syndrome and chromosomal abnormalities. Congenit Anom (Kyoto) 2007;47: 113–118.
5. Klein O, et al. Dandy-Walker malformation: prenatal diagnosis and prognosis. Childs Nerv Syst 2003;19: 484–489.
6. Harper T, et al. The fetal Dandy Walker complex: associated anomalies, perinatal outcome and postnatal imaging. Fetal Diagn Ther 2007;22: 277–281.
7. Kurdi ME, et al. Dandy Walker malformation and hypertrophic cardiomyopathy. Unusual fatal association. Neurosciences (Riyadh) 2009;14: 368–370.
8. Osenbach RK, Menezes AH. Diagnosis and management of the Dandy-Walker malformation: 30 years of experience. Pediatr Neurosurg 1992;18: 179–189.
9. Kölble N, et al. Dandy-walker malformation: prenatal diagnosis and outcome. Prenat Diagn 2000;20: 318–327.
10. Kalidasan V, et al. The Dandy-Walker syndrome-a 10 year experience of its management and outcome. Eur J Pediatr Surg 1995: 5 suppl 1: 16–18.
11. Guibaud L, et al. Prenatal diagnosis of 'isolated' Dandy-Walker malformation: imaging findings and prenatal counselling. Prenat Diagn 2012;32: 185–193.

27.10 Fetal Choroid Plexus Cysts

FACT FILE

Epidemiology and associations with trisomies

- The fetal choroid plexus develops at approximately 6 weeks gestation as a cystic space which contains cerebrospinal fluid (CSF). The choroid plexus begins to produce CSF by the ninth week of gestation. This results in expansion of the posterior horns of the lateral ventricles. Quite often, fluid collects in the choroidal villi resulting in the formation of **choroid plexus cysts (CPCs)** detected on ultrasound.
- In second-trimester scans, CPCs appear as echoluscent cysts within an echogenic choroid.
- A CPC is **not** a structural or a functional brain abnormality.
- Most CPCs resolve spontaneously by 26–28 weeks gestation.[1,2]
- CPCs are detected in an estimated 0.5–3.6 % of routine 20-week anomaly ultrasound scans.[3,4,5,6]
- A CPC is a small fluid-filled structure within the choroid of the lateral ventricles of the fetal brain.
- CPCs are usually less than 1 cm in diameter and may be single or multiple, unilateral or bilateral, and occur equally in male and female fetuses.[7]
- Most CPCs are isolated and found in otherwise low-risk pregnancies.[8].
- CPCs are entirely benign when there no other abnormalities seen on scan and no abnormal maternal serum screening markers are found.
- The presence of CPCs does not affect either fetal neurodevelopment or any longer-term problems in childhood.[5,9,10]
- **The only association found with CPCs is that of trisomy 18.[11,12,13,14] Prenatal ultrasound has shown that in 44–50% of pregnancies with trisomy 18 have CPCs.[15,16,17]** The prevalence of apparently isolated CPCs at mid-trimester in fetuses with trisomy 18 is 4.3% versus 0.47% in the general population. Thus, if apparently isolated CPCs are found, the likelihood of trisomy 18 is increased ninefold. If additional anomalies are found the likelihood of trisomy 18 is increased by almost 1800-fold.[18]
- To a much lesser extent is there an association between CPCs and trisomy 21. Only 1.4% of pregnancies with trisomy 21 show CPCs.[3,19,20] This is, in fact, no different from the frequency with which CPCs are found in the general population.[18,19,20]
- When CPCs, either uni- or bilateral, single or multiple are found, a detailed anomaly ultrasound scan must be performed. An experienced ultrasonographer[21] needs to look in particular for anomalies of the fetal hands, heart, and CNS such as ventriculomegaly, CHs, neural tube defects, diaphragmatic hernia, omphalocele, clenched hands, overlapping digits, talipes, and growth restriction.
- If other fetal anomalies or abnormal biochemistry markers in maternal serum screening are found, an amniocentesis may be offered.[3,12,14,22,23,24,25,26]

Management

- There is continuing controversy regarding the management of isolated CPCs. Most studies have recommended that isolated CPCs are not an indication for amniocentesis for karyotyping, if after careful ultrasound scanning, no other structural abnormalities are detected and there are no abnormal serum screening results.[27,28,29,30] Others, however suggest that karyotyping should be offered.[3,13,14,31,32]
- An individualized risk estimation based on maternal age, presence of an isolated CPC, and serum screening markers for aneuploidy has been proposed.[33]
- The ultrasound features of CPCs such as bilaterality, number, and resolution do not seem to be linked to any greater risk of aneuploidy.[34,35,36]
- The present consensus appears to be that small CPCs (<5 mm diameter) may not be linked with trisomy 18, whereas larger cysts (>10 mm diameter) may be associated with a greater risk.[11,17,31,37,38]
- The risk estimate for trisomy 18 in an unselected population when CPC is found without any other sonographic abnormality is about 1 in 189.[39]
- Some experts[40] suggest that it is unnecessary for the doctor to discuss a finding of an isolated CPC because of the unnecessary but inevitable anxiety it is bound to create in low-risk women. However, withholding information about ultrasound findings in order to decrease maternal anxiety can be regarded as paternalistic.[41] A clear explanation to reassure the pregnant woman and partner should highlight:
  - the benign nature of CPCs
  - the lack of association with any neurodevelopmental impairment
  - the extremely low risk of trisomy 18 when other abnormalities have been excluded and no abnormal maternal serum markers have been found.
- Genetic counselling may be required, especially in women over 37 years of age, if parental anxiety persists despite such reassurances. In such cases amniocentesis or non-invasive prenatal testing may need to be considered.[33]

Information for patients

Please see Information for patients: Choroid plexus cysts (p. 557)

References

1. DeRoo T.R., et al. Fetal choroid plexus cysts: prevalence, clinical significance, and sonographic appearance. Am J Roentgenol 1988;151: 1179–1181.
2. Chitkara U, et al. Choroid plexus cysts in the fetus: a benign anatomic variant or pathologic entity? Report of 41 cases and review of the literature. Obstet Gynecol 1988;72: 185–189.
3. Kupferminc MJ, et al. Isolated choroid plexus cyst(s): an indication for amniocentesis. Am J Obstet Gynecol 1994;171: 1068–1071.
4. Chinn DH, et al. Sonographically detected choroid plexus cysts: frequency and association with aneupolidy. J Ultrasound Med 1991;10: 255–258.
5. DiPietro JA, et al. Choroid plexus cysts do not affect fetal neurodevelopment. J Perinatol 2006;26: 622–627.
6. Demasio K, et al. Isolated choroid plexus cyst in low-risk women less than 35 years old. Am J Obstet Gynecol 2002;187: 1246–1249.
7. Landy HJ. Association of sex of the fetus in isolated fetal choroid plexus cysts. J Ultrasound Med 1999;18: 769–771.
8. Bronsteen R, et al. Second-trimester sonography and trisomy 18: the significance of isolated choroid plexus cysts after an examination that includes the fetal hands. J Ultrasound Med 2004;23: 241–245.
9. Bernier FP, et al. Developmental outcome of children who had choroid plexus cysts detected prenatally. Prenat Diagn 2005;25: 322–326.
10. Dipietro JA, et al. Isolated prenatal choroid plexus cysts do not affect child development. Prenat Diagn 2011;31: 745–749.
11. Chitty LS, et al. The significance of choroid plexus cysts in an unselected population: results of a multicenter study. Ultrasound Obstet Gynecol 1998;12: 391–397.
12. Snijders RJ, et al. Fetal choroid plexus cysts and trisomy 18: assessment of risk based on ultrasound findings and maternal age. Prenat Diagn 1994;14: 1119–1127.
13. Porto M, et al. Fetal choroid plexus cysts: an independent risk factor for chromosomal anomalies. J Clin Ultrasound 1993;21: 103–108.
14. Zerres K, et al. Chromosomal finding in fetuses with prenatally diagnosed cysts of the choroid plexus. Hum Genet 1992;89: 301–304.
15. Denis E, et al. Choroid plexus cysts and risks of chromosome anomalies. Review of the literature and proposed management. J Gynecol Obstet Biol Reprod 1998;27: 144–149.
16. Lopez JA, Reich D. Choroid plexus cysts. J Am Board Fam Med 2006;19: 422–425.
17. Gray DL, et al. Is genetic amniocentesis warranted when isolated choroid plexus cysts are found? Prenat Diagn 1996;16: 983–990.
18. Gupta JK, et al. Management of fetal choroid plexus cysts. Br J Obstet Gynaecol 1997;104: 881–886.

19. Bromley B, et al. Choroid plexus cysts: not associated with Down syndrome. Ultrasound Obstet Gynecol 1996;8: 232–235.
20. Leonardi MR, et al. The apparently isolated choroid plexus cyst: importance of minor abnormalities in predicting the risk for aneuploidy. Fetal Diagn Ther 1998;13: 49–52.
21. Sepulveda W, Lopez-Tenorio J. The value of minor ultrasound markers for fetal aneuploidy. Obstet Gynecol 2001;13: 183–191.
22. ACOG Practice Bulletin. Prenatal diagnosis of fetal chromosomal abnormalities. Obstet Gynecol 2001; 97(S Part 1) Suppl 1–12.
23. Nava S, et al. Significance of sonographically detected second-trimester choroid plexus cysts: a series of 211 and a review of the literature. Ultrasound Obstet Gynecol 1994;4: 448–451.
24. Oettinger M, et al. Antenatal diagnosis of choroid plexus cyst: suggested management. Obstet Gynecol Surv 1993;48: 635–639.
25. Platt LD, et al. Fetal choroid plexus cysts in the second trimester of pregnancy: a cause for concern? Am J Obstet Gynecol 1991;164: 1652–1656.
26. Fitzsimmons J, et al. Choroid plexus cysts in fetus with trisomy 18. Obstet Gynecol 1989;73: 257–260.
27. Lilford RJ. Fetal choroid cysts. Lancet 1995;346: 1361–1362.
28. Nadel AS, et al. Isolated choroid plexus cysts in the second trimester fetus: is amniocentesis really indicated? Radiology 1992;185: 545–548.
29. Donnenfeld AE. Prenatal sonographic detection of isolated fetal choroid plexus cysts: should we screen for trisomy 18? J Med Screen 1995;2: 18–21.
30. Donnenfeld AE. Risk and benefit analysis of offering karyotyping for an isolated choroid plexus cyst. Ultrasound Obstet Gynecol 1997;9: 67–68.
31. Walkinshaw S. Isolated choroid plexus cyst—the need for routine offer of karyotyping. Prenat Diagn 1994;14: 663–667.
32. Burrows A, et al. Choroid plexus cysts in the fetal brain. Aust N Z J Obstet Gynecol 1994;34: 220.
33. Fuchs KM. Isolated fetal choroid plexus cysts. Their implications and outcomes. Contemporary Ob/Gyn 2013;58: 42.
34. Walkinshaw S. Fetal choroid plexus cysts: are we there yet? Prenat Diagn 2000;20: 657–662.
35. Shields LE, et al. Isolated fetal choroid plexus cysts and karyotype analysis: is it necessary? J Ultrasound Med 1996;15: 389–394.
36. Peleg D, Yankowitz J. Choroid plexus cysts and aneuploidy. J Med Genet 1998;35: 554–557.
37. Ostlere SJ, et al. Fetal choroid plexus cyst: a report of 100 cases. Radiology 1990;175: 753–755.
38. Sasani M, et al. A large choroid plexus cyst diagnosed with magnetic resonance imaging in utero: a case report. Cases J 2009;2: 7098.
39. Benacerraf BR, et al. Are choroid plexus cysts an indication for second trimester amniocentesis. Am J Obstet Gynecol 1990;162: 1001–1006.
40. Filly RA, et al. Choroid plexus cyst and echogenic intracardiac focus in women at low risk for chromosomal anomalies. J Ultrasound Med 2004;23: 447–449.
41. Doubilet PM, et al. Choroid plexus cyst and echogenic intracardiac focus in women at low risk for chromosomal anomalies: the obligation to inform the mother. J Ultrasound Med 2004;23: 883–885.

CARE PATHWAY

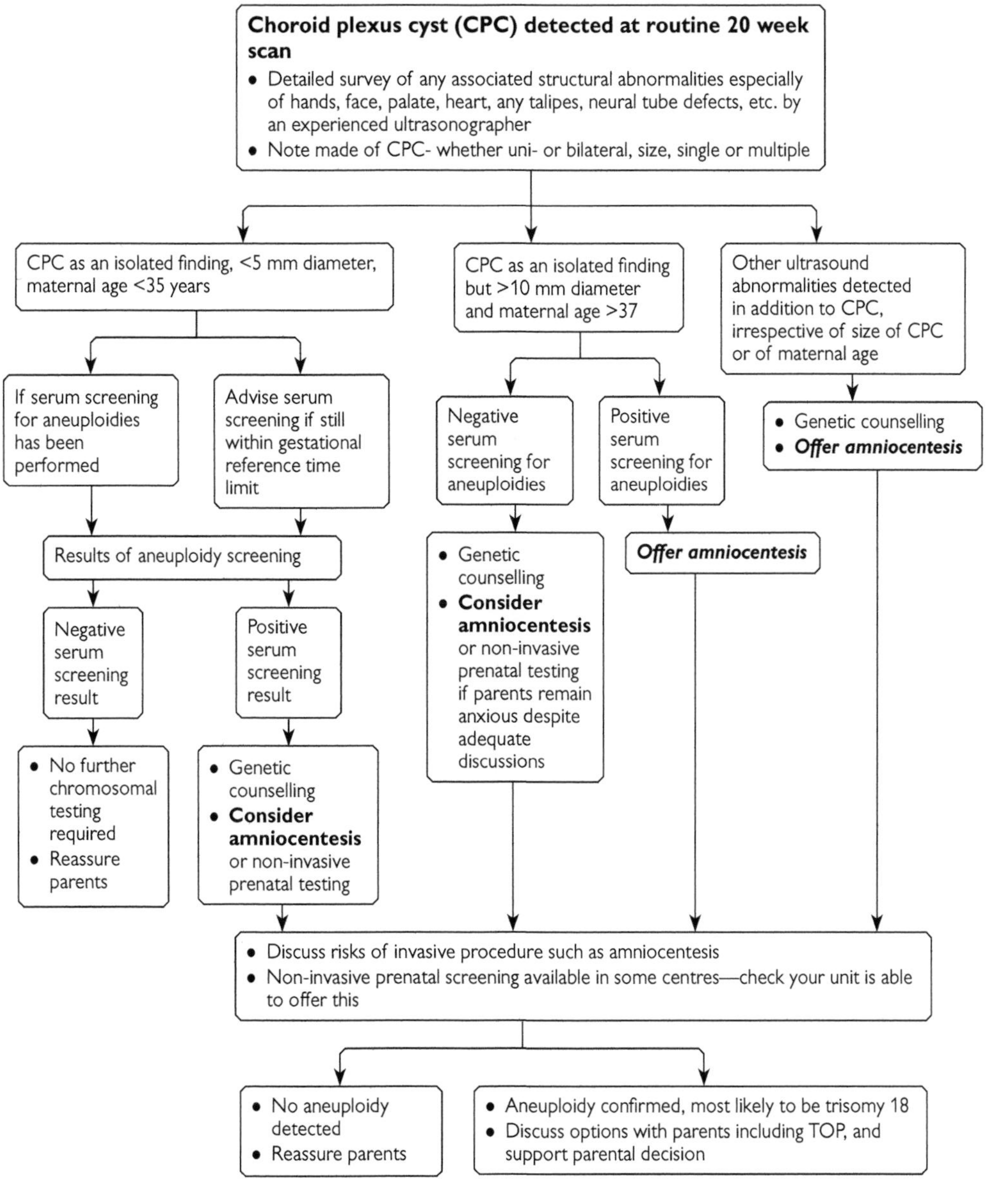
Choroid plexus cyst (CPC) detected at routine 20 week scan
• Detailed survey of any associated structural abnormalities especially of hands, face, palate, heart, any talipes, neural tube defects, etc. by an experienced ultrasonographer
• Note made of CPC- whether uni- or bilateral, size, single or multiple
CPC as an isolated finding, <5 mm diameter, maternal age <35 years
If serum screening for aneuploidies has been performed
Advise serum screening if still within gestational reference time limit
Results of aneuploidy screening
Negative serum screening result
• No further chromosomal testing required
• Reassure parents
Positive serum screening result
• Genetic counselling
• Consider amniocentesis or non-invasive prenatal testing
CPC as an isolated finding but >10 mm diameter and maternal age >37
Negative serum screening for aneuploidies
• Genetic counselling
• Consider amniocentesis or non-invasive prenatal testing if parents remain anxious despite adequate discussions
Positive serum screening for aneuploidies
Offer amniocentesis
Other ultrasound abnormalities detected in addition to CPC, irrespective of size of CPC or of maternal age
• Genetic counselling
• Offer amniocentesis
• Discuss risks of invasive procedure such as amniocentesis
• Non-invasive prenatal screening available in some centres—check your unit is able to offer this
• No aneuploidy detected
• Reassure parents
• Aneuploidy confirmed, most likely to be trisomy 18
• Discuss options with parents including TOP, and support parental decision

28 Other Fetal Conditions

28.1 Non-Immune Hydrops Fetalis

FACT FILE

- **Hydrops fetalis** is defined as abnormal fluid collection in two or more compartments of the fetus including skin oedema, ascites, pleural or pericardial effusions (heart failure of the fetus in utero). Isolated ascites, pericardial effusion, and pleural effusion have specific aetiologies and hence are not fetal hydrops.
- Hydrops fetalis may also be associated with polyhydramnios and placental oedema.
- Hydrops fetalis can be due to a variety of disparate causes. Hydrops is classified as:
  - **immune:** due to alloimmunization of the fetus caused by blood group incompatibilities
  - **non-immune** hydrops fetalis (**NIHF**).

Epidemiology

- With the significant reduction of rhesus (Rh) disease due to effective prophylaxis with Rh (D) immune globin and appropriate screening, the incidence of immune hydrops fetalis has been greatly reduced.[1]
- Nowadays over 90% of fetal hydrops is NIHF and includes all cases that are not due to red cell alloimmunization by Rh (D), Kell, or other red cell antigens.
- Overall incidence is between 1:600 and 1:4000 pregnancies, varying according to population risks of certain conditions such as alpha-thalassaemia.[2]
- Pathogenesis of NIHF depends on the underlying cause and disease process but usually involves one or more of the following mechanisms:[3]
  - disturbance of colloid osmotic pressure due to liver disease
  - fetal heart failure resulting in increased capillary permeability; this could result from both high and low output cardiac failure
  - obstruction of venous return to the heart
  - blockage of lymphatic drainage from abdominal and thoracic cavities
  - fetal myocardial injury or severe myocarditis.

Clinical presentation

- Hydrops fetalis is usually detected during ultrasound examination for conditions such as:
  - polyhydramnios
  - uterine size larger than dates
  - decreased fetal movements
  - fetal tachycardia or arrhythmia
  - abnormal serum screening results
  - maternal infections: parvovirus B19, cytomegalovirus, toxoplasmosis, etc.
- Ascites is an early feature; pleural effusion if severe and long standing can even result in lung hypoplasia.
- Skin oedema is usually a late sign of NIHF with skin or scalp oedema of more than 5 mm being pathognomonic.
- Polyhydramnios is present in most cases and can be the first indication to prompt ultrasound evaluation.
- Placental oedema can result in an unusual appearance of the placenta with a thickness exceeding 6 cm as in certain infections.

Aetiology

Aetiology of NIHF can be varied and while a cause may be found in up to 50–85% of cases, the rest are idiopathic. Structural and rhythm cardiac abnormalities are the most common cause, followed by chromosomal abnormalities; supraventricular tachycardia is therefore one of the common and treatable causes.

Chromosomal abnormalities

- Aneuploidies such as Turner's, trisomies 21, 18, 13, and triploidies.
- NIHF in such cases is thought to evolve from fluid accumulation due to cystic hygroma, obstruction of lymphatic drainage, and/or cardiac defects.
- Various studies have quoted chromosomal anomalies as the cause of 10–75% of cases of NIHF.[4,5,6]

Haematological causes

- **Haemolytic disorders** like glucose 6-phosphatase deficiency (G6PD), pyruvate kinase deficiency
- **Disorders of red cell** production, e.g. alpha-thalassaemia, hereditary spherocytosis
- **Fetal anaemia**: intracranial or intraventricular haemorrhage, fetomaternal haemorrhage, TTTS, etc.
- Some studies have indicated that as much as 25% of NIHF is due to haemolysis, haemorrhage, defective red cell production, or abnormal haemoglobin production. In some cases the NIHF may be reversible when fetal anaemia is corrected in the form of intrauterine transfusion by cordocentesis.

Fetal cardiac causes

These can account for up to 40% of NIHF either as the sole cause or as part of the pathology involved with the condition.

- ***Cardiac causes without structural cardiac abnormalities:***
  - arrhythmias—prolonged and repetitive
  - tachyarrhythmia due to uncontrolled or poorly controlled Grave's disease.
  - supraventricular tachycardia
  - congenital heart block causing bradyarrhythmias.
  - myocarditis
  - superior or inferior vena caval occlusion
  - disorders of normal lymphatic drainage
  - presence of intrathoracic or intra-abdominal masses (e.g. CCAM)
  - other fetal tumours, e.g. sacrococcygeal teratomas, cystic hygromas, rhabdomyosarcomas, cervical teratomas
  - prenatal closure of foramen ovale or ductus anteriosus.
- ***Structural cardiac and vascular abnormalities:***
  - atrioventricular (AV) septal defects
  - isolated ventricular or atrial septal defects
  - aortic valve stenosis or atresia
  - coarctation of aorta
  - truncus arteriosus
  - hypoplastic left heart
  - pulmonary valve atresia or insufficiency
  - arteriovenous malformations, haemangiomas, sacrococcygeal teratomas; these result in high-output cardiac failure due to arteriovenous shunts.

Infective causes

These can account for 8–20% of NIHF and include:

- Parvovirus B_{19}—causes hydrops because of destruction of fetal RBCs

- Cytomegalovirus
- Toxoplasmosis
- Herpes simplex
- Syphilis
- Listeriosis
- Hepatitis B
- Coxsackie viruses, adenoviruses, etc.

Metabolic and other causes

- Inborn errors of metabolism (e.g. glycogen storage disease)
- Several autosomal recessive genetic disorders
- Noonan's syndrome
- Severe fetal hypo- or hyperthyroidism
- Congenital nephrosis (where maternal serum αFP is elevated).

Evaluation and investigations[7]

- **Detailed history:** Ethnicity, history of familial genetic defects, inherited metabolic or enzymatic defects, or maternal infection.
- **Ultrasound scan:**[8] Any structural defects, Doppler assessment of peak systolic velocity in the fetal middle cerebral artery in suspected fetal anaemia, BPP if gestational age is relevant.
- **Fetal ECHO** would be helpful especially in arrhythmias.
- **Amniocentesis** to be offered with due counselling, for:
  - fetal karyotyping
  - PCR in viral infection
  - metabolic testing if relevant family history.
- **Laboratory tests:** Full blood count with red cell indices, repeat blood type and screening for any antibodies, electrophoresis, IgM and IgG serology for viruses, Kleihauer–Betke test for fetomaternal haemorrhage

Prognosis

- Prognosis in hydrops fetalis depends on recognition of the underlying cause as well as any treatment modalities that may be offered.[9]
- The prognosis differs markedly between different aetiological causes. In treatable conditions such as in parvovirus B19[9,10,11] the outcome is likely to be good whereas certain cases of hydrops fetalis carry considerable perinatal mortality and morbidity or are incompatible with life.[5,9]
- Spontaneous remission has also been noted in several cases of cardiac arrhythmias, parvovirus infection,[9,10,11] CMV infections, twin-to-twin transfusion syndrome, cystic hygromas, or idiopathic pleural or pericardial effusions.
- NIHF fetuses carry a high mortality rate, 50–90% depending on the gestation of onset (worse with early onset hydrops <24 weeks gestation), presence of pleural effusion, polyhydramnios, etc. Half of these occur antenatally and 50% after delivery.[12]
- In idiopathic NIHF the mortality rate is about 50%. When NIHF is associated with structural cardiac defect, nearly 90–100% mortality can be expected.

Management options

- Management depends on accurate identification of cause and the parental wishes regarding interventions.[7]
- Pregnancy termination is one of the options to be considered depending on the individual circumstances, especially if NIHF appears early in pregnancy without a treatable cause found.
- Therapeutic interventions are sometimes possible.
- Intrauterine intraperitoneal red cell fetal transfusions have been successfully used in the presence of severe fetal anaemia in some cases.
- Other interventions such as percutaneous laser ablation of CCAM or laser occlusion of arteriovenous anastomosis in selective cases of TTTS in monochorionic twins may be discussed, though several uncertainties prevail regarding safety and efficacy of such procedures.
- Treatment of fetal arrhythmias with drug therapy such as digoxin or adenosine[13] administered to the mother in cases of fetal supraventricular arrhythmia need to be considered. If fetal maturity has been reached, early delivery is an option in some cases of fetal arrhythmias.
- Careful maternal surveillance is recommended due to increased risks of pre-eclampsia and 'mirror syndrome' as well as of abruption and PPH in the presence of polyhydramnios,
- Continued supportive care is essential.
- Clear, sensitive, documented, discussion with the parents should take place to help them choose options such as termination or continuation of the pregnancy depending on whether the abnormality is compatible with continued survival of the fetus/neonate.[14]
- Parents must be given detailed information of possible/potential sequelae and their informed choice should guide management.
- Sensitive discussions about post-mortem etc. should also be undertaken at the same time.
- Parents will require counselling and support at such a vulnerable time.
- If the decision is made to continue the pregnancy, issues to be considered are:
  - when is 'out' safer than 'in' with reference to preterm delivery, to reduce the possibility of further fetal risk in the intrauterine environment
  - whether interventional invasive measures such as shunt placements are warranted.
- ***Every case must be treated according to an individualized plan of management. Referral to tertiary fetal medicine units will be required for second opinion or for interventional fetal therapy.***
- Frequency of ultrasound scans, of visits to the specialist antenatal clinics in the DGH or tertiary centre and continued fetal assessments including BPP and Doppler scans will need to be planned on a case-by-case basis.
- If treatment appears to be successful or the hydrops appears to be resolving spontaneously, repeat ultrasound scans may be performed at 1–2-weekly intervals.
- ***Delivery in a tertiary unit is advisable and early referral may be required for continued high-intensity fetal surveillance before a planned delivery.***
- Early referral to the local paediatric consultant is mandatory in addition to collaboration with the tertiary specialist unit, in the event that a woman whose delivery has been planned in a tertiary unit arrives at the local hospital in active labour before this.
- Coordinated care by the multidisciplinary team of haematologist, fetal medicine obstetrician, midwives, clinical geneticist, virology, microbiology, radiology (ultrasound) specialist, neonatologists, and anomaly screening coordinator is essential.
- The placenta must be sent for histology and virology and provided with clear clinical details.
- Parental screening for inherent metabolic defects should be considered in cases where the karyotype is normal and there is a history of consanguineous marriage, previous stillbirth, or recurrent hydrops.
- A postnatal follow-up should take place some 6–8 weeks after either TOP or IUD, with results of the placental histology and virology studies, as well as autopsy results (if performed) and full karyotype results obtained from cord insertion sample which might assist discussions[15] regarding aetiology and recurrence risk in a subsequent pregnancy.

Information for patients

Please see Information for patients: Non-immune hydrops fetalis (p. 557)

References

1. Wilson DC, et al. The changing pattern of fetal hydrops. Ulster Med J 1990;59: 119–121.
2. Wilkins I. Non-immune hydrops. InGreene MF, et al., ed., Creasy and Resnick's maternal-fetal medicine: principles and practice 6th ed. Philadelphia: Saunders Elsevier 2009, pp. 505–517.

3. Harahan D, et al. Clinicopathological findings in non-immune hydrops fetalis. Irish Med J 1991;84: 62–63.
4. Iskaros J, et al. Outcome of nonimmune hydrops fetalis diagnosed during the first half of pregnancy. Obstet Gynecol 1997;90: 321–325.
5. Ismail KM, et al. Etiology and outcome of hydrops fetalis. J Matern Fetal Med 2001;10: 175.
6. Has R. Non-immune hydrops fetalis in the first trimester: a review of 30 cases. Clin Exp Obstet Gynecol 2001;28: 187–190.
7. Jones DC, et al. Non-immune fetal hydrops: diagnosis and obstetrical management. Semin Perinatol 1995;19: 447–461.
8. Moise KJ. Ultrasound evaluation of hydrops fetalis. In:Callen PW, ed., Ultrasonography in obstetrics and gynecology, 5th ed. Philadelphia: Saunders Elsevier, 2008, pp. 676–697.
9. Huang HR, et al. Prognostic factors and clinical features in liveborn neonates with hydrops fetalis. Am J Perinatol 2007;24: 33–38.
10. Bhal PS, et al. Spontaneous resolution of non-immune hydrops fetalis secondary to transplacental parvovirus B19 infection. Ultrasound Obstet Gynecol 1996;7: 55–57.
11. Xu J, et al. Hydrops fetalis secondary to parvovirus B19 infections. J Am Board Fam Pract 2003;16: 63–68.
12. Sohan K, et al. Analysis of outcome in hydrops fetalis in relation to gestational age at diagnosis, cause and treatment. Acta Obstet Gynecol Scand 2001;80: 726–730.
13. Dangel JH, et al. Adenosine triphosphate for cardioversion of supraventricular tachycardia in two hydropic fetuses. Fetal Diag Ther 2000;15: 326–330.
14. Abrams ME, et al. Hydrops fetalis: a retrospective review of cases reported to a large national database and identification of risk factors associated with death. Pediatrics 2007;120: 84–89.
15. Santo S, et al. Prenatal diagnosis of non-immune hydrops fetalis: what do we tell the parents? Prenat Diagn 2011;31: 186–195.

CARE PATHWAY

Hydrops fetalis diagnosed at any gestation by ultrasound scan

Seen as urgent in specialist antenatal clinic

Hydrops due to blood group alloimmune incompatibility

Further care as in red cell antibody care pathway (Chapter 1.9, p. 39)

Non-immune hydrops fetalis (NIHF)

- Detailed history: any familial genetic/metabolic defects? Maternal infection, flu-like illness?
- Re-check electrophoresis result
- Re-check FBC, red cell indices, blood group antibodies
- Urgent serology for parvovirus, CMV, toxoplasmosis, herpes simplex, listeriosis
- Confirm negative VDRL
- Serum screening for G6PD and pyruvate kinase deficiency
- Kleihauer for evidence of fetomaternal haemorrhage

If infective cause found

- Continue close scan monitoring
- Discuss prognosis: Spontaneous remission or worsening of NIHF can occur
- Management options depend on subsequent course of NIHF
- If worsening picture, TOP may need to be discussed with and considered by mother and partner
- If pregnancy continues, refer to paediatricians during pregnancy
- Refer to tertiary unit

If TOP opted for by parents:

- Arrange to send placenta for histology, virology, microbiology studies, **document instructions on Intrapartum page of notes**
- Discuss post-mortem with parents, particularly valuable for future pregnancy counselling. Document these discussions

---

- Urgent scans by fetal medicine specialist for any structural defects especially fetal cardiac anomalies, fetal tumours, arrhythmias, supraventricular tachycardia, polyhydramnios, Doppler studies of peak systolic volume in middle cerebral artery and BPP if appropriate
- Discuss amniocentesis for karyotyping and PCR for fetal infection

- Refer to tertiary unit for fetal ECHO if indicated and further scans for arrhythmia, maternal medications for fetal treatment of arrhythmia, etc.
- Amniocentesis if patient opts for invasive testing

Chromosomal abnormality confirmed and/or serious structural cardiac defect identified

- Screening coordinator contacts mother, invites her to specialist antenatal clinic
- Review in specialist antenatal clinic to discuss very poor prognosis and management options including TOP

Normal karyotype rapid result

- Back to specialist antenatal clinic
- Discuss prognosis—mortality in idiopathic cases may be up to 50%
- Discuss other results
- Discuss and document patient's/parents views about pregnancy options
- If parents decide to continue with pregnancy, close ultrasound follow-up at a suggested frequency of 2 weekly scans and Dopplers arranged
- Refer to paediatricians at DGH and refer to tertiary centre fetal medicine unit for continued joint care
- Delivery in tertiary centre ideal. Joint discussions between tertiary unit and DGH with parents about timing and route of delivery
- Cord bloods sent for further tests

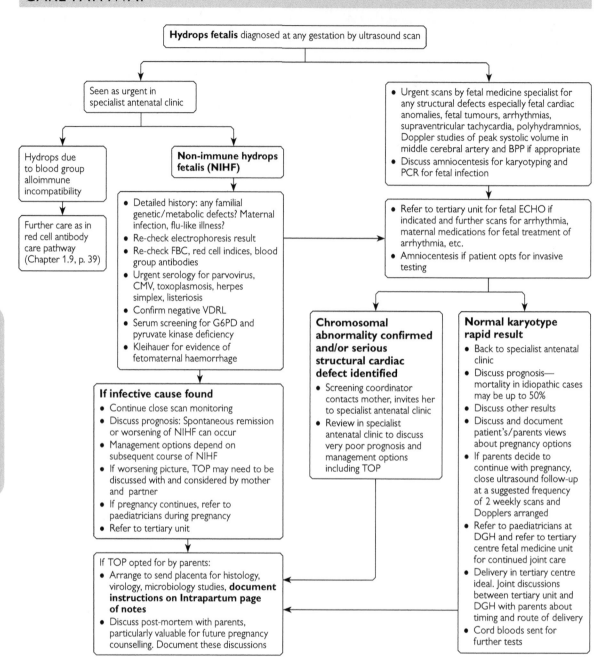

28.2 Irregular Fetal Heart Rhythm

FACT FILE

Transient irregularities of fetal heart rate

- Fetal arrhythmias are noted in only 1–2% of all pregnancies and can be categorized by rate and regularity.[1]
- Transient irregularities of the fetal cardiac rhythm are common and rarely have serious consequences.
- Infrequent ectopic beats can occur in upto 90% of normal pregnancies. Short bursts of tachycardia or bradycardia lasting for 3–4 s are often observed in normal pregnancy.
- Fetal arrhythmias are often first noted on auscultation during routine antenatal examinations.The CTG, while accurately reflecting rate and rhythm when the FHR is within the normal range, may be inaccurate when there is fetal tachyarrhythmia in excess of 200 bpm.
- In general, the pregnant mother does not notice any change in fetal activity.
- If a fetal tachycardia is heard, its rate and type must be established.
- Normal fetal heart rate accelerations are associated with fetal movements.
- **Premature atrial contractions** (**PACs** or **fetal extrasystoles** or **fetal ectopics**): The vast majority of PACs are associated with good outcomes. In less than 0.5% of cases, PACs may progress to fetal tachycardia.
- Detailed structural analysis of the heart is necessary and it is also recommended that these patients be monitored weekly to exclude the development of tachyarrhythmias.[1,4]
- Vaginal delivery is to be anticipated in isolated ectopic beats in the absence of any other features.
- Though usually of no sinister significance, sustained fetal ectopic beats can lead to heart failure and hydrops fetalis.
- Approximately 50% of fetuses referred for evaluation of fetal arrhythmias are in normal sinus rhythm, with the vast majority having isolated supraventricular systoles. Fewer than 10% of fetuses are found to have sustained tachyarrhythmias or bradyarrhythmias.[1]

Sustained irregularities of fetal heart rate

- Sustained bradycardia (<100 bpm), tachycardia (>200 bpm) or frequent irregular beats (>1 in 10 beats) constitute abnormal cardiac rhythm.[2,3]
- Fetal and neonatal arrhythmias are diverse in type and severity, including irregular tachycardia and bradycardias.
- The mechanisms of fetal and neonatal arrhythmias are similar and include a wide range of possible diagnosis.
- Abrupt and sustained changes, especially if the rate is over 200 bpm when the fetal heart rate was previously normal, need further investigation.
- Once an arrhythmia is detected by auscultation, additional evaluations are indicated.[1,4] Such evaluation is vital to plan the place, timing, and mode of delivery.
- Echocardiography, to exclude structural cardiac defects, and pulsed Doppler analysis of the fetal heart can be used to identify fetal rhythms.

Fetal tachyarrhythmias

- The most common fetal tachyarrhythmias are **atrial flutter (AF)**, **supraventricular (re-entrant) tachycardia (SVT)**, and **ventricular tachycardia (VT)**.
- **AF** accounts for approximately 50% of fetal tachycardia, and may be associated with structural abnormalities. Fetal hydrops is associated with about 43% of AF cases. AF is defined as an atrial rate ranging from 250 to 500 bpm. The diagnosis can be confirmed by fetal echocardiography, which documents the atrium beating at a faster rate than the ventricle.
- Medical management, successful in 82% of cases without hydrops, may consist of digoxin therapy administered to the mother, whereas in others a second agent such as flecainide or procainamide may be needed. Hydropic fetuses may require more medication and a longer treatment period to control the condition.
- **SVT** is reported in about 68% of cases of fetal tachycardia, and only 2% of cases are associated with structural abnormalities. SVT may be either incessant or paroxysmal in nature, may have ventricular rates varying from 250 to 300 bpm, and is associated with fetal hydrops in 64% of cases.
- Medical therapy includes digoxin as the first-line treatment. This can be maternally administered, both orally and IV, or even administered directly to the fetus by an intramuscular, intraperitoneal, or intra-amniotic route. Placental transfer is excellent but diminished in the hydropic fetus. In about 40% of cases, a second agent such as flecainide or sotalol may be needed to be more effective and reduce fetal mortality
- **Antenatal VT** is rare and can be difficult to diagnose. The fetal heart rate is often relatively normal (<200 bpm) and is usually well tolerated. The treatment of fetal VT includes propranolol, procainamide, and phenytoin. **Digoxin should be avoided as it may potentially exacerbate VT.**
- ***A viable fetus with refractory arrhythmia should, preferably be delivered in a tertiary centre with the means to provide pharmacological or electroversion immediately after birth. Delivery may need to be by Caesarean section. A planned Caesarean section at an optimal time will facilitate immediate neonatal care by the neonatologist and paediatric cardiologist.***

Fetal bradyarrhythmias

- The most significant fetal bradycardia is **congenital complete heart block (CHB).** Approximately 50% of fetuses with CHB are identified in mothers with connective tissue or autoimmune conditions like lupus (SLE) or antiphospholipid syndrome (APS) where there is transplacental transfer of two specific antibodies (anti-Ro and anti-La) that may cause cause damage to the fetal heart's conduction system.
- Diagnosis is made by echocardiography with a normal atrial rate and slower ventricular rate. Most fetal heart rates are approximately 60 bpm.
- The prognosis depends on the presence or absence of structural heart disease, and the development of hydrops secondary to the very slow rate. Sympathomimetic drugs (such as terbutaline, isoprenaline and salbutamol) administered maternally have been demonstrated to increase in heart rate with variable improvement in hydrops.
- ***A pregnancy where the baby is known to have congenital CHB should preferably be delivered in a tertiary care centre with the means to provide emergency pacing techniques, pharmacological or electroversion, immediately after birth.***

Neonatal bradyarrhythmias

- The most common cause of sustained bradycardia in neonates is CHB. This may be associated with structural congenital heart defects, with the most common being ventricular inversion and defects of the AV septum.
- When there is no structural abnormality of the heart, congenital heart block can occur in infants born to mothers with **lupus with anti-Ro and anti-La** antibodies which cross the placenta and effect the myocardium and the conduction system of the heart. Symptomatic newborns may need to have a permanent pacemaker placed which is why delivery needs to take place in a tertiary centre with paediatric cardiology and cardiac surgery facilities.

Information for patients

Please see Information for patients: Irregular fetal heart rate (p. 558)

References

1. Zaidi AL, Ro PS. Treatment of fetal and neonatal arrhythmias. US Cardiol 2006;3: 1–4.
2. Snider AR. Two dimensional and doppler echocardiographic evaluation. Clin Perinatol 1988;15: 523–565.
3. Ito S, et al. Drug therapy for fetal arrhythmias. Clin Perinatol 1994;21: 543–552.
4. Stewart PA, et al. Arrhythmia and structural abnormalities of the fetal heart. Br Heart J 1983;50: 550–554.

CARE PATHWAY

Irregular fetal heart rate auscultated in community or in hospital

↓

Referral on same day to day assessment unit for repeat auscultation and CTG

↓

If **sustained arrhythmia**, urgent same-day referral to tertiary centre for fetal ECHO, exclusion of structural cardiac defects, identification of type of arrhythmia, ± initiation of treatment as indicated

Transient arrhythmia
- Reassurance, weekly auscultation or CTG, till returns to normal rhythm
- If continues >2–3 weeks, scan for hydrops

↓ (from sustained arrhythmia)

Bradyarrhythmias

Structural defect
- Ventricular inversion
- Defects of AV septum

No structural defect
- Congenital heart block
- Check lupus, anti-Ro, anti La

↓

- Prognosis depends also on presence/absence of hydrops, signs of cardiac failure
- Sympathomimetic drugs as/if directed by fetal medicine specialist

Tachyarrhythmias

PACS | AF | SVT | VT

↓

- Detailed examination for any structural defect, hydrops/signs of cardiac failure
- Medical therapy: Digoxin, propranolol, etc. as directed by fetal medicine specialist

↓

- Early involvement of neonatologists at both local hospital and tertiary centre
- In congenital heart block or refractory arrhythmias, delivery in a tertiary unit with facilities for emergency pacing techniques or medical/electroversion immediately after birth
- Good communication and a clear management plan for timing, place and mode of delivery essential and must be well documented

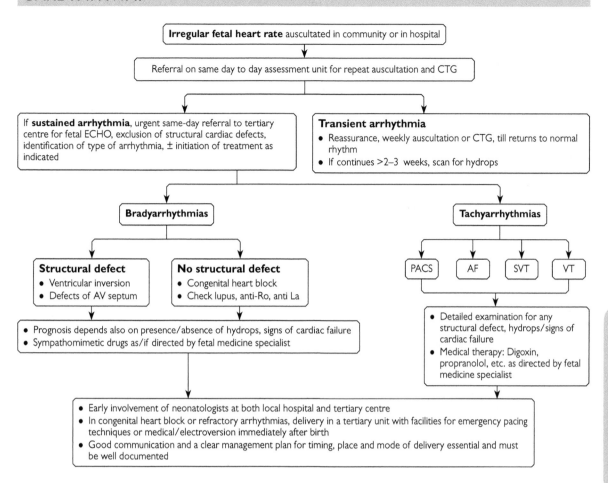

28.3 Fetal and Neonatal Alloimmune Thrombocytopenia

FACT FILE

Epidemiology and pathogenesis

- **Neonatal alloimmune thrombocytopenia (NAITP)** is the most common cause of early-onset thrombocytopenia in neonates,[1] responsible for 10% of all cases where the platelet count is less than 150 × 10^9/litre.[2]
- Reported incidence in the white population varies from 1:800 to 1:2000 live births.[3,4] About 400–600 cases of NAITP occur per year in the UK.[5]
- NAITP develops in utero, causing severe effects for the fetus and neonate but without maternal consequences, unlike immune thrombocytopenia. Maternal platelet counts are normal even in cases of severe F/NAITP.
- Severe NAITP is defined as a platelet count of less than 50 × 10^9/litre and occurs with equal frequency in both sexes.
- NAITP is associated with significant mortality (7–15%) and severe neurological morbidity (7–26%) including cerebral palsy, mental impairment, seizure disorders, and cortical blindness, due to the **high incidence of intracranial haemorrhage (ICH)**.[6,7,8]
- ICH occurs in about 10% of cases of severe NAITP.[6]
- NAITP is due to maternal alloantibodies directed against platelet-specific alloantigens that the mother herself lacks and which the fetus has inherited from the father.[9,10]
- The most frequent antibodies implicated are anti-HPA-1a (80–90% of cases) followed by anti-HPA-5b in 10–15%.[11] NAITP associated with HPA-1a is usually more severe than that due to HPA-5b. Other HPA antibodies are only detected occasionally.
- In 30% of cases, however, no maternal platelet antibodies are found.[11]
- The parents are found to be incompatible for human platelet antigens HPA-1a or 5b in 90% of cases.[12] Paternal zygosity needs to be determined in counselling parents about the recurrence risks of NAITP in a subsequent pregnancy with the same partner.[13]
- Maternal IgG alloantibodies cross the placental barrier as early as the start of the second trimester and bind to fetal platelets which are then destroyed by the fetal reticuloendothelial system.[11]
- Although the pathophysiology resembles that of red cell alloimmunization, the essential difference in F/NAITP is that even a first pregnancy can be severely affected (as it is in 40–60% of cases). **As there is no system of universal screening at present, F/NAITP is almost always diagnosed only in the next pregnancy after the birth of an unexpectedly affected first child.**
- Subsequent pregnancies are affected in 75–90% of cases, displaying either the same degree of severity or worse.
- ICH occurs antenatally in 50–80% of cases of NAITP[11,14] with about half occurring before 30 weeks gestation.[8] Intrauterine death can occur due to severe ICH.
- A purpuric rash, cephalhaematoma, bleeding into abdominal viscera, or excessive bleeding after venepuncture may be seen as first signs of NAITP at, or a few hours after birth, of a full-term, otherwise healthy neonate without signs of sepsis, systemic illness, or skeletal abnormalities.[5]
- NAITP could, however, be asymptomatic at first, with thrombocytopenia detected incidentally on a full blood count performed for some other indication.[15]

Antenatal management

- ***Although there is no universal consensus about the optimal antenatal treatment, multidisciplinary management is essential. when flnaitp is diagnosed, referral to the regional referral centre with a multispecialty team including obstetricians, neonatologists, neonatal neurologist, haematologist, neuroradiologist, and midwife is necessary.***
- There is no routine population-based screening programme; therefore it is only the birth of a first affected infant that signposts possible interventions required to reduce the risk in a subsequent pregnancy.
- The family should ideally be referred to a regional specialist centre before commencing a subsequent pregnancy.[16]
- Diagnosis depends on demonstration of maternal platelet alloantibody against the father's platelets. The platelet antigen phenotype of both parents is determined by referral to a regional reference laboratory as advised by local haematologists.
- The aim of antenatal management in F/NAITP is to try to prevent catastrophic ICH in utero.
- The practice of weekly intrauterine platelet transfusion via cordocentesis in F/NAITP was found to carry an unacceptable procedure-related risk of fetal loss and therefore abandoned.[18,19]
- Non-invasive management of F/NAITP by weekly IVIG at doses of 1 g/kg given to the mother, with or without steroids,[7,17,18,19] is now the first-line therapy.
- IVIG is required weekly starting from any time between 16 and 32 weeks[21] gestation and continued till delivery, depending on the protocols employed by the regional referral centre.
- In pregnancies where ICH as a result of NAITP is demonstrated by MRI of the fetal brain, outcomes will depend on the severity of cerebral damage, stage of pregnancy, and parental informed choice.
- TOP is an option for some couples when the fetal brain damage is severe.[21]
- In severe cases where the prognosis is expected to be poor, some couples might opt for non-intervention to allow nature to take its course, without any neonatal intervention being involved after a vaginal delivery.
- Less extensive ICH in the fetus may be managed with weekly maternal IVIG ± prednisolone and an elective Caesarean performed at around 34 weeks gestation[21] after prophylactic betamethasone/dexamethasone to accelerate fetal lung maturity.
- A **planned delivery** either by induction of labour or Caesarean section at 36–38 weeks is usually recommended.[11] During labour, fetal blood sampling, fetal scalp electrode, or ventouse delivery must be avoided, as should difficult vaginal delivery such as rotational forceps.
- Vaginal delivery is not absolutely contraindicated in pregnancies with F/NAITP where antenatal treatment with IVIG has been instituted and a previous sibling has had NAITP without ICH.[22]
- Matched platelets must be available for delivery and immediate cord blood fetal platelet count obtained after delivery.

Neonatal management

- The variable clinical course seen postnatally in NAITP may range from spontaneous resolution within 1–16 weeks after birth, to the most severe complication of ICH.[21]
- The primary goal of postnatal management of the neonate with F/NAITP is to prevent or stop thrombocytopenic bleeding by prompt transfusion of matched platelets or in severe emergencies, of serial unmatched donor platelets.
- Neonatal transfusion of compatible platelets, or in severe emergencies, of random donor unmatched platelets till matched platelets become available, must take place without delay in cases of severe thrombocytopenia, especially if less than 30 × 10^9/litre.
- Neuroradiological studies (ultrasound, CT, or MRI) of the neonatal brain must be performed as soon as possible after birth and may reveal features of porencephaly and lateral ventriculomegaly in cerebral damage caused by F/NAITP.[23]

Information for patients

Please see Information for patients: Neonatal alloimmune thrombocytopenia (p. 559)

References

1. Israels SJ. Thrombopoietin and neonatal thrombocytopenia. Pediatr Res 2000;47: 176–177.
2. Blanchette VS, et al. The management of alloimmune neonatal thrombocytopenia. Am J Perinatol 2000;5: 365–390.
3. Williamson LM, et al. The natural history of fetomaternal alloimmunization to the platelet specific antigen HPA-1a (PlAy,´Zwa) as determined by antenatal screening. Blood 1998;92: 2280–2287.
4. Turner ML, et al. Prospective epidemiologic study of the outcome and cost-effectiveness of antenatal screening to detect neonatal alloimmune thrombocytopenia due to anti-HPA-1a. Transfusion 2005;45: 1945–1956.
5. Rayment R, et al. Antenatal interventions for fetomaternal alloimmune thrombocytopenia. Cochrane Database Syst Rev 2011;5: CD004226.
6. Kamphuis MM, et al. Screening in pregnancy for fetal or neonatal alloimmune thrombocytopenia: systematic review. BJOG 2010;117: 1335–1343.
7. Knight M, et al. The incidence and outcomes of fetomaternal alloimmune thrombocytopenia: a UK national study using three data sources. Br J Haematol 2011;152: 460–468.
8. Spencer JA, Burrows RF. Feto maternal alloimmune thrombocytopenia: a literature review and statistical analysis. Aust N Z J Obstet Gynecol 2001;41: 45–55.
9. Metcalfe P, et al. Nomenclature of human platelet antigens. Vox Sang 2003;85: 240–245.
10. von dem Borne AE, Décary F. Nomenclature of platelet specific antigens. Br J Haematol 1990;74: 239–240.
11. Kaplan C. Neonatal alloimmune thrombocytopenia. Haematology 2008;93: 805–807.
12. Mueller-Eckhardt C, et al. 348 cases of suspected neonatal alloimmune thrombocytopenia. Lancet 1989;i: 366–368.
13. Davoren A, et al. Neonatal alloimmune thrombocytopenia in the Irish population: a discrepancy between observed and expected cases. J Clin Pathol 2002;55: 289–292.
14. Bussel JB, Primiani A. Fetal and neonatal alloimmune thrombocytopenia: progress and ongoing debates. Blood Rev 2008;22: 33–52.
15. Dreyfus M, et al. Frequency of immune thrombocytopenia in newborns: a prospective study. Blood 1997;89: 4402–4406.
16. Letsky EA, Greaves M. Guidelines on the investigation and management of thrombocytopenia in pregnancy and neonatal alloimmune thrombocytopenia. . Br J Haematol 1996;95: 21–26
17. Berkowitz RL, et al. Parallel randomized trials of risk-based therapy for fetal alloimmune thrombocytopenia. Obstet Gynecol 2006;107: 91–96.
18. Birchall JE, et al. European collaborative study of the antenatal management of feto-maternal alloimmune thrombocytopenia. Br J Haematol 2003;122: 275–288.
19. Kjeldsen-Kragh J, et al. A screening and intervention program aimed to reduce mortality and serious morbidity associated with severe neonatal alloimmunthrombocytopenia. Blood 2007;110: 833–839.
20. Van den Akker E, et al. Noninvasive antenatal management of fetal and neonatal alloimmune thrombocytopenia: safe and effective. BJOG 2007;114: 469–473.
21. Kamphuis MM, Oepkes D. Fetal and neonatal alloimmune thrombocytopenia: prenatal interventions. Prenat Diagn 2011;31: 712–719.
22. Van den Akker E, et al. Vaginal delivery for fetuses at risk of alloimmune thrombocytopenia? BJOG 2006;113: 781–783.
23. Dale ST, Coleman LT. Neonatal alloimmune thrombocytopenia: antenatal and postnatal imaging findings in the pediatric brain. Am J Neurol 2002;23: 1457–1465.

CARE PATHWAY

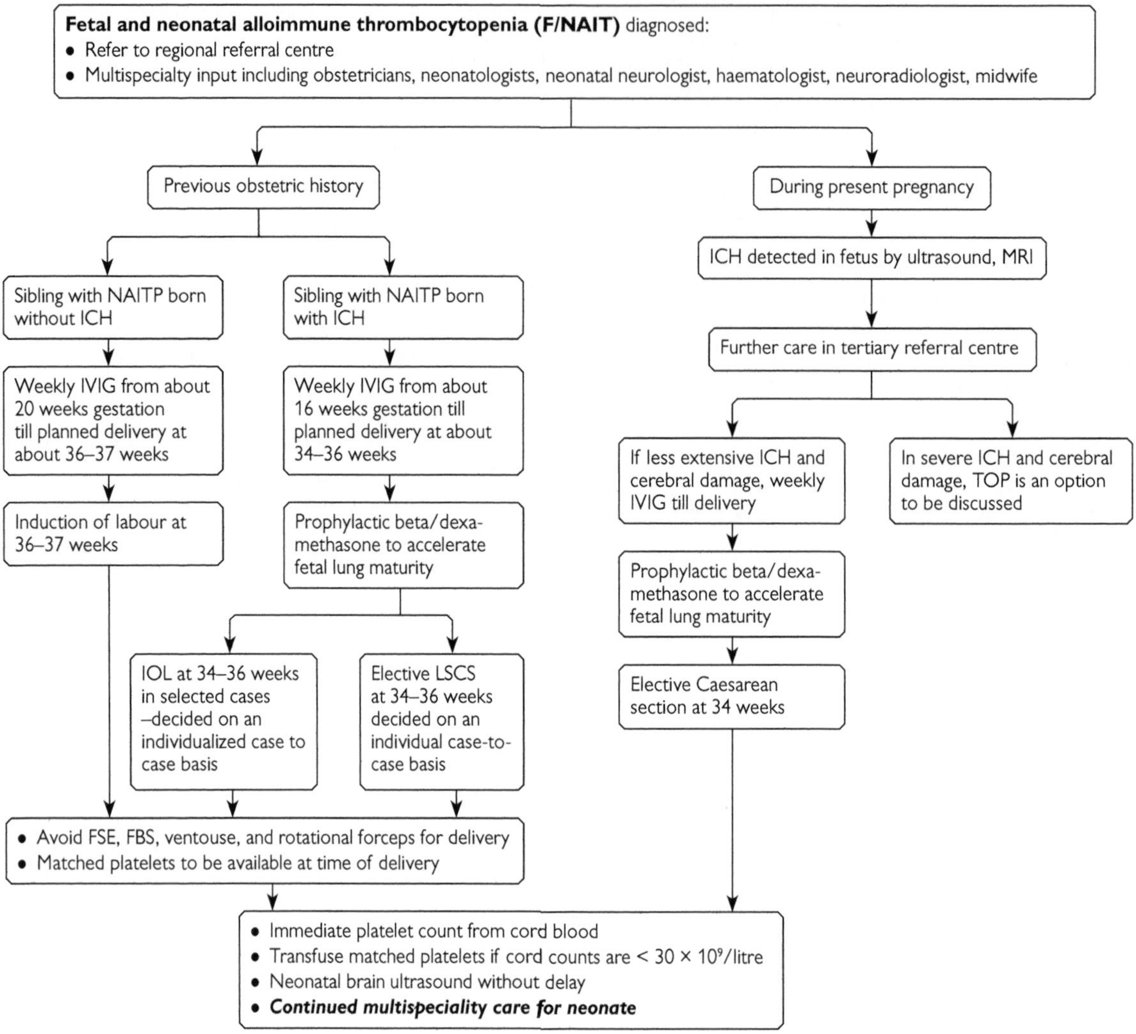
Fetal and neonatal alloimmune thrombocytopenia (F/NAIT) diagnosed:
• Refer to regional referral centre
• Multispecialty input including obstetricians, neonatologists, neonatal neurologist, haematologist, neuroradiologist, midwife
Previous obstetric history
During present pregnancy
Sibling with NAITP born without ICH
Sibling with NAITP born with ICH
ICH detected in fetus by ultrasound, MRI
Further care in tertiary referral centre
Weekly IVIG from about 20 weeks gestation till planned delivery at about 36–37 weeks
Weekly IVIG from about 16 weeks gestation till planned delivery at about 34–36 weeks
If less extensive ICH and cerebral damage, weekly IVIG till delivery
In severe ICH and cerebral damage, TOP is an option to be discussed
Induction of labour at 36–37 weeks
Prophylactic beta/dexa-methasone to accelerate fetal lung maturity
Prophylactic beta/dexa-methasone to accelerate fetal lung maturity
IOL at 34–36 weeks in selected cases –decided on an individualized case to case basis
Elective LSCS at 34–36 weeks decided on an individual case-to-case basis
Elective Caesarean section at 34 weeks
• Avoid FSE, FBS, ventouse, and rotational forceps for delivery
• Matched platelets to be available at time of delivery
• Immediate platelet count from cord blood
• Transfuse matched platelets if cord counts are < 30 × 10⁹/litre
• Neonatal brain ultrasound without delay
• Continued multispeciality care for neonate

Adapted from Kamphuis MM and Oepkes D, Fetal and neonatal alloimmune thrombocytopenia: prenatal interventions, *Prenatal Diagnosis*, 31, 7, pp. 712–719, copyright 2011, with permission from Wiley and International Society for Prenatal Diagnosis (ISPD).

28.4 Abnormal Biochemistry Markers From First/ Second-Trimester Screening

FACT FILE

There are two biochemical tests that are used to evaluate the risk for Down's syndrome. One is performed in the first trimester of pregnancy and the other in the second. These tests measure the levels of a number of substances secreted either by the fetus or the placenta These levels vary and are significantly correlated with Down's syndrome at certain weeks of pregnancy, as different quantities are secreted at specific stages of gestation (see Tables 28.1 and 28.2).

- First-trimester screening markers:
  - nuchal translucency (NT)
  - pregnancy-associated plasma protein-A (PAPP-A)
  - free beta-human chorionic gonadotropin (hCG)
- Second-trimester screening markers
  - free beta-hCG
  - inhibin A
  - unconjugated oestriol
  - alpha-fetoprotein (AFP)
- ***In certain cases, although the overall risk for trisomies is computed as low, the levels of some of the individual components of the test may be abnormal. This chapter deals with the significance of these individual markers in pregnancy if found to be abnormal.***

PAPP-A

- PAPP-A is produced by placental trophoblasts, especially the extravillous cytotrophoblasts.[1] It is a protease for insulin-like growth factor (IGF)[2] binding proteins 4 and 5. PAPP-A plays a role in the release of IGF in trophoblast invasion and thus the early development and vascularization of the developing placenta and its bed.
- A low level of PAPP-A is the most common first-trimester marker associated with adverse pregnancy outcomes.[3] Data from the **FASTER trial** (first and second trimester evaluation of the risk for fetal aneuploidy) has shown that the lower the PAPP-A result in the first trimester, the greater risk of adverse pregnancy outcomes.
- Defects in these early stages of placental formation and function, signposted by low PAPP-A levels (lowest 5% of values for gestational age or less than 0.4–0.5 MoM), may be associated with poor pregnancy outcomes that are related to abnormal trophoblast invasion. This includes miscarriage, IUGR, preterm delivery, pregnancy-induced hypertension, pre-eclampsia, preterm birth, or intrauterine death, prelabour premature rupture of membranes, all indicative of placental dysfunction.[4,5,6]
- PAPP-A levels of 0.2 MoM (multiples of the median) or less are associated with Cornelia de Lange's syndrome. Overall, fetuses with chromosomal abnormalities have low PAPP-A values. Values lower than 0.4 MoM signify an increased risk of chromosomal anomaly, making it one of the most useful biochemistry markers during the first trimester.
- Although it is a marker for adverse pregnancy outcomes, PAPP-A lacks the individual sensitivity or positive predictive value to act as a *sole* screening test.

Table 28.1 First-trimester maternal serum markers and possible adverse outcomes of pregnancy

Low PAPP-A	Miscarriage, gestational hypertension, pre-eclampsia, preterm delivery, preterm premature rupture of membranes, small for gestational age, IUD after 24 weeks pregnancy
Low free beta-hCG	Miscarriage, IUD after 24 weeks gestation, low birthweight

IUD, intrauterine fetal death.

Table 28.2 Second-trimester maternal serum markers and possible adverse outcomes of pregnancy

Elevated AFP	Miscarriage, placental abruption, abnormally adherent placenta, IUGR, IUD after 24 weeks, preterm delivery
Elevated beta-hCG	Very preterm delivery (<28 weeks), gestational hypertension, pre-eclampsia, IUD after 24 weeks gestation, low birth weight (< 10th centile)
Low unconjugated oestriol	Miscarriage, IUD >24 weeks, oligohydramnios, birth weight <10th centile
Elevated inhibin A	Pre-eclampsia, IUD >24 weeks, preterm delivery <32 weeks, IUGR

IUD, intrauterine death; IUGR, intrauterine growth retardation.

Human chorionic gonadotropin

- hCG, a glycoprotein produced by syncytiotrophoblasts, helps maintain pregnancy by stimulating progesterone synthesis by the corpus luteum. After reaching a maximum value of about 100 000 i.u/litre at 8–10 weeks gestation, the levels drop as placental steroid synthesis starts.
- The normal range is 0.2–4.5 MoM. High levels indicate a significantly raised risk of Down's syndrome, while low values are seen with an increased risk of trisomy 18. Apart from this, high levels of hCG have no correlation with specific genetic problems. High hCG levels are, of course, associated with gestational trophoblastic disease and multiple pregnancies.
- In the **first trimester**, **low levels** of free hCG (<0.5 MoM) have been associated with low birthweight and increased risk of spontaneous miscarriage, whereas **high levels** of hCG in the first trimester are not associated with such pregnancy outcomes.
- However, in the **second trimester**, while low levels of hCG have not been linked to adverse pregnancy outcomes, **elevated hCG** (>2–4 MoM) has been associated with several poor outcomes of pregnancy.[7,8]
- If there is reduced perfusion to the placenta, cytotrophoblasts proliferate as a response to hypoxic changes. This, in turn, leads to high serum hCG levels as seen in association with retroplacental haematomas, placental abruption, and low fetoplacental weight ratio.[9]
- High hCG levels may also serve as a marker for the subsequent risk for developing pregnancy complications such as pre-eclampsia (threefold increased risk)[6] and to placental dysfunction. About 10% of those with high hCG values develop obstetric complications, compared with 5% of pregnant women with a normal hCG.
- In the second trimester, an elevated serum hCG concentration has been associated with a two- to threefold increased risk of subsequent fetal growth restriction, preterm delivery, and pregnancy loss.
- As a general rule:
  - ***In trisomies 13 and 18, maternal serum free hCG and PAPP-A are decreased.***
  - ***In cases of sex chromosomal anomalies, maternal serum free hCG is normal and PAPP-A is low.***
  - ***In paternally derived triploidy, maternal serum free hCG is greatly increased, whereas PAPP-A is mildly decreased.***

- ***Maternally derived triploidy is associated with markedly decreased maternal serum free hCG and PAPP-A.***

Alpha-fetoprotein (AFP)

- AFP is a fetal glycoprotein, synthesized in early gestation by the yolk sac and then by the fetal liver. The levels normally reach a peak at 13 weeks gestation after which there is a rapid decrease. After circulation in fetal serum and extrusion into the amniotic sac by means of being passed in fetal urine, AFP then enters maternal circulation by diffusion across the placenta.[10]
- The normal range is 0.5–2.49 MoM. Elevated levels of AFP are associated with adverse pregnancy outcomes. High levels of AFP indicate an increased risk of open defects of the central nervous system and of the abdomen. Other problems that may be indicated include renal anomalies, defects of skin integrity, defects in the fusion of the anterior abdominal wall, and placental defects.
- When raised levels of this marker are found, the mother is advised to undergo an anomaly-directed ultrasound scan before the routine detailed scan at about 20 weeks gestation.
- Low levels of AFP (<0.4 MoM), are observed in certain chromosomal anomalies. In trisomies 21 and 18 serum AFP may present low values whereas in trisomy 13 it can be slightly higher than normal.
- Low AFP levels may also indicate a fetus with Down's syndrome as well as a fetus with trisomy 18. Although AFP remains one of the proteins used for screening during the second trimester it is actually one of the least useful markers. Also, screening for elevated AFP levels is a now regarded as an inferior method of screening for neural tube defects where high-quality obstetric ultrasound is available.
- An unexplained elevation of maternal serum AFP could be associated with placental conditions such as chorionic villitis as well as ischaemic or thrombotic changes in the placental vasculature.[11]
- There is a significant association between unexplained elevated levels of maternal AFP and placenta accreta, increta, or percreta.

Unconjugated oestriol

- Oestriol is an oestrogen produced in the syncytiotrophoblasts from the precursor molecule dehydroepiandrosterone sulphate (DHEAS) found in the fetal adrenals.
- This oestriol, which enters the maternal circulation, by diffusion is first detectable by about 9 weeks gestation.
- Low levels of oestriol have been found to be associated with an increased risk of Down's syndrome. In pregnancies with Down's syndrome, AFP and oestriol are lower while the level of hCG is higher. Oestriol values lower than 0.5 MoM can indicate possible trisomies of chromosomes 21, 13, or 18.
- **Chronic uteroplacental insufficiency** results in decreased DHEAS, therefore decreased oestrogen levels in both the fetus and the maternal serum. Low maternal serum oestriol levels (<0.5 MoM) are associated with adverse pregnancy outcomes.[8]
- Undetectable or absent maternal oestriol values may also indicate fetal pathology, miscarriages, growth restriction, or X-linked ichthyosis, and should lead to further investigations.[8,12]

Inhibin A

- The addition of inhibin A to the triple screen in the late 1990s resulted in the so-called **quadruple screen** (the 'quad test'). The quadruple screen can detect 70–75% of cases of fetal Down syndrome. When inhibin A values are greater than 2.5 MoM, they may be indicative of trisomy 21 or 13.
- Raised levels of inhibin A in the second trimester have been found associated with pre-eclampsia and pregnancy-induced hypertension.[7]
- Overall, the normal value for different markers is 1 MoM. Therefore, the farther away from 1 MoM the marker's level is, the worse the result.

Table 28.3 Markers and reference multiples of the median (MoM)

Marker	*MoM*
Nuchal fold thickness	>1.8–2
PAPP-A	< 0.4
hCG	<0.4, >4.5
AFP	<0.4, >2.5
Unconjugated oestriol	<0.5
Inhibin A	>2.5

Note: These are reference values, but in order to calculate the probability or risk of chromosomal anomaly different markers expressed in MoM must always be combined with the risk for the mother's age.

- Table 28.3 shows reference values, expressed in MoM. A marker is considered suspicious if its values are higher or lower than these reference values.

Antenatal surveillance of pregnancies with abnormal maternal serum markers (first or second trimester markers)

- While the association of abnormal levels of serum markers and the increased risk of adverse pregnancy outcome has been established, there is no consensus about the management of such pregnancies or of the differing modes of surveillance for varied obstetric complications that might develop.
- A balance must be achieved between creating undue anxiety in the pregnant woman with a hitherto normal pregnancy, yet informing her of possible complications and the need to maintain increased awareness of certain symptoms.
- As part of the antenatal care for such pregnancies, the pregnant woman should receive information about:
  - Being aware of fetal movements and reporting any reduction or significant change without delay
  - The symptoms and signs of pre-eclampsia; home BP monitoring may be recommended in some women
  - Reporting any bleeding without delay, whether or not it is accompanied by pain
  - Possibility of preterm contractions or preterm prelabour rupture of membranes.
- If interventions such as prescribing low-dose aspirin or extra scans are considered, adequate explanation that firm evidence is lacking those such measures would make a difference in this group. However, in practical terms such increased surveillance, once abnormal levels of serum markers have been detected, may help allay anxiety in the pregnant mother.
- The safety of low-dose aspirin during pregnancy is well established.

Surveillance and fetal monitoring

No evidence-based surveillance protocol exists to date. The following may be applicable, individualized to each case, although it must be acknowledged that these interventions or surveillance strategies are of unproven effectiveness to alter outcomes.

- **Uterine artery Doppler** has been used as a screening modality when raised serum AFP and hCG have been found in the second trimester. When a diastolic notch is found, the risk of an adverse outcome of pregnancy could be predicted with an overall sensitivity of 43%.[13] The application of this tool in routine practice in all maternity units has not been established to date.
- Consideration of interventions such as low-dose aspirin, maternal home monitoring of blood pressure.
- Regular urine checks to exclude protein from late second trimester onwards.
- Serial growth and liquor volume ultrasound scans with umbilical artery Dopplers.
- Cardiotocography ± BPP as indicated.

- If raised AFP and placenta found to be anterior and praevia, consider MRI to assess uteroplacental interface as greater chances of morbidly adherent placenta.

References

1. Handschuh K, et al. Modulation of PAPP-A expression by PPAR gamma in human first trimester trophoblast. Placenta 2006;27 suppl A: S127–134.
2. Boldt HB, Conover CA. Pregnancy-associated plasma protein-A (PAPP-A): a local regulator of IGF bioavailability through cleavage of IGFBPs. Growth Horm IGF Res 2007;17: 10–18.
3. Dugoff L, et al. First trimester maternal serum PAPP-A and free beta subunit human chorionic gonadotropin concentrations and nuchal translucency are associated with obstetric complications: a population-based screening study (the FASTER) trial. Am J Obstet Gynecol 2004;191: 1446–1451.
4. Spencer K, et al. First-trimester ultrasound and biochemical markers of aneuploidy and the prediction of impending fetal death. Ultrasound Obstet Gynecol 2006;28: 637–643.
5. Cowans NJ, Spencer K. First trimester ADAM12 and PAPP-A as markers of intrauterine fetal growth restriction through their roles in the insulin-like growth factor system. Prenat Diagn 2007;27: 264–271.
6. Dugoff L, et al. Quad screen as a predictor of adverse pregnancy outcome. Obstet Gynecol 2005;106: 260–267.
7. Lakhi N, et al. Maternal serum analytes as markers of adverse obstetric outcome. Obstetrician and Gynaecologist 2012;14: 267–273.
8. Gagnon A, et al. Obstetric complications associated with abnormal maternal serum markers analytes. J Obstet Gynaecol Can 2008;30: 918–949.
9. Liu DF, et al. Pathologic findings in pregnancies with unexplained increases in maternal serum human chorionic gonadotrophin levels. Am J Clin Pathol 1999;111: 209–215.
10. Chandra S, et al. Unexplained elevated maternal serum alpha-fetoprotein and/or human chorionic gonadotropin and the risk of adverse outcomes. Am J Obstet Gynecol 2003;189: 775–781.
11. Alkazaleh F, et al. Second-trimester prediction of severe placental complications in women with combined elevations in alpha-fetoprotein and human chorionic gonadotrophin. Am J Obstet Gynecol 2006;194: 821–827.
12. Minsart A-F, et al. Indication of prenatal diagnosis in pregnancies complicated by undetectable second-trimester maternal serum estriol levels J Prenat Med 2008;2: 27–30.
13. Elsandabesee D, et al. The clinical value of combining maternal serum screening and uterine artery Doppler in prediction of adverse pregnancy outcome. J Obstet Gynaecol 2006;26: 115–117.

CARE PATHWAY

- Combined or quadruple test performed according to NICE guidelines
- **Abnormal biochemistry markers found in otherwise 'low-risk' trisomy serum screening tests**
- Screening laboratory to fax overall trisomy risk as well as individual abnormal biochemistry result to screening coordinator in maternity unit

↓

B hCG >4.5 MoM | **PAPP-A <0.415 MoM** | **AFP >2.5 MoM**

B hCG >4.5 MoM / PAPP-A <0.415 MoM ↓

Increased risk of IUGR, abruption, pre-eclampsia, intrauterine death; degree of risk proportional to degree of deviation from median

↓

- Screening coordinator or antenatal clinic midwife informs woman of biochemistry result and possible implications.
- Appointment made to see senior obstetrician as soon as possible in a specialist antenatal clinic before 20 weeks gestation
- Contemporaneous documentation made in hospital notes

↓

- Patient seen in specialist antenatal clinic by senior obstetrician
- Discuss possible association of abnormal biochemistry markers to small increased risk of pregnancy problems including pre-eclampsia, fetal growth restriction, abruption, etc., and therefore the need for closer surveillance
- Woman advised of symptoms relating to risks (e.g. bleeding, pain, reduced fetal movements, etc.) which she needs to report directly. Contact numbers given for her to seek advice and help
- All the above to be documented in the hospital and hand-held notes
- Patient information leaflet given
- Low-dose aspirin may be considered
- Serial growth scans ± Dopplers organized from 26 weeks onwards according to individual maternity unit's protocol for serial scans. Specialist clinic antenatal checks on same day
- Community midwife to be informed of abnormal biochemistry results by screening coordinator and need for stepped-up surveillance for pre-eclampsia, clinical fetal growth assessments
- Prompt re- referral to specialist antenatal clinic if any signs of IUGR or concerns noted by community midwife

↓

- If IUGR, pre-eclampsia, or abruption suspected, refer to relevant care pathways
- If pregnancy otherwise uncomplicated, rest of care according to NICE pathway for normal pregnancy

AFP >2.5 MoM ↓

- Patient informed of possible association with neural tube fusion defects, etc. and therefore need for extra scans at 16 and 18 weeks for fetal spine, abdominal wall, and lip and palate
- Arrange preliminary scan for neural tube and abdominal wall within 3 working days, if possible
- Further scans at 16 and 18 weeks gestation
- If NAD in these scans, proceed with routine anomaly scan at about 20 weeks gestation as routine
- If NAD, antenatal care reverts to low-risk community midwife-led care according to NICE guidelines
- Any concerns—prompt referral to specialist antenatal clinic for individualized management

28.5 Reduced Fetal Movements

FACT FILE

Normal fetal movements

- Spontaneous fetal movements are generated as early as 7 weeks gestation. By the end of 15 weeks gestation, the fetus has developed all but one of the 15 distinct varieties of movements (e.g. general body movements, isolated limb movements, jaw movements, breathing movements, swallowing, sucking, stretch, yawn, hiccups, startle) that the baby will display after birth.[1] Fetal eye movement is the last to develop and can be observed from 16–18 weeks onwards.[2]
- Once developed, these movements persist unchanged during the entire course of the pregnancy. From 16 weeks to term, the fetus repeatedly performs these 15 types of movements.[1]
- Maternal perception of fetal movements usually commences at 18–20 weeks gestation, with multiparas being able to recognize movements earlier than primigravidae.
- Mothers feel only a proportion of fetal movements (37–88%), whole body movements or those lasting for more than 7 s being the ones felt most often.
- Fetal movements include discrete kicks, flutters, rolls, prods, etc.
- Fetal movements increase till 32 weeks and then plateau until labour. However, there is no decrease in the number and frequency of movements after 32 weeks gestation, although the quality of movements necessarily changes.
- Diurnal changes are seen as early as 20 weeks gestation; fetal movements are maximal in the afternoons and evenings.[3]
- Fetal sleep periods take place regularly throughout the day and night. During sleep periods there are few movements. These sleep periods usually last for 20–40 min at a time and, in a healthy fetus, rarely last for more than 90 min.
- Maternal perception of movements may be influenced by various factors:
  - She is less likely to note fetal movements when busy during the daytime. Studies have shown that when the woman focuses on fetal movements lying semi-recumbent on her left side in a quiet room, she is usually able to appreciate 10 movements within a mean time of 21 min. When not focusing on fetal movement counting, the mean time taken for her to perceive 10 movements increases to 162 minutes.[4]
  - An anterior placenta may serve to blunt the maternal perception before 28 weeks gestation, though not after.
  - Alcohol and drugs such as opioids or benzodiazepines can cause a transient reduction in fetal movements. Corticosteroids cause a decrease of fetal movements for about 48 h.[5]
  - Smoking, which increases maternal carboxyhaemoglobin, causes a decrease of fetal movements.[6]
  - Fetal neurological or skeletal abnormalities can cause a lack of vigorous fetal movements (e.g. arthrogryposis).
  - When the fetal back is anterior, maternal perception of movements may be reduced.[7]

Antenatal surveillance to prevent stillbirth

- The rate of stillbirths (excluding congenital abnormalities) in the UK is about 4 per 1000 total births.[8]
- The objectives of antenatal surveillance include detection of a fetus at risk in a pregnancy with no identified risk factors for an adverse outcome as well as the safe management of a pregnancy where there are recognized risk factors for adverse perinatal outcomes.
- Various methodologies for antepartum fetal surveillance exist, ranging from maternal awareness of fetal movement to in-depth biophysical profile with Doppler studies and cardiotocography (CTG).
- No antenatal surveillance strategy, either simple or complex, even if appropriately applied to all women (with or without risk factors), can prevent all adverse perinatal outcomes. The effectiveness of the test depends on its timely application followed by appropriate intervention, and effective clinical action if feasible.
- It is difficult to find evidence from existing research evidence that antenatal surveillance methodologies are directly responsible for improved fetal outcomes because of:
  - variations in the interpretation of fetal surveillance tests, especially the CTG
  - variations in the interventions applied when abnormal results of fetal surveillance tests are found[9]
  - lack of standardization of reporting of important adverse fetal outcomes other than perinatal death.

Relationship between maternal perception of decreased fetal movements and adverse fetal outcome

- Studies have shown that the majority of women who have suffered a stillbirth have observed a decrease in fetal movements for a varying period of time before confirmation of the IUD.[10,11]
- Yet, formal fetal movement counting in low-risk pregnancies setting a specified alarm limit, was not shown to have any advantage in a large RCT[12] conducted in the early 1980s when CTG monitoring had just been introduced into routine practice.
- **Several methodological issues have now emerged questioning the validity of this RCT of Grant et al.[12] which had concluded that formal counting of fetal movements had no advantages over an informal awareness of fetal movements by the mother in low-risk pregnancies.[8,13]** The concerns regarding this RCT[12] include:
  - Delayed reporting of reduced fetal movements. In this study patients with reduced fetal movements were assessed with a delay of up to 48 h, whereas other studies on fetal movement counts required women to report reduced fetal movements within 1–12 h.
  - 14% of these patients were managed by telephone advice alone without actually being seen once they reported reduced fetal movements. This might explain the high stillbirth rate on admission found in this study, **thus reflecting inadequate management protocols than a reflection of the inherent value of fetal movement counting**.
  - No data was collected on perinatal morbidity or neonatal mortality.
  - As approximately 60% of controls who were not meant to count fetal movements nevertheless had to sign a consent form, these controls were aware of the formal fetal movement counting system. This inevitably introduces bias due to the Hawthorne effect prejudicing outcomes. Almost 7% of women in the control group filled in fetal movement count charts. There was a high reporting rate of reduced fetal movements, which was not expected in the control group, thus making contamination of results inevitable.
  - Only 60% in the fetal movement counting arm of the study complied with charting movements and only 50% adhered to the study threshold of decreased movements.
- Numerous studies have shown a significant reduction in stillbirth rates after introduction of fetal movement counting in various pregnant populations, and several meta-analyses[15,16] analysing 24 studies have shown that:
  - In high-risk pregnancies, decreased fetal movements are associated with increased risk of adverse outcomes.
  - In low-risk pregnancies, there was a trend towards lower fetal mortality rates among those women who maintained fetal movement counts compared with controls, though this did not reach statistical significance.
  - With the setting of alarm limit on fetal movement counting, it is estimated that the number of antenatal visits would increase by 2 to 3 per 100 pregnancies.
- ***Such analyses provide support for the use of fetal movement counting in pregnancies, particularly those with risk factors for adverse perinatal outcomes.***

Fetal movement counting

The purpose of fetal movement counting is to evaluate three types of fetuses:

- **The healthy fetus:** A fetus with normal activity of 6 or more movements perceived by the mother in an interval of 2 h is generally healthy.
- **The structurally normal fetus at risk of adverse perinatal outcomes** due to maternal diseases or fetal conditions. In such cases if the mother experiences decreased fetal movements, this warrants examination and further tests such as CTG, ultrasound scanning for amniotic fluid volume, Doppler flow studies, and BPP as indicated.
- **The fetus with anatomical anomalies:** Babies with anomalies show a greater rate of reduced fetal movements when compared with those without such anomalies, varying between 16.5% vs 1% in one study [17] and 28% vs 4%[18,19] in another. In some cases, therefore, a second-look ultrasound scan may help identify previously unsuspected anomalies and thus influence management plans.

Antenatal management of reduced fetal movements

- When a woman presents with reduced fetal movements (RFM), **a careful history regarding RFM** should be taken, including enquiry into the duration of RFM, any previous such episodes, any associated pain or vaginal bleeding, and whether fetal movements are entirely absent or reduced.[8]
- **A comprehensive and systematic history** to obtain a stillbirth risk evaluation will need to include previous episodes when the patient presented with RFM, identified IUGR, maternal diabetes, hypertension, smoking, alcohol or opioid misuse, recent course of steroids (dexa-or betamethasone) within 48 h, extremes of maternal age, primiparity, maternal obesity, previous poor obstetric history (IUGR, IUD), known fetal anomaly, poor attender for antenatal checks, etc.
- **Evaluation of maternal** status including pulse, BP, urine analysis for protein, ketones, glucose, and signs of pathological oedema, should be noted. If she is diabetic, a blood sugar reading must be taken.
- **Fetal tests:** The first-line test is to auscultate for the fetal heart with a handheld Doppler, differentiating it from maternal pulse, to exclude fetal death.
- **After fetal viability confirmation, clinical assessment** of the symphysio-fundal height and fetal presentation should be performed.
- This is followed by a CTG initially for a minimum of 20 min, if the pregnancy is more than 28 weeks gestation. Rates of this initial CTG showing non-reassuring features have been found to vary between 3% and 21%.[20,21]
- Ultrasound scan assessment is indicated within 24 h preferably, if RFM persists though the CTG was reassuring in a pregnancyof more than 28 weeks gestation **or** there are additional risk factors identified for IUGR or IUD. The ultrasound scan should measure amniotic fluid volume (deepest pool), abdominal circumference, and/or estimated fetal weight is IUGR is suspected. Some studies suggest adding Doppler studies of the umbilical artery to this assessment, others have not shown addition of Doppler confers any added benefit.[22]
- If, for some reason the patient has not previously had an anomaly scan, this should be offered at the earliest opportunity.
- A BPP has mainly a negative predictive value and does not form part of the fetal assessment strategy in this context.[8]
- If all investigations are normal after the initial episode of RFM and there no risk factors for IUD or IUGR are identified, further routine CTGs are not indicated.
- Some practitioners suggest advising the woman to start formal counting of fetal movements after one episode of RFM, but there is no firm evidence to support this.[8] **The woman must be advised, however, to promptly report any recurrence of RFM to the maternity unit.**
- ***Increased risk of poor perinatal outcomes are found in those who present with repeated episodes of RFM compared with those who present with only a single episode.***[23]
- ***Detailed documentation is of paramount importance in all cases that present with RFM including the advice offered about follow-up and vigilance to directly report any recurrence of RFM to the maternity unit without delay.***
- Decisions regarding IOL in women with repeated episodes of RFM where no problems have been identified on CTG or ultrasound scan, must be ideally consultant-directed.

Information for patients

Please see Information for patients: Reduced movements of the baby (p. 559)

References

1. de Vries JIP, et al. The emergence of fetal behaviour: qualitative aspects. Early Hum Dev 1982;7: 301–322.
2. Bots RSGM. Human fetal eye movements: detection in utero by ultrasonography. Early Hum Dev 1981;5: 87–94.
3. Nijhuis J, et al. Are there behavioural states in the human fetus? Early Hum Dev 1982;6: 177–195.
4. Moore TR, Piacquadio KA. Prospective evaluation of fetal movement screening to reduce the incidence of antepartum fetal death. Am J Obstet Gynecol 1989;160: 1075–1080.
5. Mulder EJ. Antenatal corticosteroid therapy and fetal behaviour: a randomised study of the effects of betamethasone and dexamethasone. Br J Obstet Gynaecol 1997;104: 1239–1247.
6. Ritchie K. The fetal response to changes in the composition of maternal inspired air in human pregnancy. Semin Perinatol 1980;4: 295–299.
7. Fisher ML. Reduced fetal movements: a research-based project. Br J Midwifery 1999;7: 733–737.
8. RCOG Green-top Guideline No. 57. Reduced fetal movements. London: Royal College of Obstetricians and Gynaecologists, 2011.
9. Barrett JF, et al. Inconsistencies in clinical decisions in obstetrics. Lancet 1990;336 (8714): 549–551.
10. Efkarpidis S, et al. Case-control study of factors associated with intrauterine fetal deaths. Med Gen Med 2004;6: 53.
11. Saastad E, et al. care in stillbirths—a retrospective audit study. Acta Obstet Gynecol Scand 2007;86: 444–450.
12. Grant A, et al. Routine formal fetal movement counting and risk of antepartum late death in normally formed singletons. Lancet 1989; ii: 345–349.
13. Liston R, et al. Fetal health surveillance: antepartum and intrapartum consensus guideline. J Obstet Gynaecol Can 2007;29Suppl 4: S3–56.
14. Westgate J, Jamieson M. Stillbirths and fetal movements. N Z Med J 1986;99: 114–116.
15. Frøen JF. A kick from within—fetal movement counting and the cancelled progress in antenatal care. J Perinat Med 2004;32: 13–24
16. Frøen JF, et al. Management of decreased fetal movements. Semin Perinatol 2008;32: 307–311.
17. Sadovsky EJ, et al. Decreased fetal movements and fetal malformations. Fetal Med 1981;1: 62.
18. Rayburn WF, McKean HE. Maternal perception of fetal movement and perinatal outcome. Obstet Gynecol 1980;56: 161–164.
19. Rayburn WF, Barr M. Activity patterns in malformed fetuses. Am J Obstet Gynecol 1982;142: 1045–1048.
20. Saastad E, Tveit JVH. Uniform information on fetal activity is associated with reduction of stillbirth rates among primiparous mothers: an intervention study from Norway. International Stillbirth Alliance Annual Conference 2007.
21. Whitty JE, et al. Maternal perception of decreased fetal movement as an indication for antepartum testing in a low-risk population. Am J Obstet Gynecol 1991;165: 1084–1088.
22. O'Sullivan O, et al. Predicting poor perinatal outcome in women who present with decreased fetal movements. J Obstet Gynaecol 2009;29: 705–710.

CARE PATHWAY

First presentation at >28 weeks gestation

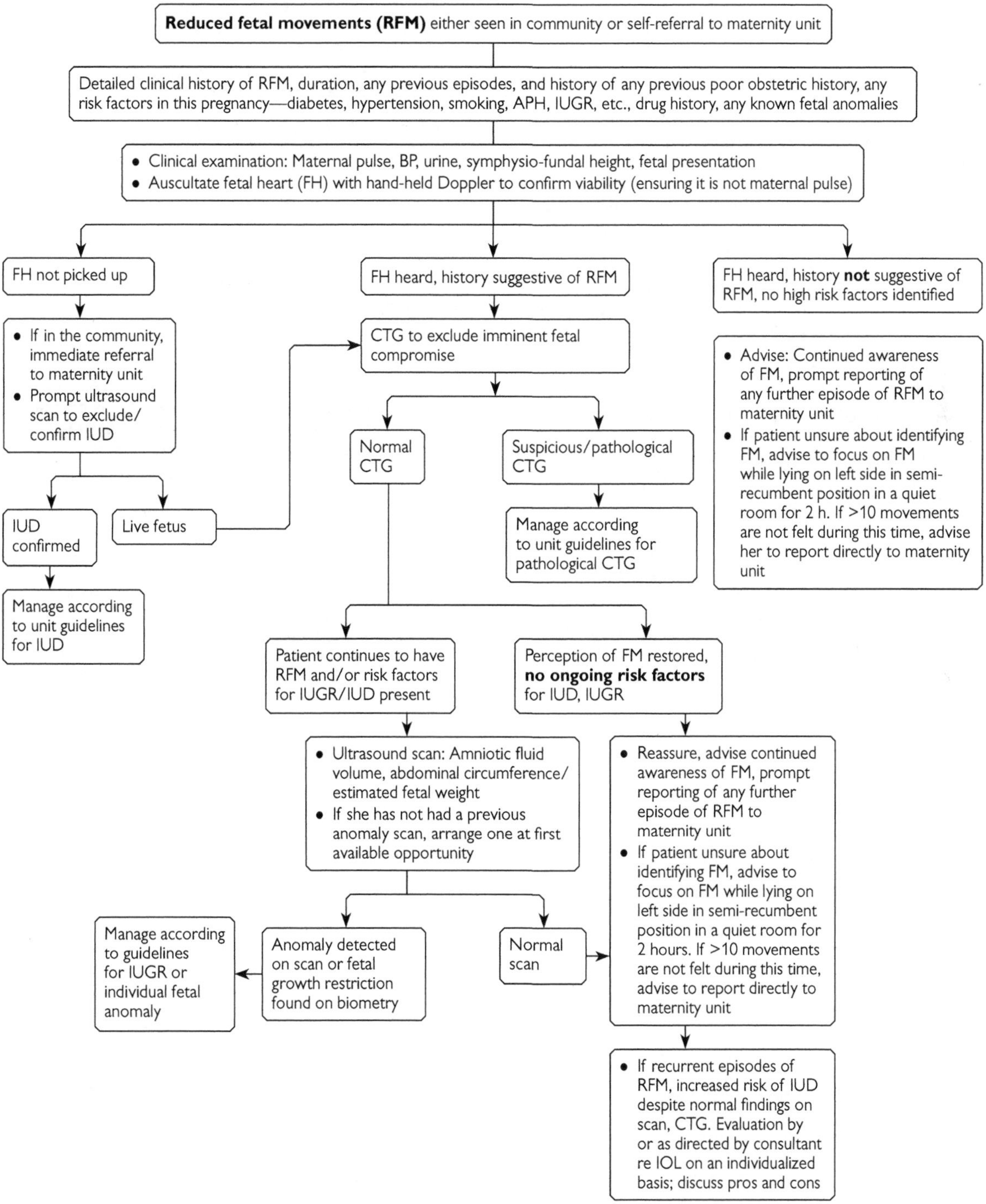

Reduced fetal movements (RFM) either seen in community or self-referral to maternity unit
Detailed clinical history of RFM, duration, any previous episodes, and history of any previous poor obstetric history, any risk factors in this pregnancy—diabetes, hypertension, smoking, APH, IUGR, etc., drug history, any known fetal anomalies
• Clinical examination: Maternal pulse, BP, urine, symphysio-fundal height, fetal presentation
• Auscultate fetal heart (FH) with hand-held Doppler to confirm viability (ensuring it is not maternal pulse)
FH not picked up
FH heard, history suggestive of RFM
FH heard, history **not** suggestive of RFM, no high risk factors identified
• If in the community, immediate referral to maternity unit
• Prompt ultrasound scan to exclude/ confirm IUD
CTG to exclude imminent fetal compromise
• Advise: Continued awareness of FM, prompt reporting of any further episode of RFM to maternity unit
• If patient unsure about identifying FM, advise to focus on FM while lying on left side in semi-recumbent position in a quiet room for 2 h. If >10 movements are not felt during this time, advise her to report directly to maternity unit
Normal CTG
Suspicious/pathological CTG
IUD confirmed
Live fetus
Manage according to unit guidelines for pathological CTG
Manage according to unit guidelines for IUD
Patient continues to have RFM and/or risk factors for IUGR/IUD present
Perception of FM restored, **no ongoing risk factors** for IUD, IUGR
• Ultrasound scan: Amniotic fluid volume, abdominal circumference/ estimated fetal weight
• If she has not had a previous anomaly scan, arrange one at first available opportunity
• Reassure, advise continued awareness of FM, prompt reporting of any further episode of RFM to maternity unit
• If patient unsure about identifying FM, advise to focus on FM while lying on left side in semi-recumbent position in a quiet room for 2 hours. If >10 movements are not felt during this time, advise to report directly to maternity unit
Manage according to guidelines for IUGR or individual fetal anomaly
Anomaly detected on scan or fetal growth restriction found on biometry
Normal scan
• If recurrent episodes of RFM, increased risk of IUD despite normal findings on scan, CTG. Evaluation by or as directed by consultant re IOL on an individualized basis; discuss pros and cons

Reproduced from: Royal College of Obstetricians and Gynaecologists. Reduced fetal movements. Green-top Guideline No. 57. London: RCOG; 2011, with the permission of the Royal College of Obstetricians and Gynaecologists

First presentation <24 weeks

Woman presents before 24 weeks gestation with RFM, having felt them in last few weeks

History, initial examination. auscultate with hand-held Doppler

FH not picked up
- Urgent referral to maternity unit for ultrasound scan

FH auscultated
- Reassure patient
- Check report of previous anomaly scan at ~20 weeks—note placental position, structural normality
- **If no risk factors**, further investigations not required
- **If risk factors present**, advise awareness of FM and to start counts from about 28 weeks gestation

- Scan confirms IUD
- Further management according to unit guidelines for IUD

- Live fetus. Check placental site—if anteriorly located may blunt maternal perception of FM till 28 weeks gestation, but not after
- Reassure patient, advise awareness of FM. **If no risk factors for IUD or IUGR**, no further investigations necessary
- **If risk factors for IUD/IUGR**, advise FM counting from ~28 weeks

Woman presents <24 weeks gestation, **not having felt FM at all in this pregnancy**

- Detailed history and clinical examination: Note any risk factors, e.g. gross obesity, primigravida, anterior location of placenta, maternal diabetes, hypertension, any vaginal bleeding or pain, previous poor obstetric history if applicable
- Check report of previous anomaly scan at ~20 weeks—note placental position, any structural abnormality noted

Auscultation with hand-held Doppler

FH not picked up: urgent referral to maternity unit for ultrasound scan

Scan confirms IUD
Further management according to unit guidelines for IUD

Live fetus on scan, movements visualized
- Reassure mother, advise awareness of FM
- **If no risk factors for IUD or IUGR**, no further investigations necessary
- **If risk factors for IUD/IUGR**, advise FM counting from ~28 weeks

Live fetus on scan, no movements visualized
- **No movements visualized** even after scanning for 15–20 min
- Check images of previous scan at 20 weeks and note findings. If consistence absence of fetal movements, suspicion of neuromuscular abnormality such as fetal akinesia
- Urgent referral to tertiary centre for further investigations

Presentation at 24–28 weeks gestation

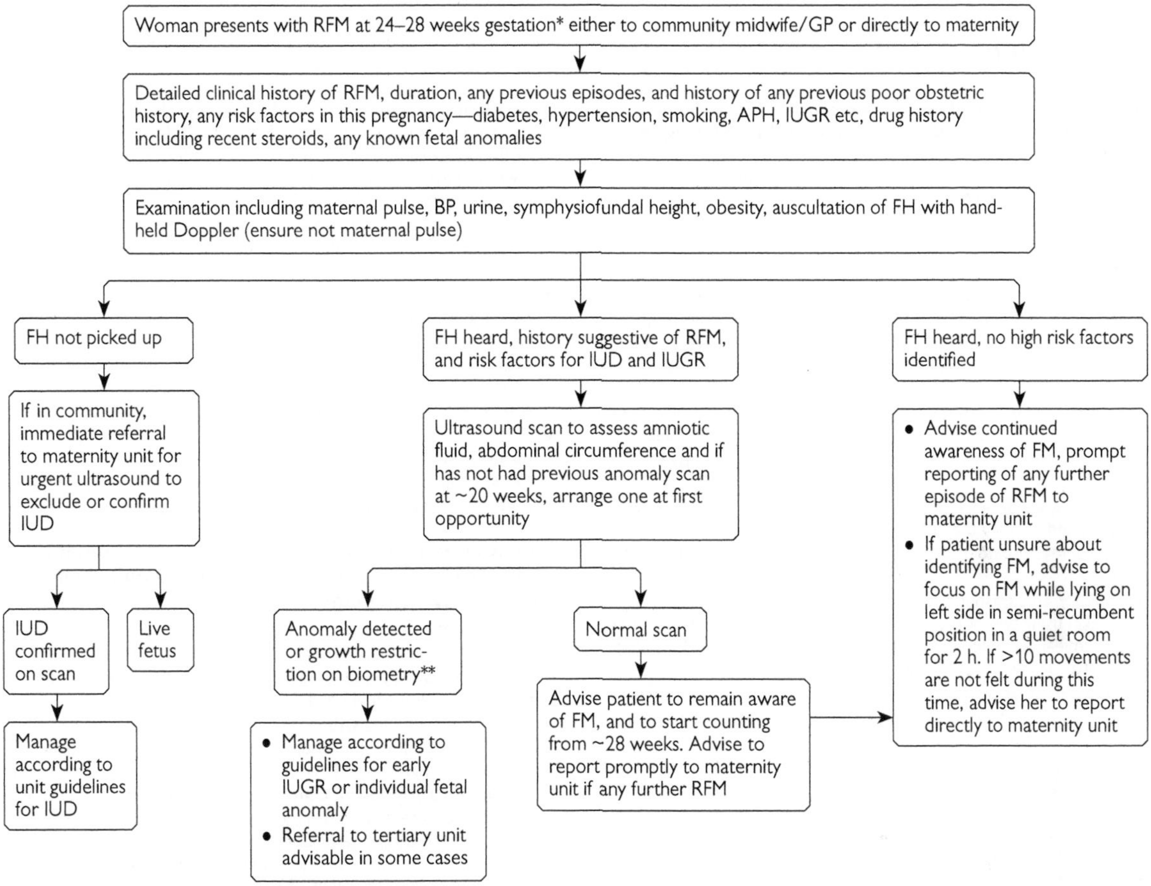
Woman presents with RFM at 24–28 weeks gestation* either to community midwife/GP or directly to maternity
Detailed clinical history of RFM, duration, any previous episodes, and history of any previous poor obstetric history, any risk factors in this pregnancy—diabetes, hypertension, smoking, APH, IUGR etc, drug history including recent steroids, any known fetal anomalies
Examination including maternal pulse, BP, urine, symphysiofundal height, obesity, auscultation of FH with hand-held Doppler (ensure not maternal pulse)
FH not picked up
If in community, immediate referral to maternity unit for urgent ultrasound to exclude or confirm IUD
IUD confirmed on scan
Live fetus
Manage according to unit guidelines for IUD
FH heard, history suggestive of RFM, and risk factors for IUD and IUGR
Ultrasound scan to assess amniotic fluid, abdominal circumference and if has not had previous anomaly scan at ~20 weeks, arrange one at first opportunity
Anomaly detected or growth restriction on biometry**
• Manage according to guidelines for early IUGR or individual fetal anomaly
• Referral to tertiary unit advisable in some cases
Normal scan
Advise patient to remain aware of FM, and to start counting from ~28 weeks. Advise to report promptly to maternity unit if any further RFM
FH heard, no high risk factors identified
• Advise continued awareness of FM, prompt reporting of any further episode of RFM to maternity unit
• If patient unsure about identifying FM, advise to focus on FM while lying on left side in semi-recumbent position in a quiet room for 2 h. If >10 movements are not felt during this time, advise her to report directly to maternity unit

* Note: No evidence to support routine use of CTG at this gestation.
** If early growth restriction suspected, more detailed ultrasound studies may be indicated.

Adapted from RCOG Green-top Guideline No. 57, *Reduced fetal movements*, 2011

28.6 Prolonged Pregnancy

FACT FILE

- ***WHO definition of a post-term pregnancy is one that has extended to or beyond 42 completed weeks (294 days) of gestation.***[1]
- In older studies, the incidence of prolonged pregnancies was reported to be 5–10%;[2] however, with the accuracy in dating pregnancies achieved by first-trimester ultrasound scans, the incidence is closer to 2–5%.[3]
- Accurate initial dating of pregnancy is crucial when decisions are made regarding interventions for 'post-term pregnancy'.[4]
- Routine use of first-trimester scans rather than last menstrual period (LMP) has been shown in several studies to have a significant impact in reducing rates of induction of labour for 'post-term' pregnancy.[5,6,7]
- First-trimester ultrasound scanning, ideally at 11–13 weeks, should be offered as it is a more accurate assessment of gestational age than the LMP, with fewer pregnancies prolonged past 41+0 weeks.[8]
- If there is a difference of more than 5 days between gestational age dated by using the LMP and the first-trimester ultrasound scan, the estimated date of delivery should be adjusted according to the scan.
- Similarly, an ultrasound scan in the second trimester (13–26 weeks) using two or more parameters such as biparietal diameter, abdominal circumference, and femur length, is accurate for dating pregnancies within ± 10 days.
- Induction of labour for 'post-term' pregnancies is decreased when gestational age is calculated using a second-trimester scan versus the LMP alone.[9]
- In units offering only a routine second-trimester ultrasound scan at about 20 weeks gestation for both dating and anomaly surveillance, if there is a difference of more than 10 days between scan derived dates and the LMP, the estimated date of delivery should be adjusted according to the scan.
- Where there has been both a first- and a second-trimester scan, gestational age should be determined by the earlier ultrasound.

Risks involved with prolonged pregnancies

- The risk of stillbirth increases from 41 weeks onwards, as shown in several studies. The rate of stillbirth increases from 0.35 per 1000 at 37 weeks to 2.12 per 1000 at 43 weeks, a six-fold increase.[7,10]
- A recent RCOG scientific opinion paper[11] highlights, in particular, the higher fetal and maternal risks faced by **older mothers** (≥40 years) including placental abruption, low birth weight, placenta praevia, pre- and post- term delivery, and PPH. The risk of stillbirth at 39 weeks gestation in women aged 40 and over is similar to the stillbirth risk at 41 weeks in those aged 25–29 years.[11,12,13]
- Prolonged pregnancy has also been shown to increase the risk of meconium staining of liquor, meconium aspiration, failure to progress in labour, increased risk of operative delivery (both instrumental vaginal and Caesarean section), macrosomia, shoulder dystocia, intrapartum fetal hypoxia, low Apgar scores, neonatal seizures, and perinatal death.[7,9,14]
- Perinatal mortality, particularly rates of antepartum stillbirths after 37 weeks gestation, have been shown to be significantly higher among women of South Asian origin (India, Pakistan, Bangladesh, Sri Lanka) in the UK, even after adjusting for confounding factors.[15]

Interventions to reduce prolonged pregnancies beyond 41+0 weeks gestation

- Women with uncomplicated pregnancies should be given every opportunity to go into spontaneous labour.[9]
- **Accurate dating of pregnancy** with a first-trimester ultrasound scan reduces the rate of 'prolonged pregnancies' dated erroneously with LMP alone.
- **Stretching of the cervix and sweeping of membranes:** If the cervical os is more than 1–1.5 cm dilated, further stretching of the cervix can be performed during an internal examination. Sweeping the membranes involves separating the membranes as high as possible from the cervix and lower uterine segment during a vaginal examination, by inserting a finger through the cervical os and circling it by 360° if possible. This procedure obviously requires the cervix to be sufficiently dilated.
- Sweeping of the membranes has been shown to release endogenous prostaglandins with plasma prostaglandin levels rising to 10% of those in active labour.[16]
- Membrane stripping has been shown to be an effective outpatient method to reduce the number of pregnancies going beyond 41+0 weeks gestation as well as the sweep-to-delivery interval.[16]
- This benefit has been mainly seen in nulliparous women with relatively unfavourable cervices.[17]
- Other studies have demonstrated that membrane stripping at term is more effective if performed on multiple occasions.[18]

Induction of labour versus expectant management at and from 41 weeks gestation in uncomplicated singleton live pregnancies

- Several studies have shown that all components of perinatal mortality are significantly increased at 42 weeks and beyond.[6,7,9,11,12]
- Uncertainty is still present regarding optimum management of pregnancies between 41 and 42 weeks gestation.
- Three large meta-analyses including the Canadian trial of Hannah et al. and the Cochrane Collaboration, each including several studies, have shown that IOL at 41 or more weeks results in:
    - a **significantly lower Caesarean section rate** than in those managed expectantly.[19] (In the Cochrane meta-analyses there was no increased rate of Caesarean section or of operative vaginal delivery in those undergoing induction compared with those managed expectantly.[20])
    - a **lower rate of fetal distress** than expectant management
    - a **lower rate of meconium staining of amniotic fluid and meconium aspiration syndrome** than expectant management
    - a **lower rate of macrosomia** than expectant management
    - a **lower rate of fetal or neonatal death** (excluding congenital malformations) than those managed expectantly. (This was statistically significant in the Canadian meta-analyses,[19] but although lower rates were found in the two other meta-analyses they did not reach statistical significance,[20,21] mainly due to inadequate numbers of women enrolled in these studies.)
- ***IOL at ≥41 weeks thus seems to reduce the need for Caesarean section or an operative vaginal delivery, or the baby to have fetal distress, meconium-stained liquor or fetal distress in labour or to die during the perinatal period.***
- These meta-analyses have influenced the current practice in most UK maternity units, especially with the benefit of accurate dating achieved by first-trimester ultrasound scanning.
- Routine induction of labour is offered to women with uncomplicated, singleton, live pregnancies after 41 weeks gestation.
- This policy does not increase the Caesarean section rate.
- A proportion of women will spontaneously deliver between 41 and 42 weeks gestation. Provided there is no indication for an earlier delivery, most units have adopted a policy of offering routine IOL at 40^{+7} to 40^{+14} according to availability of resources.
- In the largest study to date, at 37 weeks gestation, 45% of women thought that they would agree to expectant management, but this changed as the pregnancy advanced. Only 31% of women at 41 weeks gestation were agreeable to an expectant policy to await spontaneous onset of labour, even though that was the policy of that unit.[22]

Recommendation on maternal request for induction of labour

- Maternal request from healthy younger women(<40 yrs) for early IOL (<40 weeks) in uncomplicated pregnancies should be discouraged with sensitive and sympathetic explanations.[9] However, under exceptional circumstances (e.g. if the woman's partner is soon to be posted abroad with the armed forces), induction may be considered at or after 39-40 weeks.
- In applying any such policy, it must be acknowledged that some women would prefer to await natural onset of labour even beyond 42 weeks.
- Successful management of a prolonged pregnancy therefore depends on effective counselling and full involvement of women in the decision-making process.[23]
- The exact timing of induction should take into account preferences of the women and local circumstances.[9]

Fetal surveillance of pregnancies after 41 completed weeks gestation

- There are no randomized trials regarding antepartum fetal surveillance between 41 and 42 weeks gestation, though general consensus is that some form of fetal surveillance should be applied.[9]
- There is no universal consensus, either, in what type of fetal surveillance modality needs to be employed and at what frequency and whether one modality is better than another.[8,19,23,24] Options for fetal surveillance include fetal movement counting, CTG, ultrasound scan for liquor volume, modified biophysical profiles (with added CTG), and Doppler studies of the umbilical artery.
- Both observational data and a RCT[24] have shown no **clinical differences between simple and complex monitoring**.
- Amniotic fluid volume measurement usually forms part of the surveillance, either using the maximum vertical pool depth (MVPD) of amniotic fluid index (AFI).[25]
- The American College of Obstetricians and Gynecologist (2004, level III recommendation) suggests initiating fetal surveillance between 41 and 42 weeks with twice-weekly assessment of amniotic fluid volume and a CTG.[26]
- The Society of Obstetricians and Gynaecologists of Canada, based on the recommendations from the Canadian trial,[19] recommend daily fetal movement counting with thrice-weekly CTGs and amniotic fluid volume assessment 2–3 times per week.
- NICE and the Royal College of Obstetricians and Gynaecologists recommend increased fetal surveillance consisting of **twice-weekly CTG and an ultrasound scan for maximal amniotic pool depth from 42 weeks gestation** in women who decline IOL.[9,27]
- Each unit needs to formulate a system for fetal surveillance for those pregnancies prolonged beyond 41 weeks gestation, depending on the resources and facilities available.

In summary:

- At the 38-week antenatal visit, all women should be offered information about the risks with pregnancies that last longer than 42 weeks, and their options.[9] They should be informed that most women will go into labour spontaneously by 42 weeks.
- Options, as relevant, must be discussed including:
  - membrane sweeping, which makes spontaneous labour more likely, and so reduces the need for formal induction of labour to prevent prolonged pregnancy
  - what a membrane sweep involves, and that that mild discomfort and vaginal bleeding are possible from the procedure
  - induction of labour between 41+0 and 42+0 weeks
  - expectant management.
- Healthcare professionals should explain the following points to women being offered IOL for prolonged pregnancy:
  - reasons why IOL is being offered
  - when, where, and how IOL will be carried out
  - arrangements for support and pain relief
  - alternative options if the woman chooses not to have IOL
  - that IOL may not be successful, and what the woman's options then would be.
- Healthcare professionals offering induction of labour should:
  - allow the woman time to discuss the information with her partner before coming to a decision
  - encourage the woman to look at a variety of sources of information
  - invite the woman to ask questions, and encourage her to think about her options
  - support the woman in whatever decision she makes.
- Points to note before discussions or arrangements are made for 'routine' IOL for prolonged pregnancies:
  - Ensure that the pregnancy has been uncomplicated and that no high-risk factors have developed since her last antenatal visit.
  - Ensure that it is a singleton, live pregnancy.
  - Ensure that the EDD has been arrived at by means of a first-trimester ultrasound scan, with dates adjusted if the difference between scan and LMP dates is more than 5 days.
  - Recheck that the presentation is cephalic.
  - Enquire regarding fetal movements.
  - Discuss management options with the woman if the pregnancy was to go past 41 weeks gestation, and note her preferences.
  - Offer sweeping of membranes after 40 weeks gestation on a single occasion or repeated, following a discussion of risks and benefits. This could be performed by the community midwife.
  - Discuss increase in perinatal and maternal problems if pregnancy is prolonged much beyond 41 weeks.
  - Reassure the woman that IOL after 41 weeks pregnancy does not increase the overall risk of Caesarean section compared with expectant management. The policy of IOL at about 41–42 weeks gestation reduces the risk of perinatal death, meconium staining and aspiration syndrome, fetal distress in labour, and macrosomia, compared with expectant management continued to or beyond 42 weeks.
  - The exact timing of induction will depend on local circumstances and unit policy while taking maternal preferences into account.
  - If a woman chooses not to have IOL, her decision should be respected and increased fetal surveillance in the form of maximal amniotic pool depth assessment and CTG twice a week should be offered.[27]
  - Remind the woman to report any reduction of fetal movements without delay to the day assessment unit or delivery suite even if the CTG/scan has been reassuring, while anticipating spontaneous onset of labour or the agreed date of IOL.

Information for patients

Please see **Information for patients: Prolonged pregnancy** (p. 560)

References

1. WHO. International statistical classification of diseases and related health problems, 10th revision. Geneva: World Health Organization, 2006.
2. Shea KM, et al. Post term delivery: a challenge for epidemiologic research. Epidemiology 1998;9: 199–204
3. Boyd ME, et al. Obstetric consequences of postmaturity. Am J Obstet Gynecol 1988;158: 334–338.
4. Gardosi J, et al. Gestational age and induction of labour for prolonged pregnancy. Br J Obstet Gynaecol 1997;104: 792–797.
5. Bennett KA, et al. First trimester ultrasound screening is effective in reducing post term induction rates: a randomized controlled trial. Am J Obstet Gynecol 2004;190: 1077–1081.
6. Crowley P. Interventions for preventing or improving the outcome of delivery at or beyond term. Cochrane Database Syst Rev 2004; 4.
7. Treger M, et al. Post-term pregnancy: should induction of labor be considered before 42 weeks? J Matern Fetal Med 2002;11: 50–53.
8. Delaney M, et al. The management of pregnancy at 41+0 to 42+0 weeks. Clinical practice guidelines. J Obstet Gynaecol Can 2008;30: 800–810.
9. NICE Clinical Guideline. Induction of labour. CG70. London: National Collaborating Centre for Women's and Children's Health and Royal College of Obstetricians and Gynaecologists, 2008
10. Cotzias CS, et al. Prospective risk of unexplained stillbirth in singleton pregnancies at term: population based analysis. BMJ 1999;319: 287–288.

11. RCOG Scientific Impact Paper No. 34. Induction of labour at term in older mothers. London: Royal College of Obstetricians and Gynaecologists, 2013.
12. Reddy UM, et al. Maternal age and the risk of stillbirth throughout pregnancy in the United States. Am J Obstet Gynecol 2005;192: 764–770.
13. Haavaldsen C, et al. The impact of maternal age on fetal death: does length of gestation matter? Am J Obstet Gynecol 2010;203: 554.e 1–8.
14. Olesen AW, et al. Perinatal and maternal complications related to postterm delivery: a national register-based study, 1978–1993. Am J Obstet Gynecol 2003;189: 222–227.
15. Balchin I, et al. Racial variation in the association between gestational age and perinatal mortality: prospective study. BMJ 2007;334 (7598): 833.
16. Boulvain M, Irion O. Stripping/sweeping the membranes for inducing or preventing post-term pregnancy. Cochrane Database Syst Rev 2004;3: CD001328.
17. Foong LC, et al. Membrane sweeping in conjunction with induction. Obstet Gynecol 2000;96: 539–542.
18. de Miranda E. et al. Membrane sweeping and prevention of post-term pregnancy in low-risk pregnancies: a randomized controlled trial. BJOG 2006;113: 402–408.
19. Hannah ME, et al. Induction of labor as compared with serial antenatal monitoring in post-term pregnancy. A randomized controlled trial. N Engl J Med 1992;326: 1587–1592.
20. Sanchez-Ramos L, et al. Labor induction versus expectant management for postterm pregnancies: a systematic review with meta-analysis. Obstet Gynecol 2003;101: 1312–1318.
21. Gulmezoglu AM, et al. Induction of labour for improving birth outcomes for women at or beyond term. Cochrane Database Syst Rev 2006;18: CD004945.
22. Roberts LJ, Young KR. The management of prolonged pregnancy—an analysis of women's attitudes before and after term. Br J Obstet Gynaecol 1991;98: 1102–1106.
23. Luckas MJM, Walkinshaw SA. Prolonged pregnancy. Obstetrician and Gynaecologist 2000;2: 39–41.
24. Alfirevic Z, Walkinshaw SA. A randomised controlled trial of simple compared with complex antenatal fetal monitoring after 42 weeks gestation. Br J Obstet Gynaecol 1995;102: 638–643.
25. Alfirevic Z, et al. A randomised comparison between amniotic fluid index and the maximum pool depth in the monitoring of post-term pregnancy. Br J Obstet Gynaecol 1997;10: 207–211.
26. McNellis D, et al. A clinical trial of induction of labor versus expectant management in postterm pregnancy. Am J Obstet Gynecol 1994;170: 716–723.
27. National Collaborating Centre for Women's and Children's Health. NICE antenatal care: routine care for the healthy pregnant woman, 2nd ed. London: RCOG Press, 2008.

CARE PATHWAY

- At the 38 week antenatal visit, offer information about risks of prolonged pregnancies (>42 weeks) and reasons why induction is recommended at 41–42 weeks. In women aged 40yr and above, IOL can be offered at 39 wks.
- Reassure woman that most will go into labour spontaneously by 42 weeks
- Discuss management options including sweeping of membranes after 40 weeks gestation, if versus expectant management or formal induction of labour between 41^{+0} and 42^{+0} weeks
- Explain what 'stretch and sweep of cervix' involves; mild discomfort and minimal bleeding may result
- For a formal IOL between 41 and 42 weeks, explain when, where, and how induction would be carried out and options for pain relief
- Alternative options if the woman chooses not to have IOL
- That induction may not be successful and what the woman's options would then be
- Allow the woman time to discuss the information and options with her partner before coming to a decision
- Invite questions, and offer support of whatever decision she makes

If IOL chosen

- The exact timing of induction will depend on local circumstances and unit policy while taking maternal preferences into account
- Confirm the EDD has been established by means of a 1st-trimester ultrasound scan, with dates adjusted if the difference between scan and LMP dates is >5 days
- Ensure placenta is not low-lying
- Ensure presentation is cephalic
- Ensure live singleton pregnancy

If IOL is declined in prolonged pregnancy

- Recommend cervical stretch and sweep of membranes on one or more occasions, either by community midwife or in the day assessment unit in the hospital, to encourage natural onset of labour
- Effective counselling required to explain risks of prolonged pregnancy, especially in those over 40 years of age and in those of south Asian origin
- Discuss increase in perinatal and maternal problems if pregnancy is prolonged much beyond 41 weeks
- RCOG/NICE recommend increased fetal surveillance consisting of twice weekly CTG and an ultrasound scan for maximal amniotic pool depth from 42 weeks gestation in women who decline IOL
- If suboptimal or suspicious features noted, emphasize urgent need to deliver due to possible change of state of fetal well-being
- Remind women that while awaiting spontaneous onset of labour or the agreed date of IOL, she should report any reduction of fetal movements to the maternity unit without delay, even if the CTGs/scans have been reassuring

29 Placental Conditions

29.1 Placenta Praevia, Morbidly Adherent Placenta

FACT FILE

This fact file offers information pertaining only to the antenatal planning of the management of placenta praevia and of suspected morbid adherence of placenta. It does **not** deal with the actual intraoperative procedures, techniques, and options that may be involved at the time of delivery.

Definitions

- Placental conditions such as **placenta praevia** and **morbid adherence of the placenta** are associated with significant maternal mortality and morbidity[1,2,3] and with the rising Caesarean section rates, such placental pathologies are being increasingly encountered.
- Placenta praevia is classed as **major praevia** if ultrasound examination shows that it lies over the internal cervical os and as **minor praevia** (or **partial praevia**) if the leading edge is it the lower segment of the uterus but does not cover the internal os.
- A placenta is classed as being **morbidly adherent** if it penetrates into the decidua basalis (**accreta**), into the myometrium (**increta**) and through the whole thickness of the myometrium (**percreta**).

Placenta praevia

- **Antenatal diagnosis** of placenta praevia relies on ultrasound identification of the placental site and the location of its leading edge from the internal os. Certain symptoms and signs such as painless bleeding or bleeding provoked by intercourse, a high presenting part at term in a primip, or abnormal lie raise the clinical suspicion of placenta praevia but confirmation has to be achieved by ultrasound imaging.
- It is current practice to include placental localization at the 20 week gestation routine fetal anomaly scan. If on the routine abdominal scan at about 20 weeks gestation, the placenta is suspected to be low-lying, **an immediate transvaginal scan (TVS) is highly recommended as the TVS can reclassify 26–60% of such cases.[4,5,6] This will reduce the number of women needing follow-up.[3]**
- If painless vaginal bleeding is experienced at any stage in pregnancy, management needs to be on a case-by-case basis.
- All those found to have major or partial placenta praevia at the 20-week scan should have further scan follow-up.
- If asymptomatic and the placenta is found to be of a minor degree or praevia, a follow-up scan can be performed in the late third trimester at about 34–36 weeks gestation.
- If asymptomatic and the placenta is found to be of a major degree of praevia at the 20-week routine scan, a further follow-up scan should be performed at 32 weeks.
- ***In any woman with previous Caesarean section(s), if the 20-week routine anomaly scan shows that the placenta is anterior and reaches or overlaps the internal os, this raises the possibility of both placenta praevia and morbid adherence to the previous Caesarean section scar.***
- In such cases, an anterior placenta, even if only of a minor degree at 20 weeks, is more likely to remain as praevia in the later scans as seen in about 50% of cases, compared with 11% when there is no previous uterine scar.[7]
- If at the 32-week scan, **minor** praevia is identified, 73% will remain so at term. If at 32 weeks, **major** praevia is found, 90% will remain so at term.[7]
- Women with placenta praevia have an increased risk of preterm labour and major haemorrhage especially in late third trimester. Admission to hospital for those with major praevia from about 34 weeks gestation is standard practice.[3,8] For an in-patient, adequate hydration and thromboembolic stockings are recommended for thromboprophylaxis, with low molecular weight heparin injections reserved only for women at specially high risk of thromboembolism.
- If the patient declines admission despite full discussion of the risks, and if she lives close to the hospital, she should be advised to have someone available to assist at all times should an emergency develop.
- She should be advised to attend labour ward immediately if there is any bleeding, contractions or even dull period-like suprapubic pain.[3]
- In cases of partial placenta praevia, if the head is found not to have engaged in the pelvis by about 36 weeks of gestation in primips, a TVS can be employed to ascertain the distance between the fetal head and the leading edge of the placenta. The thicker the placenta (>1 cm), the less likely that a vaginal delivery is possible.

Morbid adherence of the placenta

- In women who have had previous Caesarean section(s), when the placenta in this pregnancy is found to be praevia and anterior, **morbid adherence** must be suspected.
- Colour Doppler or three-dimensional power Doppler can be used to help confirm the diagnosis and MRI can clarify the depth of infiltration in morbidly adherent placenta. MRI has been shown to correlate well with surgical findings and can therefore lead to modification of management plans.[9]
- Antenatal diagnosis and assessment of the extent of myometrial involvement can assist in planning management of surgical delivery: for example, whether to proceed with standard surgical techniques employed for any low-lying placenta at Caesarean section or to proceed directly to hysterectomy without attempting to separate the placenta in cases of extensive myometrial infiltration.
- Elective delivery is recommended by Caesarean section in asymptomatic women with placenta praevia at about 38 weeks gestation while those suspected to have a morbid adherent placenta are best delivered as a planned procedure at 36–37 weeks gestation after receiving prophylactic steroids to accelerate fetal lung maturity.[3]
- Before planning delivery in a woman with suspected morbidly adherent placenta, detailed discussion with the patient and partner should include
  - Details about what the forthcoming surgery might involve, registering their concerns, answering queries regarding management options
  - Anticipated skin and uterine incisions
  - Need for blood transfusions
  - Whether to leave the placenta behind or proceed directly to a hysterectomy
  - One in three chances of peripartum hysterectomy[10]
  - HDU/ITU admission may be necessary
  - That a hysterectomy will mean no further pregnancies.
- In cases where the woman declines any donor blood products, she should be transferred to a unit with interventional radiology and cell saver facilities.[3]

- Those with special cross-matching requirements due to atypical antibodies should be identified well ahead of time to the local blood bank service to ensure adequate supplies are on site for the planned procedure.

The Care Bundle for suspected placenta accreta

- The Care Bundle for suspected placenta accreta[10] must be clearly documented and arranged for all cases where morbid adherence of the placenta is a strong possibility, i.e. an anterior placenta praevia with previous Caesarean section scar(s).[10]
- The essentials of this Care Bundle include:
  - Multidisciplinary preoperative planning, including consultants in obstetrics, anaesthetics, interventional radiology (if available), haematology, intensive care unit (ICU) and the senior midwife in charge of labour ward.
  - Blood and blood products readily available; the amount required will depend on clinical features of each case and local blood bank facilities. The consultant haematologists should be kept fully involved in this process where high-volume blood transfusion may be anticipated.
  - Informed consent after comprehensive discussions regarding surgery, that Caesarean section for placenta praevia can involve a 12-fold increased risk of massive haemorrhage and interventions such as uterine artery embolization, hysterectomy, leaving the placenta behind, and cell salvage may be required.
  - Availability of level 2 critical care bed must be confirmed and re-confirmed before the elective procedure is commenced.
  - Consultant obstetrician(s) to plan and preferably perform the surgery or offer direct supervision.
  - Consultant anaesthetist to plan and either manage the anaesthetic themselves or directly supervise the anaesthetics for delivery.
- ***Delivery should be planned in units that can fulfil the Care Bundle criteria, otherwise plans need to be made to arrange delivery in a tertiary unit with multidisciplinary support and facilities for interventional radiology, cell salvage, etc. if required in individual circumstances.***

Information for patients

Please see Information for patients: Low-lying placenta, placenta accreta (p. 561)

References

1. Lewis, G, ed. Saving mother's lives: reviewing maternal deaths to make motherhood safer—2003–2005. The Seventh Report of the Confidential Enquiries into Maternal Deaths in the UK (CEMACH). London: RCOG Press, 2007.
2. CEMACH. Why mothers die: 2000–2002. The Sixth Report of the Confidential Enquiries into Maternal Deaths in the United Kingdom. London: RCOG Press, 2004.
3. RCOG Green-top Guideline No. 27. Placenta praevia, placenta praevia accreta and vasa praevia: diagnosis and management. London: Royal College of Obstetricians and Gynaecologists, 2011.
4. National Collaborating Centre for Women's and Children's Health. Antenatal care: routine care for the healthy pregnant woman. Clinical guideline. London: RCOG Press, 2003.
5. Smith RS, et al. Transvaginal ultrasonography for all placentas that appear to be low-lying or over the internal cervical os. Ultrasound Obstet Gynecol 1997;9: 22–24.
6. Lauria MR, et al. The use of second-trimester transvaginal sonography to predict placenta praevia. Ultrasound Obstet Gynecol 1996;8: 337–340.
7. Dashe JS, et al. Persistence of placenta previa according to gestational age at ultrasound. detection. Obstet Gynecol 2002;99: 692–697.
8. Wong HS, et al. Antenatal ultrasound assessment of placental/myometrial involvement in morbidly adherent placenta. Aust N Z J Obstet Gynaecol 2012;52: 67–72.
9. Ghourab S. Third-trimester transvaginal ultrasonography in placenta previa: does the shape of the lower placental edge predict clinical outcome? Ultrasound Obstet Gynecol 2001;18: 103–108.
10. Paterson-Brown S, Singh C. Developing a care bundle for the management of suspected placenta accreta. Obstet Gynaecol 2010;12: 21–27.

CARE PATHWAY

Major placenta praevia ± suspected morbid adherence of placenta

> **This care pathway refers only to the antenatal investigations and multidisciplinary planning required when Major placenta praevia and/or morbid adherence of the placenta is suspected and not to intrapartum details**

Routine ~20 week anomaly ultrasound scan (transabdominal) includes placental localization: shows placenta praevia (major or minor degree)

↓

Abdominal scan to be followed by transvaginal scan (TVS) at ~20 weeks for better definition of degree of praevia—TVS will re-classify degree of praevia in 26–60% of cases

↓

Major degree placenta praevia: whether anterior, posterior, or central praevia

No previous Caesarean section

Symptomatic—bleeding experienced

- Individualize management.
- Admission till bleeding settles, blood crossmatch
- Repeat scan at 32–34 weeks for leading edge of placenta
- If repeat haemorrhage later in pregnancy, anaesthetic review and Caesarean section at 37–38 weeks if no intervening major haemorrhage; otherwise earlier Caesarean section
- Document requisites for Caesarean section, blood availability, consultant obstetrician and anaesthetist to perform or directly supervise Caesarean section

Asymptomatic—no bleeding experienced

- Repeat scan (TVS) at 32 weeks, major praevia confirmed in 90%
- If no longer major degree (10%), refer to minor praevia pathway (see next care pathway)

Major placenta praevia

- Admit at about 34 weeks. In-patient till delivery by planned Caesarean section at 37–38 weeks.
- Crossmatch renewed weekly
- Anaesthetic review
- **Document** requisites for Caesarean section, blood availability, consultant obstetrician and anaesthetist to perform or directly supervise Caesarean section

Previous Caesarean section—single or multiple

Anterior/central major praevia: consider morbid adherence

Consider tertiary centre transfer if **Care Bundle** (see fact file, reference 10) requisites not available on site

↓

Further TVS/colour Doppler at 32 weeks

- Further imaging at 32 weeks: MRI, colour Doppler to assess depth of myometrial penetration to help management planning
- **Admit at 34 weeks:** Crossmatch
- Pre-op planning with multidisciplinary team including interventional radiology, cell saver, etc.
- Detailed discussions and informed consent for proposed surgery, interventions that may be required, blood transfusion, hysterectomy, ITU/HDU, possibility of leaving placenta behind
- High volume blood availability and HDU bed confirmed as ready before surgery at 36–37 weeks; steroids if <36 weeks
- Placenta accreta Care Bundle requisites documented and in place (see fact file, reference 10)

Scan at 20 weeks: **posterior major praevia** without anterior extension

Further TVS/colour Doppler at 32 weeks

Shows anterior extension involving previous scar: Consider **morbid adherence**

No anterior extension

Minor degree placenta praevia ± suspected morbid adherence of placenta

This care-pathway refers only to the antenatal investigations and multidisciplinary planning and not to the operative details or intrapartum interventions

Routine ~20 week anomaly ultrasound scan (transabdominal) includes placental localization: shows placenta praevia (minor degree)

↓

Abdominal scan to be followed by transvaginal scan (TVS) at ~20 weeks for better definition of degree of praevia—TVS will re-classify 26–60%

↓

Minor degree placenta praevia

No previous Caesarean section

Symptomatic-bleeding experienced

- Individualize management.
- Admission till bleeding settles, blood crossmatch
- Repeat scan to evaluate position of leading edge of placenta
- If repeat haemorrhage in last part of pregnancy, anaesthetic review and Caesarean section at 38 weeks if no intervening major haemorrhage; otherwise earlier Caesarean section
- Document requisites for Caesarean section, blood availability, consultant obstetrician and anaesthetist to directly supervise Caesarean section

Asymptomatic

- Outpatient management—advise to report immediately if bleeding, pain, or contractions
- Correct anaemia,
- **Repeat scan (TVS) at 35–6 weeks**

Then:

- If head engaged and thickness of encroaching tongue of placenta between fetal head and uterine wall is <1 cm and leading edge is >3 cm away from internal os, vaginal delivery feasible

or:

- If head free or abnormal lie, ± placental tongue >1 cm thickness ± leading edge of placenta <2 cm from internal os—plan elective Caesarean section at 38–39 weeks
- Anaesthetic review,
- Crossmatch,
- Experienced senior obstetrician to perform surgery

Previous Caesarean section—single or multiple

Anterior minor (partial) praevia: consider morbid adherence

- Further imaging at 32 weeks: TVS/colour Doppler/MRI to assess depth of myometrial penetration to help management planning
- If morbid adherence suggested by imaging, admit at 34–36 wks, crossmatch renewed weekly
- Pre-op planning with multidisciplinary team including interventional radiology, cell saver
- Detailed discussions and informed consent for proposed surgery, interventions that may be required, blood transfusion, ITU/HDU
- High volume blood availability and HDU bed confirmed as ready before surgery at 36–37 weeks after steroids
- Placenta accreta Care Bundle requisites documented and in place.

↓

Consider tertiary centre transfer if Care Bundle requisites not available on site

Posterior minor praevia without anterior extension in scan at 20 wks

↓

Further TVS/colour Doppler at 35–36 weeks

Then:

Head engaged and below leading edge of placenta, which is >3 cm from internal os—vaginal delivery feasible

or:

- No anterior extension, head free or abnormal lie, placental tongue >1 cm thickness and leading edge of placenta <2 cm from internal os—plan elective Caesarean section at 38–39 weeks
- Anaesthetic review
- Crossmatch
- Senior obstetrician to perform surgery

29.2 Abruptio Placenta—Previous Pregnancy, Small Antepartum Haemorrhage in Present Pregnancy

FACT FILE

This fact file deals with only the non-acute management of abruptio placenta, either repeated small **antepartum haemorrhage (APHs)** with a normally sited placenta during the current pregnancy or a past history of abruptio placenta in a previous pregnancy.

- **APH** is defined as bleeding from or into the genital tract, occurring from 24+0 weeks of pregnancy and prior to the birth of the baby. APH can occur at any time until the second stage of labour is completed.
- APH complicates 3–5% of pregnancies and is a leading cause of perinatal and maternal mortality worldwide.[1,2,3,4]
- **Abruptio placenta** is a partial or complete separation of the placenta from its uterine attachment before delivery of the baby.
- Up to one-fifth of very preterm babies are born in association with APH.
- Due to the heterogeneity of causes and pathophysiology, abruption cannot be predicted.[4] In fact, approximately 70% of cases of placental abruption occur in low-risk pregnancies.
- Placental abruption occurs in 1 in 200 of all pregnancies and accounts for 20–30% of all cases of antepartum haemorrhage.[5] Perinatal mortality rate with abruption placentae is approximately 15%.[6]
- ***Recurrence risk for abruption in a subsequent pregnancy is about 4–5%.***[7]
- ***Abruption recurs in 19–25% of women who have had two previous pregnancies complicated by abruption.***[8,9]
- ***A history of abruption in a previous pregnancy not only confers the label of 'high risk' for a subsequent pregnancy but also warrants further investigations and close antenatal surveillance.***

Risk factors

- A number[10,11,12,13,14,15,16] of clinical and epidemiological studies have identified predisposing risk factors for placental abruption, including:
  - abruption in previous pregnancy(ies)—the strongest predictor of abruption in a subsequent pregnancy
  - smoking
  - high blood pressure
  - diabetes
  - pre-eclampsia
  - uterine malformation
  - cocaine, amphetamine misuse
  - overdistension of the uterus—multiple pregnancies, polyhydramnios, large fibroids
  - prolonged rupture of membranes
  - increased maternal age and parity
  - thrombophilias,[17,18] especially heterozygous factor V Leiden deficiency, prothrombin variant, protein C or S deficiency, antithrombin III deficiency
  - autoimmune conditions, e.g. lupus and/or antiphospholipid syndrome
  - direct trauma to the uterus
  - low body mass index (BMI),
  - pregnancy following assisted reproductive techniques
  - intrauterine infection.
- The management of the subsequent pregnancy has to take those factors into consideration that continue to be relevant in this pregnancy (e.g. hypertension, diabetes, thrombophilia, age, parity, uterine malformations unless surgically corrected, smoking, etc.) when planning antenatal care and timing and method of delivery.
- The principles detailed in this chapter are equally applicable in the management of a pregnancy in a woman who has had a previous pregnancy complicated by abruptio placenta.

Recurrent episodes of APH in a current pregnancy

- Recurrent APH is the term used when there are episodes of APH on more than one occasion.[4]
- Following APH from placental abruption or unexplained APH (having excluded bleeding from placenta praevia, local causes, etc.) the pregnancy should be re-classified as 'high risk' with specialist obstetrician-led management[4] due to:
  - Increased risk of placental abruption in later pregnancy. Histological lesions of the placenta, umbilical cord, and membranes are often found in such cases, also suggesting that the final episode of abruption is the culmination of a chronic process.[19]
  - A history of repeated episodes of APH in this pregnancy with a normally situated placenta also increases the risks of intrauterine growth retardation (IUGR), oligohydramnios, premature rupture of membranes, preterm delivery, pregnancy-induced hypertension and pre-eclampsia, PPH, and even IUD.[20]
- Close surveillance during pregnancy may help reduce at least some of these risks. It is important that the patient is made aware of the risks, and maintains vigilance over daily fetal activity, symptoms such as bleeding (any amount), or pain, and that she knows how and from where she should seek immediate help and advice.
- It is essential to advise and offer support for the woman to stop smoking or misusing drugs such as cocaine and amphetamine.
- Serial ultrasound for fetal growth should be performed to assess fetal growth and liquor volume.
- Ultrasound scans cannot confirm or exclude an abruption in the majority of cases as any entrapped blood clot must be more than 200 ml in volume to be seen on scan. Ultrasonography will fail to detect three-quarters of cases of abruption.[21]
- Remember every fresh episode of APH in a Rhesus (D) negative woman must be covered with anti-D immunoglobulin.
- Elective delivery, individualized on a case-to-case basis, is usually arranged between 38–40 weeks gestation; may be warranted even earlier, if indicated by further significant APH, pre-eclampsia, IUGR, PPROM, etc.
- Following delivery after a major placental abruption, irrespective of the fetal outcome, postnatal follow-up must be arranged. Apart from debriefing of the woman and her family before discharge from the hospital, a follow-up appointment in about 6 weeks following birth should be offered. Contact numbers for access to medical and psychological support should be provided as appropriate[4] if the woman wants to access this support meanwhile.

Postnatal counselling, pre-pregnancy advice

- ***The initial postnatal appointment could also serve as an opportunity to arrange any further investigations and to provide counselling before a next pregnancy is commenced.***
- **Post-pregnancy (≥12 weeks following delivery) or pre-pregnancy investigations** should include two tests 12 weeks apart for lupus, antiphospholipid syndrome, and thrombophilias. These tests are best performed remote from pregnancy because there is an expected physiological drop in the levels of both protein C and protein S during pregnancy without indicating true thrombophilia.
- If these tests are positive for acquired or inherited thrombophilia, the patient needs to be offered a further appointment in order to to discuss additional management in a future pregnancy based on these results.

- If the patient is hypertensive, advice regarding the need for good pre-pregnancy and pregnancy BP control with medications suitable for pregnancy (e.g. methyldopa or labetalol) should be reiterated and this communicated to the GP. The patient must be advised to start low-dose aspirin from the first trimester of any future pregnancy and to continue it throughout pregnancy.
- Inter-pregnancy interval of at least 12–18 months is advisable, especially if the delivery was achieved by Caesarean section to reduce the risks of placenta praevia or placental abruption as well as morbid adherence of the placenta (see Chapter 29.1).
- Appropriate contraceptive advice must be offered, taking into account that the combined pill is to be avoided in those with identified thrombophilia, diabetes, hypertension, etc.
- If the patient is diabetic, the need for tight glucose control, both before and during the entire course of pregnancy, should be highlighted.
- If the presence of a uterine malformation such as a septum was thought to be causally linked to the abruption, it is worth considering metroplasty before the next pregnancy is commenced.
- If investigations reveal the definitive presence of lupus, antiphospholipid syndrome, or inherited thrombophilias, appropriate prophylaxis and management plans for the next pregnancy must be discussed with the patient (see Chapter 1.2 for inherited thrombophilias and Chapter 13.1 for lupus and antiphospholipid syndrome).
- In women who have had an abruption and are also known or found to have comorbidities such as diabetes, obesity, lupus, hypertension, previous pre-eclampsia, IUGR or a baby who is small for gestational age (SGA), consider low-dose aspirin starting from the first trimester of a future pregnancy to be continued throughout gestation.
- If relevant to the individual woman, reiterate advice about cessation of smoking or drug misuse and offer the necessary support.
- Routine peri-pregnancy folic acid must be advised for all women, with high-dose folic acid (5 mg per day obtained on prescription from the GP) in those with conditions such as obesity or diabetes

Information for patients

Please see Information for patients: Placental abruption (premature separation of the placenta) (p. 561)

References

1. Calleja-Agius J, et al. Placental abruption and placenta praevia. Eur Clin Obstet Gynaecol 2006;2: 121–127.
2. Cantwell R, et al. Saving mothers' lives: Reviewing maternal deaths to make motherhood safer, 2006–08. The Eighth Report of the Confidential Enquiries into Maternal Deaths in the United Kingdom. Br J Obstet Gynaecol 2011;118: 1–203.
3. Lewis, G, ed. Saving mothers' lives: reviewing maternal deaths to make motherhood safer 2003–2005. The Seventh Report on Confidential Enquiries into Maternal Deaths in the UK (CEMACH) London: RCOG Press, 2007.
4. RCOG Green-top Guideline No. 63. Antepartum haemorrhage. London: Royal College of Obstetricians and Gynaecologists, 2011.
5. Neilson JP. Interventions for treating placental abruption; Cochrane Database Syst Rev 2003;1: CD003247.
6. Pariente G, et al. Placental abruption: critical analysis of risk factors and perinatal outcomes. J Matern Fetal Neonatal Med 2010;24: 698–702.
7. Rasmussen S, et al. Outcome of pregnancies subsequent to placental abruption: a risk assessment. Acta Obstet Gynaecol Scand 2000;79: 496–501.
8. Tikkanen M.Etiology, clinical manifestations, and prediction of placental abruption. Acta Obstet Gynecol Scand 2010;89: 732–740.
9. Toivonen S, et al. Reproductive risk factors, Doppler findings, and outcome of affected births in placental abruption: a population-based analysis. Am J Perinatol 2002;19: 451–460.
10. Tikkanen M, et al. Prepregnancy risk factors for placental abruption. Acta Obstet Gynecol Scand 2006;85: 40–44.
11. Raymond EG, Mills JL. Placental abruption: maternal risk factors and associated fetal conditions. Acta Obstet Gynecol Scand 1993;72: 633–639.
12. Tikkanen M, et al. Clinical presentation and risk factors of placental abruption. Acta Obstet Gynecol Scand 2006;85: 700–705.
13. Ananth CV, et al. Evidence of placental abruption as a chronic process: Associations with vaginal bleeding early in pregnancy and placental lesions. Eur J Obst Gynecol Reprod Biol 2006;128: 15–21.
14. Ananth CV, et al. Preterm premature rupture of membranes, intrauterine infection and oligohydramnios: risk factors for placental abruption. Obstet Gynecol 2004;104: 71–77.
15. Ananth CV, et al. The normal anticoagulant system and risk of placental abruption: protein C, protein and resistance to activated protein C. J Matern Fetal Neonatal Med 2010;23: 1377–1383.
16. Deutsch AB, et al. Increased risk of placental abruption in underweight women. Am J Perinatol 2010;27: 235–240.
17. Paidas MJ, et al. Inherited thrombophilias and adverse pregnancy outcome: screening and management. Semin Perinatol 2005;29: 150–163.
18. Robertson L, et al. Thrombosis: Risk and Economic Assessment of Thrombophilia Screening (TREATS) Study. Thrombophilia in pregnancy: a systematic review. Br J Haematol 2006;132: 171–196.
19. Ananth CV, et al. Women with preeclampsia, SGA, and placental abruption in their first pregnancy-conditions that constitute ischemic placental disease-are at substantially increased risk of recurrence of any or all these conditions in their second pregnancy. Obstet Gynecol 2007;110: 128–133.
20. Harlev A, et al. Idiopathic bleeding during the second half of pregnancy as a risk factor for adverse perinatal outcome. J Matern Fetal Neonatal Med 2008;21: 331–335.
21. Glantz C, Purnell L. Clinical utility of sonography in the diagnosis and treatment of placental abruption. J Ultrasound Med 2002;21: 837–840.

CARE PATHWAY

Referral by GP or community midwife to a specialist antenatal clinic of a woman booking in a new pregnancy, who has had a **previous pregnancy complicated by abruption of the placenta, or if a woman has had recurrent bleeding after 24 weeks gestation in the present pregnancy with a normally sited placenta and no local cause has been found**

↓

Previous pregnancy complicated by significant abruption of a normally sited placenta and which warranted urgent delivery at term or pre-term

↓

First visit to specialist antenatal clinic

- Detailed history of previous pregnancy, gestational age at time of abruption and of delivery, weight of baby, fetal outcome, type of uterine incision, persistent risk factors and comorbidities
- Advice and support for smoking cessation, substance abuse (cocaine, amphetamine)
- If diabetic and/or hypertensive, aim for tight glucose and BP control
- Low-dose aspirin if hypertensive and/or previous history of pre-eclampsia, PIH and/or IUGR
- Screening for thrombophilias, lupus, APS, if not previously done
- Patient education regarding symptom recognition and plan of care

↓

- Close surveillance of serial scans for fetal growth, liquor with same day Specialist Clinic appointments from about 26 weeks
- If past h/o abruption & hypertension, close surveillance with 2-weekly BP series from 24 weeks gestation
- Advise continuation of low-dose aspirin till end of pregnancy

↓

Continued care with community midwife avoiding overlap with hospital appointments.

→

- If no IUGR noted, no APH in this pregnancy, good control of diabetes or hypertension if they coexist, plan delivery for no later than 38–40 weeks gestation, decided on a case-to-case basis
- If known diabetes, lupus, APS, or poorly controlled hypertensive, delivery advisable by 38 weeks

---

History of recurrent bleeding (APH), i.e. bleeding on more than one occasion after 24 weeks in this pregnancy with a normally sited placenta and no local causes

↓

Specialist antenatal clinic within 2–3 weeks following ward discharge, advise prompt self- referral if any further bleeding, rupture of membranes, reduced fetal movements, abdominal pain, etc.

↓

- Serial growth scans at 3–4 week intervals ± Doppler
- Same day specialist antenatal clinic reviews
- Continued routine community midwife visits meanwhile, avoiding overlap with hospital visits

↓

Evidence of significant IUGR and/or further significant APH, give steroids (if <35 weeks) and consider delivery

No evidence of IUGR, no further large APH

↓

Plan delivery at 38–40 weeks; individualized plan for delivery on a case-to-case basis

29.3 Vasa Praevia

FACT FILE

Definition and incidence

- **Vasa praevia** is a placental vascular anomaly where unprotected fetal vessels cross the internal os beneath the fetal presenting part.
- It is a rare condition: reported incidence varies between 1:1300 and 1:6000.[1,2,3,4]
- There are two types of vasa praevia:
  - Associated with velamentous insertion of cord. Incidence of velamentous insertion in an unselected population is ~1% and vasa praevia coexists in 2–6%.[5,6,7]
  - Associated with normally inserted cord but where fetal vessels traverse placental lobes in a succenturiate or bilobed placenta. Incidence of bilobed or succenturiate placenta is ~1.7% in an unselected population.[8]

Risks and mortality rate

- Unlike placenta praevia, vasa praevia carries no major maternal risk, but is associated with significant risk to the fetus.
- **Fetal mortality rates** are very high when prenatal diagnosis has not been made. Rapid exsanguination can result in fetal death within a few minutes when the unsupported fetal vessels tear with cervical dilatation or when the forewaters rupture, either spontaneously or artificially.
- ***Only a small amount of fetal blood needs to be lost in ruptured vasa praevia to cause fetal death as the total fetal blood volume at term is only about 250–300 ml (about 80–100 ml per kg of body weight at birth).***
- The mortality rate is generally quoted as around 60%,[9,10,11] although significantly improved survival rates of up to 97% have been reported where diagnosis has been made antenatally.[9,12]
- **Risk factors** associated with vasa praevia apart from succenturiate lobe and velamentous insertion are multiple pregnancies, IVF pregnancies, and where there is relative upward 'migration' of a placenta that was praevia earlier in pregnancy.[1]

Diagnosis

- **Antenatal diagnosis** of vasa praevia is usually made incidentally by ultrasound scan with colour flow Doppler in the second trimester.
- Clinically, without access to the fetal membranes, it is not possible to diagnose the intact vessels of vasa praevia. In the antenatal period, in the absence of vaginal bleeding, there is no method to diagnose vasa praevia.[12]
- Rarely, while performing a cervical assessment at term (to assess the Bishop's score prior to induction of labour (IOL) or to perform a sweep of the membranes) and if the cervix has started to dilate, these vessels may be felt digitally. It is therefore important for clinicians to have a high index of suspicion if they feel something unusual. Confirmation of the diagnosis prior to membrane rupture by using an amnioscope or by colour flow Doppler can avert the risk of fatal fetal haemorrhage.
- Colour flow Doppler via the transvaginal route has been shown to have good specificity but sensitivity has not been determined. Using both the abdominal and vaginal routes of scanning and changing maternal position can improve diagnostic accuracy.
- At present in the UK there is no routine national screening programme for identification of cord insertion or vasa praevia.

Management

- **Management of suspected vasa praevia** is difficult to standardize due to the rarity of the condition and infrequency of prenatal diagnosis.
- If vasa praevia has been identified in the second trimester, transvaginal colour Doppler ultrasound has to be repeated in the third trimester to confirm its persistence, thus reducing the need for prolonged admission and anxiety.[2]
- If vasa praevia is confirmed in the third-trimester scan, in-patient admission to a unit with appropriate neonatal facilities any time from about 28 to 32 weeks gestation till elective Caesarean is performed between 35–37 weeks gestation will facilitate quicker intervention in the event of bleeding, rupture of membranes, or labour.[2]
- It must be acknowledged that adoption of this advice could cause significant inconvenience and anxiety for the patient and her family.[1]
- Parents must be informed (and this discussion documented) that in a minority of cases, significant morbidity and even mortality may be unavoidable, despite close surveillance and prompt action in the hospital.[1]
- In the presence of vaginal bleeding, especially associated with membrane rupture and fetal compromise due to the speed at which fetal exsanguination occurs, delivery should not be delayed to try and diagnose vasa praevia.
- Rapid delivery by category 1 Caesarean section and aggressive neonatal resuscitation including the use of blood transfusion, if required, are essential.[12]
- Very rarely, fetal heart rate abnormalities may be seen even in the absence of bleeding due to compression of the fetal vessels by the presenting part.[13]
- Elective Caesarean section before the onset of labour at about 35 weeks gestation, or earlier if indicated, is advisable.[1,2]
- Prophylactic steroids are needed if preterm delivery has been planned.
- Neonatologists must be kept updated to ensure that blood is kept available for immediate transfusion of a hypovolaemic, shocked neonate if rupture of vasa praevia should occur at any time during the mother's in-patient stay.
- ***In cases of vasa praevia, irrespective of the perinatal outcome, postnatal follow-up should include debriefing and counselling regarding the events that occurred, the reasons that led to the outcomes, and any implications for future pregnancy or fertility.***

Information for patients

Please see Information for patients: Vasa praevia (p. 562)

References

1. Murray A, Murphy DJ. Vasa Praevia: Diagnosis and management. Obstetrician and Gynaecologist 2008;10: 217–223.
2. RCOG Green-top Guideline No. 27. Placenta praevia, placenta accreta and vasa praevia: diagnosis and management. London: Royal College of Obstetricians and Gynaecologists, 2011.
3. Lee W, et al. Vasa previa: prenatal diagnosis, natural evolution, and clinical outcome. Obstet Gynecol 2000;95: 572–576
4. Baulies S, et al. Prenatal diagnosis of vasa praevia and analysis of risk factors. Prenat Diagn 2007;27: 595–599.
5. Sepulveda W, et al. Prenatal detection of velamentous insertion of the umbilical cord: a prospective color Doppler ultrasound study. Ultrasound Obstet Gynecol 2003;21: 564–569.
6. Quek SP, Tan KL. Vasa praevia. Aust N Z J Obstet Gynaecol 1972;12: 206–209.
7. Paavonen J, et al. Velamentous insertion of the umbilical cord and vasa previa. Int J Obstet Gynecol 1984;22: 207–211.
8. Benirschke K, Kaufmann P. Pathology of the human placenta, 4th ed. New York: Springer-Verlag, 2000.
9. Fung TY, Lau TK. Poor perinatal outcome associated with vasa previa: is it preventable? A report of three cases and review of the literature. Ultrasound Obstet Gynecol 1998;12: 430–433.
10. Oleyese KO, et al. Vasa previa: an avoidable obstetric tragedy. Obstet Gynecol Surv 1999;54: 138–145.
11. Dougall A, Baird CH. Vasa praevia—report of three cases and review of the literature. Br J Obstet Gynaecol 1987;94: 712–715.
12. Oyelese Y, et al. Vasa previa: the impact of prenatal diagnosis on outcomes. Obstet Gynecol 2004;103: 937–942.
13. Oyelese Y, Smulian JC. Placenta previa, placenta accreta, and vasa previa. Obstet Gynecol 2006;107: 927–941.

CARE PATHWAY

Incidental finding of velamentous insertion of cord or of succenturiate placenta at routine 20 week anomaly scan

↓

- After explanation of the reason, ultrasonographer proceeds with TVS scan with colour flow Doppler to check for **vasa praevia**
- Clinical team alerted if vasa praevia confirmed

↓

- Explain the condition of vasa praevia, diagnosis, possible perinatal outcome if bleeding or rupture of membranes
- Assess associated risk factors, e.g. multiple pregnancy, IVF pregnancy, low-lying placenta in the 2nd trimester
- Arrange a further TVS Colour flow Doppler at approximately 28 weeks and clinic appointment to follow after scan
- Discuss options with patient—if the 3rd-trimester scan confirms persistence of vasa praevia, in-patient admission may be required for 6–9 weeks from about 28–32 weeks gestation till delivery by Caesarean section at about 35–37 weeks gestation, sooner if indicated. This allows time for the patient and family to make any arrangements as necessary
- Give support group website details (<http://www.vasapraevia.co.uk>)

↓

Repeat TVS scan with colour Doppler at 28 weeks

↓

If repeat scan confirms vasa praevia:

- Advise in-patient admission from this stage till delivery by 35–37 weeks by elective LSCS. In-patient admission is recommended at some time between 28 and 32 weeks
- Re-discuss risks associated with vasa praevia if membranes rupture or if contractions start or there is even minimal vaginal bleeding. These events indicate need for immediate Category 1 LSCS
- Below knee compression stockings for thromboprophylaxis, patient to remain as mobile as normal
- Prophylactic steroids
- Explain to parents that in a few cases, despite close hospital-based surveillance and prompt action, fetal mortality or severe morbidity may not be avoided if the fetal vessels rupture. **Record this discussion in notes.**
- From when the pregnant woman is admitted, keep neonatologists informed of patient's admission and to have blood available for immediate transfusion of neonate should vasa praevia vessels rupture at any time needing immediate delivery by category 1 Caesarean section.
- From point of in-patient admission, keep obstetric anaesthetists, labour ward midwifery and obstetric teams informed to anticipate category 1 Caesarean section under GA at any time
- Aim to avoid any anticipatable delays in performing category 1 Caesarean section, maternal G&S to be ready at all times.

↓

- Routine daily fetal and maternal monitoring and checks from when admitted
- If uneventful, arrange elective LSCS for about 35–37 weeks gestation
- Steroids, if not given earlier
- Inform neonatologists, anaesthetists
- Document that placenta and membranes should be sent for histological examination

If repeat scan excludes vasa praevia:

- Resolution occurs in 15%
- Reassure parents
- Routine antenatal care to resume

Appendix 1 Information for Patients

1. Maternal Haematological and Vascular Conditions

INFORMATION FOR PATIENTS Anaemia and pregnancy

If your community midwife or GP has detected that you have mild anaemia in pregnancy they will give you the appropriate advice and treatment and your pregnancy can continue to be managed by your community midwife. However, if you continue to have significant anaemia, you will be referred to one of our specialist antenatal clinics in the hospital for further tests and management of the anaemia.

What is anaemia?

Anaemia is when the level of healthy haemoglobin in your blood is lower than normal. This may range from mild to severe. You may experience tiredness, breathlessness, fainting, headaches, and your heart beating faster (palpitations).

Blood is made up of different components such as **red blood cells**, **white blood cells**, and **platelets**, which are all suspended in a fluid called **plasma**.

- **Red blood cells** contain an iron-rich pigment called haemoglobin which carries oxygen around the body. You need a certain level of healthy haemoglobin in your blood. A haemoglobin level of more than 110 g/litre during pregnancy is generally regarded as normal although this differs in different populations. (**Note**: 110 g/litre is the same as 11.0 g/dl, as it was described before March 2013 when a change was made to how haemoglobin units are expressed.)
- **Platelets** help control bleeding by making the blood clot where there is a cut or wound.
- **White blood cells** fight infection and form the body's defence system (immune system).

Anaemia is not uncommon during pregnancy, which is why your haemoglobin level will be routinely checked at your first pregnancy appointment, at 28 weeks, and between 34 and 36 weeks.

Severe anaemia is when the level of healthy haemoglobin is very much lower than normal (60–70 g/litre or less). It can make you feel very unwell, with increasing breathlessness, palpitations, fainting, and chest pain. With such severe anaemia there are considerable risks in pregnancy, during delivery, and after birth.

Causes of anaemia during pregnancy

Anaemia can develop in pregnancy for two main reasons:

- Normally, from very early pregnancy, your body starts to produce more red blood cells and plasma. Although there is a huge increase in the total blood volume (by about 50%) during the pregnancy, the amount of plasma produced is much more than the red cell volume. This causes a dilution of the blood, causing a drop in haemoglobin levels. This is a normal process, with the haemoglobin concentration at its lowest between weeks 25 and 30 of pregnancy. You would not normally experience any significant symptoms due to such a dilution effect, but if your haemoglobin at the start of the pregnancy was on the low side, you might be prescribed additional iron supplementation.
- There is an increased demand for iron and certain other vitamins needed by the developing baby and the placenta, which can be supplied only through your blood.

Other less common causes of anaemia in pregnancy include:

- A diet particularly low in iron. If you are vegetarian or vegan, or have been on a crash diet before pregnancy, you need to ensure that your diet provides you with enough iron. You should have received information about healthy eating at the very start of your pregnancy; otherwise you can discuss it with your midwife.
- Inadequate iron and/or folic acid in the diet or poor absorption from the gut.
- Loss of blood due to bleeding from any source including from the womb, from haemorrhoids (piles), or from stomach ulcers.
- If you have had several pregnancies close together, your body will not have had sufficient time to rebuild reserve stores of iron and folic acid.
- If you are carrying twins or triplets, the requirements of the babies can often outstrip supply, leaving you anaemic.
- If you are taking certain types of medication for specific medical conditions, you may need a higher dose of folic acid, prescribed by your GP or specialist doctor to prevent folic acid deficiency anaemia.
- Very rarely, a lack of vitamin B_{12} may lead to anaemia.

Symptoms of anaemia during pregnancy

If you are otherwise healthy, you might not have symptoms of anaemia unless the haemoglobin falls below 80 g/litre.

The symptoms you first notice could be tiredness, palpitations (awareness of your heartbeat), breathlessness, and dizziness. People around you may notice you are unusually pale. Severe anaemia (haemoglobin less than 60 g/litre) may cause chest pain (angina) or headaches in addition.

Ways of avoiding anaemia during pregnancy

- Be sure to eat a well-balanced and varied diet.
- If you are planning a pregnancy, talk to a doctor or midwife about food and supplements. If you are following any kind of strict diet, make sure to include iron and folate-rich sources in what you eat.
- Good sources of iron are beef, wholemeal bread, cereals, eggs, spinach, and dried fruit. To absorb the maximum amount of iron from the diet, it helps to eat plenty of vitamin C. Salads, potatoes, and citrus fruit such as oranges are all good sources of vitamin C.
- Taking 400 micrograms of folic acid daily, starting from a few months before getting pregnant and continuing this till the end of the twelfth completed week of pregnancy, is very important to reduce the chances of having a baby with spinal defects such as spina bifida. You may be advised to take a combined iron and folic acid supplement.
- Foods rich in folic acid include beans, muesli, broccoli, beef, brussels sprouts, and asparagus.

How is anaemia diagnosed during pregnancy?

Apart from the clinical symptoms you experience, anaemia is usually detected by antenatal blood tests. Blood tests are usually done at the first consultation, and repeated in the second half of pregnancy.

The blood test results include a description of the form, size, and volume of your red blood cells, which provide doctors with information about the type of anaemia a woman has and how severe it is.

In women of Afro-Caribbean, Asian, or Mediterranean origin, other additional tests are done to screen for genetic causes of anaemia, such as sickle cell anaemia and thalassaemias, which are more common in these groups.

Treatment of anaemia during pregnancy

After a clinical examination including assessment of your symptoms and the results of blood tests, the type of anaemia can be determined. Treatment can then be planned accordingly, and will also depend on how far the pregnancy has progressed.

Iron tablets can often cause constipation or diarrhoea; a few people simply cannot take them. Such side effects may be reduced by taking the iron with or after food, or by starting with a low dose and increasing gradually—talk to your midwife about this. Iron supplements can also be taken in syrup form. You may also be prescribed folic acid tablets in addition to iron to improve your haemoglobin levels.

If you cannot tolerate oral iron supplements in any form, or have a bowel disorder which causes poor absorption, you may be advised to have an iron infusion—that is, iron given through the vein as a drip. The decision to offer iron in this way depends on how far you have advanced in pregnancy and how severe your anaemia is, as well as checking that you do not have an allergic reaction to a test dose.

If you have a blood condition such as sickle cell disease or thalassaemia, it will affect your body's ability to produce healthy haemoglobin. As there is an increased risk of developing anaemia when you become pregnant, you will receive specialist care in addition to the antenatal care provided by your midwife during pregnancy.

Further information

- <www.netdoctor.co.uk/diseases/facts/anaemiapregnancy.htm>
- Blood transfusion, pregnancy and birth—information for you <http://www.rcog.org.uk/blood-transfusion-pregnancy-and-birth>.

INFORMATION FOR PATIENTS Inherited thrombophilia

The inherited thrombophilias are a group of genetic conditions that can make you prone to developing abnormal blood clots in the veins, resulting in a deep vein thrombosis (DVT) or pulmonary embolism (PE).

Blood circulates around the body delivering oxygen and removing waste products. It is normally not meant to clot within the circulation. If a blood clot does form within the circulation, this is known as **thrombosis**. When blood clots in a deep vein, this is known as a **deep vein thrombosis** (DVT for short). If a DVT occurs, there is a further risk that a piece of the blood clot might break off and travel through the circulation to lodge in the lungs. This is a dangerous condition known as a **pulmonary embolism** (PE).

There are several types of inherited thrombophilias and when considered together, about 15% of the population may have one of these conditions.

A few types of thrombophilia may be associated with causing certain pregnancy problems such as causing a baby to be small, the placenta not working well to feed the baby, or pre-eclampsia, in addition to the risk of thrombosis.

Fortunately, most women with thrombophilias have uncomplicated pregnancies with good outcomes for both the mother and the baby.

What are the different types of thrombophilia?

Some types of thrombophilia are due to a variation within an individual's genetic code which is known as a mutation. Some mutations are not uncommon, occurring in about 1 in 30 people. The two main mutations that cause thrombophilia are **factor V Leiden** (V is pronounced 'five') and **prothrombin gene** mutation.

There are other less common thrombophilias where there is a deficiency of natural anticoagulants. Such natural anticoagulants are normally found in the blood of all healthy people and help to control blood clotting. Rarely, in about 1 in 3000 people, a reduced level of one of these natural anticoagulants may occur and this may increase the risk of DVT or PE. The three main types of this kind of defect are **antithrombin deficiency, protein C deficiency, and protein S deficiency**.

What special precautions should I take if I have thrombophilia?

If you are a smoker, you should stop smoking. Similarly, if you are overweight, you should lose weight. This is even more so if you have already had a DVT or PE.

You may be at significantly increased risk of another DVT or PE in certain situations, such as pregnancy or major surgery.

If you have thrombophilia, or if you have had a previous DVT or PE you must tell the midwife about it at booking, as well as informing the medical and nursing staff who are looking after you.

What tests can be done?

A variety of blood tests are available and your doctor or thrombophilia nurse specialist will arrange these for you. These tests can help identify the type of thrombophilia you have, as well as determining the best management during your pregnancy and afterwards. Some of these tests cannot be done during pregnancy or if you are on anticoagulation medication, because the results may be inaccurate. These tests need to be done about 12 weeks after the birth of your baby, or the end of the anticoagulation treatment.

Should other members of my family be tested for thrombophilia?

If you have had a DVT or a PE and tests have shown that you have an inherited form of thrombophilia, it may then be possible to search for the same type of thrombophilia in other family members. The reason for doing this is to identify other family members who might be at risk of DVT or PE in high-risk situations.

If a close relative of yours is known to have had a DVT or PE, whether or not they have had thrombophilia tests, you should mention this to your GP so that further tests can be organized for you. You should also tell the community midwife at the time of booking in pregnancy.

Should children be tested?

In general young children do not need to be tested until they reach puberty, when their risk of blood clots due to thrombophilia may begin to increase. Teenage daughters of patients with thrombophilia may be considered for testing before oral contraception (the 'pill') is prescribed for them.

Is pregnancy safe for me?

Pregnancy is safe in most women with thrombophilia, but when you are planning a pregnancy you should request a referral from your GP to see a specialist obstetrician before becoming pregnant. This will provide an opportunity for any further investigations that are best done before a pregnancy, and to discuss the management of any future pregnancy.

If you are currently on warfarin and are planning to become pregnant, it is **essential** that your medication is immediately changed to subcutaneous injection of a form of heparin as soon as a pregnancy is confirmed.

You should inform your GP or community midwife as soon as you know you are pregnant. In some forms of thrombophilia certain precautions may be needed from very early pregnancy, to avoid problems and improve pregnancy outcomes.

Further information

- Reducing the risk of venous thrombosis in pregnancy and after birth: information for you. <http://www.rcog.org.uk/womens-health/clinical-guidance/reducing-risk-venous-thrombosis-what-you-need-know>.

INFORMATION FOR PATIENTS High platelet counts -also called thrombocytosis or thrombocythaemia

Thrombocythaemia (pronounced thrombo-cythee-mia), also known as thrombocytosis (thrombo-cyto-sis) means a higher than average platelet count.

Platelets (thrombocytes) are essential components of blood and are the blood cells that help prevent excessive bleeding by forming blood clots. Platelets are made in the bone marrow.

The normal platelet count can change during different stages of pregnancy, ranging from about 150 to 400 $\times 10^9$/litre, or 150–400 for short. If your blood has too many platelets, you may be at a higher risk of developing blood clots, especially during pregnancy and for about 6 weeks after delivery.

Low-dose aspirin and elasticated compression below-knee stockings may be advised by doctors if your platelet counts are above 450.

Platelet counts may also be high due to infection, bleeding, or inflammation, after any surgery, or in anaemia. This is known as **reactive** or **secondary thrombocythaemia**. Many of these conditions may be relevant during pregnancy and delivery, and after the birth.

Primary or **essential thrombocythaemia** (ET) is a much rarer condition and is uncommon in women of child-bearing age. Not all cases of thrombocythaemia (high platelet count) in pregnancy are due to ET.

What if I have ET?

A diagnosis of ET would usually have been made before pregnancy, following extensive tests. Although it is very rare, ET can cause serious problems during pregnancy and the specialists would discuss these with you, as well as the extra care that will be offered during pregnancy.

Further information

- Essential thrombocytopenia <http://www.mpdvoice.org.uk/about-mpds/essential-thrombocythaemia/>

INFORMATION FOR PATIENTS Low platelet counts or thrombocytopenia

Platelets are essential components in our blood and are the blood cells that help to prevent excessive bleeding by forming blood clots. Platelets are made in the bone marrow. **Thrombocytopenia** ('thrombo-cyto-peenia') means a reduced platelet (thrombocyte) count. Low platelet counts may be associated with delayed blood clotting. Symptoms can include bruising easily, abnormal bleeding, and petechiae (tiny red dots on the skin).

The normal count during pregnancy is in the range 150–400 $\times 10^9$/l (150–400, for short), but fluctuations are common at different stages of pregnancy. In general, investigations are not usually necessary if the count is above 100 and there are no symptoms.

Low platelets can occur during pregnancy for various reasons and the management differs accordingly.

- The most common variety is called **gestational thrombocytopenia**. This accounts for three-quarters of all cases of low platelet counts in pregnant women and carries no clinical risks for you or the baby. Here, other causes for low platelets have been ruled out and the platelet counts return to normal within 1–3 months after delivery.
- In about 1 in 5 of women with low platelets, especially in the second half of pregnancy, **pre-eclampsia** and a condition called **HELLP syndrome** could be associated. You and the baby will be carefully monitored, and delivery planned accordingly. Your specialist team will explain all this in detail.
- **Immune thrombocytopenia (ITP)**, otherwise known as **idiopathic thrombocytopenic purpura**, accounts for only a small number of cases of low platelets during pregnancy. Special tests and management plans for pregnancy and labour, as well as checks of the newborn baby, will be discussed with you by your specialists.

Further information

- Idiopathic thrombocytopenic purpura <http://www.patient.co.uk/health/Idiopathic-Thrombocytopenic-Purpura-%28ITP%29.htm> (UK site)
- About ITP <http://www.pdsa.org/about-itp.html> (US site)

INFORMATION FOR PATIENTS Haemophilia and pregnancy

Haemophilia is an inherited bleeding disorder which is inherited by men with women being carriers. In haemophilia, blood does not clot properly. Several components of the blood, called clotting factors, are necessary for blood to clot properly. A clotting factor is a protein in blood that controls bleeding. Haemophilia is caused when blood does not have enough of a clotting factor.

Haemophilia A, or classic haemophilia, is the most common form, and is due to the deficiency of factor VIII (eight). Haemophilia B, or Christmas disease, is an identical condition, but due to the deficiency of factor IX (nine). Haemophilias A and B are the most common severe inherited bleeding disorders.

With good management, women who carry the haemophilia gene have no more problems with delivering a healthy baby than other mothers.

Further information

- United Kingdom Haemophilia Centre Doctors Organization patients information <http://www.ukhcdo.org/patientspage.htm>. This site provides information associated with haemophilia and other bleeding disorders, and holds the National Haemophilia Database for patients and their families.
- The Haemophilia Society <http://http://www.haemophilia.org.uk>

INFORMATION FOR PATIENTS von Willebrand disease and other bleeding disorders

Von Willebrand disease (vWD) is the most common inherited bleeding disorder. vWD is a genetic condition, meaning that the child inherits an abnormal gene from one or both parents.

People with vWD either have a deficiency of a blood protein called von Willebrand factor (vWF), or the protein does not work properly. This means that blood cannot clot properly, increasing the risk of bleeding. vWF is necessary to make platelets form into clumps and thus plug damaged blood vessels.

In women with most types of vWD, the level of vWF usually increases three- to fourfold to reach near normal range by the third trimester (26–40 weeks of pregnancy) and additional treatment is not usually necessary.

As the levels of vWF fall after delivery, there is an increased risk of excessive bleeding. Special precautions are required to prevent this and further checks are needed for both you and the newborn baby for a few days after delivery.

Further information

- United Kingdom Haemophilia Centre Doctors Organization patients information <http://www.ukhcdo.org/patientspage.htm>. This site provides information associated with haemophilia and other bleeding disorders, and holds the National Haemophilia Database for patients and their families.
- NHS Choices. von Willebrand disease <http://www.nhs.uk/conditions/von-willebrand-disease>

INFORMATION FOR PATIENTS Sickle cell and thalassaemia

Sickle cell disease (SCD) is the most common inherited condition worldwide, seen most commonly in those of African descent including Afro-Caribbean, those of Mediterranean, Middle Eastern, northern Indian, or Central and South American origin.

In sickle cell **trait**, there are rarely any symptoms except for an increased risk of urine infections.

Pregnancy increases risks for women with SCD. There are also additional risks for the baby. During pregnancy, your care will be referred to a specialist centre with an expert sickle cell team.

Further information

- NHS Sickle Cell & Thalassaemia Screening Programme <http://www.sct.screening.nhs.uk> (leaflets and factsheets)
- Patient.co.uk. Sickle cell disease and sickle cell anaemia <http://www.patient.co.uk/health/Sickle-Cell-Disease-and-Sickle-Cell-Anaemia.htm>
- NHS Choices. Sickle cell anaemia <http://www.nhs.uk/conditions/Sickle-cell-anaemia>
- Thalassaemia <http://www.patient.co.uk/health/thalassaemia-leaflet>
- NHS Choices. Thalassaemia <http://www.nhs.uk/conditions/Thalassaemia/>

INFORMATION FOR PATIENTS Red cell antibodies and pregnancy

The specialist team will be happy to explain this condition in detail and will discuss options, management plans, and possible outcomes with you.

Further information

- BabyCenter. Blood test for Rh status and antibody screen <http://www.babycenter.com/0_blood-test-for-rh-status-and-antibody-screen_1480.bc>

INFORMATION FOR PATIENTS Thrombosis or embolism and pregnancy

The specialist team will be happy to explain this condition in detail and will discuss options, management plans, and possible outcomes with you.

Further information

- Royal College of Obstetricians and Gynaecologists. Reducing the risk of venous thrombosis in pregnancy and after birth <https://www.rcog.org.uk/globalassets/documents/patients/patient-information-leaflets/pregnancy/pi-reducing-the-risk-of-venous-thrombosis-in-pregnancy-and-after-birth.pdf>
- Royal College of Obstetricians and Gynaecologists. Treatment of venous thrombosis in pregnancy and after birth <https://www.rcog.org.uk/globalassets/documents/patients/patient-information-leaflets/pregnancy/treatment-of-venous-thrombosis-during-pregnancy-and-after-birth.pdf>

INFORMATION FOR PATIENTS Hereditary haemorrhagic telangiectasia

Hereditary haemorrhagic telangectasia (HHT) is a hereditary condition also known as Osler–Weber–Rendu (OWR) syndrome. There is a 50% chance that a baby will inherit the condition if one parent has HHT.

HHT can present as frequent nosebleeds, appearance of reddish-purple spots on the skin, especially on the hands, wrists and face, and on the lips, tongue, and fingertips. These tiny 'blood spots' disappear with slight pressure. People with HHT may also have been diagnosed as anaemic. In some cases there are also abnormal connections of blood vessels within certain organs such as the lungs, liver, or gut. These features do not appear at birth but are seen to develop with each decade of age.

Most women with HHT have no problems during pregnancy and it is rare for serious complications to develop. You need to be particularly aware of recurrent nosebleeds, or if you begin to cough up blood or develop any sudden breathlessness. If any of these happens you should seek immediate help.

During the pregnancy you will be under the care of a team of specialists, who will arrange any additional investigations that are needed. The specialists will help plan your care during pregnancy, labour, and delivery.

Further information

- The Hereditary Haemorrhagic Telangiectasia Self Help Group <http://www.telangiectasia.co.uk>

INFORMATION FOR PATIENTS Henoch–Schönlein purpura

Henoch–Schönlein purpura (pronounced as Heh-nawk Shurn-line pur-puh-ra) or HSP for short, is a rare condition where is inflammation and bleeding in the small blood vessels (capillaries) within skin, joints, bowels, and kidneys.

Although it can occur at any age, it is most common in children under the age of 10 years. It is rare in adults and even rarer in pregnancy. Most pregnant women would have already had a past history of HSP in childhood, although the condition may not have been active for several years. If you are known to have HSP, you can expect either an improvement of the condition or a relapse during pregnancy. It is very rare for the symptoms of HSP to appear for the very first time during pregnancy.

The exact cause of HSP is not known for certain at the present time although it is thought to be caused as an immune reaction to certain triggers. HPS is often triggered by an upper respiratory tract infection (cough, cold, or sore throat caused by various bacteria or viruses) or by exposure to certain medications. Symptoms may be triggered by cold weather.

HSP usually improves on its own within about 4–6 weeks, with no lasting problems. There may be relapses over the next few weeks but not as severe as the first time. Most cases are mild, and simple painkillers are sufficient (but remember not to take medications such as ibuprofen or diclofenac during pregnancy).

In HSP, there is a typical purplish skin rash on the lower part of both legs, sometimes extending into the buttocks and tummy. The rash resembles bruising or bleeding into the skin and is called purpura. You could also experience cramp-like tummy pains as well as nausea, vomiting, or blood in the stools as well as painful, swollen joints, especially the knees and ankles.

In about 25–50% of cases, there could be kidney problems which can sometimes persist for years. You might notice blood-stained urine, or blood and protein in the urine may be found only on testing. It is important that your doctor maintains a long-term follow-up of your kidneys, including regular blood pressure measurements and urine tests for any blood and/or protein loss.

During pregnancy, if you have not had previous kidney damage, the chances are that the course of the disease will remain mild and no specific treatment except painkillers may be needed. However, your blood pressure and urine protein should be monitored with extra care particularly in the third trimester (26–40 weeks) to exclude pregnancy-related high blood pressure, pre-eclampsia, or kidney problems. Your baby's growth will be monitored with scans, especially if you have raised blood pressure or kidney problems.

If the HSP causes significant problems you may be prescribed a course of a corticosteroid called prednisolone for about 4 weeks in gradually decreasing doses. This steroid is safe to use in pregnancy. In rare cases, a specialist may prescribe other medications to temporarily suppress the immune system, such as azathioprine or cyclophosphamide.

HSP is **not** a condition that you can transmit to your baby as the antibodies involved do not pass through the placenta. HSP is not contagious.

It is important that you have long-term follow-up visits to see your doctor, to avoid any lasting kidney damage.

Further information

- NHS Choices. Henoch–Schönlein purpura <http://www.nhs.uk/conditions/henoch-schonlein-purpura/Pages/Introduction.aspx>

INFORMATION FOR PATIENTS Hermansky–Pudlak syndrome

Hermansky–Pudlak syndrome (HPS) is a rare condition which has usually been diagnosed before pregnancy.

In this condition, a lack of pigment in the eye and skin can cause a condition called **albinism** and lead to vision defects. There are several varieties of HPS with skin colour ranging from olive to white, eye colour including blue, green, or brown, and hair colour varying from white to brown.

There is also an increased tendency to bleed, due to a defect in the function of platelets which are blood cells responsible for normal clotting of blood. Symptoms like easy bruising or bleeding from the nose and gums are not uncommon in this condition.

You should strictly avoid medications such as aspirin, diclofenac (Voltarol), or ibuprofen (Nurofen).

Most pregnancies in women with HPS proceed without any problems either for the mother or the baby.

In addition to the community midwife, your pregnancy will be cared for by a team of specialists who will help plan your care during labour and delivery in order to avoid complications such as bleeding after delivery. You will be referred to see an anaesthetic specialist doctor to consider options for pain relief during labour and delivery, because an epidural or spinal anaesthetic is best avoided in anyone with HPS.

Specific precautions will be taken to avoid or control any excessive bleeding after the baby's birth. If appropriate, platelets matched to your type will be kept available for transfusion.

Further information

- Hermansky–Pudlak Syndrome Network UK <http://www.hpsnetwork.co.uk>

INFORMATION FOR PATIENTS Hereditary spherocytosis

Hereditary spherocytosis ('sphe-ro-cy-to-sis) (HS for short) is an inherited condition where one parent has the condition and there is a 50% chance of passing it on to the baby. In most cases, there is a family history of the same condition.

The defect in HS lies in the red blood cells breaking up too quickly. Red blood cells contain haemoglobin, an iron-containing substance which carries oxygen to all parts of the body. The cells develop in the bone marrow and circulate for about 120 days in the body, after which they naturally break down and their components are recycled. Millions of new red blood cells are continuously produced every second in the bone marrow. In humans, normal mature red blood tcells are oval discs that are concave on both sides. In HS, the red cells are round in shape (hence 'sphero' appears in the name) and this changed shape makes them prone to break down easily. The lifespan of these abnormally shaped red cells decreases from the usual 120 days in the blood circulation to just a few days. This leads to a form of chronic or long-standing anaemia.

HS can vary from mild to severe. In some people there are no symptoms and the condition is only diagnosed when you have had booking bloods taken in your first pregnancy. In others, HS may be severe with significant anaemia, jaundice, and an enlarged spleen. Such cases are found in childhood and need repeated red cell transfusions.

If you have been diagnosed to have HS before pregnancy, you will be advised a high dose of folic acid to be taken throughout pregnancy. These high-dose folic acid tablets (5 mg) can be obtained only on prescription from your GP or specialist obstetrician and cannot be purchased over the counter.

If you have not had parvovirus ('slapped-cheek') infection in the past, you need to be particularly careful to avoid exposure to this in pregnancy as it may cause rapid and severe breakdown of red cells in people with HS. Emergency red cell transfusions may be required.

If you have previously had your spleen removed you will be on lifelong penicillin and this will need to continue during pregnancy. You will be advised about how best to prevent a deep vein thrombosis (DVT) as there is an increased tendency for abnormal blood clotting in people with high platelet counts after previous removal of the spleen. (Platelets are cells in the blood responsible for normal clotting.) If you have had your spleen removed it is advisable to carry a **splenectomy card** on you at all times. Ask your GP or the hospital specialist team if you need one.

Your specialists will be happy to discuss your concerns about pregnancy and HS.

Further information

- Patient.co.uk. Hereditary spherocytosis <http://www.patient.co.uk/health/Hereditary-Spherocytosis.htm>

INFORMATION FOR PATIENTS Thrombotic thrombocytopenic purpura and haemolytic uraemic-syndrome

Thrombotic-thrombocytopenic purpura (TTP) and haemolytic uraemic syndrome (HUS)are closely connected and extremely rare conditions.

Women are more prone to TTP-HUS especially during pregnancy. Some rare forms of HUS can also occur outside of pregnancy and can recur in subsequent pregnancies.

The symptoms of TTP-HUS are often not specific and include features such as fatigue, paleness, and chest, tummy or joint pains with mild fever. Several organs and tissues in the body can be affected.

Specific tests including blood tests and kidney function tests are necessary to diagnose the condition and you may need to be referred to a specialist centre for urgent treatment in pregnancy and after, in the case of an acute attack. This could include a procedure called plasma exchange. All tests and treatment options will be discussed in detail with you by the specialists involved in your care.

During pregnancy, particular care will be taken for early detection of conditions such as pre-eclampsia or growth problems of the baby. Ultrasound scans to monitor the baby's well-being will be arranged.

Further information

- Atypical haemolytic uraemic syndrome support group (aHUS): <http://ahusuk.org/ahus-is-rare-2/>
- Haemolytic Uraemic Syndrome Help support group (HUSH)<http://www.ecoli-uk.com/>
- Netdoctor. Haemolytic uraemic syndrome <http://www.netdoctor.co.uk/diseases/facts/haemolyticuraemic.htm>
- TTP Network (online support group) <http://www.ttpnetwork.org.uk>

2. Maternal Infections

INFORMATION FOR PATIENTS Bacterial vaginosis and pregnancy

Frequently asked questions

What is bacterial vaginosis (BV)?

BV is a common condition caused by an overgrowth of various bacteria. It is not caused by just one type of bacterium. BV is at least twice as common as thrush. At least 1 in 10 women have BV at some time in their child-bearing years.

What are the symptoms of BV?

- The main symptom of BV is a vaginal discharge. BV is the most common cause of vaginal discharge for women of child-bearing age. The discharge is usually white-grey in colour with a fishy odour.
- There is usually no itching or soreness.
- Up to 50% of women with BV do not have any symptoms and BV may be found by chance when vaginal swabs are taken for other reasons.

What causes BV?

Normally there are a number of different types of harmless bacteria in the vagina. When there is a change in the balance of the normal bacteria, some types multiply and thrive much more than usual. The normal lactobacilli are replaced by high concentrations of BV bacteria, thereby changing the pH of the vagina.

BV is not caused by poor hygiene, nor is it sexually transmitted. Your partner does not need any treatment.

What are the possible complications with BV during pregnancy?

Untreated BV during pregnancy can cause an increased risk of premature birth, late miscarriages (after 13 weeks of pregnancy), early breaking of the waters before labour, and prematurity.

What is the treatment for BV in pregnancy?

Clindamycin is the antibiotic most commonly used to treat BV during pregnancy. This usually involves a course of 5–7 days treatment either with a vaginal cream of clindamycin (2%) or oral tablets of clindamycin. This may need to be repeated during the course of pregnancy as BV can recur within 3 months of successful treatment. A repeat course of antibiotics will usually be sufficient. You will need further swab testing to check that BV has been eradicated.

Can further episodes of BV be avoided?

Most instances of BV occur for no apparent reason, both during pregnancy and at other times, and cannot be prevented. Avoidance of douching, which pushes water into the vagina, may help prevent upsetting the normal balance of bacteria in the vagina.

Further Information

- Patient.co.uk. Bacterial vaginosis <http://www.patient.co.uk/health/bacterial-vaginosis-leaflet>
- NHS Choices. Bacterial vaginosis <http://www.nhs.uk/conditions/bacterialvaginosis>

INFORMATION FOR PATIENTS Chickenpox and pregnancy

The specialist team will be happy to explain this condition in detail and will discuss options, management plans, and possible outcomes with you.

Further information

- Royal College of Obstetricians and Gynaecologists. Chickenpox in pregnancy <http://www.rcog.org.uk/womens-health/clinical-guidance/chickenpox-pregnancy-what-you-need-know>

INFORMATION FOR PATIENTS Cytomegalovirus infection and pregnancy

Cytomegalovirus (CMV) is one of the herpes group of viruses. About 60% of all adults in Western countries have had CMV infection at some time, usually in childhood. After the initial infection the virus remains inactive in the body for life but can become reactivated during pregnancy. Blood tests are used to detect specific antibodies to identify recent infection or reactivation of CMV.

Most infections occur without any symptoms but flu-like illness with fever, sore throat, fatigue, swollen glands, muscle and joint pains, loss of appetite, shortness of breath, diarrhoea, and painful mouth ulcers can also be experienced.

In most cases where CMV is transmitted from the mother to the baby during pregnancy, no damage is caused to the baby. In 1 in 10 cases, however, the baby could be born with symptoms that might cause long-term problems, such as learning difficulties.

If CMV infection occurs for the first time during pregnancy, in about 40% of infected mothers the infection can be transmitted to the baby **through the placenta.** There is a greater chance of the fetus being infected if the mother contracts CMV infection just before getting pregnant, or within the first trimester (the first 13 weeks of pregnancy), or early in the second trimester. This might result in growth restriction and problems with the development of the skull bones or brain.

If the mother gets infected during the second half of pregnancy, there is a greater risk of the newborn baby developing problems affecting the liver, lungs, and blood clotting.

CMV can also be transmitted due to the baby swallowing secretions in the birth passage during the birth process. Rarely, a baby can become infected after birth by CMV transmitted through breast milk.

At present there is no treatment available to treat the unborn baby if the mother contracts CMV infection for the first time during pregnancy The specialist team caring for you during pregnancy will discuss all available options with you. The paediatricians will be alerted and all the necessary tests will be performed once the baby is born.

Further information

- UK Screening Portal. Cytomegalovirus <www.screening.nhs.uk/cytomegalovirus>
- NHS Choices. Cytomegalovirus (CMV) <http://www.nhs.uk/conditions/pregnancy-and-baby/pages/pregnancy-infections.aspx#Cytomegalovirus>
- Great Ormond Street Hospital. Congenital CMV infection information <http://www.gosh.nhs.uk/medical-information/search-for-medical-conditions/congenital-cmv-infection/congenital-cmv-infection-information/>

INFORMATION FOR PATIENTS Genital herpes and pregnancy

The specialist team will be happy to explain this condition in detail and will discuss options, management plans, and possible outcomes with you.

Further information

- Royal College of Obstetricians and Gynaecologists. Genital herpes in pregnancy <http://www.rcog.org.uk>

INFORMATION FOR PATIENTS Group B streptococcus infection and pregnancy

The specialist team will be happy to explain this condition in detail and will discuss options, management plans, and possible outcomes with you.

Further information

- Royal College of Obstetricians and Gynaecologists. Group B streptococcus (GBS) infection in newborn babies <https://www.rcog.org.uk/en/patients/patient-leaflets/group-b-streptococcus-gbs-infection-in-newborn-babies/>.

INFORMATION FOR PATIENTS Hepatitis B and pregnancy

Hepatitis B virus (Hep B or HBV for short) is an infectious virus that attacks the liver. The virus is transmitted through blood and infected bodily fluids. This can occur through direct blood-to-blood contact, unprotected sex, use of unsterile needles, and from an infected woman to her newborn during the delivery process.

A hepatitis B infection is considered to be 'acute' during the first 6 months after being infected, which the average period of time is taken to recover from a hepatitis B infection. If you still test positive for the hepatitis B virus after 6 months, you are considered to have a 'chronic' hepatitis B infection, which can last a lifetime.

Most people with chronic hepatitis B can expect to live long, healthy lives. It is important, however, to know that you can pass the virus along to others, even if you are not ill. This is why it is important that you make sure that your partner and all family members are vaccinated against hepatitis B.

As it is found in highest concentrations in blood, the viral infection can be transmitted from an affected mother to the baby during childbirth.

All pregnant women should be offered the test for hepatitis B. This is included as part of the booking blood tests that are performed at the first visit by your midwife. If you test positive for hepatitis B the virus can be passed on to your newborn baby during delivery. To help to prevent the baby from getting infected, certain procedures will be followed during delivery and the proper medications and vaccines kept ready to be given to the newborn baby immediately after birth. Without such procedures, the risk of your baby getting infected is as high as 90–95%.

Once the appropriate vaccine and immune medications (as indicated by the tests you have already had during pregnancy) are given within the first 12 hours of life, a newborn has more than a 90% chance of being protected against a lifelong hepatitis B infection.

It is also very important that your baby receives the second and third dose of the hepatitis B vaccine at 1 month and 6 months of age to ensure complete protection.

Although hepatitis B infection does not generally cause any problems for you or your unborn baby during the pregnancy itself, long term follow-up of your liver by the doctors and liver specialists is recommended and appropriate referrals will be arranged.

Further information

- British Liver Trust. Looking after your liver. <http://www.britishlivertrust.org.uk/liver-information/looking-after-your-liver/viral-hepatitis/>
- Hepatitis B Foundation. Pregnancy and HBV. <http://www.hepb.org/patients/pregnant_women.htm>
- Patient.co.uk <http://www.patient.co.uk/health/hepatitis-b-leaflet>

INFORMATION FOR PATIENTS Hepatitis C and pregnancy

Frequently asked questions

What is hepatitis C?

Hepatitis C (Hep C) is a virus transmitted by infected blood or bodily fluids. Hepatitis C virus can cause serious liver damage.

There is no medication or vaccine available to **prevent** infection, which is why activities such as sharing razors, needles or toothbrushes; using dirty needles for injecting drugs, tattooing, or body piercing; or unprotected sexual intercourse should be avoided. Blood transfusion in countries where blood is not tested (unlike in the UK where it is carefully tested) can also cause infection.

At present there are certain medications available which can clear the virus in only about half of patients who are already infected, although treatments are being developed all the time.

Transmission of infection from the mother to baby is the most common way for childhood infection to be acquired. Hepatitis C is rare in children, however, and only 1 in 20 of infected mothers will pass on the virus on to their unborn baby. This occurs during pregnancy in one-third of cases and during the process of delivery in the rest.

Diagnosis is by a blood test. If the blood test shows that you do have hepatitis C, you will be referred to a specialist liver doctor.

What are the symptoms of acute infection?

In most cases (nearly 75%) there are no obvious symptoms and the person may be unaware of having been infected for several years. If symptoms do develop they are non-specific: that is, symptoms that can occur in many conditions, not only hepatitis C. Such symptoms can include:

- flu-like illness with tiredness, muscle and joint aches as well as fever
- nausea, vomiting, and loss of appetite
- weight loss
- tummy pains
- jaundice (yellowing of the skin and whites of the eyes).

At present there are no vaccines or treatment available during pregnancy.Certain precautions will be undertaken during labour and delivery to minimize the risk of infection to the baby. Delivery by a planned Caesarean section does not make a difference to the chances of the baby becoming infected. There is no contraindication for breast feeding.

You will need to have long-term follow-up with liver specialists because of the risk of developing liver damage. Many people who become infected with hepatitis C require no treatment and are able to clear the infection naturally.

Your baby will need long-term follow-up with children's liver specialists till at least 2 years of age, because it is often difficult to detect whether an infant has been infected with hepatitis C till the child is a couple of years old when a firm diagnosis can be made.

In some babies (10–25%) the virus is cleared naturally within the first 3 years of life. Hepatitis C is usually a very mild disease in children, with few symptoms, but they may be at significant risk of developing liver disease later in life.

Further information

- Hepatitis C in pregnancy. <http://www.uhs.nhs.uk/Media/Controlleddocuments/Patientinformation/Pregnancyandbirth/HepatitisCinpregnancy-patientinformation.pdf>
- British Liver Trust. Looking after your liver. <http://www.britishlivertrust.org.uk/liver-information/looking-after-your-liver/viral-hepatitis/>
- SIGN Guideline No. 133. Management of hepatitis C <http://www.sign.ac.uk/pdf/sign133.pdf>

INFORMATION FOR PATIENTS Swine flu (H1N1) and pregnancy

If necessary, your GP, community midwives, hospital doctors, and midwives will have given you information about swine flu and encouraged you to have the vaccine as soon as possible.

Further information

- NHS Choices. Swine flu (H1N1) <http://www.nhs.uk/Conditions/Pandemic-flu/Pages/Introduction.aspx>

INFORMATION FOR PATIENTS HIV and pregnancy

The specialist team will be happy to explain this condition in detail and will discuss options, management plans, and possible outcomes with you.

Further information

- Royal College of Obstetricians and Gynaecologists. HIV in pregnancy: information for you. <https://www.rcog.org.uk/globalassets/documents/patients/patient-information-leaflets/pregnancy/hiv-and-pregnancy.pdf>

INFORMATION FOR PATIENTS Listeriosis and pregnancy

Listeriosis is a rare disease caused by *Listeria monocytogenes* (mono-cyto-gen-es) which is a common bacterium found in the natural environment. Listeriosis is most often a food-borne illness.

Listeria is found in soil, water, vegetation, and faeces of humans and animals. Plants and vegetables can become contaminated with the bacteria from soil, water, or manure-based fertilizers.

Eating food contaminated with listeria may cause mild illness in pregnant women, with fever, severe headache, nausea, and vomiting. Sometimes there may be no symptoms at all. Symptoms usually appear within 2 to 30 days, and sometimes up to 90 days after consuming contaminated food.

Rarely if the pregnant woman has additional conditions that weaken her immune system such as diabetes or HIV, or is on long-term steroids, maternal infection may be severe. Pregnant women are at higher risk than other healthy adults who come into contact with listeria.

If a pregnant woman develops listeriosis during the first 12 weeks of pregnancy, she may miscarry usually after about 2 weeks.

Listeriosis later on in the pregnancy can result in a stillbirth or the birth of an acutely-ill child.

A pregnant women can pass the infection on to the fetus within the womb during pregnancy or during passage through the infected birth canal at the time of birth. The baby may develop signs of severe sepsis within 1 to 2 days after birth. In the late-onset form of the infection, the baby may become very ill 1–2 weeks after birth, with signs of meningitis.

A pregnant woman can reduce her risk of listeriosis by following advice about hygienic food preparation, storage, and consumption.

Diagnosis is confirmed by finding the infectious agent *Listeria monocytogenes* grown from blood or amniotic fluid, or from the placenta after delivery.

If a pregnant woman contracts listeriosis, high dose of specific antibiotics can be given by injection into a vein to treat the infection. This usually needs to be given for 2–3 weeks.

Your midwife and doctor as well as specialists you see in the hospital will discuss your queries in detail.

Further information

- Health Unit. Preconception/Pregnancy—Pregnancy & Listeriosis <http://www.healthunit.org/pregnancy/pregnancy/pregnancy_Listeriosis.htm>
- NHS Choices. Listeriosis. <http://www.nhs.uk/conditions/Listeriosis>
- Patient.co.uk. Listeria. <http://www.patient.co.uk/health/listeria>

INFORMATION FOR PATIENTS Malaria and pregnancy

The specialist team will be happy to explain this condition in detail and will discuss options, management plans, and possible outcomes with you.

Sources of information

- NHS Choices. Malaria—Antimalarials <http://www.nhs.uk/Conditions/Malaria/Pages/Treatment.aspx>
- Patient.co.uk. Malaria in pregnancy <http://www.patient.co.uk/doctor/malaria-in-pregnancy>
- Patient.co.uk. Malaria prevention <http://www.patient.co.uk/health/malaria-prevention>
- Public Health England. Malaria: guidance, data and analysis <https://www.gov.uk/government/collections/malaria-guidance-data-and-analysis#prevention-treatment-and-investigation>

INFORMATION FOR PATIENTS Sexually transmitted infections and pregnancy: gonorrhoea, chlamydia, anogenital warts, and trichomonas

The specialist team will be happy to explain these conditions in detail and will discuss options, management plans, and possible outcomes with you.

Further information

Gonorrhoea

- BMJ Best Practice. Gonorrhoea infection. <http://bestpractice.bmj.com/best-practice/pdf/patient>
- NHS Choices. Gonorrhoea. <http://www.nhs.uk/Conditions/Gonorrhoea/Pages/Introduction.aspx>

Chlamydia

- Patient.co.uk. Genital chlamydia <http://www.patient.co.uk>
- NHS Choices. Chlamydia treatment <http://www.nhs.uk/Conditions/Chlamydia/Pages/Treatment.aspx>
- Family Planning Association. Chlamydia <http://www.fpa.org.uk/sexually-transmitted-infections-stis-help/chlamydia>

Anogenital warts

- Patient.co.uk. Anogenital warts <http://www.patient.co.uk>

Trichomonas vaginalis

- Patient.co.uk. Trichomonas infection <http://www.patient.co.uk>
- Women's Health, UK. Trichomoniasis <http://www.womens-health.co.uk/trich.html>

INFORMATION FOR PATIENTS Parvovirus ('slapped cheek') infection in pregnancy

Parvovirus infection, caused by a virus called parvovirus B19, is also known as 'slapped cheek' infection or 'Fifth disease'. Outbreaks usually occur in nurseries or schools, with seasonal peaks in late winter or early spring.

Approximately 60% of women are immune to the virus by the age of 20 years, following infection sometime in the past. After one attack, you develop immunity for life.

The virus is spread through infected respiratory droplets transmitted from person to person. It could present as a flu-like illness with some fever, tiredness and joint pains, but 25% of parvovirus infections occur without any symptoms. A third of patients develop a rash on the face appearing like slapped cheeks.

If infection has occurred within the first 4 weeks of your pregnancy, the fetus is safe from being infected. After this stage, there is a 50% risk of transmission from an infected mother to the unborn baby in the womb. The virus does not cause any fetal malformations.

A baby infected in the womb could develop heart failure and severe anaemia with abnormal fluid collection in tissues and under the skin. In severe cases the baby can die during pregnancy some 4–6 weeks after the mother's infection.

The time from exposure to the virus till developing the rash is 2–3 weeks. The patient is infective from 10 days before the rash is visible until the onset of the rash. Once the rash appears, patients are no longer infectious.

If you have come in contact with known or suspected parvovirus infection during pregnancy, you should have blood tests done as soon as possible to check whether you are immune or not. This will help determine whether any further investigations or interventions are required.

If the baby is suspected to have developed excess fluid accumulation within tissues and skin, known as hydrops, you will be referred to the closest specialist unit for consideration of blood transfusion for the unborn baby.

At present there is no vaccine or medication to prevent infection.

Further information

- Patient.co.uk. Slapped cheek disease, fifth disease <http://www.patient.co.uk>
- Pregnancy and Childbirth Guide. Human parvovirus and pregnancy <http://www.pregnancyandchildbirthguide.com/human-parvovirus-and-preg>
- NHS Choices. What are the risks of slapped cheek syndrome during pregnancy? <http://www.nhs.uk/chq/pages/1112.aspx?categoryid=54&subcategoryid=137>

INFORMATION FOR PATIENTS Syphilis and pregnancy

The specialist doctors in the genitourinary medicine (GUM) clinic and the maternity clinic, or the specialist midwife, will be happy to answer all your enquiries.

Further information

- Patient.co.uk. Syphilis <http://www.patient.co.uk>
- NHS Choices. Syphilis <http://www.nhs.uk/conditions/Syphilis>
- NHS Choices, Syphilis treatment <http://www.nhs.uk/Conditions/Syphilis/Pages/Treatmentpg.aspx>
- Patient.co.uk. Maternal syphilis in pregnancy childbirth puerperium <http://www.patient.co.uk/.../maternal_syphilis_in_pregnancy_childbirth_>

INFORMATION FOR PATIENTS Tuberculosis (TB) and pregnancy

The specialist team will be happy to explain this condition in detail and will discuss options, management plans, and possible outcomes with you.

Further information

- Public Health England. TB, BCG and your baby leaflet <https://www.gov.uk/government/publications/tb-bcg-and-your-baby-leaflet>

INFORMATION FOR PATIENTS Toxoplasmosis and pregnancy

Toxoplasmosis(toxo-plas-mo-sis) is an infection caused by an organism called *Toxoplasma gondii*.

In adults, toxoplasmosis infection produces very few symptoms; one in 10 may experience mild flu-like symptoms with fever, fatigue and headache, and swollen glands.

Most women of childbearing age are susceptible to infection at the time of pregnancy booking in the UK. There is no routine screening of all pregnant mothers in the UK as the prevalence of toxoplasmosis is very low.

The definitive host for the infection is the cat. Consumption of inadequately cooked or raw food such as salads contaminated with cat litter, or inadequate hand-washing after gardening or contact with cats, are the main sources of infection.

Toxoplasmosis cannot be transmitted from person to person except through the placenta from mother to baby during pregnancy. It is rare for the infection to pass to the baby during early pregnancy (first trimester, the first 13 weeks of pregnancy) but, if it does, it can cause serious abnormalities.

In later pregnancy (after the first trimester), the infection more commonly passes to the baby. For example:

- If you become infected around the time of conception, there is less than a 5% chance that your baby will also develop the infection.
- If you become infected during the third trimester of your pregnancy (from week 27 until the birth), there is about a 65% chance that your baby will also be infected. However, babies infected during later pregnancy are less likely to suffer serious consequences.

The earlier in pregnancy that the baby is infected the more severe is the clinical disease and the effects in the infant. Infection is more common later in pregnancy, but infection after the first trimester (13 weeks) of pregnancy does not usually result in serious consequences for the baby.

A baby who is infected early in pregnancy can unfortunately suffer very serious developmental abnormalities and malformations including defects of the brain, eyes, or liver. Miscarriage and stillbirth are also more likely. No treatment can undo any damage and malformations that might have already resulted due to early infection of the developing baby. The doctors looking after your pregnancy will discuss the tests and options available to you under these circumstances.

If acute infection is suspected, it is diagnosed by finding increasing levels of antibodies to the condition during pregnancy. If the mother tests positive for acute infection with toxoplasmosis, continued treatment with certain medications up until delivery can help reduce the risk of transmission of infection to the baby during childbirth.

Further information

- Tommy's. Toxoplasmosis information <http://www.tommys.org/toxo>
- NHS Choices. What are the risks of toxoplasmosis during pregnancy? <http://www.nhs.uk/chq/Pages/1107.aspx?CategoryID=54...137>
- NHS Choices. Toxoplasmosis. <http://www.nhs.uk/conditions/Toxoplasmosis>

INFORMATION FOR PATIENTS Urinary tract infection and pregnancy

Urinary tract infections (UTIs) are common in pregnancy and can lead to complications for both the mother and the baby if not recognized and adequately treated.

These infections can sometimes be silent and not produce any symptoms to alert you. On the other hand, UTIs may produce symptoms such as burning sensation while passing urine, increased urgency and frequency of having to pass water, and a sense of incomplete emptying of the bladder. The urine might have a strong smell. Pain in the lower part of the tummy, sometimes also spreading to the sides and back, can occur. If infection from the bladder, known as **cystitis (cyst-eye-tis)** spreads upwards to involve the kidneys, this can result in severe pain, high temperatures, sickness, and vomiting leading to dehydration, a condition called **pyelonephritis(pye-lo-nef-ry-tis)**.

It is also not uncommon to get repeated attacks of UTI in pregnancy, especially if it has not been completely cleared the first time or if there are other conditions such as diabetes, kidney stones, or sickle cell disease. In some situations, you may be advised to continue a low-dose of a suitable antibiotic as a maintenance dose for the remainder of pregnancy

Even if the UTI is silent, problems such as premature labour, growth problems of the baby, infection spreading into the womb, or anaemia can result due to UTIs. This is why routine urine testing for the presence of bacteria even if you have no symptoms is done at the first booking visit as part of standard antenatal practice in the UK, applicable to all pregnancies.

Prompt treatment with an appropriate antibiotic is prescribed for a minimum of 5–7 days. The antibiotics used to treat urine infections in pregnant women are safe to take in pregnancy and will not harm your baby.

After the completion of the full treatment course, a repeat sample taken from the middle of the stream of urine should ideally be sent to the lab by your GP or midwife to ensure that the infection has been cleared completely. Some bacteria are resistant to some antibiotics, and this can be identified from tests done on the urine sample. A change of antibiotic is needed if the bacterium is found to be resistant to the first antibiotic.

You will invariably need to be admitted if you develop **acute pyelonephritis**. Antibiotics and fluids are often needed, through drips, as well as adequate pain relief. The antibiotics are usually required to be continued for 10–14 days after the acute infection is controlled in order to achieve complete clearance.

Further information

- Patient.co.uk. Urine infection in pregnancy <http://www.patient.co.uk>

INFORMATION FOR PATIENTS Pneumonia and pregnancy

The specialist team will be happy to explain this condition in detail and will discuss options, management plans, and possible outcomes with you.

Further information

- NHS Choices. Pneumonia <http://www.nhs.uk>

INFORMATION FOR PATIENTS Sepsis and pregnancy

The specialist team will be happy to explain this condition in detail and will discuss options, management plans, and possible outcomes with you.

Further information

- UK Sepsis Trust. Sepsis: a guide for patients & relatives <http://sepsistrust.org/wp-content/uploads/2013/10/Sepsis_A5_final1.pdf>

3. Maternal Respiratory Conditions

INFORMATION FOR PATIENTS Moderate/severe asthma and pregnancy

Asthma is not an uncommon condition; 4–7% of pregnant women have asthma.

If your asthma is mild and well controlled, it is very unlikely to pose a problem during pregnancy. Your pregnancy care will be managed by your community midwife and if there are no other problems you will not need hospital antenatal visits. Asthma improves in a third of pregnant women, remains the same in a third, and worsens in a third!

Even if asthma is moderate or severe, with good control most women will have an uncomplicated pregnancy with good outcome.

- **If you are a smoker, you are strongly advised to stop as soon as possible**. We can offer you the help and support resource to help you to do so.
- **You are advised not to stop any asthma medications during pregnancy** as these drugs have no adverse effects on the developing baby at any stage in pregnancy.

All asthma medications are safe not only during pregnancy but during breastfeeding. **This includes steroids**. (The exception is new medications like leukotriene receptor antagonist, where not enough is known, unlike with all the common asthma medications.)

There is no increased risk of miscarriage or pregnancy loss associated with steroids used in asthma. If you have been on long-term oral steroids (prednisolone), you will be offered a glucose tolerance test at about 28 weeks to exclude the possibility of a reversible and temporary diabetes during the pregnancy. If you have needed only short courses of oral steroids during the pregnancy you will not need to have this test.

The risk of poorly or inadequately controlled asthma during pregnancy can be serious and may even lead to problems such as raised blood pressure, pre-eclampsia, or premature delivery, or could affect the baby's growth.

If you have severe asthma the most likely times when it could worsen in pregnancy are between 24 and 32 weeks of pregnancy and after you have had the baby.

Asthma can actually improve during the last few weeks of pregnancy and it is very unlikely that you would have an attack during labour or delivery.

Most forms of pain relief are safe and available to you during labour. If you have severe asthma you will have an appointment during pregnancy to discuss this with a senior anaesthetist. An epidural is particularly advisable if pain and anxiety are triggers for an asthma attack.

Certain drugs commonly used for other situations during pregnancy or labour, can on rare occasions trigger an asthma attack, especially in severe or hard-to-control asthma. The medical team will ensure that these drugs are avoided during pregnancy, labour, and delivery.

The fact that you have asthma, even if severe, should not in itself influence unnecessary interventions such as early induction of labour or Caesarean section. Such interventions would be advised only if there are other problems with the pregnancy.

If a mother is asthmatic, the chances of the baby developing asthma later in life is doubled. Breastfeeding is encouraged as it can decrease chances of your baby developing asthma later in infancy and childhood. All medications for asthma are safe for breastfeeding.

Further information

- Patient.co.uk. Management of asthma in pregnancy <http://www.patient.co.uk>
- Asthma UK. Pregnancy FAQs <http://www.asthma.org.uk>

INFORMATION FOR PATIENTS Cystic fibrosis and pregnancy

Cystic fibrosis (CF) is a common inherited disease with 1 in 25 or 4% of white Europeans carrying the defective gene.

With improved care, the survival rate in CF has significantly improved so that it is no longer found only in children. More young women with well-managed CF want to have babies and pregnancy is becoming increasingly common, with the expectation of generally good outcomes for the mother and baby.

Inheritance of cystic fibrosis

If you have cystic fibrosis, that means you have two defective copies of the CF gene. You will pass one of those on to your child. Your baby will either be a carrier or have cystic fibrosis disease, depending on the gene he or she gets from your partner.

If your partner has two normal genes, your baby will have one defective gene from you and one normal gene from your partner. This child will be a cystic fibrosis carrier.

If your partner has one normal and one defective CF gene, he is a carrier. Your baby will then have a 50% chance of having cystic fibrosis disease and 50% chance of being a carrier, depending on which gene the baby inherits from your partner.

Genetic testing to find out whether you or your partner is a carrier is available and this can help you make informed decisions about having children together.

CF and pregnancy

Outcomes of pregnancy are better when the pregnancy is planned because you would receive close monitoring from the beginning.

The strain of pregnancy can complicate cystic fibrosis. Your cystic fibrosis specialists are experts on your condition and can assess and advise if you are healthy enough to withstand the additional strain of a pregnancy.

Pregnancy is better tolerated by those with the less severe forms of the disease.

Complications that are common in pregnant women with CF include:

- Increased breathing difficulty: this is the most serious risk of pregnancy for women with CF.
- Increased respiratory infections: reduced lung function can lead to respiratory infections, which will make it even harder to breathe.
- Diabetes: the risk of developing diabetes during pregnancy is increased in women with CF because of the damage CF causes to the pancreas.
- Malnutrition: pregnancy increases the body's energy requirement, and makes adequate nutrition even more difficult to accomplish. Poor maternal weight gain or even weight loss is not uncommon in pregnant women with CF.
- Once a pregnancy is planned and established, you will be looked after by your CF team who have been responsible for your care as well as healthcare professionals in both primary care and hospital-based services, with close involvement of the regional/national specialist CF units.

In general, during pregnancy and after delivery, particular care will be given to the following:

- Improving your nutrition with good nutrition and supplements of iron, folic acid, vitamin D, etc.
- Preventing or actively treating any infection of the lungs
- Intensified airway clearance techniques as well as additional oxygen therapy and physiotherapy if there is any acute breathing difficulty
- Regular assessment of fetal growth
- Extra help and support in the postnatal period, ensuring adequate hydration and nutrition and active treatment of any infection of the lungs

Your baby will be screened for CF.

Further information

- Cystic Fibrosis Trust. Information for patients <http://www.cysticfibrosis.org.uk/about-cf/publications/leaflets>
- Cystic Fibrosis Trust <http://www.cftrust.org.uk> 11 London Road, Bromley, Kent, BR1 1BY, Tel: 02084647211, Fax: 02083130472, Email: <http://enquiries@cftrust.org.uk>

INFORMATION FOR PATIENTS Sarcoidosis and pregnancy

Sarcoidosis is a condition that may affect many areas of the body such as the lungs, skin, liver, or eyes. Calcium levels are higher than usual in both blood and urine in people with sarcoidosis.

You may have experienced cough, shortness of breath, chest pain, tiredness, weakness, weight loss, and fever. Sometimes, however, there may be no symptoms and the condition may have been diagnosed only by chance on a chest X-ray.

Sarcoidosis may sometimes resolve by itself without requiring treatment. Treatment is required if there are lung or eye problems.

Pregnancy does not affect the course of the disease in people whose sarcoidosis has been stable or inactive. If you have had active disease, you may notice an improvement during pregnancy. The symptoms can, however, worsen after about 3–6 months following delivery. Rarely, sarcoidosis can worsen during the course of pregnancy.

Sarcoidosis is not an inherited condition; you will not pass it on to your baby. It does not appear to cause any problems with pregnancy outcomes. There is no increase in miscarriages, pregnancy or delivery complications, or birth defects. The management of pregnancy, labour, and delivery does not differ except where there are severe lung problems.

Treatment with steroids (prednisolone tablets) is used to achieve control of symptoms in sarcoidosis. These tablets are safe to use in pregnancy and usually only low doses are required. Sometimes other drugs are needed in people who are not responding well to steroids, or to reduce the dose of steroids required to keep symptoms under control. These drugs include hydroxychloroquine, azathioprine, or ciclosporin.

Because of the high levels of calcium in the blood in people with sarcoidosis, it is advisable to avoid both vitamin D and calcium supplements during pregnancy. The contents of any multivitamin preparation should be carefully checked. If needed, iron and folic acid supplements can be taken separately instead of a general multivitamin preparation

During pregnancy, you can expect to be cared for specialists in obstetrics and in respiratory diseases in addition to the community midwife and your GP. Your lung function tests will be checked at specific intervals during pregnancy.

Unless you have severe lung disease, a normal delivery is to be expected. Your specialists will discuss the type of delivery as well as pain relief in labour with you after due assessments.

Your specialist team will give you information about sarcoidosis and its management in pregnancy and will be happy to answer your questions.

Further information

- Patient.co.uk. Sarcoidosis <http://www.patient.co.uk>
- NHS Choices. Sarcoidosis <http://www.nhs.uk>

4. Maternal Cardiac Disease

INFORMATION FOR PATIENTS Heart disease and pregnancy

The specialist team will be happy to explain this condition in detail and will discuss options, management plans, and possible outcomes with you.

Further information

- British Heart Foundation, Greater London House, 180 Hampstead Road, London, NW1 7AW. Tel (Heart Help Line): 0300 330 3311; <http://www.bhf.org.uk>
- NHS Choices. Congenital heart disease <http://www.nhs.uk/conditions/Congenital-heart-disease>
- NHS Choices. Congenital heart disease. Pregnancy guide <http://www.nhs.uk/Planners/.../Pages/Congenitalheartdisease.aspx>
- Patient.co.uk. Congenital heart disease <http://www.patient.co.uk>
- Royal College of Obstetricians and Gynaecologists. Cardiac disease and pregnancy, Good Practice No. 13, Appendix B <https://www.rcog.org.uk/en/guidelines-research-services/guidelines/good-practice-13/>

INFORMATION FOR PATIENTS Congenital heart disease and pregnancy

If there is a history of congenital heart disease (CHD) in you, your partner, or a previous baby, or if CHD has been diagnosed in your baby in this pregnancy, you will be invited to discuss all issues with the specialists in obstetrics, paediatric cardiology, and genetics, as well as the paediatrician (baby specialist) and scan specialists.

Further information

- NHS Choices. Congenital heart disease <http://www.nhs.uk/conditions/Congenital-heart-disease>
- NHS Choices. Congenital heart disease. Pregnancy guide <http://www.nhs.uk/Planners/.../Pages/Congenitalheartdisease.aspx>
- NHS Choices. Congenital heart disease. Complications <http://www.nhs.uk/Conditions/Congenital-heart-disease/.../Complications.as>
- British Heart Foundation, Greater London House, 180 Hampstead Road, London, NW1 7AW; Tel (Heart Help Line): 0300 330 3311; <http://www.bhf.org.uk>
- Grown Up Congenital Heart Patients Association (GUCH), Saracen's House, 25 St Margaret's Green, Ipswich IP4 2BN; Tel (Helpline): 0800 854 759; <http://www.guch.org.uk>
- Patient.co.uk. Congenital heart disease <http://www.patient.co.uk>

INFORMATION FOR PATIENTS Cardiomyopathy and pregnancy

The specialist team will be happy to explain this condition in detail and will discuss options, management plans, and possible outcomes with you.

Further information

- British Heart Foundation. Cardiomyopathies <http://www.bhf.org.uk/heart-health/conditions/cardiomyopathy.aspx>
- Cardiac Risk in the Young. Hypertrophic cardiomyopathy (HCM). <http://www.c-r-y.org.uk/hypertrophic_cardiomyopathy.htm>
- Cardiomyopathy Association. Hypertrophic cardiomyopathy <http://www.cardiomyopathy.org/index.php?id=49>
- Patient.co.uk. Dilated cardiomyopathy <http://www.patient.co.uk>
- Patient.co.uk. Hypertrophic cardiomyopathy <http://www.patient.co.uk/health/Cardiomyopathy-Hypertrophic.htm>
- PubMedHealth (US). <http://www.ncbi.nlm.nih.gov/pubmedhealth/PMH0001243/>

- '**Peripartum**' in this context refers to the few weeks before the birth of the baby and about 6 months after, and '**cardiomyopathy**' means weakness and damage of the heart muscles.
- **Peripartum cardiomyopathy** refers to the development of weakness of the mother's heart leading to heart failure that can set in during the last few weeks of pregnancy and during the first 6 months after delivery of the baby in a mother without any previous heart disease. As a result, the heart muscle becomes weak and cannot pump blood efficiently, leading to heart failure. Decreased heart function affects the lungs, liver, and all other body systems.
- Peripartum cardiomyopathy is a rare but potentially life-threatening condition unique to pregnancy and the time after birth in which no other cause of heart dysfunction (weakened heart) can be identified.
- The exact cause of peripartum cardiomyopathy is not known.
- It complicates about 1 in 1500 to 1 in 4000 pregnancies.
- It may occur in childbearing women of any age, but it is most common in older mothers, those with twin or triplet pregnancies, those with high blood pressure during pregnancy, and those of Afro-Caribbean origin.
- Symptoms may initially mimic those experienced by pregnant mothers with normal pregnancy and after childbirth. These include feeling tired, feeling of racing heart beat (palpitations), shortness of breath with any activity or at night when lying flat, and swelling of the ankles.
- Clinical examination by your GP or obstetrician may reveal signs of strain on your heart which would warrant prompt assessment by the cardiologist (heart specialist). It is quite likely that you would need hospital admission to allow further tests to be done and treatment started without delay.
- Tests would include measuring your heart function by a scan called ECHO (echocardiogram), a chest X-ray to detect any enlargement of the heart or fluid collecting around the lungs, and an ECG (electrocardiogram) to detect any abnormalities in the heart rhythm.

Treatment

Immediate treatment

- Immediate treatment is the same as for anyone who has developed sudden heart strain. You might need to be admitted to the hospital until immediate symptoms subside.
- You may require oxygen, drugs to help ease the strain on your heart and to strengthen the heart's pumping ability, and diuretics (water pills) to remove excess fluid and to reduce the fluid around the lungs.

Further treatment

- A low-salt diet may be recommended. Fluid may be restricted in some cases. Activities may be limited till symptoms subside.
- Due to the increased risk that you may develop a blood clot either within the heart or in any part of the body, a daily injection of a drug to thin your blood will be advised.
- If there are signs that your heart function is worsening despite such treatment and you are still pregnant, the baby will have to be delivered even though it might be premature. This is in order to prevent further and rapid deterioration of your heart failure.

Labour and delivery

- A planned Caesarean section will probably be advised, to avoid any extra strain on your heart that labour and vaginal delivery might involve.
- However, if your heart status is satisfactory, a normal vaginal delivery may be planned, with an epidural for pain relief. The anaesthetist will explain why an epidural would be particularly beneficial in your case.
- If a vaginal delivery is planned, the effort involved in pushing in the second stage might put too much strain on your heart. The delivery of the baby may therefore be assisted by using a suction cup (ventouse or vacuum) or with forceps, so that you do not have to push for longer than approximately 20–30 minutes.

After delivery

- Breastfeeding is not advisable if there is significant heart failure, as it can impose further stress on your heart.
- Your drugs will be reviewed after delivery and changed as necessary. Certain medications that could not be used during pregnancy because of their possible side effects on the baby could now be safely used.
- After delivery you will need a lot of help with the baby. If you will require assistance for this we can help to arrange it through community care.
- Before discharge from the hospital, arrangements will be made for you to be seen by the cardiologist within the first couple of weeks, then after 6 months with an ECHO scan.
- You will be advised to continue with prescribed medications which will be reviewed at these follow-up appointments.

Expectations (prognosis)

- There are several possible outcomes in peripartum cardiomyopathy. Some women remain stable for long periods, while others get worse slowly Others get worse very quickly and may survive only with a heart transplant.
- Better survival rates are seen in women whose hearts return to normal size within 6–12 months after the baby's birth.
- Any subsequent pregnancy after peripartum cardiomyopathy has been shown to put undue stress on your heart even if your heart function recovers this time.
- **Future pregnancies are not advisable** and you will be advised to consider the most suitable contraception for you. Any oral contraceptive pill containing the hormone oestrogen is likely to increase your risk of developing a fatal blood clot and is contraindicated. The safest choices are the Mirena, which is a hormone-loaded 'coil' inserted in the GP's surgery or in a well-woman clinic and is effective for 5 years, or the progesterone implant which is inserted under the skin of your upper arm and is effective for 3 years at a time.
- Women who have developed peripartum cardiomyopathy are at high risk of developing the same problem with any future pregnancy, with an expected death rate as high as 20%. You may need to consider a permanent sterilization procedure, and you are strongly advised to discuss this with your GP and/or gynaecologist.

Further information

- Patient.co.uk. Dilated cardiomyopathy <http://www.patient.co.uk> (provides general information about the condition, not restricted to pregnancy).

5. Maternal Hypertension

INFORMATION FOR PATIENTS High blood pressure (hypertension) and pregnancy

The specialist team will be happy to explain this condition in detail and will discuss options, management plans, and possible outcomes with you.

Further information

- NICE. Hypertension in pregnancy: The management of hypertensive disorders during pregnancy (CG107), 2010 <https://www.nice.org.uk/guidance/cg107/informationforpublic> (includes information for women with pre-existing high blood pressure, those who develop high blood pressure during the pregnancy and those who develop pre-eclampsia)

6. Maternal Renal Disease

INFORMATION FOR PATIENTS Chronic kidney disease and pregnancy

Chronic kidney diseases (CKD) include a wide range of conditions that can lead to varying degrees of damage and impaired kidney (renal) function.

The effect that CKD can have on fertility as well as on pregnancy depends on the degree of kidney damage as well as whether or not you have high blood pressure.

The possible outcomes of pregnancy if you have CKD can be estimated by assessment of the degree of kidney damage—mild, moderate, or severe—before conception. The degree of damage of the kidneys is measured by blood and urine tests. The blood marker used to measure how well the kidneys work is called **creatinine**.

Creatinine is a waste product from the normal breakdown of muscle tissue. Creatinine has to be filtered through the kidneys and excreted in urine, so blood creatinine level can be used as a test of kidney function. The ability of the kidneys to handle creatinine is called the creatinine clearance rate, which is measured in a total 24-hour collection of all the urine you produce.

The milder the degree of CKD before pregnancy (blood creatinine levels of less than 125 micromol/litre), the better the pregnancy outcomes. With severe CKD before pregnancy (blood creatinine levels more than 250 micromol/litre), especially when there is severe high blood pressure that is hard to control, a successful pregnancy outcome can be expected in only 3 out of 4 cases.

It is absolutely essential that good blood pressure control is achieved and maintained both before and during pregnancy to improve outcomes for both you and the baby.

Some blood pressure control medications that are not recommended in pregnancy, but the drugs you will be prescribed will be those that are proven to be safe during pregnancy. Ideally, your GP would have switched your blood pressure medication to pregnancy-safe ones before you get pregnant.

You will be advised to start taking a low-dose of aspirin from early in pregnancy (75 mg once a day, to be continued throughout pregnancy) in order to try to reduce the chances of a condition called pre-eclampsia that is more likely to occur in women with CKD. Pre-eclampsia is a condition usually seen after 24 weeks of pregnancy where there is increased blood pressure, loss of protein in the urine, changes in blood clotting, and in the way your liver works.

If you are diabetic, it is vital to achieve good control before pregnancy, and continue it throughout, in order to improve outcomes for you and your baby.

If there is a worsening of kidney function during the course of pregnancy, causes such as urine infections need to be tested for and vigorously treated.

The growth and well-being of the baby will be monitored at regular intervals throughout the pregnancy.

After pregnancy and delivery, close monitoring and care of your CKD will continue with the kidney (renal) specialists.

Further information

- NICE. Chronic kidney disease: early identification and management of chronic kidney disease in adults in primary and secondary care (CG182), 2014. <https://www.nice.org.uk/guidance/cg182/informationforpublic>

INFORMATION FOR PATIENTS Kidney stones and pregnancy

Kidney (renal) stones are rare during pregnancy but can cause abdominal pain requiring admission to hospital. The occurrence of kidney stones is not increased during pregnancy.

Symptoms can include pain in the abdomen, flanks, and back. Sometimes the urine is blood-stained. There may be nausea or vomiting and frequency of needing to pass urine, as well as fever.

Rarely, large stones can cause severe pain, sepsis, premature contractions of the womb, and even miscarriage or premature delivery.

Most episodes of pain from kidney stones arise in the second half of pregnancy when it is more difficult for small stones to pass in the urine because of pressure from the increasing size of the womb.

You may have also had frequent urine infections in association with a kidney stone, or may have experienced pain or the actual passage of kidney stones either when you were not pregnant or during a previous pregnancy.

Diagnosis during pregnancy may be difficult not only because of the rarity of the condition but also because other complications during pregnancy can mimic the symptoms. It is therefore very important that you tell the doctor if you have ever experienced the same symptoms in the past and if previous tests have indicated a kidney stone.

The most common investigation for the diagnosis of a kidney stone is an ultrasound scan of the kidneys.

Small kidney stones that can cause problems during pregnancy are usually managed with bed rest, adequate hydration, and appropriate pain relief. Antibiotics may be indicated if infection is suspected or proven with lab tests of the urine.

Your specialists, including the obstetrician and the kidney doctors, can advise on the safest management during and after pregnancy.

Further information

- Kidney Research UK. Kidney stones <http://www.kidneyresearchuk.org>

INFORMATION FOR PATIENTS IgA nephropathy and pregnancy

- In general, any pregnancy in a woman with known IgA nephropathy is considered as complex. Your pregnancy care will be therefore be managed by a team of specialists in both kidney disease and obstetrics with experience in such conditions. You would, however, continue to see your own midwife in the community for routine pregnancy checks.
- **Before you decide to get pregnant,** we recommend you seek an assessment by the kidney specialist. This will give valuable information on which to base plans for the pregnancy and will also highlight any additional risks that may be associated with a pregnancy, such as raised blood pressure.
- If the IgA nephropathy has caused only minimal damage to your kidney function and you do not have problems with high blood pressure or leakage of too much protein in the urine, you could expect good pregnancy outcomes in general. Both you and the developing baby would still need close monitoring during pregnancy because there is an increased risk of pregnancy complications even with mild IgA nephropathies.

- There are increased risks of pregnancy complications such as miscarriage; blood pressure problems developing as a direct result of pregnancy itself (pre-eclampsia, pregnancy hypertension); premature delivery; and the baby not growing well inside the womb due to problems with the placenta.
- If your kidney damage due to IgA nephropathy is moderate to severe **before pregnancy** and/or if you have raised blood pressure or leak excessive amounts of protein in the urine, pregnancy complications become more likely and probably more severe. In this situation, pregnancy itself can cause some further worsening of your kidney function, which could, in a few cases, be irreversible. You might be advised not to plan a pregnancy.
- Some types of medication for high blood pressure—ACE inhibitors or ARBs (angiotensin receptor blockers)—can cause serious damage to the developing baby, even leading to death. If you have high blood pressure that is being managed by these medications, it is very important that they are changed, ideally at least 6 weeks before conception, to other blood pressure medications that are safe to use in pregnancy. If you are intending to get pregnant, it is essential that your GP changes your blood pressure medication to pregnancy-safe drugs before you actually conceive.
- You will be advised to start taking low-dose aspirin (or 'mini aspirin') from the start of pregnancy and to continue this throughout pregnancy to help reduce the chances of developing pre-eclampsia.
- From the time of the first clinic visit, kidney function tests and any other relevant blood tests will be done and these will also be repeated at specific times during the course of pregnancy.
- Your blood pressure will be checked regularly throughout pregnancy. Depending on the severity of the IgA nephropathy, you may be prescribed additional medications to suppress your immune system and limit kidney damage, for example medicines such as azathioprine and a steroid called prednisolone.
- Apart from the routine scans performed in the first trimester (the first 13 weeks of pregnancy) as well as the detailed scan at about 20 weeks, additional scans will be organized at monthly intervals from about 26–28 weeks of pregnancy. These are to monitor the progressive growth of your baby and to indirectly assess how well the placenta (afterbirth) is functioning.
- If there is good evidence that your kidneys are showing signs of rapid deterioration in the last few weeks of pregnancy, you may be advised to have an earlier delivery rather than going the full 40 weeks.
- Breastfeeding is not contraindicated even with the drugs you are on. The amount of the drugs in breast milk is so tiny that it is highly unlikely that there are any harmful effects for the breastfed baby.
- After you get home following the baby's birth, your kidney specialist or GP could put you back on ACE inhibitors for blood pressure control.
  - Any woman with IgA nephropathy requires good contraception to avoid an unplanned pregnancy, which could result in poor outcomes for your long-term health and for a baby. The combined pill (containing oestrogens) is not recommended for you.
  - You will continue to need long-term follow-up with the kidney specialists.
  - The kidney doctor and specialist obstetrician looking after you and your pregnancy will be able to give you pregnancy-specific information, based on your individual condition and the extent of your kidney disease.

Further information

- National Kidney Federation. IgA nephropathy <http://www.kidney.org.uk/Medical-Info/kidney-disease/Iga.html>
- Patient.co.uk. IgA nephropathy (Berger's disease) <http://www.patient.co.uk>

INFORMATION FOR PATIENTS Autosomal dominant polycystic kidney disease (adult polycystic kidney disease) and pregnancy

Autosomal dominant polycystic kidney disease (APKD) also called adult polycystic kidney disease, is the most common inherited disorder of the kidneys.

If either you or your partner is affected with APKD, there is a 50% chance of transmission to your baby. If both you and your partner have APKD, there is a 50% chance that your baby is a carrier, a 25% chance of the baby being unaffected, and a 25% chance that the fetus is affected by the condition. A fetus that has inherited the full-blown form of APKD usually dies within the womb during pregnancy.

Symptoms seen in APKD are usually evident in early adult life. Some people have no symptoms and the diagnosis is made only by family screening.

If you have been diagnosed with APKD, you may experience pain in the back and sides due to enlargement of the kidneys, frequent infections affecting the kidneys, or visibly bloodstained urine. In addition, your liver, spleen, and kidneys may be enlarged.

The main complications during pregnancy in women with APKD are the development of urinary infections, of high blood pressure and of pre-eclampsia. Pre-eclampsia is a condition unique to pregnancy, usually appearing after 24 weeks of pregnancy, where the blood pressure is raised, protein appears in the urine in significant amounts, and there are changes in the liver function and blood clotting.

Pregnancy itself does not worsen APKD either in the short or long term. The management of your pregnancy will involve input from an obstetrician, your midwife, and the kidney specialist. Genetic input, if not already obtained, will be arranged.

Your blood pressure, urine tests and baseline kidney and liver function tests should ideally be monitored in early pregnancy followed by subsequent checks at specified intervals during the course of pregnancy.

You can expect to be prescribed low-dose aspirin (75 mg) to be taken once a day throughout pregnancy to help reduce the risk of pre-eclampsia.

Your blood pressure and the baby's growth will be closely monitored with repeat scans at regular intervals.

If your blood pressure is found to be staying high, you will be prescribed medication to lower your blood pressure. Only drugs that are safe in pregnancy will be prescribed for you.

Ultrasound scans of the baby during pregnancy enable a diagnosis of kidney cysts but here the kidneys are smaller than usual and the volume of the amniotic fluid (the liquid around the baby) is may be less than usual.

Testing for the condition in the fetus during the first 13 weeks of pregnancy is possible by performing invasive tests such as chorionic villous biopsy. Your specialist obstetrician will be happy to discuss these investigations with you.

Further information

- NHS Choices. Autosomal dominant polycystic kidney disease. Complications <http://www.nhs.uk/conditions/autosomal-dominant-polycystic-kidney-disease/pages/introduction.aspx>
- NICE. Chronic kidney disease: early identification and management of chronic kidney disease in adults in primary and secondary care (CG182), 2014 <http://www.nice.org.uk/guidance/cg182/informationforpublic>
- Patient.co.uk. Polycystic kidney disease <http://www.patient.co.uk>

7. Maternal Adrenal Disease

INFORMATION FOR PATIENTS Congenital adrenal hyperplasia (CAH) and pregnancy

Congenital adrenal hyperplasia (CAH) is a rare inherited condition marked by faulty production of vital hormones from your adrenal glands. The adrenals are hormone-producing organs that sit like caps on top of each kidney in the body.

CAH is due to a deficiency in an enzyme called 21-hydroxylase (hi-droxy-lase) which is vital for the proper production of some of the sex hormones.

If you have had a previous baby affected with CAH and become pregnant again with the same partner, this baby will have a 1 in 4 chance of also having CAH. It is important you receive thorough genetic counselling before getting pregnant again. Your GP can refer you to the appropriate specialist for this.

If the baby you are carrying is female and is affected by CAH, there is a 3 in 4 chance that the baby will show significant signs of masculinization at birth due to overproduction of male hormones such as testosterone and androgens within the womb. This may cause distressing difficulties in identifying the sex of the baby at birth. An affected female child will need reconstructive surgery at several stages during childhood and adolescence.

If the baby is a boy, exaggerated development of the male genital organs may be visible at birth.

In severe cases, newborns of either sex may suffer significant salt loss, and even death can occur in babies of either sex if the condition is not recognized and promptly treated.

The determination of fetal sex as well as a diagnosis of CAH by gene tests in a subsequent pregnancy are now possible. You would be referred to a tertiary/regional specialist centre early in a subsequent pregnancy, where these tests can be performed. In addition, hormone manipulation can be put in place during this stage of pregnancy in order to reduce the effects of CAH in the unborn baby.

Further information

- British Society for Paediatric Endocrinology and Diabetes. Congenital adrenal hyperplasia (CAH) due to 21-hydroxylase deficiency <http://www.bsped.org.uk/patients/docs/CAH_21_HYDROXYLASE_revised.pdf>
- Climb CAH (congenital adrenal hyperplasia support group) <http://www.livingwithcah.com/>
- National Institutes of Health (US). Facts about CAH (congenital adrenal hyperplasia) <http://www.cc.nih.gov/ccc/patient_education/pepubs/cah.pdf>
- Patient.co.uk. Congenital adrenal hyperplasia <http://www.patient.co.uk>

INFORMATION FOR PATIENTS Phaeochromocytoma and pregnancy

The adrenal glands sit like caps, one on top of each kidney. The outer part of the adrenal gland, called the cortex, produces steroid hormones. These include:

- **aldosterone**, which helps maintain the water and electrolyte balance in the body by its action on the kidneys, salivary, and sweat glands
- **cortisol**, which is the hormone responsible for control of carbohydrate, protein, and fat metabolism
- **sex steroids** such as androgens.

The inner part of the adrenal glands is called the medulla and this is where hormones called catecholamines (cat-ay-coal-amines) are secreted. These include adrenaline (also called epinephrine) and noradrenaline (also called norepinephrine) which are both essential to help regulate the heart rate, blood pressure, heart pumping capacity, and rate of breathing. These act as part of the 'fight or flight' response in reaction to stress or danger.

Phaeochromocytoma (feo-kro-mo-cy-toma) is a rare endocrine tumour which arises from the catecholamine-producing area of the adrenal glands. This tumour is a rare cause of severe high blood pressure due to the excessive production of adrenaline and noradrenaline.

A phaeochromocytoma can cause sustained symptoms including high blood pressure (hypertension), sweating, and headaches as well as spasms of palpitations, fainting attacks, and sudden elevation of blood sugar levels.

Though phaeochromocytoma is extremely rare in pregnancy, if it is not recognized or if the diagnosis is delayed it can prove very dangerous to the mother and the unborn baby. With early clinical suspicion, prompt diagnosis, and effective treatment the outcomes are much improved.

If phaeochromocytoma is suspected in pregnancy, you can expect several specialists to become involved in your care including obstetricians, endocrine physicians, surgeon, anaesthetist, radiologist, and midwives.

Special tests of your blood and urine and imaging such as an MRI scan will be done to help diagnose phaeochromocytoma.

The primary goal of treatment is to control blood pressure as soon as possible, initially by means of powerful drugs. Once your blood pressure is stabilized, the options for surgical removal of the adrenal tumour will be discussed with you. A decision about the type of surgery and its timing will depend on many factors, such as how far the pregnancy has advanced, your response to the anti-blood-pressure medications, how accessible the tumour is during pregnancy, or any evidence of the baby not being well. These issues will be discussed fully with you and your family.

Ideally your baby would be delivered by Caesarean section with a specialist obstetrician and anaesthetist.

Long-term follow-up with your GP and endocrine specialists is recommended.

The specialists looking after you in the hospital will discuss phaeochromocytoma, its effect on pregnancy, and the treatment options, and will try answer your queries fully.

Further information

- Society for Endocrinology. You & Your Hormones. Phaeochromocytoma <http://www.yourhormones.info/Endocrine_conditions/Phaeochromocytoma.aspx>

8. Maternal Hepatobiliary Conditions

INFORMATION FOR PATIENTS Obstetric cholestasis (itching liver disorder of pregnancy)

The specialist team will be happy to explain this condition in detail and will discuss options, management plans, and possible outcomes with you.

Further information

- British Liver Trust. Obstetric cholestasis, 2011 <http://www.britishlivertrust.org.uk/home/the-liver/liver-diseases/obstetric-cholestasis.aspx>
- Obstetric Cholestasis Support Group <http://www.ocsupport.org.uk>
- Royal College of Obstetricians and Gynaecologists. Obstetric cholestasis (itching liver disorder): information for you, 2007 <http://www.rcog.org.uk/womens-health/clinical-guidance/obstetriccholestasis-itching-liver-disorder-information-you>

INFORMATION FOR PATIENTS Gilbert's syndrome and pregnancy

Gilbert's syndrome is a genetically inherited, chronic but benign liver disease, marked by jaundice and by mild elevation of the levels of bilirubin in blood. Bilirubin is the breakdown product of haemoglobin in red blood cells and is the yellowish pigment found in bile, a fluid produced by the liver.

People with Gilbert's syndrome are otherwise entirely normal, with no other signs or symptoms.

Both parents must have the gene for the offspring to express the abnormality. Gilbert's syndrome occurs in about 3–7% of the population, with more men than women being affected.

Gilbert's syndrome is most often recognized in the second or third decade of life and is rarely diagnosed before puberty.

Symptoms can range from jaundice to nausea, tiredness, and discomfort in the right upper part of the tummy and diffuse tummy pain.

Often Gilbert's syndrome is only diagnosed following routine screening blood tests, or if any other illness unmasks the abnormal levels of bilirubin. It may come to light for the first time during pregnancy.

Gilbert's syndrome does not cause any danger to you or your baby. It does not lead to liver failure or cancer in the longer term.

Apart from correction of any dehydration and calorie replacement if you have had repeated vomiting, no treatment is required and the expectation of normal outcomes for you and the baby is excellent.

No additional ultrasound scans are required in maternal Gilbert's syndrome. The management of pregnancy, labour, and delivery need not be changed and there is no call for Caesarean section or early induction of labour just because of Gilbert's syndrome.

If you have Gilbert's syndrome the only precaution to be aware of is that *you need to avoid exposure to certain medications such as paracetamol, morphine, and some anaesthetic gases and drugs*. Your doctors and midwives will make note of those medications to be avoided during pregnancy or during anaesthesia, should you possibly need an operation.

Further information

- British Liver Trust. Gilbert's syndrome <http://www.britishlivertrust.org.uk>
- NHS Choices. Gilbert's syndrome. <http://www.nhs.uk/conditions/Gilbertssyndrome>
- Patient.co.uk. Gilbert's syndrome <http://www.patient.co.uk>

INFORMATION FOR PATIENTS Gallstones and pancreatitis in pregnancy

- Gallstones are not uncommon during pregnancy as they are found in 5–10% of women between the ages of 20 and 55.
- Most gallstones are asymptomatic. This means they do not cause problems and you might not even know you have them. They do not require any treatment.
- Gallstones are more commonly found during pregnancy in women who are overweight, those who have lost weight by crash dieting, and women who have had several babies.
- Symptoms related to gallstones can occur at any stage in pregnancy but are most common in the third trimester (26–40 weeks pregnancy).
- The symptoms are mainly caused by blockage of the bile duct which results in swelling and inflammation of the gallbladder (cholecystitis) and of the pancreas (pancreatitis).
- The symptoms can vary from mild to severe. Sudden pain in the upper part of the tummy which radiates in a belt-like grip to the back with a maximum intensity reached in 15–20 minutes is a typical presentation.
- Often after a meal you may experience pain, nausea, and vomiting, especially if the meal had a relatively high fat content.
- Mild fever could also be a feature.
- Repeated bouts of such symptoms can occur during the course of the pregnancy and some can be severe with greater risks to you and the baby.
- The main effect of acute pancreatitis on the baby during pregnancy is that it could bring about premature labour and delivery of a premature baby.
- The diagnosis is usually made with ultrasound scan of the gallbladder and pancreas which may reveal the presence of gallstones. Sometimes an MRI scan is also required to get a better picture.
- Simple blood tests to measure the levels of enzymes called amylase and lipase will show that these are raised within 6–12 hours of the onset of your symptoms and remain at these increased levels for about 3–5 days.
- Once the diagnosis is made, specialists from gastroenterology(experts who deal with conditions of the liver, gallbladder, pancreas, bowels, etc.) will probably also be involved in your care along with the obstetricians and midwives.
- Treatment in most cases does not involve surgery during pregnancy.
- The type of treatment will also depend on how far pregnant you are, how severe the condition is, and whether or not there are signs of improvement with conservative treatment aimed to manage symptoms.
- To enable treatment involving controlling the pain and other symptoms, hospital admission will be advised.
- You will have a drip placed in a vein to give you essential fluids while you are requested not to eat or drink except for small sips of water. This is to ensure that your bowels are rested till the

inflammation of the gallbladder and pancreas subsides which usually takes about 3–5 days.

- In the meantime you will receive medicines to control pain and to reduce nausea and vomiting.
- If you have fever, after the necessary tests, you will be prescribed appropriate antibiotics.
- The baby will be monitored at regular intervals.
- After the acute phase (usually 3–5 days) you can resume a low-fat diet.
- A few weeks or months after you have had your baby, at the follow-up appointment with the surgeons or the gastroenterologist, there will be the opportunity for discussion and plans can be made to have keyhole surgery for removal of the gallbladder if this is the best option for you.
- In a few cases, the condition is severe enough to consider keyhole surgery to remove the gallstones or gallbladder during the pregnancy itself, usually between 13 and 26 weeks (the second trimester).

Further information

- Patient.co.uk. Cholecystitis <http://www.patient.co.uk>
- Patient.co.uk. Acute pancreatitis <http://www.patient.co.uk>

INFORMATION FOR PATIENTS Autoimmune hepatitis and pregnancy

- Autoimmune hepatitis (AIH) is a rare condition in pregnancy.
- AIH would usually have been diagnosed before your pregnancy, perhaps during investigations for fertility problems, or if you had developed jaundice, or if abnormal liver enzymes were found on blood tests.
- You might have already been on treatment for AIH with medications to suppress your immune system and have received advice about pregnancy from the liver specialist.
- If your AIH is well controlled, in most cases pregnancy can proceed without complications, and good outcomes can be expected for you and the baby.
- There is, however, a higher risk of miscarriages and premature birth associated with AIH.
- Most patients show a good response to a combination of drugs like prednisolone and azathioprine, which suppress the immune reactions that can cause flare-ups of AIH.
- There is little evidence that drugs such as azathioprine or prednisolone cause any risk of birth defects or any other ill effects.
- It is important that AIH is well controlled (kept in remission) during pregnancy by continuing the medication you have been prescribed, because the risks to the developing baby are greater if your AIH relapses during pregnancy.
- Flare-up of AIH during pregnancy is relatively infrequent though relapses can occur in the weeks following childbirth. You will be monitored closely during pregnancy and after childbirth.
- Your pregnancy will also be monitored with regular growth scans at monthly intervals from about 28 weeks.
- In well-controlled AIH, where the baby's growth appears satisfactory on scans and there are no other complications, there is little indication to induce labour early or to have a Caesarean section.
- Standard advice is that breastfeeding may not be advisable if you are taking azathioprine. However, the amount of active drug in breast milk is so tiny that the benefits of breastfeeding outweigh this theoretical risk. Several studies have not shown any ill effects for the baby if you are on small doses of azathioprine. It is best if you can breastfeed just before that day's dose of azathioprine is due.

Further information

- British Liver Trust. Support groups <http://www.britishlivertrust.org.uk/liver-disease-support-groups/>
- Livernorth. Autoimmune hepatitis <http://www.livernorth.org.uk/pdfs/3AIH%20May14.pdf>
- NHS Choices. <http://www.nhs.uk/conditions/Hepatitis>
- Patient.co.uk. <http://www.patient.co.uk/forums/discuss/browse/autoimmune-hepatitis-4>

INFORMATION FOR PATIENTS Acute porphyria and pregnancy

Porphyrias belong to a group of genetic defects called inborn errors of metabolism. The defect involved in porphyria lies in the production of the iron-rich pigment in red blood cells, called **haem** (pronounced heem). The liver produces about 15% of the body's haem and the rest is produced by the bone marrow.

Porphyrins are the raw materials needed in the manufacture of the final product, haem. During the normal process of haem production, porphyrins have to be converted from one type to another aided by several enzymes (proteins that help chemical reactions). If any one of these enzymes is deficient or defective, the process stops and there is a build-up of the porphyrin that has been produced up to that point.

Two varieties of porphyria are recognized: the acute or hepatic (liver) type and the cutaneous (skin) type. In cutaneous porphyria, there are skin lesions sensitive to light.

People with any form of acute porphyrias can have characteristic nervous system abnormalities such as peripheral neuropathy, neuropathic severe abdominal pain, and psychiatric disturbances.

Damage to the nervous system in porphyria means that communication between the brain and other parts of the body is affected. This can affect muscle movement and prevent normal sensation in the hands and feet, leading to numbness, tingling, cold, and pain. It can also cause severe tummy pains, nausea, vomiting, abdominal distension, constipation, or diarrhoea. Palpitations, convulsions, hallucinations, and anxiety are also features.

These problems appear mainly in adult life and are more common in women. The disease can remain latent but symptoms can be triggered by smoking, alcohol, certain drugs, dietary factors, hormones such as those of pregnancy or in oral contraceptive pills.

If you have previously been diagnosed with porphyria, you are encouraged to wear a MedicAlert bracelet and carry an Alert card at all times.

You are advised not to smoke or drink alcohol as these can trigger acute attacks.

You could have a one in four chance of flare-ups during pregnancy, maximal in in early weeks of pregnancy, and in the first few weeks after the baby is born. In the case of an acute attack, which is a serious emergency, immediate steps will be taken to ensure adequate carbohydrate replacement and symptomatic therapy to control pain, nausea, vomiting, and convulsions with drugs that are safe to use in porphyria.

Most attacks of porphyria in pregnancy settle with adequate supportive therapy with good maternal and fetal outcomes.

Further information

- British Porphyria Association <http://www.porphyria.org.uk>

INFORMATION FOR PATIENTS Wilson's disease and pregnancy

Wilson's disease (WD) is a disorder of copper metabolism. Copper is common in a wide range of foods, but the human body needs only tiny amounts. The rest is normally excreted. In WD, the excess copper leaves the bloodstream and settles in various organs and structures, including the brain, spinal cord, eyes, liver, and kidneys, damaging these tissues because copper is toxic in large amounts. The damaged tissues are replaced by scar tissue. Without appropriate treatment, as more and more tissue is replaced by scars, the affected organ loses its ability to function until it eventually fails.

- Mothers with WD and their babies in general do well during pregnancy and after delivery, provided medication at prescribed doses is continued throughout pregnancy. The pregnancy outcomes for both you and the developing baby depend on compliance with the prescribed medication.
- You might already have had an opportunity to discuss pregnancy and the medications for WD during pregnancy with the liver specialist or with a specialist obstetrician.
- Wilson's disease is a rare genetic disorder and occurs in 1 in 30,000 of the population.
- The risk of your baby inheriting the disorder is small (about 1 in 200) as the faulty gene that causes WD must be inherited from both parents for the child to develop WD. If only one faulty gene is inherited, the child is a carrier but will not develop any symptoms. In many cases, WD is caused by a spontaneous defective gene without any family history of the disorder.
- You will have been reminded to take folic acid from before becoming pregnant and continue it till the end of the 13th week of pregnancy.
- It is very important that you continue your medication for WD during pregnancy. Stopping these essential drugs could cause serious problems for you and the baby. Penicillamine, trientine, and zinc are the common medications used to reduce the copper levels in your body.
- During the first 13 weeks of pregnancy, the dosage of your medication will be adjusted by the liver specialist to keep your copper levels within the normal range while avoiding higher doses which could possibly effect the baby's development. Continue folic acid during the first 13 weeks of pregnancy.
- If you are on medications such as penicillamine it is advisable not to take supplemental oral iron tablets during pregnancy. An iron-rich diet with lots of green vegetables is advised instead.
- You will be prescribed vitamin B_6 by your obstetric specialist, to take throughout the pregnancy.
- You will be looked after by a team including a liver disease specialist and a specialist obstetrician who is an expert in complex pregnancies, as well as continuing antenatal care provided by the community midwife.
- Extra scans to ensure that the baby is growing well will be organized at regular intervals from about 26–28 weeks of pregnancy onwards.
- Your blood tests will also include checks of copper levels and liver enzymes at certain stages during pregnancy.
- Your routine pregnancy care should be no different from anyone else's.
- Wilson's disease in itself should not cause any change in the management of your labour and delivery. Early induction of labour or Caesarean sections are not required unless there is some other unpredictable obstetric reason, as in any other pregnant woman.
- There is no reason why you cannot have a normal delivery just because you have WD.
- The baby will be checked by the baby doctors in view of the fact that you have WD.
- There is good evidence that breastfeeding is safe for the baby with your medication, but not enough is known about long-term effects. However, the benefits of breastfeeding with normal doses of the medication, which you must continue lifelong, are greater than any perceived risk to the breastfed infant.
- Contraception choices are particularly important for anyone with WD. The combined pill which contains the hormone oestrogen, as well as any copper-containing coil are not suitable for you. The hormone progesterone either as an implant under the skin or the hormone device Mirena® inserted into the womb are safe. The implant is effective for 3 years and the Mirena® for 5 years, with the option of easy removal at any time if you want to plan another pregnancy.
- After delivery, you can expect further routine follow-up with the liver specialist.
- Remember that before any future pregnancy, your copper levels must be well controlled in order to ensure good outcomes.
- Management of Wilson's disease is lifelong. You may already have received advice about a low-copper diet. The food items you need to avoid are:
  - Chocolate
  - Dried beans
  - Dried fruits
  - Mushrooms
  - Nuts
  - Offal such as liver
  - Peas
  - Shellfish
  - Whole wheat products.

Further information

- Better Health Channel (Australia) <http://www.betterhealth.vic.gov.au/bhcv2/bhcarticles.nsf/pages/Wilson%27s_disease>
- British Liver Trust. Wilson's disease <http://www.britishlivertrust.org.uk/...diseases/wilsons-disease-updated.aspx>
- Patient.co.uk. Wilson's disease <http://www.patient.co.uk>
- Wilson's Disease UK (support group) <http://www.wilsonsdisease.org.uk/WDSG-P0.aspK>

INFORMATION FOR PATIENTS Hereditary haemochromatosis and pregnancy

Hereditary haemochromatosis (hee-mo-krome-at-osis) (HH) is an inherited genetic disorder, particularly common in white people of northern European descent.

Both parents need to carry the defective gene for the baby to inherit the condition.

In haemochromatosis, there is excessive absorption of iron from the gut. The excessive amounts of iron accumulate within tissues and organs such as the liver, pancreas, joints, skin, and heart muscle. If untreated, the condition leads to increased pigmentation of the skin, enlargement of the liver, and diabetes.

Many people with haemochromatosis have no symptoms, but symptoms may include tiredness, tummy pain, skin pigmentation, weight loss, muscle tenderness, cramps, and painful joints. Before the stage when symptoms develop, the only clue may be that others have commented on your 'healthy all-year-round tan' and you may have an increased tendency to develop bacterial infections.

It is likely that you have already been diagnosed with HH as a result of routine blood tests or family testing.

Treatment when you are not pregnanct usually involves reduced dietary iron as well as regular removal of blood from a vein (phlebotomy).

Phlebotomy is discontinued for the duration of pregnancy and a few weeks after the baby is born. Iron and vitamin C supplements should be avoided, including routine pregnancy multivitamins. Folic acid without iron must be prescribed before conception and continued for the first 3 months of the pregnancy.

Specialists in haematology (blood disorders) and hepatology (liver disorders) and well as the obstetrician and midwife will be involved in your care throughout pregnancy and will advise on necessary interventions or medications required.

An ultrasound scan of your liver will be performed and repeated during pregnancy if recommended by the specialists.

Your liver function will be checked with blood tests at regular intervals during pregnancy.

The baby's growth will be monitored with a series of scans.

Further information

- Haemochromatosis Society UK <http://www.haemochromatosis.org.uk/>
- NHS Choices. Haemochromatosis <http://www.nhs.uk/conditions/Haemochromatosis>
- Patient.co.uk. Haemochromatosis <http://www.patient.co.uk>
- Patient.co.uk. Idiopathic haemochromatosis <http://www.patient.co.uk/leaflets/idiopathic_haemochromatosis.htm>

9. Maternal Endocrine Disorders

INFORMATION FOR PATIENTS Diabetes and pregnancy

The specialist team will be happy to explain this condition in detail and will discuss options, management plans, and possible outcomes with you.

Further information

- NICE Diabetes in pregnancy: Management of diabetes and its complications from pre-conception to the postnatal period (CG63), 2008 <https://www.nice.org.uk/guidance/cg63/informationforpublic>
- <http://www.perinatal.nhs.uk/diabetes/projectd/leaflets/leaflets.htm> This source provides excellent leaflets covering a range of issues about diabetes and pregnancy including:

Pre-pregnancy leaflets

- Do you have diabetes? Planning a family? Key facts you need to know
- Do you have diabetes? Planning a family? Things to do before you get pregnant
- Contraception for women with diabetes

During pregnancy leaflets

- Healthy eating
- What is gestational diabetes?
- Glucose tolerance test
- Diabetes & breastfeeding
- How to avoid hypoglycaemia in pregnancy?
- Type 1 and diabetes 'sick days': what to do if unwell
- Metformin treatment in pregnancy

Post-pregnancy leaflet

- Postnatal care for gestational diabetes

INFORMATION FOR PATIENTS Hypothyroidism (undereractive thyroid) and pregnancy

Frequently asked questions

What is the thyroid gland?

The thyroid gland is located in the neck alongside the Adam's apple. It releases thyroid hormones into the blood, which power the cells of the body. The thyroid gland is controlled by another gland which is situated in the brain, known as the pituitary gland. The pituitary gland regulates the thyroid gland through another hormone called thyroid stimulating hormone (TSH).

What is hypothyroidism?

Underactivity of the thyroid gland is also called hypothyroidism or myxoedema. This is when the thyroid gland is not producing enough hormones.

What happens when the thyroid gland becomes underactive?

When the thyroid gland becomes underactive it produces less thyroid hormone, which may result in a general slowing down both physically and mentally.

When your thyroid gland is underactive, you may experience few or no symptoms at first. Later, however, some of the more common symptoms can include:

- Loss of energy
- General tiredness
- Dislike of cold
- Weight gain and bloating
- Slow pulse
- Constipation
- Muscle weakness
- Dry skin and hair
- Hoarseness of voice

Each patient is different and you may experience only a few of these symptoms.

What causes underactivity of the thyroid gland?

Underactivity of the thyroid gland may be caused by an autoimmune condition. This means that cells which normally protect your body (the immune system) develop a fault and begin to act against the thyroid gland. This damages the gland, making it less able to produce thyroid hormones. It is not yet known why cells develop the fault that causes them to attack the body's own tissues.

Less commonly, underactivity of the thyroid gland may also occur in people who have previously had thyroid surgery or radioactive iodine treatment for overactivity of the thyroid gland (Grave's disease or **hyper**thyroidism)

Is underactivity of the thyroid gland rare in pregnancy?

Not that rare: it occurs in approximately 1–2% of pregnant women.

What effect does underactivity of the thyroid have on my baby?

Your thyroxine levels need to be normal both **before** pregnancy and particularly **during the first trimester** (first 13 weeks) of pregnancy as this is an extremely important for the baby's normal brain development.

As soon as you have a positive pregnancy test, you should increase the dose of thyroxine you have been on before pregnancy by 25 micrograms/day, even before seeing your midwife or GP, as the amount of thyroxine needed for the baby's brain development starts to increase as early as 5 weeks of pregnancy. You can contact your GP, community midwife, or specialists at the hospital if you have any questions or concerns.

In extreme cases untreated or inadequate correction of hypothyroidism in pregnancy can result to impairment of the child's

IQ in infancy and childhood. Taking the correct dose of thyroxine will help normal development of the baby's nervous system and help avoid these developmental delays.

If the underactivity is not corrected then there is also an increased risk of miscarriage and your baby may be smaller than expected, or be born prematurely.

How is underactivity of the thyroid gland diagnosed?

A blood test is taken to measure the TSH level, which is a marker for adequate thyroid hormone levels. This test should be repeated every 6–8 weeks during your pregnancy in the GP's surgery or at the hospital. This test result will indicate whether your dose of thyroxine supplement is adequate for that stage of pregnancy or whether it needs to be changed.

How is underactivity of the thyroid gland treated?

Underactivity of the thyroid gland is treated with an artificial thyroid hormone called levothyroxine. This is very similar to natural thyroid hormones and when given in the correct dose, it has virtually no side effects either on you or on the baby.

You will be seen more frequently at the antenatal clinic for regular blood tests (TSH levels) to ensure that you are receiving the correct dose of thyroxine. The demand for thyroxine increases in the early part of pregnancy and again in the latter half of pregnancy and may require a slight increase in your thyroxine dosage, as specified in your notes by the hospital specialist team. You will be advised to revert to your pre-pregnancy dosage of thyroxine once the baby is born.

What effect does thyroxine have on my baby?

Thyroxine in the correct dose, especially in the first 13 weeks, will help the brain development of your baby. As long as thyroxine is given in the correct dose, it will have no ill effects on your baby as very little passes across the placenta to your unborn baby. Remember to take your thyroxine on an empty stomach every day.

What will happen to my thyroxine dosage in pregnancy?

Usually the dose requirements of thyroxine will increase during pregnancy and return to pre-pregnancy values after the baby is born.

Will I be able to breast feed my baby while taking thyroxine?

It is absolutely safe to breastfeed whilst taking thyroxine.

Further information

- British Thyroid Association. Underactive thyroid and pregnancy <http://www.british-thyroid-association.org/info-for-patients/Pregnancy/index.htm>
- British Thyroid Foundation Campaigns. Thyroid in pregnancy information <http://www.btf-thyroid.org>
- Patient.co.uk. Hypothyroidism-Underactive thyroid <http://www.patient.co.uk>

INFORMATION FOR PATIENTS Hyperthyroidism (overactive thyroid) and pregnancy

Frequently asked questions

What is the thyroid gland?

The thyroid gland is located in the neck alongside the Adam's apple. It releases thyroid hormones into the blood, which power the cells of the body. The thyroid gland is controlled by another gland which is situated in the brain, known as the pituitary gland. The pituitary gland regulates the thyroid gland through another hormone called thyroid stimulating hormone (TSH).

What is overactivity of the thyroid gland in pregnancy?

Overactivity of the thyroid gland is also called thyrotoxicosis or hyperthyroidism. Overactivity of the thyroid gland is found in approximately 2 in every 1000 pregnancies.

What happens when the thyroid gland becomes overactive?

When the thyroid gland becomes overactive, it produces extra thyroid hormones making you experience a number of symptoms. Some of the more common symptoms are:

- Loss of energy
- Nervousness, tremors, agitation, irritability
- Sweating, dislike of heat
- Weight-loss
- Palpitations or fast heart rate
- Diarrhoea
- Muscle weakness
- Skin changes
- Swelling in the throat
- Dry, gritty eyes; painful protruding eyes-worsened by smoking.
- Double vision

Each patient is different and you may experience only a few of these symptoms.

What effect can overactivity of my thyroid gland have on my baby?

If the thyroid activity is well controlled, you can expect to have an uncomplicated pregnancy.

If the overactivity is not well controlled, you may go into premature labour, and your baby may be not grow well during pregnancy and be smaller than expected. The baby may also rarely show signs of temporary thyroid overactivity after birth, including weight loss or poor feeding.

What causes overactivity of the thyroid gland?

Overactivity of the thyroid gland is usually cause by an autoimmune condition called Graves's disease (named after the doctor who first described it). This is due to an overactivity of part of your immune system where cells which normally protect the body from infection develop a fault and begin to recognize the thyroid gland as foreign material and attack it. This stimulates the thyroid gland to produce extra thyroid hormones. It is not yet known why cells develop the fault that causes them to attack the thyroid gland.

How is overactivity of the thyroid gland diagnosed?

A blood test is taken to measure the level of thyroid hormones in the blood, as well as thyroid stimulating hormone (TSH).

How is overactivity of the thyroid gland treated?

Certain medicines are used to control overactivity of the thyroid gland in the first instance. These medicines work by blocking the production of thyroid hormones. Propylthiouracil (PTU) or carbimazole are the medicines most commonly used for this purpose. Like all medications they may have side effects. These are usually mild and include skin rashes, itching, and a feeling of nausea. In about 1 in 1000 patients, both may cause a potentially more serious side effect whereby the white blood cells which protect against infection are no longer produced. When this occurs there is a risk of developing serious infections. The first sign of this problem is often a severe sore throat or mouth ulcers. If you develop either of these symptoms you should contact your GP at once.

What effect does PTU or carbimazole have on my baby?

Both PTU and carbimazole are safe in pregnancy although PTU may be preferable.

PTU does not have any effect on producing birth defects for the developing baby. Taking the right dose of these drugs, enough to control your thyroid gland overactivity, will also benefit your unborn baby.

Very rarely, these medications may cause your baby's thyroid gland to become underactive after birth for about 3 months. For this reason, the specialist will monitor the therapy using the lowest dose required to control the overactive thyroid. All babies will have a test of thyroid function at birth and any problems with your baby's thyroid gland will be detected at that stage. If your baby's thyroid gland is underactive then it is easily treated with thyroid hormones until the baby's thyroid activity returns to normal, which is usually within 3 months of birth.

Could my baby develop an overactive thyroid like me?

This happens very rarely. It is far more likely that your baby will have normal thyroid function after birth. Very rarely, temporary overactivity of the baby's thyroid can occur. Overactive thyroid is often the result of the mother producing an antibody (protein) in the blood which triggers the baby's thyroid to become overactive. Here the small amount of PTU or carbimazole which passes to the unborn baby from you can be useful in controlling baby's overactive thyroid. After birth the baby's overactive thyroid gland may need to be treated with carbimazole or PTU for 3 months until the mother's antibody naturally disappears from baby's bloodstream. This is not common, however, and most babies are healthy when born.

A special blood test at 28 weeks can indicate whether there is an increased chance of hyperthyroidism developing in your baby. In this case, your baby's heart rate may be monitored in the course of the pregnancy. If you notice any overactivity of the baby's movements in the womb, please report this promptly to the hospital or your own community midwife/GP.

Will I be able to breastfeed my baby while taking thyroid blocking medication?

All mothers, including those with an overactive thyroid, are encouraged to breastfeed. PTU is passed into your milk in very small quantities and is unlikely to cause any problems, especially if you are on low doses. It is best to take your PTU medication after a breast feed.

Further information

- British Thyroid Foundation Campaigns. Thyroid in pregnancy information <http://www.btf-thyroid.org>
- Patient.co.uk. Hyperthyroidism-in-pregnancy <http://www.patient.co.uk>

INFORMATION FOR PATIENTS Hashimoto's thyroiditis and pregnancy

Thyroiditis is the name given to inflammation of the thyroid gland. Hashimoto's thyroiditis is the most common cause for an underactive thyroid or hypothyroidism and it is more common in women than in men.

In Hashimoto's thyroiditis, your body's immune system fails to recognize the thyroid tissue and begins to produce antibodies against it. This causes an initial swelling which can form a lump called a **goitre** before the thyroid gland suffers damage.

Gradual destruction of the thyroid gland causes decreased production of the thyroid hormone, leading to underactivity or hypothyroidism. This is a slow process that can take several months or even years with permanently low levels of thyroid hormone. This can be treated with thyroid hormone replacement, which is usually taken for life.

Early diagnosis of Hashimoto's thyroiditis induced hypothyroidism and prompt treatment can improve pregnancy outcomes for both you and the baby, and is especially important for the neurological development of the baby.

Pregnancy complications such as anaemia, premature labour and growth problems of the baby are greater with untreated hypothyroidism.

The diagnostic sign of Hashimoto's thyroiditis is the finding of a specific antibody in a blood test. This is called the thyroid peroxidase (TPO) antibody.

After the baby is born, in most women, the dose of thyroxine required during pregnancy can be tapered down over a period of approximately 4 weeks to the doses that you were on before pregnancy.

There is an increased chance that you might have a flare-up of the disorder after delivery and might need to continue thyroxine replacement. Continued follow-up of your thyroid function should continue as directed by your GP.

Further information

- NHS Choices. Thyroiditis <http://www.nhs.uk/conditions/thyroiditis>

INFORMATION FOR PATIENTS Prolactinomas and pregnancy

The pituitary gland is a hormone-producing (endocrine) gland which is the size of a pea and found at the base of the brain. It is sometimes called the master gland because it controls several other hormone-releasing glands, such as the ovaries, thyroid, and adrenals.

The pituitary gland helps to control various functions of the body by releasing hormones (special chemical messengers) into the bloodstream. These hormones are transported by the bloodstream to their target organ where they usually regulate the release of a second hormone.

One of the hormones produced by the pituitary gland is **prolactin**, which in turn effects other hormones in the body. A **prolactinoma** is a benign (non-cancerous) tumour of the pituitary gland, which produces too much of the hormone prolactin.

Certain drugs such as bromocriptine or cabergoline are used to treat excessive prolactin production and they usually cause your periods to stop temporarily. These drugs are discontinued once pregnancy is established. The benefit of tumour shrinkage achieved by these drugs is seen to continue during pregnancy, even after the medication has been stopped.

Even if you become pregnant while on these medications, there is no evidence of their causing any problems to you or to the developing baby. There is no evidence of any increased risk of birth malformations, miscarriages, multiple pregnancies, or any other adverse effects on pregnancy. In fact, with larger pituitary tumours, the endocrine specialist may sometimes advise continuing cabergoline during pregnancy.

Normally, the pituitary gland enlarges by about one-third in size during pregnancy. If there is a pre-existing pituitary tumour such as a prolactinoma, this will also increase in size during pregnancy. This can cause pressure that can lead to symptoms such as headaches and visual disturbances. If this happens MRI scans can be used safely, even in pregnancy, to detect any enlargement.

Visual field monitoring is required at regular intervals during pregnancy if the prolactinoma is large or if symptoms develop during pregnancy.

Breastfeeding is entirely safe and does not lead to growth of underlying prolactinomas.

Further information

- Patient.co.uk. Prolactinoma <http://www.patient.co.uk>

INFORMATION FOR PATIENTS Hyperparathyroidism and pregnancy

The parathyroid glands (para-thy-roid) which are situated in the neck, secrete a hormone called parathyroid hormone, which controls the calcium levels in your body. Excessive secretion of this hormone, known as hyperparathyroidism, causes abnormally high levels of calcium in the body.

Though hyperparathyroidism occurs in both sexes, women are more commonly affected.

Although it is rare in pregnancy, hyperparathyroidism can cause serious problems for both mother and baby if it is not promptly recognized and treated.

During pregnancy, and when they are not pregnant, between 25% and 80% of women with hyperparathyroidism may be free of symptoms. In mild cases, symptoms such as fatigue, pain in the joints, muscle ache, loss of appetite, nausea, vomiting, depression, constipation, and blurred vision may be experienced.

In more severe cases, repeated miscarriages, pre-eclampsia, kidney stones, tummy pains, irregular heart rate in the mother, dehydration, and fractures may result. In the most serious cases there may be kidney failure, coma, and death.

Pregnancy complications if hyperparathyroidism is untreated can result in repeated miscarriages, premature delivery, restricted growth of the unborn baby, or seizures in the newborn infant. With appropriate treatment all these complications are significantly reduced.

Diagnosis is by blood tests, and an ultrasound scan of the neck helps to localize the enlargement of the parathyroid gland.

Once hyperparathyroidism has been diagnosed, care during the pregnancy and after the baby is born will be provided by a team of specialists including the obstetrician, endocrinologist, neonatologist (doctor who specializes in the care of newborn babies), and anaesthetist as well as the midwife.

Treatment will involve immediate lowering of the calcium levels in the blood by medication and correction of dehydration with fluids given as drips. Close monitoring will continue for both your own welfare and the baby's. Surgery, by a keyhole procedure, may be required if symptoms persist despite medication and the outcomes of such surgery during pregnancy have been shown to be excellent with minimal complications reported. Your specialists will discuss all these options with you.

Further information

- Patient.co.uk. Hyperparathyroidism <http://www.patient.co.uk>

10. Maternal Neurological Conditions

INFORMATION FOR PATIENTS Epilepsy and pregnancy

Most women whose epilepsy is well controlled will have uncomplicated pregnancies and deliveries and give birth to normal children. Most women with epilepsy do not experience an increase in seizures during pregnancy, especially if epilepsy has been well controlled before conception.

Some anti-epileptic medications, though not all, can cause a small increase in the risk of malformations of the baby, depending on the type of drug. The risk of birth abnormalities of various types in the general population (not just those with epilepsy) is about 2 in 100 births. This risk is slightly increased to 3 in 100 in babies born to mothers who are epileptic but not on anti-epileptic medication compared to 4 in 100 for those who are on anti-epileptic medication. This risk is lowered if you are on a single type of anti-epileptic medication compared to being on more than one.

If you are on certain types of anti-epileptic medications, particularly sodium valproate, carbamazepine, or phenytoin, the risk of fetal malformations can be further lowered if you start taking high-dose folic acid, 5 mg daily, from about 3 months before getting pregnant up until at least the end of 12 weeks of pregnancy. *The high-dose folic acid has to be obtained on prescription from your GP; it is not available over the counter.*

The risks of uncontrolled seizures during pregnancy such as miscarriages, pre-eclampsia, premature delivery, even loss of the baby after 24 weeks of pregnancy, outweigh any possible risks of anti-epilepsy medications. **If your epilepsy has been well controlled with medication it is very important that you do not stop the anti-epileptic medication on your own once pregnant.**

Although you may be reluctant to continue with the medication once you realize you are pregnant, because you worry that they may cause abnormalities in the developing baby, it is important not to stop the medication suddenly without specific advice from the epilepsy specialist.

Not all drugs used to control epilepsy have adverse effects, and the risks are further reduced by taking the high dose of folic acid (5 mg) mentioned earlier. The baby's organs are fully developed by the end of 13 weeks of pregnancy, and after that time medications cannot cause any malformations.

If you have not had a seizure for several years, the consultant neurologist may advise you to stop the anti-epilepsy medications gradually during pregnancy, over the course of 3–6 weeks.

It is best to seek assessment and advice from your consultant neurologist before getting pregnant. The neurologist can assess the medication you are taking to control the epilepsy, and either change it to a more suitable one for a future pregnancy or lower the dosage to keep any potential risk of abnormality to the baby to a minimum.

Once you are pregnant, you can expect to be mainly under the care of the team of specialists in the hospital as well as continuing care in the community by your midwife. In addition to the routine scans in the first trimester (first 13 weeks of pregnancy) and at 20 weeks, a scan may be arranged at 16 weeks to look at the baby's spine, the roof of the mouth, the lips, etc., and at about 22 weeks for the baby's heart. Further scans to monitor the baby's growth will be arranged to ensure that the baby is growing consistently from about 28 weeks of pregnancy.

Depending on the type of medication you are on for epilepsy control, you might be advised to take vitamin K tablets for the last 3 weeks of pregnancy to ensure normal blood clotting.

In some women with epilepsy, pain, stress, and anxiety may be triggers for seizures. An epidural for pain relief during labour and delivery is therefore recommended.

Epilepsy, especially when stable during pregnancy, is not a reason for starting labour earlier than usual or for Caesarean section, unless there are other problems.

It is generally safe to continue anti-epilepsy medications during breastfeeding as the amount transmitted through breast milk is minimal.

You will need help with baby care to assist you to get maximum rest after childbirth. Appropriate support and simple precautions, such as never bathing the baby while alone, carrying of the baby as little as possible, and sitting on the floor or at a low level to breastfeed or to change nappies, will help reduce the risk of any injury to the infant caused by you having a seizure.

If your anti-epileptic drug dosage has been increased during pregnancy, you will be advised by the specialists and your GP to reduce the dosage **gradually** to the levels you were on before pregnancy.

The pill may not be the ideal contraceptive for you as it is less effective in those who are on medications such as sodium valproate, carbamazepine or phenytoin. Your obstetrician or GP can advise alternative contraception that is more suitable for you.

Further information

- Epilepsy Action. Epilepsy and having a baby < https://www.epilepsy.org.uk/info/women/having-baby>
- Epilepsy Society. Pregnancy and epilepsy <http://www.epilepsysociety.org.uk/pregnancy-and-epilepsy>
- Patient.co.uk. Epilepsy. Contraception/pregnancy issues <http://<www.patient.co.uk>

INFORMATION FOR PATIENTS Idiopathic intracranial hypertension and pregnancy

Idiopathic intracranial hypertension (IIH, for short), previously known as benign intracranial hypertension, is a chronic condition where high pressure builds up inside the skull. This condition may develop suddenly or gradually over time.

IIH is a relatively common condition with many different causes and is more common in women than men, **particularly in those who are overweight and in their twenties**.

It is likely that the diagnosis of IIH made was made before you became pregnant, and you may also be on medication.

Symptoms can include nausea, vomiting, pain behind the eyes, and double vision. In severe cases, unless well controlled, there is a risk of permanent damage to sight in 1 in 10 cases. Headaches may be severe, throbbing in nature, and may be worse in the morning, or on coughing or straining.

IIH generally does not cause adverse pregnancy outcomes, but symptoms may worsen during pregnancy at any stage and improve after delivery.

If you have had IIH symptoms during a previous pregnancy, the chance of it occurring again in subsequent pregnancies is about 1 in 10.

During pregnancy you can expect to be referred to the neurology specialist as ongoing review is essential during pregnancy.

Almost all treatment methods used for IIH when not pregnant can be safely continued during pregnancy. These include steroids, acetazolamide, and even lumbar puncture in order to lower the pressure. Sometimes just losing weight before your next pregnancy may help avoid the symptoms.

Certain drugs called thiazide (thy-a-zide) diuretics, should only be used with great care in pregnancy due to the risk of decreased blood flow in the placenta and low platelet counts in the newborn.

Acetazolamide is the preferred medication of choice in pregnancy but it can work against folic acid synthesis from diet. High-dose folic acid 5 mg must be prescribed especially in the first trimester (first 13 weeks of pregnancy) for this reason. (This high-dose folic acid can only be obtained on prescription from your GP, not over the counter.)

If you have IIH your vision needs to be carefully monitored every 2–3 months during pregnancy. Any problems need prompt treatment with corticosteroids.

You will also be referred to the anaesthetic specialist during pregnancy to discuss options for pain relief during labour and delivery. In general an epidural is the safe and preferred option.

If you are overweight, it is important to lose weight before another pregnancy. This not only helps reduce eye symptoms but may relieve symptoms altogether without the need for medical treatment.

Further information

- IIH UK (information and support for patients and families) 31 Wellington Street, St Johns, Blackburn, Lancashire BB1 8AF;<http://<www.iih.org.uk>
- NHS Choices. <http://www.nhs.uk/conditions/intracranial-hypertension>
- Patient.co.uk. Idiopathic intracranial hypertension <http://www.patient.co.uk>

INFORMATION FOR PATIENTS Multiple sclerosis and pregnancy

Frequently asked questions

Does having multiple sclerosis (MS) affect my chances of having a baby?

Having MS does not affect fertility, nor is there any increase in miscarriage rates or fetal abnormalities.

Does having a baby alter the long-term course of MS?

Pregnancy and childbirth do not seem to have any impact on the course of MS in the long term although MS could relapse after delivery after remission during pregnancy.

How does pregnancy affect MS in the short term?

During pregnancy there is a significant reduction in MS relapses, particularly in the last 13 weeks. This may be because of higher levels of certain hormones as well as a lower level of immune chemicals in the body during pregnancy.

Immunosuppressant drugs or disease-modifying agents, such as interferon, that are used for MS outside of pregnancy must not be used during pregnancy because of the possible adverse effects on the developing baby. Ideally you would have been advised to stop these at least 3 months before pregnancy.

In the first 3 to 6 months after childbirth, there is an increased risk of relapse, seen in about 30% of women with MS. There are no specific factors that predict a relapse after delivery.

Would I expect any problems during pregnancy due to the MS?

Many studies have shown no difference in pregnancy problems in women with MS compared to those without MS.

- If you have had MS-related bladder problems these could get worse during pregnancy, leading to urinary infections. Your urine sample will be checked at each antenatal visit. If you have any symptoms, you need to inform your midwife or GP to arrange a prompt urine test and antibiotic treatment if any infection is identified.
- Tiredness and fatigue could be more noticeable; however, these could be symptoms of pregnancy itself rather than the MS.
- If you have an unsteady gait due to MS, the change in weight distribution might make you unsteady and special care to avoid trips and falls is advisable.
- If there is an acute relapse of MS during pregnancy affecting your normal functions, you can be treated with steroids. These are safe and used for a number of conditions during pregnancy.

Can I have an epidural for pain relief in labour?

MS does not pose any special risk for pain relief with an epidural or spinal anaesthetic in labour or for delivery. Having an epidural is not risky for women with MS.

What about breastfeeding?

If you are not on medications for MS, breastfeeding is encouraged. There is no evidence that breastfeeding is a problem for women with MS or their babies

If you are on prescribed immunosuppressant drugs, you are advised not to breastfeed. These drugs are usually prescribed after the baby has been weaned.

Do I need to have a Caesarean section because of the MS?

There is no evidence that Caesarean section has any benefit over vaginal delivery in women with MS. You might need to have a Caesarean section for other obstetric reasons. A Caesarean section will not cause a relapse or progression of MS any more than normal delivery would.

What are the chances of my child getting MS?

Children of women with MS have a 2% chance of developing MS, which means that they have a 98% chance of not developing MS.

Further information

- Multiple Sclerosis Trust. Pregnancy and parenthood factsheet <http://www.mstrust.org.uk/shop/product.jsp?prodid=134>

INFORMATION FOR PATIENTS Stroke and pregnancy

Frequently asked questions

What is a stroke?

A stroke means that the blood supply to a part of the brain is suddenly cut off. The brain cells need a constant supply of oxygen from the blood. Soon after the blood supply is cut off, the cells in the affected part of the brain become damaged, or die. A stroke is sometimes called a brain attack. The area of brain affected, and the extent of the damage depends on which blood vessel supplying the brain is affected.

Is all stroke the same?

No. There are two main types of stroke—**ischaemic** ('is-ke-mik') and **haemorrhagic** ('hem-o- rāh-gic').

- **Ischaemic stroke** is caused by a blood clot. In ischaemic stroke there is reduced blood and oxygen supply to a part of the brain. It is usually caused by blood clot in an artery, which blocks the flow of blood.
- Such a blocking blood clot can often form within the artery itself but could also form in another part of the body, and then travel in the bloodstream to lodge in a blood vessel in the brain. This is called an **embolus**.
- A **haemorrhagic stroke** is caused by bleeding from a damaged or weakened artery which may have burst.
- An **intracerebral haemorrhage** is when a blood vessel bursts within the brain substance. The blood then spills into the nearby brain tissue. This can cause the affected brain cells to lose their oxygen supply and become damaged or die.
- A **subarachnoid haemorrhage** is when a blood vessel bursts within the narrow space between the brain and the skull. This space is normally filled with a fluid called the cerebrospinal fluid.

How common are strokes during pregnancy?

- Strokes are not common during pregnancy. They occur in about 30 in 100,000 pregnancies.
- Pregnant women have a higher incidence of stroke than non-pregnant women of similar age.

Why is there an increased risk of stroke during pregnancy?

Many changes take place in various structures and organs of the body during pregnancy. The changes that take place in the circulating blood during any normal pregnancy can make it more prone to form clots, therefore a slightly increasing the risk of a stroke. Most strokes occur either in the last few weeks of pregnancy or in the first 6 months after the baby's birth.

Is pregnancy-related stroke more likely in some women than in others?

Yes. There are several pre-existing conditions and risk factors that make some women more vulnerable to strokes in pregnancy and after childbirth. These include:

- Age—older women are more at risk
- Being overweight or obese
- Smoking
- More than 1–2 previous pregnancies
- Afro-Caribbean ethnic group
- Alcohol or drug misuse
- Twin/triplet pregnancies
- Severe dehydration during pregnancy
- Severe pre-eclampsia (a condition where the blood pressure increases in the second half of pregnancy, protein is found in increasing amounts in the urine and there is excessive swelling)
- Certain conditions such as diabetes, high blood pressure, inherited blood clotting disorders, sickle cell disease, lupus and related syndromes, or heart disease.

What are the symptoms of stroke in pregnancy?

Symptoms of stroke are the same in pregnancy as at other times. They can vary depending on which part of the brain is affected and on the size of the damaged area. Symptoms develop suddenly and usually include one or more of the following:

- Weakness of an arm, leg, or both; this may range from total paralysis of one side of the body to mild clumsiness of one hand
- Weakness and twisting of one side of the face, which may cause you to drool saliva
- Problems with balance, coordination, vision, speech, communication, or swallowing
- Dizziness or unsteadiness
- Numbness in a part of the body
- Headache which can be so sudden and severe that it is described as a 'thunderclap headache'
- Confusion
- Loss of consciousness (occurs in severe cases).

What is a mini-stroke?

Symptoms of a mini-stroke are similar to a stroke, but last for less than 24 hours. It is due to a temporary lack of blood to a part of the brain. It is more correctly called a transient ischaemic attack (TIA). In most cases, a TIA is caused by a tiny blood clot that becomes stuck in a small blood vessel (artery) in the brain. This blocks the blood flow and a part of the brain is starved of oxygen. The affected part of the brain is without oxygen for just a few minutes, and soon recovers.

Unlike a stroke, the symptoms of a TIA soon disappear. However, you should see a doctor urgently if you have a TIA, as you are at increased risk of having a full stroke.

A quick guide for the general public to remember

Both a stroke and a TIA are medical emergencies and need immediate medical attention. As a way of helping the general public to become more aware of the symptoms of a stroke or TIA, a simple symptom checklist to remember has been devised and publicised. This is to think of the word **FAST**. That is:

- **F**acial weakness. Can the person smile? Has their mouth or eye drooped?
- **A**rm weakness. Can the person raise both arms?

- **S**peech disturbance. Can the person speak clearly? Can they understand what you say?
- **T**ime to call 999.

If any of these symptoms suddenly develop, then the person needs urgent medical help. So call an ambulance FAST. The FAST checklist does not cover every possible symptom of stroke or TIA. However, it is easy to remember and it is estimated that about 8 or 9 in 10 people with a stroke or TIA will have one or more FAST symptoms.

What are the risks associated with a stroke in pregnancy or puerperium?

- A stroke is a serious life-threatening condition whenever it occurs. During pregnancy, prompt recognition and treatment is life-saving for both the mother and her baby.
- A large haemorrhagic stroke can cause death. A small stroke, especially if it is of the ischaemic variety, may cause less severe problems, which may improve or disappear completely over time. In many cases the effects are somewhere in between these two extremes.
- About 50% of women who have a pregnancy-related stroke may continue to have some weakness of one side of the body, unsteady gait, swallowing and speech problems, confusion, tiredness, etc.
- Every stroke is different and the problems and difficulties have to be assessed for each affected woman.
- In the first few weeks after a stroke the swelling and inflammation around the damaged brain tissue will reduce. Some symptoms may then improve. Over time, other parts of the brain may sometimes compensate for the damaged part of the brain. With rehabilitation and appropriate therapy, there may be a gradual improvement.
- Of those people who survive a stroke, about 3 in 10 are fully independent within 3 weeks. This rises to about 5 in 10 within 6 months. However, it is common for some degree of disability to remain in nearly 50% of cases.
- Outcomes for the unborn baby such as stillbirth or premature delivery depend on the type, severity, and extent of the mother's stroke.

What tests are needed to confirm a stroke?

Apart from a detailed examination, tests such as special scans of the brain (MRI or CT scan) will be done to find out what type of stroke it is, ischaemic or haemorrhagic. Other tests may include an ultrasound scan of the neck blood vessels, an ECG (heart tracing), chest X-ray, and blood tests.

What is the treatment for stroke in pregnancy?

The treatment for stroke in pregnancy will be along similar lines as treatment of stroke at any time in life with a few exceptions due to pregnancy. Initial treatment will depend on whether it is an ischaemic or haemorrhagic stroke, as they are very different.

A plan for any other treatments will be devised and started as soon as possible. Treatments should be tailored to the particular needs of the women and the pregnancy. The treatment plan will depend on factors such as the severity of the stroke, the effects it has, the cause of the stroke, and other diseases that may be present. Treatments that may be considered include:

- **Antiplatelet medication** *such as low-dose aspirin*, clopidogrel, and dipyridamole. *Aspirin* is the most commonly used antiplatelet medicine, but others may be prescribed.
- **Medication to treat other conditions contributing to the stroke** such as diabetes, high blood pressure, or heart conditions like atrial fibrillation.
- **Surgery** may sometimes be required to fix a leaking blood vessel in the brain.

Good-quality rehabilitation is vital following a stroke, and can make a big difference to your eventual outcome. The aim of rehabilitation is to maximize activity and quality of life following a stroke. Hospitals that treat stroke patients have various specialists who help in rehabilitation. These include physiotherapists, occupational therapists, speech therapists, dieticians, psychologists, specialist nurses and doctors. One or more of these may be required, depending on how the stroke has affected you.

How can the risk of stroke be reduced during and after pregnancy?

The way to prevent strokes after pregnancy is very similar to the way of preventing strokes at any other time in life.

- **Smoking**. If you smoke, you should make every effort to stop. The chemicals in tobacco are carried in your bloodstream and can damage your arteries. Stopping smoking can greatly cut your risk of having a stroke.
- **High blood pressure** needs to be well controlled. High blood pressure usually causes no symptoms, but can be damaging to the arteries. If you have high blood pressure, treatment for this is likely to have the greatest effect on reducing your risk of having a stroke.
- If you are **overweight,** losing some weight is advised.
- **Exercise and healthy diet** are essential.
- **Alcohol and substance misuse** are well-known risk factors for stroke and should be avoided.
- **Diabetes** is a risk factor. If you have diabetes, treatment to keep your blood sugar as near normal as possible is important.

What are the chances of having another stroke in a future pregnancy?

There does not appear to be any increased risk of stroke recurrence in a future pregnancy, especially if the previous stroke has been of the ischaemic type, provided predisposing risk factors are eliminated or well controlled.

(Adapted with permission from Patient.co.uk, available at <http://www.patient.co.uk/health/stroke-leaflet> ©2014, Egton Medical Information Systems Limited. All Rights Reserved.)

Further information

- Brain and Spine Foundation. What is a stroke? <http://www.brainandspine.org.uk/stroke>
- Patient.co.uk. Stroke <http://www.patient.co.uk>
- Stroke Association. Women and stroke <http://www.stroke.org.uk/factsheet/women-and-stroke>

INFORMATION FOR PATIENTS Bell's palsy and pregnancy

Frequently asked questions

What is Bell's palsy?

Bell's palsy is a condition that causes temporary weakness or paralysis of the muscles on one side of the face. It is the most common cause of facial paralysis.

How do you recognize Bell's Palsy?

The symptoms of Bell's palsy vary from person to person. The weakness on one side of the face can be mild muscle weakness (**partial** palsy) or **total**, when there is no movement of the muscles at all.

The symptoms usually involve weakness felt around the muscles on one side of the face, pain around the ear, lost or altered taste, inability to wrinkle your forehead on the affected side, dribbling from one side of the mouth, or difficulty in opening or closing the eyelids on one side.

In rare cases, complete or partial palsy can affect both sides of a person's face.

What causes Bell's palsy?

The exact cause of Bell's palsy is unknown, but many researchers believe that the herpes virus is responsible. During pregnancy, it is thought that either inflammation of the facial nerve could result from silent herpes infection or as a result of excess fluid retention in the body as seen in the condition called pre-eclampsia.

Most of the muscles in our face are controlled by a single nerve, called the facial nerve. This nerve passes through a tunnel of bone on its way from the brain to the face. Bell's palsy is thought to occur because a virus, usually the herpes virus, can sometimes cause the nerve to become inflamed. This can interfere with the signals that the brain sends to the muscles in the face, resulting in the weakness or paralysis of facial muscles.

How common is this condition?

- Bell's palsy is a rare condition that affects about 1 person in 5000. Both men and women are affected.
- Bell's palsy is 3 to 20 times more common in pregnant women than in those who are not pregnant. The reason for this is not clear. It is also more common in people who are diabetic.
- Bell's palsy is more likely to occur during the last few weeks of pregnancy or after delivery.

What is the outlook?

Most people with Bell's palsy (around 8–9 out of 10 people) make a complete recovery. There is no difference in the recovery outlook between pregnant and non-pregnant women.

Most people notice an improvement in their symptoms after about 2 to 3 weeks (with or without treatment). However, a complete recovery can take between 3 and 6 months, sometimes even longer. The recovery time varies from person to person.

Around 1–2 in 10 people with Bell's palsy will experience some long-term weakness in the facial muscles. This is particularly seen in those who are diabetic, have high blood pressure, or have suffered total facial muscle paralysis rather than mild weakness alone.

What is the treatment for Bell's Palsy?

In most cases, Bell's palsy usually improves spontaneously: that is, without any treatment being required.

A short (2 week) course of a steroid medication called prednisolone is sometimes used to speed up the recovery process, if it is started early in the course of the condition, usually before 72 hours. However, this does not guarantee a full recovery.

Possible side effects of prednisolone include nausea, headache, indigestion, difficulty sleeping, thrush infection of the vagina or mouth, tiredness, and occasional dizziness.

These side effects should improve within a few days as your body begins to get used to the medication. You should not drive or operate heavy machinery if you find that your medication is making you sleepy or dizzy. Some people also experience mood changes, such as anxiety or depression, after taking steroids for a short period of time. You should report these symptoms to your GP or obstetric specialist.

Steroids may be used alone or, if herpes is suspected, an antiviral medication called aciclovir may be used as well.

Care of the affected eye during recovery is very important. The natural protection and lubrication provided by tears are very important in keeping the eyes free of dirt and bacteria, which could cause eye infections. When you have Bell's palsy you may might find it difficult to close your eye, which can cause tears to evaporate and leave the eye vulnerable to infection. Therefore, it is very important to keep the eye lubricated. Your GP may prescribe eye drops that contain 'artificial tears' for daytime use, plus an ointment that you should use at night. If you are unable to shut your eye at night time, your GP will give you some surgical tape to help keep it closed.

You might be advised to have physiotherapy. The physiotherapist will teach you a set of facial exercises aimed at strengthening the face muscles to improve their coordination and range of movements. Physiotherapy has been successful in a number of Bell's palsy cases, although it may not be suitable or effective for everyone.

If the condition does not improve in the long term, in a minority of patients other options such as Botox injections or surgery may be considered.

How will Bell's palsy affect my pregnancy, labour or delivery?

Whatever the cause of Bell's palsy, please be reassured that it has no ill-effect on your baby and no change should be required in the management of the pregnancy itself or of labour and delivery, unless you also have other problems such as high blood pressure, diabetes, or pre-eclampsia.

You can have all the usual forms of pain relief during labour and delivery, or a Caesarean section.

Further information

- Patient.co.uk. Bell's palsy <http://www.patient.co.uk (provides general information about the condition, not restricted to pregnancy)>.

INFORMATION FOR PATIENTS Myasthenia gravis and pregnancy

Myasthenia gravis (MG for short) is a rare immune condition that causes certain muscles of the body to become weak. The weakness and fatigue may affect muscles that you can control voluntarily. Involuntary muscles that you cannot control voluntarily, such as the muscles of the uterus (womb) or heart muscles, are not affected by MG.

MG most commonly affects the muscles that control eye and eyelid movement, facial expression, chewing, swallowing, and talking, as well as muscles in the arms and legs. Onset is usually seen in the twenties and thirties.

Symptoms of MG include double vision, droopy eyelids, difficulty in swallowing, and sometimes weakness of the muscles of the chest wall in severe cases. There are times when symptoms can worsen as well as improve. Pregnancy does not worsen the long-term course of MG.

Assessment of your symptoms as well as review of your medications is highly advisable before you get pregnant because certain drugs are not advisable during any stage of pregnancy whereas others are safe and essential.

In general, women with MG have uncomplicated pregnancies and childbirths. However, the course of MG during pregnancy and after delivery can be unpredictable because the symptoms can improve during pregnancy in 4 in 10 women, worsen in 3 out of 10 women, and remain unchanged in the remaining 3 out of 10.

The first trimester (first 13 weeks of pregnancy) as well as the first month after delivery are the more common times when symptoms might worsen. You may notice a distinct improvement after the first trimester which can continue till delivery.

You can get more tired simply because of the extra weight you carry in pregnancy and a change in the centre of gravity which places extra strain on some muscles.

One pregnancy can vary from the next. The way MG behaves in a first pregnancy does not predict the symptoms in subsequent pregnancies.

In women with MG, there is an increased risk of premature birth, the waters breaking prematurely, or growth problems of the baby. This is why your care during pregnancy will involve close monitoring by a team of pregnancy specialists, neurologists, anaesthetists, and midwives as well as the specialist for the newborn baby.

The dosage of medication that keeps your symptoms under control may need to be increased during pregnancy, as advised by the neurology specialist. Only those medications that are safe for you and the baby will be used to achieve control of your symptoms throughout pregnancy.

If your MG symptoms have been controlled with drugs including pyridostigmine and azathioprine or steroids these need to be continued during pregnancy, labour, delivery, and after. Your specialist will advise you about adjusting the dosage as pregnancy advances, based on your symptoms.

Rarely, in late pregnancy you could show signs of breathing problems that require immediate admission to the hospital for emergency treatment.

During pregnancy, in addition to the usual scans in the first trimester and at 20 weeks, you can expect to have more scans later in pregnancy to monitor the baby's growth.

You will be referred to see an anaesthetic specialist during pregnancy to discuss the safest options for pain relief in labour and delivery. Certain drugs need to be avoided in women with MG, but an epidural or spinal is safe.

A vaginal delivery is entirely feasible in women with MG. Procedures such as Caesarean section or inducing labour early are required only if there are other problems present, and not just because you have MG.

The first stage of labour is unaffected by MG because the powerful muscles of the uterus are involuntary muscles that are not influenced in any way by MG. It is only in the active pushing part of the second stage of labour that you might require assistance, with the ventouse cup or forceps being used to deliver your baby.

Your newborn baby will be examined by the specialist paediatrician for any signs of temporary muscle weakness that can be seen in 1–2 out of 10 babies born to mothers with MG. Before leaving hospital, you should look out for any signs that your baby has problems, such as difficulty in feeding, floppiness, weak cry, poor sucking, or breathing problems. These symptoms usually appear within the first 12–48 hours after birth. This temporary muscle weakness normally disappears by the time the baby is 4–8 weeks old, once your antibodies are cleared out of the baby's circulation. During this time the baby may need treatment with medication such as pyridostigmine, which is usually given to the baby just before a feed. The baby's specialist doctor will arrange regular checks of the baby during this time.

Further information

- Myasthenia Gravis Association (UK) <http://www.mga-charity.org> (support group and useful source of information)>
- NHS Choices. Myasthenia gravis <http://www.nhs.uk/conditions/Myasthenia-gravis>
- Patient.co.uk. Myasthenia gravis <http://www.patient.co.uk>

INFORMATION FOR PATIENTS Charcot–Marie–Tooth disease and pregnancy

Charcot–Marie–Tooth disease (CMTD) is one of the most common inherited disorders of the nervous system, affecting approximately 1 in 2500 people. It is mainly an inherited condition with a strong family history of one or both parents affected or carrying the gene. In CMTD the peripheral nerves that control movement (motor nerves) and less often, the sensory nerves (nerves than control sensation) can be affected by a process of gradual degeneration.

The condition causes muscle weakness and thinning and weakness of the muscles in the arms, legs, hands, or feet. CMTD can cause changes in gait (manner of walking or taking steps) and this can sometimes result in frequent trips and falls. In some cases, there is reduced ability to feel heat, cold, and pain.

The onset of symptoms is most often in teenage or early adulthood. The severity of symptoms varies greatly among individuals and even among family members with the disease. Pain is a feature and can range from mild to severe.

People with CMTD can expect to have a normal life expectancy. While there is no 'cure' as such for CMTD, as it is an inherited condition, physiotherapy, braces and other orthopaedic devices, and even orthopaedic surgery can help. Painkillers may be required but drugs such as aspirin, ibuprofen, and diclofenac must be avoided during pregnancy due to potential risks to the developing baby.

You would ideally have been, referred for genetic counselling before getting pregnant. given that this is an inherited condition.

Specific management in pregnancy

CVS or amniocentesis testing may be offered to detect the condition in your baby. These are invasive tests that carry a small risk of causing miscarriage. Most pregnancies proceed without problems.

Symptoms can recur in subsequent pregnancies especially if you have had CMTD from early teenage years. If the CMTD symptoms appeared only in adulthood, pregnancy does not seem to affect the course of the disease. The outcome for your baby is not affected.

Physiotherapy involving muscle-strengthening exercises or muscle and ligament stretching can continue during pregnancy. No-impact exercises, such as swimming, are particularly recommended.

During pregnancy, you will receive care from several specialists including the neurologist, specialist obstetrician, midwife, anaesthetist, and physiotherapist.

You will be referred to see the anaesthetic specialist in order to discuss pain relief during labour and delivery. If you have muscle weakness and fatigue, an epidural is advisable to provide pain relief during labour and to avoid getting overtired.

If you experience muscle fatigue and exhaustion, some additional assistance such as with the suction cup (ventouse) or forceps may be needed. Precautions will be taken to prevent excess bleeding after delivery of the placenta.

There is no reason why women with CTMD cannot breastfeed.

Further information

- CMT United Kingdom (support group) Tel 0800 652 6316; <http://www.cmt.org.uk>
- NHS Choices. Charcot-Marie-Tooth Disease. Diagnosis <http://www.nhs.uk/Conditions/Charcot-Marie-Tooth>

INFORMATION FOR PATIENTS Muscular dystrophy and pregnancy

Muscular dystrophy (dis-trophy) is an inherited genetic condition that causes progressive wasting and weakness of muscles. There are different forms of muscular dystrophy, all caused by defects in one or more genes that are control normal muscle function.

The defective gene is usually passed on to the child from one or both parents. In some forms of muscular dystrophy 50% of boys are affected due to the defective gene being passed on to them by their mother; girls who inherit the defective gene from the mother are carriers but are not significantly affected themselves.

In most cases, muscle dystrophies will have been diagnosed before a women gets pregnant. Genetic counselling is advisable before pregnancy, given that most cases are genetically inherited.

Myotonic dystrophy

In myotonic dystrophy, muscle wasting and weakness can worsen during pregnancy, usually towards the later stages.

In this type of muscle disorder, complications in pregnancy can have significant effects on both mother and baby. Problems that are seen more often in women with myotonic dystrophy include miscarriage, excess amniotic fluid around the baby, premature birth, or prolonged labour, as well as failure of the womb to remain well contracted after birth, leading to haemorrhage (excessive bleeding).

In myotonic dystrophy, 50% of children of an affected parent will have the disease with only 1 in 5 showing symptoms at birth. These symptoms may include very poor muscle tone, floppiness at birth, and difficulty breathing.

Duchenne muscular dystrophy

Duchenne muscular dystrophy (DMD) is a condition primarily seen in boys, and occurs in all ethnic groups. Here the affected boys have inherited the defective gene that is carried by the mother. Most female carriers of DMD have few or no symptoms.

Because of the devastating effect of DMD and the lack of a cure, if you have a family history of muscular dystrophy, you are strongly advised to seek genetic counselling before starting a family in order to investigate your carrier status and to discuss the probability of having an affected child. If there is such a family history, you will also be offered tests in early pregnancy to detect whether the fetus is affected.

Further information

- Muscular Dystrophy Campaign (support group) <http://www.muscular-dystrophy.org>
- NHS Choices. Muscular dystrophy <http://www.nhs.uk/conditions/Muscular-dystrophy>
- Patient.co.uk. Muscular dystrophy <http://www.patient.co.uk>

11. Maternal Uterine, Cervical, and Vulvovaginal Conditions

INFORMATION FOR PATIENTS Pregnancy following any cervical surgical procedure (excision biopsy, laser, cone, loop, etc.)

The **cervix** is the lower tubular portion of the uterus. It is about 4 cm (1.5 inches) long and has an internal opening called the **internal os** that communicates with the cavity of the womb (uterus). The outer mouth of the cervix facing the vagina is called the **external os**. The cervical canal is the passage between the internal and external os.

The internal os should normally remain nearly closed at most times. The cervical os (internal and external) allows passage of menstrual fluid from the uterus. Sperms travel upwards through the cervical canal to reach the uterus, passing through the internal os.

There is a gradual shortening of the cervix from about 24–26 weeks of pregnancy onwards as a part of the natural changes that take place during pregnancy. This shortening of the cervix close to term in pregnancy is called cervical **effacement**. When the cervix is fully effaced, that is, it is very short, it begins to gradually widen, a process called **dilatation**. When the cervix is fully dilated (10 cm) in labour, this is defined as the end of the first stage of labour and the start of the second stage.

Cervical intraepithelial neoplasia

Cervical intraepithelial neoplasia (CIN) is a condition where abnormal cells are found in the cervix as the result of a cervical smear. These cells can be precancerous. You might have previously had a colposcopy examination after an abnormal cervical smear result. A procedure to remove these abnormal areas of the cervix might have been performed either in the outpatient department or involving general anaesthesia in the operating theatre. Many women of child-bearing age undergo these treatments, so their effect on subsequent pregnancies is very important.

Procedures where a part of the cervix is actually removed are known by several terms including excisional biopsy, cone biopsy, knife cone biopsy, laser conization, LLETZ (which stands for large loop excision of the transformation zone, and loop biopsy. These are **excisional procedures**.

Other procedures such as laser treatment to cervix, laser ablation, or cold coagulation involve destroying the abnormal cells found on the surface of the cervix but not actually cutting away any part of the cervix itself. Such **ablative procedures**, which are being increasingly performed in younger women with CIN, have fewer adverse effects on a subsequent pregnancy than excisional procedures do.

Any excisional procedure where part of the cervix has been excised (cut out) could potentially cause complications such as late miscarriage (usually after 15 weeks of pregnancy), premature delivery, or the waters breaking prematurely.

The more cervical tissue has been removed, the greater the chances of such problems arising in a subsequent pregnancy.

The type of any previous cervical procedure also matters. A LLETZ or loop excision procedure (usually done in the outpatient clinic) is associated with fewer pregnancy complications in general, compared with knife cone biopsy (usually done under general anaesthetic in the operating theatre).This is because a knife cone biopsy general removes a greater depth and volume of tissue from the cervix.

If you have had more than one excisional procedure on your cervix, there is a greater likelihood of complications during pregnancy as more cervical tissue will have been removed. Also, getting pregnant within 2–3 months of a cervical excisional procedure can increase the chances of pregnancy complications resulting in poor outcomes.

In certain cases of cancer of the cervix a radical removal of the cervix called **trachelectomy** may have been performed where the cervix is removed completely, leaving only the uterus behind. During this procedure, a permanent suture (surgical stiching) is sometimes placed at the lower end of the uterus to encircle and tighten this part. Pregnancies following trachelectomy have increased chances of adverse outcomes, compared to the less radical procedures such as cone biopsy or LLETZ.

For all these reasons a pregnancy following any cervical excision procedure needs even greater care than usual, and some additional investigations and interventions may be required.

When you meet your community midwife for pregnancy booking she will ask you from details of any cervical procedure you have had. If a shallow excision or an ablative procedure has been performed, your pregnancy care can continue with the community midwife, as routine.

If a greater depth of the cervix has been removed (a depth of more than 1 cm) you will be seen by the specialist antenatal clinic team based in the local hospital, in addition to the care you receive in the community.

If you had this procedure performed in a different hospital, you should bring any letters you may have, giving details of the type of cervical procedure, to the antenatal clinic.

In the specialist antenatal clinic, details of the type of the procedure you had and depth of cervix removed will be clarified. A series of ultrasound scans (sometimes using the internal vaginal view rather than abdominal) to measure the exact cervical length and appearance of the internal os and cervical canal will be organized. These scans are generally performed on three occasions, the first at 14–16 weeks, the second 3–4 weeks later, and the third around 22–24 weeks pregnancy. If none of these scans show any worrying signs of abnormal cervical shortening or opening (called funnelling) of the cervical canal, your antenatal care can continue as routine with your community midwife. Except for one or two extra appointments to the specialist clinic later in pregnancy, no further cervical length scans or interventions will be required.

However, if any of these scans show the cervix has undergone premature abnormal shortening, or if the internal os shows signs of opening, you will need an internal examination in the specialist antenatal clinic. Further management options will be discussed with you, such as surgical insertion of a cervical suture (a stitch placed in the cervix at the level of the internal os) which when drawn together and knotted acts like a purse string. Some units may have an alternative to a cervical suture called a cervical Arabin pessary.

You may also be advised to insert a hormone (progesterone) pessary into the vagina or into the back passage once daily till about 35–36 weeks of pregnancy. Progesterone is the natural hormone which works to keep the muscles of the womb relaxed, thereby helping to prevent premature cervical shortening.

The insertion of a cervical suture is only performed in selected cases as the procedure is not without risks. The cervix could be injured during the procedure, the waters might break, or premature contractions could start, all or any of which could lead to miscarriage. These issues will be discussed in detail with you before a decision to insert a cervical suture is made. If the decision is for a cervical suture, this will be arranged as soon as possible depending on the examination findings. The procedure will be performed in the maternity theatre under a spinal anaesthetic.

After the cervical suture has been inserted you can go home the same day or the following day if all is well. You will be advised to rest for about a week. Remember to ask for a sick note before you are discharged, if you need one. You will be given an information leaflet about the suture insertion procedure.

Some units have a non-invasive alternative called the Arabin cervical pessary inserted in the antenatal clinic, which in some cases has been shown to be as effective as a cervical suture.

You will be asked to continue the suppository insertion once a day till about 35–36 weeks of pregnancy to help prevent premature contractions of the uterus.

The cervical suture will remain in place till you are 37 weeks pregnant, and will then be removed in the delivery suite. If you have had a cervical Arabin pessary inserted instead of a suture, it can be simply removed in the antenatal clinic at about 37 weeks.

If at any time after suture (or pessary) insertion, you start to experience contractions or bleeding, or if the waters break, **it is very important that you contact the hospital without delay. You will be advised to come in straightaway for the suture or pessary to be removed**. Contractions with a cervical suture in place can cause damage to the cervix. If the waters break, infection can get into the uterus.

If these events take place after 25 weeks of pregnancy, in anticipation of premature delivery, you will be offered two injections of steroids to help ripen the baby's lungs.

Following discharge after suture insertion or after the Arabin pessary insertion in clinic you will be seen 2 weeks later in the hospital specialist clinic, then at about 28, 32, and 36 weeks. No further cervical scans are necessary, but if there is any suspicion that the uterus seems smaller than expected for that stage of pregnancy, scans will be done to serially monitor the baby's growth. Routine antenatal checks with your community midwife will also continue at the usual intervals.

At the 36-week visit to the hospital specialist clinic, a date for cervical suture (or pessary) removal will be organized for about 37 weeks and you will be advised to stop the progesterone suppositories as well. At this visit you will also be given a date for labour to be induced if you have not delivered by about 10 days after the estimated due date.

Further information

- Patient.co.uk. Colposcopy <http://www.patient.co.uk>

INFORMATION FOR PATIENTS Radical trachelectomy and pregnancy

About 40% of cervical cancers are diagnosed in women of childbearing age. Until recently, treatment of early cancer of the cervix meant having to have a radical hysterectomy (removal of all the female reproductive organs) thus removing the option of having children. More recently, treatment has been modified to try to preserve childbearing capacity, without compromising overall survival.

The surgical procedure called **radical trachelectomy** (RT for short), where the uterus (womb) is left intact, offers women hope that they might bear a child even after treatment for cancer of the cervix. RT involves amputation of the cervix below the level where the cervix merges into the body of the womb. During the same operation, a permanent suture called a cerclage is placed where the cervix used to be, to help a future pregnancy to continue in the womb.

Although RT is a fertility-sparing procedure, it is important that you have received counselling that a live birth cannot be guaranteed and there are significant pregnancy risks including late miscarriages, very premature rupture of membranes (breaking of waters), and subsequent premature birth.

Pregnancy rates following RT vary between 40% and 80% and term deliveries are achieved in only about one-third of these pregnancies. In the remainder there is, unfortunately, a high pregnancy loss rate mainly due to second-trimester miscarriages (between 14 and 24 weeks), premature delivery (20%), premature breaking of the waters, and resulting infection within the womb.

It is highly advisable to wait for at least 6 months after the RT procedure before attempting a pregnancy. During this time, effective contraception is recommended.

If an assisted reproduction (IVF) route is being considered, it is important to avoid more than one embryo being transferred as miscarriages and very premature births are significantly higher with twin or triplet pregnancies. Single embryo transfer is highly advisable, to avoid multiple pregnancy in an already high-risk situation.

The care of the pregnancy should be with a team of pregnancy specialists led by a high-risk pregnancy obstetrician, in addition to routine antenatal care in the community with your midwife. You would be referred as early as possible once a pregnancy has been diagnosed to see the obstetrician specializing in high-risk pregnancies, who will maintain close communication with the gynaecological oncologist involved in the RT procedure.

If a stub of the cervix remained at the original RT operation, vaginal scans to monitor the remaining length of the cervix may be performed during pregnancy.

You may be advised to insert a daily hormone pessary in the vagina from the end of the 13th week of pregnancy up to about 34 weeks to try to keep the muscles of the uterus relaxed.

Loss of the protective mucous plug of the cervix after RT may allow infection to reach the uterus, which could lead to premature rupture of the waters and further spread of infection. This is why you may be prescribed antibiotics, both as a vaginal cream and as oral tablets to try to prevent such infection.

You should consider not having sexual intercourse between about 14 and 34 weeks of pregnancy, to avoid any possible infection and reduce the risk of premature breaking of the waters.

If there are any symptoms or signs of premature contractions or breaking of the waters between 24 and 35 weeks of pregnancy, you will be offered steroid injections to help the baby's lungs to mature, thus improving the chances of survival.

Because a permanent suture is inserted to keep the mouth of the womb closed when the cervix was removed at the RT operation, delivery can only be achieved by an operation. *If premature or full-term contractions start or if rupture of membranes at any stage of pregnancy occurs with a previously inserted cerclage, urgent delivery is required* either by Caesarean section or a similar operative procedure called hysterotomy, where the uterus is opened up by a different incision.

Further information

- Cancer Research UK: CancerHelp. Cervical cancer and pregnancy <http://www.cancerresearchuk.org>

Size and shape of the uterus

The uterus (womb) is a pear-shaped organ, which lies deep in the pelvis. It remains within the pelvis till 12–14 weeks of pregnancy, after which it gradually expands upwards into your belly as the baby grows.

The normal non-pregnant uterus is about 7.5 cm (3 inches) long, 5 cm (2 inches) wide, and 2.5 cm (1 inch) thick from front to back. It is a thick-walled muscular organ with a cavity inside, normally a single cavity. This is called the uterine cavity and it is where the fertilized egg gets to implant and grow into the baby.

The lower part of the womb projects into the vagina and is called the **cervix**. It is from the surface and mouth of the cervix (the **os**) that a cervical smear is taken. The roof of the uterus is called the **fundus**.

A small proportion (4–7%) of the general female population may have an abnormally shaped uterus. The proportion is greater in women undergoing tests for recurrent pregnancy losses, repeated miscarriages or infertility, or those who have had repeated premature deliveries. Such abnormalities of the uterus would have occurred during your own fetal development, between 8–11 weeks as an embryo in your mother's womb, triggered by unknown factors.

Many women may not be aware of a possible abnormality in the shape and structure of their womb as it has not led to any pregnancy complications or gynaecological problems.

How will having such a womb abnormality affect fertility and pregnancy?

In most cases, uterine abnormalities do not pose a problem in getting pregnant, continuing a pregnancy, and giving birth. However, certain types of womb abnormalities may make it more difficult to get pregnant or continue the pregnancy to full-term. The baby may have growth problems, may adopt an awkward position within the womb, and may need to be delivered by Caesarean section. The outcome of pregnancy is strongly influenced by the type and extent of the particular abnormality of the womb.

Types of uterine abnormalities

Your doctor, midwife, or obstetric specialist will be able to give you details of the type of abnormality of the uterus that you have. Individual types of uterine malformations are:

Uterus didelphys

This is a very rare abnormality where there is a complete duplication of the uterus. The double wombs are fused in the centre and each uterus has its own cervix. In two-thirds of such cases there is a double vagina as well.

In about 1 in 3 women with such a duplication of the uterus, there is also a duplication of some parts of the kidney system. This can be detected by special X-ray tests which can be done either before you get pregnant or 3 months after the baby is born, but **not during pregnancy**.

There is a greater than average rate of miscarriage and of premature delivery in women with uterine didelphys.

If you have uterus didelphys, the pregnancy is contained in one of the two wombs, which then expands to accommodate the growing pregnancy. As the pregnant uterus leads to its own cervix and vaginal passage, a normal delivery is possible.

Sometimes, if a thick partitioning wall in the vagina is identified during pregnancy and if the obstetric specialist suspects that this might cause an obstruction during delivery, you may be advised to have a Caesarean section to deliver the baby.

Unicornuate uterus

This is another rare abnormality, where only one half of the uterus that has developed, with one cervix and vagina, all of which are functional. Sometimes there is a small knob-like structure attached to the unicornuate uterus which represents the undeveloped half of the uterus.

Women with this type of uterine malformation can have pregnancy complications such as miscarriages, premature delivery, or the waters might break early. These usually happen because the unicornuate uterus cannot expand any more beyond this stage of pregnancy.

There is also an increased chance of a pregnancy lodging in the undeveloped 'rudimentary horn' if it connects with the main womb, causing an ectopic pregnancy.

Bicornuate uterus

The bicornuate uterus is heart-shaped instead of the usual pear-shape, with two distinct 'horns' and a deep crater or indentation at the top. There is one cervix and a single vagina. This type of uterine shape, where pregnancy takes root in one of the 'horns' of the uterus, can cause an increased chance of miscarriages after 13 weeks of pregnancy as well as premature delivery. In this type of malformation of the womb, there is also an increased weakness of the cervix.

In a bicornuate uterus, there is a greater chance of the baby not lying in a head-down position and needing to be delivered by Caesarean section.

Septate uterus

The external contour of the womb appears normal but within the cavity is a dividing wall made up of a tough sheet of muscle and fibrous tissue. This wall or septum can may either extend through the whole length of the cavity of the womb or only partway down the womb. There could also be a septum within the vagina.

Septate uterus is the most common type of uterine malformation and is associated with more pregnancy problems than average, including increased pregnancy losses and early premature labour.

Surgical removal of the dividing septum inside the womb, done under general anaesthetic before conception, can improve the outcome of subsequent pregnancies.

Arcuate uterus

There is a small dimpling of the top of the womb, with only a small septum. This type of abnormality is associated with the fewest pregnancy problems. As the shape of the womb cavity differs only slightly from the normal, you can expect to have near-normal pregnancy outcomes.

What can I expect during my antenatal care during pregnancy?

Depending on the type of uterine abnormality that has been identified, you will be offered more frequent appointments in both the antenatal clinic and for ultrasound scans. You will also receive advice about how to recognize signs of premature labour, premature breaking of waters, and so on.

If your previous pregnancy outcomes have suggested a weak cervix in association with the abnormal uterine development, you might be offered serial scans to monitor the length and closure of the cervix or you might need to have a cervical stitch inserted. Your obstetric specialist will explain this in detail.

Ultrasound scans will be done frequently to ensure that the baby's growth remains satisfactory, and at about 36–37 weeks the baby's position and presentation will be confirmed. If the baby lies in a breech or transverse position, or keeps changing its lie frequently when you are close to your dates, you might be advised to have a planned Caesarean section.

If the baby is in breech, transverse, or unstable lie and you start having contractions or if the waters break, you will be advised to go to the delivery suite without delay as there is a chance that the baby's umbilical cord could be swept down with the waters. This is a severe emergency threatening the baby's survival if the umbilical cord prolapses.

If the pregnancy is progressing normally with no concerns about the baby's growth or movements, and the baby's head is engaged in the pelvis, you can expect to have a normal vaginal delivery. A Caesarean section is needed if any other indications arise.

After delivery and before leaving hospital, you can expect to receive advice about any further investigations that may be required to detect any associated malformation of the kidney system, which is found in one-third of women with uterine malformations. You will also be given appropriate contraceptive advice, especially if you have a double cervix (uterine didelphys). If you have a double cervix, cervical smears need to be taken from each cervix each time. Remember to remind whoever takes your smears in the GP's surgery or in the hospital clinic that you have a double cervix!

Any surgical procedure to either remove the intervening vaginal septum or unify the two halves of the uterus should be considered only after adequate discussion with the specialists and at least 3 months after the end of pregnancy.

Further information

- Patient.co.uk. Female genital abnormalities <http://www.patient.co.uk>

INFORMATION FOR PATIENTS Female genital mutilation

Female genital mutilation (FGM) is any procedure that is designed to alter or injure a girl's (or woman's) genital organs for non-medical reasons. It is sometimes known as 'female circumcision' or 'female genital cutting'. It is mostly carried out on young girls.

Crime, justice, and the law

FGM is illegal in the UK. It's also illegal to take a British national or permanent resident abroad for FGM, or to help someone trying to do this. The maximum sentence for carrying out FGM or helping it to take place is 14 years in prison.

FGM procedures can cause:

- Death
- Severe bleeding
- Infections
- Problems with giving birth later in life, including the death of the baby.

What to do if you know someone at risk

If you think that a girl or young woman is in danger of FGM:

- Contact the police if she is still in the UK.
- Contact the Foreign and Commonwealth Office if she has already been taken abroad
- You can also contact: the Safeguarding Children Board at your local council.

Further information

- Female Genital Cutting Education and Networking Project <http://www.fgmnetwork.org>
- Foreign and Commonwealth Office. Tel: 020 7008 1500; from overseas: +44 (0)20 7008 1500
- Foundation for Women's Health Research and Development (FORWARD) <http://www.forwarduk.org.uk>
- Medconsumer.info. Female genital mutilation <http://www.medconsumer.info/topics/fgm.htm>
- World Health Organization <http://www.who.int/topics/female_genital_mutilation/en/>

INFORMATION FOR PATIENTS Fibroids and pregnancy

Frequently asked questions

What are fibroids?

Fibroids are very common benign tumours that are thickenings of the muscle wall of the uterus. They are classified according to their location.

- Fibroids that project into the cavity of the uterus and change its shape are called **submucous** fibroids; they sometimes grow on a stalk.
- Fibroids that lie within the wall of the uterus without either changing the shape of the uterine cavity or projecting on the uterine surface are called **intramural** fibroids.
- Fibroids that grow outwards, causing a bulge on the uterine surface and sometimes growing on a stalk, are called **subserous** fibroids.
- Fibroids may grow singly, or many fibroids of varying sizes may be found in different locations in the uterus. They can be as small as a match-head or as large as a baby's head.

How common are fibroids?

In total, 25–40% of women of reproductive age are found to have fibroids. They are more common in Afro-Caribbean women, in older women, and in those who have had fertility problems. During pregnancy, fibroids are found in about 3 out of 100 pregnant women.

Can fibroids cause problems during a pregnancy?

Most fibroids do not cause any problems during pregnancy. The vast majority of pregnant women go on to have normal deliveries of full-term healthy babies. However, in about 10–30% of pregnant women with fibroids, they can cause problems such as increasing the risk of miscarriages and bleeding during early pregnancy.

Especially if they project into the cavity of the uterus, fibroids can cause premature labour and delivery as well as causing the placenta (afterbirth) to separate from the wall of the uterus.

If fibroids are large, they can cause compression effects on the baby or, rarely, interfere with the growth of the baby. If they are large enough to distort the cavity of the uterus, they can cause the baby to lie in awkward positions, in which case the baby needs to be delivered by Caesarean section.

Most women with fibroids, even large fibroids, can deliver normally. If there are fibroids blocking the outlet of the uterus, or if the baby is not in a head-down position, a Caesarean section may be needed to deliver the baby.

Does pregnancy cause the fibroid to grow?

The hormones of pregnancy can cause an increase in size of fibroids, especially in the first few weeks of pregnancy. However, there is no evidence that fibroids continue to grow throughout pregnancy or after delivery. They invariably shrink after childbirth.

If fibroids are in such a position that they press against your bladder, you might have a problem emptying your bladder. This is called retention of urine. This is an emergency that you need to promptly report to your doctor or midwife, or to the hospital, as the bladder needs to be emptied with a catheter.

Large fibroids can sometimes cause pain because of pressure effects on nerves and other organs of the tummy and pelvis.

If the fibroid enlarges too rapidly as a result of the hormones of pregnancy it sometimes causes severe pain due to a process called 'red degeneration'. This is when the fibroid outgrows its blood supply and the cells of the fibroid start to degenerate. The pain is severe, but usually resolves in a short time without treatment and without harm to the baby. You will be advised rest, hydration, and painkillers. You might need hospital admission for a few days till the pain resolves.

Can fibroids cause any ill-effects on the baby?
Unless fibroids cause premature labour and delivery, they have little effect on the baby.

Do I need a Caesarean section because of having fibroids?
Most women with fibroids deliver normally. However, if a large fibroid is close to the lower part of the uterus or cervix, this can obstruct the birth canal and the baby needs to be delivered by a planned Caesarean section. Also, fibroids can cause the baby to lie in breech or transverse position especially if they are large, or located in the lower part of the uterus, or there are a lot of fibroids. If the baby is lying as breech with uterine fibroids, attempting to turn the baby is not an option and Caesarean section becomes necessary in such cases.

Can fibroids be removed at the same time as a Caesarean section?
It is dangerous to attempt to remove fibroids, large or small, during a Caesarean section because of the great risk of provoking uncontrollable bleeding, which can even result in loss of the uterus. If removal of fibroids (myomectomy) is to be considered, this can only be assessed several months after childbirth and you need to ask your GP to refer you to a gynaecology specialist to discuss this.

Further information

Patient.co.uk. Fibroids <http://www.patient.co.uk> (provides general information about fibroids, not restricted to pregnancy).

12. Maternal Dermatological Conditions

INFORMATION FOR PATIENTS Pruritic urticarial papules and plaques of pregnancy

Pruritic urticarial papules and plaques of pregnancy (PUPPP), also known as polymorphic eruption of pregnancy, is the most common rash in pregnant women. It normally occurs in first pregnancies during the third trimester (26 weeks onwards) with an average onset at about 35 weeks.

PUPPP does not usually affect subsequent pregnancies.

Appearance of PUPPP

What is distinctive about PUPPP is that it does not involve the navel (belly button) area, unlike other common rashes of pregnancy.

The rash of PUPPP almost always begins in the stretch marks over the tummy. The rash itself consists of small, raised pinkish-red red spots (wheals) in the stretch marks that fuse together to form larger wheals on the abdomen around the navel. There is often a pale halo around the papules. Once the papules join, they form large red, raised (urticarial) patches (plaques) which spread to involve the buttocks and thighs, and sometimes the arms and legs. Lesions on or above the breasts are rare. The rash can sometimes form little fluid-filled vesicles. It is very itchy (pruritic in medical language), hence its name.

Although extremely bothersome, this condition is harmless to both you and the baby. It can last for an average of 6–8 weeks and resolves spontaneously 1 to 2 weeks after delivery. The peak period of the severe itching normally lasts for about a week or two.

Cause of PUPPP

The cause of PUPPP is unknown. It is not associated with obstetric cholestasis, where there are liver enzyme abnormalities, or with pre-eclampsia, or with any hormonal abnormalities.

PUPPP is most common in a first pregnancy, when the abdomen is tightest. The rash usually starts around over the abdomen where stretching is greatest. There is a theory that it is the body's reaction to the stretching of the abdominal wall. This causes the underlying elastic layer of connective tissue to split, leading to an inflammatory reaction. The PUPPP rash develops as a sort of 'allergy' to the stretch marks and then spreads elsewhere on the body.

Another theory is that the small number of the baby's cells found within the mother's circulation, which appears to be increased in women with PUPPP, can trigger an allergic skin reaction.

Most cases begin in the last 3 months, especially the last 5 weeks, when the stretching is greatest. It is rare for PUPPP to begin after delivery.

Diagnosis of PUPPP

The diagnosis of PUPPP is based solely on the appearance of the rash: itchy skin and a rash that is raised, usually starting in the abdomen and spreading from there. No laboratory tests that are needed to detect PUPPP and skin biopsies are not generally required.

Treatment of PUPPP

The treatment of PUPPP is to control the symptoms of itching. Emollients (moisturisers) can be applied liberally and frequently as required.

High-strength topical steroid creams or ointments, such as clobetasol or betamethasone, may need to be applied thinly to the red itchy patches up to 2–4 times a day to relieve the itching. Once the rash is under control, changing to a lower-strength steroid used less frequently is advisable.

In very severe cases, if the application of steroid cream or ointments do not help, the doctor may prescribe steroids as oral medication to control the symptoms. This would normally involve only a short course of a low dose which would not cause any problems for you or the baby.

Oral antihistamines such as chlorphenamine are generally less effective for itching than steroids, but may be useful at night to help you sleep.

Recurrence

This is uncommon for PUPPP to recur in subsequent pregnancies. If it does happen, the PUPPP is likely to be milder.

Further information

- British Association of Dermatologists. Polymorphic eruption of pregnancy <http://www.bad.org.uk/for-the-public/patient-information-leaflets>
- DermNet NZ. PUPPP <http://www.dermnetnz.org/reactions/puppp.html>

INFORMATION FOR PATIENTS Pemphigoid gestationis

Pemphigoid gestationis used to be known as herpes gestationis. This is a misnomer because the condition has nothing to do with herpes or any herpes-related viral infection. It is an itchy skin condition that occurs during the second and third trimesters of pregnancy and around the time of delivery.

Pemphigoid gestationis is rare, occurring in 1 in 7000 to 1 in 50,000 pregnancies.

Appearance

Pemphigoid gestationis starts as extremely itchy red hives or small bumps around the navel (belly button). Within days to weeks, the rash spreads, and the hives and bumps fuse at the edges forming irregular but roughly circular patches covering a wide area of skin.

The rash then appears on the trunk, back, buttocks, forearms, palms, and soles. The face, scalp, and inside of the mouth are usually spared. After 2–4 weeks of this rash, large, tense blisters form at the edges of the rash. These blisters can also appear on hitherto uninvolved skin.

This condition usually starts during the second trimester of pregnancy (13–26 weeks) or in the third trimester (26–40 weeks), although it has sometimes been reported in the first trimester and even a short time after delivery. The average appearance is at 21 weeks.

Although some spontaneous improvement of the rash may occur later in the pregnancy, closer to the time of delivery, uncomfortable flares occur in most (75–80%) of women. The blisters heal without scarring provided they do not get infected.

Unfortunately pemphigoid gestationis can recur in subsequent pregnancies, usually recurs earlier, and may be more severe. Only 8% of women with pemphigoid gestationis do not develop it in subsequent pregnancies.

Causes

Pemphigoid gestationis is thought to have an autoimmune background where the normal immune system in the mother fails to recognize proteins of her own skin and instead attacks them with antibodies. These antibodies attach to certain types of connective tissue in the skin and cause an inflammatory response which appears as redness, itching, swelling, and blister formation.

Diagnosis

Pemphigoid gestationis is diagnosed by taking skin biopsies of different areas of the rash as well as normal-appearing skin. A special test to detect antibodies called direct immunofluorescence is performed on the biopsies to make the diagnosis.

Effect on the pregnancy

Apart from the intense itching and lack of sleep it causes, pemphigoid gestationis does not lead to any short-term or long-term problems for you.

Some studies have shown a possible association between pemphigoid gestationis and a smaller-than-average baby as well as premature delivery. This link is not strong, but your specialist obstetrician may want to arrange extra growth scans for the baby.

Effect on the baby

Because antibodies cross the placenta, the antibodies that cause pemphigoid gestationis can in some instances also cause a temporary rash of the newborn baby. A noticeable rash has been reported in 5–10% of newborn babies born to mothers with this condition. These rashes are usually mild and resolve within 3 months as maternal antibodies are cleared from the baby's system. No treatment is generally required.

There is evidence that women with pemphigoid gestationis have an increased risk of premature delivery. Current studies indicate that there is no increased risk of miscarriage or stillbirth.

Treatment

Some women with very mild cases of pemphigoid gestationis may respond to steroid creams and antihistamines. However, most women require ***oral steroids*** to control their symptoms. A high dose is usually required to get symptoms under control and is then tapered as the rash improves.

After delivery

Breastfeeding appears to shorten the length of time that these rashes persist in the weeks following delivery.

Recurrences can occur with menstruation, with the use of the oral contraceptive pill, usually if started within 1–5 months after delivery of the affected pregnancy.

Further information

- British Association of Dermatologists. Pemphigoid gestationis <http://www.bad.org.uk/for-the-public/patient-information-leaflets>

INFORMATION FOR PATIENTS Scleroderma, systemic sclerosis, and pregnancy

Scleroderma is a rare autoimmune tissue disorder, more common in women than in men. Scleroderma may be **localized** (affecting only the skin) or **systemic** (generalized, involving many tissues and organs). In the localized type of scleroderma without any organ involvement, pregnancy outcomes are good.

Scleroderma, especially systemic sclerosis, may be associated with some increased complications during pregnancy, but with careful antenatal care good outcomes can be expected. For women with mild and limited systemic sclerosis, the pregnancy and delivery can progress without complications, resulting in a healthy baby.

In diffuse systemic sclerosis, especially when there is previous kidney and lung damage, there is an increased risk of miscarriages, premature birth, high blood pressure, or growth problems of the baby. With careful planning before starting a pregnancy, close monitoring, and appropriate treatment during pregnancy, successful outcomes can be expected.

Pregnancy outcomes are directly related to the state of scleroderma at the time of conception. Pregnancy is best planned when the disease is stable or inactive (in remission), when the outcomes of the pregnancy are generally good.

In systemic scleroderma, assessment and advice by specialists **before starting a pregnancy** are highly recommended. If you have systemic scleroderma and are planning a pregnancy, in order to reduce complications it is recommended that you discuss your individual case with your GP who may refer you to specialists.

During pregnancy, you can expect a specialist team will be involved in your care including the obstetrician specialist of complex pregnancies, the immunologist looking after your scleroderma, and an anaesthetist in addition to the routine antenatal care by your midwife.

Close monitoring of disease activity, blood pressure monitoring, and prompt control of hypertension are essential. Ultrasound scans to monitor the baby's growth will be arranged at regular intervals. Your kidney and lung function tests will be kept under regular surveillance.

The obstetric specialist will discuss the timing and type of delivery with you. It will depend on several factors such as how far the pregnancy has progressed, the baby's growth, and any additional complications such as worsening blood pressure and kidney or lung damage.

Some patients with systemic sclerosis and lung disease may deteriorate after delivery. Close monitoring must therefore continue after delivery.

Further information

- Raynaud's & Scleroderma Association (support group) <http://www.raynauds.org.uk/>
- Scleroderma Society. Pregnancy in systemic sclerosis (systemic scleroderma) <http://www.sclerodermasociety.co.uk/userfiles/Pregnancy18.02.14.pdf>

INFORMATION FOR PATIENTS Neurofibromatosis and pregnancy

Neurofibromatosis (neuro-fy-bro-ma-to-sis, or NF for short) is a term for a group of conditions affecting mainly the nervous system and skin. It is a genetic condition that can be passed on in families from one generation to the next by genetic inheritance. NF occurs in all ethnic groups and affects both sexes equally.

The chance of inheritance from an affected parent is about 50%. However, in about 30–50% of those affected by NF, there is no such family history; here NF is due to a chance or sporadic mutation that occurs in one of the genes. Any offspring of such an affected parent will still have a 50% chance of having NF.

There are two main groups of NF: type 1 (NF1) and type 2 (NF2). A small third group called schwannoma is very rare.

NF1 is also known as von Recklinghausen's NF. This accounts for 90–95% of all cases of NF and is found in about 1 in 5000 of the population.

The degree to which individuals with NF are affected can vary greatly, even within the same family. Some people will be mildly affected, with very few health problems. Others will have some serious health problems that make their daily life difficult and restrict what they can do.

In NF1, there are characteristic raised dark patches or spots on the skin and freckling in the skin folds of armpits and groin. When nerves are affected in NF1, node-like lesions develop, also involving the soft tissues and bones. In some people NF1 it can result in epilepsy and learning difficulties, deafness, vision problems, or hypertension (high blood pressure).

NF and pregnancy

NF has no effect on fertility and the outcomes of pregnancy are generally very good. Compared to the general population there is a small increase in the risk of developing certain pregnancy complications such as miscarriages, premature delivery, growth problems of the baby, and hypertension/pre-eclampsia.

With close monitoring to detect such risks and with the appropriate management the outcomes for mother and baby are very good. Hypertension, in particular, needs careful monitoring during pregnancy and prompt treatment with medications that are safe to use in pregnant women.

During pregnancy you will be looked after by the specialist obstetrician and you will have an anaesthetic assessment as well as continuing routine antenatal care with your community midwife. The baby's growth will be monitored with ultrasound scans at specific intervals during pregnancy.

If the pregnancy is otherwise uncomplicated, there is every chance that you can have a normal vaginal delivery.

People with NF may have increased sensitivity to certain anaesthetics. This can be assessed during the consultation with the anaesthetist, as well as any potential problems with spinal/epidural anaesthetic or with general anaesthetic. Options for pain relief in labour and for delivery can be discussed.

After birth, the paediatricians will examine the baby for any characteristic skin spots suggestive of NF and arrange longer-term follow-up if NF is suspected.

Further information

- Genetic Alliance UK. Neurofibromatosis type 1 <http://www.geneticalliance.org.uk>
- The Neuro Foundation. NF type 1 <http://www.nfauk.org/what-is-neurofibromatosis/nf-type-1>

INFORMATION FOR PATIENTS Epidermolysis bullosa and pregnancy

Epidermolysis bullosa (EB) refers to a group of rare inherited genetic conditions that are characterized by the development of skin blisters produced by even minor degrees of friction, trauma, or heat. Even the gentlest friction, often from simple day-to-day activities, may provoke skin blistering in EB.

The skin is made up of a number of different layers. The outermost layer is called the epidermis, and EB is the breakdown and blistering of the outer skin layer.

EB is not an infectious condition. It is a genetically inherited condition, which means it can be passed on from generation to generation. About 1 person in 230 has a defective gene that causes EB. One or both parents may pass on a defective copy of the gene to the child. One in 17,000 live births will be a baby born with a form of EB. The condition affects both sexes and all racial groups worldwide.

The effects of EB are highly variable, from being life-threating in early infancy in some cases to increasing disability but a near-normal life expectancy in others.

There are many types of EB, but three main types are recognized: EB simplex, dystrophic EB, and junctional EB. The common symptom in all these forms is blistering of the skin. The degree of blistering and residual scarring may vary according to the type of EB.

Apart from skin, the mucous membranes that line body cavities such as the mouth, gullet, or urinary tract may also be affected. The blisters may occur only in specific areas of the body such as hands and feet. In the milder forms of EB the blisters heal without leaving permanent damage to the skin. In other forms scarring occurs that can lead to permanent disfigurement and disability.

Prenatal testing for EB is now available in specialist centres between 8 and 11 weeks of pregnancy to determine whether the fetus has inherited EB.

EB and pregnancy care

Pregnancy does not affect the underlying skin condition of EB and pregnant women with EB do not develop any more non-skin-related complications during pregnancy compared to the general population.

Your care during pregnancy, labour, and delivery will be with a team of specialists from obstetrics, dermatology, genetics, anaesthetics, and midwifery as well as with your community midwife.

The basic objective of care is to avoid blistering and secondary infection, and correction of any nutritional deficiency if there is involvement of the mouth and gullet. Any examination or intervention, from measuring your blood pressure to assisting your delivery, will be performed with caution to minimize chances of bruising and blistering.

The relevant specialists will assess you and the pregnancy and will have detailed discussions with you about the type of delivery and the kind of pain relief to be used. These discussions and decisions made will take place well ahead of time. All equipment, dressings, etc. would be pre-selected to reduce pressure or friction blisters.

Your baby will be examined by the specialist paediatrician after birth to detect any signs of EB.

Breastfeeding is encouraged, unless there are infected bullae at the site and the skin surrounding the nipples. Well-lubricated nipple shields will be provided.

Further information

- DebRA (support group: Tel: 01344 771961). Pregnancy and childbirth in EB <http://www.debra.org.uk>

13. Maternal Autoimmune Disorders

INFORMATION FOR PATIENTS Lupus, antiphospholipid syndrome, and pregnancy

Systemic lupus erythematosus (SLE or lupus for short) is an autoimmune disease. This means that your body's immune system fails to recognize certain tissues of your own body as 'self' and therefore produces antibodies as a reaction to them just as it would towards 'non-self' foreign antigens such as bacteria or viruses. Production of such autoantibodies, which are capable of harming some of the body's own tissues, can ultimately lead to disease.

Lupus is a condition which can affect many systems and organs of the body. It is marked by periods of flares and remissions.

Lupus is seen in about 1:750 women in white populations, higher in Afro-Caribbean and Asian populations and 90% of lupus patients are female, primarily of childbearing age.

No two lupus patients may have the same symptoms; the range of problems may range from minor skin rashes to severe kidney failure. Some may have just a few symptoms, others can have many.

Lupus is an acquired, not an inborn, condition. The defective immune response may have been present for years before actual symptoms or signs develop. Sometimes, certain environmental triggers such as infections or smoking may trigger the SLE response.

There is no 'cure' for lupus at present, but early diagnosis can make a significant difference in management and outcomes. Ideally, pre-pregnancy assessment and counselling by a specialist obstetrician as well as planning the management of a future pregnancy is highly recommended.

Pregnancy complications such as increased risk of miscarriages, especially recurrent miscarriages, prematurity, low birth weight, pre-eclampsia, deep vein thrombosis and pulmonary embolism, and premature placental separation (abruption) can be associated with lupus. Such pregnancy complications could lead to investigations that reveal lupus for the first time.

There is increased risk of such pregnancy complications when lupus has caused kidney damage or hypertension (elevated blood pressure), or when lupus is in an active state at the time of conception.

Low-dose aspirin is advisable from the start of pregnancy till the end. Regular blood pressure monitoring and effective treatment of hypertension, vigilance for pre-eclampsia, serial ultrasound scans to monitor the baby's growth, and timely delivery form the essence of pregnancy management in lupus.

Antiphospholipid syndrome

Antiphospholipid syndrome (APS or Hughes syndrome) is also an acquired autoimmune disorder, and 30–40% of lupus-positive women will also have APS.

APS causes the blood to clot too easily, which can lead to thrombosis, embolism, and recurrent pregnancy loss.

As in lupus, the presentation in APS could vary from person to person and include epilepsy, rheumatoid arthritis, Behçet's or Sjögren's syndrome, psoriatic arthropathy, or thromboembolism.

Unrecognized or untreated APS may increase the risk of miscarriages, especially late miscarriages between 14 and 24 weeks of pregnancy, recurrent miscarriages (three or more), poor growth of the baby in the womb, and even stillbirth. Blood clots in the arteries (leading to strokes or myocardial infarction) or in the veins (deep vein thrombosis, DVT) and emboli (a piece of the blood clot lodging in the lungs causing the life-threatening emergency of pulmonary embolism), high blood pressure and severe pre-eclampsia, abruption, and other problems are not uncommon in unrecognized or untreated APS. Pregnancy complications and subsequent investigations may bring underlying APS to light.

A team of specialists from obstetrics and haematology (blood disorders) as well as midwives and anaesthetists will care for you throughout pregnancy.

If you have been diagnosed to have APS, in any future pregnancy you would be advised a combined treatment with both low-dose aspirin (75 mg once a day) and daily injections of a small dose of a blood thinning agent called low molecular weight heparin (LMWH) which you can inject yourself just under the skin, commencing from 5–6 weeks after a positive pregnancy test.

The LMWH injections will need to continue till at least 6 weeks after delivery as this is the peak time for thrombosis and embolism. You will be advised to wear below-knee elasticated compression stockings throughout the pregnancy, and for at least 6 weeks after the baby is born.

Ultrasound scans to monitor the baby's growth will be performed at regular intervals from about 24–26 weeks pregnancy.

Longer-term anticoagulant medication is required if you have previously had a DVT or pulmonary embolism. The anti-coagulation nurses and the haematologist can advise you about this and help to monitor the levels of blood clotting markers.

The combined oral contraceptive pill is unsuitable for you due to the increased risk of DVT and emboli.

Further information

- Arthritis Research UK. Antiphospholipid syndrome <http://www.arthritisresearchuk.org/arthritis-information/conditions/antiphospholipid-syndrome.aspx>
- Lupus UK. The importance of planning pregnancy in SLE. <http://www.lupusuk.org.uk>
- Patient.co.uk. Antiphospholipid syndrome <http://www.patient.co.uk>

INFORMATION FOR PATIENTS Rheumatoid arthritis and pregnancy

Rheumatoid arthritis (RA) is a chronic condition affecting the joints. It has no adverse effects on pregnancy unless there is also another autoimmune conditions such as lupus.

Three out of four women with RA experience an improvement during pregnancy, but the symptoms can return after the baby is born. Improvement usually begins in the first trimester.

Pre-pregnancy counselling with a specialist obstetrician or rheumatologist is advisable. This will allow investigations to exclude related autoimmune conditions such as lupus, antiphospholipid syndrome, or anti-Ro antibodies which can have an effect on pregnancy outcomes. If any of these proves positive, this will alter the management of a future pregnancy.

Pre-pregnancy counselling will also allow re-evaluation of the medications you are on for symptom control in RA. Drugs such as prednisolone, hydroxychloroquine, sulfasalazine, or azathioprine have good safety record during pregnancy. If you are on any of these medications the baby's growth rate will be monitored with serial ultrasound scans during pregnancy. You will also be advised to take a high dose of folic acid, available on prescription from your GP or hospital specialist, as these drugs act to oppose folic acid in the body.

Other drugs used to treat RA such as methotrexate, leflunomide, and cyclophosphamide, are contraindicated in pregnancy because there a risk of increasing the occurrence of abnormalities in the developing fetus.

If you have been on long-term steroids you will be offered a glucose tolerance test at about 26–28 weeks of pregnancy, to exclude temporary diabetes in pregnancy.

Simple analgesics such as paracetamol are the first-line choice for those with RA symptoms during pregnancy. Non- steroidal anti-inflammatory drugs such as high-dose aspirin (150 mg or more), ibuprofen, or diclofenac are **not** to be used during pregnancy due to their adverse effects on the baby.

RA does not in any way prevent you from having a normal vaginal delivery. Interventions such as early induction of labour or Caesarean section are only required for other indications and not just for RA.

Further information

- Arthritis Research UK. Pregnancy and arthritis <http://www.arthritisresearchuk.org>
- National Rheumatoid Arthritis Society (NRAS). Rheumatoid arthritis and pregnancy <http://www.nras.org.uk>

INFORMATION FOR PATIENTS Sjögren's syndrome and pregnancy

Sjögren's syndrome (SS) is a common autoimmune disorder which can cause uncomfortable symptoms including dry eyes and/or dry mouth, feeling of tiredness and aching, fatigue, and symptoms relating to the stomach or gut.

An autoimmune disorder is one where your body's immune system fails to recognize certain tissues of your own body as 'self' and therefore produces antibodies as a reaction to them just as it would towards 'non-self' foreign antigens such as bacteria or viruses. Production of autoantibodies capable of harming some of the body's own tissues can ultimately lead to disease.

SS occurs more often in women (90% of those affected). SS can be either **primary** or **secondary.** In primary SS there is no associated underlying rheumatic condition, whereas in secondary SS other autoimmune diseases such as lupus, rheumatoid arthritis, or anti-Ro antibodies can coexist.

SS usually affects only the tear ducts of the eyes and salivary glands but may also cause inflammation of joints.

It is uncommon for children to inherit SS from their parents.

SS and pregnancy

Pregnancy complications in SS are mainly due to the occurrence of other autoimmune conditions such as lupus or anti-Ro antibodies.

During pregnancy, vigilance for pre-eclampsia, poor growth of the baby, low birth weight, or premature delivery will continue. Serial ultrasound scans to monitor the progressive growth of the baby will be arranged at regular intervals.

Painful joints and generalized muscle ache are not uncommon: Paracetamol is the preferred analgesic, but you need to avoid non-steroidal anti-inflammatory drugs such as high-dose aspirin (150 mg or more), ibuprofen, or diclofenac. Rarely, you might need a short course of steroids if the joints are inflamed.

SS by itself does not require early delivery or Caesarean section if there are no growth concerns for the baby or any other obstetric problems. A normal vaginal delivery is the expected route of delivery in the absence of any other problems.

Further information

- British Sjögren's Syndrome Association (support group) <http://www.bssa.uk.net/>
- LUPUS UK. Sjögren's syndrome <http://www.lupusuk.org.uk/>
- NHS Choices. Sjögren's syndrome <http://www.nhs.uk/conditions>

INFORMATION FOR PATIENTS Dermatomyositis or polymyositis and pregnancy

Dermatomyositis (DM) and polymyositis (PM) are both rare inflammatory muscle diseases with an autoimmune basis. An autoimmune disorder is one where your body's immune system fails to recognize certain tissues of your own body as 'self' and therefore produces antibodies as a reaction to them just as it would towards 'non-self' foreign antigens such as bacteria or viruses. Production of autoantibodies capable of harming some of the body's own tissues can ultimately lead to disease.

DM and PM develop over time and are not inherited conditions. They can affect both sexes and tend to appear when the person is in the forties. These conditions are therefore relatively rare in women of childbearing age. They can be also associated with other autoimmune conditions such as rheumatoid arthritis, Sjögren's, or lupus etc.

These conditions are most likely to have been diagnosed before your pregnancy. Only rarely do they appear for the first time during pregnancy or after delivery.

DM results in weakness of the muscles, especially those of the neck, upper arms, and thighs. In about 1 in 5 cases, if untreated, there could be some difficulty with swallowing or breathing. There might also be reddish skin rashes on the hands, feet, elbows, or face.

In PM, the pattern of muscle weakness is the same as in DM but there is no skin involvement.

Pre-pregnancy counselling by specialists is advisable because pregnancy outcomes depend largely on whether the disease was active or in remission at the time you conceived. Women who are in disease remission at the time of conception not only have better pregnancy outcomes but flares during pregnancy are also better controlled with medication. Women whose disease was active at the time of conception could have more problems such as miscarriages, growth problems of the baby, and premature delivery.

Although rare, these conditions have an important bearing on pregnancy; this is why your care will be referred to a specialist team although your community midwife will be continue with your routine antenatal care.

Assessment of your health and of signs of disease activity, and close monitoring of the baby's growth and well-being, will be maintained during pregnancy.

Treatment with steroid tablets is effective in most cases. The steroids used are safe in pregnancy and the initial dose will be gradually reduced depending on the response. Other drugs that help suppress the immune response, such as azathioprine or hydroxychloroquine, are safe and have also been used widely in addition to steroids.

Epidural or spinal anaesthesia are safe procedures, but some drugs routinely used in anaesthesia need to be avoided in anyone with DM or PM. During pregnancy you can expect to be seen by a specialist anaesthetist who will discuss pain relief options during labour and delivery with you.

Your specialists will be happy to discuss all aspects of the treatment plan for the pregnancy and after delivery.

Depending on your individual pregnancy and the growth of the baby, your specialist obstetrician will discuss the ideal time for delivery and the method with you.

Medications such as steroids and azathioprine are relatively safe for breastfeeding, and given the advantages of breast feeding, you are encouraged to do so. It is advisable to breastfeed just before taking that day's scheduled dose of the medication.

Further information

- Myositis Support Group <http://www.myositis.org.uk/guide_to_myositis.htm>
- Patient.co.uk. Dermatomyositis/polymyositis <http://www.patient.co.uk>

14. Maternal Connective Tissue Disorders

INFORMATION FOR PATIENTS Ehlers–Danlos syndrome and pregnancy

Ehlers–Danlos syndrome (EDS) is a rare genetic connective tissue disorder characterized by hypermobile joints, increased elasticity of skin, thin semi-translucent skin, increased fragility of tissue and blood vessels, which can cause easy bruising.

EDS is caused by a defect in a protein called collagen which is the main building block of the body, providing strength and support to ligaments, tendons, and many organs including the uterus (womb) and cervix. This means that if the collagen itself is defective, it can produce many problems throughout the body.

ED affects both men and women females and all ethnic groups. It is estimated that 1 person in 5000 is affected by EDS. If one parent is affected with EDS there is a 50% chance (1 in 2) that the baby will inherit it.

There are six different types of EDS and they are classified according to characteristic signs and symptoms. Diagnosis is based on the family history as well as presenting symptoms. There can be overlapping of certain symptoms in some types of EDS and diagnosis is sometimes difficult. The diagnosis is confirmed by biochemical or molecular testing of a skin biopsy to determine the type of EDS.

The disease course and long-term outcomes depend largely on the type of EDS. With the exception of the vascular type of EDS (formerly type IV), affected individuals have a normal life expectancy. Life expectancy in vascular type EDS is generally only around 40–50 years due to the increased incidence of rupture of large blood vessels and major organs.

EDS and pregnancy

The type of EDS determines any potential complications during pregnancy. Not all types are associated with significant risks. In general terms, the pregnancy-associated complications are increased risk of cervical incompetence and late miscarriages, pelvic pain, premature birth, and restricted growth of the baby, as well as the risk of very early breaking of the waters.

Antenatal care focuses on the early detection of such problems, with serial scans to monitor the length of the cervix and later, the baby's growth; early referral to see the anaesthetic specialist for evaluation of potential anaesthetic-related risks; and precautions to reduce the risk of severe bleeding after delivery.

Pregnancy can be life-threatening in severe classic EDS (type I) and vascular EDS, which are the most severe forms, because the variety of collagen which is defective forms the main structure of large blood vessels, the gastrointestinal tract, and the womb (uterus). This can cause major obstetric complications.

If you have been identified as having either the severe classic type (type I) or vascular (type IV) EDS, you may already have been advised to avoid a pregnancy; or, if you are already pregnant, that management needs to be in a tertiary/regional referral centre.

If you have mild classic EDS (type II) you can expect relatively few problems: pregnancy is usually well tolerated, with successful vaginal delivery, although there is an increased risk of cervical incompetence and late miscarriages. You will be offered regular monitoring of the length of the cervix using internal ultrasound scans to detect premature shortening of the cervix or opening-up of the inner mouth of the cervix, in which case a cervical suture may be considered.

In the hypermobility type of EDS (type III), pregnancy outcomes for both the mother and baby are generally good although back pain is a significant feature.

Because of the risks associated with pregnancy, and the potential for transmission of EDS to the baby, the ideal time to determine genetic risk is before pregnancy, especially if EDS has already been diagnosed in the family. Genetic counselling for affected adult women is essential. Identification of the type of EDS is therefore crucial before pre-pregnancy discussions take place.

Further information

- Ehlers-Danlos Support UK, PO Box 748, Borehamwood WD6 9HU; Tel: 0208 736 5604; <http://www.ehlers-danlos.org>. Useful booklets published by the support group include Pregnancy & childbirth in Ehlers-Danlos syndrome; Ehlers-Danlos syndrome; The management of Ehlers-Danlos syndrome

INFORMATION FOR PATIENTS Marfan's syndrome and pregnancy

Marfan's syndrome is a genetic abnormality, with a transmission risk of 50% to the offspring. If either parent has Marfan's syndrome any child will have a 1 in 2 chance of inheriting the condition.

The main areas of the body affected in Marfan's syndrome are the skeleton, eyes, heart, and the large artery carrying blood from the heart, called the aorta. Because the syndrome can involve many organ systems, the diagnosis requires various specialists in cardiology (heart), ophthalmology (eyes), radiology (X-rays and scans), and genetics.

Women with Marfans' who are considering pregnancy need to understand the medical risks and special care needed to manage a pregnancy. Pre-pregnancy assessment and counselling is essential to avoid severe risks to you and the baby in any pregnancy.

Before conception, it is vital that you have had a recent assessment by the heart specialist with updated investigations including an echocardiogram to make sure your aorta is not at a size that would make pregnancy too risky. It is also advisable to see a maternal-fetal medicine specialist or high-risk obstetrician to discuss specific issues related to pregnancy and Marfan's syndrome. Pre-pregnancy genetic counselling is essential.

If you have previously had an aortic valve replacement with a mechanical prosthesis, the essential anticoagulation needs to continue during pregnancy as well as after. The specialist obstetrician and cardiologist will discuss the appropriate anticoagulation to be used during pregnancy and the first few weeks after the baby is born.

Prenatal diagnosis can be offered, with tests such as amniocentesis or chorionic villus sampling of the fetus early in pregnancy to determine if the fetus is affected. This is possible only if the mutation causing the Marfan's in the affected parent has already been identified before conception. Similarly, provided the specific mutation has already been identified, in-vitro fertilization ((IVF) with preimplantation genetic diagnosis is another option offered in some centres. It is therefore important to undergo genetic testing before becoming pregnant and it is highly advisable to speak to the genetics counsellor about these options.

If the aortic root is found to be enlarged beyond 4.5 cm, you will be advised not to plan a pregnancy as this can worsen during pregnancy leading to life-threatening consequences. In such a situation you would be advised to have corrective surgery before considering a pregnancy.

Even with a normal-sized aorta, there is a very small risk, 1 in 100, of the serious life-threatening emergency of aortic dissection during pregnancy.

Other pre-existing risk factors such as high blood pressure, obesity, and smoking, will worsen the outcomes for you and the baby. Your blood pressure needs to be lowered with appropriate drugs before pregnancy and maintained at a stable level throughout pregnancy. You will be strongly encouraged and offered support to lose weight and to stop smoking.

Nearly 80% of people with Marfan's syndrome have some degree of abnormality of the heart and aorta. If you have had a heart defect diagnosed, there is at least a 50% chance of the baby also having a heart defect, although not necessarily of the same type.

Care in pregnancy will be with a specialist team involving the cardiologist, maternal medicine obstetrician, anaesthetist, and radiologist. Routine antenatal care of the pregnancy can also continue with your community midwife. You will be carefully reviewed by your cardiologist throughout the pregnancy, with echocardiograms performed at least every 3 months, more frequently (every 6–8 weeks) if the aorta measures close to 4.0 cm, to check for any sudden increase in the size of the aorta.

Your blood pressure will be closely monitored during pregnancy and if it too high it will be treated with drugs called beta-blockers.

If you have any heart and/or aortic involvement, you would need to be referred during pregnancy to a tertiary/regional unit with heart surgery facilities.

Special scans during pregnancy including echocardiograms of the baby's heart and aorta will be performed, as well as serial scans to monitor the progressive growth of the baby.

A detailed and individualized plan of management for pregnancy, delivery and after, will be discussed with you, including the safest method of delivery and the anaesthetic to be used for pain relief, the cardiological and paediatric assessment of the newborn baby, and care after delivery. The specialist team will be happy to answer your queries at each stage of pregnancy and will organize further follow-up after the baby is born.

Further information

- March of Dimes (USA). Marfan syndrome <http://www.marchofdimes.com//baby/marfan-syndrome.aspx>
- National Marfan Foundation <http://www.marfan.org/marfan/2448/Pregnancy-and-Reproduction>

15. Maternal Bowel Disease

INFORMATION FOR PATIENTS Inflammatory bowel disease (Crohn's, ulcerative colitis) and pregnancy

Inflammatory bowel disease (IBD) is the name for those conditions where there is inflammation of the digestive tract, as in *Crohn's disease and ulcerative colitis*. IBD is usually diagnosed in young adults.

Ulcerative colitis is more frequent in women while Crohn's occurs equally in men and women. Most women with IBD have uncomplicated pregnancies with normal vaginal deliveries if the disease is either inactive or kept in in remission with medications. Pregnancy does not cause IBD to get worse later in life.

The state of your IBD at the time of conception strongly influences the course of the disease during pregnancy as well as pregnancy outcomes. If your IBD has been under remission or inactive at the time you conceive it is likely to remain so during pregnancy, though there may be flare-ups in some women.

However, if you conceive at a time that your IBD has been active, it is more likely that you will have disease flare-ups during pregnancy and also a somewhat increased risk of some pregnancy complications such as miscarriage, premature delivery, or growth restriction of the baby. It is therefore highly recommended that you seek advice from your GP or IBD specialist before planning a pregnancy. Your GP may refer you to a specialist obstetrician for such pre-pregnancy counselling.

It is very important for you to take *a high dose of folic acid (5 mg/day)* starting from even before conception and continue this throughout pregnancy. This is *available only on prescription from your doctor and not over the counter*, unlike ordinary strength pre-pregnancy folic acid.

The normal absorption of calcium, vitamin D, and iron from the intestinal tract is hampered by IBD, so these supplements may need to be continued throughout pregnancy.

You should not stop taking the IBD medication that has kept your disease in remission for fear of any effect it might have on your developing baby. The usual medications used in IBD are widely used and safe at all stages of pregnancy and breastfeeding. Those that are unsafe, such as methotrexate, would have been withdrawn by the specialist several months before a pregnancy and replaced by a safe alternative drug. You can always check this by calling the IBD nurse Helpline number. *It is very important that you do not stop your medications unless directed to do so by the gastroenterology specialist. If you do, relapse is inevitable and pregnancy outcomes are far* worse.

If you have been on steroid medication called prednisolone for a while during pregnancy, you will be offered a blood test called the glucose tolerance test at about 26–28 weeks of pregnancy to exclude diabetes during pregnancy.

During pregnancy while you will see your community midwife as usual. You will also be seen more often by the specialist obstetric team and the gastroenterology team. You will have regular clinical assessments of your pregnancy and of your IBD symptoms, in addition to extra ultrasound scans at regular intervals during pregnancy from about 28 weeks onwards. These scans are to ensure that the baby is continuing to grow well.

If there is any flare-up of IBD during pregnancy, this will be treated vigorously to reduce risks to the baby.

Unless you have active disease around the vagina/back-passage area or have had a previous surgical procedure called ileal-pouch-anal anastomosis, you can have a vaginal delivery. Even if you have had a previous ileostomy or a colostomy, a vaginal delivery is feasible and is the preferable option. A Caesarean section is advisable only in certain cases of IBD depending on disease activity at the area around the vagina and back passage. Similarly, IBD is itself not an indication for early induction of labour unless there are other concerns such as growth restriction of the baby.

If IBD has been active in the last few weeks of pregnancy, there is a high chance that it will flare up after the baby is born. It is essential that to continue the IBD medication during the postnatal period to avoid this.

Breast feeding is encouraged as it has been shown to reduce the chances of your baby developing IBD in future. With the exception of a few drugs that you would have been asked to avoid, most drugs for IBD have a proven safety track record for breastfeeding. If you are on oral steroids (prednisolone) or azathioprine, it is best to breastfeed immediately before you take your day's medication dose, thereby allowing about 4 hours between the drug dose and breastfeeding. If you are on sulfasalazine, very rarely the breastfed baby may develop diarrhoea for a very few days.

Further information

- UpToDate. Patient information: Inflammatory bowel disease and pregnancy <http://www.uptodate.com/contents/inflammatory-bowel-disease-and-pregnancy-beyond-the-basics?source=search_result&search=ibd&selectedTitle=1~30>

16. Maternal Musculoligamental Conditions

INFORMATION FOR PATIENTS Symphysis pubis dysfunction and pregnancy

Frequently asked questions

What is SPD?

Symphysis pubis dysfunction (SPD) or pelvic girdle pain or pelvic joint pain are all terms applied to symptoms of pain experienced around the pelvis, especially the symphysis pubis (the joint where the front two portions of the pelvis meet, in the middle).

SPD refers to symptoms of pain and discomfort particularly with movement or spreading of the legs.

Symptoms of SPD include pain over the pelvic joint in the front as well as in the groins and the lower back. These can worsen during changing position—walking, getting out of a seat, reaching up, and so on. Sometimes these can be accompanied by a grinding sensation or a 'clicking' feeling in the pubic area.

SPD is not a disease. It is a pregnancy condition and can therefore only be 'managed' not 'cured'.

Your midwife and the physiotherapists are the key health care professional who will be working with you to support and advise.

What causes SPD?

SPD symptoms result from the stretched pubic ligaments having to bear the weight of pregnancy while maintaining balance and stability, which are essential for mobility.

In any pregnancy the pelvic girdle has to bear the pressure and weight of the pregnant womb and its contents, which increase as the pregnancy advances. In addition, the pelvic ligaments become softer and more stretchy as a result of hormone changes starting from the early weeks of pregnancy.

SPD is not a 'disease of pregnancy'. It affects every pregnant woman, although to varying degrees. It can range from being a discomfort to being debilitating enough to affect day- to-day activity.

Also, after any previous pregnancy, whichever way you have delivered the previous baby/babies, your pelvic ligaments never resume the pre-pregnancy dimensions. This means they are left permanently stretched to some degree before any subsequent pregnancy.

When can symptoms of SPD start?

Most women notice increasing symptoms of SPD from around the middle of pregnancy. However, because the hormones of pregnancy that cause softening of the ligaments are released from early pregnancy, some women may start to experience symptoms as early as the start of the second trimester of pregnancy (from about 14 weeks). In others, symptoms worsen after delivery. This is, in itself, enough reason not to regard early induction of labour (that is, artificially starting labour before time) or doing a Caesarean section, as a 'cure' for SPD.

What can I expect after delivery?

The symptoms of SPD can disappear within a varying length of time following delivery. Some women notice an immediate improvement, for others it is more gradual over several days or weeks. Most women (more than 95%) are fully recovered within 3 months of delivery. Neither early induction of labour nor Caesarean section can speed up this process of recovery.

At home, you will need extra help with your newborn baby, perhaps from family or friends. Enrol help before your labour starts!

SPD does not hinder breastfeeding and the usual painkillers used for the symptoms of SPD, such as paracetamol, are safe for breastfeeding.

Can I get SPD again in future pregnancies?

There is no way of predicting whether SPD will recur in a subsequent pregnancy. After the completion of any pregnancy, irrespective of the type of delivery, the pelvic ligaments are left permanently more stretched than before your first pregnancy.

You could avoid pelvic girdle problems by working on exercises to strengthen your core muscles. From 6 weeks onwards, postnatal exercise classes, Pilates, core stability exercise, yoga, or tai chi are all appropriate. The physiotherapist can give further advice on this.

The symptoms of SPD may recur in a subsequent pregnancy in up to 65–85% of women. However, early recognition with appropriate referral to physiotherapy can alter the course of SPD symptoms in a subsequent pregnancy.

The general advice is for new mothers to try to avoid starting the next pregnancy until your baby is walking independently, as lifting a child will be especially difficult if you develop SPD symptoms again in a subsequent pregnancy.

Advice for pregnant women with SPD

- Try to avoid activities that cause discomfort, such as lifting, carrying, prolonged standing, or strenuous exercise such as pushing a heavily loaded supermarket trolley.
- Rest more frequently and regularly: sit reasonably upright with your back well supported.
- Mild to moderate exercise, including abdominal wall and pelvic floor exercises, is allowed.
- Avoid straddling or squatting movements, especially when getting in or out of the car or bath.
- Support pelvic girdles or Tubigrip ± pelvic muscle stabilizing exercises, which the physiotherapist can provide, as well as antenatal exercises are found to be very beneficial.
- Some women report improvement with the use of alternative therapies such as acupuncture.
- Avoid bending and twisting.
- Adopt a good posture.
- Roll in and out of bed, on your side and with both legs together.
- Aquanatal exercises are helpful, especially after 20 weeks of pregnancy.
- Swimming is beneficial but avoid the breast stroke.
- When dressing, sit down to put on clothing. Pull the clothing on. Do not try to put your legs into trousers, pants, or skirts while standing.

- Regular pain killers such as paracetamol and codeine can help, but avoid other painkillers such as ibuprofen or diclofenac during pregnancy.
- Codeine can sometimes make you constipated, which in itself can worsen your discomfort. Make sure you drink plenty of water and increase the fibre content of your diet.
- Ice packs can be applied for 5 minutes at a time to the lower back and sacroiliac joint—or try rubbing an ice cube on the symphysis pubis, over your pubic bone, for 20–30 seconds.
- When climbing stairs, do it one step at a time.
- Rarely, elbow crutches or a walking frame may be required to maintain stability.
- If you have been booked during pregnancy under the continued care of your community midwives, in the absence of any other complications, SPD is not something that puts you into a high-risk category needing medicalization of care in the hospital.
- There is no reason why a normal vaginal delivery cannot be achieved however severe your SPD symptoms have been, neither is there any evidence that vaginal delivery makes SPD any worse in future pregnancies.
- You will be encouraged to devise a birth plan taking SPD into account.
- You may find labour and delivery in a birthing pool particularly helpful, provided there is no other reason why you should not have a pool birth.
- You can also choose to deliver in a birthing unit as well, if there is no other reason why you should not.
- When admitted in labour, inform the midwife that you have SPD so she can assess how far you can comfortably widen your legs without experiencing pain. Your midwife will ensure that the legs are not excessively spread at the time of delivery.
- You can also choose to have an epidural for pain relief in labour.

Further information

- Association of Chartered Physiotherapists in Women's Health (ACPWH) <http://www.acpwh.org.uk>
- Mumsnet. Pelvic girdle pain (SPD) <http://www.mumsnet.com/pregnancy/spd>
- Well Mother. Pelvic girdle pain in pregnancy <http://www.wellmother.org/parents/pregnancy/pelvic-girdle-pain>

INFORMATION FOR PATIENTS Fibromyalgia, chronic fatigue syndrome, and pregnancy

Fibromyalgia syndrome (FMS) and chronic fatigue syndrome (CFS) are not related to pregnancy. Though you might notice that during pregnancy there could be a slight worsening of your long-standing symptoms, neither FMS or CFS causes any adverse outcomes to you or the baby during pregnancy, labour and delivery. The management of the pregnancy, labour, and delivery will therefore, not need to be any different from other pregnant women.

Your midwife will look after the antenatal care of your pregnancy in the community. The course of your pregnancy, labour, and delivery will not be affected by the FMS or CFS.

Interventions such as Caesarean sections or early induction of pregnancy just for the sake of FMS or CFS are not only unnecessary but have the potential for creating complications.

Certain painkillers such as ibuprofen or diclofenac tablets must not be used during pregnancy. Local application of these drugs in the form of a gel to the pain spots is relatively safe, within the limits of prescribed dosage. Application of warmth to the pain spots may also prove beneficial.

If you take any painkillers, check that these are safe to use during pregnancy. Simple painkillers such as paracetamol within recommended doses are as effective in FMS and safe to use.

Further information

- Fibromyalgia Association UK (information and support group), PO Box 206, Stourbridge, DY9 8YL; <http://www.ukfibromyalgia.com>

17. Maternal Skeletal Disorders

INFORMATION FOR PATIENTS Achondroplasia and pregnancy

Achondroplasia is the most common form of short-limbed dwarfism or disproportionate short stature, which means the legs and arms (particularly the upper arms and legs) are short compared to the trunk (body). Achondroplasia is a genetic condition that affects all ethnic groups and both sexes equally; it occurs in 1 in 15,000 to 1 in 35,000 births.

In more than 80% of cases, achondroplasia occurs as a chance mutation: that is, a change in the genetic code that has occurred out of the blue and without any reason. Achondroplasia is due to a change in a gene called fibroblast growth factor receptor 3, which is responsible for normal bone formation. This mutation results in the typical features seen in people with achondroplasia.

Most infants with achondroplasia are born to parents of normal stature. However, if either parent is affected there is a 50% chance in each pregnancy of having a child with achondroplasia.

If both partners have achondroplasia, there is a 25% chance that a baby will be of average stature, a 50% chance that the baby will have the same condition as the parents, and a 25% chance of having a double risk or homozygous achondroplasia, where unfortunately the baby is stillborn or dies shortly after birth. The difference between the non-lethal type and the lethal homozygous form can usually be diagnosed during pregnancy.

The risk of recurrence in a brother or sister of a child affected by achondroplasia born to unaffected parents is approximately 1 in 443. The recurrence risk in a sibling of a child affected by achondroplasia born to one affected parent is 50%.

Typically, the average male adult height in achondroplasia is 131 cm (4 feet 4 inches) and for adult females it is 124 cm (4 feet). Mental and sexual development are normal and unless there are childhood complications such as hydrocephalus (water on the brain), seen in about 1 in 10 infants, normal lifespan can be expected. Children with achondroplasia may reach motor milestones more slowly than children without the condition.

Apart from the short limbs, other signs are a prominent forehead, a protruding jaw, flattened area between the eyes, occasionally crowded teeth, bowed legs, short hands, and feet that are flat and broad.

Spinal problems are the most common complications of achondroplasia in adults.

Prenatal testing for pregnancies at increased risk (where one or both parents are affected) is possible by a procedure called chorionic villus sampling (CVS) between 9 and 12 weeks of pregnancy.

Prenatal diagnosis from a sample of amniotic fluid (amniocentesis) can also be offered in 'low-risk' pregnancies of normal statured parents where routine ultrasound scans have unexpectedly revealed short fetal limbs (usually not apparent till the third trimester or after 26 weeks of pregnancy).

If you have achondroplasia and are planning a pregnancy, you would ideally have been offered assessment and counselling, including baseline lung function tests as well as genetic counselling, before getting pregnant.

Your pregnancy will be cared for by a specialist team of the obstetrician, midwives, lung physician, physiotherapist and anaesthetist.

Women with achondroplasia may have an increased risk of problems such as pre-eclampsia, breathing problems, or premature birth, which is why you will be monitored at regular intervals.

As breathing problems could worsen somewhat, especially in the third trimester, repeat lung function tests and review by the lung specialist (respiratory physician) will be arranged at regular intervals during pregnancy.

Because of the contracted size and shape of the pelvis, delivery is invariably by a planned Caesarean section. You can expect a referral to anaesthetic high-risk clinic for review by a senior anaesthetist during pregnancy, when the type of anaesthetic to be used for the Caesarean section will be discussed with you.

Further information

- Achondroplasia UK (support group) <http://www.achondroplasia.co.uk>
- Genetic Alliance UK <http://www.geneticalliance.org.uk>
- Restricted Growth Association (RGA). Achondroplasia (http://www.restrictedgrowth.co.uk/Achondroplasia.html>

INFORMATION FOR PATIENTS Osteogenesis imperfecta and pregnancy

Osteogenesis imperfecta (OI), also known as *brittle bone disease*, is an inborn disease causing fractures in childhood and adults. OI is a genetic disorder usually resulting from abnormalities of the genes that control the production of a protein called collagen. This is the main protein that is the major building brick of bone essential for its strength. In OI, there is defective or abnormal structure of collagen.

The degree to which an individual is affected by OI can vary from mild to severe, sometimes being even lethal.

OI is a genetic condition that is present from the time of conception. Fractures might take place even while the baby is in the womb. Others have their first fractures soon after birth or in infancy.

While mild cases of OI can pass down from one generation to another, in severe cases of OI, it arises without any family history. In the majority of these cases, the cause is a new mutation—in other words the abnormality in the genes arises due to an error in the genetic code that has occurred out of the blue without any reason and has not been passed on from a parent.

If you or your partner has OI, there is a 50% chance in each pregnancy of the baby having OI.

Advice from a specialist in genetic problems (clinical geneticist) will help in identifying the inheritance pattern and clarify the risk of passing on the condition to a child.

When the gene mutation has been identified, other relatives may be offered tests for the disease itself or for the carrier state. Similarly, if you have OI, testing to determine whether the baby has inherited the condition can be performed by analysing cells drawn by procedures called chorionic villus sampling (CVS) or amniocentesis.

OI typically involves bones, teeth, ligaments, and eyes and is characterized by fragile bones that break easily. The joints may be lax, the whites of the eyes may be blue or grey, and there may be an increased liability to bruising.

Other features of OI may include excessive sweating, teeth that may be discoloured or fragile, deafness, hernias, and poor growth.

If you have OI

If you have OI, especially of a severe type, the normal changes that are expected during pregnancy could be very challenging. In severe forms of OI, pregnancy could worsen bone abnormalities with stress fractures due to weightbearing, as well as putting strain on the heart and lungs.

Certain pregnancy complications that are more common in women with OI are premature breaking of the waters, premature delivery, pre-eclampsia, anaemia, calcium deficiency, growth problems of the baby, and excess bleeding at the time of childbirth.

If you have OI, the care of your pregnancy will be offered by a team of several specialists including the obstetrician, cardiologist (heart specialist), lung physician, and anaesthetist as well as your own midwife. If you have severe OI, you would need referral to a tertiary/regional centre for the rest of the care during pregnancy and for delivery.

You will be offered several scans to monitor the baby's growth as well as serial measurements of the length of the baby's bones.

Delivery will most likely need to be by Caesarean section especially, if you have sustained previous fractures of the pelvis and bones of the lower spine. There could significant anaesthetic challenges, which is why the anaesthetist will assess you in detail during pregnancy and discuss the type of anaesthetic and pain relief with you.

Plans for delivery, anaesthesia, and care after childbirth will be discussed and agreed with you ahead of time.

If the baby is suspected to have OI with unaffected parents

Detailed genetic counselling will be offered and the specialist obstetrician can discuss your options with you. In the severe forms of OI (types II and III), ultrasound scans during pregnancy may show fractures of the bones. In type II the baby can die during childbirth or in early infancy and in type III the life expectancy is reduced due to complications.

In the milder forms of OI, the diagnosis may not be made during pregnancy by ultrasound scans as the fractures may develop for the first time only in infancy or childhood rather than when the baby is in the womb. In such cases, life expectancy can be normal.

In babies with OI, breech presentation (baby lying bottom-down) is more common. Depending on the individual situation and the type of suspected OI in the baby, the specialists will discuss the options for the best type of delivery with you.

Further information

- Brittle Bone Society <http://www.brittlebone.org>
- NetDoctor.co.uk. Brittle bone disease (osteogenesis imperfecta) <http://www.netdoctor.co.uk/diseases/facts/ brittlebones.htm>
- Patient.co.uk. Brittle bone disease/osteogenesis imperfecta <http://www.patient.co.uk>

Kyphoscoliosis (KS) describes an abnormal curvature of the spine both front-to-back and side-to-side. It is a combination of kyphosis and scoliosis. KS is a bony spinal deformity characterized by excessive posterior curvature (kyphosis) and lateral curvature (scoliosis).

Kyphosis, also called roundback or hunchback, is a condition of over-curvature of the thoracic vertebrae (upper back). The upper vertebrae of the spine naturally curve outwards from the middle of the back and toward the neck. When this curve exceeds 40 degrees, a person begins stooping and can eventually develop a hunched back, experience pain and trouble breathing, and have weakness or paralysis in their legs. This causes a bowing of the back, seen as a slouching posture.

Scoliosis is a condition in which a person's spine is curved from side to side. When seen on an X-ray, the spine of a person with scoliosis may look more like an 'S' or a 'C', rather than a straight line.

The combined effect of kyphosis and scoliosis (KS) is worse than either abnormality on its own. Most cases (70%) of KS occur without any known reason. Rare causes include tuberculosis, severe osteoporosis (thinning of the bones), neuromuscular disease such as polio, or syndromes such as Marfan's or Ehlers–Danlos.

KS can occur at any age but becomes most obvious at periods of rapid growth. Thoracic (upper back) KS can affect the lungs, leading to stress on the lungs and the heart. In severe untreated cases of KS, there is increased risk of respiratory problems which can in some cases be life-threatening.

Both women and men are affected, but it is more common in women. KS has been reported in 1 in 1500 to 1 in 12,000 pregnant women.

Effects of KS on pregnancy

The effects of KS on pregnancy most commonly include an increased risk of premature labour.

Effect of pregnancy on KS

Women with a stable curvature do not usually worsen in pregnancy whereas those with unstable curvatures show a worsening.

Respiratory complications such as increasing breathlessness are seen in about 17% of women during pregnancy. In severe KS, with very compromised capacity and function of the lungs, the advice may be to avoid a pregnancy because it could lead to a life-threatening crisis.

The bony pelvis is normal in women with idiopathic scoliosis alone and the likelihood of vaginal delivery is often good.

Pre-pregnancy assessment by the respiratory physician and subsequent counselling by the specialist obstetrician are therefore extremely important.

Management of pregnancy

Your pregnancy care will be provided by a team of specialists including the obstetrician, respiratory physician, cardiologist if required, and anaesthetist as well as the midwives. These experts will have input in your ongoing assessments and management advice.

Ideally, you will be assessed routinely in the respiratory medicine unit at least once in 2 months during pregnancy for lung function tests as well as having an ECG (electrocardiogram) to check for any effects on the heart. If such an effect on the heart is suspected in severe cases, you will need to be urgently assessed by the heart specialist.

Similarly, you can expect to be referred to a senior anaesthetic specialist in the anaesthetic high-risk clinic for assessment and consultation during pregnancy, well ahead of your due date. This is because in more severe cases of KS, there may be significant anaesthetic challenges during labour and for delivery, either vaginal or Caesarean section. The specialist anaesthetist will have the opportunity for a thorough assessment and for management plans to be discussed and drawn up long before the estimated date of delivery. If you have had prior surgical correction of KS with insertion of a metal rod such as the Harrington rod, or a spinal fusion operation, this will be taken into account in the anaesthetic management plan.

The baby's growth and well-being will be regularly monitored with serial scans.

If your breathing problems and lung compromise worsen in the last part of pregnancy (26–40 weeks), or there is evidence of restricted growth of the baby, early delivery may be required, probably by Caesarean section.

Further information

- eHow.com. What is kyphoscoliosis? <http://www.ehow.com/about_5127857_kyphoscoliosis.html>
- Patient.co.uk. Kyphoscoliosis <http://www.patient.co.uk>

18. Maternal Obesity

INFORMATION FOR PATIENTS Obesity and pregnancy

Although most pregnancies are uncomplicated in women who are overweight or obese, there are certain increased problems.

Many women feel uncomfortable with their weight and it can be especially hard if you require special care because of your weight during pregnancy. This information leaflet is not designed to make you feel uncomfortable or upset. It is to make you aware of some facts associated with being pregnant that you may have been unaware of. It is also designed to help you understand why extra care is taken, and the basis for any advice given.

Being overweight or obese may cause complications for both you and the baby. Such problems may occur while you are pregnant, during labour, and after your baby is born.

The most important thing is that you and your baby are cared for properly. Our aim is to look after any pregnancy which may be more complicated than usual, with extra care to achieve the safest outcomes.

Allied services can also support you with special advice about weight management, diet, and exercise programmes.

How is overweight or obesity measured in pregnancy?

The body mass index or BMI is the internationally accepted practical way of assessing overweight or obesity and it provides a good guide to the risk of health problems. BMI is the best way of making sure that all women who are possibly at more risk are getting the right care treatment.

The BMI is calculated by dividing your pre-pregnancy or early pregnancy weight in kilograms by your height in metres, squared (m^2) (see table). This will be calculated by your community midwife at the time of your first booking appointment.

A healthy BMI is between 20 and 25 (before or during early pregnancy). A result above 25 and below 30 is defined as overweight. A result above 30 is classified as obese, which has three different degrees.

The risks associated with pregnancy and birth to both you and your baby increase proportionately with the degree of obesity.

Definition of obesity

Classification	*Early pregnancy BMI (kg/m²)*	*Risk of obstetric/anaesthetic complications*
Normal range	18.5–24.9	No increased obstetric or maternal risk
Overweight	25–29.9	No increased obstetric or maternal risk
Obese I	30–34.9	Mildly increased risks
Obese II	35–39.9	Moderately increased risks
Obese III	40+	Significant/serious risks to mother and baby

The category Obese III is also known as morbid obesity.

Reproduced with kind permission from the World Health Organization. <http://apps.who.int/bmi/index.jsp?introPage=intro_3.html>.

What are these risks?

With obesity there are increased risks of the following problems, although most pregnancies are uncomplicated.

Risks when you are pregnant

- **Gestational diabetes:** a form of diabetes that develops during pregnancy. You will be offered a special test called a glucose tolerance test (GTT) at approximately 28 weeks pregnancy because of this risk as gestational diabetes is more common in obese women.
- **Pre-eclampsia:** a condition that only occurs during pregnancy, characterized by high blood pressure, presence of protein in your urine, and an abnormal degree of swelling.
- **High blood pressure:** you might have high blood pressure before pregnancy or it might worsen during the pregnancy.
- **Problems with the baby's growth, development, or health:** You will receive extra scans later in your pregnancy to get an idea about baby's growth. However, the heavier you are, the less accurate the scan measurements can be.
- Greater chance of your scans not being able to provide clear views: therefore you might be asked to return for further scans.
- You might not be able to appreciate the baby's movements well: contact your healthcare team if you have any worries!
- It may be more difficult to monitor the baby's heart rate pattern using the external monitor.

Risks during birth

- Increased risks of induction of labour.
- Labour may be slow to progress or induction of labour may not work.
- If you have had a previous Caesarean section, the chances of a successful vaginal birth this time are reduced.
- Increased risk of needing an emergency Caesarean section.
- Increased risks of problems related to the Caesarean section operation itself, both surgical and anaesthetic. This is why you will have been referred to see an anaesthetist during your pregnancy as a safeguard so that proper assessment can take place.
- If the baby is too big, the shoulders can unexpectedly get stuck during birth. This is a serious condition called shoulder dystocia. All the staff looking after you are trained in the management of this emergency. If you have a good epidural working, it makes management of such an unexpected situation easier and safer.
- Difficulties monitoring the baby's heart and problems with positioning or movement in cases of an emergency may occur.

Risks after birth

- Increased risk of wound infection.
- Increased risk of blood clots in the veins of the legs (deep vein thrombosis) which if they find their way to the lungs (pulmonary embolus) can be very dangerous and life-threatening.
- This is why you will receive an injection of a blood-thinning drug once a day till you are discharged from the hospital. You will be advised to wear anti-thrombosis stockings as well, especially after a Caesarean section, and advised to continue wearing them for several weeks after delivery.
- Problems with wound healing may occasionally cause Caesarean or episiotomy wounds to break down. The risk is greater if you are diabetic as well.
- Breastfeeding is the ideal way to feed your newborn baby. It will also help you lose some weight after the pregnancy. Breastfeeding also helps reduce the likelihood of childhood obesity and protects the baby from a range of infections and allergies

Despite all these risks, most of our overweight/obese mothers and babies have happy outcomes with few complications. Staff are dedicated to making sure that you and your baby receive close monitoring and the very best care. Both midwifery and the medical staff will discuss all aspects of your pregnancy with you when planning your care.

Frequently asked questions

How much weight gain is 'normal' during pregnancy?

The typically quoted figure is 12–14 kg (25–30 pounds) for a woman of normal BMI (18.5–24.9) which is the average weight gain associated with the safest outcome of pregnancy. The recommendations for the ideal total weight gain during pregnancy depends on what your BMI was at the start of pregnancy (see table 18.2 or view it at: http://iom.edu/~/media/Files/Report%20Files/2009/Weight-Gain-During-Pregnancy-Reexamining-the-Guidelines/Report%20Brief%20-%20Weight%20Gain%20During%20Pregnancy.pdf). Of this, 2–6 kg is an increase in the mother's body fat.

So, a modest weight gain is essential during pregnancy. You should therefore not go on a 'crash diet' programme or seriously reduce your food intake while you are pregnant. If you do so you will not only fail to meet the extra energy requirements of the growing baby but also deprive you and the baby of essential minerals and vitamins like iron, zinc, calcium, and folate.

The advice is to eat a healthy diet during pregnancy and then lose weight after childbirth and before your next pregnancy.

I am pregnant with my third baby. Why is my weight in early pregnancy much more than in my previous pregnancies, though my diet or lifestyle has not changed a lot?

Good question! Remember, the more the weight gained during each pregnancy (over and above the baby's weight and that of the womb contents), the greater will be the weight retained after pregnancy. This is why successive pregnancies make it harder to lose weight in between and the BMI progressively increases.

As a rough guide, if weight gain during a pregnancy is in an average range of 12–14 kg, then about 2–6 kg of this is the increase in your body fat. You will keep this after the baby's birth, but breastfeeding will help reduce the excess fat stores.

Exercise and a healthy programme of diet changes after pregnancy will go a long way towards ensuring that only the minimum weight gained during a previous pregnancy is retained before you start the next pregnancy.

Further information

- Royal College of Obstetricians and Gynaecologists. Information for you. Why your weight matters during pregnancy and after birth <http://www.rcog.org.uk>

INFORMATION FOR PATIENTS Pregnancy after gastric band or gastric bypass procedure

Gastric banding or gastric bypass procedures are types of bariatric surgery (BS) that you may have to enable you to lose weight. You will have already received information about these procedures, and you will have been told how to contact the unit where the BS was performed for further follow-up or to report any problems after the surgery.

Pregnancy after BS

- It is best to try to avoid getting pregnant within 12–24 months after having BS, as this is the time of the most rapid weight loss.
- You would have probably been informed that oral contraceptive pill is less effective after BS and to consider using an alternative method of contraception such as a progesterone (hormone) implant in the arm or a hormone-containing coil instead.
- Following BS you could develop deficiencies of certain essential nutrients and vitamins due to the decrease in stomach capacity restricting food intake as well as poor absorption from the gut.
- You are advised to take multivitamins including iron, folic acid, vitamin D, calcium, and B_{12} starting even before you become pregnant and continuing throughout the pregnancy.
- You will be referred to see a dietician to discuss a healthy and varied diet that gives you and the developing baby essential nutrients and vitamins.
- If you are found to have vitamin B_{12} deficiency after BS, you will be given regular supplements as injections at your GP's surgery.
- When you get pregnant following BS there are some additional factors that may require input from different specialists such as the bariatric surgeon, the obstetric specialist, community midwife, endocrinologist, etc.
- When you are booked for this pregnancy by your midwife, she will require details of what kind of BS procedure you have had. Try to get as much information as possible about this (hospital letters, etc.) from the centre where you had your BS.
- You will need to take particular care during the first 13–16 weeks of pregnancy as the symptoms of morning sickness such as nausea, vomiting, or abdominal pain may be just the same as complications related to the previous BS, such as internal hernia or obstruction of the bowels. You should report any such symptoms to your midwife/GP or the specialist hospital staff in the antenatal clinic at any stage of pregnancy.
- At certain stages of pregnancy due to the increasing size of the womb, there can be further 'squeezing' of the stomach and gut. This could result in persistent, severe vomiting leading to significant dehydration with nutrient loss. If you have had an adjustable gastric band inserted with a small port placed under the skin, the band can be loosened temporarily by withdrawing some of the fluid that has been used to inflate it—this is a minor outpatient procedure.
- If you are on any prescribed medication for whatever reason, please let your midwife and the hospital specialist team know.
- Many women who have had BS will remain overweight or obese during pregnancy. It is therefore important that a test is performed at about 26–28 weeks of pregnancy to detect the condition of diabetes in pregnancy (gestational diabetes).
- If you have had gestational diabetes in a previous pregnancy followed later by BS, you will still be advised to have this glucose challenge test.
- Apart from the scan in the first 13 weeks of pregnancy and the detailed scan at about 20 weeks to look for any abnormalities in the baby, additional scans will be arranged after about 28 weeks. These scans are to monitor the growth of the baby.
- At some stage of pregnancy, you may be referred to see the anaesthetist to discuss choices for pain relief in labour.
- Previous BS should not in itself, alter the course of your labour or delivery. A Caesarean section or induction of labour (to start labour early) are not required just because you having had previous BS. They are only indicated if there is any other reason connected with your pregnancy.
- You will be supported and encouraged to breastfeed.
- Previous BS does not mean that your stay in the hospital after giving birth has to be any longer than what is routine after the type of delivery you have had.
- If you have had gastric banding deflated during pregnancy, you can have it re-inflated a few days after delivery. Your BS unit can provide you with details of how you need to go about having this done.

Further information

- NHS Choices. Weight loss surgery <http://www.nhs.uk/conditions/weight-loss-surgery/Pages/Introduction.aspx> (provides information about the procedure in general terms).

19. Maternal Malignancy

INFORMATION FOR PATIENTS Cancer and pregnancy

- It is relatively rare for pregnancy and cancer to coexist.
- With modern treatment and improved care good outcomes can generally be expected for such a pregnancy.
- When cancer occurs during pregnancy, it is a time of great anxiety and concern for you and your family. The healthcare providers will have to consider that two patients are involved in each case: you and the unborn baby. This is why every patient's care plans will be made on an individual basis.
- In particular, the doctors (the cancer specialists and the obstetrician) will discuss the following issues with you:
  - The impact of continuation of the pregnancy on the cancer
  - The effects of the cancer and its treatment on you and on the unborn baby
  - Whether the pregnancy could have an effect on your long term cancer outcome and health
  - Whether treatment for cancer could affect your long-term fertility.
- The type of treatment will depend on the type and stage (extent) of the cancer, how far you are advanced in pregnancy, and the various treatment options available. You and your family will be able to discuss these issues in detail with the doctors and review all options.
- The decision to have any further tests or to start cancer treatment rests entirely with you. You will get all the information, the various choices and their individual risks and benefits before any decision is required of you.
- The doctors will explain:
  - What the tests or treatment will involve, why it is recommended, the risks and side effects
  - Available alternatives and any modifications of standard procedures, if relevant
  - The advantages and disadvantages of one treatment over another.

Investigations (tests)

- Any X-rays, ultrasound scans, MRI scans, biopsies, or blood tests will be discussed. Only low-radiation X-rays are used in pregnancy, with a lead shield to cover your tummy area to give additional protection for the baby. Ultrasound and MRI scans do not use radiation, making them safe in pregnancy.
- Tests or treatment using radioactive liquid iodine will not be used in pregnancy as it can have an adverse effect on the baby.

Treatment

- Treatment for cancer may be delayed in some situations till the baby has reached viability(a stage at which survival is possible). If cancer has been diagnosed relatively late in pregnancy, there may be an option not to start treatment until after the baby has been born, or even to induce your labour early.
- If delivery is planned for less than 36 weeks pregnancy, you will be offered a course of steroid involving two injections 24 hours apart, given into your muscle, which will help the baby's lungs to develop ahead of time.
- The commonly used treatments for cancer in pregnancy involve surgery and/or chemotherapy. Radiotherapy is not generally used in pregnancy and is delayed until after the birth of the baby.
- After careful evaluation, a treatment plan will be designed based on your individual circumstances.
- Before treatment is started, you will be informed of what symptoms and side effects you could expect to feel. The obstetrician who will look after your pregnancy will be a specialist in complex pregnancies. He/she will discuss whether any additional investigations are required for the baby, whether the cancer treatment could have any effect on the type and timing of your delivery, whether you could breastfeed, and any other questions you may have.
- You will be informed about symptoms you need to be aware of, and how to access help and get advice whether it is related to your treatment or to the pregnancy. You will be given details of the schedule of further appointments from both the cancer and pregnancy specialists.
- **Surgery** after the first trimester (the first 13 weeks of pregnancy) if appropriate to your type and stage of cancer is the safest option because there is little impact on the baby.
- **Chemotherapy** uses drugs which destroy cancer cells but which can also cause a fall of your red and white blood corpuscles and platelets. This can produce anaemia and make you more prone to infection.
- This is why your blood counts will be monitored closely and the next course of chemotherapy timed appropriately. You will be advised to take iron and folic acid supplements and to maintain a healthy and nutritious diet.
- Chemotherapy is usually avoided in the first trimester due to effects on the developing baby which might produce abnormalities or cause miscarriage. In certain situations, for example in acute leukaemia, it may be unavoidable.
- Chemotherapy drugs can be used in the second and third trimesters (from the 13th week to the end of pregnancy) without causing abnormalities in the baby, as the baby's organs are already fully formed by then.

Pregnancy management during cancer treatment

- Your blood tests will reveal any anaemia (low red cell count), low platelets (which can cause problems with blood clotting), or low white cells (making you more prone to infection). You will receive appropriate advice.
- The pregnancy will be monitored for any problems like premature labour and growth problems of the baby as well as infections.
- Different people have different reactions to chemotherapy. You may experience tiredness between treatments. You may have nausea, vomiting, bowel changes or mouth ulcers, and hair loss.
- Chemotherapy affects all rapidly dividing cells of the body. Cells that are affected are usually those of the digestive tract, bone marrow, skin, and hair. Most side effects are temporary.
- You will be asked to report any fever, bleeding gums, vaginal bleeding, early contractions, or if your waters break.

Frequently asked questions

Does ending the pregnancy increase chances of surviving cancer?

In many cancers, continuing the pregnancy will have little effect on cancer survival. Only in a few types and stages of cancer could continuation of the pregnancy limit the kind of treatment that can be offered and thus compromise survival.

Can chemotherapy harm the baby?

Most of these drugs can be used safely after the baby's organs are fully developed, that is after 12 weeks of pregnancy. Chemotherapy after this stage does not cause malformations. Later in pregnancy there might be a slowing of baby's growth but this can be picked up on scans. Sometimes the chemotherapy drugs cause a temporary drop in the baby's blood cell count which will soon recover. The paediatricians (baby doctors) will monitor this closely after baby's birth.

Can the cancer spread to the baby?

The vast majority of cancers do not. In rare cases of a particular cancer called malignant melanoma, the cancer could unfortunately affect the baby as well.

What about breastfeeding?

Unless you have had only surgery as treatment for cancer, you are generally advised not to breastfeed because chemotherapy drugs can be transferred to the baby in breast milk. If you receive radioactive iodine for thyroid cancer, this can harm the baby. In fact if you receive radio-iodine therapy after the birth, you will be advised to have no contact with the baby for several days as you will be radioactive!

There are so many specialists involved, I'm confused!

There are indeed many people involved in the care of the pregnancy and the cancer but please be assured that there will be close communication between all specialists and all plans will be jointly made after discussion with you. The normal aspects of the pregnancy will continue to be looked after by your own midwife as well.

INFORMATION FOR PATIENTS Breast cancer and pregnancy

- The specialist breast team will discuss all aspects of the breast cancer and explain how it can be managed during your pregnancy. There are obviously some differences in the choices of treatments available to a pregnant woman.
- The choices available and the discussions to be had, as well as any decisions made, will centre around you. The various specialists involved in your care will be happy to answer your questions.
- In addition, more information about the pregnancy, labour, delivery, and what is expected following your baby's birth will be provided by the specialist obstetrician and midwives who you will meet in the antenatal clinic.
- Information about breast cancer in general, e.g. from the internet, may not relate specifically to pregnancy with breast cancer. The treatments and options available might well be different for a pregnant woman with breast cancer.

Further information

- NICE. Breast cancer quality standard (QS12), 2011. <https://www.nice.org.uk/guidance/qs12/informationforpublic>
- Patient.co.uk. Breast cancer <http://www.patient.co.uk>

20. Pregnancy in the Mother Post Organ Transplant

INFORMATION FOR PATIENTS Pregnancy after kidney transplant

You will already have received information from both your kidney transplant team and the obstetric specialist team.

Further information

- Edinburgh Royal Infirmary Renal Unit (EdRen). Pregnancy and contraception in renal disease <http://www.edren.org /pages/edreninfo/pregnancy-and-contraception-in-renal-disease.php>
- National Kidney Federation. Are there sexual problems after a transplant? <http://www.kidney.org.uk>
- North Bristol NHS Trust. After your kidney transplant: advice for women <http://www.nbt.nhs.uk/sites/default/files/attachments/After%20Your%20Kidney%20Transplant_NBT002098.pdf>

INFORMATION FOR PATIENTS Pregnancy after a transplant operation

You will receive a lot of information from the transplant team and specialist obstetrician about preparing for a pregnancy, management options during a pregnancy, outcomes, drugs used in pregnancy and those to be avoided.

The doctors will be happy to answer questions about your pregnancy.

Further information

- International Transplant Nurses Society (USA) Pregnancy and parenthood after transplant <http://www.itns.org/uploads/ITNS_Pregnancy_English.pdf>
- Queen Elizabeth Hospital Birmingham. Information for patients who have had a kidney transplant <http://www.uhb.nhs.uk/Downloads/pdf/PiAfterKidneyTransplant.pdf>

21. Maternal Enzymatic Abnormalities

INFORMATION FOR PATIENTS C_1 inhibitor deficiency and pregnancy

C_1 inhibitor (C_1 INH) deficiency is a condition in which there are repeated episodes where some of your body's soft tissues can swell up. This soft tissue swelling is called **angio-oedema**.

- In most cases, the condition is genetically inherited with 50% of children inheriting the condition from an affected parent.
- In a smaller number of people the disorder happens by chance in the affected person without inheriting it from a parent.
- C_1 INH deficiency is diagnosed by blood tests which are also used to monitor treatment.

Features of C_1 INH deficiency

- Soft tissue swellings are not present all the time but can come and go.
- The swellings most commonly affect the face or the limbs, although any part of the body could be involved, including the mouth, tongue, throat, and bowel.
- Sometimes there may be flat red marks on the skin before the swellings begin.
- The swellings are often relatively painless, although this will depend on where on the body they occur.
- The swelling can progress for 24–48 hours before gradually subsiding, but this can sometimes take several days.
- The swellings are not usually accompanied by local heat, itching, or wheals on the skin (urticaria).

Urgent problems

- ***Always wear a MedicAlert, in case of emergencies.***

There are some serious presentations of C_1 INH deficiency, **all of which need urgent treatment:**

- Swelling of the throat can cause difficulty in breathing, a change in the quality, hoarseness or even loss of the voice.
- Swelling of the mouth or the tongue can lead to breathing obstruction in severe cases.
- If there is swelling of the bowel walls, this can result in very severe abdominal pain and vomiting.

Triggers for the swelling

- Common triggers are any local injury (often mild, such as a bump or a knock) or surgery of any kind, especially if the operation involves the mouth, tongue, or throat, such as dental procedures or removal of tonsils.
- It is vital that your dentist or the anaesthetist and surgeon are aware of your condition. You can then be given certain essential medicines and/or interventions to prevent problems arising.
- Other triggers include prolonged pressure on any area of the body surface, infection, emotional stress, excess exposure to sunlight, and exposure to vibrations.
- *The oral contraceptive pill with oestrogen (the combined pill) is not suitable for you*, as they can aggravate your symptoms.
- A few medications that are generally used for treatment of high blood pressure may trigger attacks and need to be avoided.

Pregnancy and C_1 INH deficiency

- During pregnancy, symptoms may improve for some women, but for others they may get worse.
- Certain drugs that are used for long-term prevention of swellings, such as danazol or tranexamic acid, cannot be used in pregnancy because of their effects on the developing baby.
- Early in your pregnancy your community midwife or GP will refer you to a specialist antenatal clinic at the hospital, where you can expect to be seen by the obstetric specialist.
- Your care will be multidisciplinary, that is, it will involve input from various healthcare professionals in order to ensure the safest care for you and the baby.
- During pregnancy you will be referred to see a senior anaesthetist. They will discuss with you issues such as the choices you have for pain relief in labour, the type of anaesthetic if a Caesarean section becomes necessary, safety of anaesthetic drugs, and intravenous injection of C_1 INH concentrate during labour and delivery.

- It is likely that you have already met the genetics team to discuss inheritance risk to your offspring. If not, you will be offered the opportunity to do so during this pregnancy.
- C_1 INH concentrate, which is derived from a blood product, is the treatment of choice in cases of emergency situations such as swelling in the mouth or throat, as well as for severe abdominal pain.
- *You may already have been issued with a supply of C_1 INH concentrate and both you and your partner may have been trained in administering it. If not, please let the obstetrician and anaesthetist know during your hospital appointments so that arrangements can be promptly made.*
- If you develop any swelling of the mouth, throat, or tongue or severe excruciating abdominal pain during pregnancy, you need to go immediately to the hospital Emergency Department by ambulance if necessary, just as you would if you were not pregnant.
- If you have to go into hospital, remember to take your hand-held pregnancy notes as well as this information sheet, which you should keep attached to your hand-held pregnancy notes. If you have been given a dose of C_1 INH concentrate to keep at home, take this with you too.
- Very occasionally, if C_1 INH concentrate is not immediately available, you may be offered a dose of fresh frozen human plasma (FFP). This will provide some C_1 INH.
- Remember: specific treatment must be started early to prevent progression.
- The swellings in C_1 INH deficiency do not respond to the antihistamines commonly used for hayfever or allergies.

Labour and delivery

- There is no evidence that normal vaginal delivery is associated with increased complications in women with C_1 INH deficiency
- The fact that you have this condition is not in itself a reason for either early induction of labour or a Caesarean section, if there are no obstetric indications.
- If you have a severe attack during pregnancy, labour, delivery, or after the baby's birth it will be treated in exactly the same way as usual, with C_1 INH concentrate given as an injection into a vein.
- To prevent attacks during labour and delivery, you will receive C_1 INH concentrate in the form of a slow drip at the start of active labour or for a planned Caesarean section. This is effective for 24 hours, so a second dose is rarely required unless you have not delivered by then.
- If an emergency Caesarean section becomes necessary during the course of labour, a spinal anaesthetic is preferable to a general anaesthetic.
- Attacks could recur after you have had the baby, so you will be advised to remain as vigilant for symptoms as always.
- The baby will be examined by the baby doctors after delivery. If the baby has inherited the C_1 INH deficiency, the C_1 INH concentrate, with dose adjusted for the baby, will be kept available.

Further information

- Patient.co.uk. C_1 inhibitor deficiency <http://www.patient.co.uk>

INFORMATION FOR PATIENTS Mastocytosis and pregnancy

Mastocytosis is a rare condition caused by excessive accumulation of mast cells. These cells have an important role in the immune system and they are found in many areas of the body, such as the skin, liver, spleen, bone marrow, and the lining of the lungs and stomach. When triggered by exposure to allergens, mast cells release histamine and other chemicals as an immune response. These chemicals cause symptoms such as a skin rash, itchy skin, and hot flushes. In severe cases a fall in blood pressure and even shock can result.

Although the exact cause of mastocytosis is unclear at present, the mechanism involved in most patients is a genetic change in a protein called KIT which is situated on the mast cell, resulting in too many mast cells accumulating in various parts of the body. Most cases of mastocytosis occur as a result of a genetic mutation called the c-KIT mutation. A genetic mutation happens when normal instructions carried in certain genes become scrambled, causing some of the body's processes to work abnormally.

There are two main types of mastocytosis: the cutaneous variety and the systemic variety.

Cutaneous mastocytosis

The **cutaneous** variety of mastocytosis, which is due to overaccumulation of mast cells in the skin, usually only affects children. Three-quarters of cases develop in children aged 1 to 4 years. It is therefore also known as paediatric mastocytosis. The most common symptom is blisters and spots which can form a rash on the body. This variety of mastocytosis usually settles without any specific treatment by the time puberty is reached.

Systemic mastocytosis

The **systemic** type of mastocytosis, also known as *mast cell disease*, mainly affects adults and is estimated to occur in about 1 in 150,000 people in England. There are three subtypes of systemic mastocytosis:

- In the **indolent** subtype (90% of all cases of systemic mastocytosis), symptoms are usually mild to moderate. Typical signs are reddish-brown skin rashes called macules or papules. Itching, flushing of the skin, tummy upsets with pain, vomiting and diarrhoea, pain in muscles and joints, tiredness, mood changes, and headaches are also experienced. People with this condition experience attacks, lasting 15–30 minutes, when their symptoms are severe. Triggers for such attacks may include physical exertion, stress or emotional upset, and certain medications such as aspirin or antibiotics. The indolent variety of systemic mastocytosis has no effect on life expectancy.
- In the **aggressive variety** of systemic mastocytosis mast cells invade organs such as the spleen, liver, and digestive system, so symptoms are wide-ranging and severe although skin lesions are less common. If mastocytosis has been diagnosed affecting you or your child, you may need to carry an adrenaline injection kit, which can be used to prevent the symptoms of anaphylaxis from getting worse.
- A third subvariety is where **systematic mastocytosis coexists with associated haematological (blood) disease**. Enlargement of the liver, spleen, and lymph nodes may develop. If the bone marrow is involved, anaemia and chronic leukaemia can occur. Due to large amounts of histamine being released into the bloodstream, there is an increased risk of a severe and life-threatening allergic reaction known as **anaphylaxis**.

In the systemic type of mastocytosis, triggers for attacks in different patients include:

- Physical stimuli, such as heat, cold, friction, sunlight, perfumes
- Stress
- Certain foods, such as shellfish, cheese, preservatives, flavourings
- Alcohol
- Insect bites
- Certain infections which may be bacterial, viral, or fungal
- Drugs/medications such as aspirin, ibuprofen, certain anaesthetic agents, morphine or pethidine, and even some antibiotics.

Diagnosis

- In people with cutaneous mastocytosis, skin lesions become red, swollen, and itchy when stroked or rubbed, due to excessive release of histamine.

- Diagnostic tests include skin biopsy and testing of blood or urine to find elevated levels of certain chemicals.
- In systemic mastocytosis, depending on your symptoms, other tests such as kidney and liver function tests, blood clotting tests, ultrasound of abdominal organs, or a chest X-ray may be required.
- Investigations such as skeletal X-rays, bone marrow biopsy, endoscopy, or bone density scan are always avoided during pregnancy.

Treatment

- There is no cure for mastocytosis. Treatment is based on trying to avoid exposure to known allergens and by relieving symptoms.
- You are encouraged to wear a **MedicAlert bracelet** and carry an emergency treatment protocol card from your specialist.
- If you have frequent anaphylactic episodes, you are advised to carry injectable adrenaline (epinephrine) in the form of a pen for emergencies. Early symptoms of anaphylaxis could include sudden breathing difficulties, lip/throat swelling, hives, or wheezing/heaviness in your chest.
- For most cases, treatment with medications called H_1 and H_2 antagonists, such as chlorphenamine and cimetidine, is most effective.
- Any drug known to trigger an anaphylactic reaction must be scrupulously avoided. Certain types of blood pressure medication are also to be avoided. Your GP and allergy specialist will inform you about these.

During pregnancy

- Your care during pregnancy will follow the above general advice.
- Steroid medications such as oral prednisolone may be required to control mastocytosis-related symptoms. If you have had oral steroids for longer than 2 weeks at any time during pregnancy, you will be advised steroid top-up injections at intervals during labour and to cover delivery.
- You will be referred to a specialist anaesthetist to discuss pain relief during labour and delivery as well as to assess those anaesthetic drugs that should be avoided in your case. Local anaesthetics and drugs used for a spinal or epidural for pain relief are safe.
- If you have been taking antihistamines, these will generally be continued during labour and delivery. In case of an anaphylactic attack, immediate treatment with an injection of epinephrine into the vein will be given.
- During pregnancy, flu or MMR vaccines can be given unless you have had an allergic reaction previously. Usually most reactions are mild with low-grade fever which responds to paracetamol. You will be advised to take an antihistamine on the day of the vaccination and to continue this for a few days after the vaccination in order to dampen symptoms such as itching or flushing.

Further information

- NHS Choices. Mastocytosis <http://www.nhs.uk>
- UK Mastocytosis Support <http://www.ukmasto.co.uk>

INFORMATION FOR PATIENTS Phenylketonuria and pregnancy

- *Phenylketonuria (PKU) is a* rare inherited condition caused by a deficiency in the enzyme phenylalanine hydroxylase (fee-nile-ala-neen hide-roxy-lase). A deficiency of this enzyme causes a build-up of phenylalanine in the body.
- Phenylalanine is a natural substance; it is a building block of protein. This essential amino acid is necessary for normal growth and development, but when too much of it accumulates it is harmful.
- In the UK all newborn babies are tested for PKU by measuring phenylalanine levels in the heel-prick blood test. All babies should have this test as it allows treatment to start early in life.
- PKU is a treatable condition. Phenylalanine is found in the protein part of the food we eat, so the treatment is to maintain a low-protein diet. This means that high-protein foods such as meat, cheese, poultry, eggs, and milk need to be avoided. Instead the diet is supplemented with artificial protein which contains no phenylalanine.
- If untreated, PKU can result in mental retardation. Strict dietary restrictions must be maintained throughout the lifetime of an affected person to ensure a good outcome.

Further information

- National Society for Phenylketonuria (support group: Tel 0845 603 9136) Pregnancy in women with phenylketonuria <http://www.nspku.org/publications/publication/maternal-pku>

INFORMATION FOR PATIENTS Alpha-1 antitrypsin (AAT) deficiency and pregnancy

- If you have had the alpha-1 antitrypsin (AAT) deficiency diagnosed in the last few years, you will have already been seen by the lung or liver specialists. Before becoming pregnant you might have also been referred to the obstetric specialist to discuss issues about pregnancy.
- You will have received advice to have a yearly flu jab including swine flu vaccine each autumn to protect against possible flu and any chest infection that may develop as a result of this.
- Immunization against pneumococcus (a germ that can cause serious chest infections) is also important. This is a one-off injection and not yearly unlike the flu jab.
- Because AAT deficiency is a condition that get worse rapidly in smokers, it is absolutely essential that you stop smoking. Your medical team will offer you help and support to do this. It is even more important during pregnancy, to reduce serious risks to you and your baby.
- Normal pregnancy puts extra demands on your lungs. Breathlessness is not uncommon in the later stages even of normal pregnancies.
- If you have AAT deficiency, your lungs have reduced capacity and function. As your pregnancy advances you will notice that your lungs are working extra hard. Most women with mild to moderate AAT deficiency have fairly smooth pregnancies, but in severe cases there could be serious problems.
- Your care during pregnancy will therefore be managed by specialists in different fields, nurses, and midwives, all working with you and your partner/family.
- If emphysema is a feature of your condition, the management will be similar to when you are not pregnant. This will involve using an inhaler. The medication within the inhaler is in a powdered form which you breathe in. These may include:
  - A bronchodilator to relax the muscles in the airways to open them up as widely as possible

- A steroid inhaler, which may not have much effect on the usual symptoms of emphysema, but may help to prevent flare-ups. Sometimes a short course of steroids in the form of tablets may be required. This is safe in pregnancy for both you and the baby.
- You might also be prescribed antibiotics if you develop a chest infection, when your symptoms could otherwise flare up.

- It is important that you and your baby's well-being are monitored closely throughout pregnancy:
    - The lung and liver specialists will assess how well these organs are working at each stage of pregnancy.
    - The obstetric specialist and midwives will see you more frequently in the hospital antenatal clinic to check on your and your baby's well-being.
    - Regular scans will be performed at monthly intervals after about 26 weeks of pregnancy to ensure that the baby is growing well. If there are any concerns, more frequent and detailed scans will be performed.
    - You will also be invited to meet the anaesthetist to discuss pain relief for labour and for delivery, whether it is a vaginal delivery or a Caesarean section.
- The timing and type of delivery depends on how your lungs are coping with the advancing pregnancy as well as whether the baby is growing well or not.
- Certain drugs that are commonly used in labour cannot be used in your case, and your medical team will ensure that these medications are avoided.
- Pethidine and morphine are avoided for pain relief, but an epidural is a safe option for pain relief in labour.
- An epidural also prevents any involuntary urges to push.
- Pushing in the second stage of labour can cause a potentially serious problem called pneumothorax (collapsed lung) in someone with AAT deficiency. A collapsed lung is a condition in which the space between the wall of the chest cavity and the lung itself fills with air, causing all or part of the lung to collapse. **If plans are for a vaginal delivery, to avoid such problems, we can help delivery by using either the suction cup or forceps.**
- After delivery your lung function will continue to be monitored closely.
- The baby will be examined by the paediatricians after birth and longer term follow-up arranged, as required.
- There is no contraindication for breastfeeding unless you feel too poorly to do so.
- You will require a lot of help looking after the baby after you get home. Make sure you have this support!
- Before discharge you will be offered advice about **contraception**. It is very important that you use effective and safe contraception to avoid an unplanned pregnancy, especially if your lung function deteriorates in future.
- You must not take any contraceptive pill containing the hormone oestrogen. The minipill (progesterone-only pill) if chosen must be taken at the same time every day without fail, to be effective. The safest methods of contraception for you would be either an implant inserted under the skin in your arm, which is effective for 3 years, or the Mirena®, a hormone-loaded coil that is effective for about 5 years.
- With AAT deficiency, smoking can cause severe and rapid deterioration of your lung function, so **please do not smoke**. The AAT deficiency also targets your liver and you could develop cirrhosis of the liver. You need to avoid alcohol to prevent this.
- Although there is no cure for AAT deficiency at present, the outlook with good management both in pregnancy and at other times can help to slow down the rate of progression of the disease. With regular monitoring and careful management of the condition, many people with AAT deficiency can stay well and healthy.

Further information

- Alpha-1 UK Support Group <http://alpha-1foundation.org/what-is-alpha-1/>
- British Lung Foundation <http://www.blf.org.uk/Page/support-and-information>
- Patient.co.uk. Alpha-1 antitrypsin deficiency <http://www.patient.co.uk>

22. Previous Pregnancy Problems

INFORMATION FOR PATIENTS Pregnancy after previous Caesarean section

The specialist team will be happy to explain this in detail and will discuss options, management plans, and possible outcomes with you.

Further information

- Royal College of Obstetricians and Gynaecologists. Birth after previous Caesarean. Information for you <http://www.rcog.org.uk>

INFORMATION FOR PATIENTS Previous third- and fourth-degree tears

The specialist team will be happy to explain this in detail and will discuss options, management plans, and possible outcomes with you.

Further information

- Royal College of Obstetricians and Gynaecologists. A third- or fourth-degree tear during childbirth. Information for you <http://www.rcog.org.uk>

INFORMATION FOR PATIENTS Previous postpartum haemorrhage and/or retained placenta

If you have had postpartum haemorrhage (excessive bleeding after birth of the baby) or a retained placenta (a placenta that did not separate on its own from the wall of the womb after the baby was delivered and you had to have it removed as a separate procedure) in any previous pregnancy, you have a greater change of the same happening again in this pregnancy. That is why your community midwife will have referred you to one of the specialist antenatal clinics in the hospital to have a consultation with the specialist obstetrician.

Frequently asked questions

What is postpartum haemorrhage?

Postpartum haemorrhage (or PPH) is excessive bleeding after the birth of your baby. This bleeding is of two types:

- **Primary PPH** is when you have excessive bleeding immediately after or within the first 24 hours after the birth of the baby. This occurs in about 5% of all deliveries. The amount of bleeding differs according to the type of delivery (vaginal or Caesarean).
- **Secondary PPH**, which occurs in about 1–3% of all births, is when there is abnormally heavy bleeding which occurs **after** the first 24 hours following delivery and within 6 weeks of the birth. Most secondary PPH occurs in the second week after delivery of the baby.

What causes PPH?

There are several causes, but PPH usually occurs when the womb does not contract well and remain well-contracted after the delivery of the placenta. This is called **atony** of the uterus (womb), meaning that the muscles of the uterus have weakened tone (power) to remain tightly contracted.

PPH may also be caused if the placenta is retained, in part or in whole. This often warrants a procedure called **manual removal** when the placenta needs to be removed from the womb by a doctor after ensuring you have adequate pain relief. The placenta may have been found to be abnormally attached to the wall of the uterus in a few cases.

PPH can also be caused by tissue injury sustained at birth to the lower genital tract, for example vaginal tears, tears of the cervix, or very occasionally rupture of a previous Caesarean section scar on the womb.

If you have a known disorder of blood clotting or a coagulation disorder, you might have an increased tendency for PPH.

Other factors such as having twins/triplets, excess amniotic fluid, having had more than four previous deliveries, fibroids in the uterus, previous caesarean section, induction of labour, a long labour especially in a first pregnancy, antepartum haemorrhage (bleeding during a pregnancy), or a placenta being implanted low in the womb(placenta praevia) can all increase the risk of PPH. A short interval (less than 1 year) between a previous Caesarean section and starting a new pregnancy can also increase placental problems.

Can a retained placenta or PPH recur in subsequent pregnancies?

There is a higher risk of recurrence of PPH (2–4 times as high), in women who have had previous PPH or a retained placenta compared to those women who have not had such a history.

The risk of recurrence of PPH in a subsequent pregnancy is generally about 1 in 4 to 1 in 5 for primary PPH and about 1 in 5 for secondary PPH.

If you have had a previous retained placenta, the chance of it happening again in this pregnancy is about 20%, that is, a 1 in 5 chance.

Why am I being referred to a specialist clinic?

The specialist team in the antenatal clinic will be able to discuss aspects of your previous delivery and identify any risk factors for the PPH with the details available from your previous notes.

How can the risk of recurrence of PPH be reduced?

You will be given care and advice to help improve your iron stores. You will also be advised of certain precautions needed to prevent or reduce the risk of recurrence of PPH or retained placenta in this delivery. Such advice will include:

- Having a Venflon (needle in the arm) at the time of labour.
- Recommendation for an 'active' third stage when an injection of a drug called syntocinon is given after the delivery of the baby to help the womb to contract well and to stay contracted. An actively managed third stage reduces the risk of PPH by 75–80%.
- If you have any known coagulation disorder, the relevant coagulation factor will be kept available for the labour and this will be documented in your notes.
- Any anaemia during pregnancy needs prompt correction as this makes you less able to deal with PPH, should it recur. Iron supplements will be prescribed if you have iron deficiency anaemia.
- You will be advised to have the delivery in the hospital because of the 25% risk of recurrence of PPH.
- After this initial visit to the specialist clinic, the rest of your antenatal care can take place with your midwives in the community.
- If any fresh problems should arise during the course of this pregnancy, your community midwife will refer you to the specialist for further review.

If you have any questions, please do not hesitate to ask either your community midwife or any of the specialist team in the hospital.

Further information

- Royal College of Obstetricians and Gynaecologists. Heavy bleeding after birth (postpartum haemorrhage) <https://www.rcog.org.uk/en/patients/patient-leaflets/>

INFORMATION FOR PATIENTS Previous pre-eclampsia

The specialist team will be happy to explain this condition in detail and will discuss options, management plans, and possible outcomes with you.

Further information

- NICE. Hypertension in pregnancy: The management of hypertensive disorders during pregnancy (CG107), 2010 <http://www.nice.org.uk/guidance/cg107/informationforpublic>

INFORMATION FOR PATIENTS Previous birth complicated by shoulder dystocia

Further information

The specialist team will be happy to explain this condition in detail and will discuss options, management plans, and possible outcomes with you.

- Royal College of Obstetricians and Gynaecologists. A difficult birth: what is shoulder dystocia? Information for you, 2007 <http://www.rcog.org.uk>

INFORMATION FOR PATIENTS Previous premature birth or late miscarriage

- You will naturally be worried about this pregnancy given your previous experience. Your medical team will aim to help and support you to have a better outcome in this pregnancy.
- Remember that there are several different reasons for a premature delivery or a late miscarriage. What might be relevant to one patient might not apply to another.

- In more than 50% of cases, **no single factor** which has provoked the premature labour or late miscarriage can be found. Also, quite frequently, there is more than one factor that has caused the outcome.
- You might have already been seen by the obstetric specialist after the previous pregnancy to discuss risk factors and results of investigations as well as plans for any subsequent pregnancy.
- If you have had a previous preterm birth, there is a slightly higher chance (about 15%) that this will happen again. This risk is higher if you have had two or more premature births or late miscarriages, especially if the interval between pregnancies is short.
- If you are a smoker, you will be advised to try to stop as this is a well- recognized risk factor for premature delivery or late miscarriages.
- Your community midwife will refer you to the hospital specialist antenatal clinic at or before 12 weeks pregnancy. You can expect to see the same specialist team throughout this pregnancy.
- You might not have had a chance to discuss the details of your previous pregnancy with a consultant. Therefore, at your first visit to the specialist clinic in this pregnancy, we would ask you certain details of your previous pregnancy to help narrow down any contributing factors.
- Certain blood tests will be done to exclude conditions like lupus if this has not been tested previously.
- Depending on individual circumstances you might be advised to take one tablet of low-dose aspirin (75 mg) from the early few weeks of the pregnancy till the end of the pregnancy. If you have a condition called antiphospholipid syndrome, in addition to the low-dose aspirin, a daily injection of a blood-thinning drug called dalteparin might be advised.
- You may also be given a prescription for a vaginal antibiotic cream and advised to use this for 5–7 days at 16 weeks and for 7 days at 22 weeks of pregnancy.
- If your previous pregnancy events suggest a problem with the cervix, a set of scans will be arranged to monitor the length of the cervix and how well closed the cervical canal is. These scans may be performed through a vaginal route (like an internal examination).
- In a small number of women, these cervical scans may reveal a problem of premature shortening of the cervix with opening of the inner mouth of the canal. In most women, however, no worrying features are seen.
- If it is relevant in your case, you may also be advised to insert a pessary or suppository containing progesterone (the hormone that helps to keep your womb muscles relaxed) every day till about 28 to 30 weeks, sometimes even up to 35 weeks.
- If the cervix has shortened too soon, depending on the individual conditions you might be offered a procedure called a **cervical suture insertion**, or **cervical cerclage**. This is a surgical procedure performed under a spinal anaesthetic in the operating theatre. If you have had a cervical suture insertion, no more cervical scans are needed.
- If you start having pain or contractions, or if your waters break later in pregnancy, you are advised to report this straightaway to delivery suite and come in as soon as possible so that the suture can be removed. If all remains well till 37 weeks of pregnancy, suture removal in the delivery suite will be arranges.
- You will continue to see your own community midwife as normal.
- You will be offered scans at regular intervals to ensure your baby is growing well and if possible these appointments will be on the same day as your clinic visits in the hospital.
- If you have not delivered by the time you get to your estimated date of delivery, you will be offered a date for induction of labour.
- If you have had no cervical problems and have not needed to have a suture insertion you will be seen at regular intervals in the specialist antenatal clinic, with a scan on the same day if possible, at 28, 32, and 36 weeks. Remember to apply the vaginal antibiotic cream at 16 and 22 weeks of pregnancy as mentioned above.
- If you are on low-dose aspirin, you can continue this till the end of pregnancy.
- If you are on dalteparin injections along with aspirin, it is advisable to induce labour at about 38 weeks pregnancy. You would then be asked to stop the aspirin and the dalteparin injections 24 hours before your induction date.

Further information

- BMJ Best Practice. Premature birth. <http://bestpractice.bmj.com/best-practice/pdf/patient-summaries/en-gb/533043.pdf>
- NHS Choices. Miscarriage <http://www.nhs.uk/Conditions/Miscarriage/Pages/Causes.aspx>
- Babycentre. Understanding late miscarriage <http://www.babycentre.co.uk/a1014773/understanding-late-miscarriage>

INFORMATION FOR PATIENTS Stillbirth

The specialist team will be pleased to talk with you about this and will dis cuss future options and management plans.

Further information

- Royal College of Obstetricians and Gynaecologists. When your baby dies before birth. Information for you <http://www.rcog.org.uk>

23. Fertility-Related Issues

INFORMATION FOR PATIENTS Pregnancy conceived by IVF or related techniques

- **Congratulations!**
- Your community midwife will have referred you to one of the specialist antenatal clinics in the hospital in order that your pregnancy care can be 'stepped up'.
- If you have a twin or triplet pregnancy resulting from IVF or other related procedures like ICSI, you will be referred to the multiple pregnancy clinic and will receive information leaflets relating to multiple pregnancy.
- This information leaflet has been prepared specially for those whose successful IVF treatment has resulted in a single baby developing in the womb. This leaflet is to help you understand why you need to be seen in the hospital antenatal clinic at certain stages of your pregnancy, whether any extra tests will be needed and if so, why. It will explain what you can expect from these antenatal visits and how your antenatal care will continue to be shared with your community midwife.
- You may have already received some information about pregnancies following IVF/ICSI from the fertility centre where you had your treatment.

Frequently asked questions

Why do I need to be seen in a specialist antenatal clinic?

Pregnancies resulting from IVF, even singleton pregnancies, have a few increased risks when compared to spontaneous conception, such as:

- A small increased risk of abnormalities in the baby
- Increased incidence of premature delivery
- Growth restriction of the baby
- Increased risk of you developing blood pressure problems, especially if donor eggs have been used
- Increased risk of you developing diabetes during pregnancy.

Are any extra tests or monitoring required during this pregnancy?

- We would like to keep your pregnancy care as normal as possible, with a few extra precautions.
- In order to monitor the growth of the baby, in addition to the two routine pregnancy scans (one before 13 weeks and the other scan at about 20 weeks), you will be offered growth scans at regular intervals from about approximately 28 weeks onwards. These scans are to monitor how well the baby is growing at each stage.
- You will have routine checks of your blood pressure and urine at each antenatal visit both in the hospital and with your community midwife. If there are any signs of high blood pressure, further tests and visits may be organized. If the scans and routine pregnancy checks are reassuringly normal, the care of your pregnancy will be managed mainly by your community midwife.
- You should be extra vigilant about the baby's movements in the last few weeks of pregnancy and to promptly report any reduction in movements. Your baby's heart rate pattern will then be monitored to ensure that the baby is well.

Will I need to have a planned Caesarean section because this is an IVF pregnancy?

- *Not routinely*: not unless there are other complications such as a poorly functioning placenta affecting the baby's growth or if you develop severe pre-eclampsia or blood pressure problems and induction of labour either does not work or is not feasible.
- If all has been well during pregnancy with you and the baby and if you have not delivered by the time you reach your estimated date of delivery, **induction of labour around the time of your due date** may be advisable. This is because there is some evidence that after 40 weeks in an IVF pregnancy, the placenta may not continue to work as well as compared to that of a spontaneously conceived pregnancy. Your medical team will discuss this with you.
- During labour you can expect the same level of care that is offered to any spontaneously conceived pregnancy.

24. Other Maternal Conditions

INFORMATION FOR PATIENTS Stopping smoking in pregnancy

The specialist team will be happy to explain this in detail and will discuss options, management plans, and possible outcomes with you.

Further information

- NHS Pregnancy Smoking Helpline number: 0800 1699 169
- NHS SmokeFree. Pregnancy and smoking<http://www.nhs.uk/smokefree/why-quit/smoking-in-pregnancy>
- Patient.co.uk. Pregnancy and smoking <http://www.patient.co.uk>

INFORMATION FOR PATIENTS Alcohol and pregnancy

The specialist team will be happy to explain this in detail and will discuss options, management plans, and possible outcomes with you.

Further information

- Patient.co.uk. Pregnancy and alcohol <http://www.patient.co.uk>
- Royal College of Obstetricians and Gynaecologists. Alcohol and pregnancy. Information for you <http://www.rcog.org.uk>

INFORMATION FOR PATIENTS Substance misuse and pregnancy

The specialist team will be happy to explain this in detail and will discuss options, management plans, and possible outcomes with you.

Further information

- Barking, Havering and Redridge University Hospoitals NHS Trust. Neonatal abstinence syndrome (NAS): information for you <http://www.bhrhospitals.nhs.uk/Downloads/services/bhrut-maternity-neonatal-abstinence-syndrome.pdf>
- Patient.co.uk. Pregnancy and street drugs <http://www.patient.co.uk/showdoc/27000496.htm>
- Southampton University Hospitals NHS Trust. Methadone and pregnancy <http://www.uhs.nhs.uk/Media/Controlleddocuments/Patientinformation/Pregnancyandbirth/Methadoneandpregnancy-patientinformation.pdf>

INFORMATION FOR PATIENTS Hyperemesis gravidarum

Although 80–90% of all pregnant women will experience some nausea and vomiting starting from 4 weeks pregnancy and lasting up to about 16 weeks or so, only a small minority will develop the condition called hyperemesis gravidarum. This is the term used for nausea and vomiting of pregnancy that that is so persistent and severe that it could lead to dehydration and metabolic imbalance.

Further information

- Hyperemesis Education and Research (HER) Foundation (US) <http://www.helpher.org/>
- Patient.co.uk. Hyperemesis gravidarum <http://www.patient.co.uk>
- Pregnancy Sickness Support <http://www.pregnancysicknesssupport.org.uk>

INFORMATION FOR PATIENTS Domestic violence during pregnancy

If you or someone you know is suffering domestic violence, the following sites can provide more information and support. You can also speak to your midwife, health visitor, GP, obstetrician or nurse in complete confidence.

Further information

- Best Beginnings. Domestic abuse against pregnant women <http://www.bestbeginnings.org.uk/domestic-abuse>
- Leeds City Council Domestic Violence Team. Free online training on identifying and responding to domestic abuse <http://www.seeabuse.com/>
- NHS Choices. Domestic abuse in pregnancy. Pregnancy and baby guide. <http://www.nhs.uk/conditions/pregnancy-and.../domestic-abuse-pregnant.aspx>
- Refuge. National domestic violence helpline 0808 2000 247 (Freephone 24 hour) <http://refuge.org.uk/>
- Womens Aid <http://www.womensaid.org.uk/default.asp>

25. Multiple Pregnancies

INFORMATION FOR PATIENTS Multiple pregnancies

Congratulations! You've found out you're having twins or more! No doubt you will have a number of questions to ask about the antenatal treatment, once you get over the initial surprise.

Frequently asked questions

What's the difference between identical and non-identical or fraternal twins?

- Twins may be identical (30%) or non-identical (70%).
- Identical twins are formed from one fertilized egg which splits very early in its embryonic development, giving rise to two embryos with identical genes. These babies will be monozygous and share one placenta (monochorionic) in 70% of cases, but if the division has happened early in the embryonic period, in 30% of identical twin pregnancies there may be two placentas with the twin occupying separate sacs.
- Fraternal (dizygous) twins are the result of two separate eggs being fertilized by two sperms at the same time, so that two embryos implant and develop with two placentas. These twins are non-identical, may look different, and be of different sexes or of the same sex.

What is meant by chorionicity, dichorionic, diamniotic, and monochorionic?

- Dichorionic means there are two placentas, which could appear as discrete or fused.
- Diamniotic means there are two sacs of amniotic fluid.
- *A non-identical twin pregnancy is always dichorionic diamniotic, but 30% of dichorionic diamniotic twin pregnancies can be identical twins!*
- Monochorionic monoamniotic (MCMA) twins are identical, share a single sac and have the same placenta, and have no separating membrane. They are obviously of the same sex. These twins are at a higher risk of various complications of pregnancy. MCMA twins are fortunately, rare.
- Monochorionic diamniotic (MCDA) twins have a very thin membrane separating the babies. This is the most common type of identical twins.

What kind of antenatal care can I expect during my twin pregnancy?

- You should receive more than the standard antenatal appointments and more than the two routine ultrasound scans of an uncomplicated singleton pregnancy.
- As multiple pregnancies are more complicated, you will be referred to the hospital multiple pregnancy clinic, run by a specialist team led by a senior consultant, for most of your antenatal care. You will also be seen by your community midwife or GP in between.
- Depending on the type of your twin pregnancy and on any medical conditions that develop during pregnancy, you will be requested to attend the hospital multiple pregnancy clinic at 2–4 week intervals, usually to coincide with the scan appointments arranged for the same session.
- It is extremely important not to miss any appointments, for the sake of your babies' health and your own in this 'higher risk' pregnancy. You and the multiple pregnancy specialist team will work together to ensure the safest and best possible outcome.

How will my medical care differ in my twin pregnancy?

- The antenatal care you will receive depends partly upon the type of twin pregnancy you are carrying, either identical (also called monozygotic) or non-identical (also called fraternal or dizygotic) twins.
- If your twin babies share the outer membrane and are within one sac (MCMA) or have a shared placenta (MCDA), you can expect increased scans (every 2 weeks or even weekly) and monitoring, mainly because of the risk of a condition called twin-to-twin-transfusion syndrome (TTTS). This occurs because shared blood vessels in the placenta allow blood from one twin (the donor) to flow into the other (the recipient).
- In any type of multiple pregnancy, you will be offered more ultrasound scans than if you were carrying only one baby, especially after 26 weeks of pregnancy. This is to check the growth and position of the babies as well as the fluid around them.
- Twins are much more likely to be born prematurely than single babies: 37 weeks is considered full-term for a non-identical twin pregnancy compared to a singleton pregnancy when 40 weeks is considered full-term. In uncomplicated non-identical twins, delivery

is usually advised by 37 to 38 weeks and in uncomplicated identical twins in different sacs with a single membrane between the two sacs, delivery is recommended at about 36 weeks. There is greater risk of babies not surviving if the pregnancy is prolonged beyond 37 weeks in identical twins and 38 weeks in non-identical twins. Depending on the type of the twin pregnancy and other factors such as growth problems identified in one or both babies or if you develop any complications such as pre-eclampsia, even earlier delivery may be advised. This advice will of course be individualized to your pregnancy.

- The type of delivery will depend on how the first baby is lying. If the leading baby is in any position other than head-down there are greater risks, including cord accidents, during vaginal delivery. The specialist will therefore advise a Caesarean section. In the case of identical twins sharing the same sac, or triplets, delivery by Caesarean section will certainly be advised due to the very big risks involved with labour and vaginal (normal) delivery for each of the babies.
- Local Twins/Triplets Groups or the National TAMBA-run support groups will be happy to help you understand the care you receive, to answer your questions however insignificant you might think they are, and to share in the experience of pregnancy and delivery with others who have multiple pregnancies or are already mothers of twins or triplets. You will be invited to join the group with your partner, if you choose.

When and how is my twin pregnancy found?

- Your twin/ triplet pregnancy is usually diagnosed when you have your first scan in the 1st trimester (the first 13 weeks of pregnancy). This scan will not only establish the number of babies but also identify the type of twin pregnancy.
- This is very important in order to plan the subsequent care and management of your twin pregnancy.
- Once a multiple pregnancy has been detected, you will be referred to the specialist multiple pregnancy clinic within 1–2 weeks. This clinic has a specialist team led by a consultant obstetrician, all of whom have extensive experience and expertise in the specific care of multiple pregnancies.

What happens at my first appointment?

- The first appointment should be fairly early in your pregnancy, at about 11–13 weeks. You will be given information about the pregnancy, your urine sample and blood pressure will be checked, and plans for future scans and appointments will be discussed. Routine blood tests will be discussed and performed, unless you have had them already.
- In twin pregnancies, the 'triple test' (the blood test at 15 weeks which is available to screen for chromosomal defects like Down's syndrome) is not as reliable as in a singleton pregnancy. If you opt for screening for Down's syndrome or other chromosomal abnormalities, the screening coordinator midwife will discuss which options are available to you.
- Before deciding whether or not to have Down's syndrome screening for twins, you need to consider what you would do if one baby has a high risk and one has a low risk for Down's syndrome. The only way to confirm whether the babies have normal chromosomes or not, is to have an amniocentesis. The risk of miscarriage of this invasive procedure is doubled with twins, to 1 in 75. Also, if one baby has Down's syndrome and the other does not, you will be faced with some difficult decisions. If the twins are identical, both will either have Down's syndrome or else both will not have Down's syndrome.

Common concerns with twin pregnancies

- **Nausea and vomiting**. You may have these symptoms appear earlier in the pregnancy and last longer than in a singleton pregnancy because twice as much hormone is being produced from the placenta.
- **Varicose veins, haemorrhoids**. Due to the increased size of the womb as well as the weight you have to carry in a multiple pregnancy, you might be more uncomfortable in the later weeks of pregnancy with varicose veins of the legs and sometimes of the vaginal outlet (the vulva) as well as haemorrhoids (piles). Your midwife can advise ways of reducing the discomfort.
- **Blood pressure and pre-eclampsia**. Multiple pregnancies lead to more problems with high blood pressure and pre-eclampsia. Your midwife as well as the specialist hospital clinic team will see you more frequently during pregnancy to detect these signs which include raised blood pressure, protein appearing in the urine, and an abnormal degree of swelling as well as changes in your blood.
- **Anaemia**. Because you have to meet the requirements of two babies rather than one, you can develop both iron and folic acid deficiency anaemia. You might need supplements to provide enough iron and folic acid (higher dose 5 mg/day, available on prescription only).
- **Excess fluid around the babies in the womb**. In twin pregnancies, depending on the type of twins, there could be an abnormally large amount of fluid surrounding the babies. If this develops in a very short space of time—which is more common with identical twins—it could result in acute discomfort and increased breathlessness as well leading to premature contractions. These are symptoms that you need to report immediately to your midwife or contact the maternity unit directly.
- **Premature labour / preterm birth**. This is the greatest of all risks associated with multiple pregnancies, *leading to problems with* survival of the premature twins. The earlier in pregnancy that labour starts, the greater the fetal loss rate due to prematurity. Labour starts early in 20–50% of twin pregnancies compared to 5–10% in singletons. If labour starts early, either with contractions or breaking of the waters, you need to get to hospital straightaway as labour could progress very rapidly. If you are less than 36 weeks pregnant, you will be offered a first dose of an intramuscular injection of corticosteroid which is to help ripen the lungs of the premature babies, thus improving their chance of survival. If there is time you will receive the second dose of steroids some 12–24 hours later to complete the course. This course of steroids does not cause you or your babies any harmful effects even if the threatened premature labour does not progress.
- If you go into premature labour between 24 and 34 weeks, your babies should be delivered in a hospital with special care beds for the premature babies. If the special care baby unit is full at that time, there is a possibility that you might be transferred to any neighbouring unit with these facilities. If you are already far advanced in labour and transferring you is not practical or safe, please be aware that the babies might need to be transferred after birth to other units. This is in order to give them the best care they need because of their prematurity. The specialist team will do their best not to separate you from your babies.
- **Bleeding**. Any bleeding in pregnancy might be a sign of trouble. This could be due to early preterm labour or to an abnormally early separation of the placenta from the wall of the womb (a condition called abruption) which is more common in twin pregnancies. Abruption can be a serious risk to you as well as to the well-being of the babies. It is therefore very important to contact the hospital delivery suite if you have any bleeding and come in straight away to allow appropriate assessment and examination.
- **Pain and contractions**. Abruption of the placenta could be accompanied by pain which is often severe and constant. Pain could also be a feature of the start of premature labour. You need to report such symptoms immediately by phoning the delivery suite.
- **Growth problems in one or both babies**. The reason you can expect more scans during a twin pregnancy is because growth problems can affect one or both babies as there is competition for blood supply and nutrition supplied by the placenta and your womb. This can happen in both identical and non-identical twins. You will have more detailed scans (including specialized Doppler scans) if your babies are not growing according to their own growth curves. If the problem is significant, the specialist team may advise early delivery.

Further information

- NICE. Multiple pregnancy: The management of twin and triplet pregnancies in the antenatal period (CG129), 2011 <http://www.nice.org.uk/guidance/cg129/informationforpublic>
- TAMBA <http://www.twinsuk.co.uk>; <http://www.twins-store.co.uk>

26. Fetal Growth Issues

INFORMATION FOR PATIENTS The small baby

You might have been informed that either your previous baby was 'small for gestational age' (SGA) or had signs of 'intrauterine growth restriction' (IUGR).

Alternatively you might have been told that your baby in this pregnancy is showing signs of the growth tailing off, or that the baby's measurements within the womb are below the 10th centile.

What do these terms mean?

Small for gestational age (SGA)

SGA is a term used to describe a baby whose birth weight is less than what is expected for the number of weeks of pregnancy. SGA babies have birth weights below the 10th centile, which means that they weigh less than 90% of all other babies of the same gestational age.

SGA babies may be **proportionately small** (equally small all over, **symmetrically small**), or can have a **disproportionately small** abdominal (tummy) circumference measurement (**asymmetrical**) on scan.

Most SGA babies are small but healthy. This is called being **constitutionally small** and is influenced by the relative size of the mother's own small build or by racial differences (for example, Asian babies are usually smaller than white babies).

Intrauterine growth restriction (IUGR)

However, some SGA babies have a condition called IUGR. This occurs when the fetus does not receive the necessary nutrition and oxygen required for proper growth and development in the womb, or because of infection. IUGR can begin at any time in the pregnancy and a fetus with IUGR may be born at term (after 37 completed weeks of pregnancy) or prematurely (before 37 weeks).

Newborn SGA babies who have had IUGR in the womb often appear thin and pale and have loose dry skin. Others may not have this malnourished appearance but are small all over.

What causes IUGR?

IUGR can result due to a variety of causes. Sometimes there is more than one risk factor.

Factors relating to the mother (maternal)

- Smoking
- High blood pressure
- Diseases of the kidneys, heart disease, advanced diabetes, severe anaemia, malnutrition
- Substance abuse (drugs, alcohol)
- Infection
- Some essential medications that are required to treat certain diseases in the mother.

Factors related to the womb itself and placenta (afterbirth)

- Decreased blood flow in the tiny blood vessels that supply the placenta and thereby the baby
- Increased stickiness of the blood flowing in the end-capillaries (the tiniest blood vessel branches) of the placenta, thereby reducing blood flow and gas exchange to the baby
- Partial placental abruption (when the placenta partially detaches from the wall of the womb)
- Infection in the tissues around the baby
- Placenta praevia (a placenta attached low in the womb).

Factors related to the developing baby (fetus)

- Multiple pregnancy (twins, triplets, etc.)
- Infections
- Birth defects
- Chromosomal abnormality

Why is IUGR a concern?

When the fetus does not receive enough oxygen or nutrients during pregnancy, its overall body growth and organ sizes are limited. Tissue organ cells may not grow as large or as numerous. Some of the conditions that cause IUGR restrict blood flow through the placenta. This can cause the fetus to receive less oxygen than normal, increasing the risks for the baby during pregnancy, delivery, and afterwards. In a few severe cases, the restriction of nutrients and oxygen can even lead to a slowing of the baby's heart.

Babies with IUGR may have problems at birth, including:

- Decreased oxygen levels
- Low Apgar scores (an assessment that helps identify those babies with difficulty adapting after birth)
- Meconium aspiration (inhalation of the first stools passed within the womb which could lead to breathing difficulties).
- Hypoglycaemia (low blood sugar)
- Difficulty in maintaining a normal body temperature
- Polycythaemia (too many red blood cells).

Severe growth restriction may result in stillbirth. It may also lead to long-term growth and developmental problems in babies and children.

How is growth restriction diagnosed?

During pregnancy the size of the fetus can be estimated clinically by feeling and measuring the womb size. However, ultrasound measurements are more accurate, especially if there is a series of them (serial scans).

Ultrasound measurements (biometry scan) of the baby's head and abdomen and the amount of fluid around the baby are taken and compared with charts showing comparative growth and amount of liquor (fluid around baby). The abdominal circumference measurements can be used to estimate birth weight as well as being a helpful indicator of fetal nutrition.

Another way to interpret and diagnose IUGR during pregnancy is **Doppler flow**, which uses sound waves to measure blood flow. The sound of the blood movement through a blood vessel produces wave patterns that reflect how much blood is flowing, and how fast. Blood vessels in the umbilical cord and in the fetal brain can be checked in this way.

The **biophysical profile** is not designed to measure the baby and therefore diagnose IUGR. It is an ultrasound scan combined with monitoring of the baby's heart rate (CTG) used to predict fetal well-being. When combined with the findings of a growth scan, it provides better information about the baby's well-being and, indirectly, indicates how well the placenta is coping.

Heart rate pattern monitoring (cardiotocography or CTG) provides information about the condition of the baby at that time. A reassuring pattern indicates that the baby is not likely to be oxygen deprived at the time of the monitoring. This is a snapshot view of that point in time, which can't predict the future.

Your awareness of the baby's movements is very important. A sudden decrease in the number of kicks or movements may mean that the baby is not getting enough nutrients and oxygen and may be 'under stress'. In such situations you will have been advised to contact the hospital right away. You will then be invited to come in to have the baby checked. ***Please do not ignore a decrease in movements below 10 in any 12 consecutive hours.***

It is dangerous to believe that the baby will move less frequently when you are approaching term. You can expect to feel more squirms and wriggles than thumping kicks (more baby and less space!), but the frequency of movements should not decrease. You should call the hospital at once if you are worried in any way.

Management of IUGR

- If you smoke or use illicit drugs you are advised to stop.
- If you have had a previous SGA baby, certain special blood tests to exclude an immune basis for poor placental function may be offered at your first hospital visit.
- You might be recommended low-dose aspirin 75 mg tablets to take from the end of 12 weeks of pregnancy until the end of the pregnancy to reduce the stickiness of blood in the end-capillaries of the placenta, thus improving transfer of oxygen and nutrition to the fetus.
- A programme of scan monitoring perhaps with additional Doppler studies to monitor the baby's growth will be discussed with you.
- If this pregnancy is the first time IUGR has been suspected, you will have scans to either confirm or exclude it. If IUGR is confirmed, further investigations to exclude abnormalities or infections will be offered. Serial scans, Doppler flow studies, and biophysical profiling may be part of the overall plan of monitoring baby's growth and well-being at regular intervals. You may be advised admission to hospital for closer monitoring and to be given steroids if early delivery (before 36 weeks of pregnancy) is planned.
- Delivery by the safest and most expedient route will be advised if IUGR is suspected of endangering the health of the baby. This may be even before 37 weeks of pregnancy, depending on the individual situation.
- After birth, the baby will be observed for the signs described previously. Breastfeeding will be encouraged at the earliest as these babies have been hungry in the womb! Support and feeding advice will be provided. In severe cases the baby may have to be transferred to the special care baby unit for additional feeding, temperature-controlled bed, monitoring of oxygen levels, etc.

Prevention of IUGR

SGA babies may be born even when the mother is in good health. However, some risky factors that play an important part in causing IUGR, such as smoking, poor nutrition, and alcohol and drug abuse can only be stopped by the pregnant mother—**that's you!**

Eating a healthy diet and seeking specialist advice before a pregnancy may help decrease the risks of IUGR recurring for the next baby.

Further information

- Royal College of Obstetricians and Gynaecologists. Having a small baby <https://www.rcog.org.uk/en/patients/patient-leaflets/>

INFORMATION FOR PATIENTS The large baby

When is a baby termed 'big'?

- The average newborn weighs about 3.4 kg (7 lb 8 oz).
- **Large for gestational age** refers to a baby in the womb (fetus) whose estimated weight appears to be greater than the 90th centile for a given gestational age (i.e. larger than 90% of babies in that week of pregnancy).
- If the newborn baby's weight is greater than 4.5 kg (9 lbs 15 oz), regardless of the gestational age at birth, this is termed **macrosomia**.
- In the last 2–3 decades, there has been a significant increase of 15–25% of women delivering large babies. This trend is thought to be due to increases in women's height, body mass, weight gain during pregnancy, and diabetes.
- The prevalence of babies born with a birth weight of more than 4 kg (8 lb 12 oz) is about 10% and continuously rising.

What factors can make a baby 'big'?

- Birth weight is influenced by genetic and racial factors. White babies are usually heavier than Asian babies.
- Other risk factors associated with having a large baby include maternal obesity, excessive weight gain during pregnancy, going more than 2 weeks past your due date, and having diabetes before pregnancy or developing it during pregnancy.
- Most big babies are constitutionally large, simply reflecting the overall build of their parents.
- Boy babies are more often larger than girls.
- If you have already had a large baby, you are more likely to have large babies in future pregnancies.
- However, even if any of the above factors apply to you, you are still more likely than not to have a baby of average size.
- Most newborn babies who weigh more than 4.5 kg (9 lb 15 oz) are born to women who do not have any of the risk factors listed above.

Determining the expected size of the baby before birth

- It is very difficult to determine whether your baby is truly macrosomic while he/she is still in the uterus (womb). It can only be confirmed after birth.
- Prediction of macrosomic babies may be difficult as there may be no identifiable risk factors.
- Estimation of fetal weight by clinical examination as well as with ultrasound measurements is not completely accurate and shows considerable variation.
- The distance between the top of the pregnant womb and the top of the pubic symphysis joint is known as the symphysio-fundal height. It is measured as part of every routine antenatal check. If it is measured by the same person each time, this may reduce the variation that naturally occurs with such measurements.
- If your midwife or GP suspects your baby may be big because you are 'large for dates', you may be referred to have an ultrasound scan and/or see a specialist obstetrician.
- An ultrasound scan can give an idea of how big your baby really is. However, this is not always accurate. In the third trimester (26–40 weeks pregnancy) there can be a difference of up to 20% either way between your baby's weight predicted by ultrasound and the actual weight at birth.
- The larger the fetus, the more inaccurate the ultrasound prediction of the estimated birth weight. Also, the more obese the mother the more inaccurate the estimation of expected birth weight by either clinical or ultrasound measurements.
- There does not seem to be much difference between ultrasound estimation of expected birth weight and clinical examination by an experienced doctor or a senior midwife.
- If the scan shows that your baby is large for dates, a test called a glucose tolerance test may be advised to see whether you are developing gestational diabetes.

- A large fetus may be associated with increased complications for the mother, fetus, and newborn baby:
  - **Risks for the mother** associated include injury to the birth canal, obstructed labour, increased chances of Caesarean section, and excessive bleeding after birth.
  - **Risks for the fetus and newborn baby** include problems resulting from any difficulty that may arise during delivery of a large baby's shoulders (shoulder dystocia). Long-term risks include childhood obesity and type 2 diabetes.

Planning delivery

- The specialist obstetrician will discuss the difficulty of estimating fetal birthweight accurately, and predicting the very small chance of difficulty in delivering the baby's shoulders (shoulder dystocia).
- Interventions such as early induction of labour or Caesarean section for a suspected large baby have each their own risks while not necessarily avoiding the problem of shoulder dystocia.
- For most women with a large baby, except those who are diabetic or who have developed diabetes during pregnancy, inducing labour early does not have any proven benefit for the mother or baby.
- A planned Caesarean section seems to be beneficial only if the baby is suspected to weigh more than 5 kg in a non-diabetic mother. Elective Caesarean section cannot therefore be justified if suspected macrosomia is the only indication.
- The risks and benefits of both expectant management ('wait and see') and of any interventions, as well as the precautions advisable in labour and for delivery, will be discussed with you.
- Studies have shown that the vast majority (88%) of women who labour with a large-for dates baby have a successful vaginal delivery.
- The progress of labour will be monitored by regular assessments.
- An epidural for labour and delivery is advisable if the baby is suspected to be large and if shoulder dystocia is anticipated. An epidural will help to relax your pelvic muscles, which helps with safe delivery of the baby.

27. Fetal Abnormalities

INFORMATION FOR PATIENTS Antenatal fetal hydronephrosis

What is hydronephrosis?

- Hydronephrosis (fluid-filled enlargement of the kidney) is detected in the fetus by ultrasound studies at either the 20-week detailed scan or later in pregnancy. Although the kidneys start to function in producing urine before 12 weeks of pregnancy, the detailed structure of the kidneys and the rest of the urinary tract is best visualized when the baby is of at least 18–20 weeks gestational size.
- **Renal** is another term for 'relating to the kidneys'. The outer part of the kidney is known as the **cortex** and the inner part is called the **pelvis.** This is not to be confused with the bony pelvis (hip bones). The renal pelvis is the part of the collecting system that collects urine produced by the kidney cells called **nephrons**. Each kidney is connected at its pelvis with a tube called the **ureter** that allows an uninterrupted flow of urine downwards to the bladder.
- The bladder in turn has an outlet called the **urethra** that allows the passage of urine to the outside when the muscle wall of the bladder contracts.
- Hydronephrosis in the developing baby may be caused by a number of causes including a **blockage** or obstruction at various levels of the entire urinary system: for example a blockage at the junction between the renal pelvis and the ureter on one side or at the junction of the ureter and the bladder on either side. A blockage in the urethra seen in male fetuses called the posterior urethral valves can cause backpressure and thus dilatation of the bladder and ureters on both sides as well as the renal pelvis of each kidney.
- When there is an obstruction in any part of the renal tract and the ability of the fetus to pass urine is reduced or blocked entirely, the amount of amniotic fluid (the liquid in the bag of membranes or sac surrounding the baby) is reduced. This is a condition called **oligo-hydramnios**. Normal development of the baby's lungs depends on a normal amount of amniotic fluid being present, so **hypoplasia** (underdevelopment) of the baby's lungs is a result of reduced amniotic fluid from early second trimester as seen in obstructions in the urinary tract.
- Hydronephrosis can also be caused due to **non-obstructive causes**: for example, a condition called **vesicoureteral reflux** which occurs when the valve between the bladder and the ureter is incompetent permitting urine to backflow to the kidneys, whenever the bladder fills or empties. Most children (75%) outgrow this during childhood but need close surveillance and antibiotics to try to prevent kidney infections as these can damage the kidneys before the child outgrows the reflux. Only a minority of children with such reflux need surgery, either because of failure to outgrow the reflux or because of frequent urinary tract infections.
- Hydronephrosis can often be associated with defects in the development of other organs such as the heart, brain, and spine or a result of chromosomal abnormalities. While ultrasound scanning will attempt to detect any other structural abnormalities, diagnosis of chromosomal defects at this stage of pregnancy will require an amniocentesis which your doctor will discuss with you.

Management during pregnancy and after birth

- In most cases of fetal hydronephrosis, the condition is mild and does not change the pregnancy care except that you will need more scans. Labour and delivery can be performed normally. The baby after birth will require ultrasound scans to see whether the renal dilatation is still there. Follow-up is by the paediatricians (doctors for infants and children). In a small percentage of cases surgery may be needed during infancy and childhood.
- In very rare cases a fetus with severe obstruction of both kidneys and insufficient amniotic fluid might have the kidneys or bladder drained by insertion of a tube or even antenatal surgery. These procedures are technically possible, but the outcome of the babies has not, to date, been improved. These babies are likely to have very little normal kidney tissue remaining and these abnormal kidneys do not function well. The reduction or even absence of amniotic fluid also causes inadequate lung development.
- In very rare cases, obstructed kidneys may be so enlarged as to require Caesarean section to deliver the baby, although in the case the outlook for the baby might be very poor.
- Postnatal ultrasound is usually performed on the third day after birth. If hydronephrosis persists, further tests to rule out reflux or obstruction may be required, usually when the baby is 1 month old. Most infants who have persisting reflux are managed by antibiotics and close follow-up including scans at regular intervals.
- Most blockages require surgical correction. In some babies the degree of obstruction is mild and serial tests in a few months are all that is required.
- The specialists in your local hospital or at a tertiary/regional referral hospital will be happy to discuss any aspect of the diagnosis, management, and outcomes with you.

Further information

- Great Ormond Street Hospital. Hydronephrosis information sheet <http://www.gosh.nhs.uk/medical-information/>

PATIENT INFORMATION: Sacrococcygeal teratoma

Frequently asked questions

What is a sacrococcygeal teratoma?

- An ultrasound scan may detect a rare abnormality in the baby called sacrococcygeal ('say-crow-cox-e-jee-al') teratoma (SCT for short). This is a tumour (a growth) found on the lower back and the buttocks of the developing baby. This condition will require ongoing monitoring throughout your pregnancy and the baby will most likely need to have an operation to remove the tumour after birth.
- SCT is a rare condition, found in only 1 in 35,000 to 40,000 babies. Baby girls are four times more likely to be born with this than baby boys.
- SCT is a tumour which is made of three types of tissue cells. In most cases it is a benign (innocent) tumour but in some cases it may contain cells that can develop into a cancerous variety later on.
- After birth, when the tumour is removed it will be tested to see what type of cells it contains. Most SCTs are not cancerous.

What caused this to happen?

- We do not know exactly why SCTs develop, but we do know that they contain several types of cells that grow in a disordered manner. Nothing you did or did not do during your early pregnancy caused this to happen.

How does this affect the rest of my pregnancy?

- You can expect to be referred to the fetal medicine unit at a large central referral hospital where you will not only have more ultrasound scans but also meet experts such as paediatricians (baby doctors), paediatric surgeons, and specialist obstetricians. A special type of scan (MRI scan) may be done and both you and the baby will need to be monitored regularly for the rest of your pregnancy. These tests are to detect development of any complications that can change the outcome.

What are the complications that can develop during my pregnancy to change the outlook for the baby?

- The SCT usually has a large supply of blood vessels, sometimes enough to cause a strain on the baby's heart. The baby's heart has to pump harder to cope with the unusual demand placed on it by the SCT. Ultrasound scans can detect signs of such stress on the baby's heart. These include development of a condition called **hydrops** where there is swelling under the skin and scalp surfaces due to abnormal fluid retention, **ascites** (fluid accumulating in the baby's abdomen), **effusions** (fluid collecting around the outer linings of the lungs and heart). There is also an excess of amniotic fluid (the liquid in the bag or sac that contains the baby) which may provoke premature labour.
- If these signs of impending heart failure are found, the outcome for the baby is not so good, even if surgical removal of the tumour is performed after birth. You might be asked to consider an early Caesarean section to deliver the baby if the signs of heart strain are getting worse. In such a situation, you might be offered two injections of a steroid to help accelerate the maturity of the premature baby's lungs.
- The delivery will be planned to take place in a tertiary/regional centre with facilities and experts available for such complex surgery in the newborn.
- Surgery to remove the baby's tumour while it is still in the womb may rarely be attempted in the UK. The SCT specialists can discuss such possibilities with you.

What will happen around the time of the baby's birth?

- If your baby's teratoma is small (2–5 cm or 1–2 inches), you will most likely be able to deliver naturally. If the teratoma is larger (usually more than 10 cm in diameter), you will most likely require a Caesarean section in order to avoid birth becoming obstructed by the large tumour and to prevent the tumour bursting during the birth process. The specialist team will review and discuss what options will be best for you and your baby for the actual birth, including the place, the timing and mode of delivery, anaesthesia, and so on. The paediatric surgeons will also explain what will happen after delivery regarding initial stabilization of the newborn baby before any operation to remove the tumour.

What about the future?

- When the tumour is small (2–5 cm) and without features of hydrops or ascites, the overall long-term outlook for the baby is very good once the tumour is completely removed after birth. However, regular follow-up will be maintained till the child is at least 3 years old, as even benign tumours can recur in a few cases. The baby will have scans and blood tests to ensure that there has been no such recurrence.

What are the chances that my next baby will also have SCT?

- This is not an inherited condition and the chances of a next baby being affected by SCT are very small indeed. There is only a tiny number of families where more than one member has some form of SCT.

Are there any risks to me during pregnancy with a baby with SCT?

- Very rarely, if there is significant hydrops in the baby and excess fluid in the birth sac, this can cause a so-called 'mirror syndrome' where you can develop high blood pressure, considerable fluid retention, and swelling as well as losing protein in your urine. These signs mimic severe pre-eclampsia and resolve once the delivery is complete. You will be therefore be assessed at regular intervals during the pregnancy.

Further information

- Birmingham Children's Hospital. Sacrococcygeal teratoma (SCT). <http://www.networks.nhs.uk/>

INFORMATION FOR PATIENTS Cystic hygroma

The specialist team will be happy to explain this condition in detail and will discuss options, management plans, and outcomes with you.

Further information

- Cystic Hygroma Support Group <http://www.chalsg.org.uk> Tel: 01293 571545 (24 hour answerphone)
- Great Ormond Street Hospital. Cystic hygroma <http://www.gosh.nhs.uk>
- NHS Networks. Cystic hygroma <http://www.networks.nhs.uk/nhs-networks/staffordshire-shropshire-and-black-country-newborn/documents/Cystic_Hygroma.pdf>

INFORMATION FOR PATIENTS Exomphalos and gastroschisis

The specialist team will be happy to explain these conditions in detail and will discuss all options, management plans, and outcomes with you.

Further information

- NHS Fetal Anomaly Screening Programmes. Exomphalos (omphalocele)—information for parents <http://fetalanomaly.screening.nhs.uk/>
- NHS Fetal Screening Programmes. Gastroschisis—information for parents <http://fetalanomaly.screening.nhs.uk/>

INFORMATION FOR PATIENTS Congenital diaphragmatic hernia

Frequently asked questions

What is a congenital diaphragmatic hernia (CDH)?

- The diaphragm is the tough sheet of muscle that separates the chest (containing the heart and lungs), from the abdomen (which contains the liver, kidneys, bowels, spleen, etc). In the early weeks of pregnancy the muscle layers that form the diaphragm grow from the sides of the chest wall, meet, and join together to form a complete sheet of muscle.
- Congenital diaphragmatic hernia (CDH) is an abnormality in the baby's early development whereby a defect (hole) develops because of the muscles of the diaphragm do not join up completely. This defect occurs at about 8 weeks of pregnancy. This is also the time at which the baby's lungs are starting to develop and there is a knock-on effect causing disturbance of lung growth as well.
- The precise cause of CDH is not known.
- The hole in the diaphragm is usually on the left side.
- When there is a hole in the diaphragm, the abdominal organs like the bowels, stomach, or liver can slide through into the chest, causing compression of the developing lungs and restricting their growth. The position of the heart may also be shifted. It is the poor development of the lungs (called **lung hypoplasia**) and the effect on the heart that causes the main problems in CDH.
- CDH may be the only abnormality detected on your scan or it could be part of a whole cluster of abnormalities affecting various organs or structures in the baby.

How common is this defect?

- It is a rare defect which occurs in about 1 in 2500 babies.

What happens after CDH has been found?

- Once CDH has been detected, doctors will check all other organs of the baby with ultrasound scans to exclude any other abnormalities. They will also discuss amniocentesis with you to see whether the baby's chromosomes are normal or not.
- Amniocentesis is a procedure whereby some amniotic fluid is drawn from around the baby and the cells are grown in the lab so that the chromosomes can be studied. This invasive procedure carries a 1 in 150 risk of miscarriage.
- In 10–30% of CDH, there are chromosomal abnormalities like Down's syndrome, Edward's/Patau's syndrome, or the rare Killian–Pallister tetrasomy. These chromosomal abnormalities can only be confirmed by amniocentesis.
- Most cases of CDH are diagnosed before birth at either the time of your 20-week scan or if a scan has been performed later to find why there is excess fluid around the baby. However, despite careful scanning, some cases of CDH are detected only late in pregnancy or only after birth. These babies have a mild form of CDH and tend to do better than when the defect is identified early on in pregnancy.

What is the outcome for the baby?

- Each case of CDH is different and though there is an overall survival rate of only 50–60%, individual factors in each case will point to possible outcomes and options for further management. For example, if the CDH is on the left side only or is not associated with other chromosomal abnormalities or malformations, and there is no excessive fluid accumulation, the outcome is better.
- Generally, the earlier in pregnancy that the CDH is detected, the worse the outcome. If CDH is detected before 24 weeks pregnancy for instance, the chances of the baby's survival are about 40%, meaning that only four out of ten of such babies will survive.
- You will be offered repeated scans both in your local hospital and at a tertiary/regional referral unit during your pregnancy to assess the condition of the baby. However, at present there is no 100% reliable test that will predict whether a baby will survive or not. If a number of signs indicating a very poor prognosis are found on scans, you will be counselled in detail about your options, including the possibility of terminating the pregnancy.
- If there are good prognostic signs and/or you wish to continue the pregnancy anyway, the series of scans will continue throughout pregnancy. You will also get to meet the team of paediatric surgeons and neonatologists at the tertiary/regional centre to discuss the baby's treatment/management after birth.

What else may be done?

- A procedure called FETO is currently being evaluated in Europe to see whether by temporarily blocking the baby's windpipe by inserting a small plug while the baby is still within the womb (fetal surgery), lung development will improve and the baby's survival chances will therefore be better. This procedure has shown some promising results and may be discussed with you, although it is not a standard practice as yet.
- You will also be referred to the paediatricians at the local hospital.
- After joint discussions with you and the tertiary/regional unit, your medical team will recommend the ideal time, place, and type of delivery individualized to the baby's requirements. It is advisable for delivery takes place in a tertiary/regional unit as these units have neonatal surgical facilities. Your baby will need intensive care as soon as he/she is born and, once stable, an operation to repair the defect in the diaphragm.
- Sometimes there an excess amount of amniotic fluid that develops around the baby. If severe, this can cause premature labour and delivery.
- When you see the paediatric surgeon at the tertiary/regional centre you will have the opportunity to discuss the type of operation that the baby will require, and the long-term care.

What happens after the baby is born?

- After the birth, the baby specialist team will stabilize the baby by inserting a breathing tube to supply oxygen before the baby is taken quickly to the special care baby unit.
- The first 48–72 hours after birth are critical. During this time the neonatal specialists will assess how much of the baby's lungs are developed. The better developed the lungs, the easier it is to maintain normal oxygen levels in the baby's blood. Usually, surgery to close the defect can be done after the first 2–4 days.

- Most babies stay in the tertiary/regional hospital for about a month after corrective surgery. You will be encouraged to express breast milk for the baby.
- Most babies with CDH who survive grow up to be healthy and normal. A small number, however, will have continuing lung disease and/or development problems.

Can this defect occur again in a future pregnancy?

- The risk of having further babies with CDH is very small in most cases. A recurrence risk of 1–2% is quoted. In a tiny proportion of cases, there could be family clusters of CDH. If this is the case you will have the chance to discuss it in greater detail with the genetics team.

Further information

- NHS Fetal Anomaly Screening Programmes. Congenital diaphragmatic hernia (CDH)—information for parents <http://fetalanomaly.screening.nhs.uk/>

INFORMATION FOR PATIENTS Congenital cystic adenomatoid malformation

Frequently asked questions

What is congenital cystic adenomatoid malformation of the lung?

- Normally, the right lung has three lobes and the left lung has two. Each lobe is made up of normal lung tissue.
- Congenital cystic adenomatoid malformation (CCAM) is an abnormal formation of a part of the baby's lungs. This problem occurs during the baby's development within the womb, where instead of normal lung tissue, one of the lobes of either the right or the left lung contains a cluster of fluid or air-filled spaces (cysts). The CCAM can appear as a solid or a cystic mass on ultrasound scan.
- CCAM often occurs only in one lung, either the right or the left.
- The cysts are usually found only in one lobe of a lung but occasionally more than one lobe can be affected. These cysts can be found on the baby's ultrasound scan during pregnancy The cysts can vary in appearance, from a small number of large cysts to a large number of small cysts.
- This is a very rare abnormality, occurring in only about 1 in 11,000 to 1 in 35,000 babies.

What causes CCAM?

- CCAM is a result of abnormal formation of part of the lung tissue. We do not know what triggers the abnormal development of the lung tissue in CCAM. It is not a chromosomal abnormality, it is not related to the age of either parent, and it is highly unlikely to be passed on in families. CCAM is not an inherited condition, neither is it due to any infection caught in early pregnancy. The risk of a next child also being affected with CCAM is negligibly small.
- There is no evidence to suggest that it is caused or prevented from developing by anything the parents could have done or not done.

Can it affect my baby before delivery?

- The cysts can grow during pregnancy, reaching a large size by about 28 weeks of of pregnancy. In some 20% of affected babies there is a tendency for CCAM to become smaller after this stage of growth. In some cases, the cysts may actually completely disappear without any intervention before birth, and the baby will be born with no apparent immediate problems.
- Occasionally, however, the cysts can enlarge quite rapidly during pregnancy, resulting in major problems for the baby's survival before birth. More often, however, the cysts do not grow rapidly and they may not grow at all. This is the reason why you will be offered repeat ultrasound scans throughout the pregnancy, once the CCAM has been detected.
- The scans enable the medical team to assess the size of the CCAM on each occasion, the nature of the cysts, whether there are any other abnormalities present, whether the baby is showing evidence of undue fluid retention in the tissues, and any other signs pointing to the overall outcomes that could be expected.

What are the features on ultrasound scan that may suggest a poor outcome for the baby?

- It is important to note that the course of CCAM can vary a lot during pregnancy.
- The development and worsening of the following signs could indicate a poor outcome for the baby during pregnancy or after birth:
  - The appearance of **hydrops,** which is abnormal fluid retention under the baby's skin and scalp, within the abdomen, or around organs such as the heart and lungs
  - When the baby's heart is pushed to the right side of the chest due to a large CCAM in the left lung
  - If there is excess amniotic fluid (too much liquid in the bag of membranes in which the baby is contained)
  - A large CCAM tumour which interferes with normal development of the rest of the lung tissue on both sides (**lung hypoplasia**).
- If such features are found, the specialist team in the tertiary/regional referral centre will discuss all the available options with you.

Can it affect me during the pregnancy?

- Usually the mother carrying a baby with CCAM experiences no effects.
- Very rarely, when the baby has CCAM, this might have an effect on the health of the mother. If the fetus develops hydrops (massive fluid retention), the mother may 'mirror' the sick baby, becoming ill with signs of pre-eclampsia, a condition called maternal mirror syndrome. Close monitoring of the signs and symptoms of pre-eclampsia are needed in such circumstances.

What about my antenatal care and the delivery?

- Once a CCAM has been detected, specialists from the local hospital and the experts in the tertiary/regional unit will work together in caring for you and the baby throughout pregnancy, along with the general antenatal care provided by your community midwife.
- Providing all goes well during the pregnancy, then there should be no need to alter the timing or method of delivery. You could deliver in either the local hospital or the tertiary/regional unit you have booked into, unless the scan signs have suggested there may be breathing problems for the baby following delivery, in which case delivering in a specialist tertiary/regional unit is best.
- Further information and plans about the care of your baby after delivery will be discussed in detail with you by the specialist team including the paediatric surgeon and paediatricians.
- Following birth, a CT scan should be done to assess the extent of the tumour. Surgery is the most important method of treatment, aiming to remove the tumour completely in order to avoid recurrence. Repeat surgery may also be required at a later stage.
- In a small number of cases, the CCAM may become cancerous. Close follow-up of the infant will therefore be maintained.

Can it happen again in future pregnancies?

- CCAM is not an inherited condition. It is a sporadic abnormality in lung development. The risk of a next child also being affected with CCAM is negligibly small.

Further information

- Patient.co.uk. Congenital cystic adenomatoid malformation <http://www.patient.co.uk>

INFORMATION FOR PATIENTS Autosomal recessive polycystic kidney disease

- Autosomal recessive polycystic kidney disease (ARPKD), previously known as infantile PKD, is a genetically inherited condition where both kidneys of the baby develop cysts and suffer kidney (renal) damage. In some cases, the liver can also have cysts within it, causing liver damage.
- ARPKD occurs in about 1 in 10,000 to 1 in 40,000 babies, with a carrier rate between 1 in 50 and 1 in 70.
- If only one parent carries the abnormal gene, the baby cannot get the disease. If both parents carry the gene there is a 1 in 4 chance that the baby will be affected by the disease.
- Both parents are carriers, not disease sufferers. Finding ARKD in the baby does not have any effect on the mother's health either during pregnancy or long term.
- ARPKD runs a very variable course. In severe cases of ARPKD, the baby may unfortunately not survive during pregnancy, or may die in the first few days or weeks after birth. In milder forms, symptoms might not appear until adolescence. Older children with ARPKD may develop progressive damage of both kidneys leading to kidney failure.
- The earlier the symptoms of ARPKD develop in a child's life, the more severe they usually are and the worse the outlook for survival.
- In the first type, when features of ARPKD are found in the baby during pregnancy or at birth, it is called Potter's syndrome and babies invariably die within the first week or two after birth.
- In the second variety of ARPKD, obvious features of kidney enlargement there may not be seen during pregnancy and there is less risk of underdeveloped lungs. Unfortunately there is progressive kidney failure resulting in the baby dying within a few months after birth.
- In the third category, symptoms may present only after several months in an affected infant which then progresses to end-stage renal failure, usually in adolescence.
- In a fourth category, symptoms appear for the first time during childhood (usually between 6 months to 5 years of age). There is less chance of kidney damage but greater risk of significant liver damage. In this fourth category around 80% of those affected can survive beyond the age of 15 years.
- It is only in the first and second type of ARPKD that a diagnosis is possible during pregnancy by ultrasound scan appearances. Antenatal diagnosis is unlikely before the second half of pregnancy unless there are strong reasons to suspect the condition, such as an affected older child. Early ultrasound is not very reliable at detecting the condition.
- Members of the same family can be born with different categories of the condition at different stages
- If there is a strong suspicion of ARPKD, you will be referred during pregnancy to meet the paediatricians to discuss what the outlook is likely to be in the immediate postnatal period as well as in the medium to longer term.
- The specialist team will discuss the various options and management plans on an individualised basis and would be happy to answer your queries.

Further information

- NHS Choices. Autosomal recessive polycystic kidney disease <http://www.nhs.uk>

Important: When searching the internet, only look for information about autosomal recessive polycystic kidney disease (ARPKD) otherwise known as infantile polycystic kidney disease (IPKD). This is because there is another variety of polycystic disease called adult polycystic kidney disease (APKD), which is different from the one your baby has.

INFORMATION FOR PATIENTS Tuberous sclerosis

Frequently asked questions

What is tuberous sclerosis?

Tuberous sclerosis (TS) is also known as tuberous sclerosis complex (TSC), as the condition can affect many different organs and systems of the body. It is also known as *Bournville's disease*. TS is classified as a neurocutaneous disorder. 'Neuro' refers to neurological issues that have to do with the brain, spine, and peripheral nerves (in the arms and legs). 'Cutaneous' refers to the skin. Skin lesions are the most common symptom of this disorder.

The symptoms of TS are very variable between different people who are affected by it, even within the same family. Some people are so mildly affected that they are not even aware of it whereas others have major difficulties from early life.

TS derives its name from the tuber-like growths that can be seen in the brain. These growths are not cancerous and can be seen as small white patches on a brain scan. Apart from the brain, similar benign growths can occur in many other organs of the body, particularly the heart, skin, eyes, kidneys, and lungs.

How common is TS?

TS affects about 1 in 6,000 people.

What causes TS?

TS is caused by an alteration in a gene. A gene contains the information necessary to determine our personal characteristics. We know of two genes that can result in TS, called **TSC1** and **TSC2**. Affected people are found to have an alteration in one of these genes. About 70% of people with TS are the first in their family to be affected. The remaining 30% of people with TS will have inherited it from an affected parent who may be mildly affected and unaware that they have TS. When a person with TS has children each child has a 50:50 chance of inheriting the altered gene.

How is it TS diagnosed?

It is now possible to analyse a blood sample for the **TSC1** and **TSC2** gene alteration. The test finds the alteration in most affected people, but not all. Gene testing is not necessary for everyone but can be offered to people in whom the diagnosis is uncertain, or who are at risk in a family, or to those who might wish to have prenatal diagnosis (a test on a pregnancy). Prenatal diagnosis and family gene testing can only be offered if the gene alteration has been identified in an affected family member.

TS may be diagnosed at any time throughout life depending on the severity of the symptoms. There are a number of different signs of TS, and a combination of some of these signs is necessary to make the diagnosis.

What are the symptoms of TS?

The symptoms include skin lesions, epilepsy, and mental developmental and behavioural problems. Benign tumours of the kidneys and heart may also be found.

- **Skin lesions:** White skin patches may be present from birth. A characteristic facial rash (facial angiofibroma) across the nose and cheeks often appears during childhood. Small lumps of skin (fibromas) around the finger or toe nails may appear later in childhood/adolescence. A fleshy lump (shagreen patch) can often appear on the lower back.

- **Epilepsy:** Approximately 70% of people with TS have seizures (fits). They may start at any time, but typically start in childhood, often during the first year. Babies may have infantile spasms that need to be treated promptly. People with TS may have different types of seizures at different times of their lives and seizures can sometimes stop altogether.
- **Developmental delay:** About 40–50% of people with TS have normal intelligence. Others have learning difficulties that vary from mild to severe.
- **Kidney problems:** Approximately 70–80% of people with TS will have kidney problems. Occasionally, multiple cysts in the kidneys are detected and most people have fatty growths in their kidneys (angiomyolipomas). The fatty growths are detectable later in childhood or adulthood. They frequently do not cause problems, but can sometimes bleed and therefore need to be monitored. Very occasionally, malignant tumours of the kidney may develop.
- **Heart:** Benign heart tumours (cardiac rhabdomyomas) are an early sign of TS which are seen in about 60% of children. They may be detected before birth on a routine ultrasound scan. They rarely cause any problems, and usually disappear very early in life.
- **Behaviour problems:** Behavioural problems are common. About 25% of people with TS are autistic, and another 25% show some autistic features. Attention deficit disorder and hyperactivity are common in childhood. Anxiety and depression are seen more in adults. Sleep disturbance can also occur in people with TS.

Is there a treatment available for TS?

There is no cure for TS, but many of the different aspects of the disorder can be treated. Treatment will involve a number of different professionals, depending on symptoms. For example, epilepsy should be managed by a neurologist and skin problems can be treated by a dermatologist. Kidney problems may require the input of a kidney specialist.

What is the outlook?

TS is a variable condition, so the long-term outlook depends on symptoms and severity of the disorder in any individual. About 50% of people will be intellectually normal and lead normal lives. Others will have a degree of intellectual impairment, but many of these people will have a normal lifespan.

Further information

- NHS Choices. Tuberous sclerosis <http://www.nhs.uk/conditions/>

INFORMATION FOR PATIENTS Arthrogryposis

- Arthrogryposis (ar-thro-gry-posis), means 'curved joint' and is a rare abnormality which develops in the baby while it is in the womb during pregnancy. It is also called arthrogryposis multiplex congenita (AMC). This condition, which is seen at birth, is characterized by several joints of the baby becoming contracted. AMC occurs in approximately 1 in 2000 to 1 in 3000 live births, occurring equally in boys and girls
- AMC results because of any condition that causes severe reduction or absence of the baby's movements in the womb.
- The developing baby begins to move from about 7 weeks of pregnancy. In AMC, although there is no problem in the actual formation of the joint or limb, there is joint contracture, meaning that the joint does not have a full range of movements. This is because extra connective tissue develops around the joint at about 8–10 weeks of pregnancy.
- The tendons around the affected joint cannot stretch to their normal length, making joint movement after birth even more difficult. When movement is limited for a period of several months, the limb does not grow as it should. Underdeveloped, weak, and contracted muscles can be associated problems.
- Anything that prevents normal movements of a baby in the womb will lead to a contracture. Many conditions can cause reduction or even absence of movements in the developing baby.
- Certain abnormalities of the central nervous system are the most common causes of AMC accounting for 70–80% of all cases. Other abnormalities of the connective tissue or muscles, and certain chromosomal abnormalities can also lead to poor or no fetal movements. These are called **intrinsic factors** causing AMC.
- Certain **extrinsic factors** can also result in AMC. For example, if the space in the womb is very cramped because of conditions such as severe reduction of amniotic fluid around the baby, large fibroids, or abnormal uterine shape the baby cannot move normally. Diseases such as diabetes and myasthenia gravis of the mother can also rarely lead to AMC.
- AMC is usually diagnosed either at the time of the 20-week ultrasound scan or by a scan prompted by the pregnant mother complaining that she cannot feel the baby move even after 22 or 24 weeks of pregnancy.
- The joints most often affected are the shoulders, elbows, and wrists. The legs may be curved and bowed (talipes). In severe cases, almost all joints are affected and AMC may be diagnosed even earlier than 20 weeks by ultrasound scan. The scans may also reveal other associated abnormalities of the face, jaw, spine, heart, or kidney system.
- The **outlook** for the baby depends on how severe the condition is. In general, the outlook for AMC caused by intrinsic factors is worse due to the central nervous system involvement compared to AMC due to extrinsic factors such as space limitation. A small chest with lack of movement of the chest cage or curvature of the spine can adversely affect the development of baby's lungs, which will determine outcomes after birth.
- While a near-normal independent life with a normal lifespan is seen with mild cases, in severe cases many affected individuals will remain partially or totally dependent on others for life.
- If your baby has been found to have AMC, your pregnancy care will be mainly with a team of specialists including an obstetrician who is an expert in high-risk pregnancies, a paediatrician, and genetics experts, as well as your midwife.
- The specialist team can advise you about extra tests that may be required, for example to detect chromosomal abnormalities, and will discuss the outlook for the baby with you. The options available during pregnancy will be discussed in detail as well as the type of delivery. This choice will be influenced by the degree of AMC and the position adopted by the baby in late pregnancy.
- During pregnancy you will meet the paediatric specialist who will discuss likely outcomes, and various therapies, as required, in infancy and childhood, as well as any additional long-term care that the child may require.
- The genetics team will assess the family histories of you and your partner to determine whether there is a genetic basis for the baby's AMC. If the AMC has a genetic basis, there is more chance that a future pregnancy will also be affected, compared to when the AMC in this baby has occurred as a sporadic abnormality and has no genetic inheritance pattern.
- If there are ongoing extrinsic conditions, for example if you have myasthenia or diabetes or there are womb malformations or large fibroids affecting the space within the womb cavity, there are is obviously a chance that the same factors could apply in a future pregnancy as well.

Further information

- The Arthrogryposis Group (TAG), PO Box 5336, Stourport-on-Severn, DY13 3BE; Tel: 0800 028 4447; <http://www.taguk.org.uk>; <http://www.tagonline.org.uk>

INFORMATION FOR PATIENTS Dandy–Walker syndrome

The specialists caring for your pregnancy will be happy to discuss all aspects of the condition diagnosed in your unborn baby.

Further information

- Contact a Family. Dandy–Walker syndrome <http://www.cafamily.org.uk/medical-information/conditions/d/dandy-walker-syndrome/>

INFORMATION FOR PATIENTS Choroid plexus cysts

Frequently asked questions

What is a choroid plexus cyst?

- The choroid plexus is the area of the brain that makes the cerebrospinal fluid which is the fluid that surrounds, bathes, and protects the brain and spinal cord.
- In about 1–2% of normal babies (1 in 50 to 1 in 100), a tiny bubble of fluid is pinched off as the choroid plexus forms. This appears as a cyst inside the choroid plexus at the time of the 20-week ultrasound scan. A choroid plexus cyst (CPC) is not considered a brain abnormality.
- Cysts can be found on one side or on both sides and they vary in size.
- A choroid plexus cyst does not cause learning problems or mental retardation in the child or in adulthood.
- When you hear the phrase 'cyst within the brain', this is bound to cause worry and anxiety. Please be assured that when no other abnormalities are seen on the ultrasound scan, these CPCs are not known to cause any problems for the baby.

How common are CPCs?

- CPCs are seen in approximately 1% (1 in 100) of all second or third trimester (from 14 weeks onwards) ultrasound scans. In the vast majority of cases, the cyst resolves or disappears by 28–30 weeks and has no further consequences. CPCs are relatively common in normal pregnancies and most babies found to have a CPC while in the womb are entirely normal.

Are CPCs important? If so, why?

- If, in addition to CPC, the ultrasound scan shows other abnormalities, or if the screening blood test you might have had in order to exclude chromosomal defects such as Down's syndrome or Edward's syndrome is positive, this might be significant.
- When CPC is not the only defect or the screening blood test is positive it may suggest that the baby has a higher chance of having the chromosomal abnormality called **trisomy 18**, otherwise known as **Edward's syndrome**. If this is the case, after detailed explanations, you would be offered further tests such as amniocentesis.
- Trisomy 18 is a rare serious chromosomal defect caused by an extra copy of chromosome number 18. It occurs in less than 1 in 3,000 newborn babies. Most babies born with trisomy 18 cannot survive long term. A small number of developing fetuses with CPCs have the chromosome disorder trisomy 18.
- More than a third of fetuses who have been diagnosed to have trisomy 18 are found to have CPCs.
- Most fetuses with trisomy 18 are stillborn or rarely survive beyond infancy. They usually have severe abnormalities involving almost any organ such as the heart, brain, and kidneys. These features of trisomy 18 are obvious and detectable on detailed ultrasound scanning. In fact, fetuses with trisomy 18 almost always demonstrate abnormalities on ultrasound in addition to CPCs, although some of these abnormalities can be quite subtle. If no additional abnormalities are detected by a thorough ultrasound scan performed by an experienced ultrasonographer, the likelihood that the baby has trisomy 18 is very low.

Does the size of the cyst matter?

- If the CPC is the only feature, the size does not matter. Only if the cyst is more than 10 mm do any further tests need to be considered.

What should I do?

- Even if you do nothing further, you should be confident that your baby most likely has normal chromosomes. If you have had the triple or quad screening blood test for chromosomal defects such as Down's or Edward's syndrome, this may help further evaluate the chance of trisomy 18. A targeted scan should be done, if it has not been done already, to look for other features characteristic of trisomy 18.
- If you remain anxious about the CPC even in the absence of any other abnormalities found on scan, and feel you need to be certain, we can do amniocentesis. The risk of miscarriage or premature delivery following an amniocentesis is about 1 in 100 to 1 in 200.
- Your decision should depend on what you would do with the information from an amniocentesis, whether you can accept the risk of miscarriage associated with the procedure, and how sure you need to be to enable you to continue with the pregnancy without persisting anxiety.

Further information

- University of California San Francisco. Choroid Plexus Cysts <http://www.ucsfhealth.org/education/choroid_plexus_cysts/index.html>

28. Other Fetal Conditions

INFORMATION FOR PATIENTS Non-immune hydrops fetalis

Frequently asked questions

What is hydrops fetalis?

- Hydrops fetalis is a serious condition in which abnormal amounts of fluid collects in two or more areas of a fetus (an unborn baby in the womb) causing extreme swelling of the tissues and organs. Hydrops fetalis can be life-threatening. Hydrops fetalis can be diagnosed before or after birth.
- About half of unborn babies with hydrops fetalis do not survive.

What are the types of hydrops fetalis?

There are two types of hydrops fetalis, immune and non-immune.

- **Immune hydrops fetalis**, which occurs due to blood group incompatibility, is far less common nowadays in the United Kingdom. It occurs when the mother's immune system causes the baby's red blood cells to breakdown.

- **Non-immune hydrops fetalis (NIHF)** occurs in about 1 in 1,000 to 1 in 4,000 births in the United Kingdom. It occurs when certain diseases or other complications interfere with the baby's ability to manage fluid

What causes NIHF?

Many different diseases and other medical complications disrupt the baby's ability to manage fluid.

- Severe anaemia in the fetus (such as severe thalassaemia)
- Certain infections present during pregnancy
- Heart or lung or liver defects in the fetus
- Chromosomal abnormalities such as Turner's syndrome and birth defects.

Is NIHF common?

Non-immune hydrops fetalis occurs in approximately one of every 1,000–4,000 births.

What are the features of NIHF?

Symptoms and signs of hydrops fetalis can occur during pregnancy or after the baby is born. During pregnancy, feature of NIHF may include:

- Excess amniotic fluid that can cause the uterus to appear larger than expected for that stage of pregnancy
  Ultrasound tests may show:
- large amounts of amniotic fluid (polyhydramnios)
- thickened placenta
- fluid that leads to swelling in the unborn baby's belly area and enlarged organs, including the liver, spleen, heart, or lung
- abnormal rhythm of the baby's heart
- fluid build-up in the baby's abdomen.

An **amniocentesis**, which is drawing out of some fluid from the pregnancy sac and analysing it, as well as frequent ultrasound scans may be required to try to find the cause and to determine the severity of the condition

After birth, symptoms depend on the severity of the condition and baby may show overall swelling, especially in the belly with enlarged liver and spleen. In more severe forms, the baby shows signs of:

- breathing problems
- bruising or purplish bruise-like spots on the skin
- heart failure
- severe anaemia
- severe jaundice
- total body swelling.

What is the treatment and care of NIHF?

Treatment and care depends on the cause.

During pregnancy, hydrops fetalis is treatable only in certain situations. If there is worsening hydrops with heart defects and no treatable cause is found, the chances of the baby not surviving is close to 90–100%. This outlook will be discussed in detail with you and your views will be respected. Depending on the individual circumstances, the following options may need to be considered:

- Ending the pregnancy with the use of medications to cause early labour and delivery of the baby
- In mild cases where there may be a better expectation of survival if the baby is delivered early, delivery by Caesarean section may be recommended.
- Transfusing blood through the umbilical cord during pregnancy by an invasive intervention called ' intrauterine fetal transfusion' may be relevant in certain situations where anaemia in the fetus is suspected.
  After birth, treatment of the newborn may include:
- Help for difficulty breathing using extra oxygen or a mechanical breathing machine
- Medications to help the kidneys remove excess fluid and to control heart failure
- Removal of extra fluid from around the lungs and belly area
- Direct transfusion of packed red blood cells (compatible with the infant's blood type) and an exchange transfusion to rid the baby's body of the substances that are destroying the red blood cells.

Unfortunately, hydrops fetalis often results in death of the infant shortly before or after delivery. The risk is highest among the most premature babies and those who are severely ill at birth.

Further information

- Patient.co.uk. Hydrops fetalis <http://www.patient.co.uk>

INFORMATION FOR PATIENTS Irregular fetal heart rate

Frequently asked questions

What are irregular heartbeats?

- Occasionally when the baby's heart rate is listened to, an irregular rhythm can be heard. This is quite common in pregnancy.
- This irregularity is, most often, just a temporary feature caused due to little extra heart beats in the baby called **atrial ectopic beats**.
- These are of little significance for the baby's well-being, either during pregnancy, after birth, or in later life.

What causes these irregular beats?

- A small area in the heart sends out electrical impulses that regulate the normal rhythm of heart beat in the fetus or newborn as well as in adults.
- Sometimes another area of the heart, for a short period of time, could also send out an extra impulse which in turn produces an extra early heartbeat. Following this little spurt there is a momentary resting phase during which time the heart beat appears to have a tiny pause before returning to the normal rhythm.
- Most often this is just part of the normal development of the impulse centre within the heart as well as the 'conducting' muscle fibres that spread these impulses to keep the heart beating at a normal pace and rhythm.
- Despite this temporary irregularity, the heart is working efficiently. These atrial ectopic beats are **not** associated with abnormalities of the heart structure.

What will happen now?

- The irregularity will settle on its own to resume a normal rhythm as the pregnancy progresses. Your community midwife will continue to listen to the baby's heart beat once a week, or you may be invited to have the fetal heart monitored weekly in the hospital till the irregularity settles back to a normal rhythm.
- An irregular heartbeat rhythm is unusual and therefore worrying. However, in nearly all instances, this is just part of the normal development of the heart and will settle spontaneously without needing any treatment. The normal course and care of your pregnancy and labour need not be changed in almost all instances of temporary irregularity of the baby's heartbeat.
- Only very occasionally does the baby's heart beat develop further into a continual and sustained very fast rhythm, which if left untreated for a long time could cause problems for the baby in the womb.
- If the irregular heart beat persists for longer than a few weeks, further investigations may be required and you will be kept fully informed. In the unlikely event that the irregularity persists after the baby is born, the paediatricians (baby doctors) will investigate this further.

INFORMATION FOR PATIENTS Neonatal alloimmune thrombocytopenia

The specialist team will be happy to explain this condition in detail and will discuss options, management plans, and possible outcomes with you.

Further information

- National Blood Service. Platelet groups and antibodies in pregnancy <http://hospital.blood.co.uk/library/pdf/platelet_leaflet.pdf>

INFORMATION FOR PATIENTS Reduced movements of the baby

- As the mother, you are in the best position to get to know your baby before birth. During your pregnancy, feeling your baby move gives you reassurance of his or her well-being.
- You begin to first feel the baby move at about 18–20 weeks of pregnancy, although this could vary. If you have had a baby previously you will usually be able to recognize movements earlier than in a first pregnancy
- Pregnant mothers feel only a proportion of the baby's movements in the womb. Some feel only a third of all movements, while others can feel over 80% of all movements the baby makes.
- Fetal movements include discrete kicks, flutters, rolls, prods, etc.
- If you are less than 22–24 weeks pregnant and have not yet felt movements, especially if this is your first pregnancy, it is unlikely to signal that there is a problem, as there is a wide variation in the normal time of feeling the baby's movements.
- In some cases, a baby may move less because he or she is unwell. Rarely, a baby may have a condition affecting the muscles or nerves that causes him or her to move very little or not at all.

Pattern of baby's movements

- By around the 24th week of your pregnancy, you will be well aware of your baby's movements. Movements can be large, such as kicks or changes in position, or small, such as stretching or hiccups.
- Healthy babies vary greatly in how often and how strongly they move and kick. Some mothers feel kicks less obviously than others.
- Babies sleep frequently during the day and normally will not move much during their sleep. Towards the end of pregnancy sleep periods get longer, but even near your due date it is rare that a baby will sleep for more than an hour at a time.
- Fetal movements increase steadily till 32 weeks and then stay stable until labour.
- However, there is no decrease in the number and frequency of movements after 32 weeks of pregnancy, although the quality of movements will necessarily change later on in pregnancy as there is less room for big kicks.
- The baby's sleep periods take place regularly throughout the day and night. During sleep, periods there are few movements. These sleep periods usually last for 20–40 minutes at a time. Towards the end of pregnancy sleep periods get longer, but even near your due date it is rare that a baby will sleep for more than an hour at a time.

Your ability to feel movements

This may be influenced by various factors:

- You are less likely to note fetal movements when you are busy during the daytime. When you focus on fetal movements by lying on your left side in a quiet room and focus on your baby's movements for the next 2 hours, you will usually be able to appreciate 10 movements in less than a half-hour.
- If you do not feel 10 or more separate movements within 2 hours, always seek professional help immediately.
- If the placenta is situated on the front wall of the uterus, this may act as a cushion making it harder for you to appreciate the baby's movements before 28 weeks of pregnancy. After this time, you should be able to feel fetal movements normally.
- Alcohol and certain drugs can cause a temporary reduction in fetal movements.
- Smoking causes a decrease of fetal movements because of more carbon dioxide binding with your haemoglobin (the red pigment of blood which carries oxygen), thereby supplying less oxygen to the baby.
- When the baby's back faces the front of the womb, your perception of movements may be reduced because the baby's limbs face away from your tummy wall.
- If you are very overweight, it may be more difficult for you to feel fetal movements.

How many movements are enough?

- There is no specific number of movements which is normal. During your pregnancy, you need to be aware of your baby's individual pattern of movements. A reduction or a change in your baby's movements is what is important.
- Most babies are more active in the evening or early morning.
- You will become aware of your own baby's pattern of movement each day. For the most part, the day-to-day patterns of movement for your baby will be quite similar, with daily rhythms of sleeping and waking. There could be a change in this biorhythm at about 28 weeks and again at about 36 weeks.
- As you to get to know your own baby's movement patterns you will come to know what is normal activity for your baby, and you can notice any changes.

What to do if you notice a reduction in the baby's movements

If you notice your baby is moving less than usual or if you have noticed a change in the pattern of movements, it may be the first sign that your baby is unwell. It is very important that you seek professional advice without delay.

- Do not rely on any home kits you may have for listening to your baby's heartbeat
- Never go to sleep ignoring a reduction in your baby's movements

If by 24 weeks of pregnancy you have never felt your baby move at all, you should contact your midwife, who will check your baby's heartbeat. An ultrasound scan may be arranged and you may be referred to see the specialist obstetrician. Rarely, a baby may have a condition affecting the muscles or nerves that may cause very restricted movements or none at all.

After 28 weeks of pregnancy, you are advised to act without delay if, compared to the normal levels of activity for your baby, you notice that:

- The baby has stopped moving completely, in which case you need to report this immediately to the maternity unit
- There is a significant decrease in your baby's movements
- There is a continuous decrease in movements over a few days.

You need to seek advice straight away from your maternity unit without waiting until the next day. You can avoid any delay in waiting to contact your community midwife or to see the GP by contacting your maternity unit at any time of the day or night.

A reduction in movements does not always mean that the baby is unwell, but it could be a sign that there is a problem. For example the placenta may not be providing sufficient nutrients or oxygen. This is why your baby needs to be checked without delay.

When you get to your local maternity unit, you can be sure that the doctors and midwives will take your concerns of reduction in the baby's movements seriously. Apart from an immediate assessment of the baby, any associated risk factors associated with an increased risk of stillbirth would be noted including:

- If you have previously reported a reduction in your baby's movements
- If it is known that there have been concerns about your baby's growth
- If you are obese
- If you smoke
- If you are under 20 or over 40
- If this is your first pregnancy
- If you have had pregnancy complications or have coexisting problems such as hypertension or diabetes.

The initial assessment of the baby will involve identifying the baby's heartbeat with a handheld Doppler device (a portable ultrasound device) or with the electronic fetal heart rate monitor (a cardiotocograph or CTG monitor)

Your baby's heart rate will be monitored, usually for at least 20 minutes. This should give you reassurance about your baby's wellbeing. You should be able to see your baby's heart rate increase as he or she moves.

An ultrasound scan to check on the growth of your baby, as well as the amount of amniotic fluid around your baby, may be arranged if:

- Your uterus measures smaller than expected
- Your pregnancy has risk factors associated with stillbirth
- The heart-rate monitoring is normal but you still feel that your baby's movements are less than usual.

The scan is normally done within 24 hours of being requested.

After a full antenatal check including your blood pressure and urine examination, you will usually be able to go home once you are reassured. These investigations usually provide reassurance that all is well. Most women who experience one episode of reduction in their baby's movements have a straightforward pregnancy and go on to deliver a healthy baby.

If there are any concerns about your baby, your doctor and midwife will discuss this with you.

Follow-up scans may be arranged. In some circumstances, you may be advised that it would be safer for your baby to be born as soon as possible. This will depend on your individual situation and how far you are in your pregnancy.

If you continue to have reduced fetal movements

- If the CTG is normal but you are still experiencing reduction in movements, or if there are any of the additional risk factors, a full ultrasound assessment will be made.
- If all the investigations show that everything is normal and you are sent home, but you continue to experience a reduction in movements soon after, or days or weeks later, you should not hesitate to seek immediate advice again.
- You will not be considered to be an unnecessary worrier no matter how many times this happens, because midwives and doctors know that a mother's concerns about her baby's movements are important.

Further information

- Royal College of Obstetricians and Gynaecologists. Your baby's movements in pregnancy: information for you <http://www.rcog.org.uk>

INFORMATION FOR PATIENTS Prolonged pregnancy

- Prolonged pregnancy usually refers to one that has extended to or beyond 42 completed weeks.
- The most accurate way to date a pregnancy is by use of an ultrasound scan performed within the first 13 weeks of pregnancy (first trimester) rather than by calculation from the last menstrual period (LMP). Using the dates derived from a first trimester scan only, about 2–5% of all pregnancies are prolonged.
- Although you may be sure about the date of the first day of your last menstrual period or when you think you got pregnant, remember that the time of ovulation during the cycle can be variable. If there is a difference of greater than 5 days between the gestational age dated by using the last menstrual period and the first trimester ultrasound scan, the estimated date of delivery would be adjusted according to the scan.
- Similarly, an ultrasound scan in the second trimester (13–26 weeks) is accurate for dating pregnancies within 10 days either way. If your maternity unit offers only a routine second trimester ultrasound scan at about 20 weeks of pregnancy and if there is a difference of more than 10 days between scan-derived dates and the LMP, the estimated date of delivery should be adjusted according to the second trimester scan.
- If you have had both a first and a second trimester scan, the gestational age should be determined by the **earlier** ultrasound scan as this is the most accurate.

Are there any risks involved with prolonged pregnancies?

- If there are clear medical indications for an earlier delivery, these reasons will be discussed in detail with you.
- In an uncomplicated, singleton pregnancy, provided there is no medical indication for an earlier delivery and you if you have not delivered by around 41 weeks, plans for continued management of the pregnancy will be discussed with you.
- Several studies have shown an increase of failure of the placenta functioning to serve the baby with enough nutrition and oxygen and therefore an increase in the risk of stillbirths if a pregnancy is prolonged.
- Prolonged pregnancies have also been shown to increase the risk of the baby opening its bowels (meconium) within the womb and of swallowing amniotic fluid with meconium, leading to problems after birth. Other risks associated with prolonged pregnancies include slow or no progress in labour, a large baby, difficulty in delivering the baby's shoulders, and increased chances of needing a Caesarean section.

How can the chances of having a prolonged pregnancy be reduced?

- The first step is the **accurate dating of pregnancy** with a first-trimester ultrasound scan which reduces the rate of 'prolonged pregnancies' dated erroneously using just the date of the last menstrual period.
- **'Stretching of the cervix and sweeping of membranes':** This involves your midwife or obstetrician examining you internally, and if the cervix (neck of the womb) is sufficiently open, gently inserting a finger through the mouth of the cervix and circling it right round (by 360°) if possible. This is intended to separate the membranes as high as possible from the cervix.
- Such a procedure helps to release your own natural prostaglandin, a hormone which helps start active contractions.
- Membrane stripping has been shown to be an effective and gentle method to reduce the number of pregnancies going beyond 41 weeks. Sometimes membrane stripping at term is more effective if done on more than one occasion.

Induction of labour

- A significant proportion of women will spontaneously deliver between 41 and 42 weeks of pregnancy. Of women at 40 weeks pregnancy, 65% will go into labour spontaneously within the next week. Of those at 10 days over their dates, 60% will enter spontaneous labour within the next 3 days.

- While it is well established practice to try to avoid prolonging a pregnancy beyond 42 weeks, the best way to manage an uncomplicated pregnancy between 41 and 42 weeks is not entirely clear-cut.
- Based on the results of large studies, most maternity units in the UK have adopted a policy of offering routine induction of labour between 41 and 42 weeks for women with uncomplicated, singleton pregnancies, provided there is no medical indication for an earlier delivery.
- This policy has been shown not to increase the Caesarean section rate or of instrumental vaginal delivery.
- In applying any such policy, it is acknowledged that you may prefer to await natural onset of labour even beyond 42 weeks. This is why any decision about inducing labour will only be made with your full involvement.
- The exact timing of induction would take into account both the local circumstances as well as your preferences.

Monitoring the baby's well-being beyond 41–42 weeks of pregnancy

- Various methods of monitoring the baby's well-being beyond 41–42 weeks such as kick charts, fetal heart monitoring, ultrasound scans to check for amniotic fluid volume, and Doppler assessment of blood flow in the cord have been widely used. *None of these is perfect*, and even with intensive monitoring, such as a scan at 42 weeks, then twice-weekly fetal heart monitoring, one baby in 1000 will die before it is born. The underlying problem is that the placenta starts to show signs of 'ageing' as pregnancy progresses, and eventually does not work as well as it did previously. At present, there is no direct scientific test that can predict precisely when the placenta is likely to fail altogether.
- These are the reasons why, in general, we recommend induction of labour after 41 weeks and before 42 weeks of pregnancy. Trying to inducing labour, much before 41 weeks, especially if this is your first pregnancy, is less likely to succeed. The cervix may not be ready to dilate and earlier induction carries an increased risk of caesarean section. After 41 weeks, however, it is unlikely that induction of labour will alter the final mode of delivery.
- The Royal College of Obstetricians and Gynaecologists, which advises on maternity policies and practice, recommends a stepped-up programme of monitoring. This consists of having the baby's heart rate monitoring (CTG) as well as an ultrasound scan for measuring the amount of amniotic fluid done twice a week from 42 weeks of pregnancy onwards in women who decline induction of labour.
- In addition, each maternity unit will have a system for monitoring your baby's well-being between 41 and 42 weeks of pregnancy, depending on the resources and facilities available. This might involve advice for you to remain vigilant about the baby's movements and promptly report any sudden change or decrease in the number of movements. It may also involve CTG monitoring and amniotic fluid measurements.

Further information

- NICE. Induction of labour (CG70), 2008 <https://www.nice.org.uk/guidance/cg70/informationforpublic>

29. Placental Conditions

INFORMATION FOR PATIENTS Low-lying placenta, placenta accreta

The specialist team will be happy to explain this condition in detail and will discuss options, management plans, and possible outcomes with you.

Further information

- Royal College of Obstetricians and Gynaecologists. A low-lying placenta (placenta praevia) after 20 weeks: information for you <http://www.rcog.org.uk>

INFORMATION FOR PATIENTS Placental abruption (premature separation of the placenta)

The placenta (the afterbirth) should normally detach from the wall of the womb after the delivery of the baby. If either partial or complete separation of the placenta takes place at any time in pregnancy or even during labour before completion of the second stage, i.e. after the baby is born, this is a serious condition known as **placental abruption** or **premature separation of the placenta**. The older name for this condition is '**accidental haemorrhage**'.

While most isolated episodes of bleeding may not cause immediate problems and complications, placental abruption, if severe, can quickly become a life-threatening condition for both the mother and baby.

Placental abruption occurs in 1 in 200 of all pregnancies. In severe cases, the baby unfortunately often dies within the womb and the mother can be seriously ill as well, needing urgent resuscitation and stabilization before delivery.

The exact cause of placental abruption is mainly unknown although there are several risk factors such as smoking, high blood pressure, diabetes, twin or triplet pregnancies, pre-eclampsia, older mothers, those who have had several previous babies, those who have previously had a Caesarean section, history of abruption in a previous pregnancy, excessive amniotic fluid around the baby, direct injury to the abdomen and certain conditions where there is a greater chance of abnormal coagulation of the blood, or substance abuse of cocaine and amphetamines.

Placental abruption can occur with sudden severe abdominal pain, uterine contraction which is continuous with no relaxation in between.

Ultrasound scans may not be able to demonstrate an abruption as the blood clot is not easily distinguishable from the placenta. However, if you have had more than one episode of significant bleeding during pregnancy suggestive of abruption (recurrent bleeding), a series of scans will be performed to ensure that the baby is growing well and that there is normal amount of fluid around the baby.

If you are Rhesus (D) negative, each episode of vaginal bleeding during the second or third trimester of pregnancy must be covered by an injection of Anti-D.

You will be advised to be vigilant of the baby's movements from about 30 weeks onwards on a daily basis.

If you have suffered repeated and significant bleeding during pregnancy, depending on the gestational age and your and your baby's condition, an early delivery may be advised. If you are less than 35 weeks pregnant, and an early delivery has been planned, you will be offered two steroid injections, 24 hours apart, that will help speed up baby's lung maturity and therefore improve survival and reduce problems after birth.

You would be advised to recognize and promptly report symptoms suggestive of premature separation of the placenta such as

- Sudden severe abdominal pain
- Vaginal bleeding, which may occur in 80% of cases, but the bleeding could be concealed within the uterus in 20% and pain could be the only symptom
- Too frequent uterine contractions with little relaxation of the womb in between.

If you experience any such symptoms you are requested to contact the delivery suite immediately and would be advised to come in straightaway. **In case of severe haemorrhage, contact 999 for the ambulance to bring you in**.

If you have suffered an abruption in a previous pregnancy you have an increased chance of this happening again. **This risk is about 5 per 100 (5%) in a future pregnancy**. If abruption has occurred in two previous pregnancies, the risk of it taking place once again in the next pregnancy is 20%.

The risk can be reduced by better control of diabetes or of high blood pressure if you have these conditions. If you smoke or use street drugs, stopping these can also decrease the risk of abruption occurring again.

In this pregnancy, if you have had a previous history of placental abruption, a detailed history including all the above risk factors will be taken and certain extra blood investigations may have been performed.

You can expect that your antenatal care in this pregnancy will be mainly based in one of the specialist antenatal clinics in the hospital although you will be advised to see your community midwife at regular intervals for routine antenatal checks.

Your blood pressure will be closely monitored and if it is high it will be treated with appropriate medications. If there are conditions such as diabetes or hypertension, the medical team will work with you to achieve as good control as possible. If you have high blood pressure or diabetes, the better the control, the less likely that placental abruption will occur.

A series of scans will be arranged to ensure that the baby is growing well and that there is normal amount of fluid around the baby.

Delivery may be advisable between 38 and 40 weeks of pregnancy, depending on individual circumstances. If there are problems with blood pressure control, diabetes, or the development of pre-eclampsia or poor growth of the baby, delivery may need to take place even earlier. The specialist team looking after you will discuss this fully and will be happy to answer all your queries.

Further information

- NHS Choices. What complications can affect the placenta? <http://www.nhs.uk/chq/pages/2596.aspx>
- Patient.co.uk. Antepartum haemorrhage <http://www.patient.co.uk>

INFORMATION FOR PATIENTS Vasa praevia

Frequently asked questions

What is vasa praevia?

Vasa praevia is a condition where one or more of the baby's blood vessels lies within the membranes at the mouth of the cervix. These blood vessels have their origin within the main placenta (afterbirth) but instead of being entirely contained within the placenta, they extend across the membranes that form the bag of waters at the mouth of the cervix. These blood vessels are not protected by any tissue support so that when the cervix dilates or the membranes break, the unprotected vessels can tear, causing rapid loss of the baby's blood.

Most cases of vasa praevia are not or cannot be diagnosed before labour actually starts and some blood loss is noticed at the time that the waters break. If the condition is not diagnosed before labour, this unfortunately carries a high risk of the baby dying within a very short time, literally minutes, once the blood vessels in vasa praevia tear.

When vasa praevia is strongly suspected during pregnancy with the aid of imaging techniques such as colour-flow ultrasound scan or by MRI scan, a planned delivery by Caesarean section before labour starts or the membranes break, can prevent such a disaster.

How common is this condition?

Vasa praevia occurs in approximately 1 in 2,500 births except in IVF (in-vitro fertilization) pregnancies where the frequency is as high as 1 in 300.

What are the warning signs?

Vasa praevia is usually entirely silent until the point when the membranes break and then there is a sudden onset of painless vaginal bleeding in late pregnancy. When the cervix starts to dilate or when the forewaters break either spontaneously or artificially, the baby's blood vessels in vase praevia can tear. The resulting blood loss is not your blood but that of the baby. The baby rapidly develops severe anaemia and can die within minutes. Only a small amount of fetal blood needs to be lost in ruptured vasa praevia to cause the baby's death as the total blood volume of a term baby is only 250–300 ml (about half a pint).

Who is at risk?

Women with painless bleeding (at any stage in pregnancy but particularly after about 26 weeks) are at risk. Vasa praevia is particularly associated with a placenta that is lying low in the uterus (low-lying placenta or placenta praevia).

It is also more common when, in addition to the main body of the placenta, an additional lobe or lobes (called **succenturiate lobes**) exists and the baby's blood vessels lie in the fold of membranes connecting these to the main placental body.

The umbilical cord is normally attached to the centre of the inner surface of the placenta. Rarely, the umbilical cord is found to be attached to the peripheral margin of the placental body, a condition called **velamentous insertion of the cord**. Vasa praevia is associated with velamentous insertion of the placenta in about 2–6% of cases.

Vasa praevia has also been noted to occur more frequently with IVF pregnancies, as well as with twin/triplet pregnancies.

How can vasa praevia be diagnosed antenatally (before labour starts)?

Diagnosis is usually made by chance at the time of the routine 20-week anomaly scan using ultrasound scan with colour flow Doppler.

During your 20-week scan, the position of the placenta and the site of insertion of the umbilical cord into the placenta will be recorded. If the placenta is found to be low lying and/or the insertion of the umbilical cord is not central, or in multiple pregnancies, further imaging techniques are warranted. This may include internal scanning (transvaginal scan) with colour Doppler ultrasound, for which you might be referred to a consultant ultrasonologist/obstetrician.

If vasa praevia is suspected at about 20 weeks of pregnancy, a colour Doppler ultrasound scan needs to be repeated in the third trimester (26–40 weeks),usually around 32–34 weeks to confirm its persistence, thus reducing the need for prolonged admission and anxiety.

What happens once vasa praevia has been diagnosed?

If confirmed in the third trimester scan, you may be advised to come into hospital as an in-patient till the baby is delivered by a planned Caesarean section at about 35 weeks, earlier if indicated. The reason for this recommendation is to aid quicker delivery in case the waters break or any bleeding occurs.

A prolonged in-patient stay could cause significant inconvenience and anxiety for you and your family and it will only be suggested because the risks involved for your baby are so serious and unpredictable.

In a small number of cases, significant risks may be unavoidable, even when the mother is in the hospital with close monitoring and prompt action is taken for immediate Caesarean delivery.

If delivery has been planned for earlier than 35 weeks, you will be offered two injections of steroids to help accelerate the premature baby's lung maturity.

The paediatric doctors (neonatologists) who will look after your newborn baby will be kept updated to ensure that appropriate blood is kept available for immediate transfusion to the baby, if needed in the event of rupture of vasa praevia at any time during the mother's in-patient stay.

Recent studies have shown that when vasa praevia is diagnosed before labour and a proper management plan is followed, the baby's survival rate is near 100%, provided no other abnormalities or problems are present.

Further information

- UK Vasa Praevia Awareness Group <http://www.vasapraevia.co.uk>

INDEX

IP indicates Information for Patients

Index

Index

Index

Index